Pet-Specific Care for the Veterinary Team

Pet-Specific Care for the Veterinary Team

Lowell Ackerman, DVM, DACVD, MBA, MPA, CVA, MRCVS
Global Consultant, Author, and Lecturer
Editor-in-Chief, Pet-Specific Care

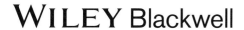

Registered Office
John Wiley & Sons, Inc., 111 River Street, Hoboken, NJ 07030, USA

Editorial Office
111 River Street, Hoboken, NJ 07030, USA

For details of our global editorial offices, customer services, and more information about Wiley products visit us at www.wiley.com.

Wiley also publishes its books in a variety of electronic formats and by print-on-demand. Some content that appears in standard print versions of this book may not be available in other formats.

Library of Congress Cataloging-in-Publication Data

Names: Ackerman, Lowell J., editor.
Title: Pet-specific care for the veterinary team / [edited by] Lowell Ackerman.
Description: Hoboken, NJ : John Wiley & Sons, Inc., [2021]
Identifiers: LCCN 2020023653 (print) | LCCN 2020023654 (ebook) |
    ISBN 9781119540663 (cloth) | ISBN 9781119540694 (adobe pdf) |
    ISBN 9781119540700 (epub)
Subjects: MESH: Animal Diseases–prevention & control | Animal
    Diseases–therapy | Pets | Precision Medicine–veterinary | Risk
    Assessment–methods
Classification: LCC SF745 (print) | LCC SF745 (ebook) | NLM SF 745 | DDC
    636.089/6–dc23
LC record available at https://lccn.loc.gov/2020023653
LC ebook record available at https://lccn.loc.gov/2020023654

Cover Design: Wiley
Cover Images: © VGstockstudio / Shutterstock, © Monty Rakusen / Getty Images, © michaeljung / Shutterstock

Set in 9.5/12.5pt STIXTwoText by SPi Global, Pondicherry, India
Printed in Singapore

M093252_260221

On a personal note, I'd like to dedicate this book to my incredible family – to my wonderful wife, Susan, and to my phenomenal children – Nadia, Rebecca, and David.

On a professional note, I'd like to dedicate this edition to my colleagues who participated in this book – to the authors who gave generously of their time and talents to help produce this incredible resource for the veterinary healthcare team.

Lowell Ackerman, DVM, DACVD, MBA, MPA, CVA, MRCVS

Contents

Contributors

Lowell Ackerman, DVM, DACVD, MBA, MPA, CVA, MRCVS
Global Consultant, Author, and Lecturer
Editor-in-Chief, Pet-Specific Care
www.lowellackerman.com

Peter Alberti, BSBA
CEO, Inulogica, Northborough, MA, USA
www.inulogica.com
peter@inulogica.com

Helen Ballantyne, PG Dip, BSc (Hons), RN, RVN
Cambridge University Hospitals NHS Foundation Trust,
Addenbrookes Hospital, Cambridge, UK
helen_ballantyne@yahoo.com

Marty Becker, DVM
Founder and CEO, Fear Free, LLC, Denver, CO, USA
www.fearfreepets.com

Jerold S. Bell, DVM
Adjunct Professor of Clinical Genetics, Department
of Clinical Sciences, Cummings School of Veterinary
Medicine at Tufts University, North Grafton, MA, USA
jerold.bell@tufts.edu

Gary Block, DVM, MS, DACVIM
Ocean State Veterinary Specialists, East Greenwich, RI, USA
GBYLC@AOL.com
www.OSVS.net

Nan Boss, DVM
Best Friends Veterinary Center, Grafton, WI, USA
drboss@bestfriendsvet.com

Jane Brunt, DVM
Cat Hospital At Towson(CHAT), Baltimore, MD, USA
jbrunt@catdoc.com
www.catdoc.com
CATalyst Council, Inc., Annapolis, MD, USA
www.catalystcouncil.org

Kara M. Burns, MS, MEd, LVT, VTS (Nutrition)
Independent Consultant, Author, and Lecturer,
Lafayette, IN, USA
karamburns@gmail.com

Betsy Choder, JD, MS
VetCounsel, LLC, Crown Pointe Parkway,
Atlanta, GA, USA
www.vetcounsel.net

Mary Craig, DVM, MBA, CHPV
Gentle Goodbye Veterinary Hospice and At-home
Euthanasia, Stamford, CT, USA
www.gentlegoodbye.org

Caitlin Dewilde, BS, DVM
Consultant, Author, and Lecturer, Founder and CEO,
The Social DVM, LLC, Webster Groves, MO, USA
www.thesocialdvm.com
cdewilde@thesocialdvm.com

Michael R. Dicks, PhD
President of AE Consulting, Arvada, CO, USA
Chief Data Human for Erupt, LLC, Kodak, TN, USA
aecnslt@gmail.com

Amanda L. Donnelly, DVM, MBA
ALD Veterinary Consulting, LLC,
Nashville, TN, USA
www.amandadonnellydvm.com
www.onecallatatime.com
adonnelly@aldvet.com

Patricia Dowling, DVM, MSc, DACVIM (LAIM), DACVCP
Professor, Veterinary Clinical Pharmacology
Western College of Veterinary Medicine, Saskatoon,
Canada
trisha.dowling@usask.ca

Robin Downing, DVM, MS, DAAPM, DACVSMR, CVPP, CCRP
Fear Free Certified Professional, Speaker, Author, Clinical Bioethicist
Hospital Director, The Downing Center for Animal Pain Management, LLC, Windsor, CO, USA
www.downingcenter.com

Ryane E. Englar, DVM, DABVP (Canine and Feline Practice)
Associate Professor, College of Veterinary Medicine, University of Arizona, Oro Valley, AZ, USA
renglar@arizona.edu

Mark E. Epstein, DVM, DABVP (Canine/Feline), CVPP
Medical Director, TotalBond Veterinary Hospitals, Gastonia, NC, USA
mark.epstein@totalbondvets.com

Maria Inês Ferreira, DVM, MTB
Veterinarian, journalist, and author, São Paulo, Brazil
mvmariaines.ferre@gmail.com
linkedin.com/in/maria-inês-f-1914852b

Tamara Grubb, DVM, PhD, DACVAA
Washington State University, Pullman, WA, USA
tamaragrubb@wsu.edu

D. J. Haeussler, Jr., BS, MS, DVM, DACVO
The Animal Eye Institute, Cincinnati, OH, USA
www.animaleyeinstitute.com

Randy Hall
4th Gear Consulting, Huntersville, NC, USA
www.4thgearconsulting.com

Tara Harmon, APR
Personal Lines Marketing Director, Illinois & Wisconsin
The Cincinnati Insurance Companies, Fairfield, OH, USA
www.cinfin.com
tara_harmon@cinfin.com

Donna L. Harris, DVM, MBA, MS(Strategic Foresight)
Veterinary Special Services, College of Veterinary Medicine, Michigan State University
East Lansing, MI, USA
harrisko@msu.edu
vssmich@sbcglobal.net

David Haworth, DVM, PhD
President, Vidium Animal Health, Phoenix, AZ, USA
vidiumah.com

Brandon Hess, CVPM, CCFP
VetSupport Inc., Cincinnati, OH, USA
Brandon@vetsupport.com
www.vetsupport.com

Alicea Howell, LVT, VTS (Behavior), KPA, CTP
Owner, Barks and Rec Animal Training and Behavior, Traverse City, MI, USA
www.BarkRanger.net

Jessica Johnson, DVM
Main Street Veterinary Dental Clinic, Flower Mound, TX, USA

Anna Katogiritis, BSc, DVM
Independent SA and Wildlife Emergency Veterinarian and NGO Consultant
www.DoctorAnnaK.com
DoctorAnnaK@gmail.com
Social media:@DoctorAnnaK

Kim Kendall, BVSc, MANZCVS (Cat Medicine and Animal Behaviour)
Clinical cat veterinarian and behavioural consultant, Roseville, NSW, Australia
www.felinefriendlycare.com

Chand Khanna, DVM, PhD, DACVIM (Onc), DACVP (Hon)
Veterinary Oncologist and Chief Science Officer, Ethos Veterinary Health, Woburn, MA, USA
ckhanna@ethosvet.com

Patricia Khuly, VMD, MBA
Independent veterinary journalist and owner, Sunset Animal Clinic, Miami, FL, USA
khulyp@bellsouth.net

Jacqui Ley, BVSc (Hons), PhD, DECAWBM, FANZCVS (Veterinary Behaviour)
Registered Specialist in Veterinary Behaviour, Melbourne Veterinary Specialist Centre, Glen Waverley, Victoria, Australia
behaviour@melbvet.com.au

Heidi B. Lobprise, DVM, DAVDC
Main Street Veterinary Dental Clinic, Flower Mound, TX, USA
HeidiDent93@gmail.com

Mark J. Mcgaunn, CPA/PFS, CFP®
McGaunn & Schwadron, CPA's, LLC, Medfield, MA, USA
www.mcgaunnschwadron.com

Brennen Mckenzie, MA, MSc, VMD
Adobe Animal Hospital, Los Altos, CA, USA
www.skeptvet.com

Emma Goodman Milne, BVSc, MRCVS
Independent Veterinary Surgeon
www.vetsagainstbrachycephalism.com

Jason C. Nicholas, BVETMED (Hons)
Independent Consultant, Author and Speaker,
Co-founder, Preventive Vet
www.DrJasonNicholas.com
www.linkedin.com/in/drjasonnicholas
DrJVet1@gmail.com

Anita M. Oberbauer, PhD
Professor and Associate Dean, Department of Animal
Science, University of California, Davis, CA, USA
amoberbauer@ucdavis.edu

Kurt A. Oster, MS, SPHR, SHRM-SCP
Bay State Veterinary Emergency and Specialty Services,
Swansea, MA, USA
www.kurtoster.com

Joanna Pendergrass, DVM
Freelance Medical Writer
Founder and owner, JPen Communications, LLC, Sandy
Springs, GA, USA
www.jpencmc.com
joanna@jpencmc.com

Saya Press, BVSc, MS, DACVECC
The Veterinary Specialty Hospital of San Diego, Sorrento
Valley, San Diego, CA, USA
spress@ethosvet.com

I. Craig Prior, BVSc, CVJ
Independent Consultant, Lecturer, and Practitioner,
College Grove, Brentwood, TN, USA
ausivet@gmail.com

Krystle L. Reagan, DVM, PhD, DACVIM (SAIM)
Assistant Professor, Department of Veterinary
Medicine and Epidemiology,
Small Animal Infectious Disease Fellow,
School of Veterinary Medicine,
University of California, Davis, CA, USA
kreagan@ucdavis.edu

Sarah Rumple
Veterinary Writer and Editor, Owner and Chief
Creative Officer of Rumpus Writing and Editing LLC,
Denver, CO, USA
rumpuswriting.com

Suzanne Russo, DVM, MS
Associate Dean of Clinical Education, College of
Veterinary Medicine, Midwestern University,
Glendale, AZ, USA
osudvm92@gmail.com

Robert Sanchez
CEO, Digital Empathy, San Diego, CA, USA
digitalempathyvet.com

Kymberley C. McLeod, DVM
Conundrum Consulting, Toronto, Ontario, Canada
kymberley-stewart@idexx.com

Samuel Stewart, DVM, DACVECC
Veterinary criticalist and commercialization scientist,
Ethos Veterinary Health, Woburn, MA, USA
sstewart@ethosvet.com

Natalie Stilwell, DVM, MS, PhD
Southeastern Cooperative Wildlife Disease Study,
College of Veterinary Medicine, University of Georgia,
Athens, GA, USA
nkstilwell@gmail.com

Jane Sykes, BVSc, PhD, DACVIM (SAIM)
Chief Veterinary Medical Officer and Professor,
Department of Veterinary Medicine and Epidemiology,
School of Veterinary Medicine, University of California,
Davis, CA, USA
jesykes@ucdavis.edu

*Lori Massin Teller, DVM, BS (Vet Sci), DABVP
(Canine/Feline Practice)*
Clinical Associate Professor, Telehealth, Department of
Small Animal Clinical Sciences, College of Veterinary
Medicine & Biomedical Sciences, Texas A&M University,
College Station, TX, USA
http://vetmed.tamu.edu

Cindy Trice, DVM
Founder/CEO, Relief Rover, Bradenton, FL, USA
reliefrover.com

Ernie Ward, DVM, CVFT (Certified Veterinary Food Therapist)
Founder, Association for Pet Obesity Prevention, Ocean Isle Beach, NC, USA
PetObesityPrevention.org
DrErnieWard.com

Linda Wasche, MBA, MA
LW Marketworks, Inc., Sylvan Lake, MI, USA
Lindaw@LWmarketworks.com
www.LWmarketworks.com

Peter Weinstein, DVM, MBA
PAW Consulting, Irvine, CA, USA
PeterWeinsteinDVMMBA@gmail.com

Preface

This book was designed to provide a valuable resource for all things related to pet-specific care, from prevention, to early detection, to evidence-based treatment, guidelines, and facilitated compliance. It is an appropriate source of information to foster consensus building and a team approach to delivering excellent healthcare to animals.

The concept of pet-specific care is relatively new in veterinary medicine (while the equivalent "personalized medicine" is now considered *de rigueur* in human medicine) and involves selecting appropriate services for pet and owner, based on both subjective and objective criteria, including breed predisposition, age, level of care requested by owner, risk assessment, appropriate guidelines, financial considerations, and many more aspects. While much of veterinary medicine has been reactive in the past, waiting for pets to develop problems before veterinary teams got involved, pet-specific care is more proactive, focuses on keeping pets healthy, and considers approaches that span a lifetime rather than from one veterinary visit to the next. It also involves managing pets in a truly team-based fashion, so throughout the book emphasis is given to the roles of team members in delivering excellent healthcare, communication, and client service. In addition to specific topics covered within the book, there is also a rich collection of appendices that provide additional resources, abbreviations, glossary, and breed tables of heritable conditions organized by canine and feline breeds, conditions, and breed attributes.

Whether you want to know how to provide genetic testing and counseling in practice, find out more about guidelines and standards of care, or the meaning of the term "incremental care" as it applies to healthcare options for clients who couldn't otherwise afford services, you'll find it within the pages of this book.

The intention is to provide as much information as is available that pertains to pet-specific care for both dogs and cats, and that can be somewhat challenging because there tend to be more resources in the veterinary literature on dogs than cats. That does not detract from the importance of cats and their owners, but recognizes that at this time there are more guidelines, genetic tests, and conditions recognized with a breed predisposition in dogs versus cats. Still, every effort has been made to include as many feline resources as possible, including topics primarily or exclusively dedicated to cats. This isn't just a nod to practices dedicated to cats. In many countries, the majority of pets are cats, and yet cats often represent a much smaller percentage of office appointments and often significantly less hospital revenue. Thus, improving pet-specific care for cats and their owners also represents a major opportunity for veterinary practices. Most of the content of this book applies equally to cats as to dogs, and there are additional cat-specific topics in the book as well. It is a sincere hope that there will be even more feline resources available in future editions as the profession develops more of such content because everyone (practices, pet owners, and cats themselves) will benefit from such developments.

The veterinary marketplace has changed dramatically from only a few decades ago. Pets are considered as family members, more so than at any time in the past, and it is imperative to recognize the human–animal bond in all of our efforts. Specialization within the profession has become more commonplace and the creation of specialty and referral hospitals has been robust on a global basis. Partially as a result of this, we also have more published guidelines for veterinary care than were available previously and many are referenced within the pages of this book. Corporate practices are also coming into their own, as are retail-anchored practices, and we are also witnessing the role this plays in delivering a more market-driven approach to healthcare. It is also important to recognize the evolution of the veterinary healthcare team and the critical role each healthcare team member provides in the delivery of excellent healthcare, and consistent healthcare.

Yes, things are changing, and change is often difficult to assimilate, especially within the veterinary profession. Veterinary practice often stood as an anachronism, an attempt to hold back the escalation in healthcare costs as pertains to animals. There was a belief that these costs needed to be kept artificially low, because pet owners would be unwilling to pay those costs for the sake of an animal. Yet, study after study has shown that this is not the case and owners do understand the high cost of healthcare and are often receptive to such realistic costs . . . as long as they see the "value" in those expenditures and reasonable expectations have been established for them by veterinary teams. That being said, it is also important to realize that not all clients can necessarily afford the care they would otherwise wish to select, and there are still ways to deliver reasonable and acceptable care without sacrificing quality. Thus, in this book there are also several topics that deal with this challenging subject.

The profession is indeed changing, and clients have changed, and the services available for pets have changed, but primary care veterinary practices are still very much as they have been in the past, and face many challenges ahead. It is the goal of this book to provide veterinary practices and teams with the information necessary to compete effectively in the marketplace and to deliver exceptional pet-specific healthcare in a truly team-based fashion.

Compiling all this information in one volume was an immense task, and I am eternally grateful to my gifted colleagues who contributed to this incredible resource. It wasn't that long ago that the delivery of healthcare was entirely veterinarian focused, and pet-specific care was a self-taught discipline based on personal experience, and often by trial and error. That has changed, and I am very proud to be involved in a project, along with the many authors of this book, that helps deliver this much-needed resource for veterinary healthcare teams.

Lowell Ackerman, DVM, DACVD, MBA,
MPA, CVA, MRCVS

Editor-in-Chief

Lowell Ackerman, DVM, DACVD, MBA, MPA, CVA, MRCVS

Dr Lowell Ackerman is a board-certified veterinary specialist, an award-winning author, an international lecturer, and a renowned expert in veterinary practice management. He is a graduate of the Ontario Veterinary College and a Diplomate of the American College of Veterinary Dermatology. In addition to his veterinary credentials, he also has a Masters in Public Administration from Harvard University, a Masters in Business Administration from the University of Phoenix, and a Certificate in Veterinary Practice Administration from Purdue University/American Animal Hospital Association. Dr Ackerman is a Certified Valuation Analyst (CVA) through the National Association of Certified Valuators and Analysts and is a Fear Free Certified Professional. Throughout his career, Dr Ackerman has been engaged in specialty practice, primary care practice, academia, consulting, industry, and teaching. Dr Ackerman is the author or co-author of several books, and he lectures extensively on a global basis on topics relative to both medicine and management.

Section 1

Overview

1.1

Overview of Pet-Specific Care

Lowell Ackerman, DVM, DACVD, MBA, MPA, CVA, MRCVS

Global Consultant, Author, and Lecturer, MA, USA

 BASICS

1.1.1 Summary

Pet-specific care is a practice philosophy in which veterinary care is transformed from a reactive model to a more proactive version in which veterinary teams provide solutions rather than just services, and pet owners become more engaged with the veterinary team in the pet care process. Pet-specific care encourages active, ongoing veterinary care throughout a pet's life as a continuum of care, rather than just a passive transaction-based process. The approach can result not only in happier, healthier pets, but also healthier families, practices, and communities.

For veterinary medicine to provide real value to pet owners and derive real success for veterinary practices, there is a need to focus on being proactive, appreciating risk factors, detecting problems early, closing compliance gaps, and managing through evidence-based guidelines.

1.1.2 Terms Defined

Care Pathway: A step-by-step approach to the management of specific conditions in specific patient populations.
Companion Diagnostics: A method to test safety and efficacy of a drug specific to a target patient group, breed, or otherwise identified individual (biomarkers, genetic markers, etc.).
Continuum of Care: The delivery of healthcare over a period of time, such that intervention at any point on the timeline affects quality of life in the period afterwards.

Healthspan: The portion of a pet's life in which it is considered generally healthy, in contradistinction to lifespan which is the quantity of time a pet is alive.
Level of Care: The intensity, appropriateness or competence of care provided.
P4 Medicine: The clinical face of systems medicine, P4 medicine is Predictive, Preventive, Personalized, and Participatory. Its two major objectives are to quantify wellness and demystify disease.
Pet Parent: A term used to designate that the relationship between individuals and their pets is more than just ownership. Such individuals endeavor to do what is best for their pets and seek to maximize the benefits of the human–animal bond for both parties.
Spectrum of Care: The availability and accessibility of veterinary medical care regardless of the socioeconomic status of the pet owner.
Stratified Medicine: An approach to medical care designed to segment or stratify patients into groupings with similar disease profiles, attributes, or presumed response to specific therapies.
Theranostics: A combination of diagnostics and therapy in which specific targeted therapy is based on specific targeted diagnostic tests.
Toxgnostics: The identification of genetic variants that predict adverse reactions to specific drugs.

 MAIN CONCEPTS

Pet-specific care is about providing customized care for pets (based on breed, lifestyle, medical history, other risk factors, etc.), and constitutes an important and value-added healthcare experience for pet owners. It could be considered as "the right care, for the right pet, at the right time."

Pet-specific care involves approaches that allow predictions to be made as to an individual's susceptibility to disease, its possible prevention, prospects for early detection, the course of that disease, and the disease's likely response to treatment.

The goal of pet-specific care is to prevent disease, if at all possible, or to decrease the impact of the disease on the patient, thereby improving the pet's quality of life. This is typically accomplished by identifying risk factors so that veterinary teams and pet owners can be proactive in instituting lifestyle modifications and increased veterinary surveillance so that problems can be detected at the earliest opportunity, hopefully while they are still subclinical, and when there are typically the most options available for successful management.

Pet-specific care is also known by several other terms, including:

- Personalized medicine
- Precision medicine
- Pet-centric care
- Client-centric care
- Lifelong care
- Theranostics
- Stratified medicine
- Predictive medicine
- Patient-specific medicine
- P4 medicine
- Genomic medicine
- Individualized medicine.

1.1.3 Why Pet-Specific Care?

The fundamental premise of pet-specific care is that each pet has unique attributes (genetic and otherwise) that make them susceptible to health issues and that by better understanding this uniqueness, we can more specifically tailor care to the needs of the specific pet and owner. At the present time, most of the research has focused on being able to predict susceptibility to disease, but the potential exists to also predict which medical treatments are most likely to be safe and effective, and which are best avoided in an individual. It might even be possible to predict which diets would be most appropriate for specific pets.

Pet-specific care has the potential to change the way we consider, identify, and approach medical management issues and it can not only streamline evidence-based care, but can help us minimize harmful side effects, ensure more

beneficial outcomes, and even help clients save money on their veterinary care by avoiding processes less likely to be successful.

In the current veterinary business model, most veterinary practices engage in routine examinations, vaccinations, and parasite control, but otherwise assume a reactive posture to healthcare issues, waiting for the onset of clinical disease before intervening. Once a clinical disease condition is recognized, the prudent approach would be to recommend an evidence-based approach to management (see 2.1 Evidence-Based Veterinary Medicine and Personal Bias) with facilitated compliance, but in many hospitals, the approach, even for very basic conditions, is left up to the individual clinician. The problem with this approach is that veterinary businesses like to tout the exceptional level of care they provide to their clients, but without consistency of care (see 9.8 Ensuring Consistency of Care), there can be no assurance to clients about the level of care provided; it will vary based on the experience and expertise of each individual veterinarian in the practice.

Pet-specific care adopts a more comprehensive approach to the situation, concentrating preferentially on health management, risk assessment, prevention, early detection, appropriate treatment, facilitated compliance and then patient management over the long term (concentrating on healthspan rather than lifespan).

Let's illustrate this philosophy with a common example – osteoarthritis. Most veterinarians diagnose osteoarthritis when a pet has lameness or displays discomfort when getting up or lying down. Diagnostic testing at this stage may indicate fairly advanced osteoarthritis evident on radiography. We might be content that we have correctly diagnosed the problem, but our human physician counterparts would likely consider this a Pyrrhic victory – their goal would have been to identify the problem much earlier and seek to change the course of the disease process, preferably so the individual never goes on to have chronic pain and mobility issues. At that point, the physician would make recommendations according to accepted guidelines, and if the patient was not responding as anticipated, would refer the patient to a specialist in a systematic fashion.

Could we do a better job in veterinary medicine? Absolutely! The first step is to create a risk profile for each individual pet during puppy and kitten visits, using information at our disposal but that often does not get the attention it deserves (see 2.7 Risk Assessment). For example, while osteoarthritis can be recognized in virtually any dog or cat, there are many breeds that have a higher prevalence of the condition, and underlying conditions that increase risk, so such pets should have screening to identify cases earlier, hopefully when they are subclinical and we have the most options for changing the trajectory of the disorder.

Are there other situations that should make us more vigilant for the increased probability of osteoarthritis in our clinic populations? Yes! In addition to underlying problems that may be heritable (such as hip dysplasia), pets with prior history of trauma, those with co-morbidities that may predispose to osteoarthritis and even those with weight management issues may be at increased risk and would benefit from early screening. These risk factors should prompt us to evaluate for osteoarthritis earlier and more consistently, but since all pets can develop osteoarthritis, and it usually presents in young adult to middle-aged pets, routine screening should also be done for all pets earlier than typical profiles that get initiated in senior patients.

Interestingly, pet-specific care is about much more than just medical competence, since it also impacts customer satisfaction and retention. It should not be surprising that pet owners actually expect this level of care from veterinary teams, and believe they are already paying for this level of excellence. Consider for a moment the pet owner who dutifully brings in their pet for evaluation and pays for that visit. Is it fair that they expect the veterinary team they are entrusting with their pet's care to actually know the problems to which their pet is prone, and act accordingly? Is it fair that the pet owner of a Cavalier King Charles spaniel expects the veterinary team to know that their pet is prone to a variety of ills, including mitral valve disease, keratoconjunctivitis sicca, macrothrombocytopenia, primary secretory otitis media, and syringomyelia (among others), and that the veterinary team is prepared to counsel and assess accordingly (see 11.4 Heritable Health Conditions – by Breed)? While most veterinary practices will admit that they are not actually providing this level of service, most will reluctantly acknowledge that it is fair for paying clients to expect it. It is a commitment to pet-specific care that creates the framework in which this can happen consistently.

Similarly, is it reasonable for clients to expect that the veterinary team will take every precaution to determine if certain drugs could cause adverse effects in their individual pet (toxgnostics) or know that a pet that travels with its owners warrants different preventive care strategies, or that pets that engage in specific activities might have altered risk profiles? In the future, we will also likely be able to engage in what is currently being referred to as companion diagnostics, which is a way to test safety and efficacy of a drug specific to a target patient group, breed, or otherwise identified individual (biomarkers, genetic markers, etc.). So, there may come a time when we are able to screen individuals at risk (for example, for potential idiosyncratic reactions such as to nonsteroidal antiinflammatory drugs). We just need a system in place to take advantage of these developments, and pet-specific care can be that system.

Pet-specific care is also client centric since decisions are ultimately made by caregiving pet owners. While it is important that veterinary teams focus on standards of care (see 9.4 Standards of Care), care pathways (see 9.6 Care Pathways), and regarding intervention on a continuum of care (see 9.7 Continuum of Care and Convergence Schedules), it takes more than that to deliver pet-specific care. To deliver pet-specific care effectively, veterinary teams need to also provide a specified level of care, which in turn is dependent on consistency of care (see 9.8 Ensuring Consistency of Care) within the practice. In addition to standards of care and level of care, veterinary teams also need to be aware that not all clients can afford recommended services, so a spectrum of care may be needed. Affordability of veterinary services is a real concern for some pet owners (see 2.10 Affordability of Veterinary Services), but options are still available (see 10.14 Providing Cost-Effective Care for Those in Need; 2.2 The Role of Incremental Care; 7.8 Providing Care for Those Unable or Unwilling to Pay; and 6.5 Opportunities and Challenges of Providing Services for Low-Income Families).

1.1.3.1 Why Pet-Specific Care Rather than Pet-Specific Medicine?

While the goal of pet-specific care is better health outcomes, and there are many medical aspects to healthspan, it is also true that some of the most important aspects of success with pet-specific care involve owner engagement in health management rather than disease management. Pet owners need to play an active role in keeping their pets healthy, not just bringing those pets in for veterinary care when something goes wrong.

The nomenclature is not yet fixed, but pet-specific care suggests that there are many important aspects to care that are not necessarily medical in nature. A commitment by pet owners to feed a nutritious and balanced diet, to promote appropriate behaviors, to ensure their pet remains within a normal body condition score, and to provide regular at-home oral care are all very important health factors. So is ensuring pets have regular exercise, socialization, and access to enrichment in their environments. Some may even say that promoting behavioral health is one of the best ways of ensuring medical health, since behavioral issues are more likely to result in relinquishment than medical problems (see 6.9 Preventing Behavior Problems).

Pet owners need to consider home issues such as fencing and shelter, pet-proofing their home to avoid mishaps, making plans for someone to care for their pets when they are away, as well as making financial decisions for how to care for their pet in sickness and in health. They also need to do more than just go to the veterinarian and buy recommended products. Compliance and adherence are critical factors, and owners need to be prepared to follow veterinary recommendations at home, when they are not under direct medical supervision (see 9.17 Improving Compliance and Adherence with Pet-Specific Care). For all these reasons and many more, the term *pet-specific care* is preferred (at least currently) over the variety of other synonyms that are being used.

Veterinary healthcare teams definitely facilitate pet-specific care, but owners must be engaged in the process and willingly accept their healthcare guardian role and take the responsibility seriously.

While all pet owners should aspire to pet-specific care, it is reasonable to predict that not all will embrace the topic initially, as well as be prepared to pay for it. Early adopters are likely to be owners of new pets, and the market segment known as pet parents. These are the early adopters, but when success is achieved with these individuals, it is possible to leverage that success across the entire hospital population. However, even a small contingent of proponents can have a powerful impact on pets and the teams that care for them. According to Pareto's principle, if 20% of clients embrace pet-specific care, they can contribute to 80% of positive outcomes (see 10.2 The Importance of Practice Differentiation).

1.1.4 Risk Assessment

Pet-specific care is all about managing risks, so the very first step typically involves assessing pets for risks based on their individual circumstances (see 1.2 Providing a Lifetime of Care). In most cases, this first happens during puppy and kitten visits, often at around 8 weeks of age.

All animals have certain risks that pertain to their individual circumstances. By acknowledging and prioritizing risks, we can craft meaningful personalized action plans for our patients (see 1.3 Personalized Care Plans). In addition, once we have identified risks, pet owners can decide how they might best manage the financial aspects of those risks, including pet health insurance (see 10.16 Pet Health Insurance).

For most pets, family history, genotype, and breed predisposition are significant contributors to disease susceptibility (see 11.4 Heritable Health Conditions – by Breed). This is true whether the pet is purebred, hybrid, or mixed-breed. In many instances, when a pet is mixed-breed and the parents have not been identified with certainty, it may be difficult to discern any type of predisposition without

performing breed composition genetic testing. Whether purebred, hybrid or mixed-breed, both genotypic and phenotypic testing are important to detect disease susceptibility (see 3.11 Integrating Genotypic and Phenotypic Testing).

Exposure risks constitute another significant contributor to disease susceptibility. For example, a pet exposed to many other pets will be at increased risk for infectious diseases and, potentially, parasite transmission. A pet that is taken for walks in wooded areas may be exposed to ticks that are enzootic to the region and may introduce tick-related infections to the pet.

Susceptibility to medical problems is also influenced by life stages and preexisting conditions. For example, an umbilical hernia is more likely to be congenital and evident in a juvenile pet, while most cases of hypothyroidism present during adulthood. Regarding preexisting conditions, a pet with early evidence of hip dysplasia will be more likely to develop osteoarthritis later in life.

A pet's gender as well as its neuter status also influence risk (see 4.2 Gender-Related Considerations). Some diseases are sex-limited in nature (such as prostatic disease in males or pyometra in females), but there are also sex predispositions for a variety of disorders. For example, there may be a modest sex predisposition in females regarding cutaneous lupus erythematosus, while adrenal sex hormone imbalance (also known as alopecia X) may be more commonly diagnosed in males. This is different from disorders that are transmitted genetically on the sex chromosomes. For example, hemophilia is more often clinically evident in males because the condition is transmitted on the X chromosome as a sex-linked recessive condition, and since males only have one X chromosome (they are said to be hemizygous; the other is a Y chromosome), they are more likely to manifest the condition. Neuter status also affects risk. Bitches spayed before their first estrus have a reduced prevalence of mammary cancers; neutered males have a lowered risk for prostatic hyperplasia. New guidelines even suggest the most appropriate age for neutering on a pet-specific basis.

Geography also plays a significant role in disease susceptibility, partially because it influences infectious diseases that are present in the area or the vectors that are associated with their transmission. Accordingly, when creating health plans, it is important to take into consideration whether or not the pet may travel outside its residential region.

Even conformation and nondisease traits can be associated with predisposition to disease. For example, cats with white fur may be at higher risk for developing squamous cell carcinoma; color dilution alopecia is more common in dogs with diluted coloring patterns, such as "blue" Dobermans, etc.

1.1.5 The Need

It makes sense for veterinary teams to embrace a pet-specific care model, in which diseases that can be prevented are prevented, especially through comprehensive vaccination and parasite control protocols, diagnostic screening is done as part of a sensible surveillance system, preferably even identifying animals in a subclinical state when there are the most options available for management, and finally, treating animals over an appropriate time period and according to evidence-based guidelines, and helping to facilitate owner compliance. In this manner, acute diseases may be treated over days or weeks, while chronic problems, such as osteoarthritis, atopic dermatitis, diabetes mellitus. and many others. are managed on a continuum of care over the remainder of the pet's life (see 9.7 Continuum of Care and Convergence Schedules).

To be successful in this regard, standards of care are critically important for hospitals (see 9.4 Standards of Care). While personal freedom for veterinarians to treat as they wish is aspirational, it may not allow practices to deliver consistent quality of care to pets and their owners. At least when it comes to basic preventive care, there is value in determining protocols for vaccination and parasite control, and care pathways for the best evidence-based approaches to the most common chronic conditions managed by the practice, such as osteoarthritis, atopic dermatitis, periodontal disease, etc. Diligence is particularly important for these chronic diseases, since how these conditions are managed when an animal is young will greatly affect its quality of life as it gets older.

A suitable starting point is to consider what risk factors might influence the decision-making process through use of health risk assessments (see 2.7 Risk Assessment), which involve client-focused questionnaires, taking a thorough medical history, and performing a skilled physical examination. The process can then continue by evaluating which strategies should be employed for prevention, early detection, appropriate treatment, and optimized compliance for an individual pet. Ongoing monitoring of the process is critical to determine gaps in the anticipated quality of care provided by the hospital.

Our major preventive strategies include vaccination, parasite control, optimal nutrition, and physical activity for each life stage, behavior counseling, sensible exercise programs, breeding recommendations (to help prevent heritable conditions), optimal reproductive control, oral hygiene, and even counseling on pet selection to minimize the risk that a pet will later be relinquished to a shelter, abandoned, or euthanized for nonmedical reasons.

Currently, many pet owners only associate the need to see a veterinarian with vaccination or serious illness. This failure to grasp the true value of preventive medicine and regular pet-specific care and the positive impact both can have on pets and pet owners can adversely affect the health of pets and the financial health of veterinary practices.

Diagnostic screening tests should provide baseline values and facilitate long-term monitoring to establish trends that may help to identify subclinical disease. Without early detection and management, many of these conditions can lead to a significant decrease in a pet's quality of life. Such periodic testing of otherwise healthy animals is indicated to help identify affected individuals before clinical manifestations become evident. Selecting appropriate tests can be facilitated by performing health risk assessments periodically and screening for conditions that might be considered higher risk because of breed predisposition, family history, lifestyle, or geographic considerations.

Early therapeutic intervention tends to offer the best chance of successful long-term management of many conditions. Clearly distinguishing between curing a medical condition and long-term management is important when discussing the many benefits of intervention and management of disease states with pet owners.

Early intervention in primary conditions can also reduce the risks of secondary problems. Periodontal disease is among the most common conditions affecting dogs and cats, yet it is often ignored by pet owners or undertreated by veterinary teams. When existing periodontal disease is comprehensively managed, the risk of debilitating sequelae is often reduced (see 4.9 Periodontal Disease).

In addition, prevention, detection, and treatment of pain (as well as ensuring compliance and adherence) should be provided to all patients. Through this process, patient quality of life, pet owner satisfaction, and perceived value of veterinary care are more likely to improve while patient stress, recovery time, and potential for exacerbation of co-morbidities will likely decrease.

1.1.6 Fundamental Drivers of Pet-Specific Care

To facilitate the adoption of pet-specific care principles in practice, veterinary teams need to understand the major "drivers" of pet owner engagement in the process – the human–animal bond, communication skills, value, and customer service – in addition to maintaining a high level of clinical competence (see 8.1 Delivering Pet-Specific Care as a Team).

EXAMPLES

Bella is an 18-month-old spayed female golden retriever who presented to ABC Animal Hospital with evidence of licking and chewing at her paws. Her owners recognized that this might be early evidence of atopic dermatitis, because the veterinary team had described this during puppy visits as something relatively common in the breed. When the owners asked if anything could be done prior to problems being recognized, the hospital team introduced them to behavioral approaches to condition Bella to willingly accept bathing and ear cleaning, so the medicated baths now recommended were not going to be an issue. A DNA panel taken at 12 weeks of age indicated that Bella was a carrier for a specific form of progressive retinal atrophy seen in golden retrievers, but since it is a recessive trait it was not a clinical concern, and since Bella had been spayed, it would not affect future generations. Bella was due for orthopedic screening in a few months, and the owners were very dutiful about providing care according to the health schedule recommended by the veterinary team.

 TAKE-AWAYS

- Pet-specific care provides customized care for pets and constitutes an important and value-added healthcare experience for pet owners.
- Pet-specific care involves approaches that allow predictions to be made as to an individual's susceptibility to disease, the course of that disease, and the disease's likely response to treatment.
- The goal of pet-specific care is to prevent disease if at all possible, or to decrease the impact of disease on the patient, thereby improving the pet's quality of life.
- The fundamentals of pet-specific care involve prevention, early detection of issues, appropriate management, and facilitated compliance.
- The ultimate success of pet-specific care relies on pet owner engagement in the healthcare process, and a commitment to play an important role in their pet's care.

 MISCELLANEOUS

Abbreviation

DNA   Deoxyribonucleic acid

Recommended Reading

Ackerman, L. (2011). *The Genetic Connection: A Guide to Health Problems in Purebred Dogs*, 2e. Lakewood, CO: AAHA Press.

Ackerman, L. (2019). An introduction to pet-specific care. *EC Vet Sci* 4 (1): 1–3.

Ackerman, L. Personalized medicine improves outcomes. Today's Veterinary Business, 2018. https://todaysveterinarybusiness.com/personalized-medicine-improves-outcomes

Ackerman, L. (ed.) (2020). Pet-specific care. In: *Five-Minute Veterinary Practice Management Consult*, 3e, 260–263. Ames, IA: Wiley.

Ackerman, L. (2020). Proactive pet parenting: Anticipating pet health problems before they happen. Problem Free Publishing.

American Animal Hospital Association (2012). *Evolving to a Culture of Prevention: Implementing Integrated Preventive Care*, 1–23. Lakewood, CO: AAHA.

Hamburg, M.A. and Collins, F.S. (2010). The path to personalized medicine. *New England Journal of Medicine* 363 (4): 301–304.

Harris, D.L., Rosenthal, K., and Hines, A. (2019). Thinking like a futurist could help the veterinary profession. *Journal of the American Veterinary Medical Association* 255 (5): 523–524.

Mealey, K.L., Martinez, S.E., Villarina, N.F., and Court, M.H. (2019). Personalized medicine: going to the dogs? *Human Genetics* 138 (5): 467–481.

Stull, J.W., Shelby, J.A., Bonnett, B.N. et al. Barriers and next steps to providing a spectrum of effective health care to companion animals. *Journal of the American Veterinary Medical Association* 253 (11): 1386–1389.

1.2

Providing a Lifetime of Care

Lowell Ackerman, DVM, DACVD, MBA, MPA, CVA, MRCVS

Global Consultant, Author, and Lecturer, MA, USA

 BASICS

1.2.1 Summary

Much of veterinary care delivered today is based on short-term goals, either providing care for a defined period (e.g., puppy and kitten care) or addressing issues as they present themselves, and often defaulting to treating conditions when they arise rather than trying to be proactive. In fact, it is not unusual that pet owners are seen regularly for puppy and kitten visits and then there is a drop-off in regular care until pets become senior or otherwise develop medical issues that bring them into the veterinary hospital.

Veterinary teams would be well advised to spend time with clients, understanding their needs and concerns, explaining in advance what the likely healthcare process will be, including expenses to be anticipated along the way and when changes in healthcare requirements will likely occur. Then, the entire healthcare team should endeavor to deliver lifelong pet-specific care on an evidence-based schedule.

1.2.2 Terms Defined

Adherence: The extent to which patients take medications as prescribed, which involves the pet owner in filling and refilling the prescription, administering the correct dose, timing and use, and completing the prescribed course.

Advocate: Someone who speaks or takes action on behalf of another.

Compliance: The extent to which pets receive a treatment, screening, or procedure in accordance with veterinary healthcare recommendations.

Continuum of Care: The timespan over which all care is provided.

Convergence Schedule: In veterinary medicine, the coming together of different processes into the same continuum of care

Genotype: The underlying genetic constitution of an individual.

Healthspan: That portion of the lifespan during which the pet remains in good general health.

Pet-Specific Care: An approach that tailors veterinary care to individual pets based on their predicted risk of disease and likely response to intervention.

Phenotype: The outward observable characteristics of an individual, resulting from the interaction of its underlying genetic constitution with environmental factors.

Telomere: Structure at the end of a chromosome that protects DNA data. Telomere shortening is associated with aging.

 MAIN CONCEPTS

To provide care that will last a lifetime, the veterinary healthcare team needs to be able to consider the needs of the individual across that lifetime, not just at specific points in time that correspond to scheduled office visits.

It is now possible to predict the needs of pets, from the time of puppy and kitten visits well into their senior years, realizing that this is a dynamic process and the model will need to be updated and tweaked throughout the pet's life (see 6.4 Creating a Pet-Specific User's Manual).

When considering pet-specific care across a pet's lifetime, it is also important to keep in mind that the goal is somewhat different from that of the standard model of disease treatment. In pet-specific care, the goal is to keep the pet healthy, focusing on prevention and early detection, just as is done in human healthcare. Thus, our goal is not just to treat animals when they are sick, but to guide owners on the path to keeping their pets healthy and optimizing their pet healthspan, not just their lifespan (see 9.7 Continuum of Care and Convergence Schedules). The process starts with understanding the factors that most affect health, and that begins with appreciating risk.

1.2.3 Risk (Needs) Assessment

To truly appreciate an animal's need for appropriate care, it is important to first discern which factors may impact its healthcare risks, either positively or negatively (Figure 1.2.1). Some of these risks can be determined very early in an animal's life (some even before birth) by evaluating genotypic and phenotypic assessment of the animal, its parents, and/or close relatives.

Other assessments can be made based on local risk factors in the particular geographic area in which the animal lives. Location typically impacts the prevalence of many infectious diseases, environmental risks (snakebite, heat stroke, frostbite, toxicities, etc.), and other factors of significance. It is important not only to appreciate risks in the place of residence, but also in other environments in which the pet may find itself (e.g., travel, boarding, grooming, activities, etc.).

Assessing lifestyle information helps a practice determine the relative risks of one animal versus another in the same locale. Given a pet's risk factors from genetics, family history, and lifestyle, it is possible to discuss a lifelong customized healthcare plan that can be shared with the pet owner, so they can better anticipate the healthcare intervention that will be needed throughout a pet's life (see 2.7 Risk Assessment). A personalized pet profile can then be created to customize care for animals on an individualized basis (see Figure 1.3.1).

1.2.4 Risk Management

Once owners can appreciate the veterinary care that will be needed by animals over their anticipated lifespan, they can also better plan how they are going to pay for such services. Owners can use several risk management strategies to financially prepare for such veterinary care, including pet health insurance (see 10.16 Pet Health Insurance), payment plans (see 10.17 Payment and Wellness Plans), and third-party payers (see 10.18 Financing Veterinary Care).

It is important for the veterinary healthcare team to reiterate that if pet owners want the most benefit from pet health insurance it should be initiated as quickly as possible, typically by 8 weeks of age, before there are any issues that could be considered preexisting.

1.2.5 The First Visit

Ideally, the first veterinary visit might be made even before the new pet is acquired (see 3.10 Advising Clients on Selecting an Appropriate Pet). If a specific breed has been selected, the veterinary team should be able to counsel the owners on possible breed-related conditions to be aware of (see 11.4 Heritable Health Conditions – By Breed), and what documentation would be worthwhile from the provider of the animal (e.g., hip joint certification of parents, DNA testing of parents, etc.). Armed with this information, the situation is established where the veterinary team is the healthcare advocate, and this helps cement an appropriate doctor–client bond.

The veterinary practice will also want to evaluate the previous healthcare that the animal received. For example, many young animals are "dewormed," have had some initial vaccinations, and perhaps other treatments. As the healthcare advocate, the veterinary team will want to safeguard the owner from any zoonotic conditions, protect any animals at home from infectious diseases (quarantine may be needed), and determine the appropriateness of any treatments to date.

Apart from thorough physical examination, the first visit is a great time to discuss overall healthcare strategies for the months and years ahead. Sometimes this is easier to discuss if the subject matter is broken down into routine healthcare, breed-related concerns, behavioral counseling, neutering, dental care, nutrition, life stage issues, and unexpected care (emergencies, specialist consultations, etc.). Providing a written healthcare plan streamlines the process and means that the client can listen to instructions and appreciate the "big picture" without trying to take exhaustive notes. Although this might seem overwhelming to the client at first, it does set the stage for the anticipated care of the pet that will span a lifetime. This also helps owners budget accordingly and consider other ways to manage the costs of pet healthcare such as buying pet health insurance (see 10.16 Pet Health Insurance).

Many pet owners have unrealistic expectations of pet care because they have never been exposed to optimal care and never had anyone detail pet-specific care guidelines for them (see 9.3 Guidelines). Most are appreciative of these clear-cut guidelines and the ability to plan in advance for realistic costs as well as which risk management strategies might be most appropriate.

Canine Risk Assessment Form

Name: Date of Birth:

Breed: Neutered   ☐ Y   ☐ N

Has genetic testing been run on your pet or its parents?   ☐ Y   ☐ N
If so, what were the results?

Has this pet or its parents been included in a breed registry
screening for heritable diseases (hip dysplasia, eye diseases, etc.)?   ☐ Y   ☐ N

What other diagnostic testing has been done to date?

Any family history of the following (please check all that apply)?
☐ Atopic (allergies)   ☐ Glaucoma   ☐ Heart disease   ☐ Kidney disease
☐ Osteoarthritis   ☐ Seizure disorders   ☐ Thyroid issues   ☐ Urinary tract "stones"

Is there a family history of any other specific medical conditions?   ☐ Y   ☐ N
If so, which condition(s)?

What food are you currently feeding?

What medications/supplements arc you currently giving?

What parasite control are you providing?

Are you doing any home dental care (brushing, rinses, etc.)?   ☐ Y   ☐ N

Do you consider your pet: ☐ Below ideal weight   ☐ Ideal weight   ☐ Above ideal weight

                                                     Comments
Does your pet ever sleep with you, or share your bed?   ☐ Y   ☐ N
Does your pet ever travel outside this immediate region?   ☐ Y   ☐ N
Does your pet come in contact with other people's pets?   ☐ Y   ☐ N
Does your pet ever visit a groomer or boarding facility?   ☐ Y   ☐ N
Does your pet ever go to dog shows or pet events?   ☐ Y   ☐ N
Does your pet ever go to parks/fields/gardens?   ☐ Y   ☐ N
Does your pet go to any other veterinary hospitals?   ☐ Y   ☐ N
Does your pet ever experience motion sickness?   ☐ Y   ☐ N
Does your pet ever have an opportunity to drink from water
outdoors. such as ponds, puddles. water bowls. rivers, or creeks?   ☐ Y   ☐ N
Is there wildlife in your area, including mice, deer, squirrels,
birds, raccoons. possums. hedgehogs, skunks, etc.?   ☐ Y   ☐ N

What other types of pets do you have in your household?
☐ Dogs   ☐ Cats   ☐ Birds   ☐ Rabbits   ☐ _____

Which of the following exist in your area?
☐ Fleas   ☐ Ticks   ☐ Mosquitoes   ☐ Lice   ☐ Slugs   ☐ _____

Figure 1.2.1   Example of a canine risk assessment form.

1.2.6 Subsequent Visits

Subsequent visits are opportunities to reinforce the healthcare plan and make any alterations needed on the basis of those visits, diagnostic testing, or treatments. Healthcare plans are dynamic and flexible and may be changed to reflect the realities of the situation. For example, if a Doberman pinscher is screened for von Willebrand disease and found to be at significant risk, this will likely change the process at the time of surgery, as well as the charges associated with such surgery. The identification of cardiomyopathy will change the previous plan regarding the interval between scheduled clinical examinations, and recommendations for ongoing monitoring.

Throughout the process, it is important to have ongoing conversations with pet owners about the important concepts of compliance and adherence. It is not enough that clients be prepared to purchase products from us for use in their pets. They need to understand the critical importance of following directions at home. There is often a lot to discuss with pet owners, and typically limited time during office visits, so successful veterinary teams often rely on convergence schedules to ensure effective communication and owner engagement (see 9.7 Continuum of Care and Convergence Schedules).

Care is often delivered on the basis of life stages, and while this varies considerably between individuals, it can be helpful to use approximations based on age and weight (Tables 1.2.1 and 1.2.2); in the future there will likely also be ways to assess genetic aspects of aging (e.g., telomeres, DNA methylation, etc.).

EXAMPLES

Mrs Stewart presented Brodie, an 8-week-old Border collie, for examination. Brodie had an uneventful physical examination, but given his breed and family history, a few recommendations were made.

Mrs Stewart was surprised to learn that Border collies were at increased risk for hip dysplasia, as she had mistakenly assumed it was only a large-dog disease. Brodie's parents had not been screened for hip dysplasia, so any family history was uncertain. A recommendation was made to do a preliminary assessment of hip laxity at 6 months of age during neutering surgery, and then a more complete radiographic evaluation at 2 years of age.

A sample was also collected to submit for genetic testing. The single panel was capable of screening Brodie for a variety of disorders, including black-haired follicular dysplasia, cobalamin (vitamin B12) malabsorption, collie eye anomaly, degenerative myelopathy, malignant hyperthermia, hereditary myotonia, ivermectin sensitivity (mdr1 mutation), neuronal ceroid lipofuscinosis, primary lens luxation, trapped neutrophil syndrome, and others. The staff discussed other phenotypic testing that would be done in the future, and provided a link to the website where Brodie's personalized pet profile would be created.

The staff also discussed pet health insurance options with Mrs Stewart, and reiterated that it would be important to select a policy in the very near future if she wanted to ensure that there would be no preexisting problems that could be excluded from coverage.

TAKE-AWAYS

- Client engagement is heightened when the client plays an active role in their pet's health, and is committed to the prospect of keeping their pet healthy.
- By examining risk factors for specific pets, it is possible to plan for a lifetime of care on the basis of their specific risk factors.
- Genotypic screening (DNA testing) is typically done early, often around 12 weeks of age, and phenotypic testing is then conducted throughout the pet's lifetime according to a sensible schedule.
- Health is a dynamic process, so action plans need to be updated on a regular basis.
- Veterinary healthcare teams are critical to being able to provide a lifetime of care, and are often the driving force behind such efforts.

MISCELLANEOUS

Pet owners are at a disadvantage compared to parents of children, who tend to have a large variety of resources at their disposal for the anticipated care and expenses of child dependents. Armed with this knowledge, emphasis is placed on routine medical visits, preventive care, proper socialization, education, and risk management to mitigate the costs of medical care. For too many years, pet owners have been trained to expect that a one-time neutering surgery, occasional vaccinations, and periodic veterinary visits are all that is needed unless their animal is ill. Ensuring continued excellence in pet healthcare requires engagement of pet owners and a veterinary team committed to pet-specific care, education, and advocacy (see 8.1 Delivering Pet-Specific Care as a Team).

Table 1.2.1 Approximation for converting "dog" years to relative human years, as well as matching life stages based on adult weights

Age	<10 kg		10–20 kg		20–30 kg		30–40 kg		40–50 kg		>50 kg	
	Life Stage	Relative Human Age (Years)	Life Stage	Relative Human Age (Years)	Life Stage	Relative Human Age (Years)	Life Stage	Relative Human Age (Years)	Life Stage	Relative Human Age (Years)	Life Stage	Relative Human Age (Years)
3 months	Puppy	4	Puppy	4	Puppy	3	Puppy	3	Puppy	3	Puppy	3
6 months	Puppy	7	Puppy	7	Puppy	6	Puppy	6	Puppy	6	Puppy	6
9 months	Young	11	Young	11	Puppy	9	Puppy	9	Puppy	9	Puppy	9
12 months	Young	15	Young	15	Puppy	12	Puppy	12	Puppy	12	Puppy	12
18 months	Young	19	Young	19	Young	16	Young	16	Puppy	16	Puppy	16
2 years	Young	24	Young	24	Young	19	Young	19	Young	19	Young	19
3 years	Mature	28	Mature	28	Mature	25	Mature	26	Mature	26	Mature	27
4 years	Mature	32	Mature	32	Mature	30	Mature	32	Mature	33	Mature	35
5 years	Mature	36	Mature	36	Mature	36	Mature	38	Mature	40	Senior	42
6 years	Mature	40	Mature	40	Mature	42	Senior	46	Senior	47	Senior	50
7 years	Mature	44	Senior	45	Senior	48	Senior	53	Senior	54	Senior	56
8 years	Senior	48	Senior	49	Senior	53	Senior	57	Senior	58	Senior	61
9 years	Senior	52	Senior	53	Senior	58	Senior	62	Senior	64	Senior	68
10 years	Senior	56	Senior	57	Senior	63	Senior	67	Senior	69	Senior	75
11 years	Senior	61	Senior	62	Senior	68	Senior	72	Senior	74	Senior	82
12 years	Senior	66	Senior	67	Senior	73	Senior	77	Senior	79	Senior	89
13 years	Senior	71	Senior	73	Senior	78	Senior	82	Senior	83	Senior	91
14 years	Senior	76	Senior	78	Senior	83	Senior	87	Senior	88	Senior	96
15 years	Senior	81	Senior	83	Senior	89	Senior	92	Senior	94	Senior	101
16 years	Senior	86	Senior	88	Senior	95	Senior	98	Senior	100	Senior	106
17 years	Senior	92	Senior	94	Senior	100	Senior	103	Senior	105	Senior	111
18 years	Senior	98	Senior	100	Senior	104	Senior	107	Senior	111	Senior	116
19 years	Senior	104	Senior	105	Senior	108	Senior	111	Senior	113	Senior	121
20 years	Senior	108	Senior	109	Senior	112	Senior	116	Senior	118	Senior	
21 years	Senior	112	Senior	114	Senior	116	Senior	120	Senior		Senior	
22 years	Senior	116	Senior	120	Senior	122	Senior		Senior		Senior	
23 years	Senior	120	Senior		Senior		Senior		Senior		Senior	
24 years	Senior		Senior		Senior		Senior		Senior		Senior	
25 years	Senior		Senior		Senior		Senior		Senior		Senior	

Table 1.2.2 Approximation for converting "cat" years to relative human years and applicable life stages. Life stages are based on AAFP-AAHA Feline Life Stage Guidelines

Age of Cat	Life Stage	Relative Human Age (Years)
3 months	Kitten	4
6 months	Kitten	10
9 months	Junior	12
12 months	Junior	15
18 months	Junior	21
2 years	Junior	24
3 years	Prime	28
4 years	Prime	32
5 years	Prime	36
6 years	Prime	40
7 years	Mature	44
8 years	Mature	48
9 years	Mature	52
10 years	Mature	56
11 years	Senior	60
12 years	Senior	64
13 years	Senior	68
14 years	Senior	72
15 years	Geriatric	76
16 years	Geriatric	80
17 years	Geriatric	84
18 years	Geriatric	88
19 years	Geriatric	92
20 years	Geriatric	96
21 years	Geriatric	100
22 years	Geriatric	104
23 years	Geriatric	108
24 years	Geriatric	112

1.2.7 Cautions

It is not possible to predict all health outcomes for pets, and this needs to be explained to owners. The purpose of planning is to detail anticipated needs and expenditures and to allow owners to plan accordingly. It is also possible that some clients will be overwhelmed with the information provided and elect to only engage with a very basic level of service. This does not negate the value of informing clients about what to logically expect but it might serve as a reminder that different approaches might be needed for different clients.

Abbreviation

DNA   Deoxyribonucleic acid

Recommended Reading

Ackerman, L.J. (2011). *The Genetic Connection*, 2e. Lakewood, CO: AAHA Press.

Ackerman, L. (2020). Proactive pet parenting: Anticipating pet health problems before they happen. Problem Free Publishing.

American Animal Hospital Association/American Veterinary Medical Association Preventive Health Guidelines Task Force (2011). AAHA/AVMA Preventive Healthcare Guidelines. *J. Am. Vet. Med. Assoc.* 239 (5): 625–629.

Bartges, J., Boynton, B., Vogt, A.H. et al. (2012). AAHA canine life stage guidelines. *J. Am. Anim. Hosp. Assoc.* 48: 1–11.

Giuffrida, M.A., Brown, D.C., Ellenberg, S.S., and Farrar, J.T. (2018). Development and psychometric testing of the canine owner – reported quality of life questionnaire, an instrument designed to measure quality of life I dogs with cancer. *J. Am. Vet. Med. Assoc.* 252 (9): 1073–1083.

Landsberg, G., Hunthausen, W., and Ackerman, L. (2013). *Behavior Problems of the Dog and Cat*, 3e. Edinburgh: Elsevier.

Partners for Healthy Pets: www.partnersforhealthypets.org

Urfer, S.R., Wange, M., Yang, M. et al. (2019). Risk factors associate with lifespan in pet dogs evaluated in primary care veterinary hospitals. *J. Am. Anim. Hosp. Assoc.* 55: 130–137.

Vogt, A.H., Rodan, I., Brown, M. et al. (2010). AAFP-AAHA Feline Life Stage Guidelines. *J. Am. Anim. Hosp. Assoc.* 46: 70–85.

1.3

Personalized Care Plans

Lowell Ackerman, DVM, DACVD, MBA, MPA, CVA, MRCVS

Global Consultant, Author, and Lecturer, MA, USA

BASICS

1.3.1 Summary

Conventional veterinary medicine sometimes considers all pets to have the same needs on a species basis. So, by this reckoning, all dogs might warrant the same medical approach based on life stage and where they reside, and the same might be considered true for cats. However, this does not even begin to appreciate the differences between mixed-breeds and purebreds, between different breeds, and even between individuals of the same breed.

Today's pet owners are educated consumers, and with access to the internet, it doesn't take much time for them to discover that the medical needs of a golden retriever are significantly different from those of a shih tzu, a Siberian husky, or a Cavalier King Charles spaniel. It's time for the profession to acknowledge and convey that pets deserve personalized care plans for their specific care – owners value them, and practices can benefit from providing the customized care that pets need and deserve.

1.3.2 Terms Defined

Adherence: The extent to which patients take the medications prescribed, which requires the pet owner to fill and refill the prescription, administer the correct dose, timing and use, and complete the prescribed course.

Compliance: The extent to which pets receive a treatment, a screening, or a procedure in accordance with accepted veterinary healthcare practices.

Epigenetics: The study of heritable changes in genetic expression caused by mechanisms other than those attributable to underlying DNA sequences.

Mixed-Breed: An animal of unknown or mixed parentage. Mixed-breed dogs are sometimes referred to as mutts or mongrels; mixed-breed cats are sometimes referred to as moggies or mutt-cats.

Off-Label: Pharmaceuticals prescribed, dispensed, or administered for an unapproved indication. Also referred to as extra-label drug use.

Pedigreed: An animal whose ancestry is recorded by a registry organization.

Pet-Specific Care: An approach that tailors veterinary care to individual pets based on their predicted risk of disease and likely response to intervention.

Purebred: An animal bred from parents of the same breed or variety; one whose ancestry contains members of the same breed.

MAIN CONCEPTS

1.3.3 Premise of Pet-Specific Care

All pets have risk factors pertaining to their specific circumstances. Pets have genetic risks associated with their genotypic predispositions to a variety of disorders [1]. In some cases, genetic testing is available. Like humans, pets can also have family histories in which there are breed predilections, even if genotypes cannot be identified (Table 1.3.1). The environment can also affect expression of traits, and certain environmental "shocks" can leave imprints on the genetic material in eggs and sperm, which

Table 1.3.1 Some common breeds and a few of the conditions to which they are predisposed [1]

Breed	Breed predispositions
Labrador retriever	Centronuclear myopathy[a], cystinuria[a], degenerative myelopathy[a], elbow dysplasia, exercise-induced collapse[a], hip dysplasia, nasal parakeratosis[a], osteochondrosis dissecans, progressive rod-cone degeneration[a], skeletal dysplasia type 2[a], tricuspid valve dysplasia
German shepherd dog	Acral lick dermatitis, elbow dysplasia, degenerative myelopathy[a], exocrine pancreatic insufficiency, hemophilia A[a], hip dysplasia, hyperuricosuria[a], masticatory myositis, perianal fistula[a], renal cystadenocarcinoma/nodular dermatofibrosis[a]
Golden retriever	Atopy, elbow dysplasia, hemophilia A, hip dysplasia, hypothyroidism, ichthyosis[a], juvenile cellulitis, muscular dystrophy[a], patella luxation, progressive retinal atrophy (GR_PRA1 and GR_PRA2)[a], progressive rod-cone degeneration[a], sensory ataxic neuropathy
English bulldog	Anasarca, brachycephalic syndrome, entropion, factor VII deficiency, fold dermatitis, hip dysplasia, hyperuricosuria[a], hypothyroidism, laryngeal paralysis, multifocal retinopathy (CMR1)[a], pulmonic stenosis, sacrocaudal dysgenesis, ventricular septal defect
Beagle	Cataracts, cryptorchidism, diabetes mellitus, factor VII deficiency[a], glaucoma (POAG)[a], hip dysplasia, juvenile polyarthritis, Musladin–Leuke syndrome[a], night blindness[a], patellar luxation, pulmonic stenosis, pyruvate kinase deficiency[a], retinal dysplasia
French bulldog	Atopic dermatitis, brachycephalic syndrome, cataracts[a], corneal ulcers, factor VIII deficiency[a], factor IX deficiency[a], histiocytic ulcerative colitis, necrotizing meningoencephalitis, hyperuricosuria[a], multifocal retinopathy[a], cone-rod dystrophy I[a]
Poodle	Cataracts, epilepsy, factor VIII deficiency, Legg–Calvé–Perthes disease, mucopolysaccharidosis[a], neonatal encephalopathy[a], organic aciduria, oxalate urolithiasis, progressive rod-cone degeneration[a], sebaceous adenitis, von Willebrand disease[a]
Rottweiler	Cervical vertebral instability, cruciate ligament rupture, fragmented coronoid process, gastric dilation/volvulus, leukodystrophy, membranous glomerulopathy, myotubular myopathy[a], patent ductus arteriosus, polyneuropathy and neuronal vacuolation[a], short tail[a]
Yorkshire terrier	Atlantoaxial instability, cataracts, cryptorchidism, L2-hydroxyglutaric aciduria[a], lymphoproliferative disease, necrotizing meningoencephalitis, patellar luxation, patent ductus arteriosus, primary lens luxation[a], progressive rod-cone degeneration[a]
Boxer	Brachycephalic syndrome, cardiomyopathy[a], cystinuria, factor II deficiency, hyperadrenocorticism, neoplasia, progressive axonopathy, pulmonic stenosis, short tail[a], sphingomyelinosis, subaortic stenosis, ulcerative colitis

[a] DNA testing is available.

can be passed on to future generations (so-called epigenetics). Epigenetic marks can switch genes on or off, affecting disease risk, and they can be passed on to offspring [1].

Lifestyle also plays a role in determining risk for pets, including the part of the country in which they live, their exposure to other animals (boarding, grooming, social activities, etc.), the protection they are already being provided (e.g., parasite control, vaccination, etc.), and their role in the family – pets in close contact with family members need more rigorous preventive care (for parasite control, etc.) than animals without such contact. This is often best determined by risk assessment (see 1.2 Providing a Lifetime of Care).

Testing can also identify risk (see 4.7 Embracing Early Detection). In some cases, it is genetic testing as previously mentioned, but in many other cases we rely on phenotypic testing to identify risk. Thus, if we perform radiographs as part of routine patient screening and identify that a pet has hip dysplasia, we know this increases the risk that the pet will develop osteoarthritis later in life.

Armed with all this information, the veterinary team is in a much better position to determine pet-specific care that is relevant to the pet and client and allows for earlier intervention, when the best clinical outcome is typically achievable (see 5.10 Discussing Pet-Specific Care).

1.3.4 Practice Pet Populations

To personalize care for clients, it is first necessary to determine the breeds most represented in a practice, and this can be achieved through appropriate fields in the practice management software system. In the United States, approximately 54% of dogs are purebreds and 46% are mixed-breeds [2]. For cats, the vast majority seen in practice are mixed-breeds, often referred to by terms such as domestic shorthair or domestic longhair (see 3.19 Mixed-Breed Considerations). Although many purebred animals might be pedigreed and have their family lineage documented with a registry organization, many others are purebred in name only and are without such documentation. Others might have documentation from a breed registry but bear little resemblance to the breed standard.

Among the mixed-breed dogs in a practice, it is often tempting to identify them based on perceived physical characteristics (e.g., beagle x) but this practice is to be discouraged because it is wrong at least as often as it is right, and it might lead to inappropriately associating risk factors that don't belong and missing ones that do belong [3]. Within the medical record, if the owners don't know with certainty which breeds contributed to their pets and if DNA testing has not been done to determine likely heritage, then the pet should be recorded as a mixed-breed or other suitable term. This should only be done proactively with new pets, and the medical record not changed for existing clients unless DNA testing has been done and there is a valid reason to change the medical record, with a copy of the DNA results maintained in the medical record to substantiate a medico-legal reason for amending the record.

1.3.5 Components of Personalized Pet Care Plans

Prevention is the cornerstone of personalized pet care and fundamental to the concept is that diseases should preferably be prevented whenever possible, on a risk/benefit basis (see 1.1 Overview of Pet-Specific Care). Not only is it easier to prevent problems than it is to treat them, but from a client perspective it is also more cost-effective to prevent disorders than to try to manage them. For example, heartworm can be effectively prevented with either injectable medications (with ensured compliance) or with monthly oral or topical medications (which practices should remind clients to administer to improve adherence). Compliance and adherence are critical in this regard, because prevention is only as good as the assurance that the pet has received the medication as directed (see 9.17 Improving Compliance and Adherence with Pet-Specific Care).

Vigilance is involved in the early detection component of our personalized pet care (see 4.7 Embracing Early Detection). As a wellness initiative, vigilance involves reviewing the risk factors for an individual pet and performing screening tests to identify problems while still subclinical and before more permanent damage has taken place (see 11.4 Heritable Health Conditions – By Breed). For example, in an animal with a family history of hip dysplasia, radiographic assessment is warranted, typically by 2 years of age at the latest, to determine if the animal shows

early evidence of the disease. An animal with a breed predisposition for von Willebrand disease (vWD) would benefit from DNA testing during puppyhood, and certainly clotting evaluation before any surgeries might be performed. A kitten with genetic testing suggesting risk of polycystic kidney disease will warrant enhanced scrutiny for kidney disease and monitoring of renal function. For all animals, it is worth performing routine testing from time to time (e.g., hemogram, biochemistries, urinalysis, radiography, blood pressure, etc.) just to be aware of unanticipated risks that might be developing, even if still subclinical. Recommended tests to consider on a breed basis are available for both dogs (www.ofa.org/browse-by-breed) and cats (https://icatcare.org/advice/cat-breeds).

Management of diagnosed conditions must also be personalized. Practices should have protocols for dealing with the most common entities treated, and care pathways for sensible management of chronic disorders, such as diabetes mellitus, osteoarthritis, atopic dermatitis, and others (see 9.4 Standards of Care and 9.6 Care Pathways). However, for many conditions, treatments are customized to the needs of a particular patient. For example, for a pregnant English bulldog, natural delivery may not be possible and cesarean section is often needed. Avermectins might be considered for the management of some conditions, but should be used only cautiously in animals with multidrug resistance (MDR1) genetic mutations.

1.3.6 Genetic Testing and Personalized Care Plans

With pet-specific care, the goal is to be proactive and address potential issues at the earliest possible opportunity, preferably when problems are still subclinical. DNA testing can be very useful for this purpose, as it can be run very early in life, even as early as 1 day of age (see 3.4 Predicting and Eliminating Disease Traits).

Genetic testing is a useful tool as long as veterinary teams have realistic expectations. The purpose of genetic tests is not necessarily to confirm a diagnosis, but to understand risk factors that could be relevant for an individual pet, even issues that may develop much later in life [4]. So, it is extremely important that veterinary team members understand the difference between *association* and *causation* when it comes to such testing.

The vast majority of DNA tests are not absolutely predictive because any one variant detected may not actually be causing the disease in its entirety (see 11.3 Heritable Health Conditions – By Disease). Most often, they just indicate suspected "risk" based on the statistical association of a variant to clinical disease, and it is up to the veterinary team to put such risks in perspective. For example, the skin condition dermatomyositis is often described as being autosomal dominant with variable expressivity (more on this term later), and confirmation of the diagnosis in affected individuals (usually collies, Shetland sheepdogs and their crosses) is based on biopsy. There are at least three different genetic variants "associated" with dermatomyositis risk, and when considered in aggregate, pets can often be classified as high risk, moderate risk, and low risk for developing dermatomyositis. This can be extremely useful for counseling owners of at-risk pets, even if the predictive ability is not absolute. For some conditions in which there is genetic risk, there can also be future testing indicated. For example, a pet that has a relevant glaucoma variant detectable on genetic testing (in a breed at risk for this variant) doesn't mean that the pet will necessarily develop glaucoma, but it does suggest that further glaucoma screening by periodically evaluating intraocular pressure (IOP) is warranted for consideration. Based on the breed, a personalized care plan can incorporate such testing at appropriate intervals.

In most instances, it is practical to perform genetic screening at about 12 weeks of age. At that time, the pet should be well into vaccination and parasite control protocols, and hopefully enrolled in pet health insurance. Once again, the goal is not to try to diagnose disease in a healthy puppy or kitten with such screening, but to help prepare a risk profile for the animal so that pet-specific recommendations can be made regarding prevention and early detection programs. For example, knowing a pet's multidrug resistant (mdr1) genetic status can help inform whether certain medications might be problematic if administered. Knowing the genotypic status for vWD can prove very useful if surgical intervention is being considered (including neutering). If veterinary teams consider that the point of genetic testing is to better appreciate potential risk, they will be able to relay more appropriate information to pet owners, and determine what future screening should be taking place in the personalized care plan.

1.3.7 Putting DNA Testing in Perspective

Whether a practice decides to embrace the concept of genetic testing depends on its strategy for delivering healthcare. There is no doubt that more validation is needed in both human and pet genetic health screening, but that doesn't negate the real value in providing such a proactive resource for pet owners.

When it comes to matching DNA from an individual with the likelihood of disease development in the future, it very much depends on the specificity of the genetic variant being measured, and the individual being tested. That's why it takes a veterinary team to help interpret DNA test results, counsel pet owners accordingly (see 3.8 Genetic counseling), and develop a relevant personalized care plan.

Part of the reason that disease detection is not simple is that diseases and traits can be influenced by a variety of different genes, as well as environmental factors. Atopic dermatitis (environmental allergy), for example, is a skin condition that tends to run in families and there are definite breed predispositions, but that doesn't mean that any one DNA test developed will be able to predict onset with any certainty in all pets and all breeds. The body has a lot of redundant systems in place, so even if there is a genetic issue somewhere, it may be possible for the body to compensate through mechanisms elsewhere. Another important point to consider is that genes themselves don't cause diseases. Genes provide the blueprint for creating proteins, and it is typically defective and poorly functional proteins that lead to the clinical picture that we interpret as disease ... often with significant environmental influences.

At this point in time, there are a few hundred genetic variants known to affect the health of pets, but new associations are being uncovered on a regular basis. The important thing to remember with such testing is that the most predictive tests will be for medical conditions controlled by a single gene pair (such as vWD type I in the Doberman pinscher, progressive retinal atrophy-rcd1 in the Irish setter, or ichthyosis-A in the golden retriever). The vast majority of diseases seen in pets (such as atopic dermatitis, heart disease, diabetes mellitus, obesity, periodontal disease, seizure disorders, etc.) actually have a more complicated pattern of inheritance, and may involve multiple genes as well as environmental influencers, and genetic tests developed for these types of conditions should be expected to be less predictive, even if they still contribute useful information [4]. Even for conditions such as hip dysplasia, heritability is important, but environmental influences often have more impact on clinical expression of the disorder than does genetics (heritability ~0.25). Genetic variants may also have some association with disease in one breed but not necessarily in others and this is not a fault of the testing, but just a reality of pet-specific care and breed-specific risk.

Because of the complexity of biological systems, just because there is a genetic mutation that leads to a poorly functional protein doesn't mean that the animal will definitely develop disease. We often describe this as *penetrance*, the likelihood that a given mutation in an animal will result in clinical disease. Not surprisingly, we don't have enough of this information for many genetic tests, nor for those tests in different breeds. Yet another form of variation is known as *expressivity*. This refers to the variability in clinical presentation that can be seen in individuals, with some animals with the same genotype being more severely affected, and others less so.

Part of the complexity of such testing is also a great opportunity for veterinary teams. If genetic testing didn't require any expertise or interpretation, there would be little reason for pet owners to want to work with veterinary teams to keep their pets healthy. It is this ability to counsel and coach that makes the veterinary team critical to the success of such programs, and to the evidence-based creation of personalized care plans.

1.3.8 Putting It All Together

The personalized care plan is just a customized maintenance schedule that helps pet owners see the type of veterinary intervention that is anticipated over a pet's lifetime (see 6.4 Creating a Pet-Specific User's Manual). Part of that schedule will be based on life stages (see 1.2 Providing a Lifetime of Care); those life stages should reflect the pet's breed or, in the case of mixed-breed animals, their adult weight (see 11.5 Life Planning by Breed). Cats tend to be of more uniform size, so more generalizations can be made based on life stages alone.

Without genetic testing, a personalized care plan will start out with just basic recommendations relevant to all members of a species within the practice locale, as well as predispositions that can be inferred based on breed, conformation, lifestyle, etc. Superimposed on that will be information from health risk assessment (see 2.7 Risk Assessment), which might include pertinent risks on the basis of exposure (travel, boarding, grooming, activities, etc.) and history (preexisting issues detected that could lead to other co-morbidities in the future). Even without genetic testing, a certain amount of risk information can be inferred on the basis of breed predisposition (see 11.4 Heritable Health Conditions – By Breed). Even in a mixed-breed, if likely breed composition can be determined, potential genetic risks can be predicted, and certain early detection screening can be added to the personalized care plan. In general, there are also likely to be nutritional recommendations made specific to each pet (see 9.15 Nutritional Counseling).

It's important to remember that while genetic testing provides some objective criteria on which to base further diagnostic recommendations, it is possible to build personalized care plans just from information available based on history, physical examination, signalment, and risk assessment. That alone could prompt recommendations that could populate a personalized care plan (Table 1.3.2, Figure 1.3.1).

While veterinary teams want to provide the right recommendations to pet owners, it is very difficult to accomplish this without having a plan in place to match risk to action items (see 9.7 Continuum of Care and Convergence Schedules).

EXAMPLES

Rocky Goodwin is a young Doberman pinscher and his owners would like to plan for his anticipated healthcare needs. As part of your assessment, you create a personalized pet care profile for Rocky. The owners are impressed but also a bit worried, because there seems to be a lot that could go wrong with Rocky that they had not considered.

You explain that most of the issues are fairly routine and common for all pets, such as parasite control and vaccinations, but that each pet does carry some unique risks for health issues, and that the best way to deal with these is to diagnose them as early as possible, when there is the best chance for effective management. The owners consent to a lifetime of optimal care for their pet, and decide that pet health insurance is a good mechanism for managing some of their concerns regarding the costs of Rocky's healthcare (see 10.16 Pet Health Insurance).

TAKE-AWAYS

- A personalized pet care plan or profile is just a maintenance schedule of anticipated care expected for a pet over its lifetime.
- Other than routine preventive care, early detection screening is added to the plan based on risk factors specific to the individual pet.
- The care plan should be dynamic and will be altered as new medical findings (including medication monitoring) are added to the schedule.
- The pet care plan can act as a sort of user's manual, alerting the pet owner to care anticipated for a pet over its lifetime.
- Genetic screening during puppy and kitten visits can help inform both veterinary teams and pet owners about additional testing to be considered in a pet's future.

Table 1.3.2 Further testing that might be indicated based on perceived risk

Disorder	Testing indicated
Oral care	Periodic periodontal score; radiography; charting; occlusion assessment
Orthopedic conditions (hip dysplasia, etc.)	Radiography; distraction; palpation; gait assessment
Infectious diseases; parasitism	Heartworm testing, fecal assessment, antigen testing, titers
Clotting abnormalities	Buccal mucosal bleeding time, DNA testing (vWD, hemophilia, etc.), activated coagulation time, prothrombin time, activated partial thromboplastin time, thrombin time, clotting factors
Baseline values	Periodic hemograms, biochemistries, urinalysis
Hypothyroidism	Thyroid profile (e.g., cTSH, free and total T4, T3, autoantibodies, etc.)
Glaucoma	DNA testing (some breeds); periodic intraocular pressure determination
Keratoconjunctivitis sicca	Schirmer tear test
Progressive retinal atrophy	DNA testing (some breeds), electroretinogram, indirect ophthalmoscopy
Kidney disease	DNA testing (polycystic kidney disease, hereditary nephropathy, etc.), urinalysis, urea, creatinine, SDMA, imaging, etc.
Urolithiasis	Periodic urinalysis; DNA testing (e.g., cystinuria 2,8-dihydroxyadenine, etc.)
Heart disease	DNA testing (some breeds), electrocardiogram, Holter monitoring, wearable technology, biomarkers (troponin 1, NT-ProBNP, etc.)
Hypertension	Periodic blood pressure determination
Adverse drug reactions	DNA testing (e.g., mdr1, malignant hyperthermia, etc.)
Inflammation	Biomarkers (C-reactive protein, serum amyloid A, homocysteine[?], etc.)
Senior status	Age-specific screening (laboratory, imaging, cardiac assessment, etc.)

NT-ProBNP, N terminal pro B-type natriuretic peptide; TSH, thyroid-stimulating hormone.

MISCELLANEOUS

1.3.9 Cautions

No matter how vigilant we are, it is impossible to identify all risk factors for an animal, and it is important not to misrepresent this situation to clients. Personalized care plans are meant to address the most common disorders likely to affect an individual. Routine veterinary visits and vigilant screening and monitoring are critical to ensuring that even unanticipated disorders can be diagnosed and managed with some expediency.

Abbreviation

DNA Deoxyribonucleic acid

Personalized Pet Profile: Marilyn

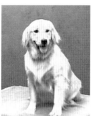

Age	Human Age (Approx.)	Needs
2–8 weeks		Fecal parasite testing; parasite control
		Congenital disease screening (cataracts, umbilical hernia, malocclusion, patellar luxation, heart murmur, persistent pupillary membranes, etc.); Risk Assessment; Start monthly parasite prevention;
8 weeks		Microchipping; Start pet health insurance
6–16 weeks		Initial vaccination series
		Genetic screening (including GR-PRA 1 & 2, progressive rod-cone degeneration, Ichthyosis A, dystrophic epidermolysis bullosa, neuronal ceroid lipofuscinosis, osteogenesis imperfecta, skeletal
12 weeks		dysplasia, degenerative myelopathy, etc.)
16 weeks		Create Personalized care plan based on risk assessment, genotypic and phenotypic assessment
26 weeks	6 years	Coagulation function testing, fecal parasite testing; heartworm prevention
36 weeks	10 years	Neutering surgery, dental evaluation, congenital disease screening
		Adult re-evaluation; vaccine boosters/titers as needed; parasite check; baseline hemogram,
1 year	12 years	biochemistry, thyroid screening and urinalysis; cardiac evaluation; ophthalmic evaluation
1.5 years	16 years	Mid-year evaluation; dental evaluation with radiographs/cleaning as needed
		Adult re-evaluation; vaccine boosters/titers as needed; parasite check; orthopedic screening (hips,
2 years	19 years	elbows), cardiac and ophthalmologic evaluation; blood pressure determination
2.5 years	24 years	Mid-year evaluation; dental evaluation with radiographs/cleaning as needed
		Primary re-evaluation; vaccine boosters/titers as needed; parasite check; baseline hemogram,
3 years	26 years	biochemistry, thyroid screening and urinalysis; cardiac evaluation; ophthalmic evaluation
3.5 years	28 years	Mid-year evaluation; dental evaluation with radiographs/cleaning as needed
4 years	32 years	Primary re-evaluation; vaccine boosters/titers as needed; parasite check; ophthalmic evaluation
4.5 years	36 years	Mid-year evaluation; dental evaluation with radiographs/cleaning as needed
		Primary re-evaluation; vaccine boosters/titers as needed; parasite check; baseline hemogram,
5 years	40 years	biochemistry, thyroid screening and urinalysis; cardiac evaluation; ophthalmic evaluation
5.5 years	44 years	Mid-year evaluation; dental evaluation with radiographs/cleaning as needed
		Primary re-evaluation; vaccine boosters/titers as needed; parasite check; senior evaluation; blood
6 years	48 years	pressure determination
6.5 years	52 years	Mid-year evaluation; dental evaluation with radiographs/cleaning as needed
7 years	54 years	Primary re-evaluation; vaccine boosters/titers as needed; parasite check; senior evaluation
7.5 years	56 years	Mid-year evaluation; dental evaluation with radiographs/cleaning as needed
8 years	60 years	Primary re-evaluation; vaccine boosters/titers as needed; parasite check; senior evaluation
8.5 years	63 years	Mid-year evaluation; dental evaluation with radiographs/cleaning as needed
9 years	66 years	Primary re-evaluation; vaccine boosters/titers as needed; parasite check; senior evaluation
9.5 years	69 years	Mid-year evaluation; dental evaluation with radiographs/cleaning as needed
10 years	72 years	Primary re-evaluation; vaccine boosters/titers as needed; parasite check; senior evaluation
10.5 years	75 years	Mid-year evaluation; dental evaluation with radiographs/cleaning as needed
11 years	78 years	Primary re-evaluation; vaccine boosters/titers as needed; parasite check; geriatric evaluation
11.5 years	80 years	Mid-year evaluation; dental evaluation with radiographs/cleaning as needed
12 years	82 years	Primary re-evaluation; vaccine boosters/titers as needed; parasite check; geriatric evaluation
12.5 years	84 years	Mid-year evaluation; dental evaluation with radiographs/cleaning as needed
13 years	86 years	Primary re-evaluation; vaccine boosters/titers as needed; parasite check; geriatric evaluation
13.5 years	88 years	Mid-year evaluation; dental evaluation with radiographs/cleaning as needed
14 years	90 years	Primary re-evaluation; vaccine boosters/titers as needed; parasite check; geriatric evaluation
14.5 years	92 years	Mid-year evaluation; dental evaluation with radiographs/cleaning as needed
15 years	94 years	Primary re-evaluation; vaccine boosters/titers as needed; parasite check; geriatric evaluation
15.5 years	96 years	Mid-year evaluation; dental evaluation with radiographs/cleaning as needed
16 years	98 years	Primary re-evaluation; vaccine boosters/titers as needed; parasite check; geriatric evaluation
16.5 years	100 years	Mid-year evaluation; dental evaluation with radiographs/cleaning as needed
17 years	102 years	Primary re-evaluation; vaccine boosters/titers as needed; parasite check; geriatric evaluation

Figure 1.3.1 Example of a personalized care plan.

References

1 Ackerman, L.J. (2011). *The Genetic Connection*, 2e. Lakewood, CO: AAHA Press.
2 American Veterinary Medical Association (2012). *US Pet Ownership & Demographics Sourcebook*. Schaumburg, IL: AVMA.
3 Simpson, R.J., Simpson, K.J., and VanKavage, L. (2012). Rethinking dog breed identification in veterinary practice. *J. Am. Vet. Med. Assoc.* 241 (9): 1163–1166.
4 Ackerman, L. What veterinary healthcare teams should know about genetic testing. AAHATrends, 2019.

Recommended Reading

Ackerman, L. (2011). *The Genetic Connection: A Guide to Health Problems in Purebred Dogs*, 2e. Lakewood, CO: AAHA Press.

Ackerman, L. Personalized medicine improves outcomes. Today's Veterinary Business, 2018. https://todaysveterinarybusiness.com/personalized-medicine-improves-outcomes

Ackerman, L. (2019). An introduction to pet-specific care. *EC Veterinary Science* 4 (1): 1–3.

Ackerman, L. (2020). Personalized pet profiles. In: *Five-Minute Veterinary Practice Management Consult*, 3e (ed. L. Ackerman), 268–271. Ames, IA: Wiley.

Ackerman, L. (2020). Proactive pet parenting: Anticipating pet health problems before they happen. Problem Free Publishing.

American Animal Hospital Association (2012). *Evolving to a Culture of Prevention: Implementing Integrated Preventive Care*, 1–23. Lakewood, CO: AAHA.

Bell, J.S., Cavanagh, K.E., Tilley, L.P., and Smith, F.W.K. (2012). *Veterinary Medical Guide to Dog and Cat Breeds*. Jackson, WY: Teton New Media.

Hamburg, M.A. and Collins, F.S. (2010). The path to personalized medicine. *N. Engl. J. Med.* 363 (4): 301–304.

World Small Animal Veterinary Association. Hereditary diseases. https://wsava.org/global-guidelines/hereditary-disease-guidelines/

1.4

Opportunities for Pet-Specific Care

Nan Boss, DVM

Best Friends Veterinary Center, Grafton, WI, USA

BASICS

Tailoring your healthcare recommendations to the wants and needs of individual patients and clients is good medicine and good business. It is easier (and less expensive) to make the most of the clients you already have than it is to find new ones. Chances are good you have the potential to grow your practice by offering more to your current clients – services that can increase the healthspans of the pets they love. As a bonus, clients who have been made to feel special and unique tend to refer others with a similar philosophy to pet care.

1.4.1 Terms Defined

Healthspan: The portion of a pet's life in which it is considered generally healthy, in contradistinction to lifespan which is the quantity of time a pet is alive.

MAIN CONCEPTS

1.4.2 Veterinary Teams are Teachers

There are dozens of factors that influence how an individual pet will be cared for. Most of these are out of our control. We don't choose the genetics of the animals (but we can counsel; see 3.4 Predicting and Eliminating Disease

Traits), their lifestyles or how the client was raised to treat or care for pets. However, we do have influence over how we deliver information to our clients, and we choose the services and products we promote and market to them. We have hundreds of opportunities every week to teach our clients about what is available to them, why it's important for their pets, and how we can deliver it. The better the care we offer and the more customized it is to the needs of the specific pet, the longer our patients will live and the greater their healthspans will be.

We are responsible for the health and well-being of our patients. If a pet dies from a disease for which we had a preventive or a treatment that we never told the client about, that pet's death is at least partially our responsibility. It is our job to tell the client what products or services would benefit their pet – without judging, prejudging or making assumptions about what the pet owner wants or doesn't want done. It is their job to decide which services and products they want. We should be giving them enough information to make sound decisions. We create opportunity for ourselves by giving pet guardians choices as to levels of care. Ways to personalize care for each client and patient include:

- breed-specific programs and DNA testing (see 3.13 Breed Predisposition)
- Fear Free™ strategies (see 6.6 Fear Free Concepts)
- customized healthcare plans (see 1.3 Personalized Care Plans)
- multiple payment options (see 10.13 Approach to Pricing)
- offering house calls or virtual care (see 2.5 Virtual Care (Telehealth))
- offering compounded medications and home delivery (see 9.10 Dispensing and Prescribing)

- fostering personal relationships between clients and individual team members (see 5.1 Pet-Specific Customer Service)
- providing classes or seminars for clients
- developing good relationships with specialists or utilizing mobile specialists within your practice (see 10.10 Making Referrals Work)
- performing health risk assessments (see 1.2 Providing a Lifetime of Care and 2.7 Risk Assessment)
- customizing client education materials (see 5.14 Client Education Materials).

We waste opportunities to better care for our patients when we worry about rejection, being too assertive or spending too much of the client's money. Instead, we should be providing choices and giving every pet guardian the chance to take the best care possible of their furred or feathered family members.

By and large, our clients don't know all that much about medicine, whether animal or human. Nearly half of US adults are considered medically illiterate [1]. Many clients have difficulty following even simple instructions on a drug label or understanding a doctor's diagnosis and instructions. The majority of human patients don't know the names of their own medications. Even otherwise intelligent, well-educated people can become confused when dealing with information outside their area of expertise, particularly in times of stress.

Clients who don't understand the complexity of a problem or its solution will question the expense. This certainly applies to treating sick or injured animals but fear influences decisions about wellness care as well. Fear of anesthesia, fear that the pet won't be able to chew if you extract those teeth, fear of medication side effects, of overvaccinating, of chemicals in pet food and many other things.

Clients don't know how to judge risks and benefits, they don't understand the causes of diseases their pet might get ("Where would he have gotten THAT?" "He's an indoor cat, he doesn't need to see the vet every year") They don't know which of those medications they are giving is the one for the cough and which is the one for pain. They think that blood testing is a waste of money because they don't understand that we have medications or special diets to treat what we find.

Our clients are paying for our knowledge and guidance. They did not attend veterinary school, so it is our obligation to communicate that knowledge to them. Practicing medicine means being a teacher to pet owners. *Every* client interaction is an opportunity to teach about pet care, including what problems their pet might have or be susceptible to and how we could address them. Just think – we each have the opportunity to teach and influence thousands of people over our careers!

1.4.3 Wellness and Prevention are Key

Clients won't buy products and services if they don't know they are available or don't fully understand the benefits they provide. It is rare that a Great Dane owner comes into the practice whose previous veterinarian discussed gastric dilation volvulus (GDV) and gastropexy with them, nor bulldog owners who already are aware of brachycephalic syndrome and the availability of surgery for elongated soft palate. Many owners of senior pets still have never heard of senior screening and most have never received a specific nutritional recommendation. Most adult cats are overweight but only a fraction of those cats' owners have been told their cats are overweight.

Whose responsibility is it to teach them about these things if not ours? Every client should be given the opportunity to learn, and every pet should have an owner who knows how to take care of it for a long, healthy lifetime.

This is a different mindset from what we learned in veterinary school. We learned normals and then abnormals, typically from specialists. We learned very little about maintaining normal. Preventive care focused mostly on vaccinations and parasite control, with a bit of dentistry thrown in. We were not told that it was our responsibility to provide in-depth client education to every client in a pet-specific fashion.

Yet the general practitioner spends more than half of his or her time on wellness and preventive medicine: puppy and kitten visits, annual examination visits, spay/neuter services, dental prophylaxis, heartworm testing, etc. We pride ourselves on doing a good job working up cases yet often neglect the bread and butter of our profession – keeping pets from getting sick. There is nothing more awesome than a successful surgery. Yet, other than specialty surgical practices, only a small percentage of clients will benefit from our surgical expertise, compared to the number that will benefit from working on weight management, helping clients choose a good pet food, and preventing behavior problems.

1.4.4 Components of Individualized Care

Answer questions, give written materials or refer clients to credible websites. We cannot deliver pet-specific care until we have delivered client-specific care. What we are recommending should always be what we believe is in the best interests of the patient. Your body language, eye-contact, and speech patterns need to project a caring message. It may be your 20th appointment today – it may be the client's only visit all year. To you it's another patient – to them it's a family member. These are important conversations!

In general, the vast majority of pet owners consider their pets to be members of the family. They consider their pets' health to be an important issue. They want veterinarians to help them do the right things right. For example, most pet owners actually want and expect nutritional advice from their veterinarian.

More specifically, though, every client has a different learning and communication style, different experiences with pets, and a different level of understanding. We have clients who are physicians and those who are truck drivers or office workers. The way we explain things to a medical professional is not the same as the way we would explain for someone with only a high school diploma. The majority of our clients may want nutritional advice – but the rest don't, and if you insist on talking about it anyway your advice may not be well received. We have to get a feel for who each person is, what level of knowledge they already have about pet health care, and what information and help they want from us.

This means we have to ask questions and listen to the answers. What has been your past experience with dogs? What role does your pet play in your family? How can I help you to feel more comfortable with this decision? Have I explained this well enough or do you still have questions?

What we choose to recommend or educate our clients about at a given visit is a combination of what the pet owner wants from us and what we want to discuss, based on our risk assessment for the pet (see 2.7 Risk Assessment). We often have to prioritize and we also need to be brief. Most people don't have the time or the attention span for a 40-minute discussion on flea control. However, you must also keep in mind that the vast majority of pet owners want their veterinarian to tell them about all the recommended diagnostic and treatment options for the pet, even if they cannot afford them.

1.4.5 Pet-Specific Care Takes Extra Time and Effort

The opportunity to deliver pet-specific care comes with an obligation to present care recommendations well. Take the time to explain and to coach your clients, whether the pet is well or ill. Clients will take better care of their pet if they understand its disease and treatment needs.

It takes thought and practice to change the way we work. Remembering a new protocol can be hard. Investing more time in each individual client may mean scheduling more time over the course of a year, team training, developing tools and doing performance evaluations and coaching. The opportunity to deliver pet-specific care comes at a cost. You cannot necessarily deliver high-quality care while remaining a low-cost provider, so some consideration is warranted.

Medical record keeping is very important if you are initiating a new program and a good electronic medical record (EMR) system can facilitate this (see 9.1 Medical Record Entries). We have been taught since childhood to fill in the blanks. Providing a place to document recommendations helps us to remember to make them. For example, let's say I want to start offering Schirmer tear testing (STT) for all my senior canine patients, to catch keratoconjunctivitis sicca (KCS) at an early stage. If an item is added to the exam template where the STT results are recorded, team members will remember to obtain that information.

If we want to offer a STT or a blood pressure screening to senior pet owners, we also need a handout or laminated sheet or some other tool to be sure we don't forget to do so. That's how we become consistent with client presentations and the care we deliver.

In addition, we need a plan or program for every type of routine visit. Protocol development includes not just how you will treat a particular patient but also how you will educate the client about the pet's care. You need to document every recommendation and provide written materials. Give your clients all their instructions in writing – every disease or problem, every diagnosis, every medication, every recommendation.

People comply better with their own physician's recommendations when there is sound education on why a medication or procedure is needed, and there is follow-up and follow-through. You have to do these things too, and train your staff to do these things.

1) Explain the recommendation, and why it is your standard of care.
2) Solidify the recommendation, by selling the product, scheduling the appointment for the procedure if you can, or calling back later.
3) Remember the 3 Rs. For every patient and every disease process there should be one of these: a Reminder entered for the next exam, vaccination or blood test; a Recheck appointment scheduled; or a Recall to contact the client again.
4) The client education, call-back and follow-up should be done in a kind, gentle, and professional manner by well-trained employees.

EXAMPLES

- Include STT with senior wellness panels for dogs.
- Include blood pressure measurement for every senior feline exam.
- Offer preanesthetic ECG screening for every patient, not just blood testing.
- Monitor blood pressure every six months for dogs on phenylpropanolamine.
- Offer ECG screening annually for every large-breed dog with genetic risk for cardiomyopathy, including boxers and Doberman pinschers. VPCs often precede heart failure in dogs of these breeds when cardiomyopathy is developing.
- Offer NT-ProBNP screening for giant breeds, which don't usually develop VPCs with their cardiomyopathy.

TAKE-AWAYS

- We have hundreds of opportunities every week to teach our clients about what is available to them, why it's important for their pets, and how we can deliver it.
- What we choose to recommend or educate our clients about at a given visit is a combination of what the pet owner wants from us and what we need to discuss, based on our risk assessment for the pet. We have to prioritize, and we also need to be brief.
- We need a plan or program for every type of routine visit, in order to maximize our opportunities.

- The pet owner has the right to make the decisions for their pet's care. It's our job to give clients the information they need to make responsible choices.
- The opportunity to deliver pet-specific care comes at a cost. You cannot necessarily deliver high-quality care while remaining a low-cost provider.

MISCELLANEOUS

Abbreviations

DNA	Deoxyribonucleic acid
ECG	Electrocardiogram
NT-proBNP	N-terminal pro B-type natriuretic peptide
VPC	Ventricular premature contraction

Reference

1 Institute of Medicine Committee on Health Literacy, Board on Neuroscience and Behavioral Health, and Institute of Medicine of the National Academies (2004). *Health Literacy: A Prescription to End Confusion*. Washington, DC: National Academies Press.

Recommended Reading

Baldwin, K., Bartges, J., Buffington, T. et al. (2010). AAHA nutritional assessment guidelines for dogs and cats (Canine & Feline). *Journal of the American Animal Hospital Association* 46: 285–296.

1.5

Feline-Friendly Care

Jane Brunt, DVM

Cat Hospital At Towson (CHAT), Baltimore, MD, USA

 BASICS

1.5.1 Summary

Cats are the most unique and ubiquitous household pet. As a species, they are obligate carnivores and normally exhibit behaviors related to being both predators *and* prey, hunters *and* hunted. As such, cats are frequently lumped together as if they are all the same when, just like people, they are individuals with different experiences, different responses to external stimuli, and therefore different needs. A variety of so-called personalities are frequently described, including the widely used "scaredy-cat" descriptor. Pet-specific care is a practice philosophy involving transformation from the current reactive model to a proactive version of care. This must start with understanding normal behavior for cats as a species and recognizing individual expressions of behavior. This is the foundation for being both feline friendly and pet specific.

1.5.2 Terms Defined

Body Language (Feline): Communicating nonverbally through movements or position. When properly reading a cat's body language, veterinary team members and cat parents can recognize how cats feel. Body posture and facial expression, including ear set and whisker positions, provide significant information on a cat's level of arousal, distress, and pain. This is a key feature of being feline friendly because an astute observer of cats' body language can alter their interaction with the cat accordingly *in advance of* any necessary physical contact.

Environment Enrichment (Feline): Availability of resources for a cat to exhibit normal behavior where it lives, including physical, nutritional, elimination, social, and behavioral resources. Examples include providing adequate space and locations for eating and drinking, resting and sleeping, playing and perching, hiding and personal space, and elimination. Thoughtful, open-ended client queries can explore the number and location of food and water stations, toys, perches and resting areas, and litter box number, location, and substrate(s).

Ethos: The distinguishing character, sentiment, moral nature, or guiding beliefs of a person, group, or institution. An ethical appeal using credibility and character.

Handling (Feline): The term and mindset which should replace the concept *and* the word "restraint" in all veterinary practices. Scruffing has been shown to be detrimental in handling cats due to the stress and distress it can cause.

Heightened Arousal (Feline): Arousal is a state of heightened activity in mind and body that makes individuals more alert. It manifests along a spectrum from low to high. An individual can be slightly aroused or extremely highly aroused. Arousal is the result of stimulation related to a change in places, people, and patterns with which a cat is familiar and is an outcome of stress, anxiety, fear, or a combination of all three. Fear aggression is a common sequela in cats, and it is important to avoid labeling it as mean and understand the cat is *scared*, which allows us to act with empathy.

Medicalization: The process by which conditions and problems come to be defined and treated as medical conditions, and thus become the subject of medical study, diagnosis, prevention, or treatment. Medicalization can be driven by new evidence or hypotheses about conditions; by changing social attitudes or economic considerations; or by the development of new medications or treatments. Medicalization is also a term used to describe the percentage of animals receiving veterinary care over a 12-month period.

Pet-Specific Care for the Veterinary Team, First Edition. Edited by Lowell Ackerman.
© 2021 John Wiley & Sons, Inc. Published 2021 by John Wiley & Sons, Inc.

MAIN CONCEPTS

1.5.3 The Data is for the Dogs

Companion cats outnumber dogs in the US, Canada, and many other nations, yet comprise only 25–40% of patients in typical companion animal veterinary practices. This trend was first recognized after the release of the 2007 AVMA US Pet Owner and Demographics Sourcebook [1] which showed a decline in the number of veterinary visits and expenditures for pet cats. Furthermore, compared to dogs, cats were twice as likely not to visit a veterinarian at all. At that time, it was also noted that households considering their cats as family members had a higher average number of veterinary visits (2.0) compared to households that viewed their cats as pets/companions (1.4) or as property (0.7). This insight is one of the reasons that supporting the human–animal bond is critical for cats (see 2.14 Benefits of the Human–Animal Bond). Unfortunately, the declining trends have continued and the 2017–2018 edition of the AVMA Pet Owner and Demographics Sourcebook [2] reported that 45.7% – nearly half of all cats – did not visit a veterinarian in the year the study was conducted. Of those, 41% cited the reason as their "cats did not get sick or injured." Only 16% cited "did not have the money. . ." to pay for a veterinary visit as the reason their cats didn't receive veterinary care.

While this and other data seem daunting, it creates a tremendous opportunity for the veterinary profession. To make this happen, hospital teams need to commit to creating, implementing, and sustaining a knowledgeable, feline-friendly mindset and environment. This will allow cat owners to feel comfortable and committed to getting their cats veterinary care, irrespective of their age or perceived health status.

Fortunately, as the realization of this opportunity occurred, several organizations began or increased their efforts to improve cat health. The CATalyst Summit brought together more than 50 people and organizations representing all stakeholders in cat care, including animal welfare organizations. Subsequent to the summit, the CATalyst Council was created, representing a unique coalition of cat health and welfare organizations, companies, foundations, and the media. The American Association of Feline Practitioners (AAFP) and American Animal Hospital Association (AAHA) developed Feline Life Stage Guidelines [3]. The AAFP and International Cat Care (ICC, known as Feline Advisory Bureau at the time) both began their efforts for their Cat-Friendly Practice and Cat Friendly Clinic initiatives. These organizations have robust online resources that practices should visit and take the needed steps to acquire the related designations and certifications. The tools provided by the AAFP and ICC as well as those from the Canadian initiative Cat Healthy and the Ohio State University's Indoor Pet Initiative for Cats [4] offer resources for veterinary teams, animal shelters, and pet owners.

As a profession, we must understand consumers' desires, for without them, companion cats will not benefit from evidence-based, feline-friendly, health and welfare knowledge that we have, must implement and share. Consumers become clients when the 45.7% of cat owners not currently obtaining veterinary care do so.

1.5.4 Cat Concepts in the Veterinary Clinic

Cats are unique pets because they are both predators and prey, hunters and hunted. When pet parents and healthcare providers understand that concept, everything else becomes obvious. Cats prefer familiar places, people, and patterns, and when faced with anything unfamiliar, they become fearful and may exhibit heightened arousal. To avoid (potential) conflict, their instinct is to flee (flight) and when they have no means of escape, as in a closed exam room, this heightened arousal may manifest as fear aggression. Unfortunately, this normal behavior has caused many cats to be labeled as "AGGRESSIVE" – which is frequently captured on the medical record in upper case letters and even numbers of exclamation points. Approaching cats with quiet observation, nonthreatening postures, and expressions (get low, turn and look sideways) and slow movements is less likely to cause additional arousal. Largely due to the lack of habituation to travel and carriers, most cats are far less accepting of transport and travel than dogs. As such, they are frequently aroused before they come in our doors. What would it look like if we could have a warm, quiet and calm exam room ready for a cat so they could bypass the reception area that has the sounds, sights, and scents of their most common and feared predators – unfamiliar dogs and people?

Preventive care for all ages includes health and lifestyle-appropriate vaccines, nutrition, parasiticides, and especially regularly scheduled wellness visits, annually at a minimum and semi annual or quarterly examinations are in the "well" cat's best interest, including juveniles and young adults with weight gain or red gums. Addressing changes early in the process to prevent future problems like obesity, diabetes mellitus, and oral disease is paramount to pet-specific and client-centered care (see 4.7 Embracing Early Detection). If verbiage used in veterinary practices includes some version of "She only has a tiny bit of tartar so she might need a dental next year," there is an immediate opportunity to ask your co-workers why, and as a team explore how that cat, their owners and even the veterinary practice could be better helped with earlier care (see 4.9 Periodontal Disease). A single, simple circumstance such as that could provide the pivot point for all team members including owners and managers, veterinarians and veterinary nurses, assistants and caregivers to be aligned and on board with pet-specific care.

1.5.5 Feline Friendliness Starts at Home

The educated and engaged veterinary team is knowledgeable about helping owners understand cats' needs and environment enrichment by engaging in conversations using open-ended questions such as "How many litterboxes do you have. . . where are they. . .how often are you able to clean them. . .?" and "Tell me about mealtimes in your home. . ." Note: the most important part of asking open-ended questions is listening to the answers (see 9.2 Asking Good Questions). Therein are the clues for true patient status.

Regarding mealtimes, we know that cats are solitary hunters and as such, their normal feeding preference is without oversight or interruption by other animals, including cat housemates. If a client describes feeding their cats within eyesight of each other, during the nutritional assessment and recommendation, information on *how* to feed (location, frequency, puzzle/foraging feeders) is as important as *what* to feed.

It is also important to know that simple changes in a cat's routine have been shown to induce stress-related illnesses. Sickness behaviors have been documented and include gastrointestinal (vomiting, diarrhea) and lower urinary tract signs (feline interstitial cystitis) [5]. All are common presentations to veterinary clinics and environmental stress should be carefully explored in these cases.

Many cats will benefit from anxiety abatement in advance of collecting the cat for travel. Having carriers out in advance of transport, using synthetic facial pheromones in and around the carrier and bedding, nutritional supplements and diets to promote calmness, and even antianxiety therapeutics are examples of tactics and treatments used widely (see 6.6 Fear Free Concepts). Gabapentin can help prevent and diminish arousal and is routinely used in advance of travel for this purpose. It is important to recognize that tranquilizers merely diminish the cat's ability to respond to fear and arousal, and do not help the cat feel less stressed or fearful.

1.5.6 It's All About the Cat, and Their Person

As knowledgeable advocates for cats, veterinary teams that have made the sustained commitment to understanding cat behavior and handling cats appropriately represent the ethos of feline-friendly, client-centered, and pet-specific care. That, along with celebrating the bond between people and their cats, will help ensure lifelong care for cats with your practice.

EXAMPLES

Sunshine, a 12-year-old spayed female brown tabby DSH, presented for the first time to a feline-exclusive veterinary practice. She had received no veterinary care after her kitten vaccines and sterilization. She was reported to have a "good appetite and thirst," and the owner brought her in because she noticed she was losing weight. On subjective observation, she was emaciated, agitated, and vocalizing. On examination, she had a 2/9 body condition score (BCS), stage 3 periodontal disease, a grade 2/6 systolic murmur, and a unilateral thyroid nodule. The owner was counseled on the likelihood of hyperthyroidism, which is treatable, and could be the primary reason for her weight loss and heart murmur. Since the condition was treatable, the owner agreed to laboratory work to confirm the presumptive diagnosis. Sunshine was taken to the inpatient area of the clinic where the veterinarian and assistant performed a jugular venipuncture while holding the cat in sternal recumbency. Immediately upon completing the sampling, Sunshine collapsed, and did not respond to resuscitation.

It is important to consider that if Sunshine had been handled in a more feline-friendly manner, a better outcome might have been achieved.

TAKE-AWAYS

- The current undermedicalization of companion cats presents a significant opportunity for veterinary practice teams.
- Recognizing and understanding normal cat behavior is a critical skill in companion animal practice. Cats thrive when they can exhibit normal cat behaviors including hunting and hiding.

- Because of cats' unique relationships with their environment, feline-friendly care is the foundation of pet-specific care for companion cats.
- Transitioning our mindset from "diagnose and treat" to "predict and prevent" will enhance cats' well-being, health, and longevity, as well as client compliance and satisfaction.
- Caring for cats in feline-friendly ways enhances the human–cat bond, and it is the right thing to do.

MISCELLANEOUS

1.5.7 Cautions

1) "Look all ways before crossing…" In the context of cats – observation in advance of any intervention.
2) Think twice before laughing at viral videos showing cats and cucumbers.

Abbreviations

AVMA	American Veterinary Medical Association
DSH	Domestic short hair

References

1 AVMA (2007). *US Pet Owner and Demographics Sourcebook*. Schaumberg, IL: AVMA.

2 AVMA (2017–2108). *Pet Owner and Demographics Sourcebook*. Schaumberg, IL: AVMA.

3 Hoyumpa Vogt, A., Rodan, I., Brown, M. et al. (2010). AAFP/AAHA feline life stage guidelines. *Journal of Feline Medicine and Surgery* 12: 43–54.

4 Ohio State University Indoor Pet Initiative for Cat Owners. https://indoorpet.osu.edu/cats

5 Stella, J., Lord, L., and Buffington, C. (2011). Sickness behaviors in response to unusual external events in healthy cats and cats with feline interstitial cystitis. *Journal of the American Veterinary Medical Association* 238: 67–73.

Recommended Reading

American Association of Feline Practitioners. Cat Friendly Practices. https://catvets.com/cfp/cfp

Cat Healthy. http://www.cathealthy.ca

International Cat Care. Cat Friendly Clinic. https://catfriendlyclinic.org

Rodan, I. and Heath, S. (2016). *Feline Behavioral Medicine: Prevention and Treatment*. St Louis, MO: Saunders.

1.6

Adapting to a New Normal

Lowell Ackerman, DVM, DACVD, MBA, MPA, CVA, MRCVS

Global Consultant, Author, and Lecturer, MA, USA

 BASICS

1.6.1 Summary

Life has changed for veterinary practices, the hospital team, clients, and even pets. Periodically, the world experiences events considered "shocks" that change the fundamental way we do things. These events can include such diverse things as war, terrorist attacks, financial crises, climate change, and pandemics. Even though the event may only occupy a finite span of time, the after-effects can last significantly longer. As economic shocks appear to be occurring with some regularity, it is important to adapt to the realities that follow.

1.6.2 Terms Defined

Economic Shock: An event that has a major impact on economic indicators, such as unemployment, inflation, consumer confidence, or consumption.

Formulary: An approved list of medications that may be stocked in a practice or are allowed to be prescribed.

New Normal: The changed state recognized following the occurrence of a major or catastrophic event that alters our routines.

Pet-Specific Care: An approach that tailors veterinary care to individual pets based on their predicted risk of disease and likely response to intervention.

 MAIN CONCEPTS

1.6.3 Client Experience

The occurrence of COVID-19 may have been the latest notable economic shock, but there are bound to be others. In the immediate post-COVID era, even with vaccination, clients may continue to be wary of their interactions with staff, so it is a great opportunity to innovate. This includes rethinking how we engage with clients (even hand shaking), and how we articulate the value of our services. Clients have experienced new ways of dealing with their own physicians and the healthcare system and are bound to question why dealing with veterinary teams should be any different. It is important to consider the long-term applications of appropriate principles, because there are bound to be future pandemic concerns as well as other economic shocks that will affect the profession. It is important to adapt to such shocks and learn from them.

Immediately following a pandemic, clients are likely to have expectations when it comes to routine wellness visits, conditions that they believe could be handled virtually, preference for "curbside" services rather than coming into the hospital, home delivery of products, and much more. For a service industry such as veterinary medicine, it is important to articulate the value proposition in ways that make sense to consumers. This is a particularly great opportunity to consider pet-specific care, in which we take a more proactive and transparent approach to the care that pets will need over their lifetimes, and do so on a customized basis. It will also be important to curate resources used for client education, so we can be sure that pet owners are receiving consistent messaging about the care of their pets. We also need to ensure that such resources are deliverable in paperless forms and even contact-less, so direct contact can be minimized.

Clients are quite aware when their world has changed, and it is likely that they have experienced stay-at-home isolation, so their attitudes toward social contact will likely be affected for some time. Expect that they will continue to be looking for assurances that they, their pets, and their families will be safe in their interactions with the veterinary team. Many of them will have been working from home, teleconferencing with work colleagues, family, and friends, doing much of their shopping online, downloading their entertainment, and receiving many of their purchases by home delivery.

Clients have also changed dramatically in terms of their knowledge of infectious disease transmissibility, hand washing, physical (social) distancing, premise disinfection, contact tracing, and the wearing of facemasks. This type of vigilance and anxiety tends to continue until they feel completely safe, and pet owners will be looking for some assurance that the veterinary hospital is a safe place to visit.

Some clients will have prolonged trepidation about visiting businesses, including their own physicians, and so veterinary hospitals should not consider themselves unaffected by this. Client anxiety may be heightened if they do not have access to a vehicle but are still hesitant about the inherent risks of using public transportation or ridesharing. This apprehension can be allayed if teams explain all the protocols in place to keep those anxious clients and their pets safe, and this might include telehealth options based on telephone triage with clients.

For pets that need to be seen in hospital, clients should receive instructions on how this can be done safely, and expectations should be established for how the visit will be conducted in a step-by-step manner. This might include instruction for the pet owner to wear a facemask (if indicated), access they may or may not have to the facility, whether they are allowed to accompany their pet for its veterinary visit, communication options with the veterinary team, and what is being done to ensure their safety. Even long after a pandemic has passed, some clients will likely have developed habits around hand washing, physical distancing, and the use of hand sanitizers, and everything possible should be done so they can feel comfortable seeking veterinary care for their pets.

In the immediate aftermath of a pandemic, there is also a great opportunity to introduce topics that might not have garnered much attention previously, such as One Health (see 2.19 One Health). This initiative that links the health of animals, humans, and the environment is a great way to highlight the interrelatedness of such concerns, and the need for clients to appreciate the "big picture" of caring for our pets, ourselves, and our planet.

1.6.4 Changing Practice Protocols

Veterinary staff are typically well educated and dedicated to animal health, but at the same time they want to protect themselves and their families from transmissible diseases, and their concern is legitimate. For the foreseeable future, we should expect that they will appreciate ongoing instruction on practice safety protocols, patient flow, and access to appropriate personal protective equipment (PPE). Because veterinary teams work collectively, there should be protocols in place for monitoring the health of individual staff

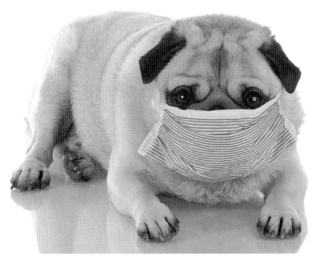

Source: Creative Commons. Public Domain.

members, having policies for isolation and quarantine, and supporting unambiguous and generous policies about which situations should prompt team members to leave the premises to preserve the health of others. It is also important to be aware of the additional stress experienced by staff and how that can take an immeasurable toll on productivity, commitment, and teamwork. Most veterinary hospitals have a relatively small contingent of team members, so without careful and considerate policies, staff could wrongly interpret that their physical and mental health is not a major concern of the hospital, which would be a very unfortunate conclusion.

While they were always appropriate, protocols for personal hygiene were not always followed in periods prior to pandemics, but are definitely critical afterwards. There should be hand washing between each patient visit and adequate time allowed not only for sanitization of the examination rooms, but also for more thorough disinfection. This includes not only surfaces used for pets, but also those that might have contact from owners as well. This will add time to appointments which might eventually need to be recouped through increased fees.

Veterinary staff are extremely valuable and their health is an important concern, so there should be ongoing dialogue about what steps the hospital is taking to keep everyone safe. Whenever possible, such protocols should be institutionalized as standards of care (see 9.4 Standards of Care) and staff should be counseled and coached as to what they should be doing to keep themselves and each other safe. It is important to consider even minor risks and work collectively to address concerns. When staff appreciate that their ongoing health is a major priority, and when it is reinforced by other team members, they can be confident that things are being done to mitigate their risks for getting sick. It is important to realize that fear is likely to persist long after a pandemic, so relaxing standards should only be contemplated after robust team discussions and the best available evidence.

1.6.5 Expectations for Telehealth

An increasing number of our clients have become quite familiar with teleconferencing in their daily lives. This comfort has extended to dealing with their physicians, and telehealth consulting with veterinary teams should be presumed to become a routine matter and perhaps even a preference for many clients (see 2.5 – Virtual Care (Telehealth)). The interaction can be synchronous (real-time) or asynchronous (respond following review) but the expectation of clients will likely be that there are many times when dealing with pet care virtually is preferred. It is

not just a matter of personal safety, but many clients have found this to be convenient as well.

We should anticipate that many clients will be receptive to the practice of telehealth, and this is also a great way for pets to be triaged before exposing them to our facilities and hospital teams. Some conditions will be more amenable to virtual care than others, and clear guidelines should exist as to what can be attempted through this platform, and what should prompt a recommendation for the animal to be seen in the hospital.

Remote monitoring is also available for our patients, and a variety of clinical attributes can now be measured at home. This includes collars that can measure activity, heart rate, respiratory rate, and some aspects of body temperature, but other devices such as glucometers can also be used. This can be very helpful for hospice patients, postsurgical patients, and those with a need for routine monitoring.

Many clients are familiar with a variety of options for virtual connection, but hospitals should be comfortable with the privacy protections for any type of telehealth attempted, and it is best if the hospital designates only a few programs with which they are comfortable in this regard, and at which teams can gain proficiency. Because telehealth is likely to become a routine part of veterinary practice going forward, one of the most important things for veterinary teams to have in place are the criteria for telehealth visits, the structure of those visits, and the fees associated with telehealth consults. Telehealth need not be a money-losing proposition for the practice and can be as or more profitable than other types of services if instituted correctly.

1.6.6 Economic Insecurity

The impact of the pandemic was not felt equally across populations, as is often the case with economic shocks. Many clients had interruptions in their ability to work and earn money, some may have had to deal with personal tragedies, and the uncertainty of what might come next often influences spending decisions for many years. Thus, it is reasonable to expect that clients might be hesitant when it comes to large expenditures for their pets, typically for several years or until they no longer feel vulnerable. Others may prefer to postpone procedures that are not considered essential and immediate until they feel more financially secure.

Following any economic shock, such consumer attitudes are inevitable, and veterinary practices should anticipate this and plan their client messaging accordingly. There should be unequivocal communication about what services should be prioritized and which can be delayed, not to scare clients but to help them make informed decisions for the care of their pets. It may also be advisable to consider credit terms for procedures that might be preapproved by the hospital, as well as payment plans that allow clients to do the work recommended but spread payment out over a longer interval (see 10.17 Payment and Wellness Plans). This is also a great time to promote pet health insurance as one way of "flattening the curve" when it comes to veterinary expenditures (see 10.16 Pet Health Insurance). If done correctly, these strategies can be profitable for the practice, as well as convenient for pet owners.

In times of turmoil, people often safeguard their cash reserves and postpone everything that is not considered essential. In an emergency situation, that might also necessitate postponing things that are actually essential, including rent, mortgage, groceries, and even healthcare. Because veterinary care is often considered a discretionary expense, it can become a low priority if there is not a system in place to help ensure funding for such care.

If at all possible, this is a time to consider the best ways to help pet owners manage their financial insecurity around pet expenditures. This can be done by recommending pet health insurance, if feasible, and also by considering payment plans (also known as wellness or concierge plans), which offer established fees charged intermittently (often monthly) for a defined basket of services. As mentioned previously, pet health insurance helps "flatten the curve" when it comes to unanticipated expenses, while payment plans "smooth the curve" for anticipated expenses (vaccines, parasite control, etc.). Both allow pet owners to budget more effectively for veterinary care without having to contend with periodic "spikes" in expenditures. Because most consumers will be anxious about pet care expenses, this can help pet owners plan for needed care without adversely affecting practices. If positioned correctly, both insurance and payment plans can be profitable for veterinary hospitals and a convenient and anxiety-reducing approach for pet owners.

1.6.7 Retail Considerations

If your clients were not used to making online purchases before the pandemic, that has likely changed, and they have now established a new comfort level for dealing with e-commerce and home delivery. Expect that this will continue, and many clients will also be considering and researching making online purchases for their pet supplies, foods, and medications.

This is the time to consolidate and promote online retail, as this is not only convenient for your clients but increases the safety of your staff as well (see 9.10 Dispensing and Prescribing). Veterinary hospitals might consider aligning with an online veterinary pharmacy and directing clients toward such purchases. It is important that veterinary practices price their products competitively, so clients can make a seamless transition to online purchasing without having to price shop for better deals elsewhere. It is possible for veterinary hospitals to do this profitably, because with online pharmacies and retailers there are no inventory costs for the practice. While it might seem that veterinary hospitals could stock and dispense products and keep a larger share of the revenue, it can actually be more satisfying to earn a profit margin without having to deal with all the costs of maintaining inventory.

In some countries, veterinary medicine still involves actual cash exchange, but following a pandemic expect that most customers will prefer cashless transactions, and even more likely contactless transactions, where there is not even the handling of credit or debit cards, or even receipts. It is important to consider payment options carefully, and this type of retail experience is likely to continue long into the future.

1.6.8 Vendor Relationships

Economic shocks can be extremely challenging, but they also provide opportunities to improve operations, and this is very true of our relationships with vendors. Rather than treat vendor visits as intrusions and assigning front office teams as gatekeepers, this is a great time to establish systems for prescheduling vendor visits (or even televisits), streamlining inventory to just those products needed, and leveraging vendor relationships to bring the most value to clients, the hospital team, and the hospital itself. This does not necessarily always favor the vendor with the lowest price, since value can be conveyed in other ways such as hospital support, continuing education, expedited delivery, and prioritization when supplies are in high demand but short supply.

As new products become available, rather than sales representatives visiting with any staff member who might be available, they can be requested to provide a packet of information to a formulary evaluation committee, in charge of making recommendations for what might be included in inventory. In general, if a product is recommended to be included in the hospital formulary, then the committee should also recommend which product in the same class of medications should be removed from the formulary, or only made available through the hospital's online pharmacy. If the committee evaluates a product and finds that it is not suitable to be included in the practice formulary, those reasons should be recorded and conveyed to the hospital staff so the product does not need to be reevaluated every time a representative makes a sales call.

1.6.9 Changing Business Models

With every new economic shock comes opportunities for improving the veterinary business model to be more responsive to current market pressures. Following the most recent pandemic, some of the most acute problems to be addressed include embracing pet-specific care so that clients better understand the lifelong needs of their pets without requiring prompting by in-hospital visits; making it easier for virtual care to be delivered to clients; facilitating e-commerce and home delivery; and constructing a more profitable business model better able to withstand such economic shocks. Such crises should also convince practice owners of the importance of financial metrics and dashboards that allow clinics to be resilient and thrive despite challenging events. Veterinary care may be an essential service, but all veterinary practices are not recession proof.

Pet-specific care allows clients to understand the lifelong needs of their pets in advance, and to financially prepare for dealing with them (see 1.2 Providing a Lifetime of Care). Even in the case of economic shocks, clients can appreciate where care needs to restart when situations normalize, what is to be prioritized, and discussions to be had with the veterinary team either virtually or in person. There is no need to wait for regular appointments to resume before instituting appropriate care.

TAKE-AWAYS

- Economic shocks tend to have an impact on consumer behavior long after the actual shock has concluded.
- Consumer spending habits are often dramatically changed by an economic shock, and tend to persist as long as individuals feel vulnerable.
- It should be expected that clients will have a heightened sensitivity to hygiene following a pandemic, and will be concerned for their own health and that of their family.

- Hospital protocols need to change to reflect evidence-based standards of care, including ways to keep everyone in the hospital safe.
- Clients are likely to be receptive to services that allow them to interact with the hospital remotely, including telehealth, online purchasing, and home delivery.

MISCELLANEOUS

1.6.10 Cautions

Economic shocks are difficult to predict, but often have profound effects that last long after the precipitating event has concluded. Because most shocks are not anticipated, it is difficult for veterinary teams to be completely prepared from one crisis to the next. Each crisis tends to provide its own lessons for the future, and veterinary practices need to consistently adapt to remain relevant and vital.

Recommended Reading

Ackerman, L. (2019). Why should veterinarians consider implementing virtual care? *EC Veterinary Science* 4 (4): 259–261.

Ackerman, L. (2019). Why pet health insurance is important for the profession. *EC Veterinary Science* 2: 6–7.

Ackerman, L. (2019). Ready to partner with an online pharmacy? *AAHA Trends* 35: 49–53.

Ackerman, L. (2020). Bracing for the new normal. *EC Veterinary Science*. 5(9): 49–52.

Ackerman, L. (2020). The new e-commerce: E-commerce is more than just selling products online. AAHA Trends; 36(11): 51–54.

American Animal Hospital Association (2012). *Evolving to a Culture of Prevention: Implementing Integrated Preventive Care*, 1–23. Lakewood, CO: AAHA.

Hamburg, M.A. and Collins, F.S. (2010). The path to personalized medicine. *New England Journal of Medicine* 363 (4): 301–304.

Zigrang, T. and Bailey-Wheaton, J.L. (2020, March/April). Healthcare valuation implications of COVID-19. *Value Examiner*: 28–34.

Section 2

Concepts and Prospects

2.1

Evidence-Based Veterinary Medicine and Personal Bias

Brennen McKenzie, MA, MSc, VMD

Adobe Animal Hospital, Los Altos, CA, USA

BASICS

2.1.1 Summary

Evidence-based veterinary medicine (EBVM) is a set of tools for generating reliable research evidence, disseminating it to clinicians, and using it to support clinical decision making. Through the practical application of the philosophy and methods of science to medical problems, and the explicit and judicious integration of research evidence, clinical experience, and the goals and resources of pet owners, EBVM can promote more effective, proactive patient care.

Veterinary professionals use information intensively in their work. Meeting the goals of pet-specific care, to identify health risks and to intervene with preventive and therapeutic measures to improve health, we must have accurate, relevant information. EBVM provides a system for ensuring that the information clinicians need is not only accurate and relevant but available and easy to use. More efficient information management supports easier and more reliable decision making, more effective client communication, and ultimately better outcomes for patients.

2.1.2 Terms Defined

Bias: Any systematic deviation of research results from the true state of the subject being studied. Most often, bias is an unintentional result of how research studies are designed and conducted.

Clinical Practice Guideline: Management recommendations for specific health conditions. To be considered evidence based, guidelines must be produced using systematic methods to reduce bias.

Critically Appraised Topic: A brief summary and appraisal of the evidence concerning a narrow clinical topic which resembling a systematic review but is shorter and less comprehensive.

Primary Literature: Published reports of original research studies.

Synthetic Literature: Published summaries and critical analyses of primary research studies.

Systematic Review: A comprehensive summary and critical appraisal of primary research studies conducted according to established procedures for minimizing bias.

MAIN CONCEPTS

2.1.3 What Is EBVM?

Evidence-based veterinary medicine is a comprehensive system for generating reliable scientific evidence and getting it to those who need it in clinical practice and then integrating this evidence into clinical decision making.

In the research environment, EBVM guides the design and conduct of scientific studies to minimize bias and ensure the data generated are reliable. This element of EBVM is useful for researchers, but it is also critical for clinicians who use scientific research to inform their patient care.

EBVM tools also support the reporting of research studies in a manner that minimizes bias and ensures the reliability and utility of research evidence for the end-user, the veterinary clinician. EBVM also facilitates the dissemination of research evidence, through reporting guidelines and support for open-access publishing, to get evidence to those who need it to make healthcare decisions.

Synthetic literature sources, such as systematic reviews, critically appraised topics, and clinical practice guidelines, are practical ways of translating research into useable information for clinicians. EBVM provides standards for generating these resources and making them accessible to veterinarians in practice. This reduces the time and effort needed to find and critically evaluate needed information in the scientific literature.

Finally, EBVM includes techniques and training for clinicians to help identify their information needs and then find relevant and useful evidence. Knowing what information is most important for assessing risk and guiding treatment, and knowing how to find this information and how to judge whether it is reliable and applicable to a given patient, is a key part of providing consistent, effective pet-specific care.

2.1.4   Why Do We Need EBVM?

In the absence of EBVM practices, clinicians typically base their decisions on sources of evidence other than scientific research, especially the opinions of colleagues and perceived experts. When clinicians do use research findings to guide their practice, this involves an informal, haphazard consultation of textbooks, journal articles and other sources, often without critical assessment for bias. Veterinarians often rely most heavily on their own experience and intuition in making patient care decisions. This collection of strategies is referred to as opinion-based medicine.

Unfortunately, personal experience, even that of highly trained and experienced individuals, is subject to many cognitive biases and other sources of error that make it less reliable than is generally believed. Such biases lead to erroneous conclusions which undermine the safety and efficacy of medical interventions. The success of modern, science-based medicine in reducing suffering and improving health rests mostly on shifting reliance away from idiosyncratic personal observations and opinion and toward formal scientific research evidence.

We cannot provide effective pet-specific care without reliable information. We cannot assess health risks without understanding the causes of illness and the relationship between risk factors and health outcomes. We cannot provide effective preventive or therapeutic interventions without evidence showing which methods are effective and which are not. We cannot minimize the adverse effects of our treatments without understanding what the risks are

and why they occur. EBVM makes effective care possible by generating the needed information and helping clinicians find and use it.

Evidence-based veterinary medicine is also useful in meeting our ethical obligations to pet owners. These include not only providing the most effective care possible but also obtaining informed consent for our interventions. When we recommend a treatment to a pet owner using an evidence-based approach, we can confidently identify the potential risks and benefits of the treatment and the degree of uncertainty about these based on reliable scientific information, rather than anecdote or opinion. We will not always be certain about the outcome, but we can give an informed estimate of the degree of uncertainty. This is an important element in gaining informed consent from clients.

Pet owners have an ethical and often a legal right to be informed about the possible risks and benefits of medical interventions. EBVM helps veterinarians fulfill our ethical obligations to clients by ensuring that the information we provide is as accurate and reliable as possible. Even when the evidence is limited and the level of uncertainty is high, as is often the case in veterinary medicine, EBVM helps the clinician to be transparent about this with pet owners and to provide the information needed for fully informed consent.

2.1.5   How Does EBVM Work in Practice?

Ideally, EBVM methods should be a core part of veterinary medical training. The habits of identifying specific information needs and then finding and critically evaluating scientific evidence are extremely useful once established, but some formal training and practice are required to develop these habits.

The basic steps in the process of integrating research evidence into clinical decision making are as follows.

1) Ask specific, answerable questions.
2) Locate relevant evidence.
3) Assess the reliability and applicability of this evidence.
4) Draw a conclusion.
5) Assign a level of confidence to this conclusion.

This is an iterative process that must be repeated as information needs change and new evidence becomes available.

Of course, in a busy clinical practice it is not possible to apply such a formal method to every question for every patient in real time. The goal of applied EBVM is to develop a personal knowledge base derived from explicit, critical assessment of scientific evidence which the veterinarian can then apply to individual patients as appropriate, guided by the unique circumstances of each case, the goals and resources of the owner, and the judgment of the clinician. The meaningful difference between this process and opinion-based medicine is that the knowledge base a clinician uses to make recommendations is not a haphazard collection of information gleaned from sources of uncertain reliability but a set of conclusions with known provenance and a clearly established degree of uncertainty.

Figure 2.1.1 illustrates common types of evidence used to guide clinical decisions. Such evidence pyramids are helpful in establishing a degree of confidence in our conclusions. A recommendation based only on low-quality evidence at high risk of bias, such as clinical experience or expert opinion, should be qualified, and the inherent uncertainty of the supporting evidence must be disclosed to clients. Recommendations based on more reliable evidence, such as systematic reviews or clinical practice guidelines, can be presented with much greater confidence.

Clinicians must always use their individual judgment in drawing conclusions from scientific evidence and applying these to specific patients. However, the hierarchy of evidence makes it easier for veterinarians to identify the reliability of specific types of evidence and of conclusions

based on this evidence and to then communicate the degree of uncertainty to pet owners.

EXAMPLES

Charlie is a 4-year-old neutered male Cavalier King Charles spaniel. His owner is seeking your opinion because another veterinarian recently told her Charlie has a heart murmur. The owner was told that because Charlie is young and has no clinical issues, there is no need to do any tests or start any treatment. However, her breeder has told her that Charlie should be on a medication called "enalapril."

You are aware of the breed predisposition for mitral valve disease (MVD) in Cavaliers, and you tell the owner that this is the most likely diagnosis based on Charlie's signalment and physical exam findings. You have also recently reviewed the American College of Veterinary Internal Medicine guidelines for diagnosis of MVD [1], and you explain that Charlie has stage B MVD, meaning he has a murmur but no clinical signs.

You explain that while enalapril was once commonly recommended for dogs with preclinical MVD based on

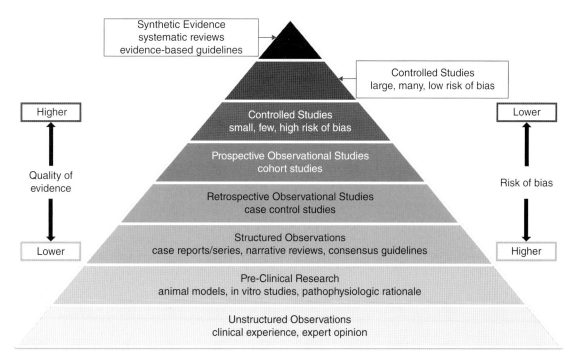

Figure 2.1.1 An evidence pyramid illustrating the variable reliability and risk of bias of different types of scientific evidence.

low-level evidence (pathophysiological reasoning and clinical experience), higher quality evidence (clinical trials) [2, 3] has since shown that it does not delay the onset of congestive heart failure (CHF), so you recommend against this medication.

In association with another case, you recently investigated whether there are any useful treatments for dogs with stage B MVD. You discovered the EPIC study, a high-quality clinical trial investigating the use of pimobendan in dogs with MVD [4]. This trial included a lot of Cavaliers, so you believe the results are applicable to Charlie. You tell the owner that this study found a dramatic delay in the onset of CHF in dogs using pimobendan if they were in stage B2 MVD, meaning they had enlarged hearts. You explain that you could stage Charlie using radiographs, but the EPIC study suggested measurements from an echocardiogram are more reliable, so you recommend this test.

The owner is impressed with your detailed scientific knowledge and happy to have something she can do to keep Charlie healthy. You arrange an echocardiogram and agree to manage Charlie's MVD based on the results.

TAKE-AWAYS

- EBVM is a comprehensive system for producing and disseminating reliable scientific evidence and for integrating this evidence into clinical decision making.
- EBVM methods make identifying, finding, and using needed information easier for veterinarians.
- Integrating research evidence with clinical experience and the needs and resources of owners helps reduce medical error and supports more proactive, effective pet-specific care.
- EBVM also facilitates our ethical obligations to provide the most effective care for patients and to support informed consent for clients by providing the most accurate information and a clear assessment of relevant uncertainty.
- EBVM helps veterinarians provide better care and better client communication with greater confidence and less time and effort.

References

1 Atkins, C., Bonagura, J., Ettinger, S. et al. (2009). Guidelines for the diagnosis and treatment of canine chronic valvular heart disease. *Journal of Veterinary Internal Medicine* 23 (6): 1142–1150.

2 Atkins, C.E., Keene, B.W., Brown, W.A. et al. (2007). Results of the veterinary enalapril trial to prove reduction in onset of heart failure in dogs chronically treated with enalapril alone for compensated, naturally occurring mitral valve insufficiency. *Journal of the American Veterinary Medical Association* 231: 1061–1069.

3 Kvart, C., Haggstrom, J., Pedersen, H.D. et al. (2002). Efficacy of enalapril for prevention of congestive heart failure in dogs with myxomatous valve disease and asymptomatic mitral regurgitation. *Journal of Veterinary Internal Medicine* 16: 80–88.

4 Boswood, A., Häggström, J., Gordon, S.G. et al. (2016). Effect of pimobendan in dogs with preclinical myxomatous mitral valve disease and cardiomegaly: the EPIC study – a randomized clinical trial. *Journal of Veterinary Internal Medicine* 30 (6): 1765–1779.

Recommended Reading

Best BETs for Vets – A collection of CATs for veterinary species. http://bestbetsforvets.org

Cockroft, P. and Holmes, M. (2003). *Handbook of Evidence-Based Veterinary Medicine*, 210. Oxford: Blackwell.

McKenzie, B.A. (2014). Veterinary clinical decision-making: cognitive biases, external constraints, and strategies for improvement. *Journal of the American Veterinary Medical Association* 244 (3): 271–276.

McKenzie, B.A. (2014). Evidence-based veterinary medicine: what is it and why does it matter? *Equine Veterinary Education* 26 (9): 451–452.

Schmidt, P.L. (ed.) (2007). Evidence-based veterinary medicine. *Veterinary Clinics of North America: Small Animal Practice* 37 (3): 409–417.

VetSRev – A database of all systematic reviews in veterinary medicine. www.nottingham.ac.uk/cevm/evidence-synthesis/systematic-review/vetsrev.aspx

2.2

The Role of Incremental Care

David Haworth, DVM, PhD

Vidium Animal Health, Phoenix, AZ, USA

BASICS

2.2.1 Summary

Veterinary medicine has made incredible strides regarding the sophistication of care that can be provided by veterinarians in practice. The training of veterinary students by board-certified specialists, usually in tertiary care facilities, has had numerous advantages but has also resulted in generations of veterinarians trained to only provide the very best options, which are usually also the most expensive. When other options are given, it is only at the behest of the client, and is clearly considered a compromise.

There is a different approach that could yield multiple benefits. By establishing that there are many diagnostic and treatment choices that fall along the cost spectrum for almost all conditions, and that responsible pet owners are those that seek out care for their pet, we can increase the number of pets that receive medical attention as well as the satisfaction of clients and veterinary team members.

2.2.2 Terms Defined

Gold Standard Care: Focusing on the most successful, most complete course of action for a given health condition, irrespective of cost.

Human–Animal Bond: The emotional connection between a person or family and their pet. This is sometimes expanded to include any emotional connection between a human and an animal.

Incremental Care: The philosophy of providing all options for treating or diagnosing a specific condition,

along with the costs of those options. This is juxtaposed to providing only the best option and then negotiating "down" to what the client can afford.

MAIN CONCEPTS

In practice, incremental care has been a part of veterinary medicine since its founding. However, cementing the practice into daily management philosophy is a relatively new development. The effort to do so stems from the belief of many that the pendulum has swung to a point where only advanced care, involving the best (and most expensive) diagnostics and therapies, is being offered to pet parents. This becomes an issue when financial or other constraints cause those owners to ask for other options and they are made to feel as though they have compromised their pet's health (see 7.8 Providing Care for Those Unable or Unwilling to Pay). This results in a negative interaction between the owner and the veterinary health team, and sometimes in the pet receiving no care whatsoever. Incremental care offers an alternative approach.

The veterinary healthcare team are informed service providers. This means that they have more information and can better contextualize information about the health of an animal than the vast majority of their clients. That is where the added value of seeking out veterinary care should be created. All too often, team members are led to believe that client value derives from the amount of money they bring into a clinic, or how many high-margin procedures or products they can provide. This is misguided and has led to an erosion of the credibility of veterinarians in the eyes of the public, and several high-profile discussions of how veterinary medicine has become a profession driven by profit instead of compassion. Pet owners often do not fully comprehend how expensive it is for teams to actually provide veterinary services, or that profitability of such services is often quite modest, but this is not their primary concern. Additionally, it can lead to emotional stress in veterinarians and other team members, forcing them to feel that the reason they pursued veterinary medicine in the first place – the healing and comforting of animals – has been subsumed by the need to make money (see 8.17 Dealing with Compromise Fatigue).

Against this backdrop, veterinary medicine faces a real revenue crisis. There are many reasons driving this, but one is an overall decrease in the number of client visits. It can be postulated (and survey data bear this out) that the significant and unexpected costs of veterinary care drive many to put off taking their pet to the veterinarian until disease has progressed. If this pattern can be reversed, if steps can be taken to decrease average invoice prices for clients but increase the number of times they come in, then the lifetime value of a client will be maintained or increased along with the overall revenues to the profession. This can partially be addressed by incremental care. Additionally, there is a very large percentage, some surveys place it as high as 50%, of pets that do not see a veterinarian after their initial series of vaccinations, largely due to real or perceived financial constraints.

There are both ground-up and top-down approaches to implementing incremental care practices in the profession.

The first step is to raise awareness of and in some cases change perception of responsible pet ownership. Pets in society are seen as a right, and the profession cannot allow pet ownership to become a privilege of the wealthy. Veterinary medicine is paid for directly, and pet health insurance is almost exclusively reimbursement based, so all costs are carried by the owners themselves except in rare and specific programs subsidized by governments or charities. This means that the responsible owner is the one who seeks out medical help in the first place. They are responsible when they pick up the phone or walk in the door. Specifically, when they cannot or do not choose to pursue a treatment or diagnostic because of cost, clients need to be reminded that they are doing the right thing for them, their pet and the rest of their family, and should not be made to feel in any way negative. While this may be frustrating to some on the veterinary health team (because there are available treatments) and some may even be tempted to absorb the costs into the organization, this is ultimately a losing proposition because it weakens the viability of the practice and cannot be scaled to meet the true need (see 8.17 Dealing with Compromise Fatigue).

What can be done if the gold standards of care are not affordable to a client (see 2.10 Affordability of Veterinary Services)? Everything else. Diagnostic and treatment options exist on a spectrum – from a complete physical examination costing only time and skill to the most expensive courses of treatment costing many thousands of dollars (see 10.14 Providing Cost-Effective Care for Those in Need). Understanding all options, their relative costs, and relative efficacies is a critical part of veterinary medical training. While veterinary schools are typically poorly equipped to do that – faculty selection, size of veterinary teaching hospitals and the multitude of specialty services would make this very difficult – early career mentors need to make sure recent graduates are given the time, tools, and exposure to better understand the variety of treatment plans available for any given condition. It is likely unreasonable to expect this to be part of the curriculum pursued at most veterinary schools, but is, anecdotally, an area where the "distributed" model of veterinary education (in which actual veterinary practices are used as places of training as opposed to a centralized veterinary teaching hospital) exceeds the more traditional teaching model. By being exposed to a wide variety of practices, clientele, and treatment plans early in their career or education, veterinarians will be more comfortable offering those plans to their clients.

Organized veterinary medicine also has a role to play. Clinical guidelines that include all options should be developed for the major health conditions of dogs and cats (see 9.3 Guidelines). The full spectrum of care choices should be elucidated and discussed, understanding that more sophisticated and expensive treatments may yield more favorable outcomes, but that more cost-effective, lower-probability-of-success options should also be included and offered, if needed. In the absence of clinical guidelines provided by national organizations, state or local organizations could produce such documents, and they could even be generated by individual practices. The most important aspect is that veterinary health professionals collectively agree upon a set of options to offer for the most commonly encountered health concerns.

Lastly, it should be recognized that some conditions do not have low-cost options available. In these circumstances, it is doubly important for the owner to understand that financial limitations are valid reasons for not pursuing treatment. Humane euthanasia is always an option when quality of life concerns are present. This may feel unsatisfactory at the moment but by incorporating incremental care philosophies into a practice, clients will feel they are an integral part of healthcare decisions, which in turn helps bind them to a practice regardless of ultimate outcome for this pet.

TAKE-AWAYS

- Incremental care is a philosophy that holds that there are medical options falling along the entire cost spectrum for most health conditions and that all the available options should be discussed with pet owners.
- This is in contrast to "gold standard care," in which only the most effective and (usually) most expensive treatment options are, at least initially, presented.
- This philosophy recognizes that responsible pet ownership is demonstrated when a veterinary care team is contacted and is not dictated by the subsequent healthcare decisions, which may be constrained by financial or other factors.
- By engaging in a conversation about the range of possible options, pet parents are more likely to consider themselves a partner in their pet's care, as opposed to a customer simply paying for a service.
- It is recognized that there are some conditions that do not have low-cost options available and therefore humane euthanasia must always be considered an acceptable course of action if quality of life could deteriorate to an unacceptable level.

MISCELLANEOUS

2.2.3 Cautions

Licensing boards and legislatures are inconsistent in their approach to standards of care in veterinary medicine (see 9.5 Better Understanding Standard of Care). Be sure to understand the current interpretations of standards before offering any healthcare option that may be considered "substandard."

Recommended Reading

Stull, J.W., Shelby, J., Bonnett, B. et al. (2018). Barriers and next steps to providing a spectrum of effective health care to companion animals. *Journal of the American Veterinary Medical Association.* 253 (11): 1386–1389.

2.3

Prevalence and Incidence

Samuel Stewart, DVM, DACVECC and Chand Khanna, DVM, PhD, DACVIM (Onc), DACVP (Hon)

Ethos Veterinary Health, Woburn, MA, USA

 BASICS

2.3.1 Summary

Prevalence and incidence are both terms used to describe the occurrence of a disease over a period of time. Prevalence is defined by the number of individuals alive with a disease, while incidence is defined by the number of newly diagnosed cases of a disease divided by the population at risk of developing that disease. Incidence is often not able to be described in veterinary medicine as the population at risk of developing a given disease process is generally not known and would require a pet census. Additionally, it assumes that there is a steady rate of disease occurrence over a specified period of time, which is not always true of disease states. In veterinary studies prevalence is more commonly used as it does not require definition of the at-risk patient population.

2.3.2 Terms Defined

Epidemiology: The study of how diseases occur in given patient populations and why.
Incidence: The rate of newly diagnosed cases of a given disease process in a specified period of time.
Prevalence: The number of cases of a disease process that occur in a specified period of time.

 MAIN CONCEPTS

2.3.3 Introduction

Epidemiology is the study and analysis of diseases in a given population of people or animals. It focuses on factors of disease, such as cause, risk factors, frequency, and distribution/pattern. The purpose for the study of these factors is the goal of achieving control of the disease process (i.e., means to reduce its occurrence) or to define the size of a market before developing and commercializing an innovation for disease.

Prevalence and incidence are terms commonly used when describing the study of epidemiology. Prevalence is the actual number of cases that are alive and affected by a specific disease in a given period of time. Incidence is the calculated risk of an individual acquiring a disease in a given period of time. Both variables can be defined as disease occurrence within a certain amount of time (rate) or within a specified population (proportion).

Prevalence and incidence are expressed as fractions, which allows for the estimation between the probability of disease and the various factors that can influence that probability. The numerator of the fraction represents the number of patients that have the disease (for prevalence) or the number of newly diagnosed cases of disease (for incidence). The denominator represents the size of the population from which the individuals were drawn (for prevalence) or the size of the at-risk group of individuals (for incidence). The denominator can also be expressed in relation to time (e.g., cases of disease/population time).

2.3.4   Key Differences

Prevalence can be expressed over a period of time, referred to as period prevalence, and can also be expressed at a specific point in time, known as point prevalence. Point prevalence does not provide as good a measurement of disease as period prevalence as it is only accounting for cases alive with that disease at a given point in time and does not look at new cases and deaths over a defined time period.

Incidence refers to the number of newly diagnosed cases of a given disease. It is expressed as a fraction of the number of new cases of disease divided by the population at risk of developing the disease (e.g., 100 cases per 100 000 people = 0.001). In essence, incidence allows for determination of an individual's probability of being diagnosed with a disease during a given period of time.

There are two ways in which incidence can be expressed: incidence risk and incidence rate. Incidence risk (also known as cumulative incidence) refers to number of at-risk individuals in a given population that become new cases of disease during the defined follow-up period (e.g., 30 cases per 1000 individuals per three years). There are multiple ways in which the follow-up period can be defined, such as a fixed duration (e.g., three years), the lifetime of the individual (e.g., lifetime incidence risk of kidney disease), or based on the duration of a given epidemic. Incidence rate (also known as incidence density) refers to the number of new cases of a disease per person-time in the at-risk population. This approach requires dividing the number of new cases by the number of years being evaluated. Using the example above, an incidence risk of 30 cases per 1000 individuals per three years would equal an incidence rate of 10 cases per 1000 individual years.

The natural progression of a disease greatly defines the relationship between incidence and prevalence. Diseases that have a high rate of spontaneous resolution will result in high incidence of disease but possibly low prevalence as the disease will be resolved in many of the patients depending on the period of time being evaluated. Likewise, in diseases that have low cure rates but have treatments that provide prolonged survival rates, the incidence will contribute to a continuous growth of the prevalence.

2.3.5   Why is Incidence So Much Harder to Determine?

Incidence is defined by the population at risk of developing a disease. In human medicine there is often stringent monitoring and reporting of disease, so the at-risk population is able to be defined. Therefore, the value of incidence data is directly related to the accuracy of disease diagnosis and its subsequent reporting. While there are reporting requirements for certain disease processes in veterinary medicine that have a potentially high impact on public health, many of these cases can be misdiagnosed or fail to be reported. Furthermore, diseases outside the reportable conditions do not have any requirement for monitoring and the at-risk patient population is even more difficult to define.

The incidence of a disease is a variable that is constantly in flux. It is affected by numerous factors, such as changes in the environment of the investigated population and improvements in preventive measures to prevent the occurrence of disease. Defining incidence as a rate, rather than pure incidence, allows for this context to be taken into consideration. This approach, however, also makes the assumption that disease occurrence is evenly distributed over that period of time, which is not necessarily an accurate reflection of the true disease occurrence.

It is also not always appropriate to report the incidence of untreated cases, as the actual determination of this rate is often difficult to achieve. This would require the differentiation of new and old cases of disease and whether an individual is from the at-risk population. It is generally more appropriate to report the number of new cases that are treated as this is a known number.

2.3.6   When/Why Do We Really Need Incidence?

In general, when studying disease, it is ideal to investigate incidence rate as it is not affected by extraneous factors related to the disease, such as the type of care a patient receives or the disease's fatality rate. This removal of influence makes it easier to compare different patient populations and be able to define differences. Incidence is also more valuable when evaluating diseases that occur over short periods of time. Prevalence does not account for the number of survivors and deaths, and therefore can underestimate the severity of the issue.

2.3.7   Always Prevalence in Veterinary Medicine

Since the calculation of prevalence does not require determination of the at-risk population, it is more commonly used in veterinary medicine. It does allow for more variability in outcomes due to extraneous factors, which can complicate the interpretation of the prevalence data collected. Prevalence, however, is more useful in determining the weight of chronic diseases, whereas incidence is solely focused on new cases of disease.

EXAMPLES

Hemangiosarcoma is an aggressive form of cancer that is most commonly encountered in German shepherd dogs, Labrador retrievers, and golden retrievers. There are an estimated 75 000 cases of hemangiosarcoma diagnosed in dogs in the US per year. There are around 78 million dogs in the US, with the breeds most commonly affected by hemangiosarcoma representing around 20% of these (15.6 million). The incidence rate would be defined as the number of new cases per year (75 000) divided by the at-risk population per unit time (15.6 million/year), which would give an incidence rate of 0.005. Most dogs with hemangiosarcoma succumb to their disease within 6–12 months of being diagnosed, depending on the treatment that is pursued. Looking at a one-year period, you can make the assumption that around one quarter of hemangiosarcoma cases from the previous year will still be alive (18 750). Add this to the number of new cases that will be diagnosed that year (75 000 + 18 750 = 93 750). If this was to be defined based on the total population, the prevalence would be 0.001.

TAKE-AWAYS

- Epidemiology is the study of disease in a population for the purposes of disease control as well as to define the market for the development and commercialization of diagnostics and therapeutics for that disease process.

- Prevalence is defined by the number of individuals alive with a given disease, while incidence is the number of newly diagnosed cases of disease divided by the population at risk of developing that disease.
- Incidence is difficult to accurately determine as it overlooks the potential for unreported disease events and misdiagnosed disease, and assumes that new cases of disease occur at a steady rate over a given period of time.
- Prevalence is more commonly utilized in veterinary medicine as it does not require defining the population that is at risk of developing that disease.
- Prevalence is preferred for the evaluation of chronic disease conditions as it does not account for survivors and deaths, which are important for the evaluation of shorter term impacts of disease.

MISCELLANEOUS

Recommended Reading

Noah, D. L., & Ostrowski, S. R. Basic Principles of Epidemiology. www.merckvetmanual.com/public-health/public-health-primer/basic-principles-of-epidemiology

Perez, A.M. (2015). Past, present, and future of veterinary epidemiology and economics: one health, many challenges, no silver bullets. *Frontiers in Veterinary Science* 2: 60.

Stevenson, M. (2008). An Introduction to Veterinary Epidemiology. www.massey.ac.nz/massey/fms/Colleges/College%20of%20Sciences/Epicenter/docs/ASVCS/Stevenson_intro_epidemiology-web_2008.pdf

Thrusfield, M. (2013). *Veterinary Epidemiology*. Weinheim, Germany: Wiley.

2.4

Checklists in Veterinary Practice

Ryane E. Englar, DVM, DABVP (Canine and Feline Practice)

College of Veterinary Medicine, University of Arizona, Oro Valley, AZ, USA

 BASICS

2.4.1 Summary

When medical teams fail today, it is less often a case of not knowing any better. More often, errors occur because medical team members are human. Care providers know what to do and how to do it; however, do they always intervene appropriately, every time, in the same manner? Despite our best efforts, patients can receive incomplete or inadequate care. Our knowledge has burdened us: the breadth and depth of what we know have exceeded our capability to deliver upon it reliably. We can overcome our shortcomings by implementing a strategy that reminds us what to do, in the proper order. Veterinary medical checklists are an effective strategy to reduce avoidable errors. Although checklists can be applied to any facet of veterinary practice, anesthesia and surgery are practical starting points for initiating change.

2.4.2 Terms Defined

Checklist: A tool that is intended to reduce human failure by drawing the user's attention to key tasks that must be performed in a particular order and allowing the user to mark off each task as it is performed to prevent missed steps.

Medical Error: An adverse effect of patient care that may or may not be harmful to the patient but could have been prevented.

 MAIN CONCEPTS

2.4.3 The Need

Failures occur in every industry, including veterinary medicine. However, few industries have been able to reduce human-based error to the degree that the aviation industry has reported. Between 1993 and 2013, the number of worldwide flight hours doubled from 25 to 54 million, yet fatalities decreased from 450 to 250 per year [1]. By comparison, 200,000 people in the United States alone are estimated to die preventable deaths annually at the hands of human healthcare [2]. This rate of deaths equates to three fatal airplane crashes per day and would be considered unacceptable to the aviation industry: "Airlines would stop flying, airports would close . . . [and] no one would be allowed to fly until the problem had been solved" [3].

Comparisons are more difficult to make between veterinary medicine and the aviation industry due to the paucity of studies in the veterinary literature [4, 5]. Most veterinary publications examine anesthetic or surgical complications, not all of which stem from human error. In companion animal medicine, these include hypotension [6–8], dysphoria [9–11], cardiac arrhythmias [8], aspiration pneumonia [12], cerebellar dysfunction [13], blindness or deafness in cats [14–16], and death [17].

A retrospective study examined medical records from 98,036 dogs and 79,178 cats that underwent anesthetic procedures between June 2002 and 2004 in the United Kingdom. Brodbelt et al. determined the overall risk of anesthetic death to be 0.17% and 0.24% in dogs and cats respectively [18]. When categorized by health status, healthy dogs and cats experienced anesthetic death at the diminished rate of 0.05% and 0.11% compared to 1.33% and 1.40% in ill dogs and cats [18]. These percentages are much higher than 0.02–0.05%, which is the range reported for anesthetized people [19–21]. However, how much death is the result of medical error is unknown. Most of what is known is largely anecdotal, which begs the questions "How much error occurs that we don't know about and what can we do to prevent it?"

2.4.4 The Tool

How might healthcare professionals learn from aviators to reduce preventable error, thereby improving safety? There is one tool in particular that the aviation industry has relied upon that has gradually trickled into various facets of human healthcare: the checklist. Checklists may seem too simplistic an approach for the complexities of medical cases but by guarding against two common pitfalls in healthcare, distractions and human fatigue, they are perhaps more important than ever for safeguarding those for whom caregivers are responsible. Checklists are tangible reminders of steps that we may have forgotten to take; steps that we may remember, but fail to carry out to completion; and steps that we may take but execute improperly [2].

In aviation, checklists may be used for ordinary procedures, such as take-offs and landings, as well as for malfunctions and emergencies. Healthcare as a whole has been slow to adopt this tool; however, human medical providers have gradually piloted, tested, and refined checklists in the following arenas [2, 22–33]:

- anesthetic equipment prechecks
- communication between team members
- emergency codes
- infection control
- medication dosing
- patient diagnosis
- patient identification
- patient tracking, from admission to discharge
- patient transfer from the operating room to the intensive care unit
- shift changes and communication between outgoing and incoming nursing staff
- surgical planning
- surgical procedures.

The World Health Organization (WHO) Surgical Safety Checklist was published in 2008 and remains one of the most widely used checklists in human healthcare today [2, 34].

The adoption of checklists and their success inherently depend upon staff training and resource management; that is, how team members interact with and influence one another [2]. Effective communication with opportunities for debriefing fosters teamwork and the opportunity to learn from mistakes, rather than hide from them [35, 36].

2.4.5 Checklists in Veterinary Medicine

Much of what we know about human-based errors in veterinary medicine stems from an analysis of liability insurance claims. Surgical errors are overrepresented, including retained surgical tools [5, 37–45]. Because these errors have the potential to increase morbidity and mortality among patients, particularly when their diagnosis is delayed, measures ought to be taken to reduce the incidence.

Checklists in veterinary surgery are an appropriate tool to address surgical instrument retention, among other surgical errors. For instance, a surgical checklist should require a pre- and postoperative count of gauze squares, swabs, and sponges [37]. If these numbers are incongruent, then the surgery cannot be completed until all missing items are accounted for. Counting swabs and gauze squares is not immune from human error but it is an appropriate starting point prior to body cavity closure; in human healthcare, the sensitivity is 77% and specificity is 99% [46]. An additional safety measure would be the use of radiopaque swabs [47]. In the event that a discrepancy persists, radiographing the area of the body that was operated on should confirm accidental retention of the missing item within a body cavity.

In addition to surgical errors, medical errors may occur in veterinary practice (see 8.14 Appropriate Handling of Medical Errors). Among these, overdoses of medication and the administration of the wrong medication appear to be most common [5]. Checklists are also important aspects of convergence schedules, to ensure that client communication is managed appropriately (see 9.7 Continuum of Care and Convergence Schedules) and as preanesthetic safeguards (see 9.13 Preanesthetic Considerations).

Checklists are therefore advisable in veterinary healthcare for many reasons, all of which promote patient safety. There is currently no standard checklist to which all veterinary practices subscribe; however, a variety of formats are available in the popular press and can be custom-fit to suit an individual practice's needs (see Table 2.4.1).

Table 2.4.1 Sample surgical safety checklist for use by veterinary practices as a tool to guard against human error. This checklist can be modified for completeness and to suit each individual hospital's needs

Surgical Safety Checklist

Procedure:

Attending Veterinarian:

CPR Code (Green / Red / Yellow)

Patient Identification	Client Information
Patient ID#:	Client Name:
Patient Name:	Client Phone Number:
Patient Signalment:	Client Emergency Contact:
Body Weight (Pounds):	Emergency Contact Number:
Body Weight (Kilograms):	Other Client or Patient-Specific Notes:
Microchip Number:	
Identifying Features: (Coat Color, Eye Color, etc.)	

Patient Drop-Off Procedures

☐ Confirm patient's identity.

☐ Confirm procedure to be performed, with client.

☐ If sterilization surgery, confirm patient's sex.

☐ Review procedure with client, including risks.

☐ Obtain client contact information, including emergency contact.

☐ Confirm the client's wishes concerning CPR code status for the patient in the event of an emergency.

☐ Invite the client to ask questions or share concerns.

☐ Make a plan with client concerning who from the practice will get in touch with them and when, relative to the end of the procedure.

☐ Place identification (i.e., neck ID collar) on patient.

☐ Weigh patient and record weight in pounds (lbs) and kilograms (kgs).

☐ Record values for the patient's vital signs: T _____ / P _____ / R _____

☐ Place patient in cage or kennel and label the housing appropriately.

Prior to Patient Induction

☐ Confirm patient's identity

☐ Review patient's chart:

Are there any preexisting conditions that may complicate anesthesia, surgery, or recovery? If so, alert the attending clinician and create a plan for management of each condition.

☐ Confirm procedure.

☐ Confirm surgical site.

☐ Perform physical examination.

☐ Design patient's anesthetic protocol and confirm with the attending clinician:

Include perioperative antibiotics (if necessary), analgesics, and other pre-medications.

Include calculations for induction agent and plans for maintaining anesthesia.

☐ Check anesthetic machine and circuitry. Troubleshoot any potential problems.

☐ Check monitoring equipment. Troubleshoot any potential problems.

☐ Check patient warming devices. Troubleshoot any potential problems.

(Continued)

Table 2.4.1 (*Continued*)

Surgical Safety Checklist

Patient Induction

☐ Double-check premedications, including route of administration.

☐ Administer premedications.

☐ Place intravenous catheter.

☐ Double-check induction agent.

☐ Induce the patient.

☐ Attach monitoring devices to the patient.

☐ Prepare surgical site.

☐ Transport patient into operating suite.

Prior to First Incision

☐ Confirm patient, procedure, and incision site.

☐ Confirm sterility of surgeon.

☐ Complete patient prep, i.e., draping.

☐ Counting of gauze squares, sponges, and swabs.

☐ Surgeon to communicate with anesthetist about patient's vital signs prior to making the first incision.

During the Procedure

☐ Patient's vital signs to be monitored and documented at predetermined intervals.

☐ Prior to surgical wound closure, gauze squares, sponges, and swabs should be recounted. Compare this number to the presurgical count. If both numbers agree, then the patient can be closed.

After Surgery / During Patient Recovery from Surgery

☐ Communication must take place between the OR surgeon/staff and those who will be tending to the patient in the postoperative period, including instructions concerning when to reassess patient and which medications to administer (how much? how often?)

☐ Any samples that were taken intraoperatively need to be accounted for, labelled, stored appropriately, and/or submitted to the laboratory.

☐ Surgeon to prepare surgical report. Any unexpected findings or complications should be documented in the patient's medical record.

☐ Client communication should take place concerning the procedure.

☐ Patient discharge instructions should be prepared.

 EXAMPLES

Retention of surgical instruments is not the only error in veterinary surgery. Performing the wrong procedure on the wrong patient is of real concern, particularly because veterinary patients cannot themselves confirm their own identity. Consider, for example, two orange tabby cats of roughly the same build and body weight, one of which presents for onychectomy and one for tendonectomy. These are two very different procedures, with two very different patient outcomes. Failure to accurately identify each individual may result in the correct procedure being performed on the wrong patient.

Another surgical error that the author witnessed as a veterinary student stems from failure to confirm the feline patient's sex prior to sterilization surgery. Attempting to spay a tomcat will continue to happen in clinical practice so long as clinicians and support staff put blind faith in the client's ability to sex the cat, particularly in this era of pediatric neutering.

TAKE-AWAYS

- As scientific advances expand our knowledge base, it becomes increasingly difficult for healthcare providers to manage the volume and complexity of clinical cases based upon memory alone.
- Human-based errors in medicine and surgery can and will happen to some degree to every veterinary practice and every healthcare provider.
- Veterinary medicine can benefit from a risk management tool that has long been employed by the aviation industry – the checklist.
- Checklists may seem like "to do" lists that are too simplistic to be of assistance in veterinary practice; however, human healthcare has paved the way in demonstrating that their use helps to reduce medical and surgical errors.
- Although checklists are imperfect, they open the door for dialogue about how providers can lessen the chance that an error will occur and jeopardize patient outcomes.

MISCELLANEOUS

2.4.6 Cautions

Checklists are an imperfect science. At their best, they are concise reminders of key aspects of care; at their worst, they can be cumbersome and inefficient. Checklists must therefore strike a balance between including every step of a task and including too few. Even then, the best checklist can fail. No checklist can prevent every human error from occurring.

So why is it that checklists fail? Checklists require buy-in from the entire team to be effective [48]. If the team leader has a poor attitude towards the implementation of a given checklist, then it is likely to fail. For a checklist to be effective, it must be consistently used. This means that team members must be properly trained to complete the checklist if it is to become part of practice procedure. Team members must understand the nuances of what they are being asked to do so that completion of the checklist

facilitates rather than hinders care. Checklist makers must be open to modifications based upon shared concerns, which means that teams need to be able to speak freely and openly about both the process and their expectations. What is it that the hospital is trying to achieve and why? Is this checklist the best answer to an ongoing hospital problem or is there a better way? Open dialogue will help everyone to get on the same page so that the checklist is customized in a way that suits that individual practice's needs. There is rarely a one-size-fits-all approach to practice management. The checklist can be an effective strategy in the right setting with the right team, provided that there is room for flexibility in its design. Flexibility breeds room for acceptance.

Abbreviation

TPR   Temperature, Pulse, and Respiration

References

1 Aviation Safety, Boeing Commercial Airlines (2014). Statistical summary of commercial jet airplane accidents: worldwide operations 1959–2014. In: *Boeing Commercial Airlines*. Seattle, Washington: Aviation Safety.

2 Kapur, N., Parand, A., Soukup, T. et al. (2016). Aviation and healthcare: a comparative review with implications for patient safety. *JRSM Open* 7: 2054270415616548.

3 Sullenberger, C.B. and Chesley, B. (2013). "Sully" Sullenberger: making safety a core business function. *Healthc. Financ. Manage.* 67: 50–54.

4 Jones, R.S. (2001). Comparative mortality in anaesthesia. *Br. J. Anaesth.* 87: 813–815.

5 Oxtoby, C., Ferguson, E., White, K. et al. (2015). We need to talk about error: causes and types of error in veterinary practice. *Vet. Rec.* 177: 438.

6 Iizuka, T., Kamata, M., Yanagawa, M. et al. (2013). Incidence of intraoperative hypotension during isoflurane-fentanyl and propofol-fentanyl anaesthesia in dogs. *Vet. J.* 198: 289–291.

7 Mazzaferro, E. and Wagner, A.E. (2001). Hypotension during anesthesia in dogs and cats: Recognition, causes, and treatment. *Comp. Cont. Educ. Pract. Vet.* 23: 728–737.

8 Gaynor, J.S., Dunlop, C.I., Wagner, A.E. et al. (1999). Complications and mortality associated with anesthesia in dogs and cats. *J. Am. Anim. Hosp. Assoc.* 35: 13–17.

9 Becker, W.M., Mama, K.R., Rao, S. et al. (2013). Prevalence of dysphoria after fentanyl in dogs undergoing stifle surgery. *Vet. Surg.* 42: 302–307.

10 Vaisanen, M., Oksanen, H., and Vainio, O. (2004). Postoperative signs in 96 dogs undergoing soft tissue surgery. *Vet. Rec.* 155: 729–733.

11 Light, G.S., Hardie, E.M., and Young, M.S. (1993). Pain and anxiety behaviors of dogs during intravenous catherization after premedication with placebo, acepromazine or oxymorphone. *Appl. Behav. Anim. Sci.* 37: 331–343.

12 Ovbey, D.H., Wilson, D.V., Bednarski, R.M. et al. (2014). Prevalence and risk factors for canine post-anesthetic aspiration pneumonia (1999–2009): a multicenter study. *Vet. Anaesth. Analg.* 41: 127–136.

13 Shamir, M., Goelman, G., and Chai, O. (2004). Postanesthetic cerebellar dysfunction in cats. *J. Vet. Intern. Med.* 18: 368–369.

14 Barton-Lamb, A.L., Martin-Flores, M., Scrivani, P.V. et al. (2013). Evaluation of maxillary arterial blood flow in anesthetized cats with the mouth closed and open. *Vet. J.* 196: 325–331.

15 Jurk, I.R., Thibodeau, M.S., Whitney, K. et al. (2001). Acute vision loss after general anesthesia in a cat. *Vet. Ophthalmol.* 4: 155–158.

16 Son, W.G., Jung, B.Y., Kwon, T.E. et al. (2009). Acute temporary visual loss after general anesthesia in a cat. *J. Vet. Clin.* 26: 480–482.

17 Clarke, K.W. and Hall, L.W. (1990). A survey of anaesthesia in small animal practice: AVA/BSAVA Report. *J. Vet. Anaesth.* 17: 4–10.

18 Brodbelt, D.C., Blissitt, K.J., Hammond, R.A. et al. (2008). The risk of death: the confidential enquiry into perioperative small animal fatalities. *Vet. Anaesth. Analg.* 35: 365–373.

19 Kawashima, Y., Seo, N., Morita, K. et al. (2001). Annual study of perioperative mortality and morbidity for the year of 1999 in Japan: the outlines – report of the Japan Society of Anesthesiologists Committee on Operating Room Safety. *Masui.* 50: 1260–1274.

20 Biboulet, P., Aubas, P., Dubourdieu, J. et al. (2001). Fatal and non fatal cardiac arrests related to anesthesia. *Can. J. Anaesth.* 48: 326–332.

21 Eagle, C.C. and Davis, N.J. (1997). Report of the Anaesthetic Mortality Committee of Western Australia 1990–1995. *Anaesth. Intensive Care* 25: 51–59.

22 Haynes, A.B., Berry, W.R., and Gawande, A.A. (2015). What do we know about the safe surgery checklist now? *Ann. Surg.* 261: 829–830.

23 Pronovost, P.J., Goeschel, C.A., Colantuoni, E. et al. (2010). Sustaining reductions in catheter related bloodstream infections in Michigan intensive care units: observational study. *BMJ* 340: c309.

24 Ely, J.W., Graber, M.L., and Croskerry, P. (2011). Checklists to reduce diagnostic errors. *Acad. Med.* 86: 307–313.

25 Winters, B.D., Aswani, M.S., and Pronovost, P.J. (2011). Commentary: reducing diagnostic errors: another role for checklists? *Acad. Med.* 86: 279–281.

26 Catchpole, K.R., de Leval, M.R., McEwan, A. et al. (2007). Patient handover from surgery to intensive care: using Formula 1 pit-stop and aviation models to improve safety and quality. *Paediatr. Anaesth.* 17: 470–478.

27 Low, D.K., Reed, M.A., Geiduschek, J.M. et al. (2013). Striving for a zero-error patient surgical journey through adoption of aviation-style challenge and response flow checklists: a quality improvement project. *Paediatr. Anaesth.* 23: 571–578.

28 Federwisch, M., Ramos, H., and Adams, S.C. (2014). The sterile cockpit: an effective approach to reducing medication errors? *Am. J. Nurs.* 114: 47–55.

29 Schelkun, S.R. (2014). Lessons from aviation safety: "plan your operation – and operate your plan!". *Patient Saf. Surg.* 8: 38.

30 Clay-Williams, R. and Colligan, L. (2015). Back to basics: checklists in aviation and healthcare. *BMJ Qual. Saf.* 24: 428–431.

31 Levy, M.M., Pronovost, P.J., Dellinger, R.P. et al. (2004). Sepsis change bundles: converting guidelines into meaningful change in behavior and clinical outcome. *Crit. Care Med.* 32: S595–S597.

32 Lingard, L., Regehr, G., Orser, B. et al. (2008). Evaluation of a preoperative checklist and team briefing among surgeons, nurses, and anesthesiologists to reduce failures in communication. *Arch. Surg.* 143: 12–17; discussion 18.

33 de Vries, E.N., Prins, H.A., Crolla, R.M. et al. (2010). Effect of a comprehensive surgical safety system on patient outcomes. *N. Engl. J. Med.* 363: 1928–1937.

34 Sivathasan, N., Rakowski, K.R., Robertson, B.F. et al. (2010). The World Health Organization's 'Surgical Safety Checklist': should evidence-based initiatives be enforced in hospital policy? *JRSM Short Rep.* 1: 40.

35 Gillespie, B.M., Chaboyer, W., Longbottom, P. et al. (2010). The impact of organisational and individual factors on team communication in surgery: a qualitative study. *Int. J. Nurs. Stud.* 47: 732–741.

36 Leonard, M., Graham, S., and Bonacum, D. (2004). The human factor: the critical importance of effective teamwork and communication in providing safe care. *Qual. Saf. Health Care* 13 (Suppl 1): i85–i90.

37 Forster, K., Anderson, D., Yool, D.A. et al. (2011). Retained surgical swabs in 13 dogs. *Vet. Rec.* 169: 337.

38 Teague, H.D., Alsaker, R., Braden, T.D. et al. (1978). Two cases of foreign-body osteomyelitis secondary to retained surgical sponges. *Vet. Med. Small Anim. Clin.* 73: 1279–1286.

39 Rayner, E.L., Scudamore, C.L., Francis, I. et al. (2010). Abdominal fibrosarcoma associated with a retained surgical swab in a dog. *J. Comp. Pathol.* 143: 81–85.

40 Putwain, S. and Archer, J. (2009). What is your diagnosis? Intra-abdominal mass aspirate from a spayed dog with abdominal pain. *Vet. Clin. Pathol.* 38: 253–256.

41 Pardo, A.D., Adams, W.H., McCracken, M.D. et al. (1990). Primary jejunal osteosarcoma associated with a surgical sponge in a dog. *J. Am. Vet. Med. Assoc.* 196: 935–938.

42 Frank, J.D. and Stanley, B.J. (2009). Enterocutaneous fistula in a dog secondary to an intraperitoneal gauze foreign body. *J. Am. Anim. Hosp. Assoc.* 45: 84–88.

43 Haddad, J.L., Goldschmidt, M.H., and Patel, R.T. (2010). Fibrosarcoma arising at the site of a retained surgical sponge in a cat. *Vet. Clin. Pathol.* 39: 241–246.

44 Lamb, C.R., White, R.N., and McEvoy, F.J. (1994). Sinography in the investigation of draining tracts in small animals: retrospective review of 25 cases. *Vet. Surg.* 23: 129–134.

45 Mai, W., Ledieu, D., Venturini, L. et al. (2001). Ultrasonographic appearance of intra-abdominal granuloma secondary to retained surgical sponge. *Vet. Radiol. Ultrasound* 42: 157–160.

46 Egorova, N.N., Moskowitz, A., Gelijns, A. et al. (2008). Managing the prevention of retained surgical instruments: what is the value of counting? *Ann. Surg.* 247: 13–18.

47 Merlo, M. and Lamb, C.R. (2000). Radiographic and ultrasonographic features of retained surgical sponge in eight dogs. *Vet. Radiol. Ultrasound* 41: 279–283.

48 Low, D., Walker, I., Heitmiller, E.S. et al. (2012). Implementing checklists in the operating room. *Paediatr. Anaesth.* 22: 1025–1031.

Recommended Reading

Gawande, A. (2010). *The Checklist Manifesto: How to Get Things Right*. New York: Metropolitan Books.

Oxtoby, C., Ferguson, E., White, K. et al. (2015). We need to talk about error: causes and types of error in veterinary practice. *Vet. Rec.* 177 (17): 438.

2.5

Virtual Care (Telehealth)

Lowell Ackerman, DVM, DACVD, MBA, MPA, CVA, MRCVS

Global Consultant, Author, and Lecturer, MA, USAr

 BASICS

2.5.1 Summary

Today's consumers want their healthcare on their own schedules, and at their own convenience. Since most have smart devices, they typically have access to online messaging, images, and even video, and are used to these devices playing a central role in their lives.

Telehealth (or virtual care or connected care or even healthcare on demand) is the umbrella term used for healthcare consulting delivered remotely, and can be subdivided based on the parties involved in the consultation.

Veterinarians providing telehealth must comply with all laws and regulations associated with their license to practice veterinary medicine. The standard of care is the same regardless of whether telemedicine or in-hospital care is provided.

Telehealth has the potential to enhance animal care and the delivery of veterinary services, and regulations are evolving accordingly.

2.5.2 Terms Defined

Electronic Prescribing (E-Prescribing): The use of digital electronic prescriptions rather than providing a printed prescription or faxing a prescription.

Mobile Health (mHealth): Subclassification of telehealth in which mobile applications (apps) and wearables are used to provide healthcare information for pets.

Teleadvice: Subclassification of telehealth in which only general advice is provided that is not specific to a particular patient's situation.

Teleconsulting: Subclassification of telehealth in which the consulting takes place between a primary care veterinarian and a specialist.

Telehealth: Broad term to describe healthcare consulting delivered remotely. Sometimes referred to as virtual care or connected care.

Telemedicine: Telehealth delivered between a veterinarian and an animal-owning client, under the auspices of a veterinary–client–patient relationship (VCPR).

Telemonitoring: A form of telehealth in which patients are monitored remotely.

Teletriage: Subclassification of telehealth in which assessment is made remotely regarding the need for urgent veterinary visitation. Teletriage does not include rendering any diagnosis, just advising regarding the potential urgency of the situation based on the information provided.

Veterinarian-Client-Patient Relationship: A legal relationship between veterinarian and animal owner in which the veterinarian has assumed responsibility for making clinical judgments and the clients has agreed to follow the veterinarian's instructions, the veterinarian has sufficient knowledge of the patient to make such judgments, continuing care is provided or available, the veterinarian provides oversight of treatment, compliance and outcome, and patient records are maintained.

 MAIN CONCEPTS

Telemedicine has had a place in veterinary medicine for decades, and yet changes in technology, and advances in human medicine, have changed the landscape in recent years. Regulatory changes, however, have not always kept pace.

Human medicine functions on a different business model from veterinary medicine, and consumers may see programs in human health that have telemedicine more completely integrated into overall care. Thus, there might be programs integrated with insurance groups, public health, and other endeavors that increase patient access and lower healthcare costs. Technologies can also be used to establish a valid physician–patient relationship in human medicine without the need for an in-person examination.

It is important to realize that most veterinary regulations do not permit the establishment of a VCPR by electronic means alone. Clients may be exposed to such human programs and infer that it should be possible for those same services to be provided by veterinarians. It should not be inferred that because a type of service is available in human health that it is legally permissible to provide the same or similar service in the veterinary business space. The American Association of Veterinary State Boards (AAVSB) has expanded the definition of the VCPR to include establishing a VCPR using telehealth tools but since the AAVSB does not dictate licensing requirements, veterinarians are advised to consult with their applicable organizations to determine what is allowed in their specific circumstances. The field and its applications are clearly evolving.

Veterinarians have often given advice by telephone, email and even text (SMS) for years; most of this has occurred within the bounds of a VCPR, but some advice is likely to have also been offered to prospective clients with whom such a relationship may not have been legitimately established.

Veterinarians with a valid VCPR have professional discretion to confer with specialists and consultants, but they remain the physicians of record and do not transfer that VCPR to the specialist or consultant. Most telehealth services with experts are not a replacement for specialist referral, but may increase accessibility, and may possibly be the only alternative for some clients who do not have a specialist within a reasonable referral area.

2.5.3   The Marketplace

Most demographic groups have embraced technology that allows instant gratification and do-it-yourself (DIY) applications. There is a growing trend among pet owners to access information online, purchase products online, encourage the monitoring of their pets with wearable technology, and seek medical opinions online.

Pet owners want applications that allow them to be in contact with veterinary professionals at the time and via the medium of their choosing, even if veterinary practices

have some qualms with this, may have concerns about the legalities of such actions, and have even more concerns about how to be compensated for such services.

Clients may attempt to contact veterinary hospitals by email or text (SMS), through social media and through online resources, including sending images and video; veterinary hospitals need to have a strategic plan for how to deal with such contact. Primary care veterinarians may try to use the same strategies with specialists, hoping for insights without having to refer the patient, and are faced with the same limitations.

Clients may have reasonable or unreasonable expectations that the veterinary hospitals with which they do business should be responsive to such contact. In some cases, it may be a follow-up question to services that have already been provided (e.g., "Sheba chewed out one of the stitches from the procedure she just had, but it isn't bleeding. Do I need to bring her in?"). In other instances, it might be an attempt to save money or avoid the necessity of bringing a pet into the hospital ("Lily has had a bout of vomiting. Can I just give her the medicine I use when I have an upset stomach, and I'll bring her in if she doesn't get better?").

2.5.4   Professional Considerations

Telemedicine consultations should only occur within a valid VCPR; this is true regardless of whether the consultation occurs by telephone, email, or other medium. If it is allowed by a jurisdiction to create a virtual VCPR, it is still important to check with the appropriate authorities if prescribing is allowed under such a telehealth relationship.

Veterinary hospitals should be careful not to inadvertently provide telemedicine to new or prospective clients, since there is legal liability when a legitimate VCPR is absent.

In the United States, there is considerable variability between states as to laws for the provision of telemedicine services, so veterinarians should consult with their state licensing boards about what is permitted in the state Practice Act. It is particularly important to be aware of jurisdictions that require a physical examination or temperature/pulse/respiration notation for visits, or every time a patient is presented for a new clinical problem. It is also important to be aware if a jurisdiction requires some form of informed consent by the client for telehealth consultations. These rules can make telemedicine extremely challenging.

If no VCPR exists, it still might be possible for veterinarians to answer basic questions that would not constitute providing specific medical advice for any specific pet (e.g., "what is mange?," "can dogs get chicken pox?," "my cat is bleeding. Should I bring her in, or go to an emergency clinic?," etc.).

Consultations with pet owners for which a VCPR has not been established are generally considered as either teleadvice or teletriage, rather than telemedicine. Both are still a subset of telehealth, even if they are not telemedicine. Teletriage might include providing advice for a pet that has consumed poison, whether that involves having them call a poison control hotline or advising them to go to the nearest emergency clinic. There are also now a variety of applications for pets using wearables, including remotely measuring pulse, respirations, temperature, position, and activity level, and this also constitutes teletriage, but this typically happens within a sanctioned VCPR.

Veterinarians providing telehealth must be legally authorized to practice veterinary medicine. Depending on the local jurisdiction, licensing requirements, and Practice Act, they may also be required to be licensed to practice in that specific state where the patient is located.

2.5.5 Implementation

Most veterinarians are already providing some forms of telehealth, but it is worthwhile creating hospital guidelines regarding the delivery of such services. It is also important to ensure that all aspects of the telehealth consultation are recorded appropriately in the medical records.

There are essentially two different ways in which virtual health can be delivered – synchronous and asynchronous. Synchronous consultations occur on a real-time basis and technology is typically used to provide an audiovisual encounter. In most cases the client is using their own smart device to communicate, but in some cases visiting paraprofessionals may be remote and act as telepresenters on the client's behalf, providing more hand-on evaluation. With asynchronous telemedicine, sometimes referred to as "store-it-forward" care, the consultations do not happen in real time. The client can submit questions, images, videos, laboratory results, etc. for the veterinary team to comment on and respond at a later time. While this lacks the personal touch of synchronous consultations, it is often much easier for both busy clients and veterinary team members to accommodate in their schedules.

Other than teleconsultations, the most common forms of telehealth relate to things like provision of prescriptions based on VCPR, recheck evaluations, after-hours care, postsurgery check-ups, patient monitoring through wearable devices and other technologies, and even following up on hospice care patients and others for which in-hospital visits are not possible or not convenient.

Telehealth can be provided directly by a hospital (e.g., telephone, teleconferencing, email, etc.), but there are now several companies, programs, platforms, and applications that facilitate the interaction and monetization of the process.

2.5.6 Remote Monitoring

Technology is now available that allows remote monitoring of pets, and this can be an important resource when considering virtual care. The most common forms of remote monitoring are wearable collars, but other options for remote monitoring include glucometers, blood pressure devices, Holter monitors, and even sensors that can allow auscultation and other features.

Wearable collars with sensors are the most common form of remote monitoring. These collars can typically measure position (lying, sitting, standing), activity, pulse, respiration, and even heart rate variability. The measurements are generally collected continuously and in real time. For many of the devices, the veterinary healthcare team can access the information any time of the day or night through a cloud-based server.

There are many reasons why practices would choose to monitor pets remotely. For pets with existing medical issues, especially chronic problems, wearables allow measurements to be taken continuously and analyzed in real time. For certain devices, systems can be set up to send alerts when specific thresholds are exceeded. This can alert the pet owner and the veterinary team when action is required, including bringing the pet in for a visit or taking it to an emergency facility.

One of the most useful features of wearable collars is that they can allow the team to determine actual resting heart and respiration rates for pets, which may be difficult if not impossible to collect during office visits. Many pets are anxious or stressed during visits to a veterinary hospital, and heart and respiratory rates taken during those visits may be significantly altered. However, in the comfort of a pet's own home, such measurements are much more likely to be indicative of actual resting rates. It might also be possible to use wearables to infer relative stress levels in pets in different circumstances, including shelters and other environments.

Another important development in remote systems is continuous glucose monitoring, which is available for both dogs and cats. Glucometers are available that can be used to sample interstitial blood for glucose determinations, but it can be difficult to collect enough samples over time to approximate a glucose curve in pets on insulin therapy. Similar to the human devices, veterinary continuous glucose monitors have a sensor that is inserted under the skin to read blood glucose levels. A garment is typically used to cover the device so that it is not dislodged. In general, the devices sample the capillary fluid every five minutes or so, and once analyzed can provide a more complete picture of glucose status. Without such home testing, it would typically take hospitalization of the pet and sampling of the blood glucose every few hours to determine glucose peak and nadir. Older remote systems offered only retrospective analysis of the glucose concentrations after disconnecting the sensor and uploading the data. Newer systems measure and display glucose reading in real time, allowing direct intervention and altering insulin doses accordingly.

Remote monitoring can also play a key role in wellness care. With overweight and obese animals constituting a near-epidemic in small animal practices, exercise is often recommended as part of the solution. Fitness wearables, in most cases accelerometers, can be used to track effectiveness of a prescribed regimen, and additional devices such as connected scales can be used to monitor weight at home between office visits. Wearable devices with accelerometers can also be used in rehabilitation after surgery or injury and can provide the veterinary healthcare team with real-time data.

Expect that in the years ahead remote monitoring will become an even more important part of pet-specific care, and clients will expect this option from veterinary teams.

2.5.7 Financial Aspects of Virtual Care

Pricing for telehealth services will vary depending on how the telehealth service is to be integrated into the practice workstream, vendor-associated charges, and the costs associated with offering telehealth solutions

Telehealth pricing can be used to drive other health-related services. For example, it might be included with payment (wellness) plans (see 10.17 Payment and Wellness Plans) as a less costly way of honoring the ongoing provision of services in a bundled care plan. It could also be priced in an à la carte fashion based on a time-based teleconsultation (either the length of the consultation or how quickly the response is needed). As a variation on a bundled service, teleconsultation could also be subscription priced. The opportunities are only bounded by one's imagination and clients' requests for services.

Virtual care services do not need to be problematic for the hospital team, and there is much flexibility that can be built into the system. Initially, teams may determine when in the schedule there are more likely to be gaps not filled by regular appointments, and those times can be allocated for virtual care. When clients cannot be immediately accommodated when they request same-day appointments, they can be offered a telehealth option in its place. It is important to realize that times that may be inconvenient for clients to bring their pets in to the clinic are not necessarily times when the client cannot make themselves available for a virtual consult.

Veterinarians may initially have some worries that offering telehealth services will cannibalize their office visits, but such fears are generally unfounded. In most cases, clients request virtual visits for assurances on whether in-clinic visits are needed. In many situations, clients will request telehealth consults so they have a better appreciation for what may be needed, but probably 70% or so of virtual care visits eventuate in the clients bringing their pet to the clinic. If human telehealth is any indication, making access to healthcare more convenient triggers new use of medical services rather than a loss of doctor office visits.

For practices that already offer payment (wellness) plans for their clients, virtual visits are a very effective way to leverage those plans, as well as to triage patients online or over the telephone to determine if the care required is part of the plan or actually constitutes a level of care that is not covered by the plan. In many cases, clients are prepared to have access to a veterinary expert just to allay their fears or to justify the need to actually bring their pet into the hospital. Virtual visits can either be incorporated into existing payment plans or clients could be asked to pay an additional fee to the payment plans to entitle them to pose questions by email, text or telephone as part of a monthly or prepaid subscription plan.

Part of the triage system that can be useful for both pet owners and veterinary teams is to allow doctors and/or nurses to screen potential emergency calls to determine whether a pet really needs to go to an emergency center, or whether the problem could be dealt with the next day at the clinic on a nonemergency basis. Pet owners know that emergency clinics can be expensive, but without being able to speak with someone they trust, they may make the decision (to go or not to go to the emergency facility) without the benefit of appropriate advice. It is important to appreciate that such monitoring does not need to be constantly available, and that such teletriage can be provided when teams have the time and inclination to provide such services.

There are many other situations when virtual care is indicated. Monitoring pets receiving hospice care often lends itself to telehealth options. Nursing visits to the home of patients can also be augmented with such consultations, and nurses/technicians can add an additional level of expertise since they can provide hands-on evaluation. For pets that cannot be easily brought in to the clinic for any number of reasons, telehealth provides one more way for them to still benefit from veterinary advice. Finally, nearly half of all pet owners are not currently bringing their pets to the veterinary clinic with any regularity, so virtual care removes one barrier to them being able to seek veterinary advice, as long as appropriate VCPRs are in place.

When considering fee options for virtual care, it is best to approach this in a team-based manner so value can be built into the system from the start. Initially, virtual care might be offered during certain time slots in the day when there are appointment gaps. The fee can be based on what the time slot would typically command as a 10-, 15-, or 20-minute appointment. Other options might include prioritizing a virtual visit over an in-clinic appointment for a premium, if such a call could be accommodated in such an interval. For example, a client may want to hear from a doctor or nurse quickly, and be prepared to pay a premium for someone to schedule a virtual visit within a certain time frame (such as two hours, etc.). The same rationale can be used for premium pricing on consults after hours, on weekends, and in other instances where the client is being accommodated. Pricing can also reflect technology used, such as telehealth platforms, accessing wearables, etc.

Finally, not all telehealth consults need to be provided exclusively by doctors. For some virtual care, nursing staff may be appropriate experts.

For clients with pet health insurance (see 10.16 Pet Health Insurance), pet owners should check with the insurance provider to determine telemedicine coverage.

EXAMPLES

Blair Donaldson is a 3-year-old neutered male Dalmatian, who has been previously diagnosed with atopic dermatitis. He has been well controlled for the past several months with a daily Janus kinase inhibitor, but started scratching significantly in the last few hours. Since Blair had previously experienced pyotraumatic dermatitis (a hot spot) from his scratching, Mrs Donaldson immediately telephoned ABC Veterinary Hospital to bring him in without delay.

Julie, the customer service representative who answered the phone, was very concerned about Blair and recalled how tragic Blair seemed after his hot spot. Julie would book Blair for an appointment the next day, which was the first availability, but asked if Mrs Donaldson might be interested in a telehealth consult that could be scheduled for that afternoon, when Julie would try to create some time between existing appointments.

When Dr Green and Mrs Donaldson connected on that telehealth call, it was very apparent that Mr. Donaldson was concerned and was afraid of what Blair might do to himself if the scratching could not be curtailed.

Dr Green suggested that the likely culprit was ragweed pollen in the environment, which was wreaking havoc with many pets in the practice as the pollen count was at an all-time high for the season. He advised that Blair be given a cool-water soak for at least 10 minutes, gently toweled dry, and then a mild antipruritic spray be used on affected areas. During the bathing, Mrs Donaldson was to do a thorough check for fleas and other parasites, and verify with her husband that Blair's parasite control product had been administered on schedule. It was advised that Blair remain indoors with windows closed and air conditioner on and it was recommended that an over-the-counter antihistamine be considered (suitable products and doses were provided). It was unlikely that the antihistamine would have a major impact on the pruritus, but it might help a bit and also have some sedating effects which might make Blair more sleepy and less likely to do damage to himself. The plan was to repeat the cool-water soak and spray before bedtime, but if Blair was not significantly more comfortable by then to give another dose of his allergy medication just this once to keep him comfortable overnight, and they would address whatever issues remained at the appointment scheduled for the next day.

Mrs Donaldson was relieved that there was now a plan in place, and felt the telehealth consult provided her with peace of mind, and she was more than happy to pay for the service.

TAKE-AWAYS

- Most aspects of virtual care must be carried out under the auspices of a veterinary–client–patient relationship.
- Ideally, guidelines should be created for telehealth consults so that the entire hospital team is aware of what they are, how they should be scheduled, payment terms, and standardized medical record entries.
- Remote monitoring will be an increasingly important aspect of virtual care, allowing veterinary teams to track certain pet indices from a distance.
- All indications are that clients are prepared to pay for virtual care options, if veterinary teams make them aware of the possibilities.
- Charging for virtual care is more a lack of a "will to bill" rather than unwillingness of clients to pay for such services.

MISCELLANEOUS

2.5.8 Cautions

Telehealth solutions are still evolving, and regulations have not caught up with many of the applications that are possible with today's technologies.

Without a valid VCPR, any advice provided should be considered general and not specific to any patient, and should not imply any intended diagnosis or treatment recommendation.

Veterinarians considering being telehealth providers should be prepared to present their particular credentials, provide any service disclaimers, and specify what services they are able to provide, and the limitations of such telehealth consultations. If clients have pet health insurance and are hoping to be reimbursed for virtual care, they should verify that telehealth services are covered by the policy.

Practices preparing to offer telehealth solutions should seek legal advice before providing such services, or affiliating with companies providing those services. It is also worth checking with the insurance provider regarding any liability issues that could be associated with telehealth solutions.

The majority of human physicians engage in different forms of telehealth. It should be anticipated that this same trend will eventually happen with veterinary medicine as well.

Recommended Reading

Ackerman, L. (2019). Why should veterinarians consider implementing virtual care? *EC Veterinary Science* 4 (4): 259–261.

Ackerman, L. (ed.) (2020). Telehealth. In: *Five-Minute Veterinary Practice Management Consult*, 3e, 310–311. Wiley.

Ackerman, L. (2020). The new e-commerce: E-commerce is more than just selling products online. *AAHA Trends* 36 (11): 51–54.

American Animal Hospital Association, (2018) American Veterinary Medical Association. The real-life rewards of virtual care – how to turn your hospital into a digitally connected practice with telehealth. www.aaha.org/globalassets/05-pet-health-resources/virtual_care.pdf or https://www.aaha.org/practice-resources/pet-health-resources/virtual-care-and-telehealth/

American Veterinary Medical Association. Telehealth & telemedicine in veterinary practice. www.avma.org/telehealth

Duncan, S. (2018). Redefining the risks and rules for telehealth services. www.veterinarypracticenews.com/redefining-risks-rules-telehealth-services/print

Green, E. (2017). Veterinary telemedicine: are we leading? https://todaysveterinarybusiness.com/veterinary-telemedicine-leading

Katayama, M., Kubo, T., Mogi, A. et al. (2016). Heart rate variability predicts the emotional state in dogs. *Behav. Processes* 128: 108–112.

Miller, M.C. (2019). The Telehealth Trend. *AAHA Trends* 35 (4): 29–34.

Surman, S. and Fleeman, L. (2013). Continuous glucose monitoring in small animals. *Vet. Clin. North Am. Small Anim. Pract.* 43: 381–406.

2.6

Generational Considerations

Kurt A. Oster, MS, SPHR, SHRM-SCP

Bay State Veterinary Emergency and Specialty Services, Swansea, MA, USA

BASICS

2.6.1 Summary

Pet-specific care is a concept that can revolutionize our approach to providing veterinary healthcare. However, in order to obtain client buy-in, we must raise their awareness and understanding of this new approach. In veterinary medicine, we would typically refer to this as client education; all other industries would call this marketing. When marketing veterinary services, it is important to know the client signalment as well as the patient signalment.

Much research is available about marketing to different generations. From the aging Traditionalists and retiring Baby Boomers to the social-media savvy Millennials and Gen Zers, with the Gen Xers in the middle, each generation requires significantly different marketing techniques. Each generation contributes its unique value to practice, but they all need to be pampered in different ways. Once you know the best way to attract each group, the next step is to gain their loyalty. Differentiated marketing can be done in ways that are simple and affordable and yield tremendous results.

2.6.2 Terms Defined

Traditionalists, Silent, Greatest Generation: Born before 1945, the "Depression Babies" influenced by the Depression and World War II.

Baby Boomers: Born 1946–1964, the "Woodstock Generation" influenced by Vietnam War, the 1960s and postwar social change.

Generation X: Born 1965–1981, the "Latchkey Generation," products of divorced parents and major corporate scandals.

Generation Y, Echo Boomers, Millennials: Born 1982–1999, the "Entitled Generation" influenced by technology and doting parents.

Generation Z: Born after 2000, the "Facebook Crowd" influenced by a media-saturated world.

MAIN CONCEPTS

The most effective way to market veterinary services is to customize the marketing strategy to target client demographics. Until a few years ago, you would have been right in thinking that differentiated marketing is for big business with big budgets. However, that is no longer true. The internet has become the great marketing leveler, allowing you to effectively customize your approach to marketing to different generations at affordable costs.

Client demographics are a major influence in buying behavior (see 5.4 The Changing Nature of Pet Owners). Individuals born at different points in time have distinct preferences in what they value, how they spend their money, and what advertising channels they use. Recognizing these behavioral differences in your clients is essential for maximizing treatment recommendation compliance. There are five distinct American demographics and although Generation Z has just begun to flex its consumer potential, they are in your practice today as new team members and will be the pet parents of tomorrow.

- **Traditionalists**: Respect authority, loyal, patriotic, excellent work ethic, stubbornly independent, dependable, advanced communication and interpersonal skills.

Pet-Specific Care for the Veterinary Team, First Edition. Edited by Lowell Ackerman.
© 2021 John Wiley & Sons, Inc. Published 2021 by John Wiley & Sons, Inc.

- **Baby Boomers**: Well-educated, question authority, excellent teamwork skills, fiercely competitive, thrive on adrenaline-producing assignments.
- **Generation X**: Independent, family-focused, intolerant of bureaucracy, critical, hardworking, and socially responsive.
- **Generation Y**: Highly socialized, loyal, technologically savvy, socially responsible, and require work/life integration.
- **Generation Z**: Technologically dependent, closely tied to parents, tolerant of alternate lifestyles, involved in green causes and social activism.

2.6.3 The Silent Generation

This generation has 50 million consumers in the US. They displayed tremendous resolve to overcome the impact of the Great Depression and World War II. They seek value for money, comfort, and a sense of belonging. Many of them are active seniors and do not like to be regarded as old or dependent.

They did not grow up using computers and probably retired before using them in the workplace; many are still lairy of technology. Therefore, the best marketing tools are the traditional ones that are printed, on the radio, or via telephone as many of them still answer their phone when it rings. They are the least likely to make an impulsive purchase. They respond best to traditional marketing tools such as flyers, newsletters, and postcards. These materials should be in larger font for ease of reading, use proper grammar, avoid slang and contain a single image (one that conveys emotions) rather than a collage. They should contain polite greetings with sir, madam, Mr or Mrs. And provide them with a phone number to call rather than a website to visit.

2.6.4 Baby Boomers

Baby Boomers grew up during the American-dream, white-picket-fence era post World War II. Comprising 76 million consumers in the US, this second largest demographic group represents individuals who focused on hard work, individualism, and social activism. They value trust, loyalty, and sense of community. Many Baby Boomers are retired or will be retiring soon. Baby Boomers have experience using technology. Most were in the workplace when computers were installed. Steve Jobs and Bill Gates are both members of the Baby Boomer generation, so members are generally comfortable using text messaging and other basic apps on their smartphones. The group still leaves and listens to voicemails. As their younger counterparts have taught Boomers how to use technology, this generation is slowly embracing it, with the vast majority utilizing Facebook to revive "dormant" relationships.

The Boomers do not enjoy Facebook ads clogging up their social media and would prefer to talk to real people. Boomers have the highest value as consumers in the market today and are more likely to splurge on items that are important to them (such as their child replacement pet as many are now empty nesters).

This group appreciates both traditional marketing (education) and twenty-first-century marketing. Baby Boomers appreciate the opportunity for face-to-face communication and having real humans answer the phone. However, when using other forms of marketing materials, it is important to include well-written content without slang or hashtags, an appeal to their youth with references to "the good old days." Solutions should simplify and improve their lifestyle. They are fiercely loyal, so having a practice app with a loyalty feature is very important, although this generation is least likely to make a purchase on their smartphone. In addition to using your smartphone app, Boomers will research product and services online and respond to email reminders and confirmations.

2.6.5 Generation X

Generation X is often referred to as the bridge between Millennials and Baby Boomers. Gen Xers number 65 million in the US and are now juggling child care, home ownership, and reaching the peak of their careers.

They grew up without the online shopping experience, so they still enjoy a trip in-store, but have fully embraced online shopping as well. Generation X also has strong brand loyalty, particularly to those brands who give back. Members of Generation X will not accept your treatment recommendations because you ask them to, and especially not if you tell them that you are the expert and know best. Gen Xers are known for their research skills and will conduct extensive research before deciding. They often will not make decisions in the exam room and pressuring them to do so will not have a positive outcome. They do want you to tell them all of their treatment options, not just your "A" Plan. They will rely more heavily on reviews and client testimonials than your recommendation.

When preparing marketing materials, note that they do not want to read large amounts of content. Some will prefer email, and some will prefer traditional mail, and all will enjoy video content.

2.6.6 Millennials

This generation has taken over the workforce and at 80 million strong in the US, out-number Baby Boomers. Millennials began entering the workforce as the economy crashed, and as a result are the largest generation of entrepreneurs. They are notoriously soft-hearted and soft-shelled, valuing social issues far ahead of economics. This generation is the most responsive to recommendations from friends and family and are motivated by shopping ease. They prefer experiences over things, so engaging them in hands-on pet care while in the exam room is critical. They are not as loyal to brands as older generations, so it can be tricky to obtain long-term buy-in.

In order to fully engage Millennials, your practice needs to have a robust online presence with blogs, use hashtags, social media posts (Instagram and Snapchat), and lots of video, but avoid email. Apps that support pet photo contests and other activities are very desirable. Discuss the experience of pet ownership and support hands-on pet care activities, rather than just "selling."

Millennials love the next big thing, such as each new technology release. They also like to do what their friends are doing which is why they decide where to eat based on Instagram pictures. A great way to market to this generation is to make sure your online reviews and customer service experiences are up to par! As difficult as it is to obtain loyalty, once you have it, they tend to stick with you, so make sure your practice app supports your loyalty program.

2.6.7 Generation Z

The youngest generation that is beginning to develop its buying power is Generation Z, the iGeneration, or Gen Z. To get their attention, your practice needs to have a website that looks great on their phones and a significant social media presence. Be socially conscious and have clients (peers) share authentic success stories. What we know about this generation will continue to grow and evolve as they age.

EXAMPLES

At ABC Animal Hospital, there was a need for a client education handout and the two doctors there, instead of working together, each created their own handout. The Boomer doctor created a handout that touted the hospital's experience and extensive research into the subject and made one very detailed and specific recommendation to the client. The handout prepared by the Gen X doctor referenced recent research that supported a change in how this condition was treated and listed several potential treatment options. It provided links to numerous resources and supplied a list of questions you should ask your veterinarian or consider while researching the option that you felt would be best for your pet. Each doctor had created a handout that reflected their generation. Consider what it would take to make such a resource multigenerational.

TAKE-AWAYS

- While generations may engage in the world differently, they all possess a common desire to be informed pet owners. It is important for us to communicate with our clients in a manner that allows them to easily absorb the information we are providing them.
- We must be accessible to our clients. When they reach out, we need to be able to respond back to them in a timely and effective manner. Many practices now have a "electronic" or "media" receptionist who is dedicated to monitoring all types of client communication whether it be via Facebook or email.
- Be authentic by thinking about what you'd want to know about if you were in their shoes. Be as open as you can, as in these times people crave transparency.
- Engage your audience and show them that you care about their opinion and feedback. Listen to their thoughts on making the pet ownership experience better and respond to them when they talk to you.
- Make sure that you have a plan in place to get important information in front of members of each generation. One topic may have a handout, a web page, and a blog post and remember to update them frequently. Not everyone responds to the same marketing approach so you must be age appropriate.

MISCELLANEOUS

Recommended Reading

Fromm, J. and Garton, C. (2013). *Marketing to Millennials*. New York: American Management Association.

Marston, C. (2010). *Generational Insights*. Mobile, AL: Generational Insights.

Marston, C. (2011). *Generational Selling Tactics that Work*. Hoboken, NJ: Wiley.

2.7

Risk Assessment

Nan Boss, DVM

Best Friends Veterinary Center, Grafton, WI, USA

BASICS

2.7.1 Summary

None of us has unlimited time and money to discuss or investigate every possible disease for every patient. When making a personalized care plan for any dog or cat, you will need to prioritize. When educating a client or screening for diseases, spend more time and effort on those problems that are most likely to be found and/or that have the highest risk for harm. When diagnosing and treating diseases, the same holds true – rule in or out what is common first. Assessing risk accurately and using that assessment to inform medical care for your patients is a skill that can be developed and improved.

2.7.2 Terms Defined

Risk: An exposure to danger, harm or loss.
Risk Assessment: A process for evaluating potential risk.

MAIN CONCEPTS

Wellness care is all about reducing risk. We vaccinate to reduce the risk for contagious diseases, we prescribe heartworm preventives to reduce the risk for parasites, and so on.

Some health risks are nearly universal, such as exposure to contagious diseases and parasites. Others are specific to a pet's species, sex, age, location (city versus rural as well as region of the country), lifestyle or breed. All of these factors must be taken into account when developing a healthcare plan for a particular patient, whether in sickness or in health.

In ill patients, our risk analysis helps to guide us toward the most likely diagnoses so that we can diagnose and treat the pet appropriately. For example, if a Boston terrier is presented for vomiting, you might consider the usual rule-outs such as foreign body, infectious or metabolic causes, or garbage ingestion. In this scenario, you would also want to consider pyloric stenosis, a reported genetic problem in the Boston terrier breed.

Risk assessment also guides our client education efforts. You wouldn't spend much time educating clients about a disease you only see a few times a year, or one a particular patient is unlikely to ever encounter. You'd spend those valuable few minutes you have with clients at wellness visits to talk about common things. You would want to incorporate the most common topics into a broad educational plan.

A simple way to do this is to choose one or two topics to focus on per visit, so you can educate every client about them. Examples would be dental care or obesity. Once that broader, more general topic has been covered, you can choose a risk or two to go over that is specific for the individual client or pet. What is likely to harm the patient and how might we prevent or treat the problem?

2.7.3 Determining Risk

There are many factors that can be used to determine and prioritize risk, so that you can offer specific laboratory tests or discuss the most important topics with your client.

Pet-Specific Care for the Veterinary Team, First Edition. Edited by Lowell Ackerman.
© 2021 John Wiley & Sons, Inc. Published 2021 by John Wiley & Sons, Inc.

EXAMPLES

2.7.4 How Common Is It?

In other words, what is the likely prevalence of each risk?

1) Most common
2) Somewhat common
3) Not very common

Sometimes this is easy to determine, but what is statistically likely in one patient may be uncommon in another. Common causes of death or injury in an indoor and an outdoor cat, for example, are completely different. You need to have a signalment, history and background information on a patient, as well as exam findings, to judge risk accurately. The answers to these questions will often determine how likely certain diseases are, what level of understanding the pet's guardian has about care for the pet, and in what direction you need to steer your healthcare plan.

- When did the owner acquire the pet and from whom?
- Where does the pet go and what does it do?
- What does it eat and how much?
- What type of care does the pet get at home? Does the owner brush its teeth? Clean its ears? Administer preventive medications regularly and on time?

Some diseases are high risk for a great many dogs and cats. Universal or high-risk conditions for most pets would include:

- dental disease – 80% of pets over age 3 years
- obesity – over 50% and climbing every year
- risk due to age – a small percentage of young apparently healthy patients will have a disease diagnosed on screening bloodwork whereas a significantly larger percentage of those of senior age will do so. Risks for cancer, heart disease, endocrine disorders, and metabolic problems increase with time. Furthermore, almost all pets will eventually develop arthritis if they live long enough.

With species and breed come other lists of disorders that need to be ranked as common or uncommon, including genetically related diseases. For example, the risk for cardiac issues in a Cavalier King Charles spaniel is virtually 100% if they live long enough, and gastric dilation-volvulus (GDV) risk is significantly higher in Great Danes than shih tzus.

Moderate-risk conditions would include orthopedic disorders such as cranial cruciate ligament disease, hip dysplasia or medial patellar luxation, and many ear, eye or skin problems, among others. The actual amount of risk will vary greatly from patient to patient, depending on age,

breed, lifestyle, and many other factors. Diabetes mellitus, for example, is a high-risk disease in an obese cat eating a high-carbohydrate diet but a lower risk in a normal-weight cat eating a low-carb diet.

Low-risk conditions include many rare genetic disorders or cancers that we barely even consider when diagnosing or screening for diseases. Yet, for an individual patient the rare condition may turn out to be pertinent and worth considering or talking about. Uncommon in a Labrador retriever may be common in a toy poodle or vice versa. A disease uncommon in your part of the country may be much more likely if your patient was recently living or traveling somewhere else. There is no list of common or uncommon conditions that applies to everyone (see Recommended Reading for tools that can be useful in determining how common risks are for particular patients).

When teaching clients about pet healthcare or offering screening tests, another set of criteria comes into play.

2.7.5 How Serious Is the Problem?

The second way to prioritize risk is by seriousness of problem – a higher risk for death or illness.

1) Diseases and problems that could be fatal.
2) Diseases or problems which could cause pain, suffering or chronic damage.
3) Diseases or problems that could cause inconvenience or mild illness.

Gastric dilation-volvulus is not common except in certain breeds but it can be quickly deadly in affected individuals. Glaucoma is not a common condition in many breeds, but it is extremely painful. Any risk at all for a painful or deadly disease may justify a discussion with a client about signs to watch for and when to call a veterinarian.

Genetic forms of alopecia, on the other hand, cause no pain or suffering for the pet (though they may be extremely distressing to a pet owner) so they may not be on a top 10 list of most important client education topics.

2.7.6 How Diagnosable Is the Problem?

Is there an inexpensive, readily available test to diagnose or screen for the disease? Keratoconjunctivitis sicca (KCS) is not extremely common but it is very inexpensive and easy to screen for, so making a Schirmer tear test (STT) part of a regular screening program would be a sensible thing to do. Offering an echocardiogram to screen for cardiomyopathy for every senior cat, on the other hand, would probably not be sensible, due to high price and low availability, even though hypertrophic cardiomyopathy (HCM) is a relatively common disease in cats. Here is a link to a client education video on screening eye tests for dogs: www.youtube.com/watch?v=d_RGk2UEdgs.

2.7.7 How Preventable Is the Problem?

If prevention is easy, or the disease or problem is serious or deadly, why not prevent it? The odds of any one particular suburban dog contracting canine parvovirus or a cat in Alaska coming down with heartworm disease are low but vaccination and parasite prevention are still widely recommended. Stomach tacking (gastropexy) may be a very reasonable thing to recommend at the time of spaying for a large-breed dog, even though the odds of most dogs suffering a GDV are low, because the disease is both deadly and preventable. Even if a client declines the stomach tack surgery, we can still teach them what the clinical signs are and why pet health insurance (see 10.16 Pet Health Insurance) might be a good idea. Here is a link to a client education video on GDV: www.youtube.com/watch?v=CrX2BJ7EI-o.

2.7.8 How Treatable Is the Problem?

Many of the diseases we screen for are easy to treat once we have diagnosed them. Hypothyroidism in dogs and hyperthyroidism in cats would be easy examples. Meningiomas in elderly cats, on the other hand, are very common but not only does diagnosis require a magnetic resonance imaging (MRI), most meningiomas do not cause any clinical signs and would not need treatment. Even if a less expensive test were available, such as a meningioma chemical marker in serum, it might never become part of our standard senior screening, since it is unlikely it would change how we care for the cat.

2.7.9 Refining Risk Assessment

Although it is possible to create complex algorithms factoring in all these criteria, our own brains do much of this automatically. We know that we should be talking to every puppy and kitten owner about vaccinations, parasite control, nutrition, behavior, reproductive control, and zoonoses. We do not think much about nor mention rare recessive genetic conditions because we know we are unlikely to encounter them.

Clients, on the other hand, are by-and-large unable to accurately factor risks for their pets. They do not have enough information about the likelihood of each risk, plus many of the risks we would know about, such as blastomycosis or ehrlichiosis, are completely unfamiliar to a client. This is one of the reasons why clients researching their pets' clinical signs on the internet are so frustrating for us. They come up with diagnoses that are extremely unlikely and then may worry unnecessarily, try the wrong home remedy or get upset when we don't think it necessary to test for that disease.

Risk assessment is also difficult for recent veterinary school graduates. It is easy to get *lost in the weeds* of a long list of rule-outs. Even for wellness visits, a new graduate may struggle to prioritize. If one has not encountered a puppy of a specific breed before, one may be unsure of what breed-related disorders should be discussed with the owner or breeder (see 3.13 Breed Predisposition). In many cases, a study may never have been done that would show the prevalence of a specific disorder in a particular breed. Experience is a great teacher, whether the person is a pet owner or a new graduate veterinarian. It is always more difficult to do risk factor analysis for things with which we are less familiar.

Risk assessment is affected by our own biases. For example, we are more likely to diagnose a disease, correctly or incorrectly, that we have recently read about or seen. We are less likely to diagnose or talk with a client about a disease we have never seen, even if we know the clinical signs and likely presentation. The brain is more likely to follow a familiar path. After a personal experience with a certain disease, whether in a patient, a family member or our own pet, we develop blinders to possibilities other than the scenario we already know. For example, if a family member had a bad experience with cancer, a client is less likely to let us treat their pet for cancer. The picture they have of cancer treatment affects how they regard the risks or rewards of treatment.

Also, things that frighten us more become higher risks in our minds, as when we are more worried about air travel than traveling by car, though the risk of a car accident is far higher than that of a plane crash.

All these factors create incentives to utilize logic and systems to help with risk assessment.

2.7.10 Risk Assessment for Well Patients

When deciding what to go over with a client at a wellness visit, it may be useful to divide risks into categories. Look for risks in each and then refine your list into no more than three things to teach about. Risks are often defined by what the pet owner is not doing, such as not giving a monthly heartworm preventive on schedule or not feeding a nutritious brand of cat food. Try these common topics:

- age related
- breed specific
- contagious diseases
- oral care
- parasites
- weight/nutrition.

If a client is already giving recommended heartworm and intestinal parasite preventives as directed, educating about parasites would not be as important as teaching about something the client is not doing, for example leptospirosis vaccination. If the pet is a normal weight but has moderate tartar build-up, we obviously would be talking about dental care and not obesity management. By looking at each category individually, it is fairly simple to come up with two or three topics to discuss.

Even when we have a scenario where there is too much to discuss – say we are seeing an overweight, older golden retriever with arthritis, bad teeth, and an ear infection – we can usually manage to prioritize. Which topics could wait until the recheck visit? We could choose to talk about otitis and arthritis now and postpone the obesity, senior screening, and dental disease topics until we recheck the ear and the arthritis in two weeks. That would also give us time to get an estimate ready for the dental work needed.

A point scoring system may work better for recommending wellness screening laboratory testing. You would give one, two or three points in each of the categories. We would want to rank the most common and most treatable higher with a higher point score. So, if the disease we are screening for is uncommon, we would give the test for that disease one point. If it is a common disease, we would give three points. So, for each of these three categories, award one, two, or three points.

- More common
- More important
- More cost-effective

Let's look at the following possible tests: complete blood count (CBC), chemistry panel, thyroid profile, urinalysis, urine protein:creatinine (UPC) level.

If we are recommending laboratory testing for a senior pet and the client is willing to spend a certain amount of money, we might choose a chemistry panel, CBC, and thyroxine (T4) for an overweight Labrador retriever. The T4 would get a score of 3 for each of the three categories.

For a normal-weight soft-coated wheaten terrier, the calculation is different. We would recommend the chemistry panel and CBC but instead of the T4 we might choose the UPC ratio. In the retriever, hypothyroidism is more common and for the wheaten, glomerulonephropathy (GN) is a big concern. Here is a link to a client education video on GN in soft-coated wheaten terriers: www.youtube.com/watch?v=eTwyUbiFPbU.

If the Labrador is young, however, the T4 becomes less important – it is neither as important nor as cost-effective if there are unlikely to be clinical signs of hypothyroidism. If it's an older Scottish terrier we are seeing instead of a wheaten, our top concern might be transitional cell carcinoma, so the urinalysis is more important than the UPC.

Whether to offer clients standardized wellness care plans that are the same for everyone, or individual, customized ones is a philosophical decision that every practice must make (see 10.17 Payment and Wellness Plans). Both for wellness packages and diagnostic protocols for disease states, it is a choice whether to individualize or generalize.

Individual plans take more time and effort, but are less likely to include unnecessary tests.

Generalized plans are less expensive to administer and help to prevent missed diagnoses because of underestimated risk. It may make more sense to generalize in a large corporate practice with many recent graduate veterinarians, or in an emergency case where you do not have time to waste waiting for one test result before deciding on the next. A boutique practice in a high-end market with an experienced team may be more likely to customize.

 EXAMPLES

A health risk assessment form (see 1.2 Providing a Lifetime of Care) can assist the veterinary healthcare team in using client-provided information to guide recommendations. The comments and recommendations need to be tailored to an appropriate locale and demographic. For example, a schnauzer and a Doberman pinscher both have risk for heart disease but not the same kinds. For the schnauzer, auscultation is warranted to listen for a mitral valve murmur and perform an ECG to look for atrioventricular (AV) block. In the Doberman, the focus is on looking for ventricular premature contractions (VPCs) caused by cardiomyopathy.

In a digital report card sort of format, it is easier to choose and print those risks that applied, and the client would not see those recommendations that weren't applicable to them.

TAKE-AWAYS

- Some diseases are high risk for a great many dogs and cats. We should ensure that every client is aware of these common risks and has the opportunity to prevent or screen for these diseases when possible.
- The second way to prioritize risk is by seriousness of problem – a higher risk for death, pain or illness. We should ensure that every client is aware of these less common but serious risks and has the opportunity to prevent or screen for these diseases when possible.
- A point scoring system may be useful for recommending wellness screening laboratory testing.
- Wellness plans can be designed to be the same for every patient or individualized for each patient.
- In ill patients, our risk analysis helps to guide us toward the most likely diagnoses so that we can diagnose and treat the pet appropriately.

MISCELLANEOUS

Abbreviation

ECG Electrocardiogram

Recommended Reading

Fleming, J.M., Creevy, K.E., and Promislow, D.E.L. (2011). Mortality in north American dogs from 1984 to 2004: an investigation into age-, size and breed-related causes of death. *J. Vet. Intern. Med.* 25: 187–198.

Gough, A. (2018). *Breed Predispositions to Disease in Dogs and Cats*, 3e. Ames, IA: Wiley Blackwell.

2.8

Risk Management

Tara Harmon, APR

The Cincinnati Insurance Companies, Fairfield, OH, USA

BASICS

2.8.1 Summary

With pet ownership comes risk that the pet may require substantial healthcare services and at considerable expense. Each pet owner manages this risk differently. Pet health insurance is one of the most common ways in which pet owners mitigate pet health risk.

2.8.2 Terms Defined

Deductible: The amount of financial loss an individual agrees to pay before insurance coverage applies.
Fixed Cost: A consistent and predetermined cost.
Insurance Policy: A legal contract between an individual and an insurance company. The insurance company agrees to pay for claims in exchange for payment of premium.
Premium: Amount paid to an insurance company in exchange for insurance coverage.
Risk-Averse: Less likely to take risks.
Variable Cost: A fluctuating cost.

MAIN CONCEPTS

2.8.3 How Risk Management is Defined

Risk is the possibility of a negative consequence such as damage, injury, or loss. Risk management describes how risk is managed. Every pet owner faces financial risk due to unforeseen pet healthcare expenses. A pet that becomes ill may require repeat veterinary visits, expensive medications, and even surgery.

2.8.4 Risk Management Methods

The ways in which individuals manage risk typically fall into one of four categories: avoidance, mitigation, transfer, and acceptance.

Risk avoidance is the elimination of an exposure that has the potential to result in a negative outcome. An animal lover may decide not to acquire a pet to avert the financial strain of an unforeseen veterinary bill. Whether the decision not to own a pet is driven by the lack of financial means or simply to avoid unforeseen pet healthcare bills, this is considered avoidance.

Risk mitigation is an activity that may lessen the chance of a negative outcome associated with a particular risk. A pet owner may decide to feed their pet a more nutritious food, ensure regular exercise, and attend regular veterinary check-ups. While these actions typically lower the chances of a pet becoming ill, they do not guarantee that a pet will remain healthy. Risk mitigation is the most common risk management tool that pet owners utilize on a regular basis.

Risk transfer is when one party transfers risk to another party. The most common example of this is insurance. An individual pays a premium to transfer their risk to an insurance company. Pet owners can transfer the unforeseen risk of a sick pet generating a large veterinary bill by purchasing an insurance policy for their pet (see 10.16 Pet Health Insurance). There are differing levels of risk transfer demonstrated through policy level and deductible selected. Different levels of pet health insurance can be purchased, which represents the total amount of financial coverage for pet medical bills for one year. A deductible is also chosen, which is the amount of financial risk retained by the individual purchasing the policy. An individual who purchases a larger policy limit or a lower deductible is more risk-averse while someone purchasing a lower policy limit or higher deductible is more risk-tolerant.

Risk acceptance is the lack of action to manage a potentially negative outcome. Being unmindful of a pet's diet or regularly skipping annual healthcare visits may indicate the acceptance of pet healthcare risk. The owner may believe the chance of illness is low, so they are willing to chance high veterinary bills and out-of-pocket expenses. Or they may have already decided to euthanize a pet that becomes ill instead of spending money on care and medication. Risk acceptance is presumably the goal of those who own pets but decide not to take them to the veterinary hospital for care. Even in advanced economies, a significant proportion of pet owners may elect to forego veterinary care for their pets – their way of avoiding the expenditures associated with such care. Some of this may be attributable to the lack of resources of certain individuals, but in other situations a conscious decision is being made not to prioritize spending on pet care.

2.8.5 Why Some People are More Risk-Averse than Others

Studies show that the vast majority of people are averse to risk. When given a choice between avoiding negative risk or choosing positive risk, most individuals choose to avoid negative risk. This is explained through the Prospect Theory which was developed by behavioral economists Amos Tversky and Daniel Kahneman. This theory explains that most people perceive the pain of loss as more severe than the benefit of an equally uncertain gain.

This theory supports why most individuals decide to purchase insurance. For example, pet health insurance has been a more commonly purchased insurance product in Scandinavia, Germany, the United Kingdom, and Australia. The United States trails significantly, but is expected to increase due to heightened pet healthcare costs and increased awareness [1].

2.8.6 The True Risk for Pet Owners

Most pet owners do not understand or plan for the true financial risk that comes along with being a pet owner. The average pet owner may budget for fixed costs such as food,

grooming, and training but not for variable costs such as medical bills or prescriptions. In fact, the average pet owner plans on spending a few thousand dollars over the lifespan of a dog or cat while in reality they may spend over $20 000 [1].

Some pets are more expensive to own than others. Age, breed, and lifestyle affect the expense of an animal over its lifetime. Adopting an older pet tends to be most costly per year due to increased chances of physical and mental deterioration that come with age. Some breeds are more likely to inherit certain diseases or become affected by certain healthcare problems. Also, a sedentary animal is proven to have more medical issues tied to obesity than those that are exercised regularly.

The best way to be fully prepared for the true financial risk of pet ownership is to transfer the risk to an insurance company by purchasing pet health insurance (see 10.16 Pet Health Insurance). The cost of pet health insurance is minimal in comparison to the potential cost of unexpected medical bills.

EXAMPLES

Mr and Mrs Schmidt adopt a 3-week-old beagle, Daisy, from the local shelter. Because they are retired and on a fixed income, they decide to purchase a pet health insurance policy for the new addition to their family. Three years later while the Schmidts are running errands, Daisy eats a chicken bone out of the kitchen trash. The surgery to remove the bone costs thousands of dollars, but because they purchased pet health insurance, they only have to pay the deductible and co-pay. Mr and Mrs Schmidt are risk-averse and transferred the risk of a high pet healthcare expense to the insurance company Daisy is insured through.

The Harvey family purchase a golden retriever from a neighbor who just put a litter up for sale. They decide to neuter the puppy to prevent potential health and behavioral issues that some unneutered pets face. While neutering the new puppy does not guarantee that it will avoid all health issues, it lowers the chances of loss for at least some of them. This is an example of risk mitigation.

TAKE-AWAYS

- With pet ownership comes risk of a pet that could generate considerable healthcare bills.

- Pet owners manage this financial risk in different ways.
- The ways in which individuals manage risk typically fall into one of four categories: avoidance, mitigation, transfer, and acceptance.
- Studies show that the vast majority of people are averse to risk.
- Most people transfer risk through purchase of an insurance policy.

MISCELLANEOUS

2.8.7 Cautions

Each individual has their own risk tolerance which may not align exactly with one of the four categories outlined above.

Reference

1 Money's best friend: Growth in the number of insured pets will boost industry demand. IIBISWorld Industry Report OD4612 Pet Insurance in the US. May 2018. https:// trupanion.com/-/media/trupanion/files/linked--pdfs/2018- -pet--insurance--industry--report.pdf?la=en-ca&hash=48C C05DADE2E02029BAAC5C99A1869099760BCC7

Recommended Reading

Harley, A. Prospect Theory and Loss Aversion: How Users Make Decisions. www.nngroup.com/articles/ prospect-theory

Peters, J. How Our Brain Decides to Get Insurance. Should we invest now in something that may or may not happen later? www.lemonade.com/blog/brain-decides-insurance

2.9

Anticipated Costs of Pet Care

Sarah Rumple

Rumpus Writing and Editing LLC, Denver, CO, USA

BASICS

2.9.1 Summary

Discussing cost of care with clients is not a lesson taught in most veterinary schools, and many veterinarians prefer to avoid the subject, leaving their support staff to deal with upset clients. Owning a pet and providing appropriate veterinary care for that pet's lifetime costs more than most pet owners realize, and veterinarians need to be prepared to discuss costs at the time they make their recommendations.

Transparent and upfront cost discussions with clients based on appropriate healthcare recommendations will lead to improved relationships, happier and more trusting clients, happier team members, and better outcomes for pets.

MAIN CONCEPTS

2.9.2 Veterinarians and Cost Discussions

It's a topic few veterinarians want to discuss, and one even fewer veterinarians were taught how to discuss during veterinary school. The money conversation is so uncomfortable and awkward, veterinarians often make their recommendations without mentioning cost until a client inquires, which can instill feelings of distrust in the pet owner (see 5.11 Discussing Finances for Pet-Specific Care).

The fear of appearing to be "in it for the money" is not new for veterinarians. Conduct an online search about veterinarians and money, and you'll find countless articles and news pieces about veterinarians recommending seemingly unnecessary diagnostics and treatments in the hope of making more money. As a result, the profession is afraid of talking about money, pet owners lose faith in veterinary healthcare providers, and pets don't get the care they need and deserve.

When veterinarians avoid discussing cost of care with clients, they aren't making the uncomfortable discussion disappear. Instead, they are punting the conversation to other members of the team, who will likely be forced to have the conversation after a sticker-shocked client confronts them. This puts client care representatives and other team members on the defensive and makes pet owners feel as if the veterinary team was not upfront about the cost of care before services were rendered. When veterinarians neglect to be upfront and transparent about the cost of care, support staff and pet owners are left with a bad taste in their mouths, and that can lead to poor reviews for veterinary hospitals and negative press about the profession.

Two studies published in the *Journal of the American Veterinary Medical Association* found that pet owners expected veterinarians to initiate discussions of costs upfront, but that those discussions were uncommon [1, 2]. And, when cost was discussed, veterinarians focused on tangibles, such as time and services provided, while pet owners focused on outcome as it related to their pet's health and well-being [1, 2]. In the earlier study, veterinarians reported feeling undervalued for their efforts, while some pet owners were suspicious about the motivation behind veterinarians' recommendations [1].

This disconnect between veterinarians and pet owners clearly poses barriers for the profession. But, if veterinarians can improve communication, educate clients, and have the cost discussion every time they make a recommendation, some of these challenges can be alleviated.

2.9.3 The Do's and Don'ts of Discussing Cost of Care with Clients

DO make recommendations based on what you believe is best for the pet.

DON'T make recommendations based on what you assume the pet owner can afford.

Never assume you know what a client can or cannot afford, and don't make your recommendations based on those assumptions. Always make your recommendations based on best practices and what you believe would provide the most necessary medical information for you to make an accurate diagnosis and end in the best result for the pet.

DO initiate the cost discussion immediately while explaining your recommendations.

DON'T wait to discuss cost until the client inquires. Be transparent and upfront about costs while making your recommendations. The two should not be different conversations, but should instead be intertwined as one.

DO explain costs as they relate to the betterment of the pet and the outcome your recommendations will lead to.

DON'T attempt to justify costs based on time or services provided. Clients don't care how much a particular piece of diagnostic equipment costs, how many staff members are involved in a pet's care, or how much time you'll need to spend to diagnose a pet. They care about the health of their pets and how your recommendations will help them.

DO discuss alternative payment options and ways to plan for future veterinary costs.

DON'T devalue your expertise by changing your recommendations when the pet owner indicates cost is a barrier.

Once you've made your recommendations and discussed cost, be prepared to offer alternative payment options for clients concerned about the price. Avoid altering your recommendations to decrease the cost of care. This devalues your expertise and can make the pet owner question the motives behind your initial recommendations. To help cover the immediate need, consider recommending third-party financing (see 10.18 Financing Veterinary Care) or a payment plan (see 10.17 – Payment and Wellness Plans). Services like these allow you to offer payment plans to your clients without having to manage them in-house. To prevent cost from becoming a barrier in the first place, educate all your clients on the benefits of pet health insurance (see 10.16 Pet Health Insurance).

2.9.4 Preparing Clients for the Cost of Care Over a Pet's Lifetime

Educate your clients on the average costs of care long before you're facing an uncomfortable exam room situation. Tables 2.9.1 and 2.9.2 show the approximate costs of preventive care in the US for dogs living 12 years and cats living 15 years. (Unless otherwise noted, average costs of services are according to the tenth edition of *The Veterinary Fee Reference* [3].) These tables reflect only the cost of preventive care and do not include any costs associated with disease diagnosis or management. For additional information on likely costs of pet-specific care programs, see 10.11 The Financial Benefits of Pet-Specific Medicine.

Providing appropriate preventive and end-of-life care for a pet is only the tip of the iceberg when it comes to the total cost of pet ownership. When sick care, food, supplies, boarding, grooming, and additional products and services are considered, lifetime pet ownership costs can skyrocket to more than $42 000, according to a report from UK-based People's Dispensary for Sick Animals [4].

Don't put yourself and your team into a defensive position when it comes to explaining cost of care to your clients. Instead, be transparent and discuss costs when you make your recommendations. Your clients will be more trusting and compliant with your recommendations, your team will be happier, your patients will receive the best care, and your practice will reap the benefits.

 EXAMPLES

Jack, a 13-year-old neutered male miniature schnauzer, visited ABC Animal Hospital for his semiannual senior preventive care exam two days ago. At that time, his senior laboratory work was drawn. For the past 10 years, Jack's urine has included some calcium oxalate crystals, but this latest test revealed 4+ crystals and Jack's abdomen had been somewhat tense on palpation. Concerned, the veterinarian calls Jack's owner with the results and recommends an ultrasound, informing her about the cost of the diagnostic test.

Jack's owner expresses concern over the price and asks if ultrasound is necessary. The veterinarian informs her that because Jack is showing other early signs of potential problems, and because urinary tract "stones" are common in the breed, she believes it is important to conduct the ultrasound to make a diagnosis so appropriate treatments can begin, if needed. Since Jack was not covered by pet health insurance, the doctor offered Jack's owner two options to

Table 2.9.1 Approximate cost of preventive and end-of-life care for dogs living 12 years

Service	Average cost	Times during average lifespan	Total
Preventive care exam (adult) (0–6 years)	$45.20	7	$316.40
Preventive care exam (senior) (biannually 7–12 years)	$47.23	12	$566.76
Annual heartworm panel (in-house)	$48.83	12	$585.96
Annual fecal exam (direct smear)	$22.07	12	$264.84
Year-round parasite control[a]	$84.89	12	$1103.57
Core vaccines			
Rabies vaccination (3-year)	$23.13	5	$115.65
DA2PP vaccination	$24.81	5	$124.05
Noncore vaccines (based on lifestyle risk assessment)			
Lyme disease	$32.77	13	$426.01
Leptospirosis	$22.65	13	$294.45
Bordetella	$21.54	13	$280.02
Additional services			
Microchipping[b]	$45.00	1	$45.00
Spay/neuter	$244.74	1	$244.74
Dental cleaning[c]	$516.13	4	$2064.52
End-of-life care			
Euthanasia (30-pound canine with owner present)	$99.79	1	$99.79
Cremation (communal, 30-pound canine)	$64.02	1	$64.02
TOTAL APPROXIMATE PREVENTIVE CARE COSTS FOR DOGS			**$6006.88**

[a] According to PetCareRx.
[b] According to Petfinder.
[c] Includes preanesthetic exam, CBC with differential, chemistry panel with eight chemistries, dental radiographs, preoperative pain medication, anesthesia, IV catheter and placement, IV fluids, dental scaling and polishing, subgingival curettage, fluoride application, electronic monitoring, postprocedure pain medication, postprocedure injectable antibiotics, hospitalization, and one-week supply of antibiotics.

help with upfront costs: a payment plan or third-party financing.

Jack's owner trusts that her veterinarian is recommending the best diagnostic option, so she applies for third-party financing, enabling her to make future monthly payments on Jack's veterinary care.

TAKE-AWAYS

- Veterinarians need to be prepared to discuss cost of care with pet owners at the time recommendations are made.

- When veterinarians are not transparent and upfront about the cost of care, pet owners lose trust in them, and support staff are left to handle the brunt of client frustrations.
- Veterinarians should make recommendations based on what is best for pets, not what they think pet owners can afford.
- If cost of care is a barrier, a veterinarian should offer payment assistance options rather than modifying the recommendations.
- When veterinarians neglect to discuss price and alter their recommendations based on price objections, clients are more likely to question their motives, which can result in negative perception of the veterinary profession.

Table 2.9.2 Approximate cost of preventive and end-of-life care for cats living 15 years

Service	Average cost	Times during average lifespan	Total
Preventive care exam (adult) (annually 0–6 years)	$46.37	7	$324.59
Preventive care exam (senior) (biannually 7–15 years)	$46.15	18	$830.70
Annual heartworm panel (in-house)	$51.24	15	$768.60
Annual fecal exam (direct smear)	$22.07	15	$331.05
Year-round parasite control[a]	$84.89	15	$1273.35
Core vaccines			
Rabies vaccination (3-year)	$23.13	6	$138.78
FVRCP vaccination	$23.35	15	$350.25
FeLV vaccination	$27.03	17	$459.51
Noncore vaccines (based on lifestyle risk assessment)			
Feline immunodeficiency vaccination[a]	$15.00	18	$270.00
Feline chlamydia vaccination	$22.67	17	$385.39
Bordetella	$21.54	16	$344.64
Additional services			
Microchipping[b]	$45.00	1	$45.00
Spay/neuter	$160.77	1	$160.77
Dental cleaning[c]	$516.13	5	$2580.65
End-of-life care			
Euthanasia (with owner present)	$95.03	1	$95.03
Cremation (communal)	$58.23	1	$58.23
TOTAL APPROXIMATE PREVENTIVE CARE COSTS FOR CATS			**$8416.54**

[a] According to PetCareRx.
[b] According to Petfinder.
[c] Includes preanesthetic exam, CBC with differential, chemistry panel with eight chemistries, dental radiographs, preoperative pain medication, anesthesia, IV catheter and placement, IV fluids, dental scaling and polishing, subgingival curettage, fluoride application, electronic monitoring, postprocedure pain medication, postprocedure injectable antibiotics, hospitalization, and one-week supply of antibiotics.
FeLV, feline leukemia virus; FVRCP, feline viral rhinotracheitis, calicivirus, panleukopenia.

MISCELLANEOUS

References

1 Coe, J.B., Adams, C.L., and Bonnett, B.N. (2007). A focus group study of veterinarians' and pet owners' perceptions of the monetary aspects of veterinary care. *Journal of the American Veterinary Medical Association* 231 (10): 1510–1518.

2 Coe, J.B., Adams, C.L., and Bonnett, B.N. (2009). Prevalence and nature of cost discussions during clinical appointments in companion animal practice. *Journal of the American Veterinary Medical Association* 234 (11): 1418–1424.

3 American Animal Hospital Association (2018). *The Veterinary Fee Reference*, 10e. Lakewood, CO: AAHA Press.

4 Guzman, Z. Owning a pet can cost you $42,000, or 7 times as much as you expect. www.cnbc.com/2017/04/27/how-much-does-it-cost-to-own-a-dog-7-times-more-than-you-expect.html

2.10

Affordability of Veterinary Services

Patricia Khuly, VMD, MBA

Sunset Animal Clinic, Miami, FL, USA

BASICS

As more and more people embrace the perception of pets as family members, the veterinary profession has worked hard to meet the needs of a more demanding audience of veterinary caregivers. To wit, the veterinary industry's principal reaction to our pets' elevated status has been to make its service offerings more sophisticated and raise the overall standard of care.

This cultural shift and the resulting veterinary advancements, while welcome, have had some unintended consequences. Most notably, these otherwise agreeable trends have unearthed an acute tension between veterinary professionals and the pet owners whose desire to treat their pets like family may outstrip their ability to pay for the veterinary care available to them.

MAIN CONCEPTS

The escalating discrepancy between emotionally invested owners and the higher cost of advanced veterinary medicine has been widely characterized by industry analysts as an affordability crisis. The primary concern is that as the gap between veterinary cost and ability to pay widens, a lower percentage of pets will receive the treatments the industry has prepared for them.

Despite a rise in pet ownership, the overall number of veterinary visits has dropped, driving speculation that veterinary care may be increasingly unattainable for pet owners at the lower end of the economic spectrum [1].

At risk is not just the veterinarian–client–patient relationship the profession has meticulously nurtured over the past several decades, but the wider industry itself. Should mounting affordability concerns lead future generations of pet owners to adopt a more adversarial attitude toward veterinary medicine – or, worse, a dismissive one – the industry stands to lose more than just the reputation of its veterinarians. Nothing less than the profession's future economic viability is at stake.

Further, it is clear that affordability represents an existential threat to the veterinary profession's moral fabric. When the veterinarian's oath pledges to "promote animal health and welfare, relieve animal suffering, [and] protect the health of the public," it cannot equitably and ethically do so if it incommensurately serves the needs of the most affluent, educated or dedicated pet owners.

To examine the issues involved in more detail, it serves to categorize the relevant concerns as flowing from the demand side versus the supply side. Primary affordability factors affecting the demand for veterinary services include the following.

- Pet keeping is expensive and overall pet costs are on the rise, which can make healthcare (especially of "healthy" animals) a lower priority. Indeed, the average pet owner spends more than ever before on their pets' nutrition, effectively lowering the percentage of income available for veterinary expenses.
- Higher income pet owners expect higher quality healthcare. For this segment of the population, the notion of pets as family means they are willing to dedicate extraordinary sums to their pets' healthcare. This fuels much of the progress in veterinary medicine.
- *Income inequality*: as the gap between rich and poor widens, more and more veterinary patients are priced out of veterinary services altogether. This despite the fact that

pet keeping appears to have increased roughly proportionately across all income levels.

- Pet owners enjoy a greater emotional attachment to their pets than in previous generations, effectively increasing a pet's overall value to the household. Given that pet care costs are similar for all pets, lower income owners spend a disproportionately larger percentage of their earnings on them.
- *Wellness aversion*: for a variety of reasons, lower income pet owners tend to eschew wellness services preferentially. This only exacerbates affordability concerns given that emergent services are innately more expensive, typically unplanned, often delivered by secondary care centers, and more likely to be required when routine care is forgone.

Supply-side considerations factoring into the affordability of veterinary care include the following.

- *Higher standards of care*: the veterinary profession has responded preferentially to the higher expectations of more affluent pet owners by raising the standard of care (see 9.4 Standards of Care).
- *Uniformity of service offerings*: higher standards of care have been adopted with impressive uniformity across the profession. As a profession, veterinarians have traditionally prioritized patient needs over client needs. Veterinarians who do not keep pace risk discipline.
- *Professional liability issues*: public attitudes toward pets and concerns over legal decisions awarding damages for emotional loss have spooked the profession. This has led to more expensive defensive medicine, justification of pricing decisions, and/or refusal to treat patients at a lower standard of care.
- *Practice management philosophy*: veterinarians receive business counsel from a relatively small group of industry advisors. Their traditional emphasis on profitability has steered veterinarians toward a more affluent client base, often by recommending financial policies which may unintentionally discourage lower income clients.
- *Language and cultural barriers*: the veterinary profession suffers from a lack of ethnic diversity. Fewer cross-culturally attuned veterinarians often means fewer financial solutions for lower income pet owners.
- *Workplace stress and burnout*: financial discussions with pet owners have been cited as one of the principal drivers of veterinary stress, leading veterinarians to avoid interactions that could potentially help pet owners overcome affordability concerns (see 8.16 Dealing with Compassion Fatigue and Burnout, and 8.17 Dealing with Compromise Fatigue).
- *Secondary- and tertiary-level care*: veterinary schools and specialty centers target the most affluent of all, offering few clinical or financial options for those without the means to pay for the best services available.
- *Specialization*: the trend toward specialization in veterinary medicine continues unabated.
- *Corporatization*: the aggressive rate of corporatization and consolidation of veterinary practices has led to a decrease in diversity among practices in most major metropolitan areas. Standardization of clinical options and financial policies typically serves to discourage lower income clientele.
- *Veterinary income loss due to online pharmacy competition*: the widespread adoption of online outlets for veterinary drugs and products has helped save pet owners money on these items. Unfortunately, it has also raised the price of veterinary services (see 9.10 Dispensing and Prescribing).
- *Consolidated supplier pricing*: the muscular market power of an increasingly consolidated veterinary supply industry means higher prices on veterinary drugs and supplies for pet owners, too.
- *The cost of veterinary higher education*: higher student debt loads have translated into higher starting salaries, which are increasingly reflected in higher prices for veterinary services.

Solutions to the Pet Healthcare Affordability Crisis

Veterinarians cite financial considerations in veterinary medicine to be the principal wellspring of stress and burnout. Whether overburdened by student loan debt, bullied by suppliers or overwhelmed by clients who cannot afford to treat their unwell pets, the veterinary profession clearly has a vested interest in addressing the affordability issues that keep pet owners from caring for their pets as they would like to.

To that end, the veterinary industry has devised some strategies to help pet owners overcome their inability to pay for veterinary services, including pet health insurance (see 10.16 Pet Health Insurance), payment (wellness) plans (see 10.17 Payment and Wellness Plans), and third-party financing (see 10.18 Financing Veterinary Care). Other options include nonprofit and for-profit programs for low-income clientele, limited-service veterinary care (e.g., vaccine clinics), publicly funded veterinary clinics, and shelter medicine programs (see 10.14 Providing Cost-Effective Care for Those in Need).

Despite these earnest attempts to address the profession's incipient affordability crisis, the veterinary profession has as yet failed to achieve a sustainable solution. Meanwhile, the divide between the "haves" and "have nots" expands exponentially with no signs of moderating any time in the near future.

The following is a list of considerations devised to mitigate costs and address other affordability concerns.

- Create and standardize tiers of care based on acceptable alternatives, allowing for a variety of standards of care (see 7.8 Providing Care for Those Unable or Unwilling to Pay). In this scenario, for example, a level one, minimal care standard could be considered ethical and legally defensible for financially stressed households.
- Create a system by which individuals may be "income qualified" for lower cost services, thereby assessing affordability concerns more objectively. This qualification could provide a more practical, verifiable route for justification of a minimal standard of care.
- Provide practical instruction for students at veterinary teaching hospitals to address affordability issues by advancing a breadth of diagnostic and treatment options. This may serve to address stigma surrounding reduced standards of care so that all practices, including secondary and tertiary care practices, can more readily offer a wider variety of care options (see 2.2 The Role of Incremental Care).
- Provide practice management consultation services to low-income practices and promote the concept of for-profit community clinics to veterinarians with shelter medicine interests or public service leanings.
- Establish not-for-profit payment plan services to help those with low credit scores to finance care.
- Negotiate more aggressively with veterinary pharmaceutical companies to provide lower cost drugs and products to prequalified low-income pet owners or in shelter settings.
- Only in very specific situations will discounting be a suitable solution (see 2.11 Discounting in Veterinary Practice)
- Support and promote shelter medicine and public policy programs in veterinary schools. Establish tuition reimbursement programs for students willing to practice in low-income settings to help address these candidates' unique financial concerns.

The veterinary profession is clearly at a crossroads in its search for a meaningful, sustainable solution to this emerging crisis. The profession is undeniably well equipped with the creativity and compassion to overcome this critical issue before it affects future generations adversely, but it will need to confront it honestly and meaningfully at the highest levels of the veterinary establishment to do so. The

profession is currently engaged in the early stages of exploration of this complex issue.

TAKE-AWAYS

- Pet owners are finding it difficult to pay for the more expensive veterinary services offered by an increasingly sophisticated veterinary profession, leading to what industry analysts have described as an affordability crisis.
- National economic trends toward growing income inequality and the dearth of low-cost options for veterinary care are at odds with the increasingly widespread cultural conception of pets as family members, further inflaming affordability concerns.
- Veterinarians' drive to increase standards of care, coupled with the higher cost of drugs, supplies and education, among other factors, have led to the higher priced veterinary services pet owners are increasingly unable to afford.
- Current solutions to the affordability problem primarily include pet health insurance, wellness plans, and financial services (credit cards and payment plans) along with a limited number of privately and publicly funded low-cost veterinary service programs and practices.
- The future of veterinary affordability rests in the hands of the veterinary establishment, where a serious examination of affordability issues is currently under way.

MISCELLANEOUS

Reference

1 Volk, J.O. (2011). Executive summary of the Bayer veterinary care usage study. *JAVMA* 238 (10): 1275–1282.

Recommended Reading

ASPCA press release. Miami-Dade County Becomes 10th Community in ASPCA Partnership. (2010). www.aspca.org/about-us/press-releases/miami-dade-county-becomes-10th-community-aspca-partnership

University of Florida College of Veterinary Medicine press release. New UF and Miami-Dade County collaboration will help homeless animals. (2016). www.vetmed.ufl. edu/2016/08/18/new-uf-and-miami-dade-county-collaboration-will-help-homeless-animals

Sullivant, A., Mackin, A.J., and Morse, D. (2020). Strategies to improve case outcome when referral is not affordable. *J Vet Med Educ* 47: 356–364.

2.11

Discounting in Veterinary Practice

Mark J. McGaunn, CPA/PFS, CFP®

McGaunn & Schwadron, CPA's, LLC, Medfield, MA, USA

 BASICS

2.11.1 Summary

Professional service providers have been particularly vexed after the provision of their service with both (i) billing and (ii) collecting from their clients. Service providers, such as veterinarians, who have acquired a great deal of technical skill may not possess the administrative and financial background skills necessary to convey the importance of what they're providing to the actual explanation of value to clients. Veterinarians should not feel that they are alone in this particular skill set as many professional service providers such as attorneys, accountants, financial planners, architects and even physicians, among others, have long been deficient in this learned skill, and they fully recognize the need to acquire those skills. There are whole consulting industries whose sole purpose is to provide professional service providers with the skills and support to actually charge a "full" price without providing discounts, and buoy the self-worth of the provider.

2.11.2 Terms Defined

Discount: A deduction from the usual cost of something typically given for prompt or advanced payment or for a special category of buyers.

 MAIN CONCEPTS

The goal of being paid for professional services is not just to recognize that there needs to be payment for services rendered, but that the service in and of itself is valuable.

Discounts in and of themselves are not a particularly good method of providing clients or patients with a reward for some form of behavior. However, discounts could be allowed to various client segments upon the execution of a set of predetermined criteria.

Without a strategic plan to outline those criteria, the general provision of payment discounts by all sorts of providers and circumstances encountered by patients could potentially lead to a significant loss in gross revenue as well as the continuation of that revenue loss into successive financial periods. Discounts are actually a detractor from a veterinary practice's profitability, as not allowing a discount allows the forgone discount to flow right to the bottom line and increase profitability (except in cases of production-based pay). But even in a production-based pay environment, a high percentage of the discount would still flow to the bottom line of the income statement as profit.

Without a strategic plan in place for providing discounts to the patient base, a veterinary practice owner could potentially continue the devaluation of his or her services without the expectation of driving positive client behavior and it could also set the expectation that future continued discounts are an automatic expectation (entitlement) rather than warranted by continued good behavior.

The goal of a sound patient payment discount program should be to:

- reward for expected good behavior on the part of compliance
- reward the client for achieving strategic financial benchmarks, and
- reward intended patient intangibles such as marketing the practice to other potential clients.

If veterinarians realize that part of the delivery of service includes an explanation of the value of that service, generally most clients will accept that delivery of value and the resulting price incurred (see 5.11 Discussing Finances for Pet-Specific Care).

Practitioners with financial knowledge will also be cognisant of the fact that pets are potentially a luxury acquisition. There are many costs post acquisition that are not factored into the original purchase of a pet, including feeding, veterinary care, licensing and registration, daycare, and even dog-walking services (see 2.9 Anticipated Costs of Pet Care). These are not always fully realized at the onset of pet ownership. As record keeping, administration, accounting, and tax reporting are necessary for keeping track of investments, so are the embedded costs of pet ownership noted above. But both investors and pet owners seem to forget that these ancillary expenditures can add up over time.

There are individuals who, whatever the amount of explanation of significant delivery of high-value services to their pet, will still be expecting a discount purely because they do not want to pay the full price of the service. There really should be no expected discount for the pet owner; discounts should really be infrequent and at the discretion of the veterinary practice.

Typically, *unwarranted discounts* are unplanned discounts and are generally provided to pet owners after difficult conversations about loss, a poor prognosis or outcome, or just generally poor communication by the veterinarian or staff with a pet owner. At this point, veterinarians may just offer a discount of some magnitude to curtail a difficult conversation or experience.

Some pet owners may prey on the humanistic trait of most veterinary hospitals to emphasize patient care over finances. But, if there is indeed an unplanned event that is precipitated by the veterinarians' or staff's action or inaction, some form of discount may be warranted. However, if there is a "difficult" or strained conversation with this particular pet owner across all patient encounters, maybe this is not the right owner to be seen at this practice. Maybe this particular pet owner should be allowed to pursue other avenues for pet care. This action may have a positive benefit in that staff (including the veterinarian) may not have to dread that client entering the facility and the ensuing tense conversations that follow, the ones that always result in a discount.

In general, the "right" or ideal pet owner is somebody who:

- follows all medical direction to the best of their ability
- pays all invoices promptly and without negativity, and
- refers family, friends, and colleagues willingly to the practice.

A typical veterinary practice might subscribe to the theory that all their pet owners should be the "right" pet owners for that particular practice – they follow directions, pay promptly, and refer family friends and colleagues willingly. Anybody who does not fit these criteria may not be a core client for the practice, although they are certainly entitled to compassionate and respectful care (see 7.8 Providing Care for Those Unable or Unwilling to Pay). In a perfect world, there would not be any payment discounts except in limited circumstances.

Below are some examples of discount programs.

- *New patient referral discounts*: a new patient referral discount is a good mechanism to reward both staff and current pet owners for the referral of a new patient to the veterinary practice. This form of discount is warranted for the referral of the right patients to the practice. Many times, it is the same small group of clients that are referring to the practice and they should be rewarded as such. The level of discount that needs to be offered can be nominal, such as a reward card or gift certificate for future retail expenditure at the practice. Most pet owners would not refer family, friends, and associates to the practice purely for the discount that is offered. They are doing it because of the care and service that they receive and wish others to enjoy the same. This discount could be termed as a marketing expense and is a relatively inexpensive means to secure new compatible clients.
- *Senior citizen, military or other "target group" discount*: some practices employ senior citizen, military or other discounts targeted to groups of pet owners they wish to attract. While this form of discount is commendable, there is questionable goodwill that is generated from its provision. Tighter control of these forms of programs needs to coincide with the practice's strategic program on discounting, since many are of questionable value.
- *Daypart strategy*: in the restaurant industry, casual dining operators attempt to recapture market share lost to competitors by focusing on certain parts of the day that are weaker in forms of revenue generation and offering

discounts on low-cost, high-margin items to boost over-all revenue and profits. Fast-food casual restaurant chains use complex analytics to capture those periods of time that may require an additional boost in customer traffic. Using the same strategy, veterinary hospitals could employ the same methods to increase patient flow to slower periods in the schedule, and book low-cost, high-margin services in those weaker periods to boost profitability (even while providing a discount). Like hotels offering last-minute bargain pricing on rooms just to increase their fill rate, veterinary hospitals could offer discounts or special pricing to those pet owners who accept appointments in these slower periods of the schedule.

- *Preventive care plans*: wellness or preventive care plan packages often represent forms of discounting (see 10.17 Payment and Wellness Plans). A small discount would be welcome to pet owners adopting preventive care plans, but receiving a discount is not their primary motivation for adopting the plan. Rather, they believe it will (i) facilitate improved overall pet health and (ii) provide a budgeted expenditure for their pet's wellness care year over year.

- *Empathy or compassion discounts*: in lieu of general discounting, each veterinary care provider could be given the discretion to provide a discount when they feel a patient care encounter merits one (i.e., job loss, family tragedy, extenuating circumstances, etc.). There should be established limits for the annual (or quarterly) amount a veterinary care provider can extend, and once that limit is reached, there are no empathy or compassion discounts beyond that point. That will rein in the unlimited discounting some practices employ.

TAKE-AWAYS

- Design written protocols that all staff understand, and the practice owner enforces in allowing discounts.
- Provide a set annual limit for all providers to utilize when circumstances warrant.
- The plan should attempt to capture new patients as well as reinforce good pet owner behavior.
- Rewarding poor pet owner behavior with discounts is generally counterproductive.
- Keep the discounting plan consistent with little change between review periods.

MISCELLANEOUS

Recommended Reading

Lee, J.G. (2015). Dissecting the discount: are incentives worth cultivating new and loyal clients who may be worth 10 times the original investment? http://veterinarybusiness.dvm360.com/dissecting-discount

Smith, D.P. (2016). The Daypart Dance. www.qsrmagazine.com/menu-innovations/daypart-dance

Stewart, J.K. (2017) Patient discounts – the fine line between leniency and liability. www.medicaleconomics.com/medical-economics-blog/patient-discounts-fine-line-between-leniency-and-liability

2.12

Blockchain in Veterinary Medicine

Lowell Ackerman, DVM, DACVD, MBA, MPA, CVA, MRCVS

Global Consultant, Author, and Lecturer, MA, USA

BASICS

2.12.1 Summary

Blockchain may be a foreign concept to many, but it is an important topic because it is demonstrating real benefits in many aspects of human healthcare and is bound to gain more prominence in veterinary medicine as well.

Blockchain gained some notoriety with the introduction of Bitcoin and other cryptocurrencies, but it has been recognized as having many more applications, including its use in healthcare. It could be particularly useful in pet-specific care in which various stakeholders could have secure privileges to various aspects of the medical record.

2.12.2 Terms Defined

Blockchain: A database that is shared across a network of computers.

Hash code: A form of cryptographic security that, unlike encryption, cannot be reversed or decrypted.

MAIN CONCEPTS

Blockchain just refers to an online database shared across a network of computers, but it differs from other databases in a number of important ways. For security, once a record has been added to the chain by a legitimate entity (such as a veterinary clinic, laboratory, or specialty center), it is very difficult for others to change. For consistency, the network makes frequent checks to ensure that all copies of records are the same across the entire network.

In a blockchain, individual records are bundled together into blocks, and then linked sequentially within the chain. The three parts of the process are thus:

- the record
- the block
- the chain.

For any given transaction, the process involves recording the details of the individual transaction (record), including digital signatures for each party. The computers in the network, called nodes, then verify the details of the record to make sure it is valid. Accepted records are then added to a block and then the block of records is ready to be added to the chain. Each block contains a unique code, called a hash, that identifies where it belongs when assembled into a chain. These hash codes are created by a mathematical formula and contribute to the security of the system. In the final step, the blocks are added to the chain, and the hash codes connect the blocks in a specific order.

Any change to the original record, no matter how miniscule, would be detected and would warrant the generation of a new hash code. That change to the hash code alters the blockchain, making it extremely difficult for hackers to make changes that are not immediately detected within the network. It's not impossible but attempting to change all the hash codes within the chain would require phenomenal computing power, making it much more secure than current systems.

A blockchain database is decentralized and computers in the network are nodes, so there is no master computer in the system. With a decentralized network, all the participating nodes can access the information and compete to be the next to add to the database, so the system sets up tests of trustworthiness. These tests are referred to as consensus mechanisms and require network members to prove themselves before they are allowed to add to the chain.

To make sure only authorized users have access to the information, blockchain systems use cryptography-based digital signatures to verify identities. Account holders have private keys that are nearly impossible for hackers to discern, but public keys can be generated for information sharing. In this way, anyone with a public key can receive information (such as a disease registry or insurance company), but only those with a private key can alter that information (such as permitted medical professionals, laboratories, etc.). Third parties, such as pet owners, can be given limited access to records, while the audit trail capability of blockchain means there is complete documentation of the creation, modification, and attempted deletion of records.

2.12.3 Healthcare Applications

Current systems for sharing electronic data among doctors, patients, referral hospitals, laboratories, and insurers are still quite error prone. Incorrect information can emerge as patient data are reentered time after time by different individuals and it is difficult to conserve changes made by one party into everyone's version of the medical record. So, for example, if a patient is seen by both a primary care and a specialty clinic, changes made to the medical records at either facility are not immediately captured in the medical records of both facilities, and require multiple steps to send, receive, and enter information; errors and omissions are possible at all stages.

Blockchain can be used to provide all clients and providers with identical content. The decentralized ledger approach to information management gives all parties simultaneous access to a single record of strongly encrypted data at relatively low cost. It also creates an audit trail each time any data item in the record is changed, helping to maintain the integrity of the system and its information. Eventually, blockchain could be used to provide secure and accurate medical information for all individual patients.

With blockchain technology, clients could actually play some role in managing the medical records of their pets and permission can be given to different providers and entities to access and modify those records, where all such modification attempts are securely recorded, annotated, and largely tamper-proof.

If a pet has received treatments from multiple doctors at different facilities, all that information can be accessed from the blockchain, and there would be an audit trail for any changes made. Ultimately, the success of any such system depends on the participation of many medical providers, or there are few benefits over those seen with traditional electronic medical records.

One of the main benefits for blockchain use in healthcare is that it is decentralized, which provides enhanced security. Because the data record is replicated across many nodes rather than on one central computer, it is more resistant to a hacking attempt or manipulation. If any one computer is hacked, other separate computers in the network that are using the blockchain would still maintain accurate information.

Blockchain itself does not perform analytics, but permission could be granted for analytics to be performed on such data. This could be extremely powerful in veterinary medicine in which large numbers of small clinics exist globally, but a single database could potentially be mined for a wealth of information relative to pet-specific care (such as breed predispositions, disease prevalence, epidemiology, etc.).

Other areas where blockchain can prove very useful is with online directories of doctors and other healthcare providers. Hospitals, doctors' groups, laboratories, and insurers all try to maintain their own online listings, but these frequently become outdated or require providers to notify the entities that the information has changed or is outdated. With blockchain, providers can update their own information at will. Especially in veterinary medicine, with so many clinics unaffiliated with one another and potentially using different practice management software, there can be many islands of information with very few opportunities for data bridges. Blockchain can help address that.

Another area of importance for blockchain is the management of personal data online. With blockchain, a patient's entire medical record can be stored in a ledger and encrypted with a private key. Changes in this information can be communicated to the ledger with the patient's authorization and securely shared with various providers. Because of the audit trail feature, everyone is aware exactly who made a change, when the change occurred, and what was changed.

There are many other potential applications, from managing prescriptions through the blockchain so that all participants know when and where a prescription was filled, to tracking laboratory results through the system, to verifying veterinary licensing. and updating information directly.

EXAMPLES

The following is an example of a fictional veterinary blockchain application.

A veterinary blockchain project was established with participation of veterinary hospitals, laboratories, and pet health insurance companies. Dr Smith of ABC Animal Hospital is a participant along with many of her colleagues.

Mrs Jones first presented her spayed female labradoodle Daisy to the clinic and once she shared her public key with the clinic, they were able to access information from all the clinics that Daisy had visited previously. In those records were also entries from diagnostic laboratories, along with time codes and verified user stamps of all participants. In fact, there was even an entry from a genetic testing laboratory indicating that Daisy carried a variant for exercise-induced collapse, and that might prove very useful should she ever display evidence of weakness.

Over the next few years, Dr Smith came to appreciate the importance of blockchain to medicine. Once, after hours, Daisy needed to be seen at an emergency clinic, and Mrs Jones was able to provide that clinic with a key to access Daisy's healthcare information, including recent blood-work that had been run. Similarly, when Daisy showed some evidence of lameness, she was referred to a specialist; the specialist appreciated access to the previous medical records, including the genetic screening, and was able to append the medical record with relevant findings, accessible to Dr Smith and others who had been given permission. Laboratory testing that had been performed was similarly entered into the record, directly by the laboratory.

Mrs Jones had purchased pet health insurance for Daisy, which was in effect since Daisy was a puppy. The pet health insurance company participated in the blockchain process and the shared ledger of encrypted data allowed all parties to view the same accurate information about the insurance claim, without anyone having to send medical information back and forth. Mrs Jones found it very convenient to see that the insurance company was able to quickly acknowledge and process the claim.

TAKE-AWAYS

- One of the main advantages of blockchain is that it allows multiple permitted providers to access and append information in a medical record.
- Blockchain tends to be much more secure than other forms of databases and while it is still theoretically "hackable," it is much more difficult to do so than with most other systems.
- Blockchain maintains an audit trail, so that it is immediately obvious to all when a provider makes an entry or change to a medical record.
- The concept of blockchain may sound exotic, but it is already being very successfully employed within many physician networks.
- The main disadvantage of blockchain is that it is of limited benefit until there are a critical number of medical professionals participating in the process.

MISCELLANEOUS

2.12.4 Cautions

Blockchain is more difficult to hack, and tends to be more secure than traditional systems, but with enough computing power it is possible that even blockchains could be hacked. So, it is considered very secure but not completely impervious to hacking. One concern in this regard is that since most blockchain networks run the same code, any vulnerability detected could potentially put the whole network at risk. To keep things in perspective, though, most other systems are much less secure and tend to be easier to hack.

To be fully effective, blockchain requires that a large number of providers participate in the process. Without such participation, it loses much of its benefits of multi-user access.

As with most systems, it is also important to determine that data are accurate when first entered into the blockchain ledger. Sometimes, such as when a medical record contains information from multiple sources, it can difficult to determine the "owner" of a piece of information in the first place (e.g., a laboratory result recorded in a medical record, but without the actual laboratory that performed the testing specified).

Recommended Reading

Ackerman, L. (ed.) (2020). Blockchain. In: *Five-Minute Veterinary Practice Management Consult*, 3e, 660–661. Ames, IA: Wiley.

Casey, M.J. and Vigna, P. (2018). *The Truth Machine: The Blockchain and the Future of Everything*. New York: St. Martin's Press.

Drescher, D. (2017). *Blockchain Basics*. New York: Apress.

Geron, T. (2018). One remedy for high health costs: blockchain. *Wall Street Journal*: R14.

Kshetri, N. (2018). Blockchain could be the security answer. Maybe. *Wall Street Journal*: R7.

Murray, M. (2018). Blockchain explained. https://graphics.reuters.com/TECHNOLOGY-BLOCKCHAIN/010070P11GN/index.html

Norman, A.T. (2017). *Blockchain Technology Explained*. Createspace Independent Publishing Platform https://books.google.com/books/about/Blockchain_Technology_Explained.html?id=Z_JcswEACAAJ.

2.13

Placebo and Nocebo

Lowell Ackerman, DVM, DACVD, MBA, MPA, CVA, MRCVS

Global Consultant, Author, and Lecturer, MA, USA

BASICS

2.13.1 Summary

The concept of placebo is well known in human medicine, but it often does not get the same sort of respect when it comes to the use of medications in animals. It might be inferred that pets are the best "blinded" controls when it comes to therapeutics since pets do not know if they are being administered active medications, and yet since it is pet owners that ultimately report on what works and what doesn't, placebo is an important topic in veterinary medicine as well.

2.13.2 Terms Defined

Nocebo: A negative type of placebo effect in which being informed that there could be adverse effects associated with a therapy increases the likelihood that adverse effects will be experienced and reported.

Placebo: The beneficial effect perceived for a product without actual physiological impact.

MAIN CONCEPTS

The placebo effect is well recognized in human medicine, but it was once believed that animals could not cognitively appreciate that a medication would be of benefit to them and react accordingly. However, there are several reasons why this line of reasoning may not be correct.

A lot of work has been done on the placebo effect, including the concept of honest placebos (patients or caregivers know something is a placebo but they discern benefit regardless). It's an important concept in veterinary medicine, not because the animals can be fooled but because the owners may identify responses as positive. In our pet-specific forum, it is important to realize that just because a pet responded, this does not mean that we made the correct diagnosis and selected the appropriate medication in all cases. We also need to account for placebo and nocebo in animals.

2.13.3 Caregiver Placebo Effect

While animals may not be able to directly perceive benefits from placebo therapies, the same cannot be said of the caregivers who are administering the medications and/or assessing its effects. This includes veterinarians, who are often eager for their interventions to have documentable success. In fact, the caregiver placebo effect may be evident around 30–40% of the time regarding subjective evaluations, such as for lameness in dogs and cats.

2.13.4 The Hawthorne Effect

Another manifestation of caregiver placebo effect can be seen as a feature of being enrolled in a study, or receiving an intervention perceived as new and potentially exciting – known as the Hawthorne effect. With the extra attention potentially shown by veterinary staff, and more scrutiny and monitoring, it is quite possible that pet owners will have expectation-based placebo effects. Conceivably, they may approach their pet in a more positive manner, spend more time praising and having physical contact with it, and pets can respond to that increased attention.

Pet-Specific Care for the Veterinary Team, First Edition. Edited by Lowell Ackerman.
© 2021 John Wiley & Sons, Inc. Published 2021 by John Wiley & Sons, Inc.

If studies in human medicine are any indication, the placebo effect can also be enhanced if clients are told a medication is hard to get or expensive; the color of the tablet can also affect degree of perceived benefit. All of this supports the contention that a placebo is more than just an inert substance without physiological effects, even if those effects cannot be completely explained.

2.13.5 Regression to the Mean

When treating chronic problems, such as arthritis, allergies, inflammatory bowel disease, and others, there tends to be a progressive nature to the diseases, but attitudes and clinical signs tend to wax and wane over time – there are good days and bad days.

When patients are having "bad days" and are clinically at their worst, this is the most likely time when clients are going to be most receptive to trying something new. Since waxing and waning of clinical signs is typical, it is also not unusual that a percentage of patients will be better following the administration of anything – be it a legitimate therapy or a placebo – just because that is the fluctuating nature of chronic disease.

In other cases, even though chronic problems are by their very definition "chronic," there can be much larger cycles that can explain observed changes from placebo. For example, with atopic dermatitis, pets may be worst during peak pollination periods for specific allergens. During the worst periods of such pollination, owners are more likely to be desperate for new treatment alternatives. However, intense pollination periods tend to be relatively short-lived, so in some instances the allergen load may actually have diminished significantly on its own and the clinical benefits should really be attributed to this discontinuation of intense pollination. Just because a pet gets better on a therapy does not mean that the primary effect can be attributed to the medication.

2.13.6 Honest Placebo

One very interesting aspect of placebo studies is that sometimes they can still provide benefits even if the patient/client knows they are administering placebos. This is known as the honest placebo effect. Thus, human researchers for several years have been conducting open-label placebo studies where patients know they are receiving placebo, and still documenting benefit. We know that for some clients, there is an expectation that they will receive at least some sort of medication for whatever problem their pet might have. In fact, even some veterinarians might feel the need to dispense *something* for a client in need, even if there is not a specific medical indica-

tion. For example, sometimes clients request antibiotics for a pet when it is sick, even if there is no indication of bacterial involvement. Sometimes owners (and veterinarians) just want to feel like they are doing "something," and a percentage will report success with this "something."

2.13.7 Nocebo Effect

The nocebo effect is an interesting phenomenon in which people have negative expectations about something and that alone is enough to make them perceive an ill effect. This may account in part for people who believe that certain vaccines have deleterious effects or that certain foods are more responsible for allergies and insensitivities than would otherwise be statistically reasonable. Adverse effects to food and vaccines certainly exist and are well documented in animals, but many more people harbor beliefs about potential adverse effects than can be justified by scientific likelihood.

EXAMPLES

Mrs Jansen brought Meili, her 2-year-old spayed female shih tzu, to ABC Animal Hospital for persistent scratching, especially around her face and ears. Mrs Jansen seemed to think the problem was most likely due to a food allergy, since the problem started a few weeks after a new commercial diet was introduced and she noticed that the diet included gluten, which she herself was avoiding.

In consultation with the veterinary team, Mrs Jensen agreed to commence an elimination diet trial for a minimum of eight weeks, and if there was any question of effect, she was willing to continue for a total of 12 weeks. She was given the option of either a commercial hypoallergenic diet or a home-made recipe with novel ingredients, and she thought she would have better control with the home-made diet. An allergy medication was dispensed to be used for the first two weeks of the trial just to give Meili some relief, and then would be discontinued for the remainder of the dietary trial.

Meili was presented eight weeks later and was substantially improved. Mrs Jansen was happy that she was able to stick to the home-made diet, even though it was more work that she was doing in addition to food preparation for her other family members. She also lamented why pet food companies were able to sell foods with such ingredients that were capable of making pets sick.

Dr Green congratulated Mrs Jansen on her ability to persevere for the entire dietary trial, but had one other request just to conclusively determine a cause-and-effect relationship.

He didn't want Mrs Jansen to have to cook for Meili forever, or to try diet after diet to find an acceptable commercial option, so he asked if she would be prepared to try one other scientific trial – reintroduce the original diet to see how long it took for the clinical signs to start to recur. After all, if the problem was really the diet, they should be able to induce the clinical signs with reintroduction of the offending allergen(s), and then make them quickly go away again by stopping the diet once again. Once they had conclusively established the diet as the culprit, they would commence challenge feeding to determine which ingredient(s) were actually problematic.

Mrs Jansen was a bit unsure of the process, and didn't want Meili to suffer, but she agreed to the trial realizing that she could reverse any ill effects quickly, and that it would appease Dr Green's scientific curiosity so they could get on with more permanent solutions. However, with challenge feeding, Mrs Jansen was surprised that Meili did not get worse when she reintroduced the original diet, even after she had fed it for a full two weeks. She even fed Meili some bread and pasta, the gluten content of which she was sure would aggravate Meili's condition . . . but it didn't. Dr Green explained that the likelihood was that Meili was allergic to certain pollens which were prevalent during the period when she was symptomatic, and perhaps food was not playing a major role after all. He praised Mrs Jansen for her willingness to explore the complexity of Meili's condition, provided her with information on atopic dermatitis, and asked her to track Meili's clinical signs on a calendar and if major problems recurred, they would have some documentation to compare with allergy test results to determine the most likely allergens implicated.

TAKE-AWAYS

- Don't be fooled – the placebo effect is evident in animals.

- Caregivers are responsible for judging the impact of interventions on clinical issues and their impressions can be influenced.
- Simply enrolling in a study or taking part in a therapeutic trial can influence the perception of benefit. This is known as the Hawthorne effect.
- Most chronic conditions tend to wax and wane over time, and sometimes medication benefits can be attributed to times when clinical signs would be waning regardless.
- People can be influenced to expect that certain interventions are likely to have bad effects, even if not likely. This is known as the nocebo effect.

MISCELLANEOUS

Recommended Reading

Conzemius, M.G. and Evans, R.B. (2012). Caregiver placebo effect for dogs with lameness from osteoarthritis. *J. Am. Vet. Med. Assoc.* 241 (10): 1314–1319.

Gruen, M.E., Dorman, D.C., and Lascelles, B.D.X. (2017). Caregiver placebo effect in analgesic clinical trials for cats with naturally occurring degenerative joint disease-associated pain. *Vet. Rec.* 180 (19): 473.

McKenzie, B. (2018). What is a placebo? Animals receiving inert treatments may show improvement due to causes other than direct placebo effects. http://veterinarypracticenews.com/what-is-a-placebo

McKenzie, B.A. (2019). *Placebos for Pets? The Truth about Alternative Medicine in Animals.* England: Ockham Publishing, Newmachar, Scotland.

Munkevics, M., Munkevica, S. (2017). Why does placebo work on dogs and cats? http://pet-happy.com/why-does-placebo-work-on-pets

Sifferlin, A. (2018). Placebo's new power. *Time Magazine* 3/10: 65–69.

2.14

Benefits of the Human–Animal Bond

Jacqui Ley, BVSc (Hons), PhD, DECAWBM, FANZCVS (Veterinary Behaviour)

Melbourne Veterinary Specialist Centre, Glen Waverley, Victoria, Australia

BASICS

2.14.1 Summary

The human–animal bond (HAB) is the glue that keeps companion animals in families. The strength of the HAB affects if a pet is obtained, its management and healthcare and if it is retained and valued by its family. Many benefits arise from the HAB such as improved human physical and psychological health. Veterinary clinics and the wider community benefit from strong HABs. Understanding how the bond is expressed and how it affects owner decisions can aid veterinary practices to provide the kind of care they want while avoiding compassion fatigue.

2.14.2 Terms Defined

Attachment: The enduring emotional bond between individuals. It is characterized by behaviors such as seeking proximity to the individual and being attentive to their needs.

Compassion Fatigue: Also known as secondary traumatic stress disorder, this is the gradual loss of compassion by people who work with individuals who are ill, suffering, or victims of trauma. This includes veterinary staff working with worried clients with sick or injured animals. Signs include indifference, disengagement, withdrawal from patients and co-workers, and even physical signs relating to chronic stress.

Human–Animal Bond (HAB): A measurable psychological construct encompassing the feelings of attachment between an owner and a pet. It has been well described

from the human perspective but is not well understood from the animal's view.

Problem Behavior: Behavior exhibited by the animal that is considered undesirable. The behavior may be normal for the species or it may be due to a mental health disorder.

MAIN CONCEPTS

It can be difficult to understand why one owner will do everything for their pet and another will only do the bare minimum. The cause may be differences in the HAB. The HAB describes the connection people feel toward animals for which they care. The expression of the HAB is affected by many things but two factors important to veterinary practice, because they affect owner healthcare decisions, are owner attachment and owner commitment to the pet.

The HAB may affect owner decisions as to the choice of pet and where it is acquired, how the pet lives with them and owner lifestyle such as where they live, work, and take holidays. The bond is affected by the owner's experience of pet ownership, expectations of this pet and perceived social expression and norms, among other factors.

The human experience of the HAB is well described. Owners can be located along a continuum from highly attached (the pet is considered a valued family member) through to less attached (the pet is a thing). For example, owner attachment levels may affect an owner's willingness to accept the financial costs of treatment for a pet. Highly attached owners may also have difficulty accepting that their pet is unwell [1]. Some highly attached owners may also struggle emotionally when their pet is given a terminal diagnosis or when it dies.

The HAB is also affected by the animal. The bond is fragile and easily damaged and is especially vulnerable when owners have high expectations of a pet. Relinquishment occurs most commonly due to problem behavior by the animal. Annoying behaviors such as being boisterous or destructive and dangerous behaviors such as aggression are frequently given as reasons for surrendering dogs.

How fracture of the bond affects the animal is not well understood but it may have far-reaching effects for some. Humans report that the decision to relinquish a pet causes significant distress [2].

Communities benefit when owners have strong bonds with their pets. Interacting with pets has documented benefits for people – for their health and their psychological welfare. Strong bonds result in fewer animals being relinquished to shelters or abandoned. The HAB can also have negative effects for communities. Attached and committed owners are less likely to evacuate during natural disasters (see 2.17 Emergency Preparedness). If unable to take their pets with them, people in abusive relationships may delay leaving and seeking help. The large numbers of pets relinquished to animal shelters every year due to fracture of the HAB create community problems in caring for, rehoming or euthanizing unwanted pets. Noise from dogs and cats, feces left in public places, aggression by dogs to people and other animals, and cruelty and neglect of animals are all community issues that stem from the HAB.

The challenge for veterinary clinics is to encourage and support their clients' bonds with their pets, while accepting all levels and types of bonds. When veterinary clinic staff are aware of the HAB in general and, more specifically, the nature of their personal bond with their pets, it can help them support owners and accept different approaches to pet care. For example, many staff struggle when owners elect not to treat very treatable conditions because it clashes with their own beliefs about how animals should be treated.

Supporting client bonds with their pets must be authentic to be worthwhile [1]. How each clinic does this will be different due to the nature of their community and clinic. For some clinics, pet birthday card mailouts work while others find displaying professional photographs of staff with their pets demonstrates the HAB best for them. Genuine interest in the client's pet and their concerns is essential.

Clinics can encourage strong HABs in several ways. Managing owner expectations of pets is very important. This may be done by posting information about raising a puppy or a kitten for the first 12 months on the clinic website or blog. The value of pets to humans and communities can be written about in newsletters. Technicians and nurses can offer "Preparing for a new pet" consultations for clients before they purchase a pet. Well-run puppy and kitten classes are also great assets for supporting the HAB. Clients should be asked about problems with their pet's behavior at each consultation.

Recognizing an owner's attachment level also helps when presenting healthcare information. Highly attached owners may respond to information that emphasizes quality of life and pain relief outcomes while owners with more utilitarian attachment will respond to information that considers the costs of treatment versus benefits and prognosis.

The end of a pet's life can also be a celebration of the bond between the owner and pets (see 6.20 Quality of Life and End of Life Issues). Palliative care services can preserve animal welfare while providing time for owners to prepare for the loss of their pet (some owners find it difficult to return to the place their pet was euthanized). Some owners change vets. Offering clients home euthanasia or partnering with a veterinary palliative care and euthanasia service can help support clients (see 9.18 Hospice and Palliative Care). Offering high-quality cremation and burial services is another way clinics can help owners remember pets and support the HAB.

Highly attached owners may struggle with their grief after the death of a pet. This can be very taxing for clinic staff. Referral to a professional pet grief counselor can help these owners.

Clients' previous experience of loss can affect their approach to veterinary care for their current pets. Some owners who have cared for, treated, and nursed a chronically and seriously ill pet may decline treatment for other pets due to their perceptions of the emotional cost to themselves and the quality of life for the now deceased pet.

Staff training about the HAB can make each staff member aware of their own feelings and attitudes about animals and how this may affect their interactions with clients.

EXAMPLES

Sunnyside Veterinary Clinic educated all staff about the HAB. All staff were able to assess their attachment levels and compare them against the range and styles of HAB in literature. Understanding the different ways in which people can express their bond with their pets helped staff respond to client concerns appropriately and accept client decisions about treatment for their pets. Staff morale improved, with many reporting they felt less frustration with clients.

TAKE-AWAYS

- The HAB has benefits for owners and pets and for communities when it is strong and supported.
- The HAB is fragile and easily broken. It is very susceptible to damage from unmet expectations of the animal and problem behaviors.
- As a clinic, celebrate the HAB in ways that are authentic. Genuine interest in patient well-being and helping owners with their pets is more effective than marketing gimmicks.
- All staff must be aware of how different people express the bond they have with their pet. Accepting the range of attachment by owners helps staff accept owner decisions for their pet.
- Use other professionals to help highly attached owners cope with the loss of a pet. Some will need professional help to recover from the loss of their pet.

MISCELLANEOUS

2.14.3 Cautions

Compassion fatigue can come about in veterinary clinics when staff are dealing with highly attached pet owners who need extra attention to help them cope with sick, dying or recently deceased pets (see 8.17 Dealing with Compassion Fatigue).

Compassion fatigue can also occur when staff are interacting with clients whose attachment levels are very different from their own beliefs and attitudes about the HAB. Education of staff about the HAB and how it varies with different people can help staff accept owner decisions and minimize staff stress.

As companion animals are more highly valued, negative treatment outcomes may be less tolerated by some owners, leading to litigation. Care should be taken to cover the risks associated with treatments in writing and have the owner sign the form in all cases. Adequate professional insurance is also a necessity.

References

1 Brockman, B.K., Taylor, V.A., and Brockman, C.M. (2008). The price of unconditional love: consumer decision making for high-dollar veterinary care. *Journal of Business Research* 61 (5): 397–405.

2 DiGiacomo, N., Arluke, A., and Patronek, G.J. (1998). Surrendering pets to shelters: the relinquisher's perspective. *Anthrozoos* 11 (1): 41–51.

Recommended Reading

Blazina, C., Boya, G., and Shen-Miller, D. (2011). *The Psychology of the Human–Animal Bond: A Resource for Clinicians and Researchers*. New York: Springer.

Daley, O.M. (2009). *Made for each Other: The Biology of the Human–Animal Bond*. Cambridge: Merloyd Lawrence Paperbacks.

Human Animal Bond Research Institute: https://habri.org/

The Compassion Fatigue Project. www.compassionfatigue.org/index.html

2.15

Promoting the Human–Animal Bond

Sarah Rumple

Rumpus Writing and Editing LLC, Denver, CO, USA

BASICS

2.15.1 Summary

Veterinary professionals should play an active role in promoting the human–animal bond among their clients. At the heart of that effort is client education, with a focus on preventive healthcare and behavior. Education should be taken beyond the typical exam room discussions to include alternative methods that are easily absorbed by pet owners.

When clients understand how to keep their pets healthy and how to properly address potential behavior concerns, fewer pets will be relinquished and euthanized, the human–animal bond will continue to grow, and veterinary practices will flourish.

2.15.2 Terms Defined

Human–Animal Bond: A mutually beneficial and dynamic relationship between people and animals that is influenced by behaviors essential to the health and well-being of both.

MAIN CONCEPTS

2.15.3 The Human–Animal Bond

The human–animal bond is a mutually beneficial relationship between people and animals (see 2.14 Benefits of the Human–Animal Bond). According to the American Veterinary Medical Association (AVMA), the veterinarian's role in the human–animal bond is to maximize the potentials of the relationship between people and animals [1].

How can veterinarians maximize the potentials of the relationship between people and animals? Education is key. While pet owners usually have the best intentions, many do not understand how to provide the best care for their pets so they can enjoy longer, healthier, happier lives together. When veterinary practitioners adequately educate pet owners on how to provide exceptional care for their pets – and why they should provide this care – they are promoting the human–animal bond, which enhances the health and well-being of pets and their owners.

2.15.4 Client Education Opportunities

In addition to traditional exam room conversations, consider these opportunities to educate your clients.

- *Enhanced exam room communication*: while it's true that much of what veterinary professionals say to pet owners in the exam room is misheard, misunderstood, or later forgotten, there are resources available to aid in your exam room client education efforts (see 5.10 Discussing Pet-Specific Care). Bring visual aids to support your messaging (images of heartworms or periodontal disease will have a bigger impact on clients than your explanation of these conditions alone). Provide printouts with images, your recommendations, and more applicable information for clients to take home and read later.
- *Custom literature*: invest in brochures and other literature customized to your practice on a variety of pet health and behavior topics. While digital communication and online resources are important, many clients appreciate a tangible resource they can take home.

Pet-Specific Care for the Veterinary Team, First Edition. Edited by Lowell Ackerman.
© 2021 John Wiley & Sons, Inc. Published 2021 by John Wiley & Sons, Inc.

- *Practice blog and social media*: not only will a regularly updated practice blog do wonders for your website's search engine optimization, it can also be a wealth of credible information for pet owners to reference at the click of a button. Publish links to your blog posts on your social media channels, in e-communications to clients, and through your practice's mobile app.
- *Educational open house*: invite a veterinary behaviorist or training expert to your practice for an open house. The event could feature lessons on various training techniques or a behavior question-and-answer period. Whether your clients have dogs who pull on the leash or cats who are scratching inappropriately, your open house could prove to be priceless when it comes to nurturing the bonds between your clients and their pets.
- *Community event*: host a pet-friendly community "fun run" that raises awareness about any pet-related issue you want to promote. Or exhibit at other community events.

The entire veterinary healthcare team should contribute to educating clients on important topics that impact the human–animal bond. Ensure the team is thoroughly trained, hold regular staff meetings for updates and reminders, and empower each team member – from client care representatives to veterinarians – to educate clients when appropriate.

2.15.5 Educational Topics that Promote the Human–Animal Bond

In addition to pet-specific education, be sure to promote the bond your clients share with their companion animals by educating them on these topics.

- *Preventive care*: it's well established that regular preventive care yields longer lifespans, regardless of species. And when pet owners take exceptional care of their pets, they'll be more likely to enjoy longer, happier, healthier lives together, which strengthens the bond they share and decreases the risk of relinquishment [2]. Veterinary professionals should recommend and promote the highest quality care, including:
  - ○ regular veterinary visits
  - ○ preventive medications
  - ○ appropriate vaccinations (see 9.11 Vaccination)
  - ○ regular oral examinations and professional dental cleanings (see 4.9 Periodontal Disease)
  - ○ reproductive control (see 2.18 Population Control).

  Your clients should also understand why this level of care is important and how it affects them and their pets.

- *Fear, anxiety, and stress in pets*: fear, anxiety, and stress contribute to health and behavior problems and shorter lifespans in pets [3, 4]. Educate clients on how to reduce stress and anxiety at home, but also take steps to do the same at your practice (see 6.6 Fear Free Concepts). Methods include the following.
  - ○ Create separate entrances, waiting areas, and exam rooms for canine and feline patients.
  - ○ Limit waiting time in the lobby.
  - ○ Use high-value treats to distract pets during exams and procedures.
  - ○ Create a calm and familiar environment by using pheromone diffusers, infused towels, and wipes.
  - ○ Avoid using traditional exam room tables. Make pets more comfortable by conducting your exam on the floor at their level.
  - ○ Prescribe appropriate medications for pets with extreme anxiety, and instruct pet owners on how to administer the medication prior to the veterinary visit.
- *Positive reinforcement training methods*: dogs who have been trained using positive reinforcement methods are less likely to display behavior problems, including attention seeking, fear, and aggression, than those trained using aversive techniques [5, 6]. When pets develop behavior issues, the human–animal bond suffers, and pets are at increased risk of relinquishment or euthanasia [2]. Provide resources and guidance to help your clients properly train their pets using positive reinforcement methods (see 6.2 How Animals Learn).
- *Enrichment*: bored pets are more likely to develop behavioral problems, and studies show that environmental enrichment improves cognitive functions and reduces anxiety-related behaviors and neurodegenerative diseases [7]. Encourage your clients to strengthen the bond they have with their pets by enriching their environments (see 6.9 Preventing Behavior Problems). Create literature about ways to enrich an indoor cat's environment, including tips about scratching posts, perches, toys and games, pheromones, and alternative feeding systems. Remind dog owners about the importance of regular walks and play time.
- *Exercise and nutrition*: pets who are overweight or obese live shorter lives and are more likely to experience a number of health conditions, which adversely affect quality of life and the human–animal bond (see 6.15 Approaching Obesity on a Pet-Specific Basis). Ensure your clients understand the importance of helping their pets maintain a healthy weight through regular exercise and feeding a high-quality, safe diet that has been tested through research and feeding trials.
- *Pain in pets*: because animals cannot tell us when they are feeling pain, your clients should be aware of the

possible signs of pain in pets. Focus on behavioral changes, like decreased activity, loss of appetite, aggression, inappropriate elimination, withdrawing or avoiding interaction, hiding, and changes in grooming habits (see 2.16 Pain and Pain Management). Be sure your clients know to inform you when they notice behavioral changes in their pets so potential pain can be quickly and appropriately addressed.

● *Pet health insurance*: when a pet is facing a medical emergency or a potentially devastating diagnosis, the last thing the owner wants to think about is the cost of care. However, many pet owners are forced to choose substandard care, no care at all, relinquishment, or euthanasia when they cannot afford recommended treatments. Help take the cost of care out of the equation and keep the human–animal bond intact by educating your clients on pet medical insurance (see 10.16 Pet Health Insurance).

EXAMPLES

Leo, a 5-year-old neutered male domestic shorthair, has received regular preventive care since he was adopted as a kitten. Leo has recently begun scratching furniture inappropriately. Frustrated, his owners conduct internet research on potential remedies, including declaw. They visit ABC Animal Hospital's website, where they find a blog post about inappropriate scratching that recommends environmental enrichment, including scratching posts, interactive and engaging toys, food puzzles, climbing structures, and more frequent interaction and play with owners. The blog post also recommends regular nail trimming and pheromone diffusers.

Hoping to avoid declawing their cat, Leo's owners implement several of the blog's suggestions. Within a month, Leo stops scratching the furniture.

TAKE-AWAYS

● Client education is key to the promotion of the human–animal bond.
● In the exam room, visual aids and client handouts should be utilized to promote understanding and compliance.

● Additional opportunities for client education include brochures, blogs and social media, educational open houses, and community events.
● The entire veterinary team should be equipped to educate clients and promote the human–animal bond when appropriate.
● To promote the human–animal bond, veterinary professionals should educate clients on the importance of preventive care, fear, and stress in animals, positive reinforcement training, enrichment, exercise and nutrition, pain in pets, and pet health insurance.

MISCELLANEOUS

Abbreviation

HAB Human–animal bond

References

1 American Veterinary Medical Association. (2019). Human–Animal Bond (Policy/Position Statement). www.avma.org/resources-tools/avma-policies/human-animal-interaction-and-human-animal-bond

2 Patronek, G.J., Glickman, L.T., Beck, A.M. et al. (1996). Risk factors for relinquishment of dogs to an animal shelter. *Journal of the American Veterinary Medical Association* 209 (3): 572–581.

3 Dreschel, N.A. (2010). The effects of fear and anxiety on health and lifespan in pet dogs. *Applied Animal Behaviour Science* 125: 157–162.

4 Stella, J., Croney, C., and Buffington, T. (2013). Effects of stressors on the behavior and physiology of domestic cats. *Applied Animal Behaviour Science* 143: 157–163.

5 Blackwell, E., Twells, C., Seawright, A., and Casey, R. (2008). The relationship between training methods and the occurrence of behavior problems, as reported by owners, in a population of domestic dogs. *Journal of Veterinary Behavior* 3 (5): 207–217.

6 Ziv, G. (2017). The effects of using aversive training methods in dogs – a review. *Journal of Veterinary Behavior* 19: 50–60.

7 Sampedro-Piquero, P. and Begega, A. (2017). Environmental enrichment as a positive behavioral intervention across the lifespan. *Current Neuropharmacology* 15 (4): 459–470.

Recommended Reading

Brooks, D., Churchill, J., Fein, K. et al. (2014). 2014 AAHA weight management guidelines for dogs and cats. *Journal of the American Animal Hospital Association* 50: 1–11.

Knesl, O., Hart, B.L., Fine, A.H., and Cooper, L. (2016). Opportunities for incorporating the human-animal bond in companion animal practice. *Journal of the American Veterinary Medical Association* 249 (1): 42–44.

Todd, Z. (2017). New Literature Review Recommends Reward-Based Training. www.companionanimal psychology.com/2017/04/new-literature-review-recommends-reward.html

Todd, Z. (2016) Seven Reasons to Use Reward-Based Dog Training. www.companionanimalpsychology.com/2016/06/seven-reasons-to-use-reward-based-dog.html

2.16

Pain and Pain Management

Mark E. Epstein, DVM, DABVP (Canine/Feline), CVPP

TotalBond Veterinary Hospitals, PC, Gastonia, NC, USA

 BASICS

It may come as a disappointing surprise to some that the focus on recognition, assessment, prevention, and management of pain in dogs and cats is a relatively recent phenomenon, having gained significant traction only since the late 1990s.

Furthermore, underrecognition and undermanagement of pain is not merely an ethical problem – although it is very much that – but generates significant physiological and medical consequences leading to increased patient morbidity at the very least (protracted patient recovery, compromised quality of life), and at times possibly even mortality (including humane euthanasia).

The very good news is that pain management is now a central, and increasingly sophisticated, feature of small animal medicine and surgery, with an increasingly wide array of tools at the disposal of all members of the veterinary team.

2.16.1 Terms Defined

Allodynia: A pain response to nonnoxious stimuli such as touch and light pressure.

Dysthesia: Unpleasant or abnormal sensation, e.g., tingling, burning, itching, numbness.

Hyperalgesia: An exaggerated pain response to a noxious stimulus.

Hypersensitization: The molecular and cellular "wind-up" in peripheral tissue and dorsal horn of the spinal cord, characterized by decreased neuron firing threshold, decreased descending inhibition, recruitment of bystanding neurons and more; results in maladaptive pain.

Nociception: Pain processing with peripheral neuronal activation, transmission in the primary afferent neuron, modulation in the spinal cord, and perception in various centers throughout the brain.

Osteoarthritis (OA): A subset of degenerative joint disease that occurs when the protecting cartilage on the ends of bones wears down over time.

Pain: Multidimensional unpleasant sensory and emotional experience associated with actual or potential tissue damage. Chronic pain occurs when the pain persists for three months or longer.

Pain, Adaptive: Normal and protective pain.

Pain, Acute: Pain experienced during the expected time of posttrauma inflammation and healing.

Pain, Chronic: Pain experienced past the expected time of posttrauma inflammation and healing (in humans, defined as pain still present 2–3 months or longer after initial tissue damage).

Pain, Maladaptive: Peripheral and central hypersensitization-induced abnormal pain, characterized by increased scope, character, and field of pain: hyperalgesia, allodynia, dysthesias.

Pain, Neuropathic: Hypersensitization and maladaptive pain that has progressed to gene expression and permanent morphological and functional changes in the peripheral and central nervous system (CNS); pain as a disease at this point.

 MAIN CONCEPTS

Pain (defined by the International Association for the Study of Pain, IASP) is an unpleasant sensory and *emotional* experience associated with actual or potential tissue damage [1]. Pain is not merely the sensation or perception of it, but has an additional affective, emotional component. In other words, pain is said to be *multidimensional* (i.e., it is not just what you feel, but *how it makes you feel*). This is because pain pathways terminate not only in the frontal cortex (perception), but in deep, primitive parts of the brain (the limbic center) that control emotions such as anger, fear, anxiety, stress, even depression. And with this "stress response" comes a release of hormones such as cortisol, epinephrine, and proinflammatory cytokines; these very molecules actually then sensitize nociceptors, the specialized neurons that carry pain signals. In other words, a circular problem can be present: pain causes stress, and stress causes pain.

Chronic pain, furthermore, has been shown to elicit harmful cognitive changes: decreased learning, memory, and other features of mental acuity and agility; in humans it is also co-morbid with clinical depression (and one must wonder if this element does not also exist in dogs and cats).

Nociception involves several neurons. The "first-order" neuron transducts tissue damage (mechanical, thermal, chemical, etc.) into a signal that is transmitted via action potential up to the dorsal horn of the spinal cord (the largest cells in the body; its nucleus is in the dorsal root ganglion). There in the dorsal horn, excitatory neurotransmitters are released and carry the signal across a synapse to the "second-order" neuron which then depolarizes and carries an action potential to the brain. The body has intrinsic ways of mitigating pain, through inhibitory neurons that reside in the dorsal horn and those that descend from the brain down to the dorsal horn. It is in the dorsal horn where pain signaling can be modulated; that is, like a rheostat, it can be dialed up or down – either by the body itself or through veterinary interventions.

When pain works correctly, it is both normal and protective; this is often referred to as "adaptive" pain. If pain becomes exaggerated in some way (duration, scope, character, field), it is then said to be "maladaptive." Maladaptive pain occurs through a process called "hypersensitization": a combination of cellular and molecular processes that include lowering firing thresholds of nociceptors, recruitment of "innocent bystander" nociceptors, "cross-talk" with other neurons such as those responsible for touch, pressure, and sympathetic fibers, and diminished inhibitory control. The molecular and cellular changes of hypersensitization occur in both the peripheral tissue and the spinal cord. The result for the patient is pain that is worse than it should be ("hyperalgesia"), normally nonnoxious stimuli like touch now become painful ("allodynia"), odd sensations that accompany the pain ("dysthesias" like tingling, itch, burning, even numbness), a larger area than originally affected is now painful, pain present for longer than expected, and spontaneous pain without any obvious tissue damage present.

Maladaptive pain can occur through a variety of circumstances, but generally includes nerve injury of some type. This injury can be macroscopic and obvious, or microscopic and inobvious. Taken to the extreme, maladaptive pain of any origin becomes "neuropathic," whereby permanent changes are encoded into the peripheral and central nervous system. At this point, pain can be said to be a disease unto itself.

Maladaptive pain and/or pain with a neuropathic component can occur under both heritable and acquired, and acute and chronic circumstances. A partial list of these includes but is not limited to the following.

- CNS injury, including heritable disorders such as Chiari-like malformation (Cavalier King Charles spaniels) and acquired ones such as intervertebral disc disease and other spinal trauma, traumatic nerve injury, e.g., amputation, encephalitides.
- Any severe tissue trauma.
- Persistent postsurgical pain.
- Chronic inflammation: OA, lymphoplasmacytic gingivitis/stomatitis, otitis.
- Visceral: pancreatitis, feline interstitial cystitis ("Pandora syndrome") [2], inflammatory bowel disease, glaucoma.
- Spontaneous/idiopathic: feline hyperesthesia syndrome, feline orofacial pain syndrome.
- In humans, microneuropathies may be caused by diabetes, herpesvirus, and some chemotherapy agents, especially vinca alkaloids; some dogs and cats probably also suffer thus).

2.16.2 Recognition/Assessment of Pain

The IASP stipulates that the inability to communicate (e.g., neonates, the cognitively impaired) does not negate the possibility that an individual is experiencing pain and is in need of appropriate pain-relieving treatment. In humans, pain is what the patient says it is; in animals (as in human neonates and the cognitively impaired), the pain is what we (the veterinary team) say it is.

The astute veterinary team can prompt pet owners' awareness and recognition that their pets are exhibiting either obvious or subtle clinical (or even historical) signs of pain (see 8.13 Team Approach to Pain Management). Observations of poor patient conformation, body position, gait and mobility, or a client report – even just over the phone or other communication – of "stiffness," lameness, or reluctance to perform activities of daily living (including just getting up and down on or off furniture, etc.) can be enough to say "Sounds (or looks) like she may be uncomfortable," followed by one or more of the following.

- We'll have the doctor take a look at that.
- Tell me more about what you are seeing at home.
- Let's see if we can't improve that.

This type of introductory language can help to move the conversation, exam, and management choices forward, which can subsequently have a significant positive impact on patient quality (and perhaps length) of life. It can be initiated by front desk personnel taking calls and watching pets in reception area, technicians and veterinary assistants escorting to the exam room and talking to owners, and animal caretakers interacting with the patients under their care.

In the absence of vocalizing, lameness, and other obvious signs of pain, the veterinary team can be mindful of the following observable changes in body conformation and mobility.

- *Visible conformation*: high body condition score (BCS); kyphosis (bowing up) of back, diminished angle to stifle and hock, obvious muscle atrophy (denotes a patient that has been shifting weight forward for considerable time); cow-hock, base narrow or wide, chondrodyplasia – all evident at a glance.
- Dog sitting "square" or cheating on one hip (likely stifle pain)?
- When stands from a lying position, should be all four legs simultaneously versus rising up first on forelimbs followed by hoisting up the rear quarters.
- Gait if possible – stilted or fluid? Lameness: look for a "quick step" which suggests the contralateral limb is affected; look for classic "wiggle" of rear quarters seen as the dog rotates its pelvis to reduce painful extension of the hip.
- Jumping up or standing on back legs easily, partially, or unable/unwilling?

Several clinical metrology instruments (CMIs) are validated for both dogs and cats to assign scores for acute postsurgical pain (examples: Glasgow Composite Measure Pain Scale for dogs and cats, UNESP-Botucatu Multidimensional Composite Pain Scale for cats). They utilize the domains of observing the patient without interaction (with focus on position in cage, posture, behavior, facial expression), then with interaction (willingness to interact and move), then palpating the incision site. A nonvalidated but simple tool is to apply a global 0–10 score of those domains taken together, whereby 0 is no pain at all and 10 is the worst possible pain *for that procedure*; this is a so-called dynamic interactive visual analog scale (DIVAS) and can be quickly and easily deployed in any practice setting. It can be argued that the most important of those domains is palpation of the surgical site, and if so the simplest assessment method of all would be to assign a 0–4 score based on this maneuver alone.

Several CMIs also exist for chronic OA-related pain and disability in dogs (e.g., Canine Brief Pain Inventory, Liverpool OA in Dogs, Canine OA Staging Tool in Dogs) and cats (e.g., Feline Musculoskeletal Pain Index, Montreal Instrument for Cat Arthritis). These assess various domains of owner- (not veterinarian) observed signs of discomfort and limitations on activities of daily living.

2.16.3 Prevention and Treatment of Pain

Industry guidelines and consensus statements have been published on the highest, wisest, and safest use of modalities to prevent and control surgical and OA-related pain [3, 4]. Additional discussions are available elsewhere (see 6.14 Pain Prevention, Management, and Conditioning, and 8.13 Team Approach to Pain Management). High-level concepts include the following.

2.16.3.1 Acute Postsurgical Pain

1) Anxiolysis, to include both pharmacological and nonpharmacological measures.
   - Anxiolytics such as trazodone and gabapentin administered the morning of surgery, even by the owner at home prior to transport to the hospital.
   - Fear-free experience, low-stress handling, pheromone therapy, comfortable species-specific housing (see 6.6 Fear Free Concepts).
   - Anxiolytic administered as part of in-hospital premedication, e.g., midazolam, dexmedetomidine, acepromazine (when administered with opioids).
2) Opioid – while this remains the most effective drug class for acute pain, veterinary clinicians are advised [5] to follow the shift in human medicine to use fewer opioids, lower doses, shorter frequency, and insofar as possible shift from full mu agonists (morphine, hydromorphone, fentanyl) to partial mu agonists (e.g., buprenorphine) and mu antagonists, kappa-agonist (e.g., butorphanol). Consensus statements support the aggressive use of opioid-sparing strategies (the other modalities discussed in this section), and reserving full mu agonists for the prospectively more painful procedures and patients.
3) Nonsteroidal antiinflammatory drugs (NSAIDs).
4) Local and locoregional anesthetics and techniques – the "missing ingredient" for many if not most surgical procedures in small animal medicine (but not in large animal

or in human medicine); nevertheless industry guidelines stipulate that local anesthetics should be utilized with every surgical procedure (even if just an incisional block but there are dozens of local and locoregional techniques within the scope of any veterinarian – and veterinary technician – to master).

5) Adjunctive pain-modifying medications and modalities: these are deployed with patients undergoing predictably more painful procedures and/or are at higher risk for maladaptive pain, e.g. those with nerve injury, severe trauma (preexisting or surgical, soft tissue or orthopedic), or with long-standing previous pain and inflammation. These include but are not limited to constant-rate infusions of ketamine, systemic lidocaine, dexmedetomidine, oral gabapentin, amantadine, and others.

6) Nonpharmacological interventions such as cold compression, physical rehabilitation, possibly acupuncture, and energy-based modalities such as therapeutic laser, pulsed electromagnetic field, and others.

2.16.3.2 Chronic OA Pain

There are a variety of options for managing the chronic pain of OA (see also 8.20 Team Strategies for Arthritis).

- Weight optimization
- Antiinflammatory agents (NSAIDs and prostaglandin receptor antagonists, PRA)
- Eicosapentaenoic acid-rich (dog), docosahexaenoic acid-rich (cats) diets
- Therapeutic exercise
- Polysulfated glycosaminoglycan and nutritional supplements
- Adjunctive pain-modifying medications (e.g., gabapentin, amantadine)
- Intraarticular (IA) agents such as biologics (stem cells, platelet-rich plasma) and others
- Anti-nerve growth factor (NGF) monoclonal antibody (mAb)

2.16.3.3 Non-OA Chronic Pain

Neoplastic pain, especially osteosarcoma (OSA) and any tumor metastasizing to bone, is generally considered to include a neuropathic component facilitated in part by osteoclastic activity. In palliative care circumstances (e.g., limb-sparing OSA), multiple modalities should be deployed since undercontrolled pain will predicate the decision for humane euthanasia. As cyclooxygenase (COX) enzymes are greatly upregulated in OSA, NSAIDs are appropriate medications to deploy, along with one (or more) adjunctive

pain-modifying oral medications (among the higher effectiveness:safety ratios in human cancer-related pain are anticonvulsants like gabapentin). Oral acetaminophen and opioids are frequently deployed in humans with chronic cancer pain, and can be utilized judiciously in dogs (not cats), but the bioavailability and clinic impact of these drugs have been questioned. Long-acting (days, not weeks) parenteral opioid medications are available for off-label use in dogs and cats. Uniquely in cancer pain, bisphosphonate (pamidronate, zolendronate) infusions freeze osteoclast activity and can elicit durable (approximately one month) improvement in a majority of dogs [6].

Nonneoplastic maladaptive and/or neuropathic pain syndromes described in dogs and cats often have an identifiable cause, but not always; it may be associated with identifiable inflammation, but not always. If an underlying condition is identifiable, it should be managed accordingly. To treat pain directly, if there is a grossly inflammatory component to the condition then antiinflammatory agents (NSAIDs or, when indicated, corticosteroids) can and should be utilized. But if there is no gross inflammation then antiinflammatory agents are unlikely to be beneficial, and one would gravitate to those medications and modalities which address hypersensitization leading to maladaptive and neuropathic pain. Chief among these would be gabapentinoids and possibly amitriptyline, amantadine, serotonin and norepinephrine reuptake inhibitors (e.g., venlafaxine) among others (clinical data limited).

2.16.4 Confounders of Pain

There are a variety of other situations that can complicate the assessment and management of pain in animals.

- *Age*: young, still-growing patients have enormous "plasticity" in their CNS, and early painful experiences can elicit permanent alterations embedded in the CNS and can manifest as increased pain sensitivity later in life. Older patients are often beset by chronic inflammatory processes (OA, gingivitis, otitis, dermatitis) which can elicit a neuropathic component, and whose spinal cord is a "smoldering ember" of hypersensitization upon which a subsequent acutely painful event can cause greatly exaggerated pain.
- *Obesity*: adipose tissue is the body's largest endocrine organ and secretes a witch's brew of proinflammatory cytokines and mediators that circulate systemically and sensitize nociceptors. In humans, excess abdominal fat will double the risk for a chronic pain condition later in life [7].

EXAMPLES

Example 1: Ovariohysterectomy (OHE) in a 5-month-old mixed-breed dog. Client administers trazodone at home prior to transport to hospital. Patient admitted with fear-free and low-stress handling techniques, premedicated with buprenorphine, midazolam intramuscularly (IM), and NSAID of choice orally (PO). Induction of anesthesia, placed on intravenous (IV) fluids, incisional block with bupivacaine. OHE proceeds with lidocaine mesovarium block. Patient discharged with three days of NSAID.

Example 2: Comminuted femoral fracture resulting in hindlimb amputation of 7-year-old cat. Client administers gabapentin and NSAID at home prior to transport to hospital. Patient admitted with fear-free and low-stress handling techniques, premedicated with combination of buprenorphine, dexmedetomidine, and ketamine IM. Induction of anesthesia, placed on IV fluids with ketamine constant rate infusion (CRI), epidural with bupivacaine via lumbosacral or sacral-coccygeal approach. Post-op administered long-acting buprenorphine and discharged with NSAID and gabapentin PO.

Example 3: Cruciate repair surgery in a 6-year-old lab mix. Client administers NSAID and high-dose gabapentin at home prior to transport to hospital. Patient admitted with fear-free and low-stress handling techniques, premedicated with hydromorphone and midazolam IM. Induction of anesthesia includes loading dose of ketamine IV, placed on IV fluids with ketamine CRI. Femoral and sciatic regional nerve block performed with bupivacaine, and IA hydromorphone. Patient prepped and surgery performed. Long-acting (liposome-encapsulated) bupivacaine infused into several layers of closure. Post-op cold compression, continue ketamine ± opioid CRI for 4–6 hours. Patient discharged with NSAID, gabapentin PO, and physical rehabilitation instructions (or referral), to include therapeutic laser if available.

Example 4: 12-year-old golden retriever with a BCS of 7/9 stiff in the mornings and after exercise; owner has to help up onto the couch. Physical exam reveals straight-legged conformation and atrophy rear quarters, discomfort, physical examination, and radiographic signs consistent with hip dysplasia and advancing OA. Priority is to place patient on NSAID or PRA of choice and switched to an EPA-rich diet formulation that also promotes weight loss to BCS of 6 and ultimately a lean 5. If owners agreeable, patient is also placed on polysulfated glycosaminoglycan, or alternatively, a high-quality and reputable nutraceutical;

exercise program implemented that includes vigorous walks and inclines but unrestricted activity is limited. If and when eventually deemed appropriate and available, choice (and/or combination of) pain-modifying analgesic medication (e.g., amantadine, gabapentin) is prescribed as adjunct to the NSAID or PRA, IA biologic injections, and anti-NGF mAb treatments are implemented. Acupuncture, therapeutic laser, pulsed electromagnetic field, myofascial trigger point, referral for aggressive physical rehabilitation, and other nonpharmacological modalities can be utilized at any time.

TAKE-AWAYS

- Underrecognized and undermanaged pain inflicts very real physiological and medical consequences, resulting in significant patient morbidity and in the extreme can contribute to mortality.
- Through the process of peripheral and central hypersensitization ("wind-up"), pain becomes maladaptive, exaggerated in scope, severity, character, duration, and field; a number of factors will place a patient at risk for maladaptive pain, including (but not limited to) nerve injury, severe trauma, chronic inflammation, heritable tendency.
- Assessment of both acute postsurgical and chronic OA-related pain is possible with validated CMIs.
- Evidence-based industry guidelines and consensus statements are available to direct veterinary clinicians to the highest, wisest, safest multimodal strategies for acute and chronic pain.
- Veterinarians are advised to adopt the emerging trend of reducing, full mu agonist opioid usage, insofar as possible and still maintain patient comfort, in favor of buprenorphine and butorphanol along with multiple opioid-sparing modalities and strategies.

MISCELLANEOUS

2.16.5 Cautions

With an aggressive multimodal approach to peri-perative pain management, anesthetic requirements may be significantly reduced; adjust induction doses and vaporizer settings accordingly.

Abbreviation

BCS   Body condition score

References

1 Bonica, J.J. (1979). International for the study of pain: pain definition. The need of a taxonomy. *Pain* 6 (3): 247–248.

2 Tony Buffington, C.A., Westropp, J.L., and Chew, D.J. (2014). From FUS to Pandora syndrome: where are we, how did we get here, and where to now? *J. Feline Med. Surg.* 16 (5): 385–394.

3 Mathews, K., Kronen, P.W., Lascelles, D. et al. (2014). Guidelines for recognition, assessment and treatment of pain: WSAVA Global Pain Council. *J. Small Anim. Pract.* 55 (6): E10–E68.

4 Epstein, M., Rodan, I., Griffenhagen, G. et al. (2015). 2015 AAHA/AAFP pain management guidelines for dogs and cats. *J. Am. Anim. Hosp. Assoc.* 51 (2): 67–84.

5 Muir, W.W., Berry, J., Boothe, D.M., et al. (2018). Opioid-Sparing Pain Therapy in Animals: Working Task Force. https://ivapm.org/wp-content/uploads/2018/12/Op-Sparring-Task-Force-WP.pdf

6 Fan, T.M., de Lorimier, L.P., O'Dell-Anderson, K. et al. (2007). Single-agent pamidronate for palliative therapy of canine appendicular osteosarcoma bone pain. *J. Vet. Intern. Med.* 21 (3): 431–439.

7 Ray, L., Lipton, R.B., Zimmerman, M.E. et al. (2011). Mechanisms of association between obesity and chronic pain in the elderly. *Pain* 152 (1): 53–59.

Recommended Reading

Rodan, I., Sundahl, E., and Carney, H. (2011). AAFP and ISFM feline-friendly handling guidelines. *J. Feline Med. Surg.* 13 (5): 364–375.et al., for the American Animal Hospital Association

Yin, S. (2009). *Low Stress Handling, Restraint and Behavior Modification of Dogs and Cats: Techniques for Developing Patients Who Love Their Visits*. Davis, CA: Cattledog Publishing.

2.17

Emergency Preparedness

Lori Massin Teller, DVM, BS (Vet Sci), DABVP (Canine/Feline Practice)

Department of Small Animal Clinical Sciences, College of Veterinary Medicine & Biomedical Sciences, Texas A&M University, College Station, TX, USA

BASICS

2.17.1 Summary

Disasters, man-made or natural, can be devastating. Lives can be disrupted or lost, property damaged or destroyed. It is important to prepare yourself, your family, your clients, and your practice ahead of time for a disaster. There are some disasters that you may be forewarned about, such as hurricanes or blizzards. Others may happen without warning, such as earthquakes, tornadoes, fires, or terrorist attacks. Disaster plans should include contingencies for both local emergencies, such as a building fire or flooding from a burst water main, as well as a community-wide event, such as a chemical spill or massive flooding from a hurricane or wind damage from a tornado. It is vitally important that veterinary practices have a written disaster plan to cover emergency relocation of animals, back-up of medical records, continuity of operations, security, fire prevention, and insurance and legal issues.

2.17.2 Terms Defined

Incident Command System (ICS): Defined command and control system to manage the emergency. Activities of all responding agencies and people are coordinated through the ICS.

MAIN CONCEPTS

For disasters in which there is forewarning, such as hurricanes or blizzards, it is important for veterinarians and staff to have their personal preparations, including plans for family, animals, and property, stabilized before they can focus on the business. Take care of self, then family, then the practice, then others to ensure a successful disaster response.

For practices affected by a disaster, first and foremost there needs to be an evacuation plan for people and animals. Identify locations outside the danger zone to which animals can be relocated. These locations may need to be in multiple directions and at varying distances from the practice. If the disaster is contained to the practice facility, then animals may be located to a building next door or down the street. A disaster that affects the neighborhood, such as a chemical spill, may require relocating animals several miles away. Partner with other practices with a reciprocity agreement and/or contact local community centers. Determine ahead of time where animals will be placed within these facilities, so that dogs and cats can be separated, and animals requiring medical attention can be placed in a makeshift ward away from those which just need their basic needs met. Be prepared ahead of time for the evacuation by having plenty of leashes, carriers, and feeding supplies. Prearrange transportation to the facility. Make sure each animal has some sort of identification (ID). Have a contact list of animal owners available, preferably stored offsite. This may be part of medical records and practice management information that is stored in a remote location, not on the premises.

It can be complicated when local practices become a holding place for displaced animals that come in without an identified owner. There is not an established veterinarian client–patient relationship (VCPR) to allow for anything beyond emergency treatment or for disposal of the animal after a set time if an owner never comes forward. This comes with the potential for significant expense and legal liability risks. These expenses are not likely to be reimbursed by emergency services (such as Federal

Emergency Management Administration [FEMA] in the United States) or other governmental entity. Local veterinarians should encourage their city or county to have a disaster plan that includes the handling and housing of displaced animals. Veterinarians should be included in the larger local or state government's disaster planning, and a veterinarian should have a role in the ICS.

Disaster planning needs to include preparation for continuity of operations. It is possible that the facility may still be useable, but local utilities may not be functioning. Plans need to be in place for communication; power, including a fuel source; refrigeration; food and water, in case local supplies are contaminated; and medications and supplies.

If the facility is not safe for use, then contact an unaffected practice to use as an alternate location until the facility can repaired, replaced, or relocated. This can help eliminate the need for your clients to seek services elsewhere and avoid a gap in animal care. Also make sure the inoperable facility is safe from further damage, such as looting or theft, and remove or secure dangerous drugs and hazardous supplies. Contact insurance carriers and be sure to video and photograph inventory and damages. Insurance coverage to have in place before a disaster occurs includes property, flood/wind/fire/earthquake as appropriate for the practice location, business interruption, professional extension, loss of income, mobile loss of income (if applicable), civil ordinance coverage, debris removal/clean-up, building replacement with automatic inflation, workers' compensation, and general and professional liability.

Something that many veterinarians overlook is the importance of regular practice drills. Everyone in the practice should be involved, and the drills should include everything from identifying where fire extinguishers are located to simulated evacuation. Identify where the weak spots in the plan are and correct those, so that when a true emergency occurs, the team is ready to act appropriately.

2.17.3 Pet-Specific Advice for Clients

It is very important for the veterinary healthcare team to ensure clients are prepared for their pets in times of an emergency. Clients should have an up-to-date copy of medical records, including vaccinations and the names of any medications the animal may be taking. Clients will need to have crates and/or leashes and collars to safely transport their pets. It is of vital importance that each animal has permanent ID, such as a microchip, and to make sure contact information is current in a national microchip database. It is a good idea for the pet to also wear a collar with an ID tag, but these sometimes fall off or become damaged.

Keep a pet first aid kit handy, containing basic supplies to clean and cover wounds, pain medication as recommended by a veterinarian, a muzzle to help limit biting if the pet is in severe distress, and any medications that the pet may take regularly. Clients should keep several days' worth of food and fresh water on hand to be used in case of shelter-in-place orders or when evacuation is required.

Whenever possible, it is a good idea to have knowledge of several evacuation routes ahead of time and identify pet-friendly lodging along those routes. Sometimes clients will have to go to an emergency shelter that also allows pets. Having medical records, medications, food, and water ready to go will make the evacuation less stressful. Individuals may be less likely to evacuate if they are uncertain they can bring their pets with them, including those in abusive relationships. They may not volunteer this information to veterinary teams, so having resources available in print form and on the website may help save lives.

EXAMPLES

XYZ Animal Care Clinic is located in Smithville, a small town by the Missouri River. Because of some strong winter storms in more northern locales, the residents of Smithville have been forewarned to expect massive flooding in the next few days. The doctors and staff at XYZ implement their disaster plan. First, all employees make sure their families, pets, and personal property are secured. Those who can return to work to prepare the clinic do so. Pet owners are called and asked to pick up their animals. Those dogs and cats that require ongoing care and cannot be discharged are transferred to a colleague's office several miles away from the expected impact zone, and the clients are notified of the transfers. The practice manager confirms that all insurance policies are current and that the medical records are backed up offsite. The practice owner secures dangerous drugs and controlled substances. The staff secure valuable equipment, such as anesthesia monitors and lab equipment, at an elevated height. Two staff members volunteer to stay overnight to monitor the situation. Supplies, such as food and bottled water, as well as a couple of sleeping bags and air mattresses, are provided. Because the clinic does not have a generator, the practice manager acquires a portable one and several tanks of extra propane to use if the clinic ends up without power following the flood event. A communication plan is put into place.

Once the flood event is over, the veterinarians and staff assess the damage. The building has minor flood damage in a couple of exam rooms and the surgical suite. The town, including the clinic, lost power for several days. XYZ Animal Care Clinic moves to the postdisaster phase of its plan. They determine that they can still see patients in the undamaged exam rooms and also create a temporary exam room in one of the doctors' offices. Because of the generator, they are able to maintain electricity keep the lights on and the refrigerator running. The doctors arrange to use the surgical suite at a colleague's clinic one day each week to meet client needs. More urgent procedures are referred. The practice manager contacts the necessary insurance companies and immediately starts repairs to the damaged areas. XYZ is fully operational six months after the flood event.

TAKE-AWAYS

- Make sure all doctors and staff have their personal needs taken care of – family, pets, property – so then they can focus on the veterinary practice.
- Have a disaster plan for a localized event – building fire, water damage from burst pipe, etc.
- Have a disaster plan for a regional event – earthquake, hurricane, massive fire, chemical spill, etc.
- Keep supplies ready for evacuation, shelter-in-place orders, and postdisaster needs.

- Maintain all necessary documents for medical records, practice management, and insurance needs.

MISCELLANEOUS

2.17.4 Cautions

Some disasters come without warning. Having a plan in place and using practice drills on a regular basis will help mitigate the effects. Identify leaders ahead of time who can stay calm and think on their feet to help the practice survive the disaster and its aftermath.

Recommended Reading

American Red Cross Pet Disaster Preparedness: www. redcross.org/get-help/how-to-prepare-for-emergencies/ pet-disaster-preparedness.html

AVMA Disaster Resource Center: www.avma.org/KB/ Resources/Reference/disaster/Pages/default.aspx

AVMA Professional Liability Insurance Trust, Disaster Planning for Veterinary Practices: www.avmaplit.com/ education-center/library/disaster-planning

2.18

Population Control

Ryane E. Englar, DVM, DABVP (Canine and Feline Practice)

College of Veterinary Medicine, University of Arizona, Oro Valley, AZ, USA

BASICS

2.18.1   Summary

The need to reproductively manage owned and feral dogs and cats is the driving force behind gonadectomy. Excision of sex organs (neutering, desexing) prevents procreation, which is of particular importance when considering the sheer numbers of animals that are relinquished to animal shelters annually. There is only so much room to accommodate new arrivals, and traditional shelters are often forced to euthanize otherwise healthy patients in the face of space constraints. Sterilization surgery is considered the norm in North American dogs and cats, and is increasingly performed at young ages to (i) prevent breeding of adopted dogs, and (ii) potentially reduce behaviors that may lead to relinquishment. Early-age gonadectomy is not without risk, which has led to increasing interest in reversible contraception, as opposed to the traditional ovariohysterectomy (OVH) and castration. These methods run the gamut from extra-label use of human contraceptives to intratesticular injections.

2.18.2   Terms Defined

Gonadectomy: Technically, surgical removal of an ovary or testis; colloquially, this term often refers to excision of the reproductive tract and is therefore synonymous with ovariohysterectomy or castration.

Orchiectomy: Surgical excision of both testicles; synonymous with the term castration

Ovariectomy (OVE):   Surgical removal of one or both ovaries, leaving the uterus intact.

Ovariohysterectomy: Surgical excision of the ovaries and uterus.

Reversible Contraception: A method of preventing pregnancy that does not result in permanent sterilization, such that if pregnancy is desired at a later point, removal of this method makes this physiological state possible.

MAIN CONCEPTS

2.18.3   The Reason for Sterilization

The primary purpose of gonadectomy is to manage canine and feline populations [1]. American animal shelters collectively report an estimated intake of 6.5 million companion animals annually [2]. Permanent sterilization prevents unplanned pregnancies that yield unwanted litters, which ultimately end up at shelters [3–7].

The majority of American veterinarians advocate for elective sterilization surgery [8]. Most American dogs and cats undergo elective OVH or castration within their first year of life. The recommended age for such surgeries often varies with breed, stage of growth, and underlying risks for potential medicals conditions, such as inherited orthopedic problems.

Gonadectomy reduces the risk for mammary neoplasia, particularly if females are spayed before the first heat cycle [6, 9–14]. Male dogs that are castrated are less likely to develop hormone-dependent benign prostatic hypertrophy (BPH) [9].

Neutering also curbs unfavorable behaviors: castrated male dogs roam, mount, and urine-mark less frequently, and male cats are less likely to spray [9, 15].

2.18.4 The Rise of Pediatric Neutering

Waiting to sterilize patients until they are 6 months of age or older runs the risk that they will reach sexual maturity and procreate. Because of this concern, pediatric neutering is on the rise. Shelters also do not wish to adopt out intact patients that then may reproduce, particularly since unwanted litters are often relinquished back to shelters [1, 7, 9].

In an effort to break this cycle, OVH and castration are now routinely performed at 6–16 weeks of age [4, 6, 8, 9]. Safe anesthetic protocols have been established and patients that undergo early-age gonadectomy experience fewer perioperative complications [9, 16, 17].

2.18.5 Ovariectomy Versus Ovariohysterectomy

Ovariohysterectomy is the standard sterilization surgery for bitches and queens in the US. Removing the uterus prevents uterine pathology [18]. However, uterine tumors are infrequent. Most that occur are benign and surgery is curative [18].

Ovariectomy has replaced OVH in the Netherlands and much of Europe. Because OVE spares the uterus, the procedure is associated with smaller incisions. OVE may also be performed as a minimally invasive technique using laparoscopy [19].

2.18.6 Alternatives to Permanent Sterilization

Because permanent sterilization is not considered medically or ethically appropriate by all nations and cultures, research interest in reversible contraception has grown [6, 20]. Synthetic progestins, such as megestrol acetate (MA) and medroxyprogesterone acetate (MPA), may be administered to suppress follicle-stimulating hormone (FSH) and luteinizing hormone (LH), without which follicles will not mature to ovulation [3, 21]. Adverse effects may be significant, particularly in cats [21, 22].

Other methods of reversible contraception that are being explored include [3, 21, 23–32]:

- prolonged exposure to gonadotropin-releasing hormone (GnRH) agonists
- canine intrauterine devices (IUDs)

- chemical castration with intratesticular injectable agents such as arginine stabilized zinc gluconate, chlorhexidine digluconate, calcium chloride admixed with dimethyl sulfoxide, etc
- mechanical castration, using ultrasound to induce testicular necrosis
- vaccinations against LH and GnRH, spermatozoa, or zona pellucida proteins
- melatonin implants.

 EXAMPLES

Toblerone is a 1-year-old intact female Great Dane that presents to you for elective surgical sterilization. Given the breed's predisposition to gastric-dilation volvulus (GDV), the client is interested in prophylactic gastropexy at the time of OVH. However, he worries about intraoperative hemorrhage and the large incision. You indicate that there is an alternative to the traditional laparotomy that is required to perform both procedures. You suggest that the patient undergoes laparoscopic OVE and gastropexy.

 TAKE-AWAYS

- Pet overpopulation is a global, multifaceted, animal welfare issue.
- Sterilization surgery is considered the standard of care in the US as a means of population control.
- Early-age gonadectomy is increasingly common given that safe anesthetic protocols have been developed.
- The desire for less invasive procedures has led to the successful adoption of OVE in other countries.
- Research is growing in the area of reversible contraception.

 MISCELLANEOUS

2.18.7 Cautions

Gonadectomy is not without risk. Surgical complication rates vary from study to study; however, as many as 6.1–27% of bitches and 2.6–33% of queens experience postoperative complications [9, 33].

Obesity is common among neutered dogs and cats [6, 10]. In addition, neutered dogs are at greater risk of developing:

- prostatic neoplasia [6]
- transitional cell carcinoma (TCC) [34, 35]
- osteosarcoma [36, 37]
- cranial cruciate ligament rupture (CCLR) [14].

Timing of gonadectomy may also influence a patient's predisposition to orthopedic disease [6, 14]. A recent study of 1842 dogs suggests that dogs neutered before 5 months of age have an increased incidence of hip dysplasia [4, 14].

Interest in reversible contraceptive methods continues to build but its efficacy and the potential for adverse effects remain concerns.

References

1 Farnworth, M.J., Adams, N.J., Seksel, K. et al. (2013). Veterinary attitudes towards pre-pubertal gonadectomy of cats: a comparison of samples from New Zealand, Australia and the United Kingdom. *N. Z. Vet. J.* 61: 226–233.

2 Pet Statistics. (2019). www.aspca.org/animal-homelessness/shelter-intake-and-surrender/pet-statistics

3 Asa, C.S. (2018). Contraception in dogs and cats. *Vet. Clin. North Am. Small Anim. Pract.* 48: 733–742.

4 Spain, C.V., Scarlett, J.M., and Houpt, K.A. (2004). Long-term risks and benefits of early-age gonadectomy in dogs. *J. Am. Vet. Med. Assoc.* 224: 380–387.

5 Lieberman, L.L. (1987). A case for neutering pups and kittens at two months of age. *J. Am. Vet. Med. Assoc.* 191: 518–521.

6 Kustritz, M.V.R. (2007). Determining the optimal age for gonadectomy of dogs and cats. *J. Am. Vet. Med. Assoc.* 231: 1665–1675.

7 Alexander, S.A. and Shane, S.M. (1994). Characteristics of animals adopted from an animal control center whose owners complied with a spaying/neutering program. *J. Am. Vet. Med. Assoc.* 205: 472–476.

8 Spain, C.V., Scarlett, J.M., and Cully, S.M. (2002). When to neuter dogs and cats: a survey of New York state veterinarians' practices and beliefs. *J. Am. Anim. Hosp. Assoc.* 38: 482–488.

9 Kustritz, M.V.R. (2014). Pros, cons, and techniques of pediatric neutering. *Vet. Clin. North Am. Small Anim. Pract.* 44: 221–233.

10 Reichler, I.M. (2009). Gonadectomy in cats and dogs: a review of risks and benefits. *Reprod. Domest. Anim.* 44: 29–35.

11 Schneider, R., Dorn, C.R., and Taylor, D.O. (1969). Factors influencing canine mammary cancer development and postsurgical survival. *J. Natl. Cancer Inst.* 43: 1249–1261.

12 Hayes, H.M. Jr., Milne, K.L., and Mandell, C.P. (1981). Epidemiological features of feline mammary carcinoma. *Vet. Rec.* 108: 476–479.

13 Misdorp, W. (1988). Canine mammary tumours: protective effect of late ovariectomy and stimulating effect of progestins. *Vet. Q.* 10: 26–33.

14 Reichler, I.M. (2009). Gonadectomy in cats and dogs: a review of risks and benefits. *Reprod. Domest. Anim.* 44 (Suppl 2): 29–35.

15 Kustritz, M.V.R. (1996). Elective gonadectomy in the cat. *Feline Pract.* 24: 36–39.

16 Faggella, A.M. and Aronsohn, M.G. (1994). Evaluation of anesthetic protocols for neutering 6- to 14-week-old pups. *J. Am. Vet. Med. Assoc.* 205: 308–314.

17 Howe, L.M. (1997). Short-term results and complications of prepubertal gonadectomy in cats and dogs. *J. Am. Vet. Med. Assoc.* 211: 57–62.

18 van Goethem, B., Schaefers-Okkens, A., and Kirpensteijn, J. (2006). Making a rational choice between ovariectomy and ovariohysterectomy in the dog: a discussion of the benefits of either technique. *Vet. Surg.* 35: 136–143.

19 DeTora, M. and McCarthy, R.J. (2011). Ovariohysterectomy versus ovariectomy for elective sterilization of female dogs and cats: is removal of the uterus necessary? *J. Am. Vet. Med. Assoc.* 239: 1409–1412.

20 Salmeri, K.R., Bloomberg, M.S., Scruggs, S.L. et al. (1991). Gonadectomy in immature dogs: effects on skeletal, physical, and behavioral development. *J. Am. Vet. Med. Assoc.* 198: 1193–1203.

21 Goericke-Pesch, S. (2010). Reproduction control in cats: new developments in non-surgical methods. *J. Feline Med. Surg.* 12: 539–546.

22 Agudelo, C.F. (2005). Cystic endometrial hyperplasia-pyometra complex in cats. A review. *Vet. Q.* 27: 173–182.

23 Volpe, P., Izzo, B., Russo, M. et al. (2001). Intrauterine device for contraception in dogs. *Vet. Rec.* 149: 77–79.

24 Wiebe, V.J. and Howard, J.P. (2009). Pharmacologic advances in canine and feline reproduction. *Top. Compan. Anim. Med.* 24: 71–99.

25 Kutzler, M. and Wood, A. (2006). Non-surgical methods of contraception and sterilization. *Theriogenology* 66: 514–525.

26 Levy, J.K., Crawford, P.C., Appel, L.D. et al. (2008). Comparison of intratesticular injection of zinc gluconate versus surgical castration to sterilize male dogs. *Am. J. Vet. Res.* 69: 140–143.

27 Oliveira, E.C., Fagundes, A.K., Melo, C.C. et al. (2013). Intratesticular injection of a zinc-based solution for

contraception of domestic cats: a randomized clinical trial of efficacy and safety. *Vet. J.* 197: 307–310.

28 Oliveira, E.C., Moura, M.R., de Sa, M.J. et al. (2012). Permanent contraception of dogs induced with intratesticular injection of a zinc gluconate-based solution. *Theriogenology* 77: 1056–1063.

29 Massei, G. and Miller, L.A. (2013). Nonsurgical fertility control for managing free-roaming dog populations: a review of products and criteria for field applications. *Theriogenology* 80: 829–838.

30 Fagundes, A.K., Oliveira, E.C., Tenorio, B.M. et al. (2014). Injection of a chemical castration agent, zinc gluconate, into the testes of cats results in the impairment of spermatogenesis: a potentially irreversible contraceptive approach for this species? *Theriogenology* 81: 230–236.

31 Vanderstichel, R., Forzan, M.J., Perez, G.E. et al. (2015). Changes in blood testosterone concentrations after surgical and chemical sterilization of male free-roaming dogs in southern Chile. *Theriogenology* 83: 1021–1027.

32 Paranzini, C.S., Sousa, A.K., Cardoso, G.S. et al. (2018). Effects of chemical castration using 20% $CaCl_2$ with 0.5% DMSO in tomcats: evaluation of inflammatory reaction by infrared thermography and effectiveness of treatment. *Theriogenology* 106: 253–258.

33 Pollari, F.L., Bonnett, B.N., Bamsey, S.C. et al. (1996). Postoperative complications of elective surgeries in dogs and cats determined by examining electronic and paper medical records. *J. Am. Vet. Med. Assoc.* 208: 1882–1886.

34 Knapp, D.W., Glickman, N.W., Denicola, D.B. et al. (2000). Naturally-occurring canine transitional cell carcinoma of the urinary bladder a relevant model of human invasive bladder cancer. *Urol. Oncol.* 5: 47–59.

35 Norris, A.M., Laing, E.J., Valli, V.E. et al. (1992). Canine bladder and urethral tumors: a retrospective study of 115 cases (1980–1985). *J. Vet. Intern. Med.* 6: 145–153.

36 Priester, W.A. and McKay, F.W. (1980). The occurrence of tumors in domestic animals. *Natl. Cancer Inst. Monogr.*: 1–210.

37 Ru, G., Terracini, B., and Glickman, L.T. (1998). Host related risk factors for canine osteosarcoma. *Vet. J.* 156: 31–39.

Recommended Reading

Asa, C.S. (2018). Contraception in dogs and cats. *Vet. Clin. North Am. Small Anim. Pract.* 48: 733–742.

Goerick-Pesch, S. (2010). Reproduction control in cats: new developments in non-surgical methods. *J. Feline Med. Surg.* 12: 539–546.

Kustritz, M.V. (2014). Pros, cons, and techniques of pediatric neutering. *Vet. Clin. North Am. Small Anim. Pract.* 44: 221–233.

Wiebe, V.J. (2009). Pharmacologic advances in canine and feline reproduction. *Top. Compan. Anim. Med.* 24 (2): 71–99.

2.19

One Health

Donna L. Harris, DVM, MBA, MS(Strategic Foresight)

College of Veterinary Medicine, Michigan State University, East Lansing, MI, USA

 BASICS

The veterinary healthcare team (VHT) is on the front line of the intersection of animals and the people in their lives, and the One Health concept recognizes the interconnection between people, animals, and the environment they share. The VHT has the responsibility to recognize and educate clients about the effects (both good and bad) that come with owning, caring, and living with animals. Sometimes this responsibility extends to collaborating with other healthcare fields to achieve the best outcomes.

2.19.1 Terms Defined

Ecosystem: A system that includes all the organisms and their interactions with each other and the environment around them.
One Health: A concept or an approach that recognizes the interconnection between people, animals, and the environment and has a goal of optimal health for each.
Zoonotic disease: A disease caused by an agent that can pass between animals and people.

 MAIN CONCEPTS

The One Health concept has been evident in literature as far back as ancient times when priests and healers cared for people and animals [1]. Because our ecosystem is shared so closely between people and animals, the actions of one affect the actions of the other (Figure 2.19.1). Because of these close connections, caring for one aspect of this system means caring for all.

Animal owners come to the VHT for advice and education on keeping their pets healthy but because of these close connections, it also means keeping people and the environment healthy. The VHT should be knowledgeable about how their actions fit into the larger picture of the human/animal environment.

As pets have moved from sleeping in the yard, then the house and now, for some, the bedroom, the One Health concept has taken on more relevance. Living in close proximity with animals allows easy sharing of microbes, viruses, parasites, and toxins. In addition, animal-loving people often take action when any animal needs help, not realizing that their actions might expose themselves (and their own pets) to potentially harmful consequences. In extreme cases, the VHT might need to work with other

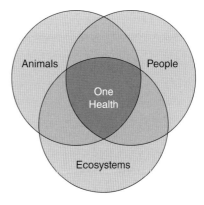

Figure 2.19.1 A graphic representation of the One Health concept.

Pet-Specific Care for the Veterinary Team, First Edition. Edited by Lowell Ackerman.
© 2021 John Wiley & Sons, Inc. Published 2021 by John Wiley & Sons, Inc.

healthcare professionals to manage a situation or uncover the cause of an illness. Examples of some of the ways in which the three systems interact are with zoonotic diseases, antibiotic use, home-made diets, and interaction with wildlife and stray animals.

2.19.2   Zoonotic Diseases

Zoonotic diseases are those that can pass between people and animals (see 4.3 Prevention and Control of Infectious Diseases). These can be microbes, viruses or parasites. Clients are often shocked to learn that the worms in their puppy's or kitten's intestines can be passed to themselves or their children. People with compromised immune systems and children are most at risk from getting sick from their animals. Worms are just one example of parasites that can affect people. External parasites like fleas, ticks, and mites can also be transmitted to people. Viruses and bacteria can also be shared between people and animals. Veterinary staff need to be aware of these potential risks and encourage owners to practice good habits that prevent transfer of disease. Simple habits such as good hand washing and keeping animal wastes out of children's play areas are helpful for clients to learn from the VHT. Regular visits to a veterinary clinic for deworming and flea and tick control medications should be encouraged. Healthy animals are much less likely to transmit diseases and parasites.

For the VHT to be effective, clients should be asked appropriate questions that might uncover connections. Open-ended questions to be posed might include:

- How is everyone else in the family feeling?
- Have you had any visiting pets or people?

- Has your pet been anywhere other than home?
- Where does your pet eliminate and how do you manage his (her) waste?

More important is what the VHT does with the answers given by clients. The workplace should have resources available to help team members make appropriate recommendations and provide education to clients. Table 2.19.1 contains some resources for educational material.

2.19.3   Antibiotic Usage

Another connection between human and animal health is the use and misuse of antibiotics (see 9.12 Judicious Use of Antimicrobials). A world without effective antibiotics is scary to imagine, but the number of bacteria resistant to antibiotics is growing and an educated VHT can be effective in educating clients about some of the causes. Antibiotics are only effective against bacteria, but some clients believe they are the cure-all for all illnesses. Antibiotic use should be restricted for appropriate bacterial diseases and education by the VHT will help clients understand this use. In addition, it is important for clients to finish using antibiotics as prescribed and not "save some for later." Clients will sometimes "try" medications that they've saved from previous use. Indiscriminate use of antibiotics contributes to the resistance problem as well. Preventing this type of antibiotic abuse takes effective communication skills by the VHT, including follow-up questions such as "Were you able to give all the medication?" It's easy to become frustrated with clients' behavior but most owners simply do not know or understand the consequences of their actions. They need education from the VHT.

Table 2.19.1   One Health resources

Resource	URL
Centers for Disease Control: One Health	www.cdc.gov/onehealth/
Public Health England: Zoonotic diseases	www.gov.uk/government/publications/list-of-zoonotic-diseases/list-of-zoonotic-diseases
Centers for Disease Control: Zoonotic Diseases	www.cdc.gov/ncezid
Herp Care Collection: Zoonotic Diseases	www.anapsid.org/worell.html
Centers for Disease Control: Antibiotic Use	www.cdc.gov/antibiotic-use
AVMA Wildlife Decision Tree	www.avma.org/resources-tools/one-health/wildlife-decision-tree
FDA Safe Food Handling	www.fda.gov/Food/ResourcesForYou/Consumers/ucm255180.htm
Centers for Disease Control: Healthy Pets, Healthy People	www.cdc.gov/healthypets/index.html

2.19.4 Home-Made Diets

Clients love their pets and want the best for them, sometimes disregarding their own safety. A distrust of commercial pet foods has led some clients to make their own pet food or sometimes veterinarians recommend homemade diets for pets with specific medical conditions. Regardless of why a client decides to make their pet's diet, handling the food properly, especially raw meat, is important for everyone in the home. Clients who embark on preparing pet foods need to be educated on proper food handling, cooking, and storage methods. They need to consider the source of their raw materials, where they are preparing the diets, and the best cleaning methods after cooking. VHTs should have good resources readily available for these clients and not hesitate to engage them in conversations. Poor food practices will endanger the pet, the owner, and especially children in the home.

2.19.5 Special Consideration for Exotic Pets and Wildlife

Clients with a love for exotic pets pose a unique challenge for VHTs. Some clients enjoy the uniqueness of owning unusual animals, including buying, selling, and breeding them. If the VHT is going to serve these clients, they need to educate themselves on the unique threats some of these species hold for people, including an increased risk of *Salmonella*, the threat of foreign animal diseases from newly imported animals, and handling the unique diets required by some. By understanding the unique issues these pets and clients have, team members can make handling, housing, and quarantine recommendations.

Wildlife poses a unique threat to pets and people. Some interactions cannot be anticipated but the most common threats come from clients with big hearts! As animal lovers, clients are often the first people to offer safe havens to stray pets and injured wildlife. If clients contact the veterinary office for advice, VHTs must be ready with references and safety advice. Wildlife often carry internal and external parasites that are potential threats to both humans and pets. Pets should be kept from "meeting" visiting wildlife or stray animals. In addition, team members should advise clients to safely transfer the wildlife to skilled, licensed rehabilitators. Sometimes, government laws dictate who can house and help wildlife.

2.19.6 Veterinary Healthcare Team Strategies

There is so much to consider when trying to educate clients about pet healthcare and safety, it's hard to be an expert in all areas. Rather than trying to "know" everything, team members should develop areas of expertise at least in the resources available. For example, one team member could have in-depth knowledge of reptile zoonotic diseases and the resources to use when questions arise. Another team member would understand the potential hazards for homemade diets and be able to consult with clients who wish (or need) to feed this way. A bit of knowledge with strong, credible resources can go a long way to keep clients and pets safe without contaminating the ecosystem.

EXAMPLES

The Joy family has two indoor cats and a terrier mix who is a house dog but also enjoys the outdoors. On a recent hike in the neighboring woods, the family came across a friendly puppy with no collar. Of course, they picked him up and brought him home to see if they could find the owner. Although the puppy had several areas of hair loss and was scratching itself, they didn't worry because their own dog had a mild case of demodicosis as a puppy and they remembered their veterinarian saying it is rarely transferable to people. They called the veterinarian's office to see if they knew of anyone that had recently lost a puppy, but were told to call the local humane society. No other issues were discussed.

After a week, the family hadn't found the puppy's owner and took the puppy to the humane society. By now, the family's dog was itching and starting to lose fur. After a veterinary visit, he was diagnosed with sarcoptic mange, likely acquired from the visiting stray puppy. Unlike *Demodex* mites, sarcoptic mites can be easily spread to other animals and people. Now all the family members were at risk. This situation might have been prevented if the staff at the veterinary hospital had advised the owners to keep the puppy isolated from the house and the other pets and children.

Mr Bay raises beagle puppies for hunting and typically takes very good care of them. He is concerned about one of the puppies he has decided to keep. The puppy is staggering and not eating well. Although the technician knows Mr Bay and all about how he raises puppies, she quizzes him about the puppy's diet, travels, and where he has been keeping him. Because of the thoroughness of her questioning, it is revealed that Mr Bay recently discovered a family of raccoons in one of his barns where the puppy plays. The veterinary team warn the owner of the risk of roundworms from the raccoon's feces, as well as rabies. They also educate him about the zoonotic potential of both of these diseases. The owner chooses euthanasia of the puppy and a necropsy confirms neurological migration of *Baylisascaris procyonis* (raccoon roundworms).

TAKE-AWAYS

- The VHT is a vitally important connection for keeping pets, people, and the ecosystem healthy.
- VHT members need to be aware of potential zoonotic diseases that will affect their clients and patients and educate clients appropriately.

- Clients preparing home-made pet diets need special instruction in safe food handling practices.
- The VHT plays an important role in preventing the misuse of antibiotics, which contributes to antibiotic resistance.
- Clients need education from the VHT about handling exotic animals and wildlife to be safe from zoonotic diseases.

MISCELLANEOUS

Reference

1 Schwabe, C.W. (1984). *Veterinary Medicine and Human Health*. Baltimore.: Williams & Wilkins.

2.20

Cancer Precision Medicine

Anna Katogiritis, BSc, DVM[1] and Chand Khanna, DVM, PhD, DACVIM (Onc), DACVP (Hon)[2]

[1] *Independent SA and Wildlife Emergency Veterinarian and NGO Consultant, USA*
[2] *Ethos Veterinary Health, Woburn, MA, USA*

BASICS

2.20.1 Summary

Cancer is a disease of dysregulated genes. Personalized cancer medicine (Pmed) is a therapeutic approach to pet-specific care that most often analyzes the molecular features of a patient's cancer, and uses this information to design treatment plans that target critical genetic alterations in that patient's tumor. In so doing, this field hopes to select approaches that may more specifically target cancer cells. This approach may also allow rapid alterations in treatment in response to patient-specific drug resistance signals that emerge during therapy and individualize monitoring of therapeutic responses. It is nearly certain that aspects of this overriding Pmed approach represent the future of cancer medicine.

2.20.2 Terms Defined

Genome: This term refers to an organism's complete sequence of DNA.
Genomics: A field of molecular biology that focuses on the structure, function, mapping, and evolution of the genome.
Mutations: Permanent alterations in the DNA sequence. These can occur due to mistakes that arise during the DNA replication process, environmental factors (e.g., ultraviolet light), or infections (e.g., viruses).
Precision Cancer Medicine: An emerging field in oncology and molecular biology through which a patient's cancer is analyzed to a molecular level with the goal of identifying unique characteristics (most often specific

mutations) that may respond more favorably to specific (targeted) treatments.

MAIN CONCEPTS

2.20.3 Cancer is a Disease of Dysregulated Genes

It is clear that cancer is a disease of dysregulated genomics. New genomic characterizations of cancer (combined with dramatic reductions in the cost of genomic analysis and computing power, and the parallel genomic and biological annotation, i.e., "naming," of cancer-associated genes) has fueled the field of precision medicine as a therapeutic approach, delivered recent drug approvals in human oncology, and is increasingly available to all species of cancer patients.

2.20.3.1 Precision Medicine for Oncology

In many disease conditions, it is well understood that conventional methods of disease characterization are insufficient to fully inform clinicians of an individual patient's needs. For the most part, the genomic characterization of many disease states can better account for these needs. As such, Pmed can allow clinicians to select better initial approaches to therapy, more rapidly alter treatment approach, and individualize plans for disease monitoring. From the perspective of need and opportunity, the field of oncology is most ready and in need of this evolution in medicine. Collectively, this has created the opportunity for relatively inexpensive genomic and molecular characterizations of disease states.

2.20.4 Cancer Precision Medicine for Individualized and Molecular Therapy

In the delivery of Pmed, a tissue biopsy or blood sample (liquid biopsy) from the patient will be used to extract nucleic acids for genomic sequencing. Altered genes are prioritized as therapeutic targets. These are then matched with specific drugs that inhibit the altered gene or its pathway. An individualized cocktail of therapeutics, matched to the patient's cancer genome, is then delivered to the patient. Adjustments can then be made after reanalysis of liquid biopsy signals.

2.20.5 Challenges and Solutions for Precision Medicine and Veterinary Oncology

Challenges to the field of precision medicine, and more generally to molecularly targeted therapy, must be addressed before this important and novel approach to cancer therapy will improve outcomes. These challenges include, but are not limited to, the following.

- *Cancer evolution.* Most precision medicine platforms analyze patient tissue from a primary tumor resection. As a consequence, subsequent molecular treatment is based on the characteristics of a patient's primary tumor. Unfortunately, metastases from a primary tumor often exhibit distinct molecular alterations compared to the initial primary tumor. Accordingly, a therapy that targets a primary tumor may not necessarily control the associated metastatic progression that is a problem for patients. Since most patients require therapeutics that target the molecular alterations that result in metastatic progression, it is very unlikely that analysis of the primary tumor or even a measurable metastatic lesion will deliver a valuable therapeutic response in that patient.
- *Cancer geography.* Within a single tumor, multiple populations of cancer cells can exist that differ in the genetic alterations they express. Because of this *geographic heterogeneity* within a tumor, it remains unclear if molecular analysis of a single portion of a tumor can sufficiently represent the tumor as a whole. As such, genetic analysis of a single biopsy sample may result in therapeutic recommendations that only target a subset of cells within a tumor. This could result in poor patient response to treatment. With this in mind, determining the most valuable and informative portions of tissue for molecular analysis

is critical for effective Pmed. Evidence from many genomic studies suggests that this problem of geographic heterogeneity is cancer specific and will require studies in specific cancers to determine optimal biopsy recommendations for Pmed.

2.20.5.1 The Liquid Biopsy Solution

A reasonable solution to the problems of cancer geography and evolution may be delivered through the identification of cell-free circulating tumor DNA. This can be accomplished through liquid biopsies, which are blood samples that contain circulating tumor DNA obtained from cancer patients. This technique is not only less invasive (only requires peripheral blood draws) but may be a more valuable approach to define the molecular events driving cancer progression, i.e., using the abundance of the mutated tumor DNA in the blood to guide optimal Pmed drug selection. Accordingly, a Pmed platform that does not include analysis of cell-free circulating tumor DNA in blood is not likely to optimally improve treatment outcomes.

2.20.5.2 Context

A critical but often ignored problem in the field of precision medicine is the growing understanding that specific genomic alterations (i.e., mutations) in a given cancer influence the biology of that cancer in the context of that cancer. In other words, a given genetic mutation may affect tumors differently depending on which type of cancer the patient has. Thus, the therapeutic value of targeting specific mutations is dependent on the cancer type in question. We should not be surprised that an understanding of context will also be species specific, and not necessarily predicted by genomic studies alone.

2.20.6 Cancer Precision Medicine for Reverse Drug Development

This is a more immediate application of cancer precision medicine than simply using it as a means to identify a specific treatment for a single patient. Pmed can also be used to form the scientific rationale for new drug development that starts with the cancer patient rather than cancer cells in tissue culture. This new approach to future cancer drug development should accelerate efforts within specific cancers. This is in contrast to a traditional and much slower drug discovery/development path which most often begins in cell-based studies and then progressively moves to cancer patients.

2.20.7 Are You Ready to Interpret a Pmed Analysis of Disease?

Considering all the factors discussed above, it is important for all veterinary clinicians to decide if they are effectively prepared to offer Pmed services to their veterinary oncology patients. As described above, a variety of Pmed offerings are commercially available and more clients will request advice on the use of these options. At this time and in the future, clinicians should assess their ability to interpret and act on Pmed data and drug reports. Ideally, practitioners should have access to a multidisciplinary team of veterinary scientists and clinicians to deliver the best value to patients from these types of complex data (see 8.26 Team Strategies for Cancer). These teams should be led by veterinary scientists with experience in molecular biology, drug development, pathology, and medicine. Leveraging this expertise within the veterinary field is paramount, since professionals in the human field will likely have insufficient background and context to deliver effective interpretations of data to veterinary clinicians and patients.

TAKE-AWAYS

- Precision cancer medicine can be utilized to improve our understanding of a patient's cancer. By identifying genetic alterations within a tumor that may be responsible for cancer progression and aggressive behavior, delivering personalized and molecularly guided therapy (i.e., targeted therapy) seeks to align effective drugs that target specific molecular alterations with patients whose tumors express those molecular alterations.
- Two patients may have the same histological type of cancer, but the genetic mutations of their cancers may differ. This can affect the response to a given therapy between the two individuals.
- Liquid biopsies, which are blood samples collected from cancer patients, can be beneficial in identifying specific cancer mutations by detecting cell-free circulating tumor DNA in the blood. These mutations can serve as targets for therapy.

- While the potential of Pmed is promising, challenges do exist that impact its widespread value. These include the changes in genetic mutations between primary tumors and metastases (i.e., cancer evolution) and the geographical genetic heterogeneity of tumors.
- As the availability of precise cancer testing increases within the veterinary field, clinicians will need to be prepared to discuss these tests with their clients as well as interpret the results, or to develop relationships with teams with this expertise.

MISCELLANEOUS

2.20.7.1 Disclosure

The authors of this topic, and our disclosed relationship with Ethos, have no commercial products for Pmed at this time. We nonetheless continue ongoing clinical research to deliver the future value of this approach to patients.

2.20.7.2 Acknowledgments

Captain Thomas R. Cotrone, DVM, PhD, for careful review and insight into this topic.

Recommended Reading

AACR Project GENIE Consortium (2017). AACR project GENIE: powering precision medicine through an international consortium. *Cancer Discov.* 7 (8): 818–831.

Haber, D.A. and Velculescu, V.E. (2014). Blood-based analyses of cancer: circulating tumor cells and circulating tumor DNA. *Cancer Discov.* 4 (6): 650–661.

Lloyd, K.C., Khanna, C., Hendricks, W. et al. (2016). Precision medicine: an opportunity for a paradigm shift in veterinary medicine. *J. Am. Vet. Med. Assoc.* 248 (1): 45–48.

Paoloni, M., Webb, C., Mazcko, C. et al. (2014). Prospective molecular profiling of canine cancers provides a clinically relevant comparative model for evaluating personalized medicine (Pmed) trials. *PLoS One* 9 (3): e90028.

Verma, M. (2012). Personalized medicine and cancer. *J. Pers. Med.* 2 (1): 1–14.

Section 3

Hereditary Considerations

3.1

Genetic Basics

Lowell Ackerman, DVM, DACVD, MBA, MPA, CVA, MRCVS

Global Consultant, Author, and Lecturer, MA, USA

 BASICS

3.1.1 Summary

When an animal is born, it receives half of its genetic blueprint from its father and half from its mother. This combination of genes is what accounts for the animal being a truly unique individual, not a clone of the parents.

3.1.2 Terms Defined

Allele: A variant or alternative form of a gene, found at the same location on a chromosome, and which can result in different observable traits.

Clone: Derivative of an animal with which it is genetically identical.

Codon: A sequence of three nucleotides that represents amino acids or start and stop commands as DNA constituents.

Exon: A segment of nucleic acid (DNA or RNA) that codes for specific proteins or peptides.

Genetics: The study of genes and how traits or conditions are passed from one generation to the next.

Genome: The complete set of genes for an animal.

Genomics: The study of the entire genome, and its combined influence on complex diseases and the impact of environmental factors such as diet, exercise, medications, and toxins on genes.

Genotype: An individual's genetic constitution.

Heterozygote: An individual with two different alleles for a given gene.

Homozygote: An individual with two identical alleles for a given gene.

Intron: A segment of nucleic acid (DNA or RNA) that interrupts the sequence within genes but does not code for proteins.

Locus: A fixed position on a chromosome for a gene or marker.

Microsatellite: A tract of DNA in which certain base pairs are repeated. They are sometimes referred to as short tandem repeats.

Open Reading Frame: A continuous stretch of amino acid-forming codons that has the ability to be translated into a protein or peptide.

Phene: A trait or characteristic that is genetically determined.

Phenotype: Observable characteristics or traits that result from the interaction of the genotype with the environment.

Polymorphism: Genetic variation within a population and with which selection pressures can operate.

Short Interspersed Element: Noncoding sequences of DNA that are useful markers of divergent evolution between species.

Single Nucleotide Polymorphism (SNP): Genetic variation in a single DNA building block (nucleotide) that occurs at a specific position in the genome and is present within the population. There are millions of SNPs in the genome, most commonly located in the DNA between genes. Most have little or no impact on health and disease, but some can predict an individual's risk of developing particular diseases, likely response to certain drugs, or susceptibility to environmental factors.

Pet-Specific Care for the Veterinary Team, First Edition. Edited by Lowell Ackerman.
© 2021 John Wiley & Sons, Inc. Published 2021 by John Wiley & Sons, Inc.

MAIN CONCEPTS

3.1.3 DNA: The Fabric of Life

DNA is a fabulous device for conserving everything that makes a living being what it is. Whether you believe in evolution or divine intervention, DNA contains a lot more than just the genes that code for all of a living thing's features.

It is the protein-coding DNA that we are most concerned with as we attempt to understand the genetics of phenes, traits, and diseases. DNA is a molecule composed of two nucleotide chains wrapped around one another in a form known as a double helix. Each nucleotide (or polynucleotide) chain is composed of individual nucleotides, which in turn are composed of four nucleobases (cytosine, guanine, adenine or thymine), a sugar molecule (deoxyribose), and a phosphate group. The nucleotides occur in chains in which the sugar of one nucleotide binds to the phosphate group in the next, and the two separate chains are bound together by the nucleobase pairs, such that cytosine (C) binds to guanine (G) and adenine (A) binds to thymine (T). The structure of the double helix resembles a ladder twisted on its long access, with the nucleobase pairs resembling the rungs and the nucleotide chains resembling the rails or stiles (Figure 3.1.1).

DNA is organized into paired structures, known as chromosomes. Each species has a defined number of chromosomes (23 pairs in humans, 39 pairs in dogs, and 19 pairs in the cat). Two of those chromosomes are known as sex chromosomes (X and Y chromosomes) and the remainder are known as autosomes. Males have one X and one Y chromosome and females have two X chromosomes.

In animals, almost all the DNA is compressed into the nucleus of cells, with a small amount found in mitochondria. The genetic information within an animal's genome is held within its genes and the genetic composition of a given animal for a specific variant is known as its genotype.

Genes represent a region of DNA that influence a particular phene, trait or characteristic. The dog genome consists of about 2.8 billion base pairs of nucleotides that represent about 19 000 protein-coding genes; cats have about 2.4 billion base pairs of nucleotides that also represent about 19 000 protein-coding genes. Humans and pets share about 85% of their genes, so it should not be surprising that many diseases found in one species may also be found in others (see 2.19 One Health).

A gene is that portion of DNA that codes for a specific sequence of amino acids, which in turn make proteins, enzymes, or polypeptides. As you might expect, DNA segments resemble but are not exactly like a passenger train, with genes end to end. Leaders and trailers occur before and after genes and within the gene, and some noncoded regions called *introns* separate coded regions of "expressed sequences" called *exons*.

For any one genetic character, then, each parent contributes one version of the gene for that character, which is called an *allele*. The location of a gene on a chromosome is its *locus*.

Given four bases (G, C, A, T) that can be arranged in groups of three (codon triplets, such as ATG, the triplet codon for the amino acid methionine), there are 64 (4^3) combinations possible, but since there are only 20 amino acid products, this provides much opportunity for redundancy in the system (e.g., the amino acid alanine can be formed from the triplet codons GCT, GCC, GCA, GCG, AGA, AGG, CGT, and CGC). The average protein the DNA codes for is about 1000 amino acids long, which also means that it is about 3000 codons in length (three codons to one amino acid). Combined with codons that initiate and complete reading (for example, ATG is a start codon, and TAA, TAG and TGA are stop codons that mark the end of a sequence), the arrangement of codons is called an *open reading frame*.

Given an alphabet with only four letters (A, G, C, T), it may seem improbable that these nucleotides could account for all the genetic diversity in the world. Given also that these nucleotides code for only 20 amino acids, it seems difficult to forge a plausible argument for all the genetic variations seen. Because those four nucleotides can occupy any position along the DNA sequence, however, even a 10-nucleotide stretch can form 4^{10} (more than 1 million) different combinations. Imagine it as a combination lock: instead of a three-number sequence, you have an amino

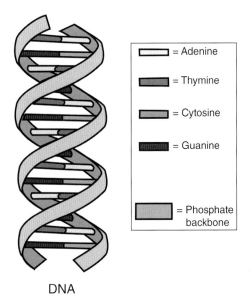

DNA

Figure 3.1.1 Double helix structure of DNA. *Source:* From Forluvoft, DNA simple2. Wikimedia Commons. Public Domain.

acid sequence of nucleotide triplets (e.g., CAT–TAG–GAC–ATT) that can code for an almost endless array of proteins.

3.1.4 Mutations

DNA stores biological information and that information is conserved and replicated as the strands peel apart and are duplicated. Just like a photocopier, cells copy the DNA throughout an animal's life as cells are replenished and, for the most part, there are very few errors in the duplication process.

Genetic diseases usually cause problems because a mutation creates a poorly functioning facsimile of the normal gene product (Box 3.1.1). Such a mutation often happens because of innocent-appearing mishaps that result in an altered product.

Even though DNA replication is remarkably efficient, mistakes occasionally do happen. A base substitution that results in a stop codon, prematurely halting the process, is called a *nonsense mutation*; the resulting polypeptide will be shorter than usual and probably not functional. Progressive retinal atrophy (PRA) in the Irish setter, for example, is the result of a nonsense mutation in the cGMP-phosphodiesterase-beta gene. A *missense mutation* occurs when one base is substituted for another, which potentially results in a different amino acid occurring in the chain.

Box 3.1.1 Story of a mutation

We know that the genetic code is actually written with triplet codons, such that three nucleotide bases together code for a single amino acid. Thus, using the four bases, adenine (A), thymine (T), guanine (G), and cytosine (C), we can construct a chain of bases that code for amino acids that will form an enzyme, a protein, or a polypeptide. DNA is read three bases at a time, and these three bases correspond to specific amino acids. Accordingly, TATAGACAACAT would be read as tyrosine (TAT)–arginine (AGA)–glutamine (CAA)–histidine (CAT).

Redundancy is built into the system. For example, both TAC and TAT code for tyrosine, so if the T in position 3 happens to be replaced by the base C, the final product is not affected (a silent mutation). Now, given the previous sequence, imagine that a point mutation occurs that deletes the third base in the sequence (T). With the bases after that point shifting one to the left, the first codon becomes TAA, which is a stop codon and arrests the process. If the deletion were to occur to the fourth base (A), the resulting peptide would be changed to tyrosine (TAT)–aspartic acid (GAC)–asparagine (AAC), which is completely different from the peptide normally produced.

In some cases, the resultant polypeptide may not be functional. In other cases, however, because of redundancy built into the system, a base substitution will not change the amino acid product (e.g., CAT and CAC both code for histidine). This substitution is referred to as a *silent mutation*. Hemophilia B is characterized by a substitution of A for G at nucleotide 1477 in the gene for canine factor IX, resulting in the substitution of glutamic acid for glycine at position 379 in the factor IX molecule, which decreases the efficiency of blood clotting.

In contrast to missense mutations, in which only one amino acid in a sequence is affected, if a base is inserted or deleted in the DNA strand, it has the potential to alter the reading of the entire coded sequence downstream because the triplet codons are now out of their original sequence. This mutation is known as a frameshift mutation, an example of which is X-linked nephritis. In simple terms, take the phrase "how are you" and insert the letter *b* after the letter *h* in *how* to see how a simple insertion of one base can change expression. The shift results in "hbo war eyo u" which doesn't communicate the same message as "how are you." You can imagine what would happen to a genetic sequence in the same circumstances.

Considering that a point mutation happens by chance, that it can affect any bases in a DNA sequence for a peptide, and it then passes to future generations, it should not be surprising that similar disorders in different breeds can result from very different gene mutations. That is why the DNA test for PRA in Irish setters will not work in miniature poodles. Although the final clinical result of PRA is similar, the underlying genetic disorder could not be more different. When the incidence of mutations is combined with the fact that about 70% of all mutations are recessive, it is not difficult to see how they can be propagated.

3.1.5 Propagation of Traits

If you have a breeding animal that has superior attributes (phenes) but inadvertently carries a recessive trait that is not clinically evident even to the trained eye (genes are read in pairs, and if one of those pairs reflects a recessive trait, then the trait will not be displayed), then the pet may be bred intensively. If that recessive trait is not present in the other breeding stock, all the offspring (F1 generation) will appear clinically (phenotypically) normal, but some of the offspring will still carry that recessive trait. If that generation is bred to unrelated stock, all the next generation (F2) will also be phenotypically normal, with even a smaller percentage being carriers. If bred to related stock that also carry the mutation, however, the recessive trait will begin to be concentrated and manifested.

3.1.6 Microsatellites

In a simple world, as described earlier, one might consider the genome as a passenger train, with the genes as railway cars coupled to one another. In reality, it is not that orderly. This unsophisticated look is what provides an opportunity to learn a lot from the genome. If the genome were arranged like a train, researchers would have to isolate each gene (passenger car) to learn anything. Fortunately, however, nature has provided spacers, known as microsatellites, that can act as markers for traits. They might be considered as dining cars spaced between groups of passenger cars.

As more and more useful microsatellites are identified, a higher resolution map of the genome will continue to be developed of which markers are inherited along with specific genes. Then, by measuring these markers, we can tell with some accuracy an individual's genetic make-up for that specific trait without having to necessarily identify the actual gene. This can be very helpful when trying to predict some disorders which are unlikely to be completely controlled by individual genes alone (e.g., hip dysplasia, atopic dermatitis, etc.).

To use the train example once more, when train cars are unhitched and transferred to other trains, which passenger cars always seem to go along with the same dining car? If you identify a specific dining car, you know which passenger cars are also likely to be found there, too. Obviously, the closer the gene (passenger car) is to the marker (dining car), the greater is the probability that the two will be transferred together. A gene that is farther away from the marker may not be transferred 100% of the time, which would affect a test's specificity and predictive ability. Thus, some microsatellite markers may be associated with increased risk of a condition, and others with decreased risk, and when considered in aggregate, they could provide an impression of the risk for such traits in individual animals.

Microsatellites have more to offer than just their role as signposts. They have considerable variability (which molecular geneticists call *polymorphism*), making them unique identifiers of individuals and their offspring. Variations in a DNA sequence are called SNPs, some of which have no impact on health while others may predispose an individual to disease or signal responsiveness to medical therapies. Microsatellites are one way to identify an individual, as well as its progeny, and have become a voluntary part of the DNA identification for the different purebred registries. If a sire has six repetitive sequences relative to a specific marker and the dam has eight, the offspring will have one copy from each parent. By comparing findings at multiple markers, the accuracy of predicting parentage becomes a virtual certainty.

Short interspersed elements are often inserted within or near genes and may regulate their expression. The pet population has thousands of short interspersed element differences, which are associated with breed differences related to behavioral and physical characteristics and also act as signposts for specific genes linked to disease susceptibility or traits.

3.1.7 Predicting Genotype

Since alleles are inherited from both parents, it would be helpful to know how they combine in individuals and the impact that has on disease susceptibility. Two terms are important in this regard – genotype and phenotype.

Genotype refers to the actual genetic sequence determined in an animal, while phenotype describes what is clinically evident, compared to the normal or typical presentation. So, for any individual genetic trait (T), in which an animal could inherit a typical (T) or variant (t) gene from its parents, there are four combinations possible (TT, Tt, tT, tt) but really only three variants (TT, Tt, tt). If the condition is recessive (such as von Willebrand disease [vWD]) and the heterozygotes (Tt) cannot be clinically distinguished from one of the homozygotes (TT), then clinically there are three variants (TT, Tt, tt) but only two clinical phenotypes – normal (TT or Tt) and abnormal (tt). In the case of a recessive disorder like vWD, we have a genetic test that can tell us genotype (the actual gene pairing in the animal), but without the test we can only determine phenotype – normal versus abnormal, by evidence of bleeding factor tests. So, for a condition like hip dysplasia where currently we cannot identify genotype, we end up making the diagnosis with phenotypic tests such are radiographs or distraction index.

Progressive retinal atrophy in the Irish setter is inherited as an autosomal recessive trait, which means that an affected individual inherits a defective gene (rcd1) from each parent, whereas dogs that inherit a defective gene from only one parent may be difficult to identify, because they appear clinically normal. The good news for veterinary teams, even without a DNA test, is that an electroretinogram can identify affected individuals (with two copies of the abnormal gene) by 6 weeks of age. This identification means the dog can be removed from a breeding program so that it will not contribute its PRA genes to future generations. The bad news for veterinary teams and breeders is that carriers of the trait, those with only one abnormal variant and one normal variant, cannot be identified clinically, even with sophisticated procedures such as electroretinography. Therefore, without genetic testing, genetic counseling is a hit-or-miss enterprise until the animal produces affected offspring and we can determine its genotype. With direct DNA testing, though, animals that are affected, clear, or carriers can be identified (see 3.4 Predicting and Eliminating Disease Traits).

That's good news for Labrador retriever breeders; labs are also prone to PRA but a clinical diagnosis cannot be made until the dogs are 4 years old, and an electroretinogram will not identify affected pups until they are 18 months old. DNA testing can identify status early, in pups as young as one day of age. Unfortunately, the specificity of DNA testing is also one of its limitations. The gene that causes PRA in Labrador retrievers (prcd) is different from the one that causes it in Irish setters (rcd1), so the same DNA test cannot be used to diagnose these two forms of the disease (and there are dozens of different genetic forms of PRA). Fortunately, DNA testing for both prcd and rcd1 is now available, and for many other forms of PRA.

3.1.8 Genetics Versus Genomics

There is a lot of attention focused on the promises of genomic medicine, and it can sometimes be confusing when we use the terms *genetics* and *genomics* synonymously. Genetics is the study of genes and how traits or conditions are passed from one generation to the next. On the other hand, genomics is the study of the entire genome, and its combined influence on complex diseases and the impact of environmental factors such as diet, exercise, medications, and toxins on genes.

3.1.9 The Impact of Breeding

With mass or individual selection, the breeder selects the animals to be bred on the basis of their superior characteristics. Whereas many breeders select their breeding stock on the basis of conformation or other physical characteristics that exemplify the breed standard, genetic counseling is intended to temper enthusiasm for physical traits with a more holistic picture of genotypic and phenotypic health (see 3.8 Genetic Counseling). Veterinarians should also exert some self-discipline by focusing not just on one health aspect (e.g., von Willebrand status) but rather on the whole animal. Otherwise, in the zeal to rid a line of one disease, another (or more) may inadvertently be fostered.

Selection works best at eliminating dominant traits from a population. After all, because all animals that carry the dominant allele develop the trait, it is theoretically possible to eliminate a dominant trait in one generation. Selection is complicated, however, by the fact that some dominant traits (e.g., dermatofibrosis) do not appear until later in life when animals may already have been bred, and by traits with incomplete dominance or variable expressivity, in which an affected animal may not be detected yet carry the trait. Fortunately, DNA testing is now available for some of these traits, including dermatofibrosis.

With recessive traits, selection can quickly remove homozygous affected animals from breeding, but if heterozygotes cannot be detected, carriers will persist in the population. The final elimination of the trait from a breed requires identifying carriers and ensuring that no carriers are bred to one another. Even though doing so does not eliminate the deleterious allele from the population, it does ensure that no affected animals are produced.

TAKE-AWAYS

- Genes don't cause diseases, but they may code for defective proteins that are associated with disease states.
- For any particular genotype, each parent contributes one allelic variant for that trait.
- Mutations can be responsible for changes along the length of a gene sequence that can have major or minor impact on the expression of that gene, depending on the mutation.
- Diseases with the same name are not necessarily caused by the same genetic mutation in all breeds.
- Genetic markers can prove useful in helping to identify disease risk, even when the specific disease gene has not yet been identified.

MISCELLANEOUS

Abbreviations

DNA Deoxyribonucleic acid
ORF Open reading frame
RNA Ribonucleic acid

Recommended Reading

Ackerman, L. (2011). *The Genetic Connection*. Lakewood, CO: AAHA Press.

Ackerman, L. (2020). *Proactive Pet Parenting. Anticipating pet health problems before they happen*. Problem Free Publishing.

Wang, W. and Kirkness, E.F. (2005). Short interspersed elements (SINEs) are a major source of canine genomic diversity. *Genome Res.* 15: 1798–1808.

3.2

Modes of Inheritance

Lowell Ackerman, DVM, DACVD, MBA, MPA, CVA, MRCVS

Global Consultant, Author, and Lecturer, MA, USA

BASICS

3.2.1 Summary

To understand genetics, we try to make it as simple as possible. We like to believe that traits have to be dominant or recessive and appear either on the sex chromosomes or the autosomes. We enjoy nice, clean statistics such as "approximately 25% of offspring will be affected." In reality, the deeper one delves into genetics and statistics, the more one realizes that, for most conditions, hard statistics do not apply unless a direct test for the genotype exists, and the condition is fully penetrant and expressed. Although people want black or white, without being able to actually determine genotype, genetics is more like shades of gray.

3.2.2 Terms Defined

Allele: A variant or alternative form of a gene, found at the same location on a chromosome, and which can result in different observable traits.

Dominant: Heritable characteristics, traits or diseases that are expressed when inherited even from one parent.

Genetics: The study of genes and how traits or conditions are passed from one generation to the next

Genome: The complete set of genes for an animal.

Genomics: The study of the entire genome, and its combined influence on complex diseases and the impact of environmental factors such as diet, exercise, medications, and toxins on genes.

Genotype: An individual's genetic constitution.

Heterozygote: An individual with two different alleles for a given gene.

Homozygote: An individual with two identical alleles for a given gene.

Locus: A fixed position on a chromosome for a gene or marker.

Phene: A trait or characteristic that is genetically determined.

Phenotype: Observable characteristics or traits that result from the interaction of genotype with the environment.

Recessive: Heritable characteristics, traits or diseases that are expressed only when inherited from both parents.

MAIN CONCEPTS

When an animal inherits the same version of an allele from both parents (e.g., TT or tt), we say it is *homozygous* for that trait. When the alleles in a gene pair differ, we say the animal is *heterozygous* for that trait (e.g., Tt). For an X-linked trait, affected males are *hemizygous* for the trait because they have only one X chromosome, which they get from their mother (they got the Y chromosome from their father). Whatever the combination, the pairing of actual genes is what constitutes the genotype.

On the basis of this pairing of genes, we have rules to determine the impact of genetic combinations on progeny. These rules are most applicable when a single gene pair determines how the trait will be expressed, which is known as *monogenic inheritance*. Progressive retinal atrophy (PRA) in Irish setters is an example of this. Other traits, such as hip dysplasia, are caused by the product of multiple gene effects, which is known as *polygenic inheritance*, sometimes also referred to as *quantitative* or *multifactorial inheritance.*

In a monogenic trait involving one pair of genes for locus A, four genotypic outcomes are possible (AA, Aa, aA, aa), but only three phenotypic expressions (AA, Aa, aa), because of how the alleles from mother and father combine in offspring. When two gene pairs are involved, 16 genotypic combinations are possible and, assuming all genotypes are expressed equally, nine possible phenotypes. For every *n* gene pairs involved in a trait, there are 4^n possible genotypic outcomes and 3^n possible phenotypic expressions.

When you realize that most traits are controlled by many gene pairs, you start to appreciate just how complicated predicting genetic outcome can be. In addition, modifiers, incomplete penetrance, epigenetics, and variable expressivity may have a significant effect on phenotypic outcome (see 3.3 The Genetics of Disease).

Because accurately predicting genotypes with polygenic traits is difficult and because the environment can have a profound influence, genetic involvement in a trait is typically expressed as heritability (h^2), which is a mathematical representation of the variance in breeding values divided by phenotypic variance. A trait's heritability can vary from 0 (no heritable component) to 1 (complete inheritance).

Dogs have 78 chromosomes (39 pairs) and cats have 38 chromosomes (19 pairs), two of which are sex chromosomes. Females are XX and males are XY. The rest of the chromosomes, which have nothing to do with sex determination, are called *autosomes.* Some traits, such as hemophilia, are transmitted on the X chromosome, but to date few if any disease traits seem to be transmitted on the Y chromosome of dogs and cats. Accordingly, a trait can be sex linked (actually almost always X linked, because few Y-linked traits have been documented) if it resides on the X chromosomes, or autosomal if it resides on one of the other chromosomes. Sex-linked traits and sex-limited traits have to be differentiated. An example of a sex-limited trait is cryptorchidism, the presence of undescended testicles, in that it can be seen only in males. This fact does not imply that a female cannot carry the gene for cryptorchidism or that it is sex linked and carried on the Y chromosome, which we know is not the case.

3.2.3 Recessive and Dominant Traits

When two copies of a disease-causing gene (one from each parent) are required to cause a specific problem, the trait is said to be *recessive.* Thus, PRA in Irish setters is recessive because, to manifest the disease, an animal must inherit a defective gene from each parent (i.e., both parents). If the parents of an Irish setter with PRA appear phenotypically normal, they must both be carriers (heterozygous for a recessive character) of the trait because each contributes a disease-causing gene to their offspring. Because the trait is recessive, both carrier parents appear normal.

When only one copy of a gene is necessary for a trait to be expressed, that trait is said to *dominant.* In our PRA example, the gene for normal retinal development is dominant, which is why carriers look outwardly normal even though they carry an abnormal allele and a normal one.

In the simplest terms, if one gene pair controls a trait, conventional use is to capitalize the dominant form and use lower case for the recessive form. For example, imagine that the coat color in a fictitious breed, the American car-chasing terrier (ACCT), is controlled by a single gene pair. The dominant presentation is black (B), and the recessive presentation is brown (b). Because black is dominant over brown in this example, individuals with a heterozygous genotype (Bb) will appear black. Those with a homozygous genotype will be either black (BB) or brown (bb).

If we did not have a genetic test to identify coat-color genotype, we would have to determine it the old-fashioned way, by progeny testing. If you were to breed a black dog (we know that at least one allele is B) to a brown dog (bb) and any of the puppies were brown (bb), the black dog would have to be a heterozygote (Bb). If all the pups were black (BB or Bb), the black parent is most likely a homozygote (BB). Similarly, if we were to breed two black dogs and any of the pups were brown, we would know that both parents had to be heterozygotes for the black color gene (Bb).

If only things were this simple! Although we could indeed give many examples of traits that are inherited in a simple fashion, many more are not nearly as easy to determine or the phenotype is the expression of more than one gene pair. Consider a genotype example for Labrador retrievers, in which nine different coat-color genotypes are possible (from 16 possible gene combinations). Some genes can affect more than one function, such as the genes affecting coat color that can also be associated with deafness, ocular anomalies, or both. When one gene affects two or more traits in the same individual, it is termed *pleiotropy.*

In addition to all the new information available on coat-color genetics, distinct mutations in three genes, *RSPO2, FGF5,* and *KRT71* (encoding R-spondin-2, fibroblast growth factor-5, and keratin-71, respectively), together account for most coat phenotypes in purebred dogs [1].

3.2.4 Cytoplasmic Inheritance

Most DNA is found in the nucleus, but mitochondria in the cytoplasm contain their own DNA, derived entirely from the mother's ovum. Sperm contain few mitochondria, and none survive fertilization. Therefore, defects in mitochondrial DNA can be passed only from the mother but are transferred to both male and female offspring.

EXAMPLES

Seamus McTigue is a 6-month-old neutered male Scottish terrier that has presented with difficulty in chewing and swallowing, and has early evidence of swelling of the mandible. A genetic panel performed at 12 weeks of age indicated that Seamus was homozygous recessive for the craniomandibular osteopathy genetic variant (SLC37A2). Mrs McTigue has confirmed that neither of Seamus' parents had been affected by the condition, which is entirely consistent with a disorder presumed to have autosomal recessive inheritance. Ordinarily Mrs McTigue would have been more alarmed, but since the veterinary team had apprised her of the likelihood of the issue, and had an action plan in place for dealing with it, she felt that Seamus was in good hands and she felt prepared to deal with the situation as needed.

TAKE-AWAYS

- Monogenic traits (those controlled by a single gene pair) are often described as being dominant or recessive, but the actual pattern of inheritance observed may not be clear cut.
- Most traits have polygenic inheritance, in which disease manifestations are controlled by a variety of genes, often with environmental influence.
- Heritability is the term used to describe how much of a condition is due to genetic influences.
- Many more conditions are caused by variants on the autosomes than on the sex chromosomes.
- Mitochondria contain their own distinct genes, and genetic diseases caused by mitochondrial DNA variants are transmitted from mothers to both male and female offspring.

MISCELLANEOUS

Reference

1 Cadieu, E., Neff, M., Quignon, P. et al. (2009). Coat variation in the domestic dog is governed by variants in three genes. *Science* 326: 150–153.

Recommended Reading

Ackerman, L. (2011). *The Genetic Connection*, 2e. Lakewood, CO: AAHA Press.

Ackerman, L. (2020). Proactive Pet Parenting: Anticipating pet health problems before they happen. Problem Free Publishing.

3.3

The Genetics of Disease

Lowell Ackerman, DVM, DACVD, MBA, MPA, CVA, MRCVS

Global Consultant, Author, and Lecturer, MA, USA

 BASICS

3.3.1 Summary

Genes do not cause diseases. They code for proteins that may have developmental or maintenance roles. When those proteins fail to function in a manner consistent with "normal," an animal may be diagnosed with a phene, trait, or disease of a genetic nature. Still, the relationship between genetics and disease is not as clear cut as one might expect.

3.3.2 Terms Defined

Allele: A variant or alternative form of a gene, found at the same location on a chromosome, and which can result in different observable traits.

Dominant: Heritable characteristics, traits, or diseases that are expressed when inherited even from one parent.

Epistasis: The situation in which the action of one gene depends on the action of another gene.

Expressivity: The extent to which a genetic variant (genotype) expresses the so-called clinical abnormality (phenotype) on an individual level.

Genetics: The study of genes and how traits or conditions are passed from one generation to the next.

Genome: The complete set of genes for an animal.

Genomics: The study of the entire genome, and its combined influence on complex diseases and the impact of environmental factors such as diet, exercise, medications, and toxins on genes.

Genotype: An individual's genetic constitution.

Heterozygote: An individual with two different alleles for a given gene.

Homozygote: An individual with two identical alleles for a given gene.

Locus: A fixed position on a chromosome for a gene or marker.

Penetrance: The likelihood of individuals in a population with a given genetic variant (genotype) fully displaying the clinical manifestations (phenotype) of that variant.

Phene: A trait or characteristic that is genetically determined.

Phenotype: Observable characteristics or traits that result from the interaction of genotype with the environment.

Recessive: Heritable characteristics, traits, or diseases that are expressed only when inherited from both parents.

 MAIN CONCEPTS

At its simplest, one would suspect that disease outcomes could be readily predicted if only the pattern of inheritance is known. However, things are rarely that simple when it comes to genetics. A few examples of genes, mutations, diseases, and modes of inheritance are in order to help explore the genetics of disease.

Fucosidosis is a rare but devastating lysosomal storage disease of English springer spaniels, transmitted as an autosomal recessive trait, meaning a dog would have to inherit an abnormal gene from each parent to be affected by the disease (see 11.3 Heritable Health Conditions – By Disease). Although the abnormal gene itself does not kill the dog, it codes for an absent or nonfunctional enzyme (alpha-L-fucosidase) that can result in clinical problems.

If the enzyme is not capable of breaking down its substrate, complex sugars collect within cells and eventually kill them. When the cells are severely compromised by this accumulated substrate, they die, and then the organs (primarily the brain) begin to be compromised, and eventually the situation will lead to the dog's demise. Carriers, who only inherited an abnormal gene from one parent, appear outwardly normal. Their levels of fucosidase enzymes, however, may be lower than normal, but not necessarily low enough to cause expression of the disease.

The same is true for many of the bleeding disorders, in which a defective gene does not produce a fully functioning protein or an enzyme important to clotting. Although carriers appear normal, their level of clotting factor may be lower than normal, just not low enough to cause spontaneous bleeding problems.

Whether a trait/phene is truly recessive depends on how hard one looks at the phenotype (see 3.2 Modes of Inheritance). A dog with fucosidosis typically shows neurological signs early in life and has an abbreviated life span. The affected dog carries two copies of the abnormal gene. If a carrier, with one abnormal gene, has no outward problems as a pup but (theoretically) suffers from dementia and is euthanized at 7 years of age, can this truly be considered a completely recessive trait without influence? If the bitch that is the carrier of one hemophilia gene has no spontaneous bleeding episodes but has complications with bleeding during surgery or whelping, is she truly phenotypically "normal"? Young Labrador retrievers with late-onset rod–cone degeneration may have measurably reduced retinal function.

In cutaneous asthenia, a disease of skin fragility, gene mutations that produce abnormal collagen are considered dominant because heterozygotes produce enough abnormal collagen to be evident, whereas procollagen-processing mutations are considered recessive because heterozygotes (those with only one abnormal gene variant) usually have enough enzyme activity to convert procollagen to collagen. Thus, as more is learned about genetic conditions and testing improves, suppositions about dominant and recessive traits will have less impact on our genetic counseling skills.

3.3.3 Dominance and Disease

Now let's take a look at dominance. A trait that is completely dominant is easy to spot because the parent is affected and so are all or most offspring. In the case of a dog that is homozygous for a dominant trait, all pups should be affected. In the case of a dog that is heterozygous for a dominant trait, that dog and 50% of its offspring should be affected. What happens in many instances is that there is incomplete dominance or expression of a dominant trait with variable expressivity. This basically means the trait has dominant features with a spectrum of possibilities in the offspring. If penetrance of a dominant gene is complete, all progeny receiving the allele will express the trait. If penetrance is 50%, only half will express the trait. With variable expressivity, some genes may produce different degrees of expression of a phenotype, ranging from severe expression to absence of the trait.

For example, dermatomyositis in collies was originally believed to be an autosomal dominant trait, but it is now believed that, although the trait has dominant features, environmental components (likely viral infection) are required for full manifestation of the disorder. Other traits may be co-dominant, each contributing to the phenotype. For dermatomyositis, the current DNA testing situation is that there appear to be at least three loci associated with an increased risk for developing the disease (*PAN2* gene on chromosome 10, *MAP3K7CL* gene on chromosome 31, *DLA-DRB1* on chromosome 12) and the three can be considered in aggregate when trying to determine relative risk. This can help identify pets that might be a low, moderate, or high risk for developing the condition. Other loci could eventually also prove to be associated with the condition.

An example of a dominant trait is merling of coat color. The normal, recessive genotype is the homozygote, mm. The heterozygous (Mm) animal has the characteristic merle coat coloring. The homozygous dominant (MM) animal is nearly all white, has blue eyes, and has a higher incidence of deafness. Although merle is a desirable feature in some dog breeds, the deafness and white coat color are completely undesirable. Breeders wishing to perpetuate merle in their lines will breed normal (mm) to merle (Mm) to achieve half typically colored offspring and half merle offspring. Fortunately, genetic testing for the merle trait is now available to facilitate that process, and avoid inadvertently creating homozygous dominant animals (MM) with health issues.

In most cases, recessive disorders are often attributable to enzyme deficiencies because heterozygotes with only 50% as much enzyme likely still have enough to perform needed functions. In contrast, dominant traits may be caused by defects in structural or substrate proteins, such that heterozygotes will be expected to be affected because these polypeptides are required in relatively large quantities. As more and more research accumulates, however, these suppositions seem to consist of more generalization than fact, and each trait is best considered individually.

A lot has been learned since Mendel began playing with peas, and new genetic tests that actually identify genotype deserve much of the credit (see 3.6 Genetic Testing). Some of the old rules just do not apply, though. For example, mitochondrial myopathy in Clumber and Sussex spaniels is believed to be a sex-linked but not an X-linked trait. The trait is passed from the mitochondrial DNA of the maternal line to both sexes. Therefore, hemophilia A is X linked and is transmitted principally from mother to son, whereas mitochondrial myopathy is believed to be passed from mother to both sons and daughters.

3.3.4 More on Penetrance and Expressivity

Genetic testing allows us to detect discrete genetic variants for diseases and traits, and yet in real life, the manifestations sometimes appear more like shades of gray than black and white (see 3.4 Predicting and Eliminating Disease Traits). If a pet has a genetic variant detected, shouldn't that mean that the clinical result is a foregone conclusion? Like much of medicine, the answer is both yes and no. Here's why.

To understand the situation, we need to go back to a basic tenet of genetics – genetic mutations/variants don't cause disease; they code for proteins that may not be fully functional and it is this dysfunction that is interpreted as disease (see 3.1 Genetic Basics). The body tends to have a lot of redundant systems, so there may be other genes, epigenetic markers, modifiers, suppressors, and environmental factors that all impact the clinical manifestations in the living patient.

Clinical diagnosis also requires that we be able to clinically differentiate between the "normal" gene and the "variant" gene in all cases within a population of animals, and this is referred to as penetrance. Penetrance can be defined as the percentage of individuals in a population with a given genetic variant (genotype) that fully display the clinical manifestations (phenotype), and this is rarely 100%. Because of this, many conditions are described as having *incomplete penetrance* and this explains why we can't fully predict the clinical situation, even with sophisticated genetic screening. Some disorders may have full (100%) penetrance, but many more do not.

In contradistinction to penetrance, which looks at genetic manifestations on a population level, expressivity measures the extent to which a genetic variant (genotype) actually expresses the so-called clinical abnormality (phenotype) on an individual level. There can be different degrees of expression of identical variants in different individuals based on other genes present or environmental factors. Because of this, we might describe that there could be *variable expressivity* for this variant in different individuals.

These features of penetrance and expressivity make genetic counseling as much an art as a science, even given the certainty of genetic screening. It is also a great reason why genetic testing favors the nuanced interpretation by well-trained veterinary teams to properly counsel pet owners on the benefits of pet-specific care and the goal of helping pets live long, healthy, and happy lives.

3.3.5 Epistasis

As if penetrance and expressivity didn't add enough variability to the equation, it's important to realize that there may be diseases, phenes, and traits caused by the effects of more than one gene. Some loci have a variety of different alleles that could participate in a gene pair. Nowhere is this more apparent than in coat coloration (Table 3.3.1). *Epistasis* is when the action of one gene depends on the action of another gene. Epistasis is wonderfully illustrated by the coat colors possible with different combinations of alleles from different loci. All breeds have all the loci mentioned, but they do not necessarily have all the possible alleles mentioned. Even within a given locus, some alleles are dominant over others.

Table 3.3.1 The genetics of coat color

Locus and allele	Effect
Agouti	
A	Solid color
Ay	Fawn/sable
Aw	Gray/wolf
as	Saddle
at	Bicolor (tan points)
a	Recessive black
Black	
B	Black
b	Liver
Color	
C	Color factor
CC	Full color
cch	Chinchilla
c_e	Extreme dilution
cd	White with dark eyes
cb	Blue eyes
c	Albinism
Dilution	
D	No dilution
d	Dilution (e.g., blue Doberman)

(Continued)

Table 3.3.1 (Continued)

Locus and allele	Effect
Extension	
Em	Black mask
E	Normal extension
e	Nonextension (yellow)
Graying	
G	Born black, turns blue
g	Born black, stays black
Intensity	
INT	Lightest tan
intm	Intermediate tan
int	Darkest tan
Solid	
K	Solid color in pigmented areas
Br	Brindle
Y	Allows yellow pigment to show
Merle	
M	Merle
m	Nonmerle
Spotting	
S	Solid color
si	Irish spotting
sp	Piebald
sw	Extreme white piebald
S-extension	
Se	Black mask
sese	No black mask
Ticking	
T	Ticking
t	Nonticking

3.3.6 Epigenetics

Although many medical conditions are the result of gene mutations that have passed from generation to generation, evidence is mounting that the environment can not only have an impact on personal health but can also be conserved in the genes. These environmental "shocks" seem to be capable of leaving an imprint on the genetic material in eggs and sperm, which can pass along new traits in a single generation.

The epigenome sits above the DNA sequence and provides a second layer of information, regulating several genomic functions, including when and where genes are turned on or off. New studies have shown that so-called epigenetic marks are associated with genes, providing instructions such as telling them to switch on or off. These marks are normal and allow cells to differentiate, but if the marks do not work properly because of an environmental stressor, cancer or cell death might result, and, worst of all, could be transmitted to descendants. So, if some stressor such as a rich diet activates an epigenetic mark, which in turn modifies histones or adds methyl groups to DNA strands, it could result in disease or susceptibility to disease that not only affects the individual but can be passed on to future generations. This epigenetic influence may not even occur equally across both alleles, in some instances depending on genotype and in other instances depending on from which parent the allele was inherited. Nutrition is likely a major factor in epigenetics, and technological advances will likely lead to the identification of nutrient-responsive genes and biological pathways, important nutrient–gene interactions, and genomic biomarkers of disease [1].

While perhaps not as well known and discussed as the genome, the epigenome is believed to be much larger and more complicated than the genome of 20 000 or so genes. Medications are even available now that exert their effects through epigenetic marks. These developments are bound to assume more significance in the years ahead.

3.3.7 Genetics and Cancer

There is no doubt that many cancers have genetic associations [2] but there is still much to learn about the genetics of cancer. Solid evidence exists that some cancers, such as those associated with dermatofibrosis, have a genetic basis, and a DNA test can even be used for that particular disorder. Pugs are predisposed to viral pigmented plaques, associated with papillomavirus. Lymphoproliferative diseases also appear to have well-defined heritable risk factors in at least some breeds. In many other instances, definite breed predispositions exist, but in many cases a definitive genetic basis is lacking. In other cases, epigenetics and environmental causes may coincide with genetics to promote cancer. For example, the incidence of transitional cell carcinoma (TCC) has been steadily increasing in dogs over the years, and the risk of Scottish terriers developing TCC is approximately 18 times the risk of mixed-breed dogs [3]. Further studies have suggested that this breed-associated risk may be due to differences in pathways that activate or detoxify carcinogens, and exposure to lawns or gardens treated with phenoxy herbicides could potentially be associated with the increased risk of TCC in Scottish terriers.

Oncogenes are genes that when mutated, or expressed at high levels, cause normal cells to transition into cancer cells. The process is typically helped along by the effects of environmental carcinogens, viruses, and other stressors. In contradistinction to oncogenes, tumor suppressor genes, or *antioncogenes* as they are sometimes called, protect normal cells from transitioning into cancerous ones. A mutation in these genes can cause a loss of or reduction in this protective function.

3.3.8 Genetics and Behavior

Similar to cancer, little doubt exists that genetics plays a key role in predicting behaviors, and yet we are very early in the process of characterizing the process. Behaviors such as herding and retrieving are firmly entrenched in some breeds, and we are getting closer to understanding the genetic bases for these traits. In addition, it appears that dogs have evolved a social–cognitive specialization that allows them unusual skill in cooperating and communicating with humans [4]. In fact, dogs and humans accept each other into a mutual social structure, which appears to have been the result of genetic selection. Behavioral traits do have a genetic basis, and a high degree of genetic correlation between traits is often found.

Some developments have occurred in identifying quantitative trait loci (QTLs) important in some behavioral conditions, but much more is to be learned in years to come. Because behaviors are often conserved within breed groups, individual qualities (e.g., retrieving ability) can often be achieved by the appropriate selection of specific breeds, especially if representative family members can be observed. For mixed-breed dogs, a rough approximation might be accomplished by discerning which breeds primarily contributed to an individual animal through commercially available genetic breed profiles.

TAKE-AWAYS

- Genes don't cause diseases, but they may code for defective proteins that are associated with disease states.
- Most traits are considered dominant or recessive, but that classification is not absolute in most cases.
- DNA testing can be used to identify risk, but may not be absolute in predictions of clinical disease due to the properties of penetrance and expressivity.
- While some diseases may be caused by a defect attributed to variants in a single gene pair, the majority of diseases are caused by an interaction of multiple genes together with environmental factors.
- Genetic diseases can be attributable to more than just variants in nuclear or mitochondrial DNA; the epigenome appears to also play a significant role in disease manifestations.

MISCELLANEOUS

Abbreviation

DNA   Deoxyribonucleic acid

References

1 Swanson, K.S. (2006). *Nutrient–gene interactions and their role in complex diseases in dogs. J. Am. Vet. Med. Assoc.* 228 (10): 1513–1520.

2 Giger, U., Sargan, D.R., and McNiel, E.A. (2006). Breed-specific hereditary diseases and genetic screening. In: *The Dog and its Genome* (eds. E.A. Ostrander, U. Giger and K. Lindblad-Toh), 249–289. New York: Cold Spring Harbor Laboratory Press.

3 Knapp, D.W., Glickman, N.W., DeNicola, D.B. et al. (2000). Naturally-occurring canine transitional cell carcinoma of the urinary bladder: a relevant model of human invasive bladder cancer. *Urol. Oncol.* 5: 47–59.

4 Hare, B. and Tomasello, M. (2006). Behavioral genetics of dog cognition: human-like social skills in dogs are heritable and derived. In: *The Dog and its Genome* (eds. E.A. Ostrander, U. Giger and K. Lindblad-Toh), 497–514. New York: Cold Spring Harbor Laboratory Press.

Recommended Reading

Ackerman, L. (2011). *The Genetic Connection*. Lakewood, CO: AAHA Press.

Ackerman, L. (2019). The skinny on genes – what you should know about genetic testing. *AAHA Trends* 35 (6): 39–42.

Ackerman, L. (2020). Proactive Pet Parenting: Anticipating pet health problems before they happen. Problem Free Publishing.

Karlsson, E.K., Baranowska, I., Wade, C.M. et al. (2007). Efficient mapping of mendelian traits in dogs through genome-wide association. *Nat. Genet.* 39: 1321–1328.

Modiano, J.F., Breen, M., Burnett, R.C. et al. (2005). Distinct B-cell and T-cell lymphoproliferative disease prevalence among dog breeds indicates heritable risk. *Cancer Res.* 65: 5654–5661.

3.4

Predicting and Eliminating Disease Traits

Lowell Ackerman, DVM, DACVD, MBA, MPA, CVA, MRCVS

Global Consultant, Author, and Lecturer, MA, USA

BASICS

3.4.1 Summary

To be able to appropriately screen pets for disease traits, it is first critical to be able to ascertain their risk of developing problems, and then intervene at the earliest possible opportunity. This is best accomplished with a combination of genotypic and phenotypic screening.

3.4.2 Terms Defined

Allele: A variant or alternative form of a gene, found at the same location on a chromosome, and which can result in different observable traits.

Dominant: Heritable characteristics, traits, or diseases that are expressed when inherited even from one parent.

Genetics: The study of genes and how traits or conditions are passed from one generation to the next.

Genome: The complete set of genes for an animal.

Genomics: The study of the entire genome, and its combined influence on complex diseases and the impact of environmental factors such as diet, exercise, medications, and toxins on genes.

Genotype: An individual's genetic constitution.

Heterozygote: An individual with two different alleles for a given gene.

Homozygote: An individual with two identical alleles for a given gene.

Locus: A fixed position on a chromosome for a gene or marker.

Nutrigenomics: The interaction of genetics and nutrition and the role the two play in the prevention and treatment of disease.

Odds Ratio: The ratio of the odds of an event in a select group (e.g., breed) to the odds of an event in a control group.

Phene: A trait or characteristic that is genetically determined.

Phenotype: Observable characteristics or traits that result from the interaction of genotype with the environment.

Recessive: Heritable characteristics, traits, or diseases that are expressed only when inherited from both parents.

Relative Risk: The ratio of the probability of a phene, condition, or trait occurring in a specific group (e.g., breed), compared to the probability of it happening in a control group.

MAIN CONCEPTS

3.4.3 Risk Factors

Pet-specific care is all about managing risks. All animals have certain risks that pertain to their individual circumstances (see 1.1 Overview of Pet-Specific Care). By acknowledging and prioritizing risks, we can craft meaningful personalized care plans for our patients (see 1.3 Personalized Care Plans).

For most pets, family history or breed predisposition is a significant contributor to disease susceptibility. This is true whether the pet is purebred or mixed-breed. In many instances, when a pet is mixed-breed and the parents have not been identified with certainty, it may be difficult to discern any type of predisposition without performing breed composition genetic testing. Whether purebred or mixed-breed, both genotypic and phenotypic testing can be done for disease susceptibility.

Exposure risks constitute another significant contributor to disease susceptibility. For example, a pet exposed to many other pets will be at increased risk for infectious diseases and, potentially, parasite transmission. A dog that is taken for walks in wooded areas may be exposed to ticks that are enzootic to the region and may introduce tick-related infections to the pet. A cat that is allowed to wander the neighborhood may be exposed to a variety of infectious diseases, as well as injury from vehicles, other pets, and wildlife.

Susceptibility to medical problems is also influenced by life stages. For example, an umbilical hernia is more likely to be congenital and evident in a juvenile pet, while most cases of hypothyroidism present during adulthood (see 4.1 Canine and Feline Life Stages).

A pet's gender as well as its neuter status also influence risk. Some diseases are sex limited in nature (such as prostatic disease in males or pyometra in females), but there are also sex predispositions for a variety of disorders. For example, there may be a modest sex predisposition to females regarding cutaneous lupus erythematosus, while adrenal sex hormone imbalance (alopecia X) may be more commonly diagnosed in males. This is different from disorders transmitted genetically on the sex chromosomes. For example, hemophilia is more often clinically evident in males because the condition is transmitted on the X chromosome as a sex-linked recessive condition, and since males only have one X chromosome (the other is a Y chromosome), they manifest the condition; in females, with two X chromosomes, it would take two copies of the hemophilia mutation before the condition would be apparent. Neuter status also affects risk. Bitches spayed before their first estrus have a reduced prevalence of mammary cancers; neutered males have a lowered risk for prostatic hyperplasia (see 4.2 Gender-Related Considerations).

Geography also plays a significant role in disease susceptibility, partially because it influences infectious diseases that are present in the area, or the vectors that are associated with their transmission. Accordingly, when creating personalized care plans, it is important to take into consideration whether or not the pet may travel outside the region.

Even conformation and nondisease traits can be associated with predisposition to disease. For example, cats with white fur may be at higher risk for developing squamous cell carcinoma; color dilution alopecia is more common in dogs with diluted coloring patterns, such as "blue" Dobermans.

3.4.4 Genotypic and Phenotypic Testing

Since pet-specific care is about anticipating problems before they happen, typically through surveillance, screening tests are paramount to the process. The main categories of screening tests are based on phenotypic and genotypic assessment (see 3.11 Integrating Genotypic and Phenotypic Testing).

Genotypic tests assess a genetic mutation or marker to determine disease susceptibility. Such genetic tests measure either the presence of an actual genetic variant or genetic markers that appear to be associated with phenes. Genetic tests typically measure a specific variant associated with disease, while genomic tests may be used for more complex diseases in which there may be interactions among genes, and between genes and the environment; information may be assessed for disease susceptibility, prognosis, or likely response to therapy.

When it comes to genetic testing, there are many DNA tests that can be run, either individually or as part of a panel (http://bit.ly/2YWXBsc). For those that are only concerned with a single medical issue, individual genetic tests can be conducted. From a medical perspective, the most valuable information typically comes in the form of genetic panels in which multiple genetic tests are run at the same time (see 3.11 Integrating Genotypic and Phenotypic Testing). This will evaluate for dozens of medical conditions, as well as for certain traits (e.g., conformation, color, etc.). Sometimes specific breed profiles are requested, evaluating only conditions common in a specific breed, although with the new "chip" technologies, it is as inexpensive to run a complete panel with dozens or hundreds of tests as it is to run a handful of tests common in a specific breed. In almost all cases, it makes more sense (financial and otherwise) to run the complete profile rather than try to guess which tests might be most relevant. However, after running such a panel, it is necessary for the hospital team to determine which tests are actually relevant for each individual pet (see 3.8 Genetic Counseling).

Phenotypic tests are those that measure a detectable abnormality or variance from normal, rather than a genetic variant. This includes most of the tests we routinely use, such as hemograms, biochemical profiles, urinalysis, radiography, etc. For example, while genotypic tests can identify some variants of primary open-angle glaucoma susceptibility at birth, phenotypic tests that rely on measurements of intraocular pressure (IOP) identify glaucoma when IOP increases above an established reference interval (range) for the breed.

Nutrigenomics will likely also play more of a role in healthcare with improved technology. There are several direct-to-consumer testing possibilities that purport to tell consumers how their eating habits could be associated with genetic predisposition and how sensitive they are to certain foods. Because of complicated environment–gene interactions, how individuals metabolize foods, and the role of the gut microbiome (see 4.6 Role of the Microbiome), this would be potentially complicated to interpret in pets.

3.4.5 History

Collecting relevant information from pet owners is critical to being able to provide truly personalized care for pets. Since pets spend much more time with their owners than with veterinary staff, pet owners must be engaged in the process and aware that such information sharing will ultimately benefit their pets.

Every hospital visit provides an opportunity to learn more about the pet, the pet owner, and how they interact with one another. In many cases, it is most efficient to use questionnaires to standardize the collection process (see 1.2 Providing a Lifetime of Care).

Important topics include understanding what other pets may co-exist in the house, activities, and exposure, diets being fed, prescription and nonprescription medications being administered, etc.

It is also important to realize that preexisting conditions may be associated with increased risk for other disorders. For example, a pet diagnosed with Cushing's syndrome likely has an increased risk for diabetes mellitus. A pet with excessive skinfolds is likely predisposed to skinfold dermatitis. A pet with early radiographic evidence of hip dysplasia is more likely to develop osteoarthritis.

3.4.6 Counseling

The benefit for veterinary practices is that pet-specific counseling is an important part of a personalized approach to healthcare, and research shows that hospitals that practice such client-centric care typically have significant growth year on year, compared to practices that do not provide this type of service (see 10.11 The Financial Benefits of Pet-Specific Medicine).

It is important to understand how early detection can influence future actions. An animal that is prone to cardiomyopathy based on genetic testing, family history or breed predisposition will potentially need regular cardiac monitoring, periodic radiographs, laboratory testing, and perhaps echocardiography, all before the condition ever becomes clinical. Once it becomes clinical, there will be pharmacological and dietary intervention, likely for the remainder of the pet's life. The client will also be more

likely to want to comply if they have some documentation of susceptibility through DNA testing.

3.4.7 Checklists

Checklists have proven to be very beneficial in human medicine, where they have helped reduce medical errors, improved patient safety, enhanced teamwork, and ensured that steps were not missed (see 2.4 Checklists in Veterinary Practice). Without mandatory adverse event reporting, or morbidity and mortality investigations, it is difficult to tell how often medical mistakes occur in animals (see 8.14 Appropriate Handling of Medical Errors).

Checklists can also be used for more basic functions, such as history taking, presurgical and postsurgical checks, and even to ensure that certain topics are addressed in client educations (Figure 3.4.1).

3.4.8 Predicting Outcomes

Most traits/phenes recognized in veterinary practice, and those that cause the most problems, do not seem to fit neatly into Mendelian patterns of inheritance. When phenes such as hip dysplasia, allergies, epilepsy, diabetes mellitus, glaucoma, and colitis are considered, no easy answers are forthcoming. If the problem is presumed likely to be caused by more than one gene, it is labeled polygenic but most of the time, it is impossible to prove this without genotype testing. If a condition such as epilepsy is seen, which might affect more than one member of a breed line, it might be described as familial without knowing precisely how the trait is passed in that family. When a disorder appears to be more common in some breeds than in others, we call this a *breed predisposition*. Once again, in most instances the exact mode of inheritance is not known.

Topic	Addressed
Pet-specific issues	☐
Vaccination	☐
Parasite control	☐
Genetic testing	☐
Nutritional counseling	☐
Oral health counseling	☐
Behavioral counseling	☐
Spay/Neuter	☐
Identification (microchipping)	☐
Risk management (Pet Health Insurance)	☐

Figure 3.4.1 Topics to be addressed in puppy/kitten client discussions.

This lack of specificity is difficult to reconcile with a desire to predict outcomes. Nearly everyone believes that German shepherd dogs are prone to hip dysplasia. We might say that the German shepherd dog has a breed predisposition or predilection for hip dysplasia. Yet, German shepherd dogs are not necessarily one of the breeds most commonly afflicted with the disorder, especially when their popularity is taken into account in terms of relative risk.

Whenever possible, risk should include a correction for a breed's prevalence in the population sampled. For example, if we were to run a hip dysplasia screening clinic and find that we had eight German shepherd dogs and four St Bernards with hip dysplasia, we might conclude that German shepherds have a higher prevalence of the problem. When these numbers are compared with the prevalence of each breed in our clinic population, however, the prevalence of hip dysplasia in St Bernards might turn out to be more than twice that in German shepherds. Because our hospital has many more German shepherd dogs, they would naturally account for a larger number of affected individuals. For many conditions, the prevalence might be high in mixed-breed dogs (mutts) and cats (moggies), just because they represent the largest segment of a hospital population.

As a fictitious example, let's say we have a clinic population of 10 000 dogs, and when we review our medical records, we see that we have diagnosed 43 cases of follicular dysplasia over the past five years. Of these, 27 cases were seen in mutts, 11 in Chinese shar pei, and five in Irish water spaniels. In this hypothetical situation, which breed has the highest prevalence of follicular dysplasia? We cannot know until we see how the hospital population breaks down by breed. Of the dogs in the practice, 3723 are mutts, 89 are Chinese shar pei, and 12 are Irish water spaniels. According to our study, then, the condition is really seen in fewer than 1% of mutts, more than 12% of Chinese shar peis, and more than 40% of Irish water spaniels. The lesson is that, without accounting for breed numbers in a population, we could easily draw inaccurate conclusions (see 2.3 Prevalence and Incidence).

Relative risk, accounting for the prevalence of issues (events) in a specified population, is a reflection of probability. Also used is an odds ratio, wherein numbers greater than 1 represent increased risk and numbers lower than 1 represent decreased risk. Thus, a canine breed with an odds ratio of 4 has four times the risk of the general canine population of developing a specific condition. For the sake of accuracy, relative risk and odds ratios are not really synonymous. Relative risk is the ratio of two probabilities, the probability (risk) of an event in a select group over the probability (risk) of an event in the control group; the odds

ratio is a ratio of two odds, the odds of an event in the select group over the odds of an event in the control group. Even with odds ratios and relative risk, breed predisposition is only a rough guide to disease prevalence. As long as individual breeders decide which qualities they wish to emphasize in their matings, overall breed statistics may not tell us much.

Finally, genetic and congenital abnormalities should be differentiated. The term *congenital* merely implies that a trait was present at birth. It does not mean that the disorder is heritable.

3.4.9 Hardy–Weinberg Law

Sometimes the magnitude of a heritable problem is not immediately obvious. It can be brought more sharply into focus with something called the *Hardy–Weinberg law*. This law helps to predict genotype frequencies with a simple algebraic formula, where p^2 is the frequency of the homozygous dominant gene pairing, $2pq$ is for heterozygotes, and q^2 is the frequency of the homozygous recessive gene pairing, with the individual gene frequencies, $p + q$, equaling 1. The Hardy–Weinberg law applies as long as no mutation (allelic changes), migration ("new blood"), or active selection for a trait occurs. Although the Hardy–Weinberg law is very useful in canine genetics, it must be remembered that dog breeding invalidates some of the basic tenets of the law because matings do not occur randomly or without selection, the way they might in nature. Also, the population is rarely in equilibrium because breeders often bring in breeding animals from outside the local population. As such, gene frequencies predicted by the Hardy–Weinberg law may not be completely accurate. Still, much useful information is provided.

Let's examine this with the American car-chasing terrier (ACCT) and the prevalence of an autosomal recessive trait, von Willebrand disease, in this breed. Although the genetic mutation associated with von Willebrand disease has been determined in many breeds, it has not yet been characterized in the ACCT, but pedigree analysis suggests that it is autosomal recessive in nature. Because von Willebrand disease in the ACCT is autosomal recessive, it is difficult to distinguish between the homozygous dominant and the heterozygote; von Willebrand factor testing does not convincingly differentiate the two in this breed, and DNA mutation testing is not yet available. The only phenotype that can conclusively be demonstrated is the homozygous recessive, those affected with von Willebrand disease.

We did a survey with the local ACCT club and found that of 1000 dogs, 53 had von Willebrand disease. The ACCT club seemed happy that the prevalence of the disorder in the breed was of the order of only about 5%. Using the figures from the survey, the actual genotype frequency for homozygous recessive (q^2) is 0.053 and the gene frequency (q) is the square root of 0.053, or 0.23. We know the sum of p and q equals 1, and q equals 0.23, so p must equal 0.77, and p^2, the proportion with the homozygous dominant genotype, equals 0.59. On the basis of these numbers, $2pq$, or 0.35 (35%), would be predicted to be the likely proportion of heterozygous carriers in the population.

What does this exercise in algebra tell us? Well, it tells us that although only 5.3% of ACCTs actually have von Willebrand disease, an incredible 35% of the ACCT population are carriers of the trait, which is not detectable by conventional means. The breed club has a potentially serious problem and would be best advised to invest money in a genetic test to detect heterozygotes. In the interim, however, the goal is to identify heterozygotes by other means so that animals that are homozygous normal can be discerned. We'll have to do the best we can with von Willebrand disease testing and progeny testing to differentiate normal homozygotes from normal-appearing heterozygotes until that DNA test becomes available.

Identifying dogs that are homozygous recessive is not a problem. They are the ones with von Willebrand disease. We also know that both normal-appearing parents of these affected animals are heterozygotes, carriers of the trait. Nevertheless, most of the other heterozygotes, which we would like to avoid breeding together, are clinically indistinguishable from the homozygous normal animals that we would like to use in our breeding program. For example, because we know that the parents of affected animals are carriers, it follows that at least one of each of their parents (grandparents of the affected animal) must also be a carrier. Inferring genotype from a family tree is known as *pedigree analysis*.

3.4.10   Preserving Genetic Diversity

Although establishing harsh criteria to rid breeds of genetic disorders by completely eliminating affected animals and carriers may seem reasonable, it is neither practical nor desirable. Because each animal carries nearly 20 000 different genes, ridding lines of all deleterious alleles is not possible. If carriers can be determined, however, breeding phenotypically normal dogs is a real possibility by never breeding two carriers together. If we are aware of heterozygotes, we can safely breed carriers with known normal individuals, and we will never see cases of the disorders we are trying to avoid. Is that not what genetic counseling is all about?

Trying to overcome polygenic traits takes longer and is more troublesome. Obviously, the higher the heritability of

a trait and the more ruthless we are in selecting superior individuals for breeding, the more successful our selection process will be. This response to selection (R) can also be described as an algebraic function, $R = h^2 S$, where R is the response to our breeding strategy, h^2 is the heritability of the condition, and S is the selection differential, the phenotypic superiority of the parents we selected versus that of the general population from which they came. The result is that the mean improves; it is not that the pups will be superior to their parents.

Hip dysplasia provides a good example of how selection pressure improves the standard, albeit slowly. Let's say we create a scoring system for hips in which 0 represents severe dysplasia and 100 represents perfect hips. In our ACCT, the mean hip score for the population is 55 and the heritability of the trait is believed to be 0.25. To try to improve hip joint morphology in the breed, we mate a stud with a hip score of 88 with a bitch with a score of 92. The average score of the parents is 90, which is 35 points higher than the mean for the breed. Should that produce terriers with great hips? The response to selection (R) is 0.25×35, or 8.75. Thus, in the litter produced, the mean hip score for the pups is predicted to be 63.75 ($55 + 8.75$). We have managed to shift the whole bell-shaped curve of hip scores to the right, but not by the magnitude you may have expected. Now you see why creating real improvement with polygenic traits takes so long, even when using superior breeding animals.

3.4.11   Bias

In scrutinizing genetic reports in the literature, one must note that study bias is rampant in clinical research, even studies published in peer-reviewed journals. *Nonselection* is defined as failure to include a subject or subjects from the population of interest in the experiment or study group; *nonresponse* is the failure to include a subject or subjects from the study population in the results and analyses of the study. Thus, for a disorder as common as hip dysplasia, prevalence data by breed are often contentious. Because submission of radiographs to most registries is voluntary, owners with dogs that are most likely to have hip dysplasia may see no reason to pay to have the radiographs submitted to the registry, which leads to substantial nonresponse bias and underestimation of the actual prevalence of hip dysplasia in these breeds.

This argument is not far-fetched. Owners with dogs that have clinical evidence of hip dysplasia are not likely to ask to have radiographs taken because they know their animal will not be certified. Other owners, who have radiographs done thinking their animal is clear and learn that it has hip dysplasia, may elect not to have those reports sent to the registry, so as not to be stigmatized by the results.

Nonselection bias also plagues hip dysplasia statistics. Even if the registry decides to petition a national breed club, such as the ACCT Club, and asks all registrants to participate in a cost-free hip evaluation plan to gather breed statistics on hip morphology, the potential for bias still exists. If the breed club has a strong policy of encouraging the breeding of only disease-free dogs, might there not be dog owners who do not agree with those policies and therefore choose to not belong to the club? Or might there not be a sizeable population of owners of the breed who do not belong to the breed club because they are pet owners, not breeders? In any case, results cannot be extrapolated to the entire breed, just the frame selected for study.

Much of the research on which breed statistics for genetic disorders have been based is subject to nonresponse and nonselection bias. When bias is not addressed, readers are left to make their own assumptions on the basis of the results reported.

A better approach is for veterinarians to take a proactive stance and to consider preventive care on a pet-specific basis whenever possible. In fact, understanding predispositions and risk profiles for individual pets allows veterinarians to create a lifetime care plan for most of their clients, based on the specific risks of each individual patient (see 1.2 Providing a Lifetime of Care), even if risk cannot be completely assessed.

EXAMPLES

A cocker spaniel breeder takes your advice and performs DNA testing for phosphofructokinase deficiency on a prospective breeding pair. The potential sire is clear, but the bitch is determined to be a carrier. What are the odds that this mating will result in affected pups?

Because the sire is clear, he must be homozygous for the normal allele (PP). The bitch, as a carrier, has the heterozygous genotype Pp. A mating of these two would produce roughly 50% homozygotes (PP) and 50% carriers (Pp), but no affected individuals (pp). Given the new technology, which allows genotypic determination for this trait in cocker spaniels, the occurrence of affected individuals can be completely eliminated even when it may be difficult to completely eliminate the recessive allele itself from a population.

TAKE-AWAYS

- The best way to predict disease is to first create a risk profile.
- The main risk factors for disease are often attributable to genetics, environmental, and lifestyle characteristics, and existing conditions that can lead to co-morbidities.
- Early detection of disease depends on both genotypic and phenotypic testing.
- It is important to realize that it is not possible, or even advisable, to use predictive tests to try to eliminate all deleterious alleles from a breeding line.
- Bias exists in most forms of research citing predisposition to disease; the information still has validity, but needs to be appreciated in context.

MISCELLANEOUS

Abbreviation

DNA   Deoxyribonucleic acid

Recommended Reading

Ackerman, L. (2011). *The Genetic Connection: A Guide to Health Problems in Purebred Dogs*, 2e. Lakewood, CO: AAHA Press.

Ackerman, L. (2019). The skinny on genes: what you should know about genetic testing. *AAHA Trends* 35 (6): 39–42.

Ackerman, L. (2020). Proactive Pet Parenting: Anticipating pet health problems before they happen. Problem Free Publishing.

Baker, L., Muir, P., and Sample, S.J. (2019). Genome-wide association studies and genetic testing: understanding the science, success, and future of a rapidly developing field. *Journal of the American Veterinary Medical Association* 255 (10): 1126–1136.

Bell, J., Cavanagh, K., Tilley, L., and Smith, F. (2012). *Veterinary Medical Guide to Dog and Cat Breeds*. Jackson, WY: Teton NewMedia.

Shaffer, L.G., Geretshlaeger, A., Ramirez, C.J. et al. (2019). Quality assurance checklist and additional considerations for canine clinical genetic testing laboratories: a follow-up to the published standards and guidelines. *Human Genetics*: 501–508.

3.5

Conformation Extremes and the Veterinary Team

Emma Goodman Milne, BVSc, MRCVS

Independent Veterinary Surgeon, France

 BASICS

3.5.1 Summary

In many countries around the world, breeds of pet animals, notably dogs, cats, and rabbits, are becoming more and more extreme in their body shapes. Examples of such extremes could be short legs, long backs, very long ears, excessive hair or hairlessness, pronounced skinfolds, bulging or sunken eyes and, perhaps the most well-recognized, the brachycephalic or flat-faced animals. All these extremes lean away from natural selection and evolution and can be associated with a wide spectrum of disease and life-altering issues. These range from very mild to immediately life-threatening. The veterinary team can make a big difference both throughout the animal's life but also by being involved right from the point of prepurchase decision making.

3.5.2 Terms Defined

Conformation: The shape or dimensions of an animal.
Entropion: An eyelid that turns inwards and rubs on the eyeball.
Exophthalmos: Abnormal bulging or protrusion of the eyeball.
Inbreeding: The breeding of closely related individuals.
Pyoderma: An infection in the skin.

 MAIN CONCEPTS

3.5.3 The Origin of the Problem

For thousands and thousands of years, humans have lived with animals. We gradually selected different types of dogs to do different jobs like herding, hunting, and guarding. We chose different sizes and selected for different temperaments depending on what the dog needed to do. Cats did what they were good at – rodent control – so have been left largely unchanged until the last century or so. When the idea of different breeds and the purity of the breed lines became popular at the end of the 1800s, body shapes started to change and inbreeding became commonplace. Over the last 100–200 years, many breeds have become more and more extreme (Figures 3.5.1 and 3.5.2). For example, pugs and bulldogs that had notable muzzles in 1900 now have very flat faces indeed. Breeds that were created to have slightly shorter legs, like dachshunds and bassets, for hunting different prey now have extremely short legs compared to their back length.

During this time, we have become more and more used to the fact that different breeds are more likely to have certain health problems than others. Many of these breed-related problems are due to unnatural and extreme body shape or conformation (Figures 3.5.3 and 3.5.4).

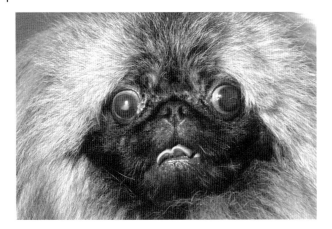

Figure 3.5.1 Flat-faced animals may experience a large number of health problems, some of which are life-threatening. *Source:* Photo courtesy of Dr David Gould.

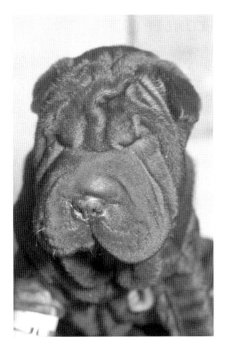

Figure 3.5.2 Excessive skinfolds cause disease and eye problems. *Source:* Photo courtesy of Dr David Gould.

3.5.4 Consequences of Extreme Conformation

We know that the more extreme the body shape or individual features become, the more likely the animal is to suffer from health issues, but it is not just the animals that are affected. The emotional and financial consequences for the owners can be huge but the whole veterinary team can also be affected. It can be emotionally difficult for members of the hospital team to see and treat animals that are suffering due to their conformation, especially when the animals are young. We can become attached to clients we see often

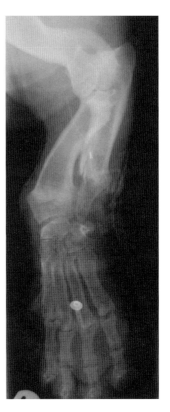

Figure 3.5.3 Short legs of a bassett compared to... *Source:* Photo courtesy of Andy Moores.

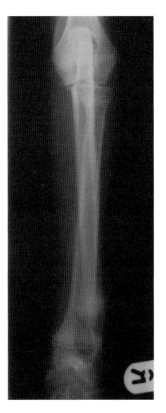

Figure 3.5.4 ...a normal straight leg. *Source:* Photo courtesy of Andy Moores.

and seeing them deal with illness and death can have a huge effect on us too.

There is also a secondary or indirect (knock-on) effect for society because many of the extreme or quirky breeds are popular in advertisements and movies so demand goes up. This can increase the number of unscrupulous breeders and production farms and the number of unwanted puppies and kittens. Equally, as these dogs and cats age and owners realize they cannot afford the increased costs of healthcare, more and more animals are abandoned or relinquished, and end up in adoption centers or simply dumped on the streets.

3.5.5 What the Veterinary Team Can Do

3.5.5.1 Make Sure You All Agree!

Many practices have policies on lots of different things like drugs, procedures, hygiene and so on but subjects like ethics and welfare can get forgotten. Some members of the team may have very strong feelings on these issues but never get the chance to air them. By having frank discussions among the whole team, you can achieve a united approach. Discuss things like the ethics of fertility services for animals that are incapable of breeding naturally. Will you offer planned cesarean sections (c-sections) or only when medically necessary? Make sure you have one or more people whose job it is to report procedures like c-sections and conformation-altering surgery if your purebred associations require it. Think about joining data-sharing schemes so that an evidence base can be gathered globally.

Remember that you can help at every stage of the animal's life, and even from before conception.

3.5.5.2 Social Media

Social media can be great for practices, but it is also a powerful tool in getting messages across both consciously and subliminally. If your team believes that conformational extremes are not to be encouraged, make sure that such animals are not prominently featured on any practice promotional materials or posts unless you are highlighting health issues. Do not do posts using words like "cute" in relation to extreme conformation and avoid sharing videos that people see as funny but are in fact signs of ill health, like dogs snoring and falling asleep sitting up. Always promote healthy animals and body shapes.

3.5.5.3 Prepurchase Advice

Many clients do little or no research before getting a pet (see 3.10 Advising Clients on Selecting an Appropriate Pet). When it comes to breeds, the decision can be an impulse buy. This can be a problem if the breed doesn't suit the family situation but also if the owner is unaware of any potential health problems. Discuss how your practice might reach more potential clients before they get their pet. This could include client evenings, booths (stands) at fun pet shows, social media drives or articles in the local paper. Reducing demand for extremes by education is one of the best ways to influence change. Encourage clients to use contracts that empower them. Talk to clients about how to avoid production farms and third-party sales. Make sure they know what health tests they should be expecting for the breed they have chosen (see 11.4 Heritable Health Conditions – By Breed).

3.5.5.4 First Visits

First visits can be difficult. The client has possibly spent hours with the breeder and may have been given spurious advice on many aspects of health and preventive medicine. It can be hard to address this in 10–15 minutes. Try and use the team effectively. Consider offering 30–60 minutes with a competent nurse as well as the veterinary visit. This way you can discuss the breed, possible health problems for the client to be aware of and look out for, as well as effective preventive healthcare and pet health insurance (see 10.16 Pet Health Insurance). It's important not to blame the client for poor choices.

Try not to think of "normal for breed." We should be open and honest about things that may be considered 'typical" for a breed but are not normal for the species. Examples would be exophthalmos, entropion, excessive skinfolds, narrow nostrils, snoring, or respiratory noise and malformed or crowded teeth. Document all abnormalities and discuss them with the owner.

3.5.5.5 Ongoing Care and End of Life

The level of intervention needed will vary greatly depending on the animal and the severity of the problems. Specialist referral may be required but there will also undoubtedly be times that the client cannot afford the treatment necessary. It can be good to discuss within the practice and with the client possible outcomes and where you might decide it is time to offer euthanasia or signing the animal over if treatment may be possible and appropriate with a new owner or adoption center.

TAKE-AWAYS

- Extreme conformation is unnatural and can lead to a variety of health issues and suffering, some of which can be life-threatening.
- The veterinary team should not normalize health problems just because they are common in a certain breed.
- Having a united approach and understanding across the whole practice team is important for client education and consistency of messaging, especially on social media.
- Try to formulate strategies for reaching prospective clients *before* they acquire a pet. Prepurchase education is key to reducing demand for extreme body shapes.
- Be open and honest with clients about their pets but remember they are not always to blame for poor choices and may have been misinformed by breeders, peers, and the internet!

MISCELLANEOUS

Recommended Reading

Gough, A., Thomas, A., and O'Neill, D. (2018). *Breed Predispositions to Disease in Dogs and Cats*, 3e. Ames, IA: Wiley Blackwell.
www.dogbreedhealth.com
www.icatcare.org/advice

3.6

Genetic Testing

Jerold S. Bell, DVM

Department of Clinical Sciences, Cummings School of Veterinary Medicine at Tufts University, North Grafton, MA, USA

BASICS

3.6.1 Summary

Genetic testing encompasses all evaluations that reveal hereditary predisposition to traits and disorders. These include physical genetic screening for disease as well as DNA tests of the genotype. These evaluations can assist with diagnosis, prognosis, treatment, and, in breeding animals, breeding recommendations. The veterinary team is increasingly presented with direct-to-consumer DNA test results for interpretation. It is up to the profession to educate itself on the types of genetic tests available, the validity of the individual tests, the applicability of each test for each breed, and what they tell you about the individual dog or cat. Genetic testing must be considered within a strategy of genetic counseling (see 3.8 Genetic Counseling).

3.6.2 Terms Defined

Allele: One copy of a gene in a gene pair.

Chromosome: The physical structure of DNA in pairs, one from the sire and one from the dam. The number of chromosomes varies between species.

Deoxyribonucleic acid (DNA): The chemical structure of the genetic instruction set containing coding and regulatory genes.

Gene: A length of DNA that codes for a specific protein, enzyme, or cellular event.

Genotype: The DNA of the animal. Usually pertaining to the two copies of a single gene, (i.e., AA, aa, or Aa).

Heterozygous: A gene pair where the two copies have different alleles (i.e., Aa).

Homozygous: A gene pair where both copies have the same allele (i.e., AA or aa).

Phenotype: What you see in the animal based on the expression of the genotype (i.e., normal, affected, coat type, etc.).

MAIN CONCEPTS

Genetic testing does not just involve breeding animals. We see genetic disease in practice every day. Every nucleated cell in the body has the same DNA instruction manual. Cells in different tissues have different genes turned on and off to control their maturation and function. Genes get turned on and off, and their effects are mitigated based on the effect of other genes, diet, drugs, inflammation, infection, and surgery.

All genes come in pairs – one from the sire and one from the dam (see 3.1 Genetic Basics). Simple Mendelian genetic diseases are caused by the effects of only one gene pair. Dominant disease can be caused by one mutated gene in the pair, and recessive disease requires two mutated genes. Sex-linked/X-linked disease involves genes on the X chromosome. As males have only one X chromosome, any mutation on the X chromosome can cause disease. Females, with two X chromosomes, can be carriers of recessive disease with one copy of a mutation, or can be affected if they have two copies (see 3.2 Modes of Inheritance).

Complexly inherited disease, also referred to as polygenically inherited traits, involves the combined effect of multiple gene pairs and usually an environmental component. The majority of genetic diseases and the most commonly seen diseases (e.g., hip dysplasia, feline inflammatory bladder disease, allergies, hypothyroidism, etc.) are complexly inherited and currently have no mutation-based DNA tests available.

Genetic tests vary on what they are able to identify, and therefore how they can be used in managing genetic disease. To understand how we can use genetic tests, we have to understand the types of tests that are available, what they can tell us, and their limitations (see 3.11 Integrating Genotypic and Phenotypic Testing).

3.6.3 Phenotypic Tests

Some tests measure the phenotype, or what can be seen in the animal. This may not directly relate to the genotype, or the genes regulating the defect that you are trying to manage. Ophthalmic screening for cataracts, auscultating for heart murmurs, hip and elbow radiographs, thyroid profiles, bile acid tests, eye examinations, urinalysis for crystals or metabolites, bladder stone analysis, skin biopsy for sebaceous adenitis, and observations on behavioral traits are all tests of the phenotype. Most tests of the phenotype only identify affected individuals from nonaffected individuals, and not carriers of disease liability genes (see 3.3 The Genetics of Disease).

3.6.4 Genotypic Tests

These tests identify specific DNA sequences and nucleotide changes. They can be run at any age, often before the onset of clinical disease. Different types of genotypic tests reflect the research that identified them. Candidate gene studies or whole-genome sequencing (WGS) usually identify specific disease-causing mutations. In genome-wide association studies (GWAS), groups of affected and normal individuals are compared at the DNA level. A SNP (pronounced *snip*) is a single nucleotide polymorphism – a single DNA letter (A, T, C, or G) that varies between individuals. GWAS utilizes gene chips that can evaluate hundreds of thousands of different SNPs. A SNP that is always present in a disease state but not in normal animals is considered a marker that lies close on the chromosome to a disease-causing gene. In some instances, the SNP is a single nucleotide substitution that actually causes the disease.

3.6.4.1 Direct Mutation-Based Tests

These tests evaluate for specific disease-causing gene mutations. For completely penetrant simple Mendelian genes, an "affected" test result is 100% accurate in predicting clinical disease. For recessive disorders requiring two copies of the

mutation to be affected, these tests allow identification of "carriers" who have one copy of the mutation, while "normal" individuals have no copies of the mutation.

If a direct mutation test does not predict disease 100% of the time, then this is considered incomplete penetrance (i.e., the genotype does not penetrate into the phenotype completely and consistently). This decreased penetrance can be due to the effect of other genes that impact their expression (complex or polygenic inheritance). For late-onset disorders, variations in age of onset can affect penetrance if the "average" age of onset is close to the average life expectancy of the individual. Examples would be late-onset cataracts, some forms of progressive retinal atrophy (PRA), and several neurodegenerative disorders.

Some direct genetic tests identify a mutation that causes increased susceptibility to a genetic disease, but is not necessarily associated with disease 100% of the time. These susceptibility or liability genes can be part of complexly inherited diseases or the cause of incomplete penetrance of (assumed) simple Mendelian diseases. Some of these mutations are required for an individual to be affected, and some just provide increased risk (increased odds ratio), if present, but are not required to produce an affected individual. An example is the susceptibility to perianal fistulae/anal furunculosis in German shepherd dogs. Dogs with the susceptibility haplotype (combination of major histocompatibility complex [MHC] genes) have a 5× odds ratio for the disease versus those without the haplotype. This means that individuals with a positive test result are five times more likely to develop the disease than animals that do not test positive. This risk factor occurs whether the susceptibility haplotype is heterozygous or homozygous, though homozygous dogs develop the disease at an earlier age. Another example is the genetic test for pug dog encephalitis, a painful, fatal disease affecting 1–2% of pugs. Dogs homozygous for an MHC susceptibility haplotype have a 15.6× odds ratio for developing the disease, but dogs heterozygous for the susceptibility haplotype have no greater risk.

3.6.4.2 Linked Marker-Based Tests

Some defective genes can be linked to a genetic marker – usually a SNP. The causative gene for the disorder in this case has not actually been identified, but a marker is available that can provide at least some predictive ability. Because the mutation and linked marker lie on the same chromosomal segment, they are usually inherited together, and the marker is relatively (but not absolutely) predictive of the presence of the disease mutation. During meiosis in the formation of eggs and sperm, the maternal and paternal paired chromosomes can cross over and exchange DNA segments. If a genetic cross-over occurs between a linked marker and the defective gene, the marker will no longer be linked to the defective gene. False-positive and false-negative results will occur and allow the marker to be passed on to offspring and descendants. Due to this phenomenon, linked marker test results must be compared with results from other family members to determine whether they correlate with their known phenotype.

3.6.4.3 Breed-Specific Genetic Testing

Due to common inheritance, different breeds of cats and dogs can be more prone to certain hereditary diseases. These can occur as a higher prevalence of common genetic diseases such as allergies, hip dysplasia, or feline urological syndrome/inflammatory cystitis. Other breed-related diseases are caused by more recent mutations that are only present in a specific breed or group of related breeds.

Several breed organizations and/or genetic testing companies list recommended breed-specific genetic tests and screening (see 3.7 Genetic Health Registries and Research Organizations). Parent-breed dog clubs in the US may list prebreeding screening tests through the OFA-CHIC program (www.ofa.org/browse-by-breed) and AKC Breed with HEART program (www.akc.org/breeder-programs/akc-bred-with-heart-program/requirements/health-testing-requirements). For cat breeds, International Cat Care lists breed-specific genetic diseases (https://icatcare.org/advice/?per_page=12&categories=cat-breeds).

3.6.5 Availability of Genetic Tests

The quantity and commercial availability of DNA-based genetic tests are rapidly increasing. A regularly updated list of available mutation-based and linked marker-based genetic tests is available at: http://research.vet.upenn.edu/WSAVA-LabSearch. For canine genetic tests, the International Partnership for Dogs has a similar database that includes quality control metrics of laboratories: https://dogwellnet.com/ctp. Unfortunately, companies offering DNA testing are unregulated and may have no established standards for quality control or validation of the genetic test results that they report.

3.6.5.1 Genetic Panel (Multiplex) Testing

Several commercial genetic testing laboratories offer breed-specific "panels" of DNA tests versus running individual tests. However, in many instances, tests may be offered that have no relevance to causing clinical disease in a specific breed. A test may be offered based on a single

published report, from a research colony, or from a related breed. Test results are of no consequence if a disease is not clinically documented in the specific breed population. Sources should be consulted to identify valid genetic tests in each breed.

Some commercial laboratories have developed gene chips that test for hundreds of SNPs from a single DNA sample (usually a cheek swab). This is far more cost and time efficient than sending out DNA samples to multiple laboratories for individual gene tests. If a SNP is the sole cause of the disease, then these are direct genetic tests. However, many of these SNPs are associated with a larger mutation and so are actually linked marker tests. These are susceptible to false-positive and -negative results. If decisions of treatment or breeding are being made, they should be based on direct mutation tests.

While multiplex (panel) testing provides a more cost-efficient way to do genetic testing, the majority of individual SNP results are of no consequence except to single breeds or subsets of breeds. There are many mutations that cause disease in one or a few breeds, however the mutation is present in many other breeds and does not cause clinical disease. This is because in the other breeds, additional mutations are not present that make the testable mutation a disease-causing gene. The *sod1* mutation for degenerative myelopathy and the *cord1* PRA mutations are examples of liability genes that contribute to disease in only a handful of breeds but may be detectable in almost all breeds. A carrier or even "affected" test result for these mutations must be ignored in breeds not prone to the specific disorder.

3.6.5.2 Mixed-Breed and Purebred Testing

Several companies offer DNA testing to identify breed heritage for pets. Unfortunately, only a few companies have actually performed the research to do this kind of analysis accurately. There are several companies that run these tests based on limited published guidelines and produce spurious results. Another issue is that these tests were designed to answer the question, "If this dog descended from only purebred ancestors, what breeds were represented?" Most mixed-breed dogs are not descended from purebred ancestors (except designer breeds) and come from multiple generations of mixed-breed ancestors. In the majority of cases the testing will identify markers that are considered breed specific and label that breed as an ancestor. It is more likely that the tested dog's ancestor and the founding members of a breed shared a marker – not that the pet's ancestor descended from the breed. For example, several "hound-type" mixed-breed dogs will be identified as being descended from rare hound breeds such as American foxhound or blue tick coonhound when the testing is just identifying markers that are present in ancestors to hound breeds. Even genetic testing companies that have done extensive research into mixed-breed testing will have conflicting results on the same DNA sample. These are "best-guess" results based on each company's algorithm of estimating breed background.

3.6.5.3 Genetic Diversity Testing

There are several genetic testing laboratories that will calculate inbreeding and genetic diversity indexes on purebred dogs or cats and make recommendations to increase heterozygosity. These are based on guidelines that are valid in endangered species preservation, but not in purebred dog or pedigree cat breeding. The gene dynamics of endangered species and purebred dog and cat breeding are directly opposite from each other.

The basis of creating a breed is selection and genetic uniformity and the basis of endangered species preservation is the randomization of genes through mating the most unrelated individuals together. Some breeds are more ancient and have larger measured genetic diversity while more recently formed breeds with smaller populations may have lower measured genetic diversity. The larger population breeds with greater measured diversity once looked like the smaller population breeds when they first began to grow their population. The size of the gene pool and measured genetic diversity does not correlate to genetic health, as this is based on the presence of disease liability genes. Some genetic testing laboratories test for MHC genes as a measurement of genetic diversity and the immune system. However, no immune-related or autoimmune diseases are shown to be caused by a decrease of MHC diversity. They are caused by specific mutations or alleles in the MHC that predispose to disease with one or two copies of a mutation.

3.6.5.4 Estimated Breeding Values

Taking a cue from large animal production methods, dogs and cats can be rated for complex genetic disease liability through the phenotypic assessment of their close relatives. This is being attempted with hip dysplasia in several dog breeds. However, valid estimated breeding values (EBVs) require the assessment of all close relatives (including all littermates), which is rarely done in dog and cat breeding. The identification of one affected relative or of one normal relative can significantly shift EBVs when full litter assessment would provide a different rating. If EBVs are being offered, they can be used as a tool in addition to direct assessment of the phenotype of the individual and its close relatives.

3.6.5.5 Genomic Breeding Values

Researchers are working on ratings for dogs and cats with complexly inherited diseases based on a panel of DNA markers that are found to differ between groups of affected and normal individuals. These panels of markers are only validated in a small group within individual breeds, and, at least at the present time, lose their validation when applied to larger populations within a breed. However, this approach to genetic testing for disease liability shows promise as the science continues to develop.

3.6.5.5.1 Tissue Testing

Advances in genetic research are providing genetic tests for pathology and biopsy specimens. These tests can provide more specific prognostic and differential treatment recommendations for many types of cancer (see 2.20 Cancer Precision Medicine), liver disease, hematological disorders, etc.

Many owners and breeders ask what tests should be done for their cats and dogs. For a pet, it is only important to know that the individual pet is not going to be affected by a specific disease. For breeding animals, it is important to know not only whether they may be affected by a genetic disease, but whether they carry validated disease liability genes that they can pass on to their offspring. Genetic testing and screening should be done for a purpose. Are the results going to change how you would treat a patient or alter your recommendations? See 3.8 (Genetic Counseling) for specific recommendations based on genetic test results.

EXAMPLES

An owner brings in an Australian shepherd puppy for its initial examination. The breed carries some increased risk relative to the *mdr1* mutation for drug sensitivity. Your veterinary team already instructed the owner to bring all paperwork they received from the breeder, and you look for evidence of parental testing for the *mdr1* mutation. If no evidence of *mdr1* testing was provided but a pedigree or registration is included, you can look up parental health testing on the OFA website (http://ofa.org). If no evidence of parental testing is found, you have the owner contact the breeder to see if they can provide official documentation of *mdr1* testing on both parents (i.e., if both parents have been tested clear, the puppies should also be clear). If this is not available by the next puppy visit or the breeder did not perform such testing, you collect a blood sample or cheek swab and submit it to a laboratory for *mdr1* mutation testing. *mdr1* status is important to document in this breed before prescribing any of the drugs that can cause seizures, coma, and death in pets that have the mutation.

A client presents a 4-year-old Abyssinian cat that they feel is having issues with vision. An eye examination shows hyperreflective retinas and attenuation of retinal vessels. You recommend an examination by a veterinary ophthalmologist but also send out a genetic test for the *rdAc* form of PRA. The genetic test result shows that the cat is affected with this simple autosomal recessive disease.

A client brings you the results of a direct-to-consumer multiplex test on their French bulldog which reports that it is homozygous for the *sod1* mutation and is "at risk" of developing degenerative myelopathy. You report to the owner that their dog has little to no risk of developing degenerative myelopathy as it has never been documented in the breed and the breed likely lacks other mutations required to cause this complexly inherited genetic disease.

TAKE-AWAYS

- Genetic testing includes physical and phenotypic examinations as well as DNA testing.
- Genetic testing is important in pet and breeding animals.
- There are many different types of genetic tests that all have different interpretations for the tested patient.
- Genetic testing should be done for a purpose, and not just because a genetic test exists.
- Genetic test results that are valid in one breed may not be valid in other breeds. That is, a genetic mutation that is associated with a specific disease in one breed may not be associated with the same disease in other breeds.

MISCELLANEOUS

3.6.6 Cautions

- Some genetic tests being offered commercially have not been validated to cause or predispose to clinical disease. Peer-reviewed publication of a mutation does not mean it is validated to cause disease in one or more breeds.
- Some genetic tests may be valid in some breeds but not in others, where the results may have no bearing on health or traits.
- Some genetic testing laboratories use unvalidated analytical techniques in running genetic tests that can produce false results.

Recommended Reading

Ackerman, L. (2011). *The Genetic Connection: A Guide to Health Problems in Purebred Dogs*, 2e. Lakewood, CO: AAHA Press.

Bell, J.S., Cavanaugh, K.E., Tilley, L.P., and Smith, F.W.K. (2012). *Veterinary Medical Guide to Dog and Cat Breeds*. Jackson, WY: Teton NewMedia.

Gough, A., Thomas, A., and O'Neill, D. (2018). *Breed Predispositions to Disease in Dogs and Cats*, 3e. Oxford, UK: Wiley Blackwell.

Mellersh, C. (2016). DNA testing man's best friend: roles and responsibilities. *Veterinary Journal* 207: 10–12.

3.7

Genetic Health Registries and Research Organizations

Anita M. Oberbauer, PhD

Department of Animal Science, University of California, Davis, Davis, CA, USA

BASICS

3.7.1 Summary

Owners want the healthiest companions they can have, and veterinary healthcare teams play a key role in achieving this goal. Predicting health characteristics is critically important for responsible pet ownership and that requires accurate health data. Veterinarians should recommend relevant health testing for all pets and then encourage owners to submit the results of those tests to existing health registries. Genetic health registries compile health data, making that information available to breeders who can then breed with intentionality, owners who can better predict the health of their individual pet, and researchers who can use that information to study disease inheritance and prevalence, and identify emerging health conditions. The value of such health information in breeding and health research cannot be overstated. It is through this type of collated information that genetic diseases are described and tools to reduce incidence discovered.

3.7.2 Terms Defined

Carrier: The animal has a normal and a mutant copy of a gene, i.e., is heterozygous.

Health Registry: Database containing the health screening information and identifying characteristics such as breed, sex, age, and pedigree of individuals.

Health Screening: The use of tests to identify individuals that do not exhibit overt clinical signs yet have risk factors or early stages of disease.

Homozygous: Both copies of a gene are the same, i.e., the DNA sequence is the same.

Linked Test: A test that targets the region of DNA that is generally associated with the disease.

Mutation Test: A test that targets the actual DNA change that causes the disease; sometimes referred to as a direct genetic test.

Phenotypic Test: A test that detects visible or measurable differences related to a disease.

MAIN CONCEPTS

3.7.3 The Need

Many veterinary organizations consider health testing an essential component of veterinary medicine. Their policies on inherited disorders often include the goals of maximizing the health and welfare of companion animals and the education of breeders, owners, and the public on the responsibilities involved to minimize inherited disorders in the pet population. In order to achieve that goal, an understanding of the inheritance and genetics underlying disease is necessary (see 3.1 Genetic Basics and 3.2 Modes of Inheritance). Such understanding requires a foundation of knowledge on disease prevalence, mode of inheritance, and, ideally, determination of the DNA mutations that cause the disease (see 3.3 The Genetics of Disease). Aggregation of descriptive health data is necessary to characterize diseases of companion animals and thereby enable the research that will lead to that fundamental knowledge of what diseases are relevant to a given breed and, importantly, the development of tests needed to reduce the incidence of those diseases.

To that end, veterinarians should encourage the use of health screening in all their clients. For the clients, screening plays a role in managing the health of an individual pet and developing a holistic, long-range health plan based upon knowledge of susceptibility to certain diseases. Adverse reactions can be avoided or preemptive care can be initiated if known disease risk is identified through screening. Additionally, screening is an important tool for the health of all companion animals in reducing the incidence of disease and discovery of trends of emerging diseases.

3.7.4 Genetic Health Registries

Many owners and veterinarians wonder if a particular medical issue observed in a companion animal is genetically controlled and related to its breed, sex, growth rate and size, age, or diet. Health registries can help answer those questions. In their simplest form, genetic health registries are repositories of the results obtained from either phenotypic or genetic health screening tests (see 3.4 Predicting and Eliminating Disease Traits). By recording and compiling the information in an accessible formant, owners, breeders, and veterinary practitioners can use that to inform decisions. Genetic health registries provide an important resource for the veterinary community by cataloging diseases of a population of animals (Table 3.7.1), permitting the development of informed treatment plans, and illuminating trends of emerging diseases.

A primary objective of a registry is to provide a resource for breeders seeking health information on potential sires or dams. Another objective is to enable prospective owners to research the health of a breed in general or the parents

and their relatives of a particular companion pet being considered. For example, Table 3.7.2 presents the health information of a dog of interest. In this example, for each dog, its registration number, birth date, and sex are listed followed by any health tests recorded. This particular dog has passed all its health clearances, as have a majority of its relatives. Health registries have the greatest value with broad participation; vast amounts of data provide the necessary power to predict outcomes and analyze trends.

Dogs are the companion species with the greatest number of health screens available; these screens range from phenotypic tests such as hip conformation, eye, cardiac, or metabolic hormonal profiles to direct genetic mutation tests (see 3.11 Integrating Genotypic and Phenotypic Testing). Depending upon the registry, any and all health information may be collected and reported along with descriptive statistics such as sex, breed, age, etc. Alternatively, a select subset of screening tests that meet particular criteria may be recorded along with the descriptors. An example of the latter is the OFA Canine Health Information Center health registry, the largest repository of canine health information in the US, which covers purebred dog breeds as well as mixed-breed dogs and some other species. The health screening data recorded and published by the OFA are limited to phenotypic results obtained through examinations and testing by professional veterinarians with the appropriate board certifications and DNA-based results from validated genetic tests (Table 3.7.3).

In contrast, some individual dog breed clubs maintain their own health databases managed by dedicated club members. These breed-specific health registries usually catalogue health conditions more typically observed within that breed as well as collecting information on a multiplicity

Table 3.7.1 The top 11 breeds with the highest prevalence of elbow dysplasia by breed for those breeds with at least 50 evaluations from 1974 thru 2018

Breed	Rank	Number of evaluations	% Normal	% Overall dysplastic	% Grade 1 dysplasia	% Grade 2 dysplasia	% Grade 3 dysplasia
Chow chow	1	1248	50	49	25	17	6
Pug	2	216	59	41	26	13	2
Rottweiler	3	20177	61	39	30	8	1
Bulldog	4	497	62	37	25	10	1
Fila Brasileiro	5	220	68	32	19	10	3
Boerboel	6	246	70	30	17	8	5
Black Russian terrier	7	767	72	27	19	7	1
Bernese mountain dog	8	17869	73	27	18	7	3
Otterhound	9	137	73	27	22	4	1
Chinese shar-pei	10	852	74	25	14	9	3
Newfoundland	11	8394	76	24	15	5	3

Source: Data from the OFA Canine Health Information Center health registry (www.ofa.org).

Table 3.7.2 Health information on a dog of interest along with that of its sire, dam, and half siblings

Dog of interest	Registration	Birthdate	Sex	Relation	Hips[a]	Elbow[b]	Eyes[c]	Thyroid[d]
Larentia di Villa Roma	DN09589103	Dec 16 2004	F	Self	BT-4753G27	BT-EL2046F27	BT-EYE316	BT-TH315/27
Sire/Dam								
Neartic de la Grande Lande	DL75874001	Mar 13 1997	M	Sire	BT-3264G32	BT-EL754M32	BT-2233	
High Clearings Zohra	DL87843301	Apr 5 2000	F	Dam	BT-3953G36	BT-EL1321F36	BT-2881	
Full sibling								
Luna di Villa Roma	DN09589105	Dec 16 2004	F	Full Sib	BT-4697G24	BT-EL1998F24	BT-3343	BT-TH299/24
Longsword di Villa Roma	DN09589104	Dec 16 2004	F	Full Sib	BT-5090E48	BT-EL2362F48	BT-3775	
Half sibling (sire)								
Touchstone's Jaiden D'Shea	DL76335705	Oct 15 1998	F	Half(Sire)	BT-3650E37	BT-EL1059F37	BT-2591	
Touchstone's Jericho Dune	DL76335702	Oct 15 1998	M	Half(Sire)	BT-3659G37	BT-EL1068M37	BT-2590	
Touchstone's Crown Jewel	DL76335701	Oct 15 1998	F	Half(Sire)	BT-3806E45	BT-EL1199F45	BSD-1372	
Half sibling (dam)								
Hufflepuff di Villa Roma	DN05032106	Oct 7 2003	F	Half(Dam)	BT-4460E24	BT-EL1781F24	BT-EYE445	BT-TH485/73
House Elf di Villa Roma	DN05032105	Oct 7 2003	M	Half(Dam)	BT-5215G71	BT-EL2476M71	BT-3162	BT-TH488/73
Humberto di Villa Roma	DN05032104	Oct 7 2003	M	Half(Dam)	BT-4486E25	BT-EL1805M25	BT-3046	
Hocus Pocus di Villa Roma	DN05032103	Oct 7 2003	F	Half(Dam)	BT-4524G28	BT-EL1833F28	BT-3544	
Hagrid di Villa Roma	DN05032101	Oct 7 2003	M	Half(Dam)	BT-4916F49	BT-EL2190M49	BT-3163	
Hex di Villa Roma	DN05032107	Oct 7 2003	F	Half(Dam)			BT-3047	
Hermione di Villa Roma	DN05032102	Oct 7 2003	F	Half(Dam)	BT-4487G25		BT-3044	
Sidekicks Masters di Villa Roma	DN15480007	Aug 16 2006	M	Half(Dam)	BT-5032G24	BT-EL2301M24	BT-EYE73	BT-TH362/13
Sidekicks Mia di Villa Roma	DN15480003	Aug 16 2006	F	Half(Dam)	BT-5103E29	BT-EL2375F29	BT-EYE101	BT-TH444/29
Sidekicks Memory di Villa Roma	DN15480004	Aug 16 2006	M	Half(Dam)	BT-5062G26	BT-EL2332M26	BT-4096	BT-TH431/26
Sidekick's Morgan di Villa Roma	DN15480002	Aug 16 2006	F	Half(Dam)	BT-5056G26	BT-EL2327F26		
Sidekicks Marquise Villa Roma	DN15480005	Aug 16 2006	M	Half(Dam)	BT-5093G28	BT-EL2365M28		
Sidekicks Marinos Villa Roma	1 096 588	Aug 16 2006	M	Half(Dam)	BT-5122G29	BT-EL2393M29		
Sidekicks Newsflash	DN21567304	May 5 2008	F	Half(Dam)	BT-5437E30	BT-EL2673F30	BT-3959	BT-TH600/39
Sidekicks Never Say Never	DN21567301	May 5 2008	F	Half(Dam)	BT-5527G37	BT-EL2762F37	BT-3983	

[a] A hip result is a two-letter breed code followed by the evaluation number, a subjective code for the hip conformation (E = excellent; G = good; F = fair), and the age of the dog in months when the hips were evaluated.

[b] An elbow result is a two-letter breed code followed by EL that indicates the number is associated with elbows, the evaluation number, an abbreviation of the sex of the dog (M = male; F = female), and the age of the dog in months when the elbows were evaluated.

[c] An eye result is a two-letter breed code followed by either the abbreviation EYE that indicates the number is associated with eyes or just the evaluation number.

[d] A thyroid result is a two-letter breed code followed by TH that indicates the number is associated with thyroid, the evaluation number, and the age of the dog in months when the thyroid was evaluated. *Source:* Data from www.ofa.org.

Table 3.7.3 Genetic test screenings recorded in the OFA Canine Health Information Center health registry

Phenotypic genetic tests	Mutation tests
Hip dysplasia	Adult-onset neuropathy
Elbow dysplasia	Adult paroxysmal dyskinesia
Cardiac disease	Basenji progressive retinal atrophy
Congenital deafness	Canine multiple system degeneration
Serum bile acid	Degenerative encephalopathy
Eye disease	Degenerative myelopathy
Legg–Calvé–Perthes	Dilated cardiomyopathy
Patellar luxation	Fanconi's syndrome
Sebaceous adenitis	Gangliosidosis
Spine	Juvenile laryngeal paralysis and polyneuropathy
Shoulder osteochondrosis	Neonatal cerebellar ataxia
Thyroid	Neuronal ceroid lipofuscinosis
Tracheal hypoplasia	Neonatal encephalopathy with seizures
Dentition	Pyruvate dehydrogenase phosphate deficiency
Kidney	Primary lens luxation
	RCD4 progressive retinal atrophy
	Spinocerebellar ataxia
	Spongiform leukoencephalomyelopathy

Source: Data from www.ofa.org.

of medical conditions. The information gathered and recorded often includes anecdotal descriptions of health issues. Although professional diagnoses are the most valuable for reliable use in decision making, sometimes aggregate anecdotal information reveals an emerging health issue.

Health screening results for cats can also be deposited with the OFA, although participation has been limited. The reduced data may be due to fewer health screens being typically employed by cat owners or that the health registration for cats is more decentralized and maintained within breed clubs. A similar breed-specific approach is seen for equine health registries. Additionally, some registries are specific for a particular condition within a specific breed, such as the International Epilepsy Register for Belgian Shepherds. Registries targeting a single condition or those more anecdotal in nature are much less valuable to the veterinary and research community than the registries that are more comprehensive and centralized with health screenings validated by professionals.

3.7.5 Research Organizations

In general, research into the inheritance and genetic basis of health conditions occurs within university laboratories, institutes, veterinary organizations, and commercial genetic testing enterprises. The research is frequently undertaken in collaboration with veterinary professionals and owners, often relying upon information contained within health registries. An emerging model in some countries as well as in large veterinary companies with multiple hospitals is the wholesale collation of health records from individual veterinary practices for the purpose of facilitating research. Financial support for research into companion animal medical conditions comes in the form of grants from private foundations including the Canine Health Foundation, Morris Animal Foundation, Winn Feline Foundation, Grayson-Jockey Club Research Foundation, and the Sport Horse Research Foundation as well as federal granting agencies when the work directly supports human health. Additionally, veterinary specialty board organizations may direct funds for the research of targeted health conditions, such as the American College of Veterinary Ophthalmologists and vision loss. Private foundations rely upon philanthropic donations to support their grant funding activities whereas commercial enterprises generally reinvest a portion of the resources obtained from marketing and sales of DNA testing.

The objective of the research is to develop predictive tools for owners and veterinarians to better manage health conditions in companion animals. Outcomes of research are phenotypic tests such as orthopedic, cardiac, ocular, and metabolic screenings that can be deployed generally once validated by healthcare professionals. Genetic mutation tests are the ultimate goal of the research as they are most predictive in disease expression or the propensity of an individual to pass genetic risk on to the next generation (see 3.6 Genetic Testing). In the absence of the mutation test, linked tests may provide guidance although caution must be applied due to the lack of accuracy of such linked tests.

Health screening diagnostics developed through research must be properly validated across many unrelated individuals living in varied locations and exposed to different environments to assess general applicability of the test. Prior to incorporating testing is an understanding of limitations that might exist for a given test in order to manage those limitations and expectations. Genetic mutation tests are usually 100% accurate; however, accuracy relies upon the generalizability of the test across breeds, the testing procedure, and the quality of the genetic testing laboratory. Ideally, researchers subject their findings to the peer review process prior to making a proposed test available.

3.7.6 Utility

Health registries provide the information background for researchers seeking to establish the genetic underpinnings of disease. With widespread owner participation, researchers can identify families or breeds having a high prevalence of a particular disease and then characterize inheritance and collect appropriate DNA samples for genetic studies.

Health testing is important for all companion animals because mixed-breed and purebred pets all have the possibility for disease. Knowledge that there is a predisposition for disease will permit the owner and veterinarian to best care for the pet long term (see 1.2 Providing a Lifetime of Care). Some diseases may be treatable or have limited impact on a dog's quality of life whereas others may require aggressive intervention. Broad-scale testing and submission of those test results to a health registry provides the needed data to permit confidence in predicting health risks.

EXAMPLES

Samson is a well-bred, accomplished German shepherd dog whose owner was approached by a friend who wanted to breed his very nice female German shepherd dog to Samson. Although Samson had quality hip conformation, Samson's uncle had poor hip conformation, so Samson's owner studied the OFA health registry for the health clearances of the female. The potential dam, and all her relatives, had good-quality hip conformation. Samson's owner agreed to the breeding because the risk of hip dysplasia in the offspring was very low and in fact, the puppies all had good hip conformation at adulthood.

The owner of Benji, a Bengal cat, read about progressive retinal atrophy in the breed, an autosomal recessive disease that causes blindness. Both carriers and homozygous normal cats will have normal vision; only if the Bengal is homozygous for the progressive retinal atrophy-b mutation will it be blind. The genetic mutation test revealed that Benji was a carrier. Benji's owner was relieved that the cat would not go blind. Furthermore, the test results were submitted to the genetic health registry and future and current Bengal cat owners could use that information in their own decisions.

TAKE-AWAYS

- Health registries serve multiple roles, all of which are designed to protect and promote the health of companion animals.
- Genetic health registries compile health data provided by owners or veterinarians and have the greatest utility with broad participation.
- Veterinarians should encourage current and future owners of all companion animals to do health screenings and submit all relevant results to health registries.
- Veterinarians and owners should explore the information in health registries and use that knowledge in selecting pets to promote overall pet health.
- Health registries form the backbone of research, which enables the development of genetic tests to reduce disease.

MISCELLANEOUS

3.7.7 Cautions

A great many of the genetic tests available have not yet been fully validated or do not apply to a given breed. With the proliferation of genetic testing companies that screen for hundreds of mutations simultaneously and the aggressive marketing directly to owners, veterinarians must counsel against the tendency to misapply or overextend results from genetic tests. Whereas many current genetic tests may be recorded in a health registry, many may have no relevance to the individual animal because the test may only be valid in a different breed. Thus, there is a growing need for understanding and interpreting test results and applying those judiciously to the pet as a whole.

Abbreviation

OFA   Orthopedic Foundation for Animals

Recommended Reading

Bell, J.S. (2011). Researcher responsibilities and genetic counseling for pure-bred dog populations. *Veterinary Journal* 189 (2): 234–235.

Farrell, L.L., Shoenebeck, J.J., Wiener, P. et al. (2015). The challenges of pedigree dog health: approaches to combating inherited disease. *Canine Genetics and Epidemiology* 2 (3).

Moses, L., Niemi, S., and Karlsson, E. (2018). Pet genomics medicine runs wild. *Nature* 559 (7715): 470–472.

O'Neill, D.G., Church, D.B., McGreevy, P.D. et al. (2014). Approaches to canine health surveillance. *Canine Genetics and Epidemiology* 1 (1): 2.

3.8

Genetic Counseling

Jerold S. Bell, DVM

Department of Clinical Sciences, Cummings School of Veterinary Medicine at Tufts University, North Grafton, MA, USA

BASICS

3.8.1 Summary

We see genetic disease in patients every day. The hallmark of genetic disease is its predictability. Therefore, we have the opportunity to intervene and lessen its impact for our patients. This includes prepurchase discussions with clients, recommendations on initial examination and throughout the life of the patient, and prebreeding evaluation. The hospital team should be knowledgeable about the genetic tests available, their proper use and interpretation, breed-specific hereditary predispositions, and proper genetic counseling for both owners and breeders of dogs and cats.

3.8.2 Terms Defined

Purposefully Bred: A description indicating the intentional breeding of two animals, compared to the random matings that tend to occur in nature.

MAIN CONCEPTS

The predisposition to genetic diseases is lifelong. Consequently, these must be treated as chronic diseases and not just requiring intermittent treatment during clinical episodes. The opportunity to genetically counsel our clients occurs throughout the pet's life (see 1.2 Providing a Lifetime of Care). The most common examples are allergies in dogs and feline lower urinary tract disease in cats.

3.8.3 On a Client Acquiring a New Pet

If a client asks about adopting or purchasing a new dog or cat, the hospital team can discuss breed or mixed-breed anatomical and behavioral expectations and whether they fit with the client's lifestyle and home environment (see 3.10 Advising Clients on Selecting an Appropriate Pet). Terrier and terrier-type dogs have very different behavioral characteristics from retrievers or shepherds. Long-haired versus short-haired cats and dogs have different grooming requirements.

If the client is purchasing a purebred dog or pedigreed cat, there are breed-specific prebreeding health screening recommendations for the parents. For dogs, these can be found at the OFA Canine Health Information Center (www.ofa.org/breedtests.html). Common genetic disorders and tests for cat breeds can be found on the International Cat Care website (https://icatcare.org/advice/?per_page=12&categories=cat-breeds).

Online resources contain information on DNA tests available in dogs and cats from multiple laboratories. One can search by breed, disease, or laboratory. Some resources also link to the original published article on each disease test, as well as which laboratories run the tests: (http://research.vet.upenn.edu/WSAVA-LabSearch). Such resources may list identified mutations, including rare mutations that may not be present in breeding populations. Many commercial genetic testing companies test and report unvalidated mutations that have no relevance to the dog or cat being tested. Caution and diligence must be exercised when providing counseling recommendations based on genetic test results (see 3.6 Genetic Testing).

Health-conscious breeders are happy to provide official documentation of the results of health screening. The results of a puppy's parents' health screening can be looked up on the OFA website (www.ofa.org). Many other countries have searchable health testing databases, although there are more for dogs than for cats.

Some pure breeds and purposefully bred mixed-breeds (designer or "bred-for-rescue" dogs) do not have specific prebreeding health screening requirements. All parents of purposefully bred litters should have prebreeding health examinations (musculoskeletal, heart, eye, etc.) and history taken for episodic hereditary disease (allergies, seizures, chronic gastrointestinal disease, etc.) to determine their suitability for breeding (see 3.4 Predicting and Eliminating Disease Traits). Prebreeding health evaluations should become as routine and commonplace as equine prepurchase examinations.

In most instances, the veterinary team is not asked for advice by a client prior to a purchase or adoption. When an appointment is being made for examination of a new purposefully bred puppy or kitten, the owner should be told to bring all paperwork provided by the breeder, pet store, broker, or agent. If evidence of health screening on the parents has not been provided, health test results that may have been performed on the parents may be looked up in online health testing databases such as the OFA.

If health screening results are not available, one can access the prebreeding health screening requirements or testable diseases and have the owner ask the breeder for health testing information on the parents. This may be the only way to educate the owner *and* breeder on the ethical obligation of health screening and health-conscious breeding. Selective pressure is the only way to reduce the frequency of genetic disorders in purposefully bred dogs and cats. Health-screened parents produce healthier kittens and puppies.

3.8.4 Genetic Counseling in Owned Animals

Veterinarians and the veterinary team should be knowledgeable about which genetic disorders have appropriate testing available, and in what patients they should be run (see 3.4 Predicting and Eliminating Disease Traits). If parental documentation of genetic testing is not available, certain breeds should undergo genetic testing early in life (see 3.6 Genetic Testing). For example, patients from breeds with an incidence of von Willebrand disease should be tested so that measures can be taken to prevent excessive hemorrhage during surgery or injury. Patients at risk of carrying the *mdr1* mutation (mostly herding breeds) should be tested before drug treatment. Owners of large-breed puppies can be counseled to feed

lower calorie "large-breed growth or puppy" foods to provide for a more uniform growth rate and better joint development. Boxers should be tested while young for the dominant arrhythmogenic right ventricular cardiomyopathy (ARVC) gene. Carriers can be auscultated for arrhythmias through life, and if they occur can be put on antiarrhythmic drugs to prevent heart failure.

As more research is being done, more disease liability genes are being identified. Some of these genes occur in only a small "familial" population of a breed or only in a research setting while some cause breed-wide disease.

The focus of molecular genetic testing is now shifting to panel (multiplex) testing that includes many mutations found across all breeds. It is much less expensive to use a gene chip that runs hundreds of genetic tests for mutations, traits, and ancestry on a single sample. This is what is found with several commercial genetic testing companies for dogs and cats. With the results of such testing, genetic counseling becomes more important. Many genetic mutations that cause disease in some breeds have no health consequences in other breeds. An example is the *sod1* mutation test for liability to develop degenerative myelopathy (DM). This is a significant clinical disease in eight breeds, although the *sod1* mutation is found across all breeds and mixed-breed dogs. The presence of the gene mutation is not predictive for clinical disease if the breed is not actually predisposed to the disease. Genetic testing companies should provide some genetic counseling based on the breed or mixed-breed status of the specific patient. Decisions based on inappropriate test interpretation may be worse than having no test at all.

The expression of some genetic disorders cannot be altered. If a genetic test is available, it should be utilized prepurchase so that owners are not burdened with predictable genetic disease. However, for owned animals, it is a personal decision whether the owner wants to know if their pet is likely to develop a nontreatable genetic condition later in life. These include polycystic kidney disease (PKD) in Persian, Himalayan and related cats, lysosomal storage diseases, and the (poorly penetrant) liability gene for DM in susceptible breeds. These genetic tests can also assist with ruling out diagnoses in clinical patients with suspected genetic disease.

Dietary recommendations should be offered for identified genetic predispositions such as feline lower urinary tract disease in cats, dogs and cats with nonstruvite bladder stones or "crystals," and obese "prediabetic" cats. Behavioral counseling and early training recommendations should be offered for breeds or individuals demonstrating aberrant or pathological behaviors.

Owners may also bring results of direct-to-consumer genetic tests or tests of ancestral breed background for interpretation (see 3.6 Genetic Testing).

3.8.5 Breeding Recommendations

As stated above, prebreeding health evaluations should be performed on all prospective breeding cats or dogs, whether for purebred or mixed-breed planned matings. Breed-specific genetic screening requirements should be performed, as well as a medical history review and thorough examination for hereditary disease. Dogs and cats affected with genetic disease where no genetic tests for liability genes occur should be selected against for breeding.

As stated above, the results of individual DNA tests should be evaluated to ensure that the genetic disease exists as a clinical entity in the breed and that the genetic test has been validated in the country's breed population. Some genetic tests were developed in one country but the DNA variation is not associated with the disease in all breed populations around the world. Genetic counseling and breeding decisions based on genetic test results need to be validated in each breed population.

Based on different modes of inheritance, there are guidelines to preserve breeding lines and genetic diversity while reducing the risk of producing carrier or affected individuals.

In the case of a simple autosomal recessive disorder for which a direct genetic test for carriers is available, the recommendation is to test breeding-quality stock, and breed *clear* to *clear* or, if necessary to preserve genetic diversity, *clear* to quality *carrier*. This prevents affected offspring from being produced. Breeders should be counseled to replace carriers in a breeding program with a quality normal-testing offspring once it is possible to do so. This will maintain breed quality and diversity. Other offspring determined to be carriers should be placed in nonbreeding pet homes. The breed frequency of disease-causing genes is usually less than the 50% produced from normal to carrier matings. It is desirable not to increase the frequency of carriers in the population.

If a breeder finds that a quality individual is a carrier, many are inclined to remove it from their breeding consideration. This is the wrong decision for the breeder and the breed. The individual dog or cat was already determined to have qualities acceptable for breeding. Genetic testing should be used to increase a breeder's choices, not limit them. Eliminating all carriers of testable disease-causing genes significantly restricts breed genetic diversity. Any quality individual that would have been bred if it had tested normal should still be bred if it tests as a carrier, at least until enough quality clear individuals are available for the breeding program. A genetic test for a simple autosomal recessive disorder should not change who gets bred, only who they get bred to. As each breeder tests and replaces carriers with normal-testing offspring, the problem for the breed as a whole diminishes.

A simple autosomal recessive disorder for which no carrier test exists allows the propagation and dissemination of inapparent carriers in the gene pool. Carrier risk must be determined based on the knowledge of affected or carrier relatives. These can be visualized through vertical pedigrees on the OFA website, or other health databases (see 3.7 Genetic Health Registries and Research Organizations). Quality carriers should be replaced with nonaffected relatives and bred to individuals with low carrier risk. This can be assessed through examination of parents and grandparents (depth of pedigree normalcy), siblings and siblings to the parents (breadth of pedigree normalcy). High carrier-risk individuals should only be bred to low-risk individuals. The high-risk parent should be replaced for breeding with a lower risk quality offspring. To further limit the spread of the defective gene, the offspring should be used in only a limited number of carefully planned matings, and then should also be replaced with one or two quality offspring. The rest of the litter should be placed in nonbreeding (pet) homes. With this mating scheme, the breeder is maintaining the good genes of the line, reducing the carrier risk with each generation, and replacing, not adding to the overall carrier risk in the breeding population.

Autosomal dominant genetic disorders are usually easy to manage. As affected individuals produce approximately 50% affected offspring, they should be replaced for breeding with normal relatives. Issues with some autosomal dominant disorders include incomplete penetrance. With these disorders, the presence of the defective gene still confers risk of producing affected offspring and should be selected against.

For sex-linked (also known as X-linked) recessive defective genes, selecting a normal male for breeding loses the defective gene in one generation. High carrier-risk females should not be used, as carrier females produce 50% affected sons. Rare sex-linked dominant disorders are managed the same way as autosomal dominant disorders.

Most complex/polygenic disorders and those with an undetermined mode of inheritance have no tests for carriers, but they do have phenotypic tests that can identify affected individuals. Controlling complexly inherited disorders involves (i) identifying traits for selection that more closely represent the expression of disease-causing genes, (ii) the standardization of nuisance factors (such as environment) that can limit selective pressure against the genes, and (iii) selecting for breadth as well as depth of pedigree normalcy as demonstrated by vertical pedigrees.

With polygenic disorders, a number of liability genes must combine to cross a threshold and produce an affected individual. A clinically normal individual from a litter that had one or no individuals affected with a complexly inherited disorder is expected to carry a lower amount of liability genes than an individual with a greater number of affected littermates. This is why it is important to screen both pet and breeding dogs and cats for complexly inherited disorders. Information on the siblings of the parents of potential breeding individuals provides additional data on which to base breeding decisions. The patient's own results represent its phenotype, but the relative's results are more representative of the patient's genotype.

If an individual is diagnosed with a genetic disorder, it can be replaced with a normal sibling or parent and bred to a mate whose risk of having liability genes is low. Replace the higher-risk parent with a lower-risk offspring that equals or exceeds it in other aspects, and repeat the process.

Genetic testing companies are increasingly providing genetic diversity measurements to breeders for individual dogs or cats and their proposed matings. As discussed in the chapter on genetic testing (see 3.6), all breeds by definition have high homozygosity which allows them to breed true. Homozygosity does not cause genetic disease. It is the presence of disease-causing mutations that cause disease, and genetic counseling recommendations should be specifically directed against specific diseases. Genetic diversity has to do with maintaining unique breeding lines in a breed. It is the genetic differences between individuals in a breed that provide breed genetic diversity, not within-individual homozygosity. It is only in rare instances when a breed suffers from high-frequency genetic disease or genetic-based infertility that a breed-rescue type of genetic diversity breeding scheme may be indicated.

Genetic tests are extremely useful tools to help manage genetic disorders. Even when there is no test or an unknown mode of inheritance, much can still be done to reduce the incidence of affected and carrier animals (see 3.4 Predicting and Eliminating Disease Traits). The use of these guidelines can assist clients in making objective breeding decisions for genetic disease management while continuing their breeding lines.

It is distressing when a genetic disorder is confirmed in an animal. The veterinary team can make positive and practical genetic counseling recommendations to maintain breed lines and genetic diversity, and improve the overall health of breeds. Each breeder will have their own rate of progress depending on the frequency of the defective gene(s) in their own breeding animals, and which desirable individuals carry liability genes.

With the increasing availability of genetic tests, there is increased risk of misusing and misinterpreting them. There is also the propensity to recommend inappropriate and unnecessary genetic testing, which can diminish client compliance. It is our responsibility to understand the proper use and interpretation of genetic tests, and to provide appropriate genetic counseling recommendations to our clients.

EXAMPLES

Example 1

A client is interested in acquiring an Alaskan malamute. You or your team discuss the grooming (and shedding) expected in the breed, as well as its exercise requirements. You look up and print out the OFA-CHIC prebreeding recommendations for the client which includes a hip evaluation for hip dysplasia, ophthalmologist eye examination, and a genetic test for polyneuropathy – a breed-specific genetic disorder. You counsel the client to ask anyone offering Alaskan malamute puppies for official documentation of the above genetic testing on *both* parents of the puppies. The OFA-CHIC also lists recommended testing for hypothyroidism and a cardiac evaluation, indicating that these diseases are also present in the breed. The client should inquire if either of the parents have any health issues, including common genetic disorders such as allergies, cruciate ligament rupture or significant arthritis.

Example 2

You remove bladder stones from a feline patient and submit them for analysis. They come back as calcium oxalate stones. You must counsel the client that this is a genetic predisposition and the cat is at high risk of forming more stones. You offer medical recommendations to minimize the risk of future stone formation. The owner desires to breed the cat. You inform the owner that there is no genetic test for oxalate urolithiasis liability. Due to the severity of the disease, affected cats should not be used for breeding.

Example 3

A French bulldog owner presents their older dog for evaluation due to clinical signs of spinal cord disease. The owner has a commercial genetic test result showing the dog is homozygous "at risk" for the *sod1* liability gene for DM. You tell the owner that no French bulldogs have been pathologically confirmed with DM and the genetic test is likely not predictive for their breed. You further inform the owner that French bulldogs have a high incidence of intervertebral disc disease, which is a treatable condition (versus the fatal prognosis of DM). Further work-up reveals spinal cord compression which is successfully treated surgically.

TAKE-AWAYS

- Genetic disease is observed every day in practice
- Genetic counseling involves the treatment of mixed-breed and purebred patients as well as prebreeding health evaluations.
- The veterinary team should be knowledgeable about breed-specific genetic disorders, especially those that can cause issues with anesthesia, surgery, and drug treatment.
- Many breed-validated disease-causing genetic mutations occur at significant frequencies in breeds so that selection against them should be done in a systematic "breed and replace" manner so as not to affect the genetic diversity of the breed.
- The veterinary team should impress upon clients that purposefully bred dogs and cats should only be obtained from health-conscious breeders who perform prebreeding health screening and genetic testing.

MISCELLANEOUS

Abbreviations

OFA   Orthopedic Foundation for Animals
WSAVA   World Small Animal Veterinary Association

Recommended Reading

Ackerman, L. (2011). *The Genetic Connection: A Guide to Health Problems in Purebred Dogs*, 2e. Lakewood, CO: AAHA Press.

Bell, J.S., Cavanaugh, K.E., Tilley, L.P., and Smith, F.W.K. (2012). *Veterinary Medical Guide to Dog and Cat Breeds*. Jackson, WY: Teton NewMedia.

3.9

Purebreds, Mixed-Breeds, and Hybrids

Lowell Ackerman, DVM, DACVD, MBA, MPA, CVA, MRCVS

Global Consultant, Author, and Lecturer, MA, USA

BASICS

3.9.1 Summary

Veterinary teams need to be prepared for a variety of patients these days, with different breed names, descriptions, and predispositions to disease. It has never been more important to ensure that such pets are properly recorded in practice management software, as this can impact risk assessment and appropriate communication with pet owners.

3.9.2 Terms Defined

Hybrid: Also known as a designer breed, this is a cross between two or more purebreds. In most cases, the cross is intentional.

Mixed-breed: This is the result of a mix of breeds, potentially some known and others unknown. In most cases, the cross was unintentional. There are a variety of other terms for this, such as mutt in dogs and moggy in cats.

Pedigree: Recorded ancestry.

Purebred: An animal of a modern breed with a documented pedigree.

MAIN CONCEPTS

In most veterinary practices, approximately half of all canine patients are mixed-breeds (and an even higher percentage for feline patients), and there are approximately an equal number of purebreds or hybrids. If the information available in practice management software is to be useful for pet-specific strategies, then it is critical that this information be correct in the medical record.

3.9.3 Purebreds

Purebred pets are those with a documented pedigree and there are literally hundreds of dog breeds and dozens of cat breeds in the world today. Many countries have organizations that recognize breed status and record pedigrees (e.g., American Kennel Club, The Kennel Club, United Kennel Club, etc.) and it is quite possible that some breeds recognized as purebreds by one organization may not be recognized by another (see 11.1 Finding More Information on Pet-Specific Care). There are also international organizations dealing with purebreds, such as the Fédération Cynologique Internationale (www.fci. be) for dogs, and the International Cat Association (TICA) (www.tica.org) and the Cat Fanciers Association (www.cfa.org) for cats.

One of the most useful features of purebreds, from a pet-specific care perspective, is that they tend to have more predictable behaviors and predispositions to disease (see 11.4 Heritable Health Conditions – By Breed). Many behaviors are highly ingrained in a breed (e.g., retrieving, herding), and pet owners may have certain expectations in this regard. It is also easier to predict features such as personality in purebreds, adult size and, as mentioned, breed predisposition to certain diseases. In addition, there are a variety of genetic screening tests now available, and most are applicable to diseases recognized in certain purebreds (although some can also be detected in mixed-breed and hybrid animals).

3.9.4 Hybrids

Hybrids are becoming more common in society, as breeders and pet owners attempt to select for specific features by crossing a variety of purebred breeds. While some breeders have attempted to create new purebred breeds from the offspring of these crosses, in general the hybrids involve the continued breeding of specific purebreds to attain the desired crosses. While there are many canine hybrids being promoted (Table 3.9.1), some feline hybrids have also been developed, and some of these are now recognized as purebreds. These include the Savannah Brown, Ocicat, Oriental Shorthair, Tonkinese, Bengal, Chausie, Savannah, Pixiebob, and Toyger.

While initial crosses were touted as being healthier than the purebreds from which they were derived (so-called hybrid vigor), it is now recognized that these crosses can still concentrate deleterious genes and may develop their own predispositions to disease. Some of these can even be detected with genetic screening in these hybrids.

Table 3.9.1 Examples of some canine hybrid crosses

Affenwich	=	Affenpinscher	×	Norwich terrier
Airedoodle	=	Airedale	×	Poodle
American Bull-Jack	=	American bulldog	×	Jack Russell terrier
Ausky	=	Australian cattle dog	×	Siberian husky
Aussiedoodle	=	Australian shepherd	×	Poodle
Baussie	=	Australian shepherd	×	Boston terrier
Beabull	=	Bulldog	×	Beagle
Belusky	=	Siberian husky	×	Belgian Malinois
Biton	=	Bichon frisé	×	Coton de Tulear
Bogle	=	Beagle	×	Boxer
Borkie	=	Bichon frisé	×	Yorkshire terrier
Bostie	=	Boston terrier	×	West Highland white terrier
Bowzer	=	Basset hound	×	Miniature schnauzer
Cadoodle	=	Collie	×	Poodle
Cairnese	=	Cairn terrier	×	Havanese
Cavachon	=	Bichon frisé	×	Cavalier King Charles spaniel
Chorkie	=	Chihuahua	×	Yorkshire terrier
Chug	=	Chihuahua	×	Pug
Cocarpoo	=	Cocker spaniel	×	Poodle
Corkie	=	Cocker spaniel	×	Yorkshire terrier
Crustie	=	Chinese crested	×	Yorkshire terrier
Daug	=	Dachshund	×	Pug
Dorkie	=	Dachshund	×	Yorkshire terrier
Double Doodle	=	Goldendoodle	×	Labradoodle
Doxle	=	Beagle	×	dachshund
Eskland	=	American Eskimo	×	Shetland sheepdog
Goldendoodle	=	Golden retriever	×	Poodle
Jack-A-Bee	=	Beagle	×	Jack Russell terrier
Jug	=	Jack Russell terrier	×	Pug
Labradoodle	=	Labrador retriever	×	Poodle
Malt-A-Poo	=	Maltese	×	Poodle
Mastador	=	Labrador retriever	×	Mastiff
Mauxie	=	Dachshund	×	Maltese
Morkie	=	Maltese	×	Yorkshire terrier

Table 3.9.1 (Continued)

Muggin	=	Miniature pinscher	×	Pug
Papastzu	=	Papillon	×	Shih tzu
Paperanian	=	Papillon	×	Pomeranian
Papichon	=	Papillon	×	Bichon frisé
Peke-A-Boo	=	Bolognese	×	Pekingese
Peke-A-Poo	=	Pekingese	×	Poodle
Peke-A-Tese	=	Maltese	×	Pekingese
Pekehund	=	Dachshund	×	Pekingese
Pinny-Poo	=	Miniature pinscher	×	Poodle
Pitsky	=	American pit bull terrier	×	Siberian husky
Pom Terrier	=	Pomeranian	×	Toy fox terrier
Pomaky	=	Pomeranian	×	Siberian husky
Pomston	=	Boston terrier	×	Pomeranian
Poochon	=	Bichon frisé	×	Poodle
Poogle	=	Beagle	×	Poodle
Pookimo	=	American Eskimo	×	Poodle
Poolky	=	Poodle	×	Silky terrier
Puggle	=	Beagle	×	Pug
Pugottie	=	Pug	×	Scottish terrier
Rotterman	=	Doberman pinscher	×	Rottweiler
Schapso	=	Lhasa apso	×	Miniature schnauzer
Schnocker	=	Cocker spaniel	×	Miniature schnauzer
Schnoodle	=	Miniature schnauzer	×	Poodle
Sharbo	=	Boston terrier	×	Chinese shar-pei
Snorkie	=	Miniature schnauzer	×	Yorkshire terrier
Spanador	=	Cocker spaniel	×	Labrador
Wauzer	=	Miniature schnauzer	×	West Highland white terrier
Yorkie-Poo	=	Poodle	×	Yorkshire terrier
Yorkinese	=	Pekingese	×	Yorshire terrier
Zuchon	=	Bichon frisé	×	Shih tzu

3.9.5 Mixed-Breeds

Mixed-breed pets have always posed a problem to disease risk prediction, since without knowing breeds, it can be difficult to predict breed predisposition to disease (see 3.19 Mixed-Breed Considerations). This has been partially offset today by the ability to determine likely breed contributions on the basis of genetic testing. Such genetic testing will often not determine ancestry with absolute precision, but perhaps with sufficient accuracy to allow veterinary teams to consider some disease predisposition in individuals. Genetic testing can also be used for disease screening

of certain entities, and may even predict a variety of traits, such as the pet's likely size as an adult.

Since medical records are also legal documents, if a mixed-breed animal is presented, it is best to identify it as a mixed-breed in the breed field within practice management software. Identifying pets as crosses based on their appearance (e.g., shepherd x, Himalayan x) is fraught with inaccuracies and likely gets things wrong as often as gets them right. Since the breed identified in a medical record can be a clue to disease predisposition, it is better not to try to "guess" what the contributing breeds might be and instead either use a generic term like mixed-breed or use genetic testing to get a better approximation, if desired. The only time more specific speculation is warranted is if the parents of the mixed-breed animal are known with certainty (e.g., neighbor's dog jumped the fence and impregnated pet owner's intact bitch).

While purebreds and hybrids tend to have higher relative risk for certain genetic disorders (especially traits attributable to single-gene mutations), it is important to realize that mixed-breed animals may still constitute a significant proportion of health concerns in a practice (e.g., diabetes mellitus, osteoarthritis, obesity, etc.).

There is a tendency to recommend mixed-breed pets to prospective owners based on the fact that there are many more of these available in shelters that need homes, and this is a very real benefit, but it is also important to realize that there are many reasons why some prefer to bring purebreds and hybrids into their homes.

TAKE-AWAYS

- Purebred animals tend to be at highest relative risk for genetic diseases, especially those attributable to disease variants associated with single-gene mutations (e.g., progressive retinal atrophy).

- In many practices, the proportion of purebreds and hybrids is roughly equivalent to the number of mixed-breed animals.
- Tracking correct breed information in practice management software is critically important and then using that information to create patient risk profiles.
- Mixed-breed animals may have lower risks for certain genetic diseases, but this can be somewhat offset by the fact that their actual disease risks are harder to predict.
- Owners often purchase purebreds and hybrids based on real or imagined benefits, but predictability of traits, behaviors, and even health risks is a real advantage.

MISCELLANEOUS

Recommended Reading

Ackerman, L. (2011). *The Genetic Connection*. Lakewood, CO: AAHAPress.

Ackerman, L. (2020). Proactive Pet Parenting: Anticipating pet health problems before they happen. Problem Free Publishing.

Gough, A., Thomas, A., and O'Neill, D. (2018). *Breed Predispositions to Disease in Dogs and Cats*, 3e. Ames, IA: Wiley Blackwell.

3.10

Advising Clients on Selecting an Appropriate Pet

Lowell Ackerman, DVM, DACVD, MBA, MPA, CVA, MRCVS

Global Consultant, Author, and Lecturer, MA, USA

 BASICS

3.10.1 Summary

Many clients acquire a pet without a good understanding of its long-term healthcare needs. Accordingly, this lack of understanding translates both to poor compliance/adherence and to improper planning for a lifetime of healthcare.

Veterinary teams would be well served to spend time with clients, understanding their needs and concerns, explaining in advance what the likely healthcare process will be, including expenses to be anticipated along the way and when changes in healthcare requirements will likely occur.

3.10.2 Terms Defined

Adherence: The extent to which patients take medications as prescribed, which involves the pet owner in filling and refilling the prescription, administering the correct dose, timing and use, and completing the prescribed course.

Advocate: Someone who speaks or takes action on behalf of another.

Compliance: The extent to which pets receive a treatment, screening, or procedure in accordance with recommended veterinary healthcare practices.

Pet-specific Care: An approach that tailors veterinary care to individual pets based on their predicted risk of disease and likely response to intervention

 MAIN CONCEPTS

3.10.3 Acquiring a Pet

Most veterinary teams play little or no role in the acquisition of a pet, so clients often begin and complete this process without appropriate healthcare advice (see 5.6 Adoption Source Options). Veterinary staff might be amused when clients come in with a "purebred cockapoo" that they purchased for a considerable sum (with papers?) and evidence of ear mites, luxating patellas, and an umbilical hernia, but most would-be pet owners have no idea how to do a better job with the process. Interestingly, these new pet owners rarely price-shop for their new pets – they typically pay in full at time of acquisition, and they often make the purchase on impulse.

In a much better process, veterinarians or trained staff could interview would-be pet owners and help them select an animal that would best fit their lifestyle (Table 3.10.1), and then counsel them on where they might find suitable animals, health guarantees that should be requested, and terms that include a no-questions-asked money-back guarantee following veterinary examination [1]. Veterinarians could even provide adoption questionnaires that inquire about health issues in the animals or their parents, and genetic testing that might have been done to mitigate healthcare risks (Table 3.10.2). Recommended tests to consider on a breed basis are available for both dogs (www.ofa.org/browse-by-breed) and cats (https://icatcare.org/advice/cat-breeds), and breed predisposition information is available (see 11.4 Heritable Health Conditions – By Breed).

Table 3.10.1 A sample of dog and cat breed selector tools found on the internet

Organization	Website
Animal Planet (dog)	www.animalplanet.com/breed-selector/dog-breeds.html
Animal Planet (cat)	www.animalplanet.com/breedselector/catselectorindex.do
American Kennel Club (dog)	www.akc.org/dog-breed-selector
DogTime (dog)	http://dogtime.com/quiz/dog-breed-selector
Hills (cat)	www.hillspet.com/cat-care/new-pet-parent/choosing-right-cat-breeds
Iams	www.iams.com/breedselector
Optimum Pet (cat)	www.optimumpet.com.au/cat-advice/cat-selector
Pedigree (dog)	www.pedigree.com/getting-a-new-dog/breed-match
Puppyfinder (dog)	www.puppyfinder.com/dog-breed-selector
Purina (dog)	www.purina.com/dogs/dog-breeds/dog-breed-selector
Purina (cat)	www.purina.com/cat-breed-selector
Select a Dog Breed	www.selectadogbreed.com
Select Smart (dog)	www.selectsmart.com/dog
Select Smart (cat)	http://selectsmart.com/CAT
Vetstreet	www.vetstreet.com/breed-finder
Whiskas (cat)	www.whiskas.co.uk/breed-selector

Unfortunately, this is not the way the situation typically evolves, so the veterinary team and client are sometimes engaged in an almost adversarial relationship in trying to determine how best to deal with the current situation. It is a much more positive relationship when the veterinary team acts as the client advocate, but for that to happen, such teams need to assume a much more proactive role in the acquisition of pets (see 5.7 Preadoption Counseling).

Preselection counseling is not only medically relevant, but it also makes good business sense. In the United States, more dogs and cats are euthanized for behavioral reasons than for all medical causes combined [2]. Accordingly, helping prospective pet owners understand the ramifications of pet ownership before they actually take on the responsibility of pet ownership is in everyone's best interest.

EXAMPLES

Mrs Stewart came to visit ABC Veterinary Hospital after hearing from a friend that the hospital offered preadoption counseling. She and her husband had a 4-year-old child, and they were thinking of getting a Siberian husky (they had seen a cute puppy of this breed in the pet store, but resisted the temptation to buy it at that time). From the selection counseling session, it was determined that the Stewarts lived in a two-bedroom apartment, both adults worked long hours, and their lifestyle was decidedly sedentary between work and childrearing. By the end of the session, Mrs Stewart had acknowledged that a Siberian husky might not be the best breed for their circumstances and narrowed their choices to a miniature schnauzer or a bichon frisé and would make the final decision with her husband while armed with the breed information provided.

A staff member also provided some resources for finding an appropriate dog of either breed, including local breed rescue, online breed-specific adoptions, and a list of breeders available from a national breeders' registry. The hospital provided a frequently asked questions (FAQ) document regarding pet adoption and basic care, forms for the prospective puppy seller to complete, and forms the practice would need once the final decision was made. A new puppy kit was provided, along with a container that the owner would use to bring a fecal sample on the first actual visit. Mrs Stewart was also invited to visit the Thursday evening "puppy kindergarten" class that was offered by one of the technicians, and they would introduce her to their basic temperament-testing regimen and go over the socialization and training classes offered. A quick introduction was made to Dr Smith, whom she would see at the first scheduled visit, and she was invited to call back with any other questions. Mrs Stewart was assured that although it wasn't quite as involved as raising a baby, ABC Veterinary Hospital would be there to help her through the process every step of the way. The client-to-be left the practice armed with a much better understanding of dog ownership and with an already considerable loyalty to ABC Veterinary Hospital.

Table 3.10.2 Golden retriever adoption questionnaire

INFORMATION TO BE PROVIDED BY SELLER				
Name of Business: Website:				
Address: Telephone:				
Name of Dog (Registered):				
Date of Birth: Weight: ☐ kg ☐ lb Color:				
Identification: Microchip _____ Tattoo _____ Collar/Tag _____				
Registration (e.g., AKC, UKC, CKC, etc.):				
☐ Show Quality ☐ Pet Quality ☐ Breeding ☐ Nonbreeding				
Question	Yes	No	Don't know	Documents provided
Did parents have prebreeding health screening?				
Are parents' health screens in a public registry?				
Are this animal's health screens in a public registry?				
Has this animal had genetic health screening?				
Have parents had genetic health screening?				
Has this animal received regular veterinary evaluations?				
Any irregularities determined by veterinary evaluations?				
Are all vaccinations current?				
Any exposure to infectious diseases?				
Is recent parasite evaluation available?				
Is this animal currently free of parasites?				
Is this animal on integrated parasite control?				
Any evidence of problem behaviors in this animal?				
Is there a history of problem behaviors in the family?				
Any evidence of allergies in this animal?				
Is there a history of allergies in the family?				
Has this animal been evaluated for orthopedic disorders?				
Have parents been evaluated for orthopedic disorders?				
Is this animal free of congenital heart diseases?				
Are both parents free of heritable heart diseases?				
Is this animal free of heritable eye diseases?				
Are both parents free of heritable eye diseases?				
Any evidence of hypothyroidism in this animal?				
Is there any history of hypothyroidism in the family?				
Any evidence of diabetes mellitus in this animal?				
Any evidence of diabetes mellitus in the family?				
Any evidence of seizure disorders in this animal?				
Any evidence of seizure disorders in the family?				
Any evidence of bleeding disorders in this animal?				
Any evidence of bleeding disorders in the family?				
Any evidence of cancer in this animal?				
Any evidence of cancer in the family?				
Medical-behavioral money-back guarantee provided?				
Signature: Date:				

About three weeks later, Mrs Stewart came in with Schnitzel, an 8-week-old miniature schnauzer, and dutifully brought in a fecal sample in the container previously provided. Schnitzel was a fine, healthy specimen, with only a minor umbilical hernia that could be fixed at time of neutering. Mrs Stewart had read most of the material provided and had some questions about which pet health insurance plan might be best for Schnitzel. Dr Smith started Schnitzel on a sensible dietary regimen and reiterated some of the breed concerns, such as pancreatitis and calcium oxalate urolithiasis. Discussions about vaccination schedules, genetic screening, parasite control, nutrition, and proper socialization ensued, and then the long-term healthcare plan was reviewed.

TAKE-AWAYS

- Most veterinary practices believe that clients should receive selection counseling before they purchase a pet, but most practices do not offer this important service.
- Clients who select an appropriate pet are less likely to relinquish it, and are more prepared for the likely care the pet will need.
- Discussing issues proactively allows the team to be regarded as advocates; when such counseling is not provided and problems ensue, the practice can sometimes appear adversarial (you never warned me about that).

- Most selection counseling can be performed by the non-veterinary team and it can be a great bonding experience even without veterinary involvement.
- It is better for veterinary teams to be involved preemptively in the selection process rather than complain about the results when they are not involved.

MISCELLANEOUS

References

1 Ackerman, L.J. (2011). *The Genetic Connection*, 2e. Lakewood, CO: AAHA Press.

2 Landsberg, G., Hunthausen, W., and Ackerman, L. (2013). *Behavior Problems of the Dog and Cat*, 3e. Edinburgh: Elsevier.

Recommended Reading

American Animal Hospital Association-American Veterinary Medical Association Preventive Health Guidelines Task Force (2011). *J. Am. Vet. Med. Assoc.* 239 (5): 625–629.

Ackerman, L. (2020). Proactive Pet Parenting: Anticipating pet health problems before they happen. Problem Free Publishing.

Fivecoat-Campbell, K. (2020). Adoption marketing. Marketing to the new adopters of shelter and rescue animals. *AAHA Trends* 36 (2): 51–55.

Partners for Healthy Pets: www.partnersforhealthypets.org

3.11

Integrating Genotypic and Phenotypic Testing

Lowell Ackerman, DVM, DACVD, MBA, MPA, CVA, MRCVS

Global Consultant, Author, and Lecturer, MA, USA

BASICS

3.11.1 Summary

In pet-specific care, there is a focus on prevention and early detection. To accomplish early detection, both genotypic and phenotypic tests are needed. Genotypic tests examine an individual's DNA for mutations (variants) or markers that may be correlated with traits and disease risk. Phenotypic tests measure observable features (e.g., blood test results, heart rhythm, body weight, etc.) and diagnostic judgments are made on that basis, and comparisons with so-called "normal" reference intervals (ranges).

Genotypic tests on their own have value, but they cannot always predict actual risk of diseases. In addition, genotypic tests are available primarily for conditions transmitted as simple Mendelian traits (e.g., von Willebrand disease, progressive rod-cone dysplasia, *mdr1*, etc.), mostly controlled by one set of genes. On the other hand, the most common hereditary conditions encountered in veterinary practice (e.g., atopic dermatitis, hip dysplasia, seizure disorders, etc.) have a more complex pattern of inheritance, often influenced by environmental factors and multiple genes, and confirmed principally through phenotypic testing. Because of this, both genotypic and phenotypic testing are needed as part of most early detection schemes.

3.11.2 Terms Defined

Genotypic Testing: Testing that determines actual genetic mutations (variants) or markers of traits or conditions.
Phene: A trait or characteristic that is genetically determined.

Phenotypic testing: Testing that determines observable features of traits or conditions and compares them to normal or typical values.

MAIN CONCEPTS

Genotypic tests, those that rely on the detection of actual genetic mutations (variants) or markers (Table 3.11.1), have a lot of benefits. They can be detected at an early age, even as early as one day of age. They don't change over time, so if a genetic mutation is present (or not present) when tested, repeat testing is not needed – the results should not change over time. In fact, if the parents have been tested for a specific variant, the status of the offspring can be inferred from such testing. So, if two Labrador retrievers are both "clear" for progressive rod-cone degeneration (prcd) and they are bred together, theoretically it should not be possible for the pups to develop that specific form of progressive retinal atrophy (PRA) if the testing has been done by a reliable genetic testing facility (http://bit.ly/2YWXBsc or https://dogwellnet.com/ctp). Of course, mistakes do happen. In this instance, the most likely cause for pups testing "affected" for prcd when the parents tested "clear" would be that the breeders made a mistake in identifying which animals were the actual parents. Theoretically, it would also be possible that the pups developed a spontaneous mutation, but this is very rare.

The other big problem with relying on genotypic testing alone is that, at the present time at least, genetic testing is only available for a relatively small number of phenes (conditions, traits, etc.), representing perhaps 20–30% of heritable conditions. Some of the most common conditions with a heritable component, such as allergies or hip dysplasia, have more complex inheritance, often influenced by

Pet-Specific Care for the Veterinary Team, First Edition. Edited by Lowell Ackerman.
© 2021 John Wiley & Sons, Inc. Published 2021 by John Wiley & Sons, Inc.

Table 3.11.1   Some of the genotypic tests currently available

2,8-Dihydroxyadenine Urolithiasis Type IA

Achromatopsia

Acral Mutilation Syndrome

Acute Respiratory Distress Syndrome

Aggression (markers)

Alanine Aminotransferase (ALT) Activity

Alexander Disease

Amelogenesis Imperfecta

Arrhythmogenic Right Ventricular Cardiomyopathy

Autoimmune lymphoproliferative Syndrome

Bardet–Biedl Syndrome

Bernard Soulier Syndrome

Brain Hypomyelination

Burmese Head Defect

Canine Leukocyte Adhesion Deficiency Types I & III

Canine Multifocal Retinopathy (CMR 1, 2 & 3)

Canine Multiple System Degeneration

Cardiomyopathy, Dilated (DCM1 and DCM2)

Cardiomyopathy, Hypertrophic

Catalase Deficiency

Centronuclear Myopathy

Cerebellar Ataxia

Cerebellar Cortical Degeneration

Cerebellar Hypoplasia

Cerobellar Abiotrophy

Chondrodysplasia

Chondrodystrophy and intervertebral Disc Disease

Ciliary Dyskinesia

Cleft Lip with Syndactyly

Cleft Lip/Palate

Cobalamin Malabsorption

Collie Eye Anomaly/Choroidal Hypoplasia

Color Dilution Alopecia

Complement 3 (C3) deficiency

Cone Degeneration

Cone-Rod Dystrophy (1, 2, 3, 4, SWD)

Congenital Hypothyroidism with Goiter

Congenital Keratoconjunctivities Sicca and Ichthyosiform Dermatosis

Congenital Macrothrombocytopenia

Congenital Myasthenic Syndrome

Congenital Stationary Night Blindness

Copper Toxicosis

Craniomandibular Osteopathy

Curly Coat Dry Eye Syndrome

Cyclic Hematopoiesis

Cyclic Neutropenia

Cystic renal Dysplasia and Hepatic Fibrosis

Cystinuria (Types I-A, II-A, II-B)

Dandy–Walker Malformation

Day Blindess

Deafness and Vestibular Syndrome

Degenerative Myelopathy

Dental Hypomineralization

Dermatomyositis

Dystrophic Epidermolysis Bullosa

Early Adult Onset Deafness

Early Onset Progressive Polyneuropathy

Ectodermal Dysplasia

Elliptocytosis

Encephalopathy

Epidermolysis Bullosa Simplex

Epidermolytic Hyperkeratosis

Epilepsy (variants)

Episodic Falling Syndrome

Exercise-Induced Collapse

Exercise-Induced Metabolic Myopathy

Factor IX Deficiency (Hemophilia B)

Factor VII Deficiency

Factor VIII Deficiency (Hemophilia A)

Factor XI Deficiency

Factor XII Deficiency

Familial Congenital Methemoglobinemia

Familial Juvenile Epilepsy

Familial Nephropathy

Fanconi Syndrome

Fucosidosis

Gall Bladder Mucocele Formation

Gangliosidosis (GM1 & GM2)

Generalized Myoclonic Epilepsy

Glanzmann's Thrombasthenia

Glaucoma

Globoid Cell Leukodystrophy/Krabbe's Disease

Glomerulopathy KIRREL2

Glycogen Storage Disease IA, II, III, IIIA

Goniodysgenesis and Glaucoma

Hereditary Ataxia

Hereditary Cataracts

Hereditary Deafness (PTPRQ)

Hereditary Footpad Hyperkeratosis

Hereditary Nasal Parakeratosis

Table 3.11.1 (Continued)

Hereditary Nephropathy

Hereditary Nephropathy (Alport Syndrome)

Hip Dysplasia (markers)

Histiocytic Sarcoma (marker)

Hyperekplexia (Startle Disease)

Hyperoxaluria

Hyperuricosuria

Hypoadrenocorticism

Hypocatalasia

Hypokalemic Polymyopathy

Hypomyelination and Tremors

Ichthyosis

Inflammatory Myopathy

Inherited Myopathy

Iron-Deficiency Anemia

Juvenile Encephalopathy

Juvenile Epilepsy

Juvenile Laryngeal Paralysis and Polyneuropathy

Juvenile Myoclonic Epilepsy

Juvenile Onset Polyneuropathy

L2- Hydroxyglutaric Aciduria

Lagotto Storage Disease

Laryngeal Paralysis

Lethal Acrodermatitis MKLN1

Leukoencephalomyelopathy

Ligneous Membranitis

Lipoprotein Lipase Deficiency

Long QT Syndrome

Lundehund Syndrome

Lupoid Dermatosis

Macrothrombocytopenia

Macular Corneal Dystrophy

Malignant Hyperthermia

Mannosidosis

May–Hegglin Anomaly

Microphthalmia, Anophthalmia, and Coloboma

Mucolipidosis II

Mucopolysaccharidosis (I, IIIa, VI, VII, VIII)

Mullerian Duct Syndrome

Multidrug Resistance 1

Multiple System Degeneration

Muscular Dystrophy

Musladin–Lueke Syndrome

Mycobacterium Avium Susceptibility

Myeloperoxidase deficiency

Myostatin Deficiency

Myotonia Congenita

Myotonia Hereditaria

Myotubular Myopathy

Narcolepsy

Necrotizing Meningoencephalitis

Nemaline Myopathy

Neonatal Ataxia

Neonatal Cerebellar Cortical Degeneration

Neonatal Encephalopathy

Neonatal Encephalopathy with Seizures

Neonatal Neuroaxonal Dystrophy

Neuroaxonal Dystrophy

Neurodegenerative Vacuolar Storage Disease

Neuronal Ceroid Lipofuscinosis 1, 2, 4a, 5, 6, 7, 8, 10, A, MFSD8

Niemann-Pick C

Oculoskeletal Dysplasia

Osteochondrodysplasia

Osteochondromatosis

Osteogenesis Imperfecta

P2Y12 Receptor Platelet Disorder

Palmoplantar Keratoderma

Pancreatitis (marker)

Pannus (marker)

Paroxysmal Dyskinesia

Periodic Fever Syndrome

Persistent Mullerian Duct Syndrome

Phosphofructokinase Deficiency

Pituitary Dwarfism

Platelet Dysfunction

Platelet Procoagulant Deficiency – Scott Syndrome

Polycystic Kidney Disease

Polyneuropathy

Pompe Disease

Porphyria

Postoperative Hemorrhage

Prekallikrein Deficiency

Primary Ciliary Dyskinesia

Primary Lens Luxation

Primary Open Angle Glaucoma

Progress Retinal Atrophy - crd4/cord1

Progressive Neuronal Abiotrophy

Progressive Retinal Atrophy - AD/RHO

Progressive Retinal Atrophy - CNGA

Progressive Retinal Atrophy - CNGB1

(Continued)

Table 3.11.1 (Continued)

Progressive Retinal Atrophy - crd (1, 2, 3, 4)

Progressive Retinal Atrophy - erd

Progressive Retinal Atrophy - Golden Retriever (1 & 2)

Progressive Retinal Atrophy - IG-PRA1

Progressive Retinal Atrophy - Late Onset

Progressive Retinal Atrophy - rcd (1, 1a, 2, 3, 4)

Progressive Retinal Atrophy - RdAc

Progressive Retinal Atrophy - Rdy

Progressive Retinal Atrophy - SAG

Progressive Retinal Atrophy - Type 1, 3, 4

Progressive Retinal Atrophy - Type A, B

Progressive Retinal Atrophy - Type III

Progressive Retinal Atrophy - X-linked

Progressive Rod Cone Degeneration (prcd)

Protein-Losing Nephropathy

Pyruvate Dehydrogenase Phosphatase Deficiency

Pyruvate Kinase Deficiency

Raine Syndrome Dental Hypomineralization

Renal Cystadenocarcinoma and Nodular Dermatofibrosis

Renal Dysplasia

Retinal Degeneration

Rickets

Rod-Cone Dysplasia 1, 1a, 3

Sanfilippo Syndrome Type A / Mucopolysaccharidosis IIIA (Dachshund Type)

Scott Syndrome

Sensory Ataxic Neuropathy

Sensory Neuropathy

Severe Combined Immunodeficiency (Autosomal)

Severe Combined Immunodeficiency (X-linked)

Shaking Puppy

Shar-Pei Inflammatory Disease

Short Tail (Brachyury)

Skeletal Dysplasia

Spinal Dysraphism

Spinal Muscular Atrophy

Spinocerebellar Ataxia

Spondylocostal Dysostosis

Spongiform Leukoencephalomyelopathy

Spongy Degeneration with Cerebellar Ataxia (1 & 2)

Stargardt Disease

Startle Disease

Subacute Necrotizing Encephalopathy

Thrombopathia

Trapped Neutrophil Syndrome

van den Ende-Gupta Syndrome

von Willebrand Disease Types I, II, and III

Xanthuria Type 1a, 2a, 2b

X-Linked Ectodermal Dysplasia

X-Linked Generalized Tremor Syndrome

X-Linked Hereditary Nephropathy

X-Linked Myotubular Myopathy

environmental factors. Such tests that get developed will likely not be entirely predictive, but may indicate whether risk is higher, lower or moderate for an individual, compared to the relevant population base.

Because the body has so many redundancies built into the system, it is also possible that an individual might have a genotypically determined risk but never develop phenotypic disease. It is also possible that a pet has a genotypically determined risk but the phenotypic presentation does not really compromise the animal's health. For example, a Labrador retriever might have a determined risk for exercise-induced collapse (EIC) but in its typical environment and with its typical exercise regimen, it never becomes problematic.

For some conditions, even though they may be predicted with a genotypic test, phenotypic tests are needed to determine when the condition becomes clinically relevant and treatment is needed, and then for monitoring. For example, the risk for some forms of glaucoma can be predicted based on genotypic testing, but it is still necessary to use intraocular pressure to diagnose clinical disease and as a way of monitoring treatment.

The best use of genotypic tests is as a health screen rather than a disease screen. Pets are typically first examined around 8 weeks of age, and during this period the veterinary healthcare team will search for evident congenital issues, such as malocclusion, umbilical hernia, and luxating patellas. On the basis of this initial physical evaluation, vaccination and parasite control typically begin, and this is also the optimal time for starting pet health insurance, before anything gets identified that would be considered a preexisting condition (see 10.16 Pet Health Insurance).

Then, at 12 weeks of age, genotypic testing is indicated. Since DNA variants and the tests that measure them don't change with age, this can provide a good indication of health, at least for the tests that can be performed at this early age. Similarly, most human infants get postnatal genetic testing, typically for a few dozen hereditary conditions (such as phenylketonuria, congenital hypothyroidism, cystic fibrosis, etc.) – not because the majority of children are expected to have these problems, but it provides peace of mind for the parents that some potential problems can be screened. Postnatal screening does not mean that there won't be any problems that develop later in life, but screening has been done for the things that can be evaluated at this young age.

Phenotypic tests are more commonly done in practice, including blood tests, urinalysis, imaging, electrocardiography, etc. (Table 3.11.2). By 16 weeks of age, phenotypic testing regimens usually begin. This might involve early evaluation for hip dysplasia, urinalysis and tests looking for evidence of "stone" or "crystal formation" in the urine, or even following up on early suspicions of potential congenital heart disease. Further phenotypic testing will likely be predicated on the results of risk assessment (see 2.7 Risk Assessment), but might include definitive screening for hip dysplasia in the mature pet, glaucoma screening based on breed or genetic susceptibility, baseline evaluation of hemograms and biochemistries, and even specialist evaluation of breeding animals by ophthalmologists and/or cardiologists. All of this can be conducted seamlessly within a personalized care plan (see 1.3 Personalized Care Plans).

Of course, phenotypic tests also have their limitations. In some cases, the disease process has to progress considerably before disease will be detected. For example, with diabetes mellitus, a diagnosis might not be confirmed until the patient is clinical and the blood glucose and urine glucose levels rise about a standard point. Prior to that, though, testing may indicate a trend toward that possible outcome. In other cases, such as with prepatent period, a pet may have a parasite, but it is not detectable until it reaches a life stage that is detectable on testing. In other situations, there may not be a single phenotypic test that can render a diagnostic result, so a panel of different tests might be needed to support a diagnosis.

One other feature of some phenotypic tests is that a particular animal (or breed) may not reflect what is considered a "normal range" for the species. For example, there is a DNA test for congenital hypothyroidism with goiter in the toy fox terrier, but no such test for the adult-onset hypothyroidism more commonly seen in practice. That requires testing with a panel of tests that might include free and total levels of thyroid hormones, thyroid-stimulating hormone and even autoantibody levels to thyroid hormones. A diagnosis can sometimes still be elusive, especially in breeds that tend not to conform to the reference interval established by the testing laboratory (see 4.8 Pet-Specific Relevance of Reference Intervals). In these cases, a better approach may be to establish a "normal range" for the individual, by assessing 3–5 tests of thyroid function in the young adult, and using that later in life to evaluate trends.

One important distinction between genotypic and phenotypic testing is that genotypic test results do not change over time and so don't need to be repeated, whereas phenotypic results do change over time so need to be periodically reevaluated. For example, diabetes mellitus is a relatively common chronic disorder in both dogs and cats. In dogs, it is likely a complex genetic disorder in which several susceptibility genes affect overall genetic risk in a breed-specific manner. Thus, some breeds might be considered at increased risk, including keeshonden, Australian terriers, golden retrievers, miniature schnauzers, pugs, Samoyeds, etc. It cannot currently be predicted with a DNA test, and phenotypic testing with blood glucose levels and urinalysis can either be used to confirm a diagnosis or, preferably, can be used proactively to screen animals at potential risk to identify the prediabetic animal and attempt to alter the course of the disease. To identify such trends regarding the slow progression of such chronic diseases (including glaucoma, hypothyroidism, etc.), veterinary teams need to determine trends by periodically reevaluating relevant phenotypic tests.

EXAMPLES

Mrs Thompson presented her 2-year-old Doberman pinscher, Brutus, for routine evaluation and vaccination. Brutus had genetic testing as a puppy and was found to be "affected" on a DNA test for dilated cardiomyopathy. Initially Mrs Thompson was quite concerned and considered relinquishing Brutus to a shelter, but the veterinary team at ABC Animal Hospital helped put things in perspective.

It was true that Brutus had the PDK4 (DCM1) mutation that was associated with an increased risk for dilated cardiomyopathy, but she now understood that the mutation did not cause the disease (it was just associated with increased risk in a certain cohort of Doberman pinschers), was not the only mutation associated with the disease, and that there were also other factors that could influence cardiomyopathy onset in a complex manner. In fact, she also read about some diets that could possibly be associated with the disease in a number of different breeds.

The team at ABC Animal Hospital helped establish a sensible ongoing screening protocol with their local veterinary cardiologist, and Mrs Thompson felt quite relieved that they had identified a risk factor, but now had a sensible program in place to make sure Brutus would have the care he needed.

TAKE-AWAYS

- In most pets, a combination of genotypic and phenotypic testing is needed for the early detection of disease conditions.
- Genotypic testing allows the earliest identification of risk, but does not always mean that the pet will develop disease.
- In most instances, genotypic testing is used as a health screen rather than a disease screen.
- Phenotypic testing can confirm a diagnosis, but typically later in the course of disease.
- Veterinary teams need to be able to effectively counsel clients as how a combination of genotypic and phenotypic testing can help deliver excellent healthcare across a pet's lifespan.

MISCELLANEOUS

Abbreviation

DNA   Deoxyribonucleic acid

Recommended Reading

Ackerman, L. (2011). *The Genetic Connection*, 2e. Lakewood, CO: AAHA Press.

Ackerman, L. (2019). An introduction to pet-specific care. *EC Vet. Sci.* 4 (1): 1–3.

Ackerman, L. (ed.) (2020). Pet-specific care. In: *Five-Minute Veterinary Practice Management Consult*, 3e, 260–263. Ames, IA: Wiley.

Ackerman, L. (2020). Proactive Pet Parenting: Anticipating pet health problems before they happen. Problem Free Publishing.

American Animal Hospital Association-American Veterinary Medical Association Preventive Health Guidelines Task Force (2011). *J. Am. Vet. Med. Assoc.* 239 (5): 625–629.

Bell, J., Cavanagh, K., Tilley, L., and Smith, F. (2012). *Veterinary Medical Guide to Dog and Cat Breeds.* Jackson Hole, WY: Teton NewMedia.

Companion Animal Parasite Council. www.capcvet.org

Partners for Healthy Pets. www.partnersforhealthypets.org

Shaffer, L.G., Geretshlaeger, A., Ramirez, C.J. et al. (2019). Quality assurance checklist and additional considerations for canine clinical genetic testing laboratories: a follow-up to the published standards and guidelines. *Hum. Genet.* 138: 501–508.

Stull, J.W., Shelby, J.A., Bonnett, B.N. et al. (2018). Barriers and next steps to providing a spectrum of effective health care to companion animals. *J. Am. Vet. Med. Assoc.* 253 (11): 1386–1389.

3.12

Orthopedic Screening

Jason C. Nicholas, BVETMED (Hons)

Independent Consultant, Author and Speaker, Co-founder, Preventive Vet, Portland, OR, USA

BASICS

3.12.1 Summary

From congenital and early-onset conditions, such as angular limb deformities (ALD), luxating patella (LP), and hip dysplasia (HD), to developmental conditions that show up later in life, like degenerative joint disease (DJD) and osteoarthritis (OA), orthopedic conditions can cause significant pain, dysfunction, and secondary complications in our canine and feline patients. Such conditions can also cause emotional distress, logistical complications, and financial strain for our clients. *Proactive* screening and early client education and intervention are crucial to help avoid or mitigate the problems associated with orthopedic conditions both for our patients and our clients.

On the other hand, a *reactive* approach typically results in affected patients suffering unnecessarily until such time that their owners recognize a problem and present their pet for evaluation. By this point, treatment options may be more limited or prognosis for the best level of return to function and good quality of life (QOL) may already be reduced.

MAIN CONCEPTS

Orthopedic conditions in cats and dogs can be more common than many people realize and they can often have a significant negative impact on the comfort and QOL of affected animals. Orthopedic conditions can cause a host of problems, both for the affected pet and also for their people. Associated problems can include:

- pain (potentially with a resulting change in behavior, including development of aggression and noise aversions)
- loss of normal function and range of motion (ROM)
- forced early retirement for a working dog
- difficulty getting into/out of owner's vehicle
- difficulty getting on/off owner's bed
- difficulty navigating stairs within/outside owner's home
- decreased jumping ability for cats
- trouble accessing litter boxes for cats (with resulting inappropriate toileting)
- overall decreased QOL
- damage to the bond between the affected pet and their people.

Earlier detection and intervention can help improve the QOL for affected pets and their people. Since many pet owners don't appreciate the prevalence of orthopedic conditions in cats and dogs, and many don't pick up on the earliest signs of such conditions, veterinary teams must be proactive in educating clients and encouraging early and appropriate screening for orthopedic issues to help advocate for and provide the best comfort and care for our patients.

3.12.2 Congenital and Acquired Orthopedic Conditions Can Be Common

3.12.2.1 Canine Hip Dysplasia (HD)

Data from the Orthopedic Foundation for Animals (OFA) puts the likelihood of canine HD at 18.3–21.2% for Rottweilers, 20.1–20.5% for German shepherd dogs, 15.5–19.9% for golden retrievers, and 8.5–12.0% for labrador retrievers [1]. (Bulldogs had the highest prevalence of HD according to OFA data, at 65.9–71.2%!)

3.12.2.2 Canine Elbow Dysplasia (ED)

OFA data also show high prevalence of ED in certain dog breeds: chow chows (48.6%), Rottweilers (38.9%), German shepherd dogs (19.1%), and golden retrievers (11.4%) [1].

3.12.2.3 Canine Osteoarthritis (OA)

In a OA screening study done on dogs undergoing dental prophylaxis, it was found that 68% had radiographic evidence of OA in at least one joint (many had more than one joint affected) [2]. It was also found in this study that 71% of the owners of the dogs that were found to have radiographic OA weren't appreciating any clinical signs of their dog's OA [2].

3.12.2.4 Feline Osteoarthritis (OA)

In one study, radiographic evidence of OA was present in approximately 30% of cats over 8 years old [3]. Another study found that 90% of cats over 12 years old had radiographic evidence of DJD [4].

3.12.3 Diagnostic Methods for Screening for Orthopedic Disease and Risk Factors

While radiographs are a central modality of orthopedic disease screening, they aren't the only diagnostic testing method to use when looking for orthopedic problems in patients.

3.12.3.1 Pain Assessment Questionnaires

Validated pet owner questionnaires exist that can help increase a clinician's index of suspicion for orthopedic (or other painful) disease in pets. When orthopedic disease is anticipated or suspected based upon breed, age, activity level, or other factors, having the client fill out one of the validated pain assessment questionnaires can help move the diagnostic process along and also assess response to interventions. Currently available pain assessment questionnaires include (see links to questionnaires in Recommended Reading section):

- Canine Brief Pain Inventory (PennVet)
- Helsinki Chronic Pain Index
- Cincinnati Orthopedic Disability Index
- Feline Musculoskeletal Pain Index (NC State CVM)
- Montreal Instrument for Cat Arthritis Testing.

3.12.3.2 Palpation and ROM

At each wellness exam, make it a part of the general physical exam to look at, palpate, and do a quick ROM evaluation of each of the patient's joints. Any abnormalities detected or suspected based on this quick assessment can be discussed with the client and further evaluated specifically.

3.12.3.3 Gait Analysis

While force plate analysis isn't available in most veterinary practices, thanks to the prevalence of smartphones, we all now typically have a rather powerful tool to help in our regular gait analyses of patients. When orthopedic or gait abnormalities are suspected, take slow-motion video using a smartphone to help in the evaluation and to show clients any abnormalities found. You can also have your client use their phone to shoot slow-motion video of their pets going up and down stairs, running, jumping, and doing other activities at home. Not only can this help you find and localize orthopedic disorders but, by using "before" and "after" videos, it can also help you and your clients appreciate any improvements with therapies instituted. *Tip:* When shooting these videos, ensure that the phone is held horizontally, in "landscape" mode, and that the lighting and background provide the right detail and contrast to get the most benefit from the videos.

3.12.3.4 Radiographs

While dedicated radiographs for orthopedic disease screening generally require and benefit from sedation or anesthesia (e.g., Penn HIP, etc.), don't forget about the orthopedic information that can be gleaned from general radiographs of patients when looking for thoracic or abdominal disease. Shoulders and hips are almost always present in thoracic and abdominal radiographic views, respectively, and elbows and stifles frequently are, too. Similarly, vertebral bodies and associated intervertebral disc spaces are also frequently present for evaluation. While thoracic and abdominal views and techniques aren't specific for evaluating joints, you can still glean a lot of initial screening information from their appearance in them. It is important to realize that all pets can develop orthopedic issues, including mixed-breeds, and so routine screening is important for all patients.

3.12.3.5 Genetic Testing

Common orthopedic disorders, such as hip and ED, patella luxation, and even cruciate disease, have been shown to have a heritable component. However, because the heritability of these conditions is complex (involving multiple mutations), truly predictive and cost-effective genetic screening isn't yet available (see 3.4 Predicting and Eliminating Disease Traits). This is an exciting area that holds good promise for future development. In the interim, it is important to recommend routine orthopedic screening of pets with known breed predispositions to such problems (see 3.11 Integrating Genotypic and Phenotypic Testing).

3.12.4 Incorporating Orthopedic Screening into Your Practice Workflow and Client Recommendations

Several suggestions for incorporating orthopedic screening into exams and practice workflows are mentioned above. Here are a few more ways to recommend and incorporate screening and monitoring of orthopedic conditions into daily practice.

- Based upon each pet's age, breed, history, and other signalment and risk factors, preplan and include orthopedic screening and monitoring radiographs into each predisposed pet's long-term care plan (see 1.3 Personalized Care Plans). Be especially forthcoming in your recommendations for these radiographs in pets that fit any of the following criteria.
  – Overweight or obese
  – Predisposed breed
  – Working dog or athlete
  – Pets that are exhibiting behavioral changes, including new aggression, decreased interaction with clients, and those exhibiting new noise aversions [5]
  – Cats with inappropriate toileting
- So long as they are stable, take advantage of any pet sedated or anesthetized for procedures (e.g., spay/neuter, dental prophylaxes, ear cleanings, laceration repairs, etc.) to do a deeper, more thorough palpation and ROM testing of joints. Since it's good practice for you and also may turn up otherwise undiagnosed conditions (providing better medicine and improving comfort for your patients, and revenue generation for your practice), do these deeper orthopedic evaluations as value-added, no-charge components of your sedated/anesthetized procedures on all patients. However, be sure to include a section on your estimates and sedation/anesthesia consent forms offering and recommending that, so long as their pet is stable under sedation/anesthesia and based on your findings and their pet's risk factors, specific orthopedic radiographs may be recommended. Provide an estimate for such and get the owner's authorization for such in advance.

EXAMPLES

Dr X loved orthopedics and made it a habit of practicing his drawer testing on anesthetized patients. Max, a 5-year-old neutered male Labrador, was in for dental prophylaxis. While Max was under anesthesia for his dental, Dr X thought he appreciated a little more laxity in Max's right stifle. He contacted Max's owner to report his concerns and recommend stifle radiographs. The owner had been advised of this possibility prior to the procedure, based on Max's breed predisposition, and consented. The radiographs were sent off for interpretation and a partial cruciate tear was suspected based on the clinical history, physical exam findings, and radiographic appearance of Max's stifles. Max's owners were counseled on weight management and Max was started on a daily joint supplement and fish oils. A referral was also made to a local veterinary physiotherapy center to aid in his weight loss and to help stabilize his stifles as much as possible. With this early detection and intervention, Max remained stable and never required cruciate surgery.

TAKE-AWAYS

- Whether they develop early in life or late, orthopedic disorders can cause significant pain, dysfunction, and decreased QOL for our veterinary patients, as well as significant financial, logistical, and emotional distress for our clients.
- Across the board, serious orthopedic disorders are going undiagnosed and therefore untreated and managed, often to the detriment of our patients, clients, and even our own businesses.
- Proactive education, screening, and appropriate interventions should be the standard of care, as they benefit all stakeholders (patients, clients, and practices).
- Radiography isn't the only method available for orthopedic disease screening in veterinary patients.
- Take advantage of any sedated or anesthetized pets to do additional screening for orthopedic conditions, with owner consent.

MISCELLANEOUS

References

1 Breed Statistics. www.ofa.org/diseases/breed-statistics
2 Mills, D. (2014). Prevalence of Osteoarthritis in Dogs Undergoing Routine Dental Prophylaxis. Presented at the

World Small Animal Veterinary Association World Congress, Cape Town, South Africa, September.

3 University of Glasgow. Cats Do Suffer From Arthritis, Study Shows. ScienceDaily. www.sciencedaily.com/releases/2007/08/070824215618.htm

4 Hardie, E.M., Roe, S.C., and Martin, F.R. (2002). Radiographic evidence of degenerative joint disease in geriatric cats: 100 cases (1994–1997). *J. Am. Vet. Med. Assoc.* 220 (5): 628–632.

5 Lopes Fagundes, A.L., Hewison, L., McPeake, K.J. et al. (2018). Noise sensitivities in dogs: an exploration of signs in dogs with and without musculoskeletal pain using qualitative content analysis. *Front. Vet. Sci.* 5: 17.

Recommended Reading

Canine Brief Pain Inventory (Canine BPI). www.vet.upenn.edu/research/clinical-trials-vcic/our-services/pennchart/cbpi-tool

Hielm-Björkman, A.K., Rita, H., and Tulamo, R.M. (2009). Psychometric testing of the Helsinki chronic pain index by completion of a questionnaire in Finnish by owners of dogs with chronic signs of pain caused by osteoarthritis. *Am. J. Vet. Res.* 70 (6): 727–734.

Valentin, C. (2009). Cincinnati Orthopaedic Disability Index in canines. *Australian Journal of Physiotherapy* 55: 288. www.sciencedirect.com/science/article/pii/S0004951409700145.

Feline Musculoskeletal Pain Index. https://cvm.ncsu.edu/research/labs/clinical-sciences/comparative-pain-research/labs-comparative-pain-research-clinical-metrology-instruments-feline-musculoskeletal-pain-index

Klink, M.P., Gruen, M.E., del Castillo, J. et al. (2018). Development and preliminary validity and reliability of the Montreal instrument for cat arthritis testing, for use by caretaker/owner, MI-CAT(C), via a randomised clinical trial. *Applied Animal Behaviour Science* 200: 96–105. www.sciencedirect.com/science/article/abs/pii/S0168159117303271.

3.13

Breed Predisposition

Nan Boss, DVM

Best Friends Veterinary Center, Grafton, WI, USA

BASICS

3.13.1 Summary

Different breeds have different predispositions to disease states caused by genetic variants. Any personalized care plan should incorporate screening, treatment plans, and client education based on susceptibility to genetic diseases. There is a large opportunity for practices to improve both patient care and professional outcomes via breed-specific programs.

MAIN CONCEPTS

A great deal of the illness seen in dogs and cats is breed related (see 11.4 Heritable Health Conditions – By Breed). All breeds of dogs and cats have genetic susceptibility to particular medical and behavioral problems. In addition, any individual pet carries genes for diseases it may never develop itself but that could be passed down to its offspring.

Many canine and feline genetic diseases have been described to date (see 11.3 Heritable Health Conditions – By Disease). Many purebred cats have serious genetic problems and even most plain old domestic shorthair or longhair cats have susceptibility to genetically related diseases.

Mixed-breed dogs are not immune to genetically related diseases either (see 3.19 Mixed-Breed Considerations). A study by researchers at the University of California-Davis [1] challenged the theory that purebred dogs are more prone to genetic disorders than mixed breed dogs.

They studied 27 254 dogs with inherited disorders over a five-year period. For 10 out of the 24 disorders studied, purebred dogs were more likely to develop the disorder. For 13 of those disorders, mixed-breed and purebred dogs had equal risk. For cranial cruciate ligament tear, mixed-breed dogs were actually at higher risk than purebreds.

Some of these diseases are very common and some are very rare. Some are common in one breed and rare in another. Breeds from similar lineages are more susceptible to certain disorders that affect closely related purebreds. Disorders with equal prevalence in purebreds and mixed-breeds seem to be more ancient mutations that are widely spread through the pet population.

Some genetic diseases are dangerous and deadly while others are minor flaws easily dealt with (see 2.7 Risk Assessment).

Some heritable diseases can be tested for, either with DNA tests or more standard types of phenotypic testing, enabling earlier diagnosis and intervention (see 3.4 Predicting and Eliminating Disease Traits and 3.11 Integrating Genotypic and Phenotypic Testing). Disorders caused by a single genetic defect can usually be more easily diagnosed and treated, and more and more genetic (DNA) tests are becoming available all the time. Collectively, early detection testing helps us tailor a pet's healthcare plan to its own particular circumstances (see 4.7 Embracing Early Detection).

Some of these genetic disorders simply require awareness on the part of the owner as to what to watch for and when to call the veterinarian. Our goal should be to make sure that every owner of an at-risk breed knows about the diseases and problems that could affect their dog or cat, both genetically related and not, and the testing or treatment that is currently available for them (see 6.4 Creating a Pet-Specific User's Manual).

Pet-Specific Care for the Veterinary Team, First Edition. Edited by Lowell Ackerman.
© 2021 John Wiley & Sons, Inc. Published 2021 by John Wiley & Sons, Inc.

3.13.2 Screening for Genetic Diseases

The fact that a pet is not a purebred does not mean that genetic diseases shouldn't be screened for. Diseases caused by recessive genes are less likely to be problems in mixed-breeds but many breeds share susceptibility to the same genetic defects, especially disorders with more complex inheritance that just a single gene mutation. Statistically, purebred dogs are not always less healthy than mixes and dominant genes can affect offspring regardless of how far from purebred they are (see link to video titled Mixed breed dogs have genetic risk too: www.youtube.com/watch?v=Ce1u_ZqwqMo).

We can sometimes infer susceptibility to genetic diseases just by looking at size or phenotype. We might expect any large or giant breed to have greater risk for hemangiosarcoma and hip dysplasia than a much smaller dog, although the risks are actually based on family history.

Gene defects may cause a direct problem every time, or they may be turned on or off by factors such as the pet's environment, diet, infection, medications or surgery. For example, a cat may have a genetic susceptibility to diabetes mellitus but may only develop the disease if it becomes overweight. A collie may have the MDR1 genetic defect that causes it to get sick from the drug ivermectin but if it never received that or other drugs implicated with this variant, the problem wouldn't be evident.

Fortunately, DNA screening can now tell us what breeds are likely in a pet's heritage as well as allowing us to test or screen for individual genetic diseases. Panels of DNA tests are available as well, so we can test for dozens or hundreds of DNA defects with a single sample of blood, saliva or cheek cells (see 3.6 Genetic Testing). These test panels are inexpensive enough to be used widely as screening tools. Unlike other types of testing, such as thyroid screening, a DNA panel typically only needs to be done once in a pet's life.

Some care must be taken when selecting a laboratory for DNA testing. Manufacturers are not required to disclose their testing methodology nor is there any oversight of the laboratory running the test. Direct-to-consumer DNA tests are popular, but the results may be suspect. The WSAVA's Canine and Feline Hereditary Disease website (https://wsava.org/committees/hereditary-disease-committee/#:~:text=The%20World%20Small%20Animal%20Veterinary,now%20and%20in%20future%20generations) lists available DNA tests by breed, disease and testing laboratory, and provides links to peer-reviewed citations. Organizations such as the Orthopedic Foundation for Animals (www.ofa.org) and the International Partnership for Dogs (www.dogwellnet.com) can provide advice on available testing. University-run laboratories are usually highly qualified, though they generally run only individual tests versus panels.

Not every genetic problem is caused by a single gene defect (see 3.3 The Genetics of Disease). Some, such as hip dysplasia, involve multiple genes and a wide range of possible presentations. Instead of a single test, radiographs for hip dysplasia look for the phenotypic evidence, not the genetic defects themselves. Some screening tests for genetic disorders, like ophthalmologist or cardiologist evaluations, or thyroid screening, must be periodically repeated (see 3.4 Predicting and Eliminating Disease Traits).

Genetic testing is especially important for anyone thinking about purchasing a purebred dog or cat, or breeding purebred or mixed-breed pets (see 3.10 Advising Clients on Selecting an Appropriate Pet). It is the responsibility of everyone who breeds animals to do so carefully and with a good understanding of the genetic risks for their breed or breeds (see 3.11 Integrating Genotypic and Phenotypic Testing). Genetic testing before breeding should be considered a standard of care today. No one should be breeding an animal without screening for genetic diseases. No one should be buying a purebred pet whose parents have not been screened. Many breed associations and clubs have genetic screening information on their websites and some offer screening clinics for common diseases present in their breed.

For the average client with a pet, we are focusing on problems that pet might develop in the future. For breeding, we also have to focus on problems that pet could pass along to its offspring. The testing then becomes more indepth.

3.13.3 Breed-Specific Risk Assessment

Much of our work in veterinary medicine hinges around the concept of reducing risk (see 2.7 Risk Assessment). Vaccinations reduce the risk of infection, parasite preventives reduce the risk for parasites, senior screening reduces the risk that we will fail to detect a disease process early, and so on. Client education follows risk assessment and management. We teach the clients about topics that pertain to their pet – for which the pet is at risk (see 10.5 Early Detection Campaigns).

When it comes to hip dysplasia in at-risk breeds, we would want to do screening radiographs and educate pet owners about arthritis diagnosis and treatment (see 3.12 Orthopedic Screening).

Breed-specific wellness is the next big leap for educating clients once all the basics have been covered. Breed tendencies for disease can jump right to the top of a "diseases or problems that could be fatal" list. For example, cardiomyopathy is common and deadly in boxers but occurs later and in a milder form in some other breeds. The more common and the more severe the risk, the more you need to talk about it early and often, so for a boxer owner annual screening should be a big priority. For a Dalmatian, one might choose something else to talk about, like bladder stones. Instead of electrocardiogram (ECG) screening, one might discuss feeding a special diet and an annual urinalysis.

Practicing high-quality medicine is all about being a better teacher. This is as simple as putting a handout in every file before the appointment, so we remember to discuss the topic with the client and send them home with written information. Preparing and preloading your patient files ahead of each visit is a very important step.

Have a system. If this is the year you want to educate every client on dental disease, load a dental brochure in every file. If you want to talk about breed-specific wellness care or healthcare plans, you need to come up with a structure for your program that makes it easy to implement. Specific recommendations and client education topics should be developed and used for every breed.

The following are links to some client education videos that can be helpful in practice. They also serve to illustrate what a breed risk discussion with a client might look like.

- Breed risks in bulldogs: www.youtube.com/watch?v=Kgz3xCzlM_c
- Eye diseases: www.youtube.com/watch?v=d_RGk2UEdgs
- Foreign body (FB) ingestion: www.youtube.com/watch?v=VYNJrVS3u8g
- Gastric dilation-volvulus (GDV): www.youtube.com/watch?v=CrX2BJ7EI-o
- GDV and von Willebrand disease in Dobermans: www.youtube.com/watch?v=7l_gL0_6cOA
- Glomerulonephropathy (GN) in wheaten terriers: www.youtube.com/watch?v=eTwyUbiFPbU
- Hemangiosarcoma: www.youtube.com/watch?v=9HBPwYG5CW4
- Hip dysplasia and arthritis: www.youtube.com/watch?v=VgAJeeSE-GA
- MDR1 testing in herding breeds: www.youtube.com/watch?v=F7D3d3Rgm7U
- Intervertebral disc disease (IVDD): www.youtube.com/watch?v=vZqXvkN67rM

3.13.4 Developing a Breed-Specific Wellness Program

Wellness programs are a lot of work, including program development, fee setting, appointment times, team training, client education, marketing and, lastly, protocols – what will you do with the information once you have it? Actually implementing a program can be challenging – it's complicated and time consuming. The more statistics you know about common disease problems, though, the more you see how early diagnosis and treatment is key to being an effective veterinarian.

Breed-specific wellness has been building in significance for a long time. Follow this link to a client education video titled What is Breed-Specific Wellness? www.youtube.com/watch?v=vDvl5L2cRNQ.

It could be started in the most basic fashion with simple laminated sheets for clients to read while waiting for the doctor that explains a single disease that their pet would be at risk for due to its breed. Then they could decide whether they wanted to do a screening test, such as an ECG screen, a Schirmer tear test or a urine protein:creatinine ratio (UPC), to diagnose it.

Such as system is simple, but the hit-or-miss approach of having such conversations may not engage many pet owners. Whenever possible, it is better to have a coherent approach to most breeds, and even mixed-breed pets (see 10.7 Breed-Specific Marketing). It often works better for a practice to put together a package that includes all the exams, tests, and vaccines we think are appropriate for the pet at its age and we factor in breed risk tests and any other services recommended because of lifestyle – so the package for a middle-aged Labrador retriever might include thyroid testing and if it has exposure to deer ticks, we would also include Lyme prevention. With pet-specific care, pet owners often select more services, so if payment (wellness) plans are being used in the practice, the client can split the larger total into monthly payments (see 10.17 Payment and Wellness Plans). A significant percentage of the client base may also elect to pay in advance for the full range of services.

Most practices market such healthcare plans through the website and social media (see 10.6 Target Marketing and Targeted Client Outreach). In time, practices will detect more problems, and earlier, so revenue from both diagnostics and therapeutics will help offset the higher costs of client service.

Every client interaction is an honest discussion about common problems that we can do something about. Our best marketing isn't what's on the screen, it's what's in our hearts and minds that we share with our clients every single day.

3.13.5 Marketing Breed-Specific Wellness

Always leave the client with something to read or watch when they have to wait. Use that time to get clients thinking about a decision they will need to make or to get exposure to a new product or service. Clients are more willing to read or watch something they know has been chosen especially for them and the needs of their particular pet (see 10.7 Breed-Specific Marketing).

Be consistent within the hospital. A patient or client should never get a greater or lesser level of care because one doctor saw them and not another, or one receptionist spoke with them and not someone else. Breed-specific care should be the standard of care throughout the practice (see 9.4 Standards of Care).

Anything you want to teach clients about has to be taught to your team first and they need to know exactly what to say or do in order to get client acceptance of any wellness recommendations, including breed risk ones. Think about and discuss scripts for breed-related testing if you want to educate clients in this area; for example, "Boxers are at risk for serious heart problems. The doctor will talk to you about ECG screening. . ."

The only way you can help your patients lead long and healthy lives is to educate their owners (see 5.10 Discussing Pet-Specific Care). Most of your clients don't have a degree in medicine or behavior. Take the time and make the effort to teach them what they need to know to care for their pets properly. It's not only good medicine – it's well worth the effort for your practice.

EXAMPLES

Here are samples of healthcare programs for two different breeds. For each item marked as needing client education, you would need to have or develop a handout or other tool to use with clients. Items in bold would become part of your screening or preventative program at the appropriate age.

Healthcare considerations for a Doberman pinscher

System	Recommendation
Behavior	Males may be aggressive; prone to flank sucking, lick granulomas
Cardiac	Dilated cardiomyopathy (DCM) very common – annual **ECG screen** to look for ventricular premature contractions (VPCs), consider annual **echocardiogram/Pro-BNP**, client education, recommend pet health insurance when young
Dermatological	Seasonal flank alopecia; lick granulomas; pemphigus; zinc-responsive dermatosis
Drug reactions	Avoid sulfa drugs which can increase risk for keratoconjunctivitis sicca (KCS) and adverse drug reactions
Gastrointestinal	Prone to foreign body, bloat. Client education. Consider gastropexy during neutering surgery. Recommend pet health insurance when young
Hemolymphatic	von Willebrand disease very common in breed. **Screen for clotting ability (DNA test, buccal bleeding time or von Willebrand factor)** before surgery or dental extractions. Recommend pet health insurance
Chronic active hepatitis	**Periodic liver function testing**
Hypothyroidism	**Periodic thyroid profiles**, starting with baseline at 1 year of age
Neurological	Intervertebral disc disease (cervical), Wobbler's, narcolepsy. Client education
Ophthalmic	Cataracts, progressive retinal atrophy – appropriate screening
Orthopedic	Hip dysplasia, anterior cruciate ligament tear. Client education, recommend pet health insurance
Infectious diseases	Potentially increased susceptibility to parvovirus vaccination. Consider vaccination booster at 5 months of age; titers
Urology	Glomerulonephropathy (GN) – consider **annual urine protein:creatinine ratio**

Healthcare considerations for a Boston terrier

Dentistry	Periodontal disease – frequent dental cleanings, client education; failure of canine teeth to erupt – check dentition at 5–6 months of age
Dermatological	Alopecia, atopic dermatitis (hyperadrenocorticism) – client education; demodicosis more common – skin scrape early if clinical presentation consistent
Reproductive	Dystocia can be an issue – client education if breeding
Gastroenterological	Pyloric stenosis more common
Neoplastic	Mast cell tumor (MCT), melanoma – fine needle aspirate (FNA)/remove all lumps
Neurological	Hydrocephalus – check for open fontanelles in puppies, monitor behavior
Ophthalmological	Prolapse of nictitating membrane (cherry eye), corneal ulcers, pigmentary keratitis, corneal dystrophy – client education; cataracts – both juvenile and late onset; iris cysts; vitreal syneresis > glaucoma and cataracts; proptosis
Keratoconjunctivitis sicca	**Schirmer tear test** routinely
Respiratory	Respiratory dysplasia, including hypoplastic trachea – client education, early surgery if needed, give estimate for soft palate surgery with spay/neuter estimate. Skilled individual to intubate at every age, to look for elongated soft palate

3.13.6 DNA Testing Recommendation Scripts

3.13.6.1 Mixed-Breed Composition

This is the test that identifies the likely breed components of a mixed-breed dog. This is a one-time investment that provides a lot of information about a dog's genetic make-up, so we know what genetic diseases are likely or possible.

3.13.6.2 Acute Ventricular Dysrhythmia Syndrome

Also known as arrhythmogenic right-ventricular cardio-myopathy (ARVC), this is a serious heart condition seen in boxers and boxer mixes. It can cause acute collapse and death. All boxers and boxer mix dogs should be DNA tested for this, ideally when they are young.

3.13.6.3 Hemophilia and von Willebrand Disease

There are quite a few different forms of inherited bleeding disorders, including von Willebrand disease. Failure of the blood to clot properly can range from mild to severe and can worsen with age. Von Willebrand disease is extremely common in several breeds, and they should be DNA tested for it. For other breeds, we usually do a less expensive buccal bleeding time instead of a DNA test whenever we are performing surgery, to make sure we don't have a problem with excessive bleeding.

3.13.6.4 MDR1

Several breeds and their crosses may possess this variant that affects tolerance for ivermectin and many other drugs. If a dog inherits two copies of the MDR1 gene, one from each parent, we must be very careful with certain medications and usually choose not to use them at all. Dogs with one copy of the gene can usually tolerate low doses of drugs if they really need to be used. We recommend all dogs from susceptible breeds be tested so we can properly prescribe medications for them.

Exercise-induced collapse (EIC) is just like it sounds – affected dogs collapse when exercising strenuously, especially in hot weather. This problem is seen especially in Labrador and golden retrievers but in other breeds as well. The problem is not common so we generally only test for it if a dog has symptoms or will be used for breeding.

TAKE-AWAYS

- A great deal of the illness we see in dogs and cats is breed related.
- Some heritable diseases can be tested for, enabling earlier diagnosis and intervention.
- Some simply require awareness on the part of the owner as to what to watch for and when to call the veterinarian.
- DNA screening is becoming an increasingly important component of pet healthcare.
- Our goal is to try to make sure that every owner of an at-risk breed knows about the diseases and problems that could affect their dog or cat and the testing or treatment that is currently available for them.

MISCELLANEOUS

Abbreviations

DNA   Deoxyribonucleic acid
MDR   Multidrug resistance
Pro-BNP Pro B-type natriuretic peptide

Reference

1 Bellumori, T.P., Famula, T.R., Bannasch, D.L. et al. (2013). Prevalence of inherited disorders among mixed-breed and purebred dogs: 27,254 cases (1995–2010). *J. Am. Vet. Med. Assoc.* 242: 1549–1555.

Recommended Reading

Ackerman, L. *The Genetic Connection: A Guide to Health Problems in Purebred Dogs*, 2. AAHA Press, Lakewood, CO, 2011.

Fleming, JM, Creevy, KE, Promislow, DEL. Mortality in north American dogs from 1984 to 2004: an investigation into age-size and breed related causes of death, *J. Vet. Intern. Med.* 2011;25:187–198.

Gough, A. *Breed Predispositions to Disease in Dogs and Cats*, 3. Wiley Blackwell, Ames, IA, 2018.

3.14

Breed-Specific Variants in Laboratory Testing

Ryane E. Englar, DVM, DABVP (CANINE AND FELINE PRACTICE)

College of Veterinary Medicine, University of Arizona, Oro Valley, AZ, USA

BASICS

3.14.1 Summary

Advances in diagnostic testing in companion animal practice have paved the way for proactive screening and early detection of disease among asymptomatic patients. Veterinarians must accurately diagnose patients in order to design appropriate healthcare plans. This task requires them to consider reference intervals (RIs) for each diagnostic test and use them to guide decision making. Historically, patient laboratory values have been compared against those that are considered "normal" for the species. However, research suggests that there is breed-specific variation in RIs among dogs and cats. Ignoring these variants may result in misinterpretation of laboratory data and misdiagnosis.

3.14.2 Terms Defined

RI: a range that has been ascribed to a population of healthy adult animals for a given diagnostic test. Synonymous with reference range or normal range.

MAIN CONCEPTS

Patients present with a wide range of ailments. Veterinarians rely upon patient data for clues that explain clinical presentations. Patient data are produced during the comprehensive physical exam and also through diagnostic testing. In situations where early detection of disease is essential for patient outcomes, data from diagnostic tests facilitate diagnosis in asymptomatic patients.

Reference intervals are established for diagnostic tests to screen patients for abnormal values (see 4.8 Pet-Specific Relevance of Reference Intervals). Abnormalities in data allow us to identify changes that may be consistent with a physiological or pathological process. For example, nonregenerative anemia, hypercholesterolemia, and mild increases in liver enzymes are consistent with a diagnosis of canine hypothyroidism in a patient with weight gain, lethargy, "ring around the collar," and rat tail.

Reference intervals facilitate interpretation of laboratory data because they capture what is considered "normal" for a given species (see 4.8 Pet-Specific Relevance of Reference Intervals). However, despite extensive guidelines that have been provided by the American Society of Veterinary Clinical Pathology, the development of RIs remains an imperfect science. There is growing awareness that certain breeds have unique clinicopathological features. Recent studies have proposed breed-specific RIs to improve clinical acumen and diagnostic accuracy.

3.14.3 Sighthounds

On complete blood count (CBC), Scottish deerhounds have lower than expected RIs for platelets and reticulocytes.

Most greyhounds have elevated red blood cell (RBC), hemoglobin (Hb), and hematocrits (Hct). They often have decreased platelets, total leukocyte counts (WBC), and absolute numbers of neutrophils, lymphocytes, monocytes, and eosinophils [1]. On blood film examination, greyhound eosinophils appear "vacuolated" and gray because they lack the orange granules that are characteristic of this cell type using Romanowsky, Wright–Giemsa, or Diff-Quik stains [1, 2].

Serum biochemistry profiles of greyhounds are also unique. Greyhounds tend to have lower "normal" values for total protein (TP), albumin, globulin, and calcium, and higher "normal" values for blood urea nitrogen (BUN), creatinine, and alanine aminotransferase (ALT) [3]. The elevation in serum creatinine is thought to reflect the build of the breed, specifically its increased muscle mass [3].

Scottish deerhounds have lower than expected RIs for chloride, bilirubin, glucose, and gamma glutamyl transferase (GGT), and higher than expected RIs for BUN, potassium, aspartate aminotransferase (AST), alkaline phosphatase (ALP), and cholesterol.

Basal serum total thyroxine (tT4) is also distinctly low in sighthounds [2]. Greyhounds that race or are in training to race have lower tT4 than retired dogs [2]. Young greyhounds may also have lower than anticipated free T4 (fT4) concentrations [2].

Greyhounds may be misdiagnosed with cardiomyopathy because of elevated serum cardiac troponin I levels [2]. This polypeptide is found in cardiac muscle, and high values have been linked to heart disease. However, greyhounds have thicker than normal left ventricular free walls and larger heart weight-to-body weight ratios that may explain elevated troponin in the absence of cardiomyopathy.

3.14.4 Akitas, Jindos, Shiba Inus, and the Chinese Shar Pei

In puppies, serum potassium is typically low compared to adults because of sodium/potassium (Na/K) pumps within the cell membrane of maturing erythrocytes [4]. These pumps pair the flow of potassium into the cell with the efflux of sodium. As dogs mature, Na/K pumps are lost [4]. This leads to high intracellular sodium and low intracellular potassium [4].

Some, but not all, dogs of particular breeds possess a high potassium (HK) mutation. These dogs have persistent Na/K pumps that cause HK erythrocytes. Roughly 20–25% of Akitas are affected. This phenotype has also been reported in Jindos, Shiba inus, and the Chinese shar-pei. HK erythrocytes may also have high intracellular aspartate, glutamate, glutamine, and glutathione. These cells are fragile and quicker to undergo hemolysis in the face of oxidative or osmotic stress.

When blood is collected from affected dogs, procedural hemolysis releases intracellular potassium. This phenomenon is termed *pseudohyperkalemia* because the patients themselves are not truly hyperkalemic; hyperkalemia is an observed artifact. Pseudohyperkalemia

may also result from marked thrombocytosis, leukocytosis, or if there is a delay in separating serum from clotted blood.

Because of erythrocyte fragility, dogs that possess the HK phenotype may be at greater risk of severe complications from hemolytic anemia.

3.14.5 Cavalier King Charles Spaniels

Many, but not all, Cavalier King Charles spaniels have moderate thrombocytopenia with larger platelets than is typical [5]. This autosomal recessive condition is referred to as macrothrombocytopenia [5]. Patients with macrothrombocytopenia are rarely symptomatic [5]. However, these patients require manual platelet counts as part of routine CBCs because autoanalyzers often mistake large platelets for erythrocytes [5].

3.14.6 Maltese Dogs

In an isolated study, over 75% of Maltese dogs without hepatic pathology had elevations in postprandial bile acid concentrations that surpassed the high end of the RI when bile acid concentrations were determined via the enzymatic spectrophotometric method [6]. The same outcome did not hold true when bile acid concentrations in the same dogs were determined via high-performance liquid chromatography. It has been theorized that this breed has a reactive substance in their serum that influences test results.

3.14.7 Canine Elliptocytosis

Mature canine and feline erythrocytes are anucleate, biconcave discs. Their shape maximizes the surface area-to-volume ratio, which facilitates gas exchange.

Variations in erythrocyte morphology may result from disease or mutations in membrane proteins. Their impact depends upon the resultant shape and its implications for gas exchange and easy passage through the vasculature.

Elliptocytosis is relatively uncommon in companion animals and is characterized by ovoid erythrocytes. Elliptocytes have been associated with myelodysplasia in dogs and hepatic disease in cats [7]. The use of doxorubicin has also been linked to elliptocytosis [7].

Elliptocytosis may also be detected as an incidental finding on blood film evaluation [7]. Recently, canine hereditary elliptocytosis has been described, and results from a mutation in the beta-spectrin gene [7]. Spectrin is one of many cytoskeletal proteins that helps maintain erythrocyte shape. Not all dogs with hereditary spectrin mutations or spectrin deficiency have elliptocytes. However, those that do are often asymptomatic.

3.14.8 Breed-Specific Hematological and Biochemical Variations in Cats

Although breed variations in RIs have been studied more extensively in dogs, certain feline breeds also have unique hematological and biochemical measurements. This should not come as a surprise, given that many cat breeds originated from a small pool of ancestors.

The following breed-specific variations are known to occur in cats [8, 9].

- Many Abyssinian cats exhibit microcytosis on CBC and elevated alpha-2 globulin.
- Some Birman cats have elevated serum creatinine, glucose, and alpha-2 globulin.
- Many Maine Coon cats have higher upper limits for BUN, ALP, and GGT.
- Norwegian forest cats tend to exhibit elevations in serum ALP and depressions in both beta-2 and gamma-globulin

Further investigation is indicated, given the high incidence of heritable disease in many breeds of cat.

TAKE-AWAYS

- Reference intervals for diagnostic tests are an essential starting point for making comparisons between individual patients and the healthy adult population of a given species.
- In some cases, values that fall well outside the RI are diagnostic for a particular disease. For example, significant hyperglycemia in a canine patient is consistent with diabetes mellitus.
- Sometimes values may fall outside the RI, but are consistent with what is expected among "normal" patients of a certain breed. For example, it is not uncommon for euthyroid greyhounds to have subnormal levels of TT4 according to the species-specific RI for dogs.
- Becoming familiar with breed-specific variations in hematological and biochemical parameters facilitates clinical communication with clients.
- When the veterinary team keeps current on breed-specific clinical pathology, patients are less likely to

be misdiagnosed on the basis of values that stray from the norm.

MISCELLANEOUS

3.14.9 Cautions

Know breed-specific tendencies concerning clinicopathological data; however, avoid the tendency to assume that all patients within a given breed follow the trends. For instance, not all Akitas have pseudohyperkalemia. Recognize that pseudohyperkalemia exists so that when a clinical scenario arises, it is familiar to you, but understand that it is not a given.

References

1 Campora, C., Freeman, K.P., Lewis, F.I. et al. (2011). Determination of haematological reference intervals in healthy adult greyhounds. *J. Small Anim. Pract.* 52: 301–309.

2 Zaldivar-Lopez, S., Marin, L.M., Iazbik, M.C. et al. (2011). Clinical pathology of greyhounds and other sighthounds. *Vet. Clin. Pathol.* 40: 414–425.

3 Dunlop, M.M., Sanchez-Vazquez, M.J., Freeman, K.P. et al. (2011). Determination of serum biochemistry reference intervals in a large sample of adult greyhounds. *J. Small Anim. Pract.* 52: 4–10.

4 von Dehn, B. (2014). Pediatric clinical pathology. *Vet. Clin. North Am. Small. Anim. Pract.* 44: 205–219.

5 Pedersen, H.D., Haggstrom, J., Olsen, L.H. et al. (2002). Idiopathic asymptomatic thrombocytopenia in Cavalier King Charles Spaniels is an autosomal recessive trait. *J. Vet. Intern. Med.* 16: 169–173.

6 Tisdall, P.L., Hunt, G.B., Tsoukalas, G. et al. (1995). Post-prandial serum bile acid concentrations and ammonia tolerance in Maltese dogs with and without hepatic vascular anomalies. *Aust. Vet. J.* 72: 121–126.

7 Di Terlizzi, R., Gallagher, P.G., Mohandas, N. et al. (2009). Canine elliptocytosis due to a mutant beta-spectrin. *Vet. Clin. Pathol.* 38: 52–58.

8 Paltrinieri, S., Ibba, F., and Rossi, G. (2014). Haematological and biochemical reference intervals of four feline breeds. *J. Feline Med. Surg.* 16: 125–136.

9 Spada, E., Antognoni, M.T., Proverbio, D. et al. (2015). Haematological and biochemical reference intervals in adult Maine Coon cat blood donors. *J. Feline Med. Surg.* 17: 1020–1027.

Recommended Reading

Battison, A. (2007). Apparent pseudohyperkalemia in a Chinese Shar Pei dog. *Vet. Clin. Pathol.* 36 (1): 89–93.

Feeman, W.E., Couto, C.G., and Gray, T.L. (2003). Serum creatinine concentrations in retired racing greyhounds. *Vet. Clin. Pathol.* 32 (1): 40–42.

LaVecchio, D., Marin, L.M., Baumwart, R. et al. (2009). Serum cardiac troponin I concentration in retired racing greyhounds. *J. Vet. Intern. Med.* 23: 87–90.

Slappendel, R.J., van Zwieten, R., van Leeuwen, M. et al. (2005). Hereditary spectrin deficiency in golden retriever dogs. *J. Vet. Intern. Med.* 19: 187–192.

3.15

Breed-Related Anesthetic Considerations

Tamara Grubb, DVM, PhD, DACVAA

Washington State University, Pullman, WA, USA

BASICS

3.15.1 Summary

There are very few true breed-related anesthetic "sensitivities," defined as an exaggerated response to a standard clinical dose of an anesthetic drug. However, individual sensitivities do exist, and more breed-related sensitivities may be identified as knowledge of canine and feline genetics expands. Breed-related anesthetic concerns definitely exist in breeds that have a tendency toward anatomical anomalies or development of pathological disease that can impact the safety of anesthesia. Regardless of breed, a good physical exam, history, appropriate diagnostic tests, and a patient-focused anesthetic plan will reduce risk for adverse effects of anesthesia.

MAIN CONCEPTS

There is an abundance of incorrect information on the internet regarding dog and cat "sensitivity" to anesthetic drugs. "Breed-related sensitivity" to anesthesia can be defined as an exaggerated response, caused by the breed of the patient, to a standard anesthetic drug administered at a standard clinical dose. Scientifically documented anesthetic breed sensitivities are uncommon. A few do exist but, more likely, exaggerated anesthetic responses are individual, not breed related, and can occur for a variety of reasons including (i) failure to identify underlying disease, either because the disease was overlooked or because the client declined diagnostic tests (e.g., underlying hepatic

disease that will compromise drug metabolism was not identified); (ii) selection of an inappropriate dose of an anesthetic drug for the particular patient (e.g., dosing a geriatric patient with a dose more appropriate for a young adult or dosing a large-breed dog with a dose more appropriate for a small-breed dog); (iii) failure to adequately support the patient during anesthesia (e.g., allowing profound hypothermia to occur); or (iv) individual patient sensitivity. The last item on the list may seem like a weak "excuse" for an adverse response to anesthesia but it is actually individual sensitivity that is the most interesting, but also the most difficult to identify prior to anesthesia.

The fields of pharmacogenomics and individualized medicine will one day dictate the way we do anesthesia by identifying the most appropriate drug and drug dose for each individual patient to be anesthetized, but, unfortunately, we don't yet have that ability.

Although true breed-related sensitivity is uncommon, breed-related concerns based on anatomical anomalies or development of pathological disease that can impact the safety of anesthesia are indeed common. In this category are breeds, like brachycephalic ("short-nosed") breeds, whose anatomical peculiarities necessitate a change in the way the patient is managed during anesthesia. Also included are breeds with any breed-related tendency for disease, especially disease of the cardiac or respiratory systems, which necessitates a change in anesthetic drugs, drug dosages, and/or management of anesthesia. Breed size can impact dosing, and utilization of a standard anesthetic drug dose for all dogs may result in underdosing of small-breed dogs and overdosing of large/giant-breed dogs. Finally, individuals or breeds with a tendency for fear, anxiety or aggressiveness can also impact management of anesthesia because a higher dose of anesthetic drugs may be needed to appropriately manage these patients and adverse effects of anesthetic drugs are generally dose dependent.

3.15.2 True Breed Sensitivities to Anesthetic Drugs

3.15.2.1 Greyhounds

Greyhounds have a decreased capacity for hepatic metabolism of some drugs [1]. The breed-related alteration leads to prolonged recovery times following large boluses – or repeat boluses – of thiobarbiturates [2]. Slightly longer recovery times may also occur in greyhounds receiving propofol or alfaxalone but these are generally clinically insignificant. The specific gene mutation causing prolonged recovery was recently determined to be CYP2B11 3′-UTR mutations causing decreased CYP2B11 enzyme expression, which is a key enzyme in hepatic metabolism of drugs and other substances [3]. This "sighthound CYP2B11 poor metabolizer phenotype" was found in almost 60% of the tested American Kennel Club (AKC) greyhounds and in a lower percentage in non-AKC greyhounds (<20%). It was also found in lower percentages in some related sight hounds including the whippet, Scottish deerhound, borzoi, Italian greyhound, and Ibizan hound but not in other sighthound breeds like salukis and Irish deerhounds. Interestingly, the gene mutation also occurred in some surprising nonsighthound breeds, although at a very low incidence (e.g., Labrador retriever, golden retriever, and English bulldog, all at <1%).

An interesting clinical note is that, before it was removed from the market, thiopental was commonly used to anesthetize greyhounds without causing prolonged recovery times. This was most likely due to the fact that the drug was appropriately used as a single low-dose bolus following premedicants. This illuminates the point that other true breed sensitivities *may* exist but are masked by the fact that clinical doses of anesthetic drugs are generally low, thus reducing the incidence of identifiable adverse effects. In addition, most of the breeds of the "sighthound CYP2B11 poor metabolizer phenotype" are commonly anesthetized without prolonged recovery, emphasizing the veterinarians' appropriate use of anesthetic drugs and drug dosages.

3.15.2.2 Collies and Other Herding Breeds

Some dog breeds, particularly collies and some other herding breeds, have a higher prevalence of a gene mutation which was called the MDR1, and is now called the ABCB-1 gene mutation (see 3.16 Breed-Related Drug Sensitivities). This gene codes for P-glycoprotein, which is a protein in the cell membrane that pumps select "foreign substances," including drugs, out of cells, including at the blood–brain barrier. With the gene mutation, the drugs are not pumped out of the cells and can accumulate, causing toxicity. In breeds with this mutation, the drugs accumulate in the brain, causing central nervous system (CNS) depression. The ivermectin toxicity that occurs in these dogs is perhaps the most well-known sequela of the mutation. The mutation can also affect anesthetic drugs that are P-glycoprotein substrates. ABCB-1 mutant collies that were sedated with high clinical dosages of butorphanol and acepromazine (0.05 and 0.04 mg/kg, respectively) developed exaggerated and prolonged sedation when compared to wild-type dogs [4]. Thus, acepromazine should be avoided, or the dose kept very low in dogs with known or suspected ABCB-1 mutation. The butorphanol dose should also be low, but the drug is not as concerning since the effects are reversible.

Breeds impacted, with the approximate percentage of dogs with the mutation, include collies (70%), Australian shepherds and miniature Australian shepherds (50%), long-haired whippets (50%), and silken windhounds (30%) [4]. Other breeds identified with the mutation at lower frequencies include Shetland sheepdogs, old English sheepdogs, English shepherds, German shepherds, and cross-breed herding dogs. Interestingly, Border collies have a <5% frequency of the mutation. Reversible drugs (like opioids or alpha-2 agonists) may be preferable in these breeds, whether or not the mutation status is known. A very important point is that other opioids (morphine, fentanyl, etc.) are transported across cell membranes by P-glycoprotein in humans but are not clinically problematic in dogs [5] and should not be avoided in herding breed dogs. If prolonged recovery does occur, the effects of the drugs are reversible.

Testing for the gene mutation can be done using blood or a cheek swab to collect oral mucosal cells. Suspect animals should be tested prior to anesthesia, if possible.

3.15.3 Controversial "Sensitivity"

3.15.3.1 Boxers

"Sensitivity" to acepromazine that results in bradycardia, hypotension, and collapse is described on every boxer internet website and has long been rumored to occur in this breed. However, in-depth review of the scientific literature yields no data on this phenomenon and few, if any, veterinarians in the US have seen this occur. One theory is that boxers with occult cardiomyopathy may become syncopal after administration of acepromazine because they are unable to compensate for drug-induced vasodilation. This, in fact, would be a sequela of their disease, not their breed, but the breed is likely to have cardiac disease so the breed-related concern is valid. The sensitivity may also be prevalent in a familial line of boxers in the United Kingdom, where more reports of the condition have originated.

In general, standard dosages of acepromazine are commonly administered to boxers without adverse consequences but avoidance of the drug may be prudent if owners insist that the drug is problematic for their particular dog(s) or if the veterinarian prefers other drugs.

3.15.4 Breeds with Common Underlying Conditions That Can Impact Anesthesia

3.15.4.1 Brachycephalic Breeds

When the term "breed-related anesthetic adverse events" is mentioned, the brachycephalic breeds (both dogs and cats) are generally at the top of the list of breeds expected to experience these adverse events. Brachycephalic patients often have difficulty breathing even without the anesthesia-induced hypoventilation and upper airway muscle relaxation with subsequent narrowing of the airway. The stenotic nares, everted saccules, redundant pharyngeal tissue, elongated soft palate, and hypoplastic trachea that define brachycephalic airway syndrome (BAS) in dogs significantly increases anesthetic risk, especially during the induction and recovery phases of anesthesia when the airway is not protected with the presence of an endotracheal tube (ET). In cats, stenotic nares and elongated soft palate occur more commonly than the other components of BAS but the risk is still significant in cats with these abnormalities. If the brachycephalic patient can breathe normally, it is likely at no or only slight increased risk over dolichocephalic (long-nosed) breeds, but BAS patients are always at high risk.

Antiemetics, like maropitant, should be administered preoperatively. Anesthetic drugs commonly cause nausea and vomiting and patients with upper airway dysfunction are more likely to aspirate vomited material. BAS patients should be lightly sedated so that they are calm and not struggling or panting and should be preoxygenated and monitored while an intravenous (IV) catheter is placed. The patient should be induced with rapid-acting drugs, like propofol, followed by immediate placement of the ET. A laryngoscope should be used for intubation so that the extent of the upper airway dysfunction can be evaluated. Expect to use a smaller ET tube than in other dogs of equal body size. Once the ET tube is in place, anesthesia is generally routine and specific anesthesia monitoring and support will be based on concurrent co-morbidities. Analgesia is an important component of the anesthetic protocol since decreasing the response to pain decreases the need for high dosages of anesthetic drugs, which will allow a faster

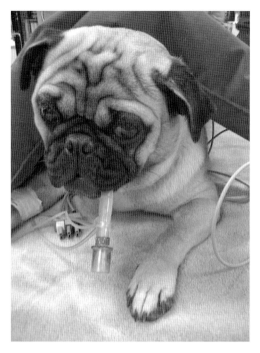

Figure 3.15.1 Fully conscious brachycephalic dog with endotracheal tube still in the airway.

recovery from anesthesia. In recovery, prior to extubation, ensure that the patient is calm and pain free. Brachycephalics generally tolerate the ET for a prolonged time and should not be extubated until they are fully awake, if possible (Figure 3.15.1).

If the patient resists the tube but is still somewhat sedated and not breathing normally following extubation, often extending the head, propping the mouth open, extending the tongue and providing supplemental oxygen via mask or the hoses on the anesthesia machine is adequate to support the patient until it is awake enough to breathe normally. Be prepared for re-nduction and reintubation if the patient cannot breathe at all. Then address the reason for not breathing and correct it. For example, the patient may need to wake up more calmly and perhaps with some pain medications to prevent hyperventilation with subsequent exacerbation of negative airway pressure, or it may need corticosteroids to decrease upper airway swelling. The pulse oximeter can be used during recovery to assess the patient's ability to oxygenate normally. If not tolerated on the tongue, the pulse oximeter probe can be put on the lip, ear, toe, vulva (female) or prepuce (male).

3.15.4.2 Breeds Prone to Other Airway Abnormalities

The list of breeds that can be at increased anesthetic risk for airway compromise should include those that are prone to collapsing trachea (e.g., Yorkshire terriers, Pomeranians, etc.) or laryngeal paralysis (e.g., Labrador retrievers, etc.). These patients can be anesthetized much like brachycephalic breeds. However, with collapsing tracheas, endotracheal intubation will not improve breathing if the patient has an intrathoracic collapse since the ET is unlikely to reach far enough to expand the collapsed area. In both sets of patients, intubation can be difficult and airway occlusion can occur at extubation.

3.15.4.3   Breeds Prone to Cardiovascular Disease

Anesthetic drugs can cause or exacerbate cardiovascular compromise. Thus, any patient with underlying cardiovascular disease is at increased risk of an adverse event during anesthesia. This includes patients with congenital malformations (e.g., subaortic stenosis in golden retrievers or patent ductus arteriosus in Yorkshire terriers) or acquired disease (e.g., mitral valve insufficiency in papillons or Cavalier King Charles spaniels; dilated cardiomyopathy in large-breed dogs like Doberman pinschers, boxers, Great Danes, and Labrador retrievers; hypertrophic cardiomyopathy in any cat but perhaps Maine Coon and Ragdoll cats are more prone).

Drug dosages, especially the inhalant dose, should be kept as low as possible. This is done by using "balanced anesthesia" which means using low dosages of several drugs rather than a high dose of any one drug. Analgesia is an important component of balanced anesthesia since decreasing the response to pain decreases the need for high dosages of anesthetic drugs. An example of balanced anesthesia would be a sedative and analgesic drug in the preanesthetic phase of anesthesia, a drug dosed "to effect" for induction and low-dose inhalants plus local anesthetic blocks and/or constant rate infusions of analgesic drugs during maintenance. Blood pressure must be measured in patients with cardiovascular disease and mean arterial pressure maintained in the normal range using support drugs like positive inotropes, with only judicious volumes of IV fluids.

3.15.4.4   Breeds Prone to Hepatic Disease

Some breeds are prone to hepatic disease or dysfunction, like congenital portosystemic shunts (e.g., cairn terriers) or acquired chronic hepatitis (e.g., Bedlington terriers, Labrador retrievers, etc.). Any patient with hepatic dysfunction may have difficulty metabolizing anesthetic drugs, resulting in prolonged recovery. Impaired clotting function, hypoglycemia, and hypoproteinemia are other potential complications, especially with severe disease. The use of reversible (e.g., alpha-2 agonists and opioids) and short-acting (e.g., propofol, alfaxalone, and inhalants) drugs is generally recommended. Oxygen delivery should be optimized through support of both oxygenation and blood pressure.

3.15.4.5   Breeds Prone to Renal Disease

Some dog (Samoyed, bull terrier, cairn terrier, German shepherd dog, English cocker spaniel, etc.) and cat (Abyssinian, Persian, etc.) breeds are prone to renal disease or dysfunction. Renal disease can result in prolonged recovery from anesthesia secondary to decreased renal elimination of certain drugs, primarily ketamine in cats. IV fluid therapy can be complicated due to the need for increased fluids to support renal function but need for decreased fluids due to hypoproteinemia and decreased ability to eliminate fluids in severe disease. The use of reversible (e.g., alpha-2 agonists and opioids) and short-acting (e.g., propofol, alfaxalone, and inhalants) drugs is generally recommended. Oxygen delivery should be optimized through support of both oxygenation and blood pressure.

3.15.4.6   Breeds Prone to von Willebrand Factor Deficiency

A deficiency of von Willebrand factor (vWF), a protein required for clotting, appears to be most common in Doberman pinschers but can also occur in German shepherd dogs, Shetland sheepdogs, golden retrievers and many other breeds (see 11.3 Heritable Health Conditions – By Disease). Excessive hemorrhage can occur in dogs with the deficiency and dogs suspected of having the deficiency should be tested prior to anesthesia. Patient support during anesthesia is impacted as blood transfusions may be necessary in hemorrhaging patients.

3.15.4.7   Others

There are other breed-related conditions or diseases that can cause anesthesia complications, for example hypothyroidism in golden retrievers and other breeds. An exhaustive list is beyond the scope of the current topic.

3.15.5   Impact of Breed-Related Size and Temperament

3.15.5.1   Breed-Related Size as a Complication of Anesthesia

Anesthetic "sensitivity" is often attributed to toy breeds and this may be very true – but it is a size issue rather than a breed issue [6]. Cats and small-breed dogs are at increased anesthetic risk for complications, and even death, when compared to medium- and large-breed dogs. This is likely due to several factors including the propensity to develop hypothermia, more likely to be overdosed (can be difficult to accurately draw up very small drug volumes), more difficult to place an IV catheter, more difficult to make anesthetic monitors work (for instance, the pulse oximeter has difficulty detecting pulses in very small arteries), can be more difficult to intubate (cats), and can more easily be overloaded with IV fluids (can be difficult to tell the exact volume of fluids administered from the commonly used 1 L fluid bags).

Giant-breed dogs may also have a size-based (not breed-based) increased risk for anesthetic complications, because drug dosing should be based on body surface area, not weight. When dosing by weight, these dogs often receive an excessively high dose of sedation and/or induction drugs. Maintenance inhalants should be dosed "to effect" so should not be a problem but sometimes the inhalants are administered as a set dose (e.g., 3% on the vaporizer), which could be extremely dangerous if combined with excessive sedation. These dogs should be dosed on body surface area (see the dexmedetomidine package insert for a good example of dosing). Body weight (BW) in kilograms can be scaled to the exponent 0.67 ($BW^{0.67}$) to convert weight to body surface area.

3.15.6 Breed-Related Temperament as a Risk Factor

Breeds or individuals prone to excitement, anxiety or aggression often need higher dosages of sedatives, and potentially induction drugs, in order to achieve adequate sedation and/or anesthesia. This can increase risk because adverse drug effects are generally related to higher dosages. However, using dosages that are too low can also be problematic since insufficient sedation can lead to struggling with the patient to control it for anesthetic drug administration, and this level of stress is also dangerous. Numerous dog and cat breeds reported to have anesthetic sensitivity are breeds also known to have high levels of excitement or anxiety and it may be the increased drug dose that creates the illusion of sensitivity. Breeds in this category include Arctic breed dogs (huskies, akitas, etc.), sighthounds (greyhounds, whippets, etc.), Bengal cats, Maine Coon cats, etc. Risk can be decreased by administering anxiolytics at home prior to travel to the hospital.

3.15.7 Decreasing Anesthetic Risk – Breed or Otherwise

Regardless of breed, a good physical exam, history, and patient-focused anesthetic plan will reduce risk for adverse effects of anesthesia (see 9.13 Preanesthetic Considerations).

EXAMPLES

The owner of a West Highland white terrier states that this breed of dog is sensitive to anesthesia as evidenced by the fact that they take longer to recover from anesthesia than other breeds. You gently point out that small dogs are more likely to become hypothermic (cold) and hypothermia is the main cause of prolonged recovery from anesthesia.

A collie is scheduled for routine dentistry in your practice. You recommend that the dog be tested for ABCB-1 gene mutation prior to anesthesia and explain to the owner that the dental procedure can be postponed while waiting for the test and that the test results will dictate the safest anesthesia for the dog.

In preparation for a bulldog that will be anesthetized today, your nurse sets out three ETs, all different sizes and all slightly smaller than would be anticipated if choosing tubes based on the patient's body size. The nurse also sets out an oxygen mask for preoxygenation and a laryngoscope so the airway can be evaluated at induction.

A Labrador retriever has low blood pressure during anesthesia. This is not because the breed has a "sensitivity" to anesthesia but because he has cardiomyopathy, which is not uncommon in this breed.

TAKE-AWAYS

- There are few scientifically proven breed-related anesthetic "sensitivities" but more proven sensitivities can be anticipated as genetic testing becomes more advanced.
- There are numerous breed-related characteristics that should be considered when designing anesthetic protocols for those breeds. These include patients with anatomical anomalies (e.g., brachycephalic patients) and tendency to develop breed-related diseases (e.g., cardiac disease in Cavalier King Charles spaniels, etc.).
- There are individual sensitivities to anesthetic drugs that can sometimes be predicted (e.g., due to body size) but are most often unknown until a concern arises. Anticipate that the response to anesthesia is individual and any patient could potentially experience an adverse event.
- In all breeds and patients, regardless of health, there is a slight inherent risk for anesthesia-related adverse events. Thus, anesthesia should always be preceded by a risk discussion with the owner. The owner should be assured that their pet, regardless of breed, will receive the best of care at your hospital (see 5.12 Discussing Anesthetic Risk).

- Regardless of breed, a good physical exam, history, and patient-focused anesthetic plan will reduce the risk for adverse effects of anesthesia.

MISCELLANEOUS

References

1 KuKanich, B., Coetzee, J.F., Gehring, R., and Hubin, M. (2007). Comparative disposition of pharmacologic markers for cytochrome P-450 mediated metabolism, glomerular filtration rate, and extracellular and total body fluid volume of Greyhound and Beagle dogs. *J. Vet. Pharmacol. Ther.* 30 (4): 314–319.

2 Sams, R.A., Muir, W.W., Detra, R.L., and Robinson, E.P. (1985). Comparative pharmacokinetics and anesthetic effects of methohexital, pentobarbital, thiamylal, and thiopental in Greyhound dogs and non-Greyhound, mixed-breed dogs. *Am. J. Vet. Res.* 46 (8): 1677–1683.

3 Martinez, S.E., Andresen, M.C., Zhu, Z. et al. (2020). Pharmacogenomics of poor drug metabolism in Greyhounds: cytochrome P450 (CYP) 2B11 genetic variation, breed distribution, and functional characterization. *Sci. Rep.* 10 (1): 69–88.

4 Mealey, K.L. (2006). Adverse drug reactions in herding-breed dogs: the role of P-glycoprotein. *Compendium* 28: 23–33.

5 Veterinary Pharmacology Laboratory http://vcpl.vetmed. wsu.edu; http://vcpl.vetmed.wsu.edu/affected-breeds; http://vcpl.vetmed.wsu.edu/problem-drugs)

6 Brodbelt, D. (2009). Perioperative mortality in small animal anaesthesia. *Vet. J.* 182 (2): 152–161.

Recommended Reading

Grubb, T.L., Albi, M., Ensign, S. et al. (2020). *Anesthesia and Pain Management for Veterinary Nurses and Technicians.* Jackson, WY: Teton New Media.

Dexdomitor package insert: www.zoetisus.com/products/dogs/dexdomitor-01/doc/dex_dex-0.1_antisedan-pi.pdf

3.16

Breed-Related Drug Sensitivities

Patricia Dowling, DVM, MSc, DACVIM (LAIM), DACVCP

Veterinary Clinical Pharmacology, Western College of Veterinary Medicine, Saskatoon, SK, Canada

 BASICS

3.16.1 Summary

The goal of rational drug therapy is to produce a desired drug effect without causing undue adverse effects. The veterinary care team is successful for the most part, but sometimes unpredicted drug effects are seen on a species or breed level. This variability in drug response may actually be due to genetic differences in pharmacokinetics (absorption, distribution, metabolism, elimination). Pharmacogenetics is the study of the genetic determinants of response to drug therapy. Although this branch of veterinary medicine is still in its infancy, it is the ultimate way to achieve our therapeutic goal of picking the "right" drug and dose for each patient while avoiding toxicities.

3.16.2 Terms Defined

Pharmacogenetics: The study of inherited genetic differences in drug pharmacokinetics and pharmacodynamics, which can affect individual responses to drugs, both in terms of therapeutic effect as well as adverse effects.

Pharmacokinetics: What the body does to a drug, including absorption, distribution, metabolism, and excretion.

 MAIN CONCEPTS

3.16.3 Basic Genetic Concepts

When a gene is expressed, DNA is transcribed into RNA which is then translated for protein synthesis (see 3.1 Genetic Basics). Three consecutive nucleotide bases form a specific codon, which specifies a particular amino acid or termination of an amino acid chain ("stop codons"). Genetic mutations alter the base sequence of DNA, which in turn alters the transcribed RNA, creating different codons. Genetic mutations are responsible for the variations seen within a population (e.g., different coat colors). Polymorphisms are genetic variations occurring at a frequency of 1% or greater in the population. Currently, the best known polymorphisms in humans and animals involve drug metabolism (mainly by the cytochrome P450 system). But drug absorption, distribution, and elimination can be influenced by polymorphisms, especially in the drug transporter proteins such as P-glycoprotein.

3.16.4 Pharmacogenetics of Drug Metabolism

Polymorphisms are known to affect phase I and phase II metabolic enzyme activity on a species and breed level. A number of polymorphisms are seen in cytochrome P450 enzymes, with many of these resulting in profound variations in clinical response (individuals range from "slow" metabolizers to "ultra-rapid" metabolizers).

Greyhounds and other sighthounds are notorious for difficulties with injectable anesthetics, particularly the barbiturates. It is now known that greyhounds have particularly low CYP2B11 activity. When anesthetized with propofol (which like barbiturates is completely eliminated through metabolism), greyhounds have sustained plasma concentrations of propofol, and delayed recovery compared with mixed-breed dogs.

The human cyclooxygenase-2 selective drug celecoxib (Celebrex®) is metabolized by CYP2D15. Elimination of celecoxib in beagles is polymorphic, with half of the dogs being extensive metabolizers and the remainder being poor metabolizers. Celecoxib has a 1.5–2-hour elimination half-life in extensive metabolizers and a five-hour half-life in poor metabolizers. The frequency and breed distribution of this polymorphism have not yet been determined since it is not a veterinary drug. But it may have clinical significance for other drugs that are CYP2D15 substrates, such as dextromethorphan and imipramine.

N-acetyltransferase is the enzyme responsible for metabolizing many drugs, including sulfonamides, procainamide, and hydralazine. The genes coding for *N*-acetyltransferase are absent in dogs, increasing the risk for hypersensitivity reactions to sulfonamides and making procainamide less effective as an antiarrhythmic as its active metabolite is not formed.

Hepatic metabolism of tramadol in humans is via the CYP2D6 system and produces the active *O*-desmethyl-tramadol (M1) metabolite. This metabolite has 2–4 times the analgesic potency of the parent compound and 4–200 times greater affinity for the mu opioid receptor. Studies in dogs show very minimal production of this metabolite, so tramadol is not as effective an analgesic in dogs as it is in humans and cats.

Thiopurine methyltransferase (TPMT) is a phase II enzyme responsible for metabolizing the immunosuppressive drug azathioprine and its active metabolites to inactive metabolites. Decreased TPMT activity has been documented to be associated with increased susceptibility to azathioprine-induced bone marrow suppression. A ninefold range in TMPT activity is documented in dogs, and seems to be related to breed. Giant schnauzers have low TPMT activity and Alaskan malamutes have high TMPT activity.

3.16.5 Pharmacogenetics and the P-Glycoprotein Drug Transporter

The best known breed-related drug sensitivity involves the ABCB1 gene that codes for a P-glycoprotein, a transmembrane protein pump. A deletion mutation of the ABCB1 gene was discovered in "ivermectin-sensitive" dogs, including collies, Australian shepherds, Shetland sheepdogs, old English sheepdogs, and other herding dogs. The deletion mutation produces a frame shift that generates a premature stop codon in the ABCB1 gene, resulting in a severely truncated, nonfunctional P-glycoprotein. Because protein synthesis is terminated before even 10% of the protein product is synthesized, dogs with two mutant alleles exhibit a P-glycoprotein null phenotype. Heterozygous dogs with only one mutant allele have reduced P-glycoprotein function.

P-glycoprotein functions as a transmembrane efflux pump, transporting chemicals from inside the cell to outside the cell. It is normally expressed in the apical border of intestinal epithelial cells, brain capillary endothelial cells, biliary canalicular cells, renal proximal tubular epithelial cells, placenta, and testes. Therefore, it affects oral absorption, distribution, and elimination of substrate drugs. Adenosine triphosphate (ATP) hydrolysis provides the energy for active drug transport, so the transporter can function against steep concentration gradients. P-glycoprotein transports a wide variety of drugs with diverse chemical structures, including chemotherapy drugs, immunosuppressants, antiparasitic agents, HIV-1 protease inhibitors, and corticosteroids. How the P-glycoprotein transporter can recognize and transport such structurally diverse compounds is not known and cannot be predicted based simply on its chemical structure. Many P-glycoprotein substrates are natural compounds, or synthetic derivatives of natural compounds, so it appears this is an evolutionary protective mechanism to decrease exposure to toxic xenobiotics.

3.16.6 P-Glycoprotein and Drug Absorption

Intestinal phase I drug metabolism and active drug extrusion by P-glycoprotein transporters are very important in determining oral drug bioavailability. Consequently, genetic variations in these processes dramatically affect oral drug absorption.

CYP 3A and P-glycoprotein are expressed at high levels in the villus tip of enterocytes in the gastrointestinal tract. CYP 3A and P-glycoprotein work in concert to prevent oral absorption of many drugs, as substrates of P-glycoprotein are often also substrates for CYP 3A.

When a substrate drug is present in the intestinal tract, it is absorbed by passive processes into the enterocyte. Once inside the enterocyte, three things can happen: the drug may be metabolized by CYP 3A to inactive metabolites, it may enter the systemic circulation, or it may be extruded by P-glycoprotein back into the intestinal lumen, where it may enter another enterocyte at a more distal site along the digestive tract, thus allowing further access to CYP 3A. So non-P-glycoprotein substrate drugs pass through the enterocyte only once, while P-glycoprotein substrate drugs may continuously cycle between the enterocyte and the gut lumen, resulting in repeated access of CYP 3A to the drug molecule, or fecal excretion of the drug because of repeated P-glycoprotein efflux.

Because so many drugs are substrates for both P-glycoprotein and CYP 3A, it is difficult to discern the individual contributions of each protein to reduced oral drug absorption. The P-glycoprotein system can be knowingly manipulated. For example, the antifungal drug ketoconazole inhibits P-glycoprotein efflux activity and CYP 3A metabolic activity and when administered concurrently with the immunosuppressant drug cyclosporine, it increases the oral bioavailability of cyclosporine. Concurrent administration of P-glycoprotein substrate drugs and inhibitor drugs must be done very carefully, or toxicity can occur.

3.16.7 P-Glycoprotein and Drug Absorption

The P-glycoprotein transporter is an important barrier to the distribution of substrate drugs to protected tissue sites, including the brain, testes, and placenta. Distribution of P-glycoprotein substrate drugs to these tissues is greatly enhanced in dogs with the ABCB1 deletion mutation. Dogs homozygous for the ABCB1 gene deletion (mutant/mutant) will show signs of neurotoxicity after a single low dose of ivermectin (120 μg/kg). Heterozygous dogs (wild-type/mutant) are not sensitive to ivermectin neurotoxicity at 120 μg/kg, but may show neurotoxicity at ivermectin doses greater than 300 μg/kg, particularly if daily doses are administered (e.g., daily treatment of demodectic mange). Dogs homozygous for the normal multiple drug resistance (MDR) allele (normal/normal) can receive 2000 μg/kg in a single dose without signs of toxicity and can receive as much as 600 μg/kg daily for months without signs of toxicity.

Distribution across the blood–brain barrier is also important for other P-glycoprotein substrate drugs. Collies are overrepresented for cases of loperamide CNS toxicity when given "normal" doses. In normal dogs, loperamide does not cross the blood–brain barrier and even in heterozygote dogs, normal doses of loperamide do not cause toxicity. The blood–brain barrier of homozygous mutant dogs is also more permeable to exogenous and endogenous steroid hormones. Collies are often considered to be "poor doers" and there is evidence that homozygous dogs have continuous suppression of the hypothalamic–pituitary–adrenal axis and cannot mount an appropriate stress response, evidenced by the lack of a stress leukogram. Such "atypical" Addisonian dogs require exogenous corticosteroid supplementation when stressed or ill.

3.16.8 P-glycoprotein and Drug Absorption

Drugs are eliminated from the body as unchanged parent drug or as metabolites (which may be active or inactive). Renal excretion and biliary excretion are the most important pathways of drug elimination. P-glycoprotein is expressed on renal tubular cells and biliary canalicular cells. Altered biliary or renal excretion plays a role in the increased sensitivity of homozygous and heterozygous ABCB1 gene deletion dogs to chemotherapeutic drugs that are P-glycoprotein substrates, such as doxorubicin and vincristine.

3.16.9 Pharmacogenetics and Hypersensitivity Reactions

Polymorphisms in metabolic pathways may also be involved in idiosyncratic (unpredictable) drug reactions. Idiosyncratic toxicity to sulfonamides is similar in dogs and people and can be manifested by a wide variety of severe clinical signs: fever, arthropathy, blood dyscrasias (neutropenia, thrombocytopenia, or hemolytic anemia), hepatopathy consisting of cholestasis or necrosis, skin eruptions (Figure 3.16.1), uveitis, and keratoconjunctivitis sicca. In dogs, sulfonamide hypersensitivity reactions tend to occur within the first two weeks after starting therapy. Doberman pinschers, Samoyeds, and miniature schnauzers appear more susceptible than other breeds. Dogs that develop hepatopathy generally have a poor prognosis.

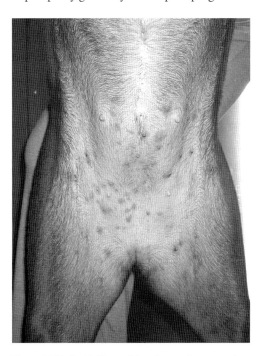

Figure 3.16.1 Sulfonamide adverse drug reaction.

TAKE-AWAYS

- Polymorphisms are genetic mutations that affect drug absorption, distribution, and elimination.
- The best known polymorphism is the ABCB1 gene deletion seen in collies and other herding breeds that impacts absorption, distribution, and elimination of a large number of substrate drugs.
- Breed-associated polymorphisms also may greatly impact drug metabolism, and can cause toxicity (e.g., delayed recovery from barbiturates in greyhounds) to inefficacy (e.g., poor efficacy of tramadol for analgesia in dogs).
- Polymorphisms in metabolic pathways may also be involved in idiosyncratic (unpredictable) drug reactions such as sulfonamide reactions in dogs.
- Knowledge of breed-related polymorphisms allows the veterinary care team to avoid certain drugs in specific breeds or to modify the dosage regimen to prevent toxicity.

MISCELLANEOUS

Recommended Reading

Mealey, K.L. (2013). Adverse drug reactions in veterinary patients associated with drug transporters. *Vet. Clin. North Am. Small Anim. Pract.* 43: 1067–1078.

Mealey, K.L. (2006). Pharmacogenetics. *Vet. Clin. North Am. Small Anim. Pract.* 36: 961–973.

Mealey, K.L. and Fidel, J. (2015). P-glycoprotein mediated drug interactions in animals and humans with cancer. *J. Vet. Intern. Med.* 29: 1–6.

Trepanier, L.A., Danhof, R., Toll, J., and Watrous, D. (2003). Clinical findings in 40 dogs with hypersensitivity associated with potentiated sulfonamides. *J. Vet. Intern. Med.* 17: 647–652.

3.17

Breed-Related Nutritional Issues

Kara M. Burns, MS, MEd, LVT, VTS (Nutrition)

Lafayette, IN, USA

BASICS

3.17.1 Summary

The veterinary team recognizes certain breeds as being at risk for specific diseases that can be nutritionally managed; for example, Dalmatians frequently develop urinary stones, Border collies are at increased risk for cobalamin malabsorption, miniature schnauzers are prone to high overall blood fat levels, Persians are at higher risk for polycystic kidney disease, and Burmese and exotic shorthair cats are at higher risk for calcium oxalate urolithiasis.

The breed should be determined in the initial patient assessment. Different breeds may be at risk for specific diseases or metabolic alterations that require nutritional management.

Additionally, dogs and cats can be prone to nutritional issues by nature of their size – small breeds vs large breeds.

MAIN CONCEPTS

Of the three components that affect the life of a pet – genetics, environment, and nutrition – nutrition is the single factor the veterinary healthcare team can affect to maximize health, improve performance and longevity, and manage disease.

The overall nutrient profiles and ingredients for specific breeds of dogs and cats may be comparable to diets recommended for all breeds or other breeds, although there may be differences in specific nutrients, the calorie content, fiber types and amounts, and even the shape of the kibble that could be beneficial for some individuals of that breed. Truly, in nutrition for animals, the important point is individualizing the diet for the pet, making it truly pet-specific care.

There may be certain characteristics in a food aimed at helping a certain breed, such as low-calorie foods for obesity-prone dogs (such as Labrador retrievers, golden retrievers, etc.) or specially extruded kibble shapes to decrease the speed at which certain breeds may eat. Another characteristic to consider would be increased fiber in foods formulated for long-haired cats which will aid in reducing hairballs. Additionally, the shape of the kibble may be formulated for flat-faced breeds such as bulldogs or Persians, thus making the food easier for these brachycephalic breeds to pick up.

When discussing breed-related nutritional issues, it is important to remember that the health issue is more important than the specific breed. This means that if a dog is overweight, it will need to be managed with a lower calorie diet regardless of the breed. Nutritional recommendations should be based on the individual pet's health and nutritional needs, regardless of breed. When choosing a pet food, the focus should be on selecting a high-quality diet from a trusted brand that meets the pet's life stage, size, and lifestyle needs. These three factors are more relevant to a dog's nutritional needs than breed.

Healthcare teams should be familiar with the nutritional feeding goals of large-breed puppies. Nutrient excesses, rapid growth rates, and excessive weight gain appear to be important factors contributing to the incidence of skeletal disorders in growing large- and giant-breed dogs. While society continues to select for increased size for many of our larger dogs, size itself is not detrimental to the dog, but management practices that allow growth rates to be maximized can cause negative consequences that we see in these dogs. It has been estimated that more than 20% of orthopedic diseases in dogs are due to dietary origins, with more than 22% of these showing up in dogs under 1 year of age [1, 2].

It is well documented that the incidence of skeletal disease, including osteochondrosis, hypertrophic osteodystrophy and hip dysplasia, is markedly increased in the growing large-breed dog if management practices are such that this maximal genetic potential for rate of growth is realized [1]. The primary management practice affecting growth rate and ultimately skeletal disease is nutritional support.

The primary nutritional considerations implicated in skeletal disease development in growing large-breed/giant-breed dogs are dietary concentrations of protein, energy, and calcium [1]. To ensure a slower growth rate, energy intake needs to be managed through measured feedings and monitoring body condition score (BCS) to maintain a lean body weight. A minimum of two meals should be fed daily, while 3–4 meals may be more appropriate for some dogs. Slight underfeeding of energy during growth will slow the overall rate but has not been shown to negatively impact the final adult size of the dog.

When looking at specific breed-related nutritional issues, the veterinary team should bear in mind specific diseases that are seen more often in certain breeds – musculoskeletal diseases in large-breed dogs, copper toxicosis in Bedlington terriers, or exocrine pancreatic insufficiency (EPI) in German shepherd dogs. It is important to consider which risks can be mitigated or managed with proper nutrition.

Proper nutrition has a positive impact on health and disease in all animals. Appropriate feeding throughout all life stages can help prevent diet-associated diseases, as well as assist in the management of other diseases. For example, diets formulated for dogs and cats with chronic kidney disease have been shown to provide significant benefits to the ill pet and to improve the pet's quality of life.

 EXAMPLES

A 3-year-old castrated male German shepherd dog presented for chronic diarrhea, polyphagia, and weight loss over four months. The stools were runny – semiformed consistency at best – and were very light colored. The owner mentioned large volumes passed multiple times per day. The pet's body weight had decreased over the past six months from 36.4 to 27.3 kg. The BCS was 1/5, and the dog's coat appearance was unkempt and dull.

Diagnostic evaluation obtained the following results.

- Complete blood count (CBC) – normal
- Serum biochemistry profile – mild elevations in liver enzyme activity

- Direct fecal smear and fecal flotation for parasites – negative
- Fecal stain for fat – positive
- Serum canine trypsin-like immunoreactivity (TLI) – decreased at 0.6 mg/L
- Serum cobalamin concentration – decreased at 150 ng/L
- Serum folate concentration – increased at 23.4 mg/L

3.17.2 Nutritional Assessment

The owner fed several commercial dry foods, ad libitum for six months. A veterinary therapeutic novel protein food had been fed for the last two months as an elimination trial for suspected food allergy. The dog was taking approximately 75% more kcals than his daily energy requirement (DER) and was still losing weight.

3.17.3 Discussion

A history of chronic diarrhea, steatorrhea, and weight loss in a young German shepherd dog suggests EPI and the decreased serum TLI confirms that EPI is present. Mild increases in hepatic enzyme activity are often seen in patients with EPI. Additionally, the decreased serum cobalamin concentration and increased serum folate concentration are consistent with small intestinal bacterial overgrowth (SIBO), often seen concurrently in EPI cases. The dull coat is representative of an essential fatty acid deficiency.

Key nutritional recommendations in patients with EPI are as follows:

- highly digestible foods (fat and digestible carbohydrate ≥90% and protein ≥87%)
- pancreatic enzyme supplements allow for nutrients to be absorbed
- excess dietary fiber should be avoided (≤5% fiber, dry matter basis)
- fat-soluble vitamins, cobalamin, and folate may be altered and must be monitored.

3.17.4 Nutritional Recommendation and Plan

- Commercial dry veterinary therapeutic food – highly digestible, moderate in fat, low in fiber.
- Supplementation with dried pancreatic extract mixed thoroughly with two cups of slightly moistened food prior to feeding, three times daily.

TAKE-AWAYS

- Nutrition is the single factor the veterinary healthcare team can affect to maximize health, improve performance and longevity, and manage disease.
- Dog and cat breeds may be at risk for specific diseases or metabolic alterations that require and can benefit from nutritional management.
- Dogs and cats can be prone to nutritional issues by nature of their size – small breeds vs large breeds.
- In nutrition for animals, the important point is individualizing the diet for the specific pet, based on the nutritional assessment of that pet.
- There are many breed inherited disease conditions which can be mitigated or managed with proper nutrition.

MISCELLANEOUS

References

1 Wortinger, A. and Burns, K.M. (2015). Growth in dogs. In: *Nutrition and Disease Management for Veterinary Technicians and Nurses*, 2e. Ames, IA: Wiley Blackwell.

2 Hazewinkel, H. and Mott, J. (2006). Main nutritional imbalances implicated in osteoarticular diseases. In: *Encyclopedia of Canine Clinical Nutrition* (eds. P. Pibot, V. Biourge and D. Elliott), 348–379. Aimargues, France: Aniwa SAS.

Recommended Reading

Ackerman, L. (1999). *The Genetic Connection, A Guide to Health Problems in Purebred Dogs*. Lakewood, CO: AAHA Press.

Bell, S., Cavanagh, K.E., Tilley, L.P., and Smith, F.W.K. (2012). *Veterinary Medical Guide to Dog and Cat Breeds*. Jackson, WY: Teton NewMedia.

3.18

Breed-Related Eye Conditions

D. J. Haeussler, Jr., BS, MS, DVM, DACVO

The Animal Eye Institute, Cincinnati, OH, USA

 BASICS

3.18.1 Summary

Many ophthalmic conditions seen in dogs and cats are more frequently observed in certain breeds. Many of these conditions have been identified as inherited within certain breeds, while other conditions are presumed to be inherited within certain breeds. It is important that the veterinary team understand and recognize these conditions with their breed predispositions, as this can help the team provide accurate diagnosis and care to each patient. While discussing each ophthalmic disease and the breeds in which they are seen is outside the scope of this text, the more common conditions and associated breed predispositions are reviewed here.

3.18.2 Terms Defined

Buphthalmia: Increased size of the globe.
Cataract: Any opacity of the crystalline lens.
Choroidal Hypoplasia: Underdevelopment of the choroid, which is a tissue layer located beneath the retina.
Coloboma: A hole in one of the structures of the eye, such as the retina, choroid, or optic disc.
Epiphora: Increased tearing.
Iridodonesis: Abnormal movement or vibration of the iris typically seen in patients with lens subluxation or luxation.
Uveitis: Inflammation of the anterior chamber.

 MAIN CONCEPTS

3.18.3 Cataract

A cataract can be defined as any opacity of the crystalline lens. Cataracts can be observed in the dog due to a variety of causes such as diabetes mellitus, nutrition, irradiation, trauma, congenital, hypocalcemia, senility, electric shock, retinal atrophy, uveitis, and inheritance. Cataracts are one of the leading causes of vision loss worldwide. Cataracts can be very minimal and not cause vision obstruction or can be extensive, causing complete blindness in the canine or feline patient. Cataracts not only cause vision loss but can lead to lens-induced uveitis, glaucoma, and retinal detachment. Many breeds develop cataracts which are presumed to be inherited (Table 3.18.1). For lists of affected cat breeds, see 11.3 Heritable Health Conditions – By Disease.

Genetic testing can be performed on several breeds, including Staffordshire bull terriers, Boston terriers, and French bulldogs, to determine if they have mutations in the heat shock transcription factor gene (HSF4–1) which leads to cataracts. A different mutation of the heat shock transcription factor gene (HSF4–2) leads to cataracts in Australian shepherds and miniature American shepherds.

If an underlying cause for a patient's cataracts cannot be determined (such as diabetes mellitus, nutrition, irradiation, trauma, electric shock, retinal atrophy, or uveitis), it should be presumed that the cataracts could be inherited.

Each patient should have a thorough ophthalmic examination at each visit, at minimum, annually. Subtle changes seen in the lens, such as cortical vacuoles, may indicate

Pet-Specific Care for the Veterinary Team, First Edition. Edited by Lowell Ackerman.
© 2021 John Wiley & Sons, Inc. Published 2021 by John Wiley & Sons, Inc.

Table 3.18.1 Some dog breeds predisposed to developing hereditary cataracts

Afghan hound	Labrador retriever
American cocker spaniel	Miniature schnauzer
Bichon frisé	Norwegian buhund
Boston terrier	Old English sheepdog
Chesapeake Bay retriever	Staffordshire bull terrier
Entlebucher mountain dog	Standard poodle
German shepherd	Welsh springer spaniel
Golden retriever	West Highland white terrier
Akita	Beagle
Alaskan malamute	Bernese mountain dog
American Eskimo	Greyhound
Australian cattle dog	Maltese
Bull mastiff	Newfoundland
Cairn terrier	Papillon
Cardigan Welsh corgi	Pekingese
Cavalier King Charles spaniel	Border collie
Great Dane	Brittany spaniel
Giant schnauzer	Brussels griffon
Pug	Samoyed
Pomeranian	Shiba inu
Toy poodle	Miniature poodle
Shih tzu	Siberian husky
Standard schnauzer	Weimaraner
Yorkshire terrier	

that the patient needs to be monitored more diligently. In order to obtain a thorough ophthalmic examination, each patient should be pharmacologically dilated with topical tropicamide. Most cataracts are not diagnosed until they are advanced due to improper examination techniques such as not dilating the patient. Each patient diagnosed with cataracts should be encouraged to obtain an opinion by a veterinary ophthalmologist. Clients should be made aware that cataracts are not benign changes to the lens. They can lead to lens-induced uveitis which in turn can lead to secondary glaucoma, retinal detachment, irreversible blindness, and loss of the eye. Topical ophthalmic anti-inflammatories can reduce the risk of these sequelae even if the client does not choose to pursue surgical options for removal of the cataract.

Genetic testing for predisposed breeds should be encouraged to allow the client to prepare for development of cataracts (see 3.4 Predicting and Eliminating Disease Traits). Genetic testing will also allow the veterinary team to provide more information to the client to advise about breeding practices.

3.18.4   Collie Eye Anomaly (Choroidal Hypoplasia)

Collie eye anomaly is a recessively inherited ocular disorder seen in a variety of breeds such as the Australian shepherd, bearded collie, berger d'Auvergne, Border collie, Boykin spaniel, English shepherd, farm collie, Hokkaido dog, Lancashire heeler, miniature American shepherd, Nova Scotia duck tolling retriever, rough collie, Shetland sheepdog, silken windhound, smooth collie, and longhaired whippet. Clinical abnormalities that can be found include choroidal hypoplasia, optic nerve coloboma, retinal detachment (partial or complete), and intraocular hemorrhage. The severity of the disease is quite variable and ranges from no visual deficits to complete blindness and can even show significant variation within each litter.

The cardinal sign of collie eye anomaly is bilateral choroidal hypoplasia. The client should be aware that these clinical signs are congenital and can be diagnosed as early as 6–7 weeks of age by a veterinary ophthalmologist. The disease is not progressive; however, retinal detachments can result in retinal tears, intraocular hemorrhage, complete blindness, and secondary glaucoma. Unfortunately, there is no treatment for dogs with collie eye anomaly. Breeders should be encouraged to maintain a breeding pair of homozygous normal individuals.

Genetic testing can identify individual dogs as normal, carrier, or affected. This is very useful information for the breeder as this will allow them to make the best breeding recommendations possible to help eliminate this disease. The client should also be counseled that each of these patients requires a yearly ophthalmic examination.

3.18.5   Lens Luxation

Primary lens luxation is a condition seen in many breeds where the lens is dislocated from its normal position in the eye caused by abnormal development of the ciliary zonules (Table 3.18.2). This condition can lead to glaucoma, corneal damage, uveitis, and retinal detachments.

If a lens luxation or subluxation is suspected in any canine patient, the client should be counseled on the potential for glaucoma, loss of the eye, retinal detachment, and uveitis. Proper medications should be prescribed, and the patient should be referred to an ophthalmologist to discuss medical and surgical options.

The patient should have a thorough ophthalmic examination at each visit, at minimum, annually. Subtle changes seen in the lens and iris such as iridodonesis may indicate that the patient needs to be monitored more diligently. In order to obtain a thorough ophthalmic examination, the

Table 3.18.2 Some dog breeds with heritable lens luxation

American Eskimo	Rat terrier
American hairless terrier	Russell terrier
Australian cattle dog	Sealyham terrier
Chinese crested	Teddy Roosevelt terrier
Chinese foo dog	Tenterfield terrier
Jack Russell terrier	Tibetan terrier
Jagd terrier	Toy fox terrier
Lakeland terrier	Volpino Italiano
Lucas terrier	Welsh terrier
Lancashire heeler	Wire-haired fox terrier
Miniature bull terrier	Yorkshire terrier
Norwich terrier	Patterdale terrier
Parson Russell terrier	Parson Russell terrier

patient should be pharmacologically dilated with topical tropicamide. Most lens subluxations are not diagnosed until they are advanced due to improper examination techniques such as not dilating the patient. A patient diagnosed with lens subluxation or luxation should be encouraged to obtain an opinion by a veterinary ophthalmologist as soon as possible as rapid medical and surgical treatment may lead to preservation of vision. Clients should be made aware that lens subluxations and luxations are not benign changes to the lens. They can lead to lens-induced uveitis which in turn can lead to secondary glaucoma, retinal detachment, irreversible blindness, and loss of the eye. An anterior lens luxation constitutes a surgical emergency and neither the veterinarian nor client should take a "wait and see" approach.

Topical ophthalmic antiinflammatories can reduce the risk of lens-induced uveitis and topical miotics such as latanoprost, demecarium bromide, or pilocarpine can be utilized in lens subluxations as well as posterior lens luxations to trap the lens in the posterior segment and prevent it from luxating anteriorly. If the patient has an anterior lens luxation, topical latanoprost, topical demecarium bromide, and topical pilocarpine should not be utilized as these are contraindicated and administration of these medications can cause the intraocular pressures (IOP) to rise rapidly, causing glaucoma and loss of the eye. If a lens subluxation or luxation is diagnosed by the veterinarian, more frequent examinations are required such as 2–3 times per year to monitor for glaucoma, uveitis, blindness, and retinal detachment. Genetic testing for predisposed breeds should be encouraged to allow the client to prepare for development of lens subluxations and/or luxation. Genetic testing will also allow the veterinarian to provide more information to the client to advise about breeding practices.

3.18.6 Progressive Retinal Atrophy

Progressive retinal atrophy is a term applied to a group of inherited diseases that result in cells of the retina degenerating prematurely, typically causing night vision loss (rod degeneration), then day vision loss (cone degeneration), and finally complete blindness. Age of onset for each breed differs significantly (Table 3.18.3). For lists of affected cat breeds, see 11.3 Heritable Health Conditions – By Disease.

Table 3.18.3 Some dog breeds predisposed to heritable progressive retinal atrophy.

American Eskimo	Entelbucher mountain dog
American hairless (rat) terrier	Field spaniel
Australian cattle dog	Finnish Lapphund
Australian cobberdog	German spitz
Australian shepherd (all varieties)	Golden retriever
Australian stumpy tail cattle dog	Golden doodle
Barbet	Jack Russell terrier
Black Russian terrier	Japanese chin
Bolognese	Karelian bear dog
Bolonka Zwetna	Kuvasz
Chesapeake Bay retriever	Lab/golden cross
Chinese crested	Labradoodle
Chihuahua	Labradoodle (Australian)
Cockapoo	Labradoodle/golden doodle cross
Cocker spaniel (American)	Labrador retriever
Coton de Tulear	Lagotto Romagnolo
Dwarf poodle	Lancashire heeler Lapponian herder
English cocker spaniel	Maltipoo
English shepherd	Manchester terrier (toy)
Markiesie	Mi-Ki
Miniature poodle	Moyen poodle
Toy poodle	Norrbottenspitz
Miniature American shepherd	Norwegian elkhound
Nova Scotia duck tolling retriever	Russian-European laika
Plott	Serbian hound
Pomeranian	Silky terrier
Portuguese Podengo Pequeno	Schipperke
Portuguese water dog	Spanish water dog
Puli	Sprocker spaniel
Standard poodle	Swedish jamthund
Swedish Lapphund	Tibetan terrier
Xoloitzcuintle	Yorkshire terrier
Giant schnauzer	

Clinical abnormalities consist of tapetal hyperreflectivity, retinal vascular attenuation, and optic nerve pallor. Secondary cataracts can form as a result of retinal degeneration.

Progressive retinal atrophy actually represents the end-result of dozens of different genetic variants, and genetic testing can be performed for several of these variants. Although there is no cure for this disease, owners should be counseled on management of a blind dog. In addition, these patients are not considered candidates for cataract surgery and should be managed and monitored for a secondary glaucoma.

The patient should have a thorough ophthalmic examination at each visit, at minimum, annually. Subtle changes observed and reported in the client's history will elucidate decreased vision in low light conditions. The client may observe this at night time outside or when the lights are low in the house in the evening. Subtle changes visualized in the retina include tapetal hyperreflectivity due to a thinning of the retina, optic nerve pallor, and retinal vascular attenuation.

Although there is no cure for progressive retinal atrophy, the patient is at risk for cataract development as well as secondary glaucoma. In order to obtain a thorough ophthalmic examination, the patient should be pharmacologically dilated with topical tropicamide. Any patient diagnosed with progressive retinal atrophy should be encouraged to obtain an opinion by a veterinary ophthalmologist. Topical ophthalmic antiinflammatories can reduce the risk of lens-induced uveitis and therefore glaucoma if the patient develops cataracts. If progressive retinal atrophy is diagnosed by the veterinarian, more frequent examinations are required 2–3 times per year to monitor for uveitis and secondary glaucoma.

Genetic testing for predisposed breeds should be encouraged to allow the client to prepare for development of progressive retinal atrophy, blindness, and secondary sequelae. Genetic testing will also allow the veterinarian to provide more information to the client to advise about breeding practices.

Client education is very important when managing patients with progressive retinal atrophy. Lights should be turned on if the patient goes outside in low light conditions, night lights can be utilized in electrical outlets to provide lights at the level of the patient, gates should be utilized near steps, and bodies of water such as creeks, swimming pools, ponds, and lakes should be avoided in patients with severe vision compromise.

3.18.7 Glaucoma

Glaucoma refers to a variety of ocular diseases that exhibit increased levels of IOP that can adversely impact vision and eye health. Glaucoma is the end-result due to inadequate drainage of aqueous humor from within the eye. It is one of the leading causes of not only vision loss but loss of the eye in animals. The only way to properly diagnose glaucoma in any species is to use a digital tonometer. Recognition of glaucoma in patients by the veterinary team is critical and time sensitive in order to delay loss of vision and manage comfort in the patient (see 8.21 Team Strategies for Glaucoma).

Primary glaucoma is typically thought to occur in dogs with a genetic predisposition for anatomical differences which cause an inadequate outflow of aqueous, thereby leading to an increase in IOP (Table 3.18.4). For lists of affected cat breeds, see 11.3 Heritable Health Conditions – By Disease.

Secondary glaucoma is typically thought to be the result of a decrease of aqueous outflow with an increase in IOP in eyes with open angles. Potential causes of secondary glaucoma include a chronically detached retina, uveitis, hyphema, hypopyon, lens luxation (both anterior and posterior), chronic progressive retinal atrophy, posterior synechia, and intraocular neoplasia. Chronically detached retinas, chronic uveitis, intraocular neoplasia, and progressive retinal atrophy result in the formation of a pre-iridal fibrovascular membrane. This membrane is a fibrovascular network that extends on the anterior surface of the iris and progresses into and over the iridocorneal angle, which can obstruct aqueous outflow resulting in increased IOPs.

Any patient that presents with increased decreased vision, buphthalmia, corneal edema, conjunctival hyperemia, episcleral injection, epiphora, or ocular pain should have their IOPs measured on examination.

A few types of glaucoma can now be genetically tested for in specific breeds. Currently, there have been four mutations to the *ADAMTS10* gene that have been responsible for primary open angle glaucoma in the beagle as well as the Norwegian elkhound. Two mutations are associated with the *ADAMTS17* gene that cause primary open

Table 3.18.4 Some dog breeds predisposed to primary glaucoma

American cocker spaniel	Great Dane
Basset hound	Siberian husky
Chow chow	Beagle
Chinese shar-pei	Samoyed
Boston terrier	Jack Russell terrier
Wire-haired fox terrier	English cocker spaniel
Norwegian elkhound	Cairn terrier
Siberian husky	Miniature poodle

angle glaucoma in the petit basset griffon Vendeen and the basset hound. Over time, it is inevitable that more genes will be elucidated that can be tested to determine risk level for glaucoma.

For the veterinary team, it is important to counsel clients as to the risk level that each of these breeds have for glaucoma. Genetic testing as well as semiannual or annual IOP testing is important to monitor for increases in IOP as well as changes in vision. It is also important to discuss the potential for heritable traits if the client has an interest in breeding the patient.

EXAMPLES

Example 1: A client brings her 9-year-old intact female Yorkshire terrier to your hospital for cloudy eyes and decreased vision. After obtaining a history, your technician obtains positive menace responses in both eyes, positive dazzle responses in both eyes, and positive direct and consensual pupillary light responses in both eyes. Schirmer tear testing is normal in the right eye at 24 mm/min and normal in the left eye at 22 mm/min. IOPs are also normal at 14 mmHg in the right eye and 16 mmHg in the left eye. Fluorescein stain is negative in both eyes. After dilating the patient with tropicamide, you perform a thorough ophthalmic examination and diagnose the Yorkshire terrier with cataracts. Since your client has an interest in breeding this dog, you discuss that Yorkshire terriers develop cataracts which are presumed to be inherited and this may affect her progeny. You recommend referral to an ophthalmologist for further discussion of medical and surgical options for this potential breeding animal.

Example 2: A client brings her 9-year-old female spayed English cocker spaniel to your hospital for decreased night vision. After obtaining a history indicating decreased night vision and potential decreased day vision, your technician obtains positive menace responses in both eyes, positive dazzle responses in both eyes, and positive direct and consensual pupillary light responses in both eyes. Schirmer tear testing is normal in the right eye at 20 mm/min and normal in the left eye at 27 mm/min. IOPs are also normal at 11 mmHg in the right eye and 13 mmHg in the left eye. Fluorescein stain is negative in both eyes. After dilating the patient with tropicamide, you perform a thorough ophthalmic examination and identify tapetal hyperreflectivity, retinal vascular attenuation, optic nerve pallor, and incipient posterior cataracts. You discuss with your client that her dog most likely has progressive retinal atrophy and will progressively lose

vision over time. You discuss that her dog's cataracts will likely progress, and the patient will need to be monitored for glaucoma in the future and offer her advice on how to care for a visually compromised dog. You refer her to an ophthalmologist for confirmation and further options to care for her beloved dog.

Example 3: A client brings his 8-year-old male neutered Jack Russell terrier to your hospital for an annual examination. After obtaining a history indicating no vision changes, your technician obtains positive menace responses in both eyes, positive dazzle responses in both eyes, and positive direct and consensual pupillary light responses in both eyes. Schirmer tear testing is normal in the right eye at 26 mm/min and normal in the left eye at 24 mm/min. IOPs are also normal at 14 mmHg in the right eye and 17 mmHg in the left eye. Fluorescein stain is negative in both eyes. After dilating the patient with tropicamide, you perform a thorough ophthalmic examination and identify a subtle lens subluxation and iridodonesis. You discuss with your client that his Jack Russell terrier most likely has a lens subluxation and that this is an inherited condition seen in this breed. You suggest that this patient is at risk for a posterior lens luxation, anterior lens luxation, uveitis, glaucoma, and retinal detachment. You recommend evaluation by a veterinary ophthalmologist for further medical and surgical recommendations. If the client does not elect to see a veterinary ophthalmologist, you initiate treatment with topical latanoprost to maintain the lens in the posterior segment of the eye and recommend a recheck examination in 2–3 months.

TAKE-AWAYS

- Many eye conditions that are diagnosed can be found commonly within specific breeds.
- Genetic testing is quickly evolving and over time will likely elucidate more genes that produce carrier and affected animals.
- Genetic testing can further help clients and breeders on improving the breed and helping to reduce or eliminate the disease in future generations.
- Diseases can be identified more readily if one is familiar with the breeds in which the disease is more commonly seen.
- Appreciating breed predisposition further enhances the education of the client and can improve overall breed quality.

MISCELLANEOUS

Recommended Reading

Davidson, M.G. and Nelms, S. (2013). Diseases of the lens and cataract formation. In: *Veterinary Ophthalmology*, 5e, vol. 2 (eds. K. Gelatt, B. Gilger and T. Kern), 1199–1233. Ames, IA: Wiley.

Mellersh C. (2015). Primary Glaucoma in Dogs – Relieving the Pressure Through Genetic Investigation and the Development of DNA Tests. www.vin.com/apputil/content/defaultadv1.aspx?id=6976366&pid=12513&

Narfstrom, K. and Petersen-Jones, S. (2013). Diseases of the canine ocular fundus. In: *Veterinary Ophthalmology*, 5e, vol. 2 (eds. K. Gelatt, B. Gilger and T. Kern), 1303–1392. Ames, IA: Wiley.

Plummer, C.E., Regnier, A., and Gelatt, K. (2013). The canine glaucomas. In: *Veterinary Ophthalmology*, 5e, vol. 2 (eds. K. Gelatt, B. Gilger and T. Kern), 1050–1145. Ames, IA: Wiley.

3.19

Mixed-Breed Considerations

Lowell Ackerman, DVM, DACVD, MBA, MPA, CVA, MRCVS

Global Consultant, Author, and Lecturer, MA, USA

BASICS

3.19.1   Summary

Mixed-breed dogs and cats constitute the majority of pets in most small animal veterinary practices, and there may be misconceptions about their health status compared to purebred animals, as well as their susceptibility to heritable diseases.

3.19.2   Terms Defined

Disease Liability Genes: The genetic factors that contribute to the manifestation of complex heritable conditions.
Hybrid Vigor: Biological enhancements that may result from outbreeding.

MAIN CONCEPTS

Mixed-breed pets are common in veterinary practice, often constituting about half of all dogs in a typical practice, and likely over 90% of cats in practice. The concept of mixed-breed animals as lower status variants of purebreds is no longer a view held by many pet owners, and the term "mixed-breed" or "cross-breed" can even be somewhat controversial, with some geneticists preferring terms like randomly bred or nonintentionally bred to designate that it is the intentional versus nonintentional actions of breeding that most determine genetic outcomes.

Most pet owners, on the other hand, are happy enough with embracing comfortable terms for the products of such matings for dogs (mutt, mongrel, xbred, etc.) and

cats (moggies, mutt cats, polycats, etc.). The terms *domestic shorthair* and *domestic longhair* are often used for cats of mixed ancestry, classified by their coat length. Such distinctions have become more important as so-called designer breeds have arisen from the intentional matings of two different breeds to achieve a hybrid.

It is important to consider that it is not the unintentional mating of two animals that confers hybrid vigor; it is the intentional act of selecting two individuals with appropriate traits and genotypes to produce offspring with desirable outcomes. This is not necessarily something that can be achieved just by chance. After all, the purebreds themselves are the result of artificial selection, using genetic pressure to create traits based on conformation, coat characteristics/colors, and behaviors. It just so happens that in some of that selection pressure, certain heritable conditions also got concentrated in those animals. Certain influential ancestors that were commonly included in pedigrees may also have served to concentrate such genes in purebred populations.

3.19.3   Hybrid Vigor

Hybrid vigor, or heterosis, implies that there are potential health benefits associated with the cross-breeding of different animals. However, it is really the advantage of having a large gene pool that confers genetic benefits, and many pets, including purebreds, mixed-breeds and hybrids, can carry liability genes for many different heritable disorders (hip dysplasia, atopic dermatitis, patellar luxation, cryptorchidism, feline lower urinary tract disease, etc.). Since many of these common diseases are associated with ancient disease liability genes, many that preceded the relatively recent evolution of current purebreds and hybrids, those genes are widely disseminated in the general pet population.

It has been mentioned that many of today's purebreds have resulted from selection pressure, concentrating the genes of certain ancient ancestors and removing individuals that do not conform to a certain standard from participating in the gene pool. However, this lack of genetic diversity does not necessarily affect genetic health. In fact, deleterious genes can become concentrated in randomly bred animals as well as intentionally bred animals, and there are many examples of nondomesticated species proceeding to extinction without any apparent benefit from hybrid vigor. In the end, it is not the purity of the breeding animals that affects health outcomes; it is the relative accumulation of disease liability genes.

3.19.4 Health Considerations

Even in pets that are of mixed heritage, the propagation of heritable diseases is a function of animals with deleterious genetic mutations having the opportunity to contribute offspring to future generations. In many cases those deleterious mutations are recessive and do not hamper the success of potential genetic influencers from disseminating both good and bad genes to descendants. Thus, if a particular animal (purebred or mixed-breed) is successful at producing offspring but has health issues that develop later in life, those beneficial and not so beneficial traits are likely to be propagated. The result is that many disease genes that were present in the ancient dog and cat populations are still present in both purebreds and mixed-breed animals. Where a difference is observed is in the purebred populations in which some of the rare genetic diseases (e.g., hemophilia, cerebellar ataxia, dystrophic epidermolysis bullosa, gangliosidosis, etc.) were inadvertently concentrated.

Because so many common conditions (atopic dermatitis, diabetes mellitus, hip dysplasia, hypothyroidism, urolithiasis, etc.) are so widely disseminated, all pets should be appropriately screened. It is true that prevalence may be higher in certain purebreds than the general population, but since the actual number of mixed-breed animals in any primary care practice is much larger than the population of any one breed, it is worth creating screening protocols that apply to all dogs and cats, not just purebreds.

Accordingly, mixed-breed pets should be screened in the same manner as purebreds and hybrids for the conditions most commonly seen in practice. Screening for the more rare and breed-specific disorders (e.g., intervertebral disc disease, cystinuria, muscular dystrophy, etc.) can be reserved for those animals at higher risk. For any of these groups, the only way to select against deleterious genes is by screening breeding animals with genotypic and phenotypic tests and using appropriate strategies (e.g., breeding carriers to normal noncarriers) to minimize the risk of offspring having genotypes in which they

manifest disease (see 3.11 Integrating Genotypic and Phenotypic Testing).

3.19.5 Practical Implications

Most mixed-breed pets are not intentionally bred, and the majority are neutered so do not typically contribute their genes to future generations. Thus, the purpose of screening is for the health benefits of the individual animal and not necessarily for the benefit of potential progeny.

Mixed-breed pets should be screened for common heritable conditions (Table 3.19.1). Most of those conditions are complexly inherited, and many do not have genetic tests available. Thus, most of the screening will be done with phenotypic tests, such as blood work, urinalysis, imaging, etc.

3.19.6 Genetic Testing

Genetic testing can provide a lot of information regarding susceptibility to disease (see 3.4 Predicting and Eliminating Disease Traits). Most of the testing, however, is directed at relatively rare single-gene disorders, which tend to be less common in mixed-breed animals. Mixed-breed animals may be carriers of a variety of genetic disorders, but are less likely to have two of those recessive alleles that would cause them to manifest clinical disease. Most of the heritable conditions clinically evident in mixed-breed animals are typically of a more complex inherited nature and most of the testing for these disorders relies on phenotypic testing (blood tests, urinalysis, imaging, etc.).

Table 3.19.1 Conditions commonly seen in mixed-breed pets

Dog	Cat
Behavioral issues	Behavioral issues
Cancer	Cancer
Mitral valve disease	Feline lower urinary tract disease
Hip dysplasia	Osteoarthritis
Cranial cruciate ligament rupture	Eosinophilic syndromes
Patellar luxation	Kidney failure
Hyperadrenocorticism	Hyperthyroidism
Hypoadrenocorticism	Inflammatory bowel disease
Hypothyroidism	Upper respiratory infections
Diabetes mellitus	Diabetes mellitus
Lens luxation	Odontoclastic resorptive lesions
Urolithiasis	Urolithiasis

Still, there are some genetic tests that can be appropriate for screening all animals. Even in mixed-breed animals, it is possible to see affected animals and carriers for a variety of monogenic traits, including cataracts, mdr1, von Willebrand disease, progressive rod-cone degeneration, and others. Some are more difficult to interpret unless there is a known gene association with clinical disease in that specific breed, including testing like SOD1 for degenerative myelopathy. In the future, it is likely that there will be marker-based genetic tests that might indicate which animals could be at increased risk for complexly inherited conditions (such as hip dysplasia, atopic dermatitis, mitral valve disease, etc.).

One other aspect of genetic testing for mixed-breed animals that is worthy of discussion is the availability of heritage tests, DNA tests that determine possible breeds that contributed to a mixed-breed individual. These tests are partially for entertainment value as much as health value, but they can provide useful information about pets, from the likely contributions of different breeds to the mix, trait characteristics such as adult size and coat characteristics, possibly some traits associated with some breeds that could provide insight into demonstrated behaviors or conformation, and potentially some information relative to disease susceptibility. It is interesting to note that while many hospital teams pride themselves on being able to determine breed contribution based on physical characteristics, they tend to get it wrong at least as often as they get it right. In medical records, it is best to use the term *mixed-breed* or something similar if the parentage is not known, or if genetic testing has not been done. Entering potentially incorrect information into the medical record is not advised and can prejudice medical judgment.

EXAMPLES

Jezebel Garcia is a 2-year-old frug (a cross between a pure-bred French bulldog and a purebred pug, also known as a Frenchie pug) who presented to ABC Animal Hospital for routine health assessment and vaccination. Dr Aronson determined Jezebel to be a healthy specimen, but recommended orthopedic screening for hip dysplasia, in addition to some other routine diagnostic testing.

Mrs Garcia seemed surprised by the recommendation, believing that not only was hip dysplasia a condition of large dogs, but that since Jezebel was a hybrid (she preferred the term designer breed), she inferred that the risk for such genetic diseases was very low. Dr Aronson and the veterinary team spent time educating Mrs Garcia that not only was hip dysplasia a condition that could be seen in any size and breed of dog, but that actually both pugs and French bulldogs were at increased risk for the condition.

They recommended orthopedic screening for all dogs at this age, and while there was a good chance that Jezebel would be clear on radiographs, it was still worth assessing her for it, so that if there were problems, they could start addressing them early.

Mrs Garcia said she would take some time to think about it, and the hospital team gave her some information on the topic and some links to online resources. They also followed up with her a few days later by telephone, and Mrs Garcia then consented and brought Jezebel back for the evaluation. As it turned out, Jezebel did have some early evidence of hip dysplasia and the team went over an action plan for how they would help the family deal with any consequences of the situation. Mrs Garcia was thankful that she had decided to act, and was appreciative that the hospital team had provided her with everything she needed to make that difficult decision.

TAKE-AWAYS

- For many common heritable disorders, mixed-breed animals have prevalence rates similar to those of many purebreds.
- In most hospitals over half of canine patients and likely greater than 90% of feline patients are mixed-breed.
- Mixed-breed pets benefit from routine screening for heritable conditions.
- Hybrid vigor is a term often incorrectly used to suggest that mixed-breed animals have fewer heritable issues than purebreds.
- Genetic testing can be used for screening pets for traits and diseases but in the case of mixed-breed animals, can also be used to infer possible contributing breeds.

MISCELLANEOUS

Recommended Reading

Ackerman, L. (2011). *The Genetic Connection*. Lakewood, CO: AAHA Press.

Ackerman, L. (2020). Proactive Pet Parenting: Anticipating pet health problems before they happen. Problem Free Publishing.

Bellumori, T.P., Famula, T.R., Bannasch, D.L. et al. (2013). Prevalence of inherited disorders among mixed-breed and purebred dogs: 27,254 cases (1995–2010). *J. Am. Vet. Med. Assoc.* 242 (11): 1549–1555.

Donner, J., Anderson, H., Davison, S. et al. (2018). Frequency and distribution of 152 genetic disease variants in over 100,000 mixed breed and purebred dogs. *PLoS Genet.* 14 (4): e1007361.

Section 4

Nonhereditary Considerations

4.1

Canine and Feline Life Stages

Sarah Rumple

Rumpus Writing and Editing LLC, Denver, CO, USA

BASICS

4.1.1 Summary

In human medicine, toddlers receive very different care from adults or seniors. The same should be true in veterinary medicine. An animal's physiology evolves as it ages, so veterinary care needs to evolve with it. While every preventive care exam should include core elements regardless of a patient's age, there are additional components to consider as pets experience different stages of life.

MAIN CONCEPTS

Unlike human medical professionals, veterinary healthcare professionals deal with patients who cannot tell them how they're feeling. You rely on the ability of pet owners to effectively convey their observations to you. You also rely on a number of scientific methods and formulas to tell you when something is wrong.

But not everything can be determined with a formula. And not every pet owner will notice changes in a pet and tell you about those changes. There is no "one size fits all" when it comes to veterinary medicine. Pets are individuals, and they need and deserve individualized healthcare. And, while you can't read minds, you can use tools to help you customize each exam so the individual needs of your patients in every stage of life are met.

4.1.2 Veterinary Care for All Life Stages

Regardless of age, all pets should receive regular preventive care. The frequency and components of each preventive care exam will vary based on life stage, but certain elements remain constant regardless of age. According to the *2019 AAHA Canine Life Stage Guidelines* [1], each exam should include the following.

- **Comprehensive physical exam**
  - Conduct a thorough physical exam, including the five vital assessments (temperature, pulse, respiration, pain, and nutritional assessment), thoracic auscultation, gait analysis, pain score, body mapping, and reproductive status.
  - Make recommendations about frequency of visits.
  - Discuss disaster preparedness and estate planning.
- **Lifestyle assessment**
  - Make recommendations concerning regular exercise, mental stimulation, and environmental enrichment (see 4.10 Environmental Considerations).
  - Ask open-ended questions to encourage discussion about the pet's lifestyle and potential safety risk factors (see 9.2 Asking Good Questions). It's important to know about the pet's home environment, whether the pet encounters other pets or wildlife, the activities enjoyed by the pet, etc.
- **Breed-specific considerations**
  - Evaluate and report findings for conditions that occur more frequently in particular breeds (see 11.4 Heritable Health Conditions – By Breed).
- **Parasite screening and protection**
  - Perform a fecal exam for intestinal parasites, and recommend year-round intestinal parasite control (see 4.5 Prevention and Control of Parasites).

- Test for heartworm, and recommend year-round heartworm preventive.
- Examine the pet for the presence of fleas and ticks, and recommend year-round flea and tick prevention.
- Discuss the importance of properly removing feces from the environment and how to do it.

● **Vaccines**
- Administer core vaccines when appropriate (see 9.11 Vaccination).
- Administer appropriate noncore vaccines based on lifestyle and risk assessment.

● **Nutritional assessment**

According to the Association for Pet Obesity and Prevention, an estimated 60% of cats and 56% of dogs in the United States were overweight or obese in 2018.
- Evaluate the pet's body condition score (BCS) and muscle condition score (MCS), and recommend diet changes if indicated.
- Discuss the feeding schedule, food choice, and quantity (see 9.15 Nutritional Counseling).
- Review the medical records to identify trends in weight.
- Discuss the risks of raw food, including the differences between commercial and home-made raw diets.
- Discuss supplement use (see 9.16 The Role of Nutritional Supplements in Pet-Specific Care).

● **Behavior evaluation**

Behavior problems are a common cause of relinquishment and euthanasia, so a behavior evaluation should take place during every veterinary visit. Life stages are also recognized based on behavioral aspects in both dogs and cats (see 6.1 Normal Development Stages of Dogs and Cats).
- Discuss normal behavior, and evaluate emotional and behavioral history (see 6.9 Preventing Behavior Problems).
- Evaluate each pet's behavior and address undesirable behaviors, such as pulling on the leash or jumping on people (see 6.10 Behavior Problems – Advice).
- Provide direction on how to teach basic manners, and refer appropriate cases to a trainer.
- Pets with serious behavior concerns, such as aggression, self-injury, or extreme phobias, should be referred to a veterinary behaviorist (see 6.11 Treating Animals with Behavior Problems).
- Provide bite prevention education (see 8.12 Preventing Animal-Related Injuries).
- Educate on the signs of fear, stress, and anxiety in animals, and provide ways to reduce fear and stress (see 6.6 Fear Free Concepts).

● **Oral exam and dental health discussion**

Most pets have some degree of periodontal disease by the age of 3 (see 4.9 Periodontal Disease).

- Conduct an oral examination, document assessment of dental condition, and develop a preliminary treatment plan.
- Determine if the patient needs to be anesthetized so you can further evaluate dental health. Anesthesia is necessary for you to complete a thorough and complete oral exam, periodontal probing, and intraoral radiography.
- Provide education on the signs of oral pain in pets and the importance of proper dental home care, including:
  ○ how to brush a pet's teeth
  ○ choosing dental care products that prevent plaque and tartar and have the Veterinary Oral Health Council (VOHC) seal of approval
  ○ avoiding hard chews, bones, and toys that can damage and break teeth

● **Reproductive health exam**
- Examine genitalia.
- Verify and document reproductive status (see 4.2 Gender-Related Considerations).
- Recommend that all pets not intended for breeding be prevented from producing unintended offspring (see 2.18 Population Control).
- Promote responsible breeding practices for pet owners who choose to breed their animals.

While some components of the veterinary appointment will remain constant, others will vary based on the pet's life stage (see 6.1 Normal Development Stages of Dogs and Cats).

4.1.3 Canine Life Stages

The four stages of life for the canine patient are puppy, young adult, mature adult, and senior. What do these life stages indicate to members of the veterinary healthcare team? The following recommendations are from the *2019 AAHA Canine Life Stage Guidelines* [1].

PUPPY

Definition	From birth through cessation of rapid growth (approximately 6–9 months of age, varying with breed and size) [1]
Frequency of veterinary visits	Every 3–4 weeks
Additional components of the physical exam	● Evaluate for congenital disorders ● Recommend microchipping and discuss the importance of maintaining the microchip registration with current contact information ● Evaluate for congenital disorders

- Recommend microchipping and discuss the importance of maintaining the microchip registration with current contact information
- Discuss increased awareness of potential hazards and how to "puppy-proof" the home and outdoor spaces
- Recommend socialization and regular handling. Encourage enrollment in an appropriate puppy class (see 7.7 Puppy and Kitten Classes)
- Discuss the importance of positive reinforcement training (see 6.2 How Animals Learn)
- Provide education on canine body language and how to prevent dog bites
- Discuss the benefits of crate training
- Recommend establishing a feeding schedule
- Recommend an appropriate diet, and discuss the dog's caloric needs (see 3.17 Breed-Related Nutritional Issues)
- Recommend appropriate, regular exercise
- Discuss the prevalence of intestinal parasites in puppies, and recommend deworming at 2 weeks of age and every 2 weeks thereafter until the dog begins regular parasite prevention (see 4.5 Prevention and Control of Parasites)
- Begin heartworm, flea, and tick preventive as early as the label allows
- Recommend core vaccines and appropriate noncore vaccines based on the anticipated lifestyle risks, finishing at 16–20 weeks (see 9.11 Vaccination). Consider antibody titer testing to determine protection from canine distemper virus, canine parvovirus, and canine adenovirus-2 infections
- Provide dental health education, including how to choose safe, appropriate chew toys and dental health products and how to provide dental home care. Emphasize the importance of avoiding negative experiences during the puppy's dental home care
- Discuss spay/neuter or breeder planning. Examine for a tattoo, or place a tattoo after spaying the pet.
  - Small-breed dogs (<45 pounds/20 kg projected adult body weight) should be neutered at 6 months of age or spayed before the first estrus (5–6 months of age) [1]
  - Large-breed dogs (>45 pounds/20 kg projected adult body weight) should be neutered after growth stops (9–15 months of age) or spayed before the first estrus (5–6 months of age) [1]
    - For male dogs at increased risk for hip dysplasia or knee ligament injuries, discuss risks with the client, and consider neutering after growth stops (9–15 months of age), regardless of projected adult body weight
    - For male dogs at increased risk of lymphoma or bone cancer, discuss risks with the client, and consider neutering at 12 months of age, regardless of projected adult body weight
    - For female dogs at increased risk of hip dysplasia, knee ligament injuries, or bone cancer, discuss risks with the client, and consider waiting to spay until after growth stops (9–15 months of age)
- Educate owners of intact animals on the hazards of roaming, appropriate breeding frequency and ages, and genetic counseling. Examine the prostate, testes, and mammary glands. Consider brucellosis testing
- Evaluate for breed-specific conditions, and discuss conditions common in the breed and the signs to watch for (see 11.4 Heritable Health Conditions – By Breed and 3.4 Predicting and Eliminating Disease Traits)
- Discuss grooming needs specific to the breed

| Additional considerations | New puppy owners should be educated on the importance of regular veterinary visits for the lifetime of the dog, and they should understand that puppies will be seen more frequently than dogs in other life stages (see 1.2 Providing a Lifetime of Care) |

New puppy owners should be educated on the importance of regular veterinary visits for the lifetime of the dog, and they should understand that puppies will be seen more frequently than dogs in other life stages (see 1.2 Providing a Lifetime of Care)

Help puppies build positive associations with veterinary visits by incorporating clinical practices that reduce fear, anxiety, and stress in animals (see 6.6 Fear Free Concepts). Encourage new puppy owners to bring their pets to your hospital frequently for "happy" visits, where the puppy can be weighed and receive treats and affection from the healthcare team

Now is the time to focus on preparing puppies for life as companion animals. Socialization is necessary for puppies to gain life skills. There is no medical reason to delay puppy classes or social exposure until the vaccination series is completed, as long as exposure to sick animals is prohibited, basic hygiene is practiced, and diets are high in quality [2]

Prepare the pet owner for the cost of veterinary care for the lifetime of the dog (see 2.9 Anticipated Costs of Pet Care), and discuss pet health insurance (see 10.16 Pet Health Insurance) and other options intended to decrease the potential financial burden of providing appropriate veterinary care.

YOUNG ADULT

Definition	From cessation of rapid growth until completion of physical and social maturation, which occurs in most dogs by 3–4 years of age [1]
Frequency of veterinary visits	At least annually
Additional components of physical exam	• Evaluate congenital disorders • Discuss continued need for increased awareness regarding hazards young dogs commonly encounter • Recommend continued training classes, which improve obedience and offer opportunities for socialization • Discuss current behaviors of concern to the pet owner, and refer to a trainer or veterinary behaviorist when appropriate • Encourage regular, appropriate exercise • Test for heartworm disease once per year beginning at 7–12 months of age • Test for tick-borne diseases annually beginning at 7–12 months of age • Examine the dog's teeth, taking note of developmental anomalies. If the pet is missing any permanent teeth, intraoral dental radiographs should be taken • Evaluate the health of the gums and the presence of plaque and calculus • Based on the condition of the teeth, consider recommending the pet's first comprehensive oral exam, full-mouth radiographs, dental cleaning, and dental charting • If the pet has not been spayed or neutered, discuss the benefits • Owners of intact animals should be educated on the hazards of roaming, appropriate breeding frequency and ages, and genetic counseling. Obtain a heat cycle history for female dogs, and discuss inherited disorders for dogs being considered for breeding • Screen for orthopedic, ophthalmic, renal, and hepatic abnormalities
Additional considerations	Between 6 months and 3 years of age, dogs mature socially and behaviorally. This time period can be challenging for owners as they face common behavior issues, including jumping and barking, and normal, breed-specific behaviors, such as digging or herding actions.

Ask open-ended questions to identify potential concerning behaviors. Set owners up for success by emphasizing the importance of meeting a dog's exercise needs and enriching the environment to prevent boredom-induced behavior problems

Continue educating owners on the importance of regular wellness exams and recommending annual visits during this life stage.

MATURE ADULT

Definition	From completion of physical and social maturation until the last 25% of estimated lifespan (breed and size dependent) [1]
Frequency of veterinary visits	Every 6–12 months
Additional components of physical exam	• Evaluate for cognitive changes, dysfunction, or any anxiety or phobias that might have developed since the pet's last wellness exam • Ask open-ended questions about house training, separation anxiety, aggression, and other common behavior problems to identify issues that may result in relinquishment or euthanasia • When appropriate, recommend continued training classes • Recommend appropriate regular exercise and emphasize the importance of maintaining a healthy weight (see 8.25 Team Strategies for Weight Management) • Evaluate and treat the progression of periodontal disease • Screen for neoplasia risk, renal, hepatic, endocrine, and cardiovascular problems
Additional considerations	Mature adults are more likely to begin developing age-related health conditions. Seeing them more frequently can help the veterinary team identify potential problems early, which can lead to a better prognosis for the pet and cost savings for the pet owner.

SENIOR

Definition	The last 25% of estimated lifespan through end of life [1]
Frequency of veterinary visits	At least every six months

Additional components of physical exam	• Conduct body mapping • If needed, discuss potential environmental adaptations for mobility, sight, or hearing (see 6.18 Aging Gracefully) • Evaluate for cognitive changes or dysfunction (see 6.19 Problem Aging) • Evaluate and treat the progression of periodontal disease • Screen for neoplasia and late-onset disorders. Manage breed-related conditions
Additional considerations	During the senior years, more frequent veterinary visits and screening tests are needed to catch changes and abnormalities, and possibly extend life (see 6.17 Senior Care) Senior dogs often experience declines in mobility, vision, hearing, and cognition. Educate owners about ways to modify a dog's environment to improve comfort and safety, including providing traction on floors and stairs, reducing the need for stair climbing, and minimizing clutter If you need to sedate or anesthetize a senior pet for any procedure, take the opportunity to conduct a more comprehensive physical exam, including an oral exam, orthopedic evaluation, etc. Provide guidance and resources to help owners deal with chronic disease and end of life issues (see 6.20 Quality of Life and End of Life Issues)

4.1.4 Feline Life Stages

The six stages of life for the feline patient are kitten, junior, adult, mature, senior, and geriatric. What do these life stages indicate to the veterinary healthcare team? The following recommendations are from the *2010 AAHA/AAFP Feline Life Stage Guidelines* [3]. Life stages are also recognized based on behavioral aspects in both dogs and cats (see 6.1 Normal Development Stages of Dogs and Cats).

KITTEN

Definition	Birth to 6 months of age [3]
Frequency of veterinary visits	Approximately every 3–4 weeks
Additional components of physical exam	• Evaluate for congenital disorders • Recommend microchipping and discuss the importance of maintaining the microchip registration with current contact information
	• Discuss breed-specific predispositions and genetic concerns (see 11.4 Heritable Health Conditions – By Breed, and 3.4 Predicting and Eliminating Disease Traits) • Provide advice on how to properly care for a cat's claws, and offer alternatives to declawing • Discuss how to socialize kittens to the carrier and to help them acclimate to traveling and visiting the veterinarian • Educate owners on elimination needs, including appropriate number of litter boxes, cleaning and maintenance, and normal elimination behaviors • Discuss appropriate cat toys and enrichment items, including scratching posts and elevated resting areas (see 4.10 Environmental Considerations) • Evaluate reproductive health, and recommend spay/neuter (see 4.2 Gender-Related Considerations and 2.18 Population Control) • Spay or neuter cats between 6 and 14 weeks of age [4] • Discuss importance of maintaining a healthy weight (see 8.25 Team Strategies for Weight Management) • Recommend an appropriate diet, and discuss the benefit of offering dry foods in foraging devices (e.g., hunting feeders or food puzzles) and in multiple small meals to encourage slower intake and increase mental and physical activity • Deworm every two weeks from three to nine weeks and monthly thereafter • Conduct fecal exams 2–4 times during the first year of life • Recommend regular parasite prevention, including heartworm prevention • Administer core vaccines as appropriate and evaluate the need for noncore vaccines based on lifestyle and risk assessment (see 9.11 Vaccination). FeLV vaccine is highly recommended for kittens because of their unknown future lifestyle • Discuss dental home care, and educate on the signs of oral pain in cats (see 4.9 Periodontal Disease). Recommend dental products with the VOHC seal of approval

Additional considerations	Because cats are excellent at hiding signs of illness, new cat owners should be educated on the importance of regular veterinary visits
	A cost-of-care discussion should take place, and the veterinary team should be prepared to offer ideas on how to mitigate the financial burden of appropriate veterinary care (see 5.11 Discussing Finances for Pet-Specific Care), including pet health insurance (see 10.16 Pet Health Insurance), and wellness plans (see 10.17 Payment and Wellness Plans).

JUNIOR

Definition	7 months to 2 years of age [3]
Frequency of veterinary visits	At least annually
Additional components of physical exam	• Social play and intercat interactions may decline as cats age. Recommend continued training to allow manipulation of the mouth, ears, and feet
	• Recommend spay/neuter if not yet complete, or discuss responsible breeding
	• Evaluate body condition score/muscle condition score, and monitor weight changes. Inform owners that caloric needs decrease after sterilization
	• Discuss litter box needs and confirm that the growing cat's litter box is large enough
	• Evaluate dental health, and examine the teeth for the presence of plaque and calculus. When appropriate, recommend the cat's first comprehensive oral examination, full-mouth radiographs, dental cleaning, charting, and scoring
	• Continue fecal exams 1–4 times per year depending on health and lifestyle
Additional considerations	By 6 months of age, intact cats can become pregnant or begin spraying, so it is important to educate clients on the benefits of spay/neuter [4]

ADULT

Definition	3–6 years of age [3]
Frequency of veterinary visits	At least annually

Additional components of physical exam	• Discuss environmental enrichment, provide techniques to increase activity level, and encourage play to help maintain a healthy weight
	• Evaluate and treat the progression of periodontal disease
	• Gather baseline data to compare to future diagnostics. Consider performing a complete blood count, urinalysis, culture and sensitivity testing, fecal analysis, blood urea nitrogen, creatinine, alanine aminotransferase, alkaline phosphatase, glucose, total calcium, total protein, albumin, bilirubin, total thyroxine, and potassium [5]
Additional considerations	Although often overlooked and assumed to be healthy, cats in this life stage would benefit from regular veterinary care.

MATURE

Definition	7–10 years of age [3]
Frequency of veterinary visits	Twice annually
Additional components of physical exam	• Monitor for changes, including increased sleeping or decreased activity
	• Discuss appropriate litter box parameters so an aging cat can enter the box easily
	• Evaluate and treat the progression of periodontal disease
Additional considerations	As cats age, they become less interested in playing and other physical activities, which makes them susceptible to weight gain.

SENIOR

Definition	11–14 years of age [3]
Frequency of veterinary visits	At least twice annually
Additional components of physical exam	• Ask open-ended questions to identify changes in behavior
	• Evaluate and treat the progression of periodontal disease (see 4.9 Periodontal Disease)
	• Provide guidance and resources to help owners deal with chronic disease and end of life issues (see 6.20 Quality of Life and End of Life Issues)

Additional considerations	Senior and geriatric cats can exhibit changes in behavior, like increased vocalization or changes in litter box use, that could be due to an underlying medical problem (see 6.19 Problem Aging).

GERIATRIC

Definition	Over 15 years of age [3]
Frequency of veterinary visits	At least twice annually
Additional components of physical exam	• Discuss and address potential changes in behavior • Evaluate and treat the progression of periodontal disease • Provide guidance and resources to help owners deal with chronic disease and end of life issues
Additional considerations	Keep potential medical conditions in mind when senior or geriatric cats exhibit behavioral changes.

4.1.5 Ensure Everyone is on Board

When you adapt your preventive care recommendations for patients in different life stages, it's important to ensure your entire team is on board. Everyone – from client care representatives and assistants to technicians and doctors – needs to understand why these recommendations are being made and should be able to discuss them confidently with clients.

Also, prepare pet owners for what to expect as their pets age (see 6.18 Aging Gracefully). When a client brings a new pet into your hospital, provide an overview of your standards of care and the healthcare recommendations you'll make as the pet gets older. Discuss the potential costs associated with this level of care, and offer suggestions on how to mitigate the financial burden. Your clients will appreciate your transparency and the customized approach to their pet's healthcare.

TAKE-AWAYS

• Every wellness visit should include a comprehensive physical exam, lifestyle assessment, breed-specific

considerations, parasite screening and protection, appropriate vaccines, nutritional assessment, behavior evaluation, oral health exam and discussion, and reproductive health exam.
• The four stages of life for the canine patient are puppy, young adult, mature adult, and senior.
• The six stages of life for the feline patient are kitten, junior, adult, mature, senior, and geriatric.
• Each life stage indicates additional components or areas of focus during the preventive care exam.
• The entire veterinary team should understand the different healthcare recommendations based on life stage and should be able to confidently discuss those recommendations with clients.

MISCELLANEOUS

Abbreviations

AAFP   American Association of Feline Practitioners
AAHA   American Animal Hospital Association

References

1 AAHA Canine Life Stage Guidelines. American Animal Hospital Association, 2019. www.aaha.org/aaha-guidelines/life-stage-canine-2019/life-stage-canine-2019

2 AAHA Canine and Feline Behavior Management Guidelines. American Animal Hospital Association, 2015. www.aaha.org/aaha-guidelines/behavior-management/behavior-management-home/

3 AAHA/AAFP Feline Life Stage Guidelines. American Animal Hospital Association, American Association of Feline Practitioners, 2010. www.aaha.org/globalassets/02-guidelines/feline-life-stage/felinelifestageguidelines.pdf

4 American Association of Feline Practitioners. AAFP Position Statement. Early Spay and Castration, 2012. https://catvets.com/public/PDFs/PositionStatements/EarlySpay&Neuter.pdf

5 American Animal Hospital Association. AAHA Senior Care Guidelines for Dogs and Cats FAQs. 2005. www.aaha.org/aaha-guidelines/senior-care-configuration/senior-care/faqs/

4.2

Gender-Related Considerations

Lowell Ackerman, DVM, DACVD, MBA, MPA, CVA, MRCVS

Global Consultant, Author, and Lecturer, MA, USA

BASICS

4.2.1 Summary

Gender can influence veterinary healthcare in a variety of ways. Some conditions may be associated with a gene on the sex chromosomes, some may just be more prevalent in one gender or the other, and others may be genetically influenced by mitochondrial DNA rather than nuclear DNA.

4.2.2 Terms Defined

Gender Predisposition: A predilection for a condition to occur predominantly but not exclusively in one gender over another.
Sex-Limited Trait: A trait that can be only seen in one gender, even though it is not transmitted on the sex chromosomes.
Sex-Linked Trait: A trait that is transmitted on the X chromosome.

MAIN CONCEPTS

In pets, there are two sex chromosomes, and all the rest are known as autosomes. Parents contribute either an X chromosome or a Y chromosome to each offspring and the combination determines whether that offspring is male (XY) or female (XX). In rare circumstances, chromosomal mistakes can occur which yield indistinct genders (such as XXY, XO, etc.), but these are quite rare.

4.2.3 Sex-Linked Traits

Sex-linked traits are those that are transmitted on the X or Y chromosomes. There are few traits transmitted on the Y chromosome, so most influence is given to X-chromosome traits, which can display either dominant or recessive inheritance depending on the trait.

X-linked dominant traits occur when an X chromosome from either parent is able to cause disease in the offspring. Males tend to be affected more often and more severely than females because they only have one X chromosome. Accordingly, affected offspring must have a least one affected parent (unless the mutation is new) and the disorder does not skip generations. Affected males mated to normal females will transmit the disorder to all of their daughters but none of their sons, since the sons only receive a Y chromosome from their fathers; the X chromosome comes from the mother. Because of the dominant nature of the trait, any normal offspring from affected parents will themselves produce only normal offspring. An example of an X-linked dominant condition is hereditary nephritis, in which the defect in the Samoyed is similar to that seen with Alport syndrome in humans.

X-linked recessive traits occur when an X chromosome from either parent is able to cause disease in the offspring, but the features are slightly different from those in which the traits are dominant. With X-linked recessive disorders, both genders can be affected, but because males only have one X chromosome (they are hemizygous), they can manifest the disease with only one variant, whereas because of the recessive nature of the disorder, females would require two copies of the defective variant to have clinically evident disease. So, with an x-linked recessive disease, males tend to be overrepresented, and affected females mated to normal males produce male offspring that are all affected, but female offspring that appear phenotypically normal. On the other hand, if two affected animals are bred, then all the offspring will be affected (since the mother will have two abnormal copies of the variant and the male will be hemizygous with one). Because of the recessive nature of the trait, the disorder is capable of skipping generations. There are a variety of X-linked recessive disorders in pets, such as hemophilia A (factor VIII deficiency) in the German shepherd dog, X-linked progressive retinal atrophy in the Siberian husky, and X-linked muscular dystrophy in both dogs and cats.

Most coat characteristics are autosomally linked, but the orange color gene is sex linked and located on the X chromosomes in cats. One of the most interesting manifestations of this orange mutation is the tortoiseshell cat. The orange allele (O) is co-dominant with nonorange (o). Thus, cats with a mosaic coat of both orange and nonorange (Oo) must have two X chromosomes, which means tortoiseshell cats are almost always female. Males, with only one X chromosome, can be either orange (O-) or nonorange (o-); the very occasional phenotypic male (approximately 1 in every 3000 male births) with Klinefelter's syndrome, with at least two X chromosomes in addition to a Y chromosome (XXY), can have this color combination. Chimerism is another mechanism for how this is sometimes seen in males.

Y-linked inheritance is theoretically possible, in which the mutated gene is located on the Y chromosome, one of the two sex chromosomes in each of a male's cells. Because only males have a Y chromosome, Y-linked inheritance can only be passed from father to son. There are relatively few genes present on the Y chromosome, so this is a rare form of sex-linked inheritance. In humans, some examples of Y-linked inheritance are Y-chromosome infertility and some cases of Swyer's syndrome.

4.2.4 Mitochondrial Inheritance

Some conditions can be sex linked but not necessarily due to problems on the X chromosome, due to mitochondrial inheritance. Most DNA is found in the nucleus, but mitochondria in the cytoplasm contain their own DNA, derived almost entirely from the mother's ovum. Sperm contain few mitochondria, and almost none survive fertilization. Therefore, defects in mitochondrial DNA tend to be passed only from the mother but are transferred to both male and female offspring. An example is mitochondrial myopathy in Clumber and Sussex spaniels.

As genetic understanding of mitochondrial DNA has advanced, it has been determined that at least some mitochondrial diseases could be inherited from either parent, because most of the mitochondrial proteins are actually encoded by DNA in the cell nucleus, rather than by mitochondrial DNA. In fact, in human medicine, it is now appreciated that mitochondrial dysfunction can play a role in many common conditions, such as diabetes mellitus, heart disease, and even Alzheimer's disease.

4.2.5 Sex-Limited Traits

In contradistinction to sex-linked traits, sex-limited traits are seen in one gender but are not transmitted on the sex chromosomes. For example, cryptorchidism refers to the presence of undescended testicles, so it is seen only in males. This fact does not imply that a female cannot carry a gene for cryptorchidism or that it is sex linked and carried on the Y chromosome, which we know is not the case. Similarly, pyometra is the accumulation of pus in the uterus, and thus can only occur in females. However, that does not imply that predisposition to the trait cannot be carried by males or that the trait resides somewhere on the X chromosome.

4.2.6 Gender Predisposition

Sex predisposition occurs when diseases are noted to have prevalence that are thought to differ between males and females. This gender predisposition does not necessarily have anything to do with the sex chromosomes, or sex-limited traits. For example, there tends to be a slight sex predisposition for males with canine dilated cardiomyopathy and females might have a slight sex predisposition for diabetes mellitus. Of course, there are also a variety of clinical entities that vary depending on whether pets are intact or neutered.

4.2.7 Abnormalities in Sexual Differentiation

Normal sexual differentiation depends on a series of three steps under genetic control: the establishment of chromosomal, gonadal, and then phenotypic sex. Thus, abnormalities of sexual differentiation can also be determined on the basis of the step at which the trait differs from normal (i.e., a chromosomal, gonadal, or phenotypic error).

Chromosomal intersex, resulting from abnormalities in chromosomal sexual differentiation, is rare in dogs and is thought not to have a genetic basis. Examples include Klinefelter's syndrome (XXY), Turner's syndrome (XO), X trisomy (XXX), chimeras, and mosaics.

True hermaphroditism can reveal chimeras with XX–XY or XX–XXY chromosome combinations, the external appearance of a female, and both internal testicular and ovarian tissue. In other cases, the testicle-determining gene may be translocated to cause development of both ovarian and testicular tissue from the undifferentiated gonads.

Gonadal intersex, resulting from sexual differentiation abnormalities in the gonads, includes XX sex reversal, which is autosomal recessive in cocker spaniels but is limited to dogs with an XX chromosome constitution.

True hermaphrodites with an XX chromosome complement (hereditary XX sex reversal) can have the external appearance of a female and ovotestes internally. Hereditary XX sex reversal has been documented in several dog breeds. In the American cocker spaniel and Norwegian elkhound, the condition is transmitted as an autosomal recessive trait.

In the XX male syndrome, the phenotype is predominantly male, and individuals are positive for the H-Y antigen, but there is an XX chromosome complement. In most cases, one of the X chromosomes has a small insertion from the Y chromosome, which includes the Sry gene. This condition has been reported in the cocker spaniel, pug, German shorthaired pointer, and Kerry blue terrier.

Phenotypic intersex, resulting from sexual differentiation abnormalities in the phenotype, includes persistent Mullerian duct syndrome and testicular feminization syndrome, which has not been conclusively demonstrated in the dog but is seen in the cat. Male pseudohermaphroditism is caused by inadequate synthesis of fetal testosterone and is seen in miniature schnauzers in association with persistent Mullerian duct syndrome, and it has also been reported in the poodle, Pekingese, and pug. Female pseudohermaphroditism is primarily caused by environmental influences (exogenous androgens, metabolic errors), and no evidence has suggested a genetic etiology. It is seen in many different breeds.

Persistent Mullerian duct syndrome is a hereditary disorder in male miniature schnauzers, transmitted as an autosomal recessive trait. In this syndrome, normal-appearing XY males have oviducts, a uterus, and a cranial vagina in addition to their male sex organs.

4.2.8 Spay/Neuter

From time to time there are controversies about the best times to perform ovariohysterectomy and neuter surgeries, from the benefits of very early surgeries (e.g., 8 weeks) to proponents recommending waiting until well after 1 year of age. Those controversies will continue into the foreseeable future, but there are some recommendations that can be made on a pet-specific basis and that are consistent with the AAHA Canine Life Stage Guidelines.

For pets without specific risk factors and predicted adult weight of less than 20 kg, the consensus seems to be that spay and neuter surgeries are best performed around 6 months of age, as has long been the custom. If there is a pet-specific risk for conditions such as hip dysplasia and cruciate ligament rupture, neutering surgery is best scheduled after growth stops, which is typically at 9–15 months of age; for pets at risk of lymphoma or osteosarcoma, it is best to schedule surgery after 12 months of age. For females at risk of mammary cancer, it is still best to perform ovariohysterectomy before the first estrus, typically around 6 months of age.

EXAMPLES

Fritz is a healthy 16-week-old German shepherd pup. At 12 weeks of age, a sample from Fritz was submitted for a genetic panel and it has identified Fritz as having sex-linked hemophilia A (factor VIII disease). To date, Fritz has appeared healthy, but one male littermate has had lameness due to bleeding into the joints and muscles and another developed a spontaneous nosebleed.

Fritz's owners are very concerned about him and although they have owned him for less than two months, they are already quite attached and committed to his care. At the urgings of the hospital healthcare team, they enrolled him in pet health insurance at 8 weeks of age, and are thankful they did that while there were no preexisting issues.

Fritz has abnormal activated partial thromboplastin time (aPTT); a factor VIII assay has also been offered to the owners, and they are considering it, but they feel confident of the diagnosis given the other findings and the family history. They are going to recommend to the breeder that the dam be tested to spare others the heartbreak of adopting a hemophiliac pet.

While the owners recognize that there are currently no cures for hemophilia, they are appreciative that the hospital has provided them with so many resources, and they will treat any minor bleeding episode as a potential emergency and bring Fritz to the hospital immediately, conceivably for substitution or replacement therapy. They are also grateful that the hospital staff introduced them to an online support group for humans with hemophilia A, and that they have been so warmly welcomed by that group.

TAKE-AWAYS

- Sex-linked traits are those in which the causative genetic variant resides on one of the sex chromosomes.
- Sex-limited traits are those that can only be seen in one gender, regardless of any mode of inheritance.

- Cytoplasmic inheritance can be seen when the genetic variant is found in mitochondrial DNA rather than nuclear DNA.
- In some instances, such as tortoiseshell coloring in cats, the coat color genetics are sex linked.
- There are many instances when conditions may seem to be more common in one gender or another (sex predisposition), even if there is not a clear-cut genetic reason for it.

MISCELLANEOUS

Abbreviation

AAHA   American Animal Hospital Association

Recommended Reading

Ackerman, L. (2011). *The Genetic Connection*. Lakewood, CO: AAHAPress.

American Animal Hospital Association. Canine Life Stage Guidelines. www.aaha.org/globalassets/02-guidelines/canine-life-stage/canine_life_stage_guidelines.pdf

Hart, B.L,, Hart, L.A., Thigpen, A.P., Willetts, N.H. (2020): Assisting decision-making on age of neutering for 35 breeds of dogs: associated joint disorders, cancer and urinary incontinence. *Front Vet Sci*, 7: 388. doi:10.3389/fvets.2020.00388

4.3

Prevention and Control of Infectious Diseases

Krystle L. Reagan, DVM, PhD, DACVIM (SAIM) and Jane Sykes, BVSc, PhD, DACVIM (SAIM)

Department of Veterinary Medicine and Epidemiology, School of Veterinary Medicine, University of California, Davis, CA, USA

 BASICS

4.3.1 Summary

Prevention and control of infectious disease requires an understanding of how infectious diseases are transmitted among pets. The most common mechanisms for transmission of pathogens are direct contact, fecal–oral, air-borne, or vector-borne transmission. Pathogen, pet (host), and environmental factors all contribute to the risk of transmission and infection. General prevention strategies include good husbandry practices, regular preventive veterinary care, and management of environmental risks. Pet-specific factors that should be considered for disease prevention include general health status, including nutrition, regular health screenings, vaccinations, and parasite prevention. Environmental control strategies include limiting contact with wildlife and disease vectors, managing social gatherings among pets and practicing responsible introduction of new pets to the household. While it is impossible to completely eliminate the risk of infectious disease in pets, following the recommendations outlined here can decrease the risk of contracting an infectious disease.

4.3.2 Terms Defined

Biofilm: A collection of microorganisms and extracellular matrix that adheres to the surface of inanimate and living beings.

Contagious or Communicable Disease: A disease caused by an infectious agent that is transmissible between hosts.

Core Vaccine: A vaccine that is considered standard and recommended for all pets.

Ectoparasite: A parasite that lives on the outside of its host, e.g. flea, tick, mosquito.

Endoparasite: A parasite that lives inside its host, e.g. roundworm, whipworm, tapeworm.

Enteropathogen: A microorganism that causes disease of the gastrointestinal tract.

Fomite: Inanimate object that can harbor microorganisms on its surface.

Herd Immunity: Concept that if a sufficient proportion of a population is immune to a pathogen, there will be resistance to spread of infection despite not reaching 100% immunization rate.

Immunity: Resistance to infection by a pathogen due to the action of the immune system including pathogen-specific antibodies and sensitized immune system cells.

Pathogen or Infectious Agent: Organism causing disease, typically referring to microorganisms or microbes such as prion, virus, bacterium, protozoan, or fungus.

Vaccine: Substance used to stimulate a prolonged immune response against an infectious agent prepared from killed microorganisms, live attenuated microorganisms or a portion of the microorganisms.

Vaccine, Noncore: Vaccines that are optional and should be administered if there is exposure risk for the individual.

Vector: An agent that carries or transmits pathogens to other living organisms.

MAIN CONCEPTS

4.3.3 Introduction

Infectious or contagious diseases can occur in dogs and cats and have a wide array of clinical signs ranging from a mild self-limiting illness to being life threatening. These diseases can be caused by a variety of pathogen types including viruses, bacteria, protozoa, and parasites. Opportunities for transmission of these organisms occur when pets are in a shared environment. By understanding how infectious diseases are transmitted between pets, one can act to mitigate the risks of spread. Factors that determine how readily a pathogen can spread from one host to another include those specific to the pathogen, general health and immune status of the pet, and exposure to vectors or contaminated environments.

4.3.4 Pathogen Factors Influencing Disease

4.3.4.1 Ability to Spread and Cause Disease

Individual pathogens have different intrinsic abilities to spread and cause disease. Pathogens that have high infectivity spread readily between hosts, while those with low infectivity may require high doses or prolonged contact with the pathogen for a new host to become infected. Pathogenicity refers to a pathogen's ability to cause disease in a host once it has become infected. High-pathogenicity organisms have the ability to cause severe disease in the host while low-pathogenicity organisms may produce no or mild clinical signs. An example of a pathogen that has both high infectivity and high pathogenicity is canine parvovirus, which is readily spread between susceptible dogs and can cause severe clinical signs.

4.3.4.2 Stability in the Environment

The ability of pathogens to persist in the environment is determined by their properties and the environment in which they are found. Survival time can range from a few minutes to several years. Organisms that are relatively hardy in the environment include spore-forming bacteria (*Clostridium* spp.), nonenveloped viruses (canine parvovirus, feline calicivirus), and fungi (*Coccidioides* spp.). Other organisms, including enveloped viruses (feline herpesvirus-1) and bacteria lacking a cell wall (*Mycoplasma* spp.), are relatively short-lived in the environment. Some micro-organisms form community aggregates with other microorganisms and a protective extracellular matrix on living or inanimate objects, which is collectively referred to as a biofilm. Biofilms in the environment can protect microorganisms from harsh conditions and be a source of infection, especially with gram-negative pathogens such as *Pseudomonas*.

4.3.4.3 Route of Transmission

Infectious agents can be transmitted in a variety of ways, and individual pathogens have varied potential to spread. Modes of transmission range from direct contact to airborne droplet exposure, and an understanding of these modes enables the planning of appropriate intervention methods to prevent transmission. For transmission to be successful, one pet must be infected and contagious and the second pet must come into contact with an adequate dose through the appropriate route and be susceptible to the infection. Some pets that are shedding pathogens may not be showing outward signs of disease, so all animals must be initially presumed to have the potential to transmit infectious agents.

Direct transmission occurs when a pathogen is transferred from one host to another by directly interacting. This can occur with greeting, grooming, fighting, or mating behaviors when there is direct bodily contact between two pets. To prevent direct transmission, it is recommended that pets not be in direct contact with healthy pets if they are suspected to have infectious diseases or have unknown histories. There are many pathogens that can be spread via direct transmission, including feline immunodeficiency virus, dermatophytes, and *Brucella canis*.

Infection via the oral route can occur when foodstuffs or water have been contaminated, typically with fecal material or other bodily fluids, and another pet ingests this material. This can also occur when pets chew on toys contaminated with bodily fluids containing pathogens from another pet (fomite transmission). To reduce oral transmission, it is recommended that pets have access to clean drinking water and safe food sources. It is also recommended that good cleaning and disinfectant practices are observed when cleaning bodily fluids or feces. Pathogens that are spread through the oral route include canine parvovirus, *Salmonella*, and *Leptospira*.

Air-borne transmission occurs when a pet produces respiratory secretions by vocalizing, coughing, or sneezing that result in particles dispersing into the air. Respiratory droplets of greater than 5 μm can spread 4–5 ft in diameter from an infected dog whereas aerosol droplets of less than 5 μm can linger in the air for much longer. Fortunately, pathogens that form aerosols are rare in veterinary medicine. These include agents of tuberculosis (*Mycobacterium tuberculosis*), pneumonic plague (*Yersinia pestis*), and tularemia (*Francisella tularensis*). Infectious agents that can be spread via droplet transmission include those that cause most common dog and cat respiratory diseases, such as canine distemper virus, feline herpesvirus 1, and feline calicivirus.

Vector-borne pathogens are transmitted via an intermediary mechanism. This can be mechanical or biological in nature. Mechanical transmission occurs when a vector such as a fly moves a pathogen from one pet to another via contaminated feet or mouthparts whereas biological transmission results in the vector becoming infected with the pathogen. Vectors such as fleas and ticks are typically infected with pathogens when obtaining a blood meal from one pet, the pathogen establishes an infection within the vector, then when the vector feeds on a second host, the pathogen is transmitted. Some common diseases caused by vector-borne infectious agents include Lyme disease (*Borrelia burgdorferi*), ehrlichiosis, and bartonellosis.

4.3.5 Pet-Specific Factors Influencing Disease

4.3.5.1 Nutrition

Proper nutrition is essential to maintain health and a proper immune system. Pets should be fed a balanced diet that has been approved for their life stage by appropriate organizations (such as the Association of American Feed Council Officials in the US) to ensure minimum nutrient requirements are met. Diets containing uncooked meat products can be contaminated with enteropathogens such as *Salmonella* and *Escherichia coli* so they are not recommended.

4.3.5.2 Preventive Veterinary Care

All pets should have routine veterinary examinations and preventive care that is tailored for each patient and the geographical location (see 1.3 Personalized Care Plans). This care aims to ensure wellness and identify healthy concerns early. Pets that are healthy are generally less vulnerable to development of infectious disease. Preventive care for infectious disease includes vaccination and thorough parasite prevention strategies.

Vaccinations stimulate the immune system to provide protection against pathogens and are one of the most valuable tools available to prevent infectious disease (see 9.11 Vaccination). Vaccines contain live attenuated ("weak") strains of a microorganism, inactivated microorganisms, or fragments of a microorganism which then induce an immune reaction when administered to a pet. Ideally, vaccinations should provide prolonged protection against infection and significantly decrease the severity of disease or prevent infection when exposed without causing adverse effects. Published guidelines (see 9.3 Guidelines) provide lists of vaccines that are considered core (recommended for all pets) and noncore (recommended only if there is significant exposure risk).

Antibody titers have become increasingly popular as a means to monitor a pet's response to vaccination and predict if it has adequate immunity to a pathogen. Minimum protective antibody titers are known for canine distemper virus, canine parvovirus, and rabies, but attainment of these titers does not guarantee that a pet is protected or indicate how long the protection will persist. There is considerable variation among laboratories in reporting results. Caution should be exercised when interpreting results for pathogens when antibody titers are not a good predictor of protection such as canine parainfluenza virus and *Bordetella* [1].

Parasite prevention is recommended for all pets, and this should be tailored to the geographical location and prevent infestation with ectoparasites, endoparasites, and heartworm (see 4.5 Prevention and Control of Parasites). Ectoparasites including fleas, ticks, and mosquitoes can induce disease directly and can serve as vectors for microorganisms. Ectoparasite control includes environmental management by eliminating ectoparasite breeding sites, in conjunction with administration of effective topical or oral flea and tick preventive medications.

Intestinal endoparasites (roundworms, hookworms, whipworms, tapeworms) can cause significant health concerns in pets and some can be zoonotic in nature. Prevention of transmission, which is typically fecal–oral in nature, involves prompt and thorough removal of feces from a pet's environment. It is recommended that pets have regular deworming and fecal testing for intestinal endoparasites as recommended by the Companion Animal Parasite Council (www.capcvet.org). Administration of heartworm prevention medication is recommended year round in endemic regions.

4.3.5.3 Reproductive Control

For pets that are not being used for breeding purposes, spay and neuter should be considered to prevent some infections (see 4.2 Gender-Related Considerations, and 2.18 Population Control). Intact female dogs and cats are at risk for development of pyometra, an infection of the uterus that occurs during times in the reproductive cycle when progesterone levels are elevated and opportunistic bacterial invasion occurs [1]. The most common infectious agent associated with pyometra is the bacterium *E. coli*, but many other bacterial species can also be involved. This condition is not transmissible among pets, because *E. coli* is a bacterium that is normally present in feces and invades the uterus opportunistically when a pet's normal defenses against pathogens are compromised. Venereal transmission can occur with some pathogens, including *Brucella canis* (the cause of canine brucellosis), and *Brucella* also has zoonotic potential [1].

4.3.6 Environment-Specific Factors Contributing to Disease

4.3.6.1 Maintaining a Clean Environment

Pets should be kept in clean environments. This includes prompt removal of fecal material, urine, and any other body fluids from the environment, because feces can harbor infectious agents such as roundworms, protozoa (e.g., *Giardia*), bacterial pathogens (e.g., *Salmonella*), and viral pathogens (e.g., canine parvovirus). If body fluids or feces are present on surfaces other than those with good drainage, the area should be physically cleaned and then disinfected to remove organic material and any infectious agents (see 7.14 Premise Disinfection). The disinfectant should be chosen based on any suspected pathogens present and application should follow the manufacturer's recommended protocol to ensure activity.

4.3.6.2 Wildlife Interaction

Wildlife and rodents are reservoirs for some pathogens that cause disease in pets. These diseases include but are not limited to leptospirosis, toxoplasmosis, rabies, plague, tularemia, and some intestinal parasitic diseases. Wildlife can also maintain ectoparasite populations (such as tick and mosquito populations), which in turn can act as vectors for disease such as Lyme disease, anaplasmosis, Rocky Mountain spotted fever, and heartworm disease. It is recommended that rodent control and prevention strategies are used in and around areas where pets are housed, including keeping food and garbage in contained rodent-proof containers. Complete prevention of interaction with wildlife is not feasible, but areas where pets are housed and exercised should have fencing to prevent wildlife from congregating and contaminating the environment.

4.3.6.3 Introducing a New Pet to the Household

When a new pet is introduced into the household, a number of precautions should be observed to prevent spread of infectious disease, especially if the new pet is being obtained from an environment with potentially high pathogen exposure such as an animal shelter. Existing resident pets should be vaccinated according to recommendations and receive appropriate preventive medications before the introduction of a new pet, and the new pet should receive a thorough physical examination, be vaccinated and treated with preventive medications before introduction. The new pet should be examined for any signs of illness and isolated from resident pets until illness has resolved. If possible, the new pet should be maintained in a separate environment from other animals in the household for 1–2 weeks after introduction to give any signs of illness that might be incubating at the time of acquisition a chance to appear.

4.3.6.4 Socialization and Group Events

To ensure proper behavioral development, pets should be socialized with other animals and humans, but precautions should be in place to prevent infectious disease spread. Socialization of incompletely vaccinated puppies and kittens should take place only in environments where extreme caution is exercised to prevent introduction of infectious agents. In one study, puppies that had received their first canine parvovirus vaccine and attended socialization classes were not at higher risk of developing disease when compared to puppies that did not attend these classes [2]. Nevertheless, strict rules should be in place to prevent ill dogs from attending classes and thorough disinfection should be practiced with use of agents active against canine parvovirus (such as potassium peroxymonosulfate, a 1:32 bleach to detergent solution, or accelerated hydrogen peroxide).

Recommendations have been published for formal gatherings of dogs such as dog shows and boarding facilities that aim to prevent spread of infections [3]. The general recommendations include having a consulting veterinarian, supplying training for event staff for methods of disease prevention, only allowing participation of dogs that are clinically well, requiring a valid health certificate for dogs traveling from out of state or country, creation and implementation of disease prevention and control protocols, and education of the dog handlers. Further recommendations are outlined including immunization requirements, parasite and vector control measures, and environmental control measures [4].

4.3.7 Conclusion

Understanding the risk factors for development of infection in pets can allow for implementation of strategies to prevent infection. The ability of a microorganism to infect a pet and cause disease depends on pathogen factors as well as host factors. Pathogen factors include inherent infectivity, pathogenicity, mode of transmission, and ability to survive in the environment. Host factors include overall health status, immune status, and potential exposure to the microorganism. It is recommended that pets have regular preventive care to ensure good general health, necessary immunizations and parasite prevention and only attend social gatherings that have procedures and protocols in place that aim to prevent the spread of infectious diseases.

EXAMPLES

A newly adopted 3-year-old female spayed Labrador retriever was examined by a veterinarian. No medical history was available for the dog including any history of vaccination or preventive care. The dog was not showing any clinical signs of disease at the visit. It was recommended to administer all core vaccines, start regular flea and tick prevention, perform a heartworm test and start monthly heartworm preventive, and perform fecal testing for intestinal parasites. A discussion with the owners took place about exposure to infectious diseases and they indicated that their dog would interact regularly with other dogs at a dog day care facility and would have wildlife exposure when hiking. It was recommended that noncore vaccines for the respiratory pathogens (*Bordetella* and parainfluenza) and leptospirosis be administered due to the exposure risk. The owners were also counseled on providing a well-balanced diet that does not consist of raw meat.

TAKE-AWAYS

- The most common mechanisms for transmission of pathogens are direct contact, fecal–oral, air-borne, and vector-borne transmission.
- Pet foods that have met minimum requirements set forth by regulatory or research organizations (such as AAFCO in the USA) are recommended. Diets containing raw

meat are not recommended as enteropathogens can commonly contaminate these foods.
- Preventive veterinary care is integral to preventing infectious disease, including regular health screenings, core vaccinations, noncore vaccinations if exposure risk is present, and regular parasite prevention.
- Socialization is an important part of development for a pet, but caution should be exercised to limit the risk of pathogen exposure especially in pets that have not completed their juvenile vaccinations.
- Formal gatherings with pets should follow published guidelines for the prevention of infectious disease spread.

MISCELLANEOUS

References

1 Sykes, J.E. (2013). *Canine and Feline Infectious Diseases*. St Louis, MO: Elsevier Saunders.

2 Stepita, M.E., Bain, M.L., and Kass, P.H. (2013). Frequency of CPV infection in vaccinated puppies that attended puppy socialization classes. *Journal of the American Animal Hospital Association* 49: 95–100.

3 Stull, J.W., Kasten, J.I., Evason, M.D. et al. (2016). Risk reduction and management strategies to prevent transmission of infectious disease among dogs at dog shows, sporting events, and other canine group settings. *Journal of the American Veterinary Medical Association* 249: 612–627.

4 National Association of State Public Health Veterinarians Animal Contact Compendium Committee 2013 (2013). Compendium of measures to prevent disease associated with animals in public settings. *Journal of the American Veterinary Medical Association* 243: 1270–1288.

Recommended Reading

American Animal Hospital Association. (2017). AAHA Canine Vaccination Guidelines. www.aaha.org/aaha-guidelines/vaccination-canine-configuration/vaccination-canine

Infectious Disease in Dogs in Group Settings. https://vet.osu.edu/sites/vet.osu.edu/files/documents/preventive-medicine/Infectious%20Disease%20in%20Dogs%20Final.pdf

Worms and Germs blog. http://wormsandgermsblog.com

4.4

Preventing Infectious Diseases in the Small Animal Veterinary Hospital

Krystle L. Reagan, DVM, PhD, DACVIM (SAIM) and Jane Sykes, BVSc, PhD, DACVIM (SAIM)

Department of Veterinary Medicine and Epidemiology, School of Veterinary Medicine, University of California, Davis, CA, USA

 BASICS

4.4.1 Summary

Infection control strategies within small animal veterinary hospitals are implemented to protect both animals and members of the public from hospital-acquired infections. Elements of infection control include prevention of pathogen entry into the patient population, standard animal handling procedures and special precautions for animals suspected to have infectious diseases, including personal protective equipment (PPE) and cleaning protocols. All small animal veterinary hospitals should have an infection control program (ICP) consisting of personnel overseeing the program, standard operating protocols, and regular training of staff members.

4.4.2 Terms Defined

Antiseptic: Antimicrobial agents that are applied to living tissues (e.g., skin) to decrease the number of microorganisms present.

Biofilm: A collection of microorganisms and extracellular matrix that adheres to the surface of inanimate and living beings.

Contagious or Communicable Disease: A disease caused by an infectious agent that is transmissible between hosts.

Disinfectant: An antimicrobial agent that is used to decrease the numbers of microorganisms present on the surface of inanimate objects.

Flora: Also known as microbiota, this refers to the community of microorganisms present on/in people or animals.

Fomite: Any nonliving surface or object that can harbor microorganisms and transfer them from one individual to another.

Hospital-Acquired Infections (HAI): Also known as nosocomial infections, these are infections that are contracted within a healthcare facility or hospital setting.

Methicillin-Resistant Staphylococci: Related species of *Staphylococcus* bacteria that have acquired antimicrobial resistance to beta-lactam antibiotics. Methicillin-resistant *Staphylococcus aureus* (MRSA) is a major health concern in people, whereas methicillin-resistant *Staphylococcus pseudintermedius* (MRSP) is more of a health concern in dogs and cats, although both species can cause infection people and animals.

Multidrug resistant (MDR): A classification of antimicrobial resistance in a microorganism characterized by resistance to three or more classes of antimicrobial drugs.

Pathogen or Infectious Agent: Organism causing disease, typically referring to microorganisms or microbes such as prion, virus, bacterium, protozoan, or fungus.

Personal Protective Equipment (PPE): Protective garments used to prevent infection or injury to the wearer.

Sterilization: A process by which *all* microorganisms are removed, deactivated, or eliminated from the object.

Zoonotic Disease: A disease that is transmissible between animals and humans.

Pet-Specific Care for the Veterinary Team, First Edition. Edited by Lowell Ackerman.
© 2021 John Wiley & Sons, Inc. Published 2021 by John Wiley & Sons, Inc.

MAIN CONCEPTS

4.4.3 Overview of Common Hospital-Acquired Infections

Hospital-acquired infections (HAI) can result in increased patient mortality and morbidity, increased cost to owners, and can have public reputation consequences. In veterinary medicine, risk factors for development of HAI are similar to those in human medicine, including placement of indwelling devices such as intravenous and urinary catheters, administration of immunosuppressant medications such as chemotherapeutics, and performance of invasive surgical procedures. Recognizing the causes and risk factors for HAI can help to develop infection control strategies.

The most common HAIs in veterinary medicine are urinary tract infections associated with catheter placement, infectious diarrhea, pneumonia, surgical site infections, infectious upper respiratory disease, and dermatophyte infection [1]. A wide range of pathogens are associated with HAI, including those that are highly infectious or readily transmitted, opportunistic infections, pathogens that are highly stable in the environment and multidrug-resistant (MDR) pathogens. The following is a discussion of infection control strategies that can be applied to decrease the risk of HAI.

4.4.4 Infection Control Program Goals

Infection control programs can decrease the rate of HAI and are integral to ensuring both patient and public health. While data surrounding the incidence of HAI in veterinary medicine are limited, one survey noted that over 80% of veterinary teaching hospitals reporting an outbreak in the preceding five years, indicating this is a common occurrence [2]. Additionally, it has been estimated that 16% of hospitalized veterinary patients will develop one or more HAI [2].

Guidelines have been developed that indicate the importance of ICPs and outline steps that small animal practices can take to implement these guidelines [1]. Small animal veterinary hospitals are recommended to have an ICP that involves personnel overseeing the program, written protocols, training for all staff members, and that is tailored to address specific practice requirements. An ICP should address prevention of pathogen entry into the patient population and procedures that dictate standard precautions when interacting with all patients and specific infectious

disease protocols for those that have potential communicable pathogens. Standard precautions include attention to hand hygiene, hospital attire, general animal handling procedures, hospital cleaning protocols, and surgery preparation. Protocols and checklists for each of these situations should be compiled into an infection control manual for easy reference. All staff members of veterinary hospitals have an ethical responsibility to adhere to these guidelines to improve patient care.

4.4.5 Prevention of Pathogen Introduction

Preventing entry of a pathogen into the hospital begins with identifying high-risk patients prior to arrival at the hospital. When appointments are made, it is recommended that staff be trained to determine the age and vaccination status of a pet and potential exposure to infectious diseases such as a recent boarding event. It is also recommended to determine if there are acute signs of vomiting, diarrhea, coughing, or sneezing that could indicate an infectious disease. A medical alert should be placed on these patients so that upon their arrival, they do not enter the reception area and mingle with other patients. A dedicated examination room that is readily able to be cleaned and barrier precautions should be utilized to assess the patient.

Patients known to be infected with MDR pathogens should have medical alerts in their patient files that are readily available to reception staff, as many of these pets may not be showing outward evidence of their infection. Similar protocols should be in place such that these patients are directed to a dedicated examination room and not allowed to enter the reception area with other pets.

4.4.6 Hand Hygiene

Hand hygiene, when utilized correctly, will remove or decrease the population of transient flora present on the hands and can reduce the incidence of HAI [3]. Hand hygiene includes hand washing with soap and water or use of an alcohol-based hand sanitizer before and after each patient interaction (Table 4.4.1). Hand washing is also indicated before and after any procedure that involves nonintact skin, before and after gloves are worn, after exposure to bodily fluids or secretions, after cages are cleaned, before and after eating, smoking or leaving the hospital and after going to the restroom [3]. Alcohol-based hand sanitizers are convenient alternatives to hand washing and stations can be easily placed throughout the hospital. Additionally,

Table 4.4.1 Hand hygiene protocols

Soap and water handwashing	Hand rub alcohol-based sanitizers
1) Wet hands with water	1) Apply ~3 cm diameter pool of product to palm of hand
2) Apply soap	—
3) Rub hands together for at least 15 seconds including backs of hands, between fingers, fingertips and fingernails	2) Rub hands together for 15 seconds including backs of hands, between fingers, fingertips and fingernails
4) Rinse under running water	3) Rub hands until dry
5) Dry hands with a disposable towel	
6) Use towel to turn off the faucet to prevent direct contact	
Total time 30–60 seconds	Total time 20–30 seconds

Source: Adapted from [1].

they are less damaging to the skin than soap and water. However, these sanitizers should be avoided in situations with gross contamination of organic material or when pathogens including *Clostridium* spp. or parvovirus are suspected as they are not readily inactivated by alcohol [3].

Proper hand-washing protocols should be posted at hand washing stations throughout the hospital and educational videos are available online that can improve the compliance of all staff members (see Recommended Reading).

Disposable gloves should be used when there is anticipated contact with broken skin or bodily fluids, disinfectants, animals with infectious diseases or immunocompromised animals. Hands should be washed immediately after glove removal.

4.4.7 General Animal Handling

Pets that visit a veterinary hospital should have a complete history collected and physical examination performed to identify those with potential infectious diseases. All pets should have either dedicated equipment or equipment that has been properly disinfected prior to use such as food bowls and stethoscopes. Rectal thermometers should only be used with disposable sleeves. Interactions between pets should be limited and pets should only be housed individually in cages that have been properly disinfected between patients. Staff interaction with pets should be limited to those directly providing patient care.

Raw food diets are becoming increasingly popular and present a concern as pets that are fed these diets can be colonized with organisms that could cause illness in people or other pets. Clients must be educated about this risk before a pet receiving a raw food diet is hospitalized. If a pet has been fed a raw food diet in the preceding one month, it is recommended that feces is handled with PPE and encountered surfaces are promptly cleaned and disinfected. Raw food diets should not be fed or stored in the hospital.

Patients that are immunocompromised, such as those receiving chemotherapy or patients that have been splenectomized, are at higher risk of HAI. Medical alerts should be placed in these patients' medical records and strict hand hygiene should be observed and procedures that have a high risk of HAI should be avoided.

4.4.8 Handling Animals with Infectious Disease

Pathogens that cause infectious diseases can be spread by several different means and infection control protocols are designed based on the biological behavior of the pathogen that a patient is suspected or confirmed to have (see 4.3 Prevention and Control of Infectious Diseases). Three broad categories of transmission-based handling procedures are used in human medicine: air-borne (aerosol), droplet, and direct contact transmission precautions.

Direct contact transmission includes direct body contact, fomite transmission and fecal–oral transmission. Direct or indirect transfer of the pathogen from one patient to another can take place through muocus membranes or abraded skin. Some common pathogens spread in this manner include *Leptospira* spp., *Salmonella* spp., parvoviruses, *Staphylococcus* spp., other MDR bacteria, and dermatophytes. Contact precautions include PPE (e.g., gloves, gown, shoe covers, facemask), limiting movement within the hospital, posting of warning signs, standard hand hygiene precautions, and proper cleaning, disinfection, and disposal of medical waste [3]. Strict isolation is recommended for patients infected or suspected to be infected with the agents listed in Box 4.4.1, as these organisms can be difficult to contain within the hospital environment. Isolation areas preferably have direct access to outside or an alternate entrance that allows for patient movement without mingling with the general patient population.

Box 4.4.1   Dogs or Cats Infected or Suspected to Be Infected with These Pathogens Should be Handled with Strict Isolation Protocols

Salmonella spp., *Francisella tularensis*, *Yersina pestis*, *Mycobacterium tuberculosis*, *Mycobacterium bovis*, *Microsporum canis*, rabies virus, enteric viruses such as parvoviruses, canine transmissible respiratory disease pathogens (*Bordetella*, canine distemper virus, influenza viruses, canine respiratory coronavirus, canine adenovirus, canine parainfluenza virus), feline upper respiratory tract disease pathogens (feline herpesvirus 1, feline calicivirus, influenza virus, *Chlamydia*) *Source:* Adapted from [3].

Movement into and out of the isolation area should be limited and materials such as treatment sheets should not be moved into and out of the area. PPE should be removed and discarded if disposable or disinfected if not disposable. Good hand hygiene should be practiced upon exit from the isolation area.

Air-borne transmission occurs when very small particles (<5 μm) are expelled by a patient through the mouth and nose when sneezing, coughing or vocalizing or during some medical procedures involving the respiratory system, such as bronchoscopy. Pathogens transmitted via this route in dogs and cats include *Mycobacterium tuberculosis* (causing tuberculosis), *Yersinia pestis* (causing plague), and *Francisella tularensis* (causing tularemia). Precautions beyond standard handling should be instituted if any of these infections are suspected, including strict isolation (preferably in a negative pressure facility), all staff wearing fit-tested respirators (e.g., N95 duckbill mask), and contact precautions as outlined above.

Some common pathogens transmitted via droplets (particles >5 μm) include infectious respiratory diseases other than those listed above, including canine distemper virus, feline herpesvirus 1, *Bordetella bronchiseptica*, and canine influenza virus. Because of the larger droplet size, these pathogens cannot be transported over long distances and do not require negative pressure isolation protocols. Transmission precautions for these agents include isolation from other pets with a 4 ft (1.2 m) radius between pets and contact precautions as listed above.

4.4.9   Environmental Cleaning

Cleaning, disinfection, and sterilization of equipment and surfaces within veterinary hospitals decrease the risk of HAI, but when performed incorrectly or inconsistently, pathogens will remain and the risk of HAI increases. Cleaning is a mechanical process that removes gross organic material using soap and is an essential first step before disinfection or sterilization. Disinfection refers to the process of removing most of the microbes from inanimate objects whereas sterilization is the complete elimination of all microbes.

A variety of chemical disinfectants are available with different properties and spectrum of action against pathogens. Several factors that impact the action of a disinfectant other than the chemical make-up include residual organic material, the number of microbes present, the presence of biofilms, and the surface that is to be disinfected. It is important that the disinfectant is applied according to the manufacturer's recommendation for the specified pathogen at the correct dilution and remains wet on the surface for the labeled contact time.

Disinfectants should be employed on surfaces after patients have been present, including exam room (floor, table) and cages. They should also be used on medical equipment that comes into contact with patients, including endotracheal tubes, otoscopes, stethoscopes, etc. Other surfaces such as the reception area floor should be cleaned and disinfected daily or if soiled with bodily fluids. It is recommended that mop heads should be laundered daily to prevent spread of pathogens.

Methods of sterilization include pressurized steam, gas sterilization with ethylene oxide or formaldehyde, and liquid sterilizers. Autoclaves apply steam and pressure to objects and are the most efficacious and commonly utilized form of sterilization in the small animal hospital. Prior to objects being placed into an autoclave, they must be cleaned with soap and detergent to remove any organic debris. All jointed items such as hemostats should be opened to allow steam to penetrate the entire object. To ensure sterilization is adequate, autoclave indicator tape should be used on the outside of a package and steam indicator strips should be included in each surgical pack and assessed prior to utilizing the instruments. It is recommended that the ICP have regular biological assessment of the practice autoclave whereby a commercially available bacterial spore impregnated strip is autoclaved then submitted for culture in a microbiology laboratory. If any bacterial growth is noted, use of the autoclave should be suspended and it should be thoroughly inspected and retested prior to use.

Laundry should be performed daily on site or by a commercial service. Laundry that is potentially contaminated with infectious organisms should be presoaked in bleach or appropriately discarded.

4.4.10   Surgical Preparation

Proper preparation of patients is essential to reduce the risk of surgical site infections. This distinct category of HAI has several known risk factors including length or invasiveness of the procedure, "dirty" procedures and placement of implants such as bone plates [4]. The most common bacterial pathogen causing surgical site infections in dogs is MRSP [4]. Proper patient and surgeon preparation protocols and checklists should be in place in every veterinary practice.

Patients should have their hair clipped at the surgical site using clippers immediately prior to moving into the operating room. The surgical site should be cleaned with an aqueous- or alcohol-based antiseptic such as chlorhexidine or povidone-iodine without inducing trauma to the skin. The surgical field should be draped with sterile drapes, with single-use disposable drapes being preferred.

The surgical team should always wear properly fitted surgical masks and caps that cover the head and clean surgical scrubs. Proper hand hygiene is critical to prevent surgical site infections. Antisepsis should be accomplished with 2–4 minutes of scrub time with an antiseptic product or an alcohol-based waterless product. Studies have found these procedures to be similarly effective, but the alcohol-based products have benefits including rapid onset of action, wider spectrum of action, fewer adverse effects, and decreased risk of contamination, making them the recommended presurgical hand hygiene scrub [3]. Sterile single-use disposable gowns are recommended and sterile surgical gloves should be changed every 60 minutes during a procedure [4].

Perioperative antibiotic prophylaxis decreases risk of HAI in veterinary patients, but there is not one accepted protocol for delivering these antibiotics. It is recommended that empiric antibiotic therapy be selected based on suspected pathogen contamination and be narrow spectrum to limit disruption of the patient's normal flora and prevent development of antimicrobial resistance [4].

4.4.11 Conclusion

Implementation of the ICP outlined here can decrease the risks of HAI. It is critical that all members of the veterinary team are educated on the importance of these principles and take a proactive approach to applying them in practice. Each veterinary hospital should have written protocols that reflect the needs of the individual hospital and personnel that are responsible for overseeing the ICP. By ensuring that all team members are trained on the principles of preventing pathogen entry into a patient population, exercising good patient handling techniques and proper cleaning and hygiene

practices, HAI can be minimized to the benefit of both patient and public health.

EXAMPLES

A 12-week-old male intact mixed-breed puppy was examined for acute onset of lethargy, vomiting, and diarrhea. The puppy was from a rescue situation and vaccination history was unknown. At the time that the appointment was made, the age, unknown vaccination status, and clinical signs were noted by the client services representative, and the owner was instructed to meet a veterinary team member in the parking lot and enter the building through a side entrance to an isolation examination room for evaluation. The veterinarian and team member who evaluated the puppy donned appropriate PPE including disposable gloves, gowns, and shoe covers. Good hand hygiene was practiced before and after each interaction with the puppy. The puppy was diagnosed with canine parvoviral enteritis and required hospitalization. The puppy was hospitalized in an isolation room and had dedicated equipment utilized. Upon recovery, the patient was discharged from the hospital and was transported out of the hospital on a gurney through the alternate exit. The isolation area was cleaned with soap and water then a disinfectant with activity against canine parvovirus was utilized once the patient was discharged from the hospital.

TAKE-AWAYS

- Hospital-acquired infections are infections associated with healthcare facilities and have significant patient and public health implications.
- Infection control protocols are imperative to limit the spread of infections within the hospital setting.
- It is recommended that designated personnel be trained in infection control and train other veterinary team members on proper protocols to limit HAI.
- Proper hand hygiene is one of the most important strategies to prevent HAI. Alcohol-based hand sanitizers are preferred over traditional soap and water hand washing protocols.
- Understanding pathogen transmission can help determine the precautions needed to prevent spread within a hospital.

MISCELLANEOUS

References

1 Stull, J.W., Bjorvik, E., Bubb, J. et al. (2018). 2018 AAHA infection control, prevention, and biosecurity guidelines. *Journal of the American Animal Hospital Association* 54 (6): 297–326.

2 Ruple-Czerniak, A., Aceto, H., Bender, J. et al. (2013). Using syndromic surveillance to estimate baseline rates for healthcare-associated infections in critical care units of small animal referral hospitals. *Journal of Veterinary Internal Medicine* 27: 1392–1399.

3 Sykes, J.E. (2013). *Canine and Feline Infectious Diseases.* St Louis, MO: Elsevier Saunders.

4 Verwilghen, D. and Singh, A. (2015). Fighting surgical site infections in small animals: are we getting anywhere? *Veterinary Clinics of North America Small Animal Practice* 45: 243–276.

Recommended Reading

Anderson, M.E.C. (2015). Contact precautions and hand hygiene in veterinary clinics. *Veterinary Clinics of North America Small Animal Practice* 45: 343–360.

Canadian Committee on Antibiotic Resistance. *Infection Prevention and Control Best Practices for Small Animal Veterinary Clinics.* www.wormsandgermsblog.com/files/2008/04/CCAR-Guidelines-Final2.pdf

Centers for Disease Control and Prevention. *Hand Hygiene in Healthcare Settings.* www.cdc.gov/handhygiene/index.html

Stull, J.W. and Scott Weese, J. (2015). Hospital-associated infections in small animal practice. *Veterinary Clinics of North America Small Animal Practice* 45 (2): 217–233.

4.5

Prevention and Control of Parasites

I. Craig Prior, BVSc, CVJ

College Grove, Brentwood, TN, USA

 BASICS

4.5.1 Summary

Prevention and control of parasites in dogs and cats is important to the concept of pet-specific care. By protecting the pet, we are in turn protecting the family, as many parasites can be zoonotic or vectors of zoonotic disease. The ultimate aim is to see every pet tested and every pet protected. Achieving this requires the commitment of the whole veterinary team to knowing the parasites, their life cycles (as it pertains to your area), the risk factors for exposure of the pet, the preventive products (including their mode of action, spectrum of action, safety profile, interactions, and costs), and compliance with the predetermined clinic protocol, which reveals the potential for improvement. Veterinary teams need to ask pointed questions and tactfully direct conversations with pet owners in order to better understand each situation and prescribe medications that will set the client up for success at home.

After a visit, it is critical that a hospital has multiple touch points with the client to follow up on the visit and set reminders regarding return visits and on time administration of medications provided. This improves client adherence to the hospital recommendations.

4.5.2 Terms Defined

Adherence: The extent to which patients take medications prescribed, involving the pet owner in filling and refilling the prescription; administering the correct dose,

timing and use; and completing the prescribed course. Adherence is a term applied specifically to medications; it does not refer, for example, to recommendations for wellness checks, diagnostic screenings, and so on.

Compliance: The extent to which pets receive a treatment, screening or procedure in accordance with accepted veterinary healthcare practices. Compliance involves both veterinary staff performing and/or recommending treatments, screenings and procedures, and pet owner follow-through.

Parasite: An organism that lives in (endoparasite) or on (ectoparasite) another organism (its host) and benefits by deriving nutrients at the host's expense

Recommendation: A suggestion or proposal as to the best course of action, especially one put forward by an authoritative body.

Vector: An organism that does not cause disease itself but which spreads infection by conveying pathogens from one host to another.

Zoonotic: Pertaining to a zoonosis; a disease that can be transmitted from animals to people or, more specifically, a disease that normally exists in animals but that can infect humans.

 MAIN CONCEPTS

4.5.3 The Need

Most pets will become infected with parasites at some point in their lives. This can include *in utero*, ectoparasitic infection, endoparasitic infection, or both – many of which may be zoonotic or involve zoonosis vectors. Parasites often cause one or more of the following more common clinical signs:

weight loss, malnutrition, anemia, vomiting, diarrhea, and respiratory signs. Vector parasites transmit diseases that may cause fever, lethargy, anorexia, weight loss, lameness, petechiae, neurological abnormalities, icterus, ocular abnormalities, epistaxis, muscle pain, and anemia.

Common parasites of dogs and cats include the following.

- *Coccidia*
- *Giardia* (some subtypes zoonotic)
- Hookworms (zoonotic)
- Roundworms (zoonotic)
- Tapeworms (some species zoonotic)
- Whipworms
- Fleas
- Heartworms (considered zoonotic in some countries)
- Lice
- Mites
- Ticks (vector zoonosis)
- *Toxoplasma* (zoonotic)

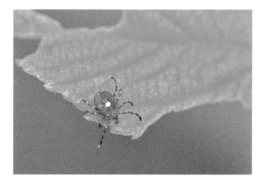

Amblyomma americanum female. *Source:* Image courtesy of Dr Michael Dryden.

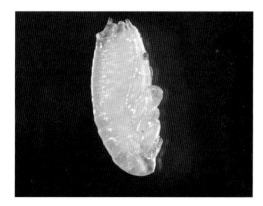

Ctenocephalides felis (flea) pupa. *Source:* Image courtesy of Dr Michael Dryden.

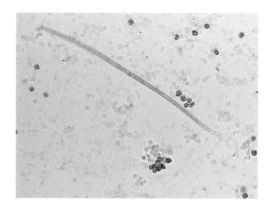

Dirofilaria immitis (heartworm) microfilaria. *Source:* Image courtesy of Dr Michael Dryden.

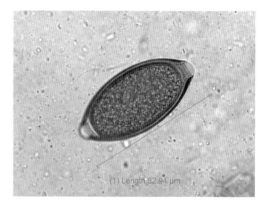

Trichuris vulpis (whipworm) egg. *Source:* Image courtesy of Dr Michael Dryden.

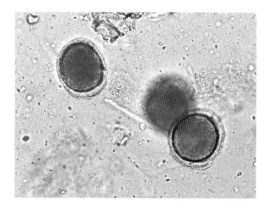

Toxocara canis (roundworm) eggs. *Source:* Image courtesy of Dr Michael Dryden.

Common vector-borne diseases of dogs and cats include the following.

- Anaplasmosis
- Babesiosis
- Bartonellosis
- Cytauxzoonosis

- Erhlichiosis
- Hepatazoonosis
- Leishmaniasis
- Lyme disease (borreliosis) (vector zoonotic)
- Rocky Mountain spotted fever (vector zoonotic)
- Trypanosomiasis (Chagas' disease)

4.5.4 The Products

There are a variety of preventive and treatment products available from many different companies. Products may be from different classes of drugs or chemical compounds. Within these unique classes, products may have different spectrums of activity, safety profiles, and indications. Most companies selling these products have local pharmaceutical representatives and professional service veterinarians available to help you better understand spectrum of activity, indications, mode of action, safety profile, drug interactions, and product costs.

4.5.4.1 Standards of Care and Recommendations

Practices should develop internal guidelines to ensure that clients receive consistent messaging and firm product recommendations (see 9.4 Standards of Care). Recommendations have a greater impact on clients compared to offering a variety of product choices. Clients are seeking expertise and knowledge from their veterinarian and want a firm recommendation whatever the subject. Parasiticides should be considered one of these medical recommendations. Standards should be determined by the veterinarians in the practice, taking into account the geographic location of the client, travel habits, parasite prevalence, and products available.

Many resources are available to aid in this endeavor. In the USA, there are several valuable resources (http://CAPCVET.org, http://petsandparasites.org, http://petdiseasealerts.org). In Europe, the European Scientific Counsel Companion Animal Parasites (http://ESCCAP.org) is available, as is the Tropical Council for Companion Animal Parasites (https://www.troccap.com) for the tropics and subtropics.

Other major parasitological societies are:

- American Society of Parasitology (http://amsocparasit.org)
- Australian Society of Microbiology (http://theasm.org.au)
- British Society for Parasitology (http://bsp.uk.net)
- European Federation of Parasitologists (eurofedpar.eu)
- German Society of Parasitology (dgparasitologie.de)
- Hungarian Society of Parasitologists (parazitak.hu)
- Japanese Society of Parasitology (jsp.tm.nagasaki, http://u.ac.jp/english)

- Science & Technology Australia (STA) (http://scienceandtechnologyaustralia.org.au)
- International Federation for Tropical Medicine (IFTM) (http://iftm-hp.org)
- World Association for the Advancement of Veterinary Parasitology (http://waavp.org)
- World Federation of Parasitologists (http://wfpnet.org)

Typically, there is no one product that can address all parasites that need to be controlled or eliminated; therefore, use of multiple products in combination may be necessary. Hospitals should be aware that although many products may provide similar coverage, there are subtle differences between them. For the economic health of the practice, not all products should be carried (product consolidation) and inventory management is an essential part of keeping clinic pharmacies profitable (see 9.10 Dispensing and Prescribing).

4.5.5 Compliance

Compliance is essential to successfully preventing and controlling parasites (see 9.17 Improving Compliance and Adherence with Pet-Specific Care). Noncompliance is the result of owners not giving or applying products on time, not refilling products, or not giving products year round (if appropriate). Results of noncompliance can be devastating to pets and can lead to potential resistance to products due to parasites being exposed to sublethal doses. Compliance is typically quantified as:

- doses/year (if using a monthly product)
- months/year (e.g., average client gives four months of heartworm preventive per year)
- percentage of clients on a preventive (e.g., 40% of clients use a heartworm product).

Most veterinary practices do not track compliance but instead rely on "guestimates," which tend to be overly optimistic. Compliance testing reveals opportunities for the practice – this could be described as "found" business or business opportunity. Increasing compliance requires staff training and consistent messaging. Some tools and strategies for achieving this include:

- "One Voice, One Message" concept
- improving reminder systems
- linking products to reminders and full use of reminder systems whether text, email, postcard, etc.
- use of client engagement strategies to remind clients of the risks of unprotected pets (see 10.3 Pet-Specific Outreach). These may include social media posts (Facebook, Twitter, Instagram, Snapchat), posters, handouts, mailings, emails,

text messages, reminders (postcard, email, text), YouTube videos, in-house seminars, etc. (e.g., Companion Animal Parasite Council (CAPC) monthly Facebook posts showing monthly county prevalence for practice chosen parasites, or http://petdiseasealerts.org to see the upcoming 30 day forecast)

- product consolidation as too many products on the shelf lead to staff and client confusion.

Compliance testing should be run promptly every six months and reviewed at management meetings to determine the effectiveness of campaigns, messaging, and execution.

4.5.6 Staff Training

Clients should receive specific, firm recommendations from the hospital team instead of a list of choices. Recommendations are based upon concepts of best medicine, and are limited, concise, and consistent. When provided with too many choices, clients can become confused, overwhelmed, and may turn to the internet for additional but noncurated information (see 9.8 Ensuring Consistency of Care). The hospital team must adhere to the "One Voice, One Message" principle – all team members, whatever their position in the practice, must be on the same page, educated on the key points, key messages, and key client "take-aways." Formulating and regularly reviewing a set of key customer questions often helps staff members lead clients to key recommendations of services or products. For example, "What's your tolerance to fleas and ticks (and mosquitoes)?" The client's answer is typically: "None." The staff member's reply should be: "Then we recommend (product X)." Additionally, asking the client what they currently use on their pet and when they last gave or applied it helps to determine the level of client adherence and allows the staff to then make better recommendations.

4.5.7 Client–Staff Interaction

Asking open-ended questions helps determine the ability, wants, and needs of the client. A few examples of open-ended questions in regard to parasiticide control and prevention follow.

- Tell me what's important to you regarding parasite control.
- Can you tell me what parasites your pet may come in contact with in this area?
- What is your tolerance for fleas and ticks (and mosquitoes)?
- What do you know about flea and tick-borne diseases?
- How often does your cat/dog go outside?

- What kind of lifestyle does your pet have?
- How often does your pet travel with you and to where?
- How do you think (pet's name) is responding to . . .?
- How many doses of XYZ parasiticide do you have left for (pet name)? This question helps identify client adherence. Asking it in this manner may help bring out the truth in a less "shaming" manner than asking them if they are giving a monthly medication on time every time.

Once the pockets of resistance are identified, then solutions may be implemented or strategies developed to overcome them. Coming to these solutions and strategies together – the veterinarian firstly with education then a medical recommendation and client with their level of comfort and ability to implement them – improves adherence and compliance to the desired treatment plan. Other solutions that improve adherence include client education resources (web-based, videos, printed handouts, brochures or longer in-person discussions), financing options for more expensive procedures, pet insurance, wellness plans, smartphone apps for medication reminders, longer acting medications and/or different administration options (included simple treat based administration), in-hospital vs home care options, house call options or even referral.

Clients should always be asked to bring all medications (including parasiticides and supplements whether prescribed by the hospital or obtained elsewhere) that the pet is on to the biannual wellness exam. This helps reveal the extent of client adherence, as well as parasiticides being purchased outside the hospital.

After a patient visit, following up with the client is crucial. The veterinary support team should call/text/email the client around the time of the next dose to remind them of the importance of on-time administration. Many reminder services are able to accomplish this now, sending either a text or email to the client with a customized message, further freeing up the hospital staff.

 EXAMPLES

Example 1: A 4-year-old pet: biannual visit with immunizations.

The customer service representative (CSR) calls the owner 24–48 hours before the appointment to remind them of their appointment, and also to remind the owner to not feed their pet (making treats and a fear-free atmosphere more enticing), bring a fresh stool sample, and all medications including any heartworm/flea/tick medications being used (and any previous medical records if new to the practice). Before checking in, the CSR has already reviewed the patient record, noting that the patient has not been seen in 14 months, and the client had only bought a six-month supply of flea/tick and heartworm preventive at that time. The CSR greets the patient, then the client, asks the client if she brought all the pet's medications with her; the client obliges, and the CSR reviews and notes all the medications in the patient file. The CSR reaffirms that the patient is here for her wellness exam and states that her parasiticide preventives are needed and recommended year round, and will be refilled today. The nurse greets the patient, then the client, and escorts them to an exam room, where he collects a history, reviews the medications the owner brought, updating the medical record as appropriate and noting client adherence to long-term medications, including parasiticides. Here, open-ended questions should be utilized to gain a better understanding of any obstacles to adherence by the client.

Recommendations should be made. A treatment plan for the visit should then be reviewed. The treatment plan encompasses all wellness care needed, including appropriate bloodwork, intestinal parasite screen (centrifugation + fecal antigen test), heartworm testing, and vector-borne disease testing, as appropriate for patient, lifestyle, and geography. The treatment plan includes 12-month refills of parasiticides. The nurse also discusses the hospital online store, with autoship and discounts, as well as the hospital reminder app, and, per client interest and request, helps the client set up both.

Vital signs are collected, and the veterinarian summoned. The doctor provides a nutritional consultation, performs a thorough examination, verbalizing it as performed, and discusses findings. Life stage and lifestyle appropriate vaccinations are administered. The doctor then reaffirms the need for year-round flea/tick/heartworm/intestinal parasite control and prevention. Products the client is using are reviewed to ensure the broadest spectrum of coverage and client adherence. When there are obvious gaps, the doctor, through open-ended questions, guides the client to the clinic's product(s) of choice according to their standards of care. If product changes are to be made, the nurse dispenses per instructions and updates the patient record.

The client is preferably checked out in the exam room by the nurse, or at the front desk by the receptionist, and at this time, reminders are updated, the hospital online store prescription completed (with autoship of doses), reminder app updated, and rebates submitted.

Example 2: An 8-week-old pet: first visit to veterinarian. The CSR calls the owner 24–48 hours before the appointment to remind them of their appointment, and also to remind the owner to not feed their pet (making treats and a fear-free atmosphere more enticing), to bring a fresh stool sample and any vaccination records. The CSR greets the patient, then the client, asks the client for any vaccination history and adds it to the patient file. The CSR reaffirms that the patient is here for her wellness exam and states that parasiticide preventives are needed and recommended year round, and will be filled today. The nurse greets the patient, then the client, and escorts them to an exam room, where he collects a history and reviews the vaccination history. A treatment plan for the visit is then reviewed. The treatment plan encompasses all wellness care needed, including vaccinations, intestinal parasite screen (centrifugation + fecal antigen test), deworming, and parasiticides. The nurse also discusses the hospital online store, with autoship and rebates, as well as the hospital reminder app, and per client interest and request, helps the client set up both. Vital signs are collected, and the veterinarian summoned.

In addition to a full exam (verbalized) with appropriate vaccinations, intestinal parasite screen, behavior counseling, nutritional consult, appropriate life stage counseling, etc., parasites and zoonoses should be discussed, including specific product recommendations. The patient should be started on a monthly heartworm preventive with potential for broad-spectrum intestinal deworming and parasite control, and an ectoparasiticide with efficacy against fleas, ticks, and mosquitoes. Often due to the patient's growth potential, single, monthly, weight-appropriate doses can be dispensed at each visit until the patient's growth potential has been satisfied, at which time larger quantities can be dispensed. The doctor then reaffirms the need for year-round flea/tick/heartworm/intestinal parasite control and prevention. The doctor, through open-ended questions guides the client to the clinic's product(s) of choice according to their standards of care as well as determining the expected adherence by the client and changing recommendations if needed. If product changes are to be made, the nurse dispenses per instructions and updates the patient record.

The client is preferably checked out in the exam room by the nurse, or at the front desk by the receptionist, and at this time, reminders are updated, the hospital online store prescription completed (with autoship of doses), reminder app updated, and rebates submitted.

TAKE-AWAYS

- Every pet is at risk of parasites, and as an extension, so are the family members. Protecting the pet is part of a One Health strategy.
- The overarching goal should be: Every pet tested, Every pet protected, Every year, All year, All their lives.
- Clients look to veterinary professionals for a recommendation, not a choice.

- Practice-specific standards of care and training help staff members to reinforce desired parasite control goals for the clinic and patients.
- Compliance testing is an essential component of a successful program as it helps to improve pet protection.

MISCELLANEOUS

4.5.8 Caution

Pets 6 months of age or older should be tested for existing heartworm infections before being started on heartworm preventives.

Recommended Reading

Bowman, D.B. (2013). *Georgis' Parasitology for Veterinarians*, 10e. St Louis, MO: Elsevier.

Foreyt, W.J. (2013). *Veterinary Parasitology Reference Manual*, 5e. Ames, IA: Wiley.

Companion Animal Parasite Council (CAPCVET.org). https://capcvet.org/guidelines/general-guidelines

4.6

Role of the Microbiome

Natalie Stilwell, DVM, MS, PhD

College of Veterinary Medicine, University of Georgia, Athens, GA, USA

BASICS

4.6.1 Summary

Microorganisms maintain complex relationships with each other that may benefit or compromise their host. Recent technological advancements have helped the medical community to study the roles that microbial communities play in health and immunity.

4.6.2 Terms Defined

Commensal: A relationship in which one organism benefits from another organism without helping or hurting it.
Dysbiosis: An imbalance of microbial communities with potential negative consequences for host health.
Microbiome: The collective populations of microorganisms inhabiting a particular environment, including body surfaces and tissues.
Probiotic: A substance or preparation that stimulates proliferation of beneficial microorganisms.

MAIN CONCEPTS

4.6.3 The Microbiome Defined

The term *microbiome* describes the collective populations of microorganisms inhabiting a particular environment, including the body's surfaces and tissues. These microorganisms include bacteria, fungi, archaea, protists, and

viruses. Each species of plant and animal is believed to harbor a unique microbiome that has evolved over time to exist with and even benefit the host.

Early attempts to characterize microbial communities in humans and animals were limited to culture-based methods, which could isolate only a small percentage of organisms. The development of the polymerase chain reaction (PCR) in 1983 revolutionized the ability to study the genetic sequence of nearly any organism. Molecular tools, which continue to be preferred over other methods for detecting microbial communities, have revealed a greater diversity of human- and animal-associated microbial populations than previously thought.

In 2007, the United States National Institutes of Health launched the Human Microbiome Project (HMP) to study populations and biological properties of microbes inhabiting five major body regions: the airway, skin, oral cavity, digestive tract, and vagina. By comparing microbial communities of healthy and diseased individuals, HMP investigators observed that key changes in microbial populations occur with certain diseases, including inflammatory bowel disease and eczema. Another ongoing effort of the HMP is to generate a catalogue of the genomes of human-associated microorganisms.

Since the innovation of the HMP, research groups around the world have followed suit to study microbial communities of plants and animals. Microbiomes from many companion animal, livestock, and wildlife species have been characterized, and some animals (particularly mice) also frequently serve as models for human microbiome work.

4.6.4 Functions of the Microbiome

Researchers are only just beginning to understand the complexity of the microbiome. Each region of the body has distinct communities of microbes that may vary even among healthy individuals of the same species, depending on age, diet, genetics, living environment, and other factors. Despite these individual differences, the microbiome has core roles in host health and immune function.

First, the microbiome modulates the immunity of the host by influencing the innate and adaptive immune responses. In many cases, commensal microbes provide a physical barrier protecting the host environment against invasion by pathogenic organisms. Some commensal microbes also competitively inhibit opportunistic pathogens from binding to specific cell receptors.

The microbiome also helps optimize nutrient assimilation by the host, particularly in the gastrointestinal tract. For example, cattle rely on healthy microbiota in the rumen for the breakdown of consumed plant material into proteins, short-chain fatty acids, and other nutrients that can be digested.

4.6.5 Microbiomes of the Body

The HMP and other studies have identified several unique microbiome regions throughout the body, including the respiratory, integument, and gastrointestinal systems.

Commensal microorganisms inhabiting the upper respiratory tract (URT) act as a first line of defense against pathogens by outcompeting them for cellular binding sites. The URT microbiome is distinct from that of the lower respiratory tract (LRT), and certain URT bacteria (such as *Staphylococcus* and *Streptococcus* spp.) may cause disease after migrating to the LRT. Human studies show that URT microbial populations in young children and the elderly differ from those of adults, which may contribute to an increased risk of respiratory infections in the very young and old. This factor likely holds true for many other mammalian species.

Microbial cells in the mammalian gastrointestinal system are so numerous that they outnumber host cells 10 to 1. Most microbes in the canine and feline gastrointestinal tract are bacteria (97–98%), while the remaining 2–3% include fungi, archaea, protists, and viruses. Species diversity and abundance are greater in the large intestine than the small intestine, while the acidic environment of the stomach favors growth of relatively few bacterial types.

Microbial populations are frequently altered in individuals with gastrointestinal diseases. Some enteric bacteria may produce toxins or trigger inflammatory processes that impair host immunity and allow for secondary bacterial invasion into the tissue. HMP studies have also determined that gut microbiota can influence the development of nonenteric diseases (e.g., allergic airway disease, obesity, and diabetes) and mental health disorders (e.g., depression and anxiety).

Each cutaneous and mucocutaneous region of the skin has a distinct microbiome affected by temperature, pH, moisture, and living environment. Canine studies show that haired areas have more diverse microbial communities compared to mucosal or mucocutaneous junctions, and disease is associated with a greater bacterial diversity [1].

4.6.6 Maintaining a Healthy Microbiome

Much attention has been given to the adverse effects of broad-spectrum antibiotic administration on the microbiome. With global pressure to reduce indiscriminate antibiotic usage, there is an urgent need to study the acute and chronic effects of antibiotics on microbial communities. As dysbiosis is a frequently reported issue, commercial tests to examine microbiome status are gaining popularity in human and veterinary medicine. While these tests are still in the early stages of development, investigators are using data from the HMP and other studies to determine if certain microbiota may be useful biomarkers for diagnosing or monitoring recovery from dysbiosis.

Several treatment options have also been developed to maintain or restore a healthy microbiome. These involve supplementing or transplanting beneficial microorganisms from a healthy to a diseased individual. Oral probiotic supplements have become increasingly popular in recent years and are largely marketed to encourage healthy microbial populations in the intestinal tract. Oral probiotics include high concentrations of "beneficial" enteric bacteria and are typically incorporated with dietary and lifestyle changes to optimize digestive health.

Various methods to transfer microbes between individuals have also been used in veterinary medicine. For example, fecal microbiota transplantation involves transferring a healthy donor's stool into the colon of an individual suffering from disease, such as *Clostridium difficile* colitis [2]. A similar procedure, rumen transfaunation, has been performed in cattle since the 1700s, long before microbial function was understood. In this procedure, rumen fluid from a healthy animal is orally administered to restore digestive function in an ailing patient.

4.6.7 The Future of Microbiome Work

Molecular technology is advancing at a rapid rate, but the exact role of the microbiome in animal health and immunity is still unclear. For example, while genome-sequencing software may identify microorganism populations within a sample, the clinical significance of these findings can be difficult to ascertain. Multiple national and international associations and meetings are now devoted to sharing and understanding the latest developments in microbiome work, and targeted research using the microbiome as a tool for overall patient health is expected to continue.

EXAMPLES

Charlie is a 12-month-old neutered male Weimaraner who presented to ABC Animal Clinic with a one-day history of diarrhea. The owners shared that Charlie had gotten into the kitchen trash and consumed leftovers from the family's chicken dinner. They admitted this was not the first episode of indiscriminate feeding for Charlie and that he regularly exhibited soft stool, despite acting otherwise healthy and active. Contrast radiography, blood work, and fecal examination ruled out parasitism or foreign body ingestion. The attending veterinarian instituted at-home treatment for intestinal dysbiosis likely due to indiscriminate feeding. The hospital team provided a probiotic paste specifically formulated for canine gastrointestinal health, which was administered orally twice daily with food until stool was normal. They advised feeding a bland diet until diarrhea resolved, after which Charlie was restricted to a diet of high-quality dry kibble that was supplemented with probiotic powder once daily. During a follow-up phone call two weeks later, the owners reported an excellent treatment response, including a complete resolution of gastrointestinal issues.

TAKE-AWAYS

- Resident microbial communities consisting of bacteria, fungi, archaea, viruses, and protists, known as the "microbiome," play an important role in patient health.
- The National Institutes of Health (NIH) HMP, a global collaborative effort using molecular methods to examine microbial populations in healthy and diseased human patients, has revolutionized understanding of the microbiome.
- Each region of the body, including the gastrointestinal tract, skin, and respiratory tract, has a distinct microbiome that can be affected by an animal's immune status, lifestyle (including diet and habitat), and medications.
- Dysfunction or dysregulation of the microbiome has been implicated in the development of many veterinary diseases, though the mechanisms are often poorly understood.
- Treatments for microbiome dysfunction that aim to supplement or transplant "good" microbiota to ill patients are becoming increasingly popular.

MISCELLANEOUS

References

1 Rodrigues Hoffmann, A., Patterson, A.P., Diesel, A. et al. (2014). The skin microbiome in healthy and allergic dogs. *PLoS One* 9 (1): e83197.

2 Van Nood, E., Vrieze, A., Nieuwdorp, M. et al. (2013). Duodenal infusion of donor feces for recurrent *Clostridium difficile*. *New England Journal of Medicine* 368 (5): 407–415.

Recommended Reading

Hoffman, A.R., Proctor, L.M., Suretta, M.G., and Suchodolski, J.S. (2016). The microbiome: the trillions of microorganisms that maintain health and cause disease in humans and companion animals. *Veterinary Pathology* 53 (1): 10–21.

Markel, M., Berghoff, N., Unterer, S. et al. (2012). Characterization of fecal dysbiosis in dogs with chronic enteropathies and acute hemorrhagic diarrhea. *Journal of Veterinary Internal Medicine* 26 (3): 765–766.

National Institutes of Health. Human Microbiome Project. www.commonfund.nih.gov/hmp

4.7

Embracing Early Detection

Lowell Ackerman, DVM, DACVD, MBA, MPA, CVA, MRCVS

Global Consultant, Author, and Lecturer, MA, USA

 ## BASICS

4.7.1 Summary

Early detection is one of the core principles of pet-specific care. The early detection of issues allows the veterinary team to provide clients the most options for veterinary care, and often with a better prognosis than waiting for the condition to become more advanced.

4.7.2 Terms Defined

Accounts Payable: Monies owed by a practice to its creditors (laboratories, distributors, etc.).

Cascade of Care: The increasing array of tests that may be attempted when trying to understand an abnormal laboratory result that may be spurious. The term is also used to describe the different sequential aspects of care in the management of a complex disorder.

Dynamic Laboratory Testing: A testing format in which multiple samples are collected over a period of time to assess function (e.g., adrenocorticotropic hormone [ACTH] stimulation testing).

Healthspan: That portion of the lifespan during which the pet remains in good general health.

Screening: Testing for disease or disease precursors in seemingly well individuals for the purposes of early detection of subclinical disease.

Subclinical: Referring to a condition which has not yet advanced to the stage where there are readily evident clinical signs.

 ## MAIN CONCEPTS

Veterinary teams should endeavor to identify potential problems at the earliest possible opportunity, when there are typically the most options available for management. Sometimes it might even be possible to change the course of disease with early intervention. For example, there are often differences between the way veterinary teams and human medicine teams approach the issue of diabetes mellitus. In veterinary medicine, a diagnosis is typically not rendered until the patient has clinical evidence of disease, often with polyuria, polydipsia, polyphagia, and perhaps the pet starts having "accidents" in the house. In human medicine, this would likely not be considered proactive medicine. The goal in human medicine is to identify the "prediabetic," when intervention is more likely to change the course of the disease, and potentially even avoid the onset of clinical signs of diabetes and its consequences.

One of the main issues that veterinary teams contend with is that most pets (at least in the United States) are not covered by pet health insurance (see 10.16 Pet Health Insurance), and so running early detection tests also involves financial discussions with pet owners (see 5.11 Discussing Finances for Pet-Specific Care). Because of this, some team members might feel that they cannot justify spending money on tests if the pet looks healthy. This is understandable in one sense, but means that it will never be possible to identify a problem when it is still subclinical . . . if it is necessary to wait for a patient to become clinical for any testing to be done. Teams need to reconcile the desire to save clients money with the very real value associated with identifying problems earlier than otherwise, and having many more medical management options available, which are very much in the best interest of clients and pets. Saving clients money is laudable, and inappropriate testing can unfairly inflate the cost of care, but this can be mitigated by reflecting on the value of proposed testing, and proceeding when there are legitimate reasons to do so.

From a hospital management standpoint, sometimes practices worry about their laboratory expenses increasing and try to limit testing as a way of decreasing accounts payable. It is always good to manage expenses, but laboratory expenses are not like utilities, where decreasing expenses can be associated with conservation. Every laboratory expense should be associated with an invoiced item, so this expense is directly related to, and offset by, revenue generation. If the laboratory expense is increasing, it means that the team is running more diagnostics, hopefully as directed by hospital standards of care (see 9.4 Standards of Care) and thus should have generated sufficient income to pay for them. As long as testing is appropriate and in the best interest of the client and pet, rising laboratory expenses are not a cause for concern as long as there is a corresponding increase in laboratory revenue.

4.7.3 Practical Applications

If the hospital goal is to detect problems early, when there are the most options available for successful management, then there should be plans in place for sensible early detection of problems in both dogs and cats, purebred, hybrid, and mixed-breed.

In purebred dogs and cats, a sensible screening plan may be based on the information gleaned from history taking, risk assessment (see 2.7 Risk Assessment), physical examination, breed predisposition (see 3.13 Breed Predisposition), and genetic testing (see 3.4 Predicting and Eliminating Disease Traits). This same approach often applies to hybrids as well, where predisposition to disease has often been documented. Such screening can be used to test for clotting disorders, glaucoma, cardiac issues, dental disorders, diabetes mellitus, hypothyroidism, and even certain cancers. In fact, if breed predisposition to disease is taken into account (see 11.4 Heritable Health Conditions – By Breed), then it is possible to incorporate sensible screening into standards of care and personalized care plans (see 1.3 Personalized Care Plans).

Another issue that is evident with purebreds and hybrids is that certain testing may be more difficult to interpret because of breed peculiarities regarding reference intervals (see 3.14 Breed-Specific Variants in Laboratory Testing,

and 4.8 Pet-Specific Relevance of Reference Intervals). In these cases, rather than relying on reference intervals, it may be preferable to evaluate the pet with 3–5 samples taken during young adulthood, or in a period prior to when clinical problems typically first appear, and use those to create a "normal" reference interval for that particular pet. This is sometimes referred to as dynamic (rather than static) laboratory testing, including such procedures as ACTH stimulation or glucose tolerance testing. For example, some breeds tend to have low thyroid hormone levels (and some have higher levels of thyroid-stimulating hormone), even when they are not hypothyroid. In these breeds, it is easier to create a normal range by taking multiple thyroid profiles during young adulthood, and using those as a reference interval for determining legitimate changes to thyroid status over time. In an ACTH stimulation test, it is appreciated that single levels of cortisol are often not diagnostic, but stimulating maximal cortisol levels with ACTH helps confirm a diagnosis of hyperadrenocorticism (Cushing's syndrome) by comparing baseline levels to levels following stimulation.

For mixed-breed dogs and cats, it is harder to predict breed susceptibility to disease, although it is possible to garner some information from heritage genetic screening (see 3.19 Mixed-Breed Considerations). Otherwise, it makes sense to establish early detection schemes based on the conditions that are most prevalent in all dogs and cats, and test accordingly.

For all dogs and cats, it is advantageous to perform orthopedic screening (see 3.12 Orthopedic Screening), determine baseline values in young adulthood for hemograms, biochemistries, and urinalysis, consider preanesthetic testing (if more regular testing is not already scheduled), and evaluate more thoroughly as pets become seniors.

Diagnostic testing should have a positive impact on diagnostic and treatment decisions made by veterinary healthcare teams, especially when they are based on sensible criteria. In doing so, it is important not to be led astray by the occasional spurious result, which may prompt some clinicians to investigate with more and more tests in what is sometimes referred to as a cascade of care. The goal is not to test for testing's sake, or to test even if it will not influence treatment approaches or outcomes, but to be proactive in keeping pets as healthy as possible for as long as possible, and testing preemptively based on a pet's specific risk factors. Accordingly, much of this testing is conducted in a pet-specific manner of trying to preserve healthspan more than lifespan. Thus, early detection can be used with lifestyle changes or surveillance to reduce the risk of disease, or to detect it early enough to treat it most effectively. As such, screening may not necessarily be diagnostic, but used to identify a subset of our patient populations who warrant further testing to determine the presence of absence of disease.

Another important feature of proactive testing is that the healthcare team typically then has access to sequential tests, the results of which might indicate trends. For example, pets do not become diabetic overnight. Their blood glucose values tend to trend upwards over time until they cross a threshold when the diagnosis of diabetes is warranted. Such testing allows teams to intervene earlier, when there are indications that the pet is trending toward becoming diabetic, when changes can be made to hopefully alter the course of the disease.

Once pets are diagnosed with some clinical disorder, they should participate in care pathways (see 9.6 Care Pathways), and this is typically associated with a different array of testing to help diagnose, treat, and monitor patients as accurately and quickly as possible. Patients with heart disease, cancer, kidney disease, and dental disorders are living longer and enjoying better health through the benefits of pet-specific care and personalized medicine. This tends to result in earlier diagnosis and treatment, better prevention, and better targeted therapy with fewer side effects.

There is no need to run every test in every circumstance. Testing is only indicated if there are actions that would be taken differently if testing results are known. However, it is also important to realize that this is the type of medicine most veterinary teams want to offer and pet owners appreciate receiving. Being constrained in our ability to provide value is what often leads to compromise fatigue (see 8.17 Dealing with Compromise Fatigue).

EXAMPLES

Percy Langston is a frisky 16-week-old intact male Persian kitten. Mrs Langston was very protective of Percy, and while she was at first hesitant to have genetic testing done according to the veterinarian's recommendations, she followed the directions of the hospital team at ABC Animal Hospital, and the testing was done at 12 weeks of age.

Mrs Langston was somewhat shocked to learn that Percy had a detectable variant for polycystic kidney disease (PKD) as she had spent a lot of money for him and he came with "papers." The veterinary healthcare team acknowledged that the result was not anticipated, but that it was the reason they recommended performing such testing in all pets at risk.

Dr Green explained that PKD is an autosomal dominant hereditary disease, so inheriting a problem gene from either parent is enough for pets to be affected. The cysts

tend to be present from birth and are small, but they can grow over time so will need to be monitored. Mrs Langston was concerned, but relieved to learn that most affected cats don't have clinical problems until middle age, and that the hospital would be monitoring the situation since the clinical course was quite variable. Dr Green provided a handout on PKD that set out an action plan for how the condition would be monitored, with laboratory testing and ultrasound, including tests that would detect the earliest hint of kidney disease.

Mrs Langston learned a lot about breed-related diseases, and also why it is so important to work with veterinary teams that are knowledgeable about such proactive care.

TAKE-AWAYS

- Early detection testing is meant to screen at-risk patients to determine problems when they are still subclinical.
- Identifying problems when they are still subclinical may provide veterinary teams with the ability to change the course of disease.
- Screening tests can be breed specific, but also can be generalized based on the early detection needs of all dogs and cats.
- Laboratory expense is not a liability that needs to be controlled; there should be offsetting revenue generated for every test run.
- Set appropriate expectations early, so clients know what type of testing is anticipated over a pet's life, allowing them to plan for it financially.

MISCELLANEOUS

Recommended Reading

Ackerman, L. (2020). Proactive Pet Parenting: Anticipating pet health problems before they happen. Problem Free Publishing.

American Animal Hospital Association. Promoting Preventive Care Protocols: Evidence, Enactment and Economics. www.aaha.org/globalassets/05-pet-health-resources/promoting_preventive_care_protocols.pdf

Dell'Osa, D. and Jaensch, S. (2016). Prevalence of clinicopathological changes in healthy middle-aged dogs and cats presenting to veterinary practices for routine procedures. *Aust. Vet. J.* 94 (9): 317–323.

Lewis, H.B. Healthy pets benefit from blood work. www. banfield.com/getmedia/1216c698-7da1-4899-81a3-24ab 549b7a8c/2_1-Healthy-Pets-benefit-from-blood-work

McKenzie, B. Why do we run diagnostic tests? www. veterinarypracticenews.com/why-do-we-run-diagnostic-tests

Paepe, D., Verjans, G., Duchateau, L. et al. (2013). Routine health screening: findings in apparently healthy middle-aged and old cats. *J. Feline Med. Surg.* 15 (1): 8–19.

Timsit, E., Leguillette, R., White, B.J. et al. (2018). Likelihood ratios: an intuitive tool for incorporating diagnostic test results into decision making. *J. Am. Vet. Med. Assoc.* 252 (11): 1362–1366.

Willems, A., Paepe, D., Marynissen, S. et al. (2017). Results of screening of apparently healthy senior and geriatric dogs. *J. Vet. Intern. Med.* 31 (1): 81–92.

4.8

Pet-Specific Relevance of Reference Intervals

Ryane E. Englar, DVM, DABVP (CANINE AND FELINE PRACTICE)

University of Arizona College of Veterinary Medicine, Oro Valley, AZ, USA

BASICS

4.8.1 Summary

Veterinary teams strive to maintain patient health, and identify and manage disease. History taking and physical examinations are important diagnostic tools but laboratory tests are often necessary for early detection of disease. Reference intervals (RIs) have been established for diagnostic tests to guide decision making and patient-specific care. Although RIs capture the majority of the population of a particular species, some patients have values that fall above or below the RI. Values may be truly abnormal or they may reflect a normal state for that particular patient – it is not always easy to decipher which is which. Establishing baselines for individual patients during times of health facilitates data interpretation when faced with clinical disease.

4.8.2 Terms Defined

Reference Interval (RI): A range that has been ascribed to a population of healthy adult animals for a given diagnostic test. Synonymous with reference range or normal range.

MAIN CONCEPTS

Reference intervals are provided for diagnostic tests to establish if a patient's result is normal, high, or low. If the patient's result is normal, is the value at the high or low end of the normal range? Values at either end may reflect preclinical disease. This patient may then benefit from serial diagnostic testing. Observing how values change over time facilitates early detection of disease among asymptomatic patients (see 4.7 Embracing Early Detection).

4.8.3 Establishing Reference Intervals

Reference intervals are established for a given species based upon extensive guidelines that have been outlined by the American Society of Veterinary Clinical Pathology. Even within a species, there can be marked variation; hence the recent trend toward breed-specific RIs (see 3.14 Breed-Specific Variants in Laboratory Testing).

Ideally, RIs are established by sampling healthy adults, taking care to include a relatively even distribution of breeds, sex, and sexual status [1]. In theory, samples should reflect the population of animals that you service. Unfortunately, establishing RIs for each clinic is impractical and cost-prohibitive. Most clinics rely upon previously published RIs, including those that are associated with in-house autoanalyzers.

4.8.4 The Statistics Underlying Reference Intervals

Reference intervals are typically reported in terms of means and standard deviations (SDs). The mean is the sum of every value in a data set divided by the number of values in the data set. It is essentially a calculated average, whereas SDs tell us how spread out the data are around the expected value, the mean.

A Gaussian distribution of data is often assumed, meaning that data are distributed symmetrically around the mean. This makes SDs easier to interpret.

Values that fall within two SDs of the RI constitute what is considered "normal" in 95% of the population [1]. Two-and-a-half percent of clinically healthy animals will fall above the high end of the RI and 2.5% of clinically healthy animals will fall below the low end of the RI [1]. In these cases, the veterinary team must decide if variations from normal are clinically relevant, and also if and when to become concerned.

4.8.5 Patient-Specific Varations in Reference Intervals

What may be "abnormal" on paper may in fact be "normal" for the patient. How do we approach patient values that stray from the RI? How do we decide if we need to take action or if it is appropriate to follow a "watch and see" approach?

Reference intervals are guidelines only. In the face of high or low values, the clinician must consider the following questions.

- Is the change in value a new finding for the patient?
- Is the change in value mild?
- Is the change in value known to be associated with pathology?
- In other words, if we do nothing, will this change be detrimental to the patient?

An isolated value, taken at a single point in time, may be diagnostic for a particular disease state. However, more often we must look at the complete clinical picture. Even better, we need to be open to performing serial testing to follow patient trends. Trends tell us if there a progressive climb or decline in one or more values of a data set.

Consider an adult domestic shorthair cat that has screening laboratory work performed at annual exams. The cat's serum blood glucose (BG) is consistently elevated (values below expressed in both mg/dL and mmol/L).

Age of cat (years)	Serum BG (mg/dL)	Serum BG (mmol/L)
1.5	198 (70–150)	11 (3.9–8.3)
2.5	205 (70–150)	11.4 (3.9–8.3)
3.5	202 (70–150)	11.2 (3.9–8.3)
4.5	193 (70–150)	10.7 (3.9–8.3)
5.5	211 (70–150)	11.7 (3.9–8.3)
6.5	352 (70–150)	19.6 (3.9–8.3)

The patient's BG has never fallen within the RI. This is not surprising for those with experience in feline practice. Stress hyperglycemia is a real phenomenon and is quite common in cats. However, at what point do we become concerned that the patient's elevated BG is a sign of something insidious, such as diabetes mellitus?

We start our investigation by asking if the patient's clinical signs match the change in value? Does the patient fit the clinical picture?

We must also consider the patient's record: what historically has been considered "normal" for the patient? In this case, serial testing provides significant clues. From 1.5 to 5.5 years old, this patient's BG was elevated, but static. The sudden spike at the cat's visit at 6.5 years old is a significant change.

4.8.6 Retest When Presented with Unusual or Unexpected Results

Retesting is an important diagnostic consideration. If ever you are in doubt that an abnormal test result is accurate, then repeat the test. Repetition will demonstrate if the identified "abnormality" persists or is progressing.

When in doubt, complete blood counts (CBCs) are often retested within 24 hours. Retesting for liver enzymes is typically delayed by 1–2 weeks.

4.8.7 The Impact of Panel Testing on Reference Intervals

Panel testing is when a group of diagnostic tests are performed on one or more samples to facilitate disease detection or patient monitoring. Common panel tests in companion animal practice include CBC, serum biochemistry, urinalysis, and thyroid profile.

In practice, panel testing is often viewed as advantageous by the veterinary team because it provides more information about the patient and attempts to paint a more complete clinical picture. In addition, panel testing offers rapid turnaround time for test results: you know all the results at once rather than waiting on outcomes from sequential tests.

Panel testing may also be more cost-effective for the client, who pays a one-time fee for a "package deal" rather than a fee for each test.

However, there is a price to pay for ordering diagnostic tests in bulk. Statistics tells us that 5% of patients that are truly "normal" for any given test will have a value that is outside the RI [1, 2]. When more than one test is performed on the same animal, the chance of having more than one "abnormal" result increases [3, 4]. One test out of every 20 on a panel for any given patient is likely to be "abnormal" on paper whether or not that "abnormality" is clinically relevant [3]. Having access to more information is therefore not always better.

False-positive results are challenging for the veterinary team to interpret. They also cause unnecessary anxiety among our clients. Clients may become focused on a small deviation from the RI that is inconsequential to the patient.

EXAMPLES

Each and every patient is unique. If we can identify what is considered "normal" for each patient early on in its life, then we will have a better sense of when to intervene and with how much urgency. There is great value to establishing baselines for individual patients before disease strikes (see 4.7 Embracing Early Detection). If we wait to perform baseline diagnostic tests until a patient succumbs to illness, then we may mismanage, if not misdiagnose, "borderline" patients.

Consider, for example, the senior cat that presents for nonspecific lethargy, reduced appetite, and intermittent vomiting. On physical examination, the patient is underweight, with muscle wasting along the epaxial muscles and caudal thighs. The patient appears to be adequately hydrated. If we have not taken care to establish a baseline in this patient in health and its serum biochemistry profile today reveals high-end blood urea nitrogen (BUN) and creatinine, then what do we do with these values? The patient's azotemia may be renal in origin and reflect early renal insufficiency. On the other hand, the elevations in BUN and creatinine may be red herrings; they may be "normal" for this patient. They may be unchanged values that he has lived with for years, rather than the root cause of his malaise.

TAKE-AWAYS

- Reference intervals are provided for diagnostic tests to help clinicians make educated decisions about whether a test result in a given patient is truly abnormal.

- Reference intervals are established using a large sample size of a given population of healthy adults of mixed ages, breeds, and sexes.
- For any given diagnostic test, 95% of the normal population is captured within two SDs of the mean for the established RI.
- Two-and-a-half percent of the normal population will have a value that falls above the RI, and 2.5% will have a value that falls below.
- Not all values that fall outside the RI are truly "abnormal"; each veterinary patient is unique. What may be considered off the chart in one individual is another individual's norm.

MISCELLANEOUS

4.8.8 Cautions

As diagnosticians, we all want access to the perfect test – the test that accurately diagnoses all disease, without false positives and false negatives. Unfortunately, no such test exists. Even tests that possess high sensitivity and specificity may not be "perfect" for the individual patient whose values just happen to fall outside the RI.

Because pet-specific variations in hematological and biochemical parameters exist, it is important to establish baselines early and revisit them regularly. In this way, you know what to expect for each patient in health, which facilitates diagnosis in the face of true disease.

References

1 Klaassen, J.K. (1999). Reference values in veterinary medicine. *Laboratory Medicine* 30: 194–197.

2 Tvedten, H.W. (1981). Hematology of the normal dog and cat. *Veterinary Clinics of North America Small Animal Practice* 11: 209–217.

3 Cornell University College of Veterinary Medicine. *Reference Intervals*. www.vet.cornell.edu/animal-health-diagnostic-center/laboratories/clinical-pathology/reference-intervals

4 Naugler, C. and Ma, I. (2018). More than half of abnormal results from laboratory tests ordered by family physicians could be false-positive. *Canadian Family Physician* 64: 202–203.

4.9

Periodontal Disease

Heidi B. Lobprise, DVM, DAVDC and Jessica Johnson, DVM

Main Street Veterinary Dental Clinic, Flower Mound, TX, USA

BASICS

4.9.1 Summary

Periodontal disease (PD) is one of the most common conditions affecting dogs and cats. The infection and inflammation associated with PD can not only cause oral discomfort and at times tooth loss, it has also been associated with systemic diseases (cardiac, renal, diabetes). Since it is for the most part preventable, dental care starting at a young age can impact the oral and dental health of our patients, as well as their overall health and quality of life. It is essential that small animal veterinary teams be able to identify and assess PD in order to provide optimal care. Preventive care with comprehensive oral cleaning, charting, radiographs, and polishing can be started at 1–2 years of age. Once disease has advanced, a variety of therapies can be provided to either help restore the health of the tissue around the tooth or to extract teeth where appropriate.

4.9.2 Terms Defined

Attachment Loss (AL): Loss of any periodontal tissues around the tooth (gingiva, bone, periodontal ligament (PDL), cementum).

Curettage: Removal of calculus, debris, and diseased soft tissue from a tooth surface using a hand instrument (curette).

Furcation Exposure (FE): Exposure of the space in between roots of a multirooted tooth that is normally covered by periodontal tissues (gingiva and bone).

Gingival Recession (GR): Loss of gingival tissue that, together with accompanying bone loss, can expose the root of the tooth and even the furcation of a multirooted tooth.

Gingivitis: Inflammation of the soft tissue immediately surrounding the tooth – the attached gingiva.

Hand Curette: Hand instrument with a rounded tip and curved back that can be safely introduced into a periodontal pocket (**PP**) to help dislodge or curette away calculus, debris, and even soft tissue from the surfaces in a PP.

Hand Scaler: Hand instrument with a sharp tip that can be used to help dislodge or scale calculus and debris from an exposed tooth/root surface; never to be used under the gum line.

Home Care, Dental: Any effort a pet parent can provide to help decrease the amount of plaque and calculus from forming on tooth surfaces; daily effective tooth brushing is optimal, with other methods including dental wipes and appropriate dental food, treats, and chews.

Horizontal Bone Loss: Loss of alveolar bone in a horizontal manner, lowering the ridge of alveolar bone across several roots or several teeth.

Periodontal Disease: Infection, inflammation, and loss of the tissues surrounding and supporting the teeth, including attached gingiva, bone, the PDL, and cementum covering the root.

Periodontal Ligament (PDL): Connective tissues that run between the tooth and bone (alveolar socket), supporting and keeping the tooth in the alveolus (socket).

Periodontal Pocket: The deepening of a sulcus depth due to the attachment loss of periodontal tissues, measured in millimeters.

Periodontal Probe: A hand instrument used to measure the depth of a pocket or amount of root exposure; marked in various millimeter increments, depending on type of probe.

Pet-Specific Care for the Veterinary Team, First Edition. Edited by Lowell Ackerman.
© 2021 John Wiley & Sons, Inc. Published 2021 by John Wiley & Sons, Inc.

Periodontitis: Inflammation of the periodontal structures.

Root Exposure: Exposure of the root of a tooth that is normally covered by periodontal tissues (gingiva and bone).

Root Planing, Closed (RP/C): Scaling, curettage, or debridement of a root without making a gingival flap to expose the area; calculus, debris, and diseased soft tissue are removed from the PP area.

Root Planing, Open (RP/O): Making a gingival flap with incisions and elevation (lifting the gingival tissue off the surface of the tooth and bone) for scaling or debridement of the exposed/visible portion of a root; calculus, debris, and diseased soft tissue are from the PP area.

Scaling: Removal of calculus and debris from a tooth surface using hand instruments (hand scaler or curette) or mechanical instruments (ultrasonic scaler).

Sulcus: The space that naturally exists between the tooth/root surface and the unattached edge of gingiva (free gingival margin).

Vertical Bone Loss: Loss of alveolar bone in a vertical manner, causing a wide separation between the root and adjacent bone.

MAIN CONCEPTS

Periodontal disease is the infection and inflammation of the tissues that surround and support teeth: attached gingiva (gums), alveolar bone (tooth socket), PDL (keeps the tooth in the socket), and the cementum on the surface of the root. The condition is mostly preventable but will be progressive if not identified and managed appropriately. Ultimately, teeth will be lost if this supporting tissue is lost, and in the process, other body organs can be affected by the inflammation and infection.

Soft plaque constantly accumulates on the tooth surfaces with bacteria that can cause active inflammation and can potentially lead to significant infection. If the plaque is not removed with home care (brushing or wipes), it hardens or mineralizes into calculus/tartar that cannot be brushed away. The tartar accumulates and has a rough surface to which more plaque can adhere. As more plaque and tartar accumulate, the infection in the periodontal tissues can lead to the destruction of these tissues around the tooth, resulting in gingival (gum) recession, bone loss, and eventual tooth loss. Often this tissue loss results in a PP, a pathological deepening of the normal space between the tooth and the gingival margin (sulcus). If this infection and inflammation affected just the periodontal tissues and teeth, that would be bad enough, but disease in the oral

cavity has been associated with disease in the rest of the body, such as the kidney, liver, lungs, and heart.

The initial oral examination of the awake patient can provide just an estimate of what may be encountered when a full exam (under anesthesia) is completed. With a cooperative patient, the amount of plaque and calculus can typically be evaluated, as can the extent of inflammation of the gingival tissue. It can be helpful to take a picture of the teeth with the owner's cellphone to point out the issues seen – plaque, calculus, discolored or broken teeth, tooth resorption, etc. Preliminary recommendations for therapy can be made on this basis (see 8.19 Team Strategies for Periodontal Disease).

The complete examination must be done with general anesthesia. Visual evaluation can more closely evaluate the extent of plaque and calculus accumulation (mild, moderate, heavy) which can be recorded by dental charting (see 8.11 Dental Charting). These observations to score the extent of the disease can be used, such as plaque index and calculus index (PI, CI). It is also important to record the extent of gingival and mucosal inflammation and ulceration (mild, moderate, extensive), including a gingival index (GI).

If there is any AL (loss of periodontal tissues), there will often be pockets formed along the teeth, between the tooth surface and the tissues, deeper than the normal sulcus (2–3 mm in a dog, 0.5 mm in a cat). PP depth is measured with a periodontal probe in millimeters (Figure 4.9.1). If roots are exposed due to loss or recession of gingival tissue and bone, this is also measured in millimeters.

When enough AL has occurred, support for the tooth is decreased. Determine if a tooth has mobility with gentle pressure. Record the extent of mobility from mild to extensive (M0–M3) and chart accordingly (see 8.11 Dental Charting). A Mobility Index (M) can be used to subjectively document the degree of movement.

Intraoral radiographs are critical to the ability to evaluate for PD. Determine the extent and type of periodontal bone

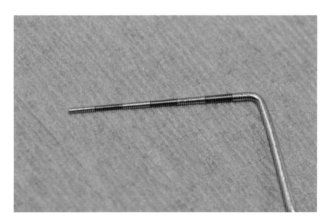

Figure 4.9.1 Periodontal probe.

loss. Use this, with other factors, to determine whether to treat periodontally or extract, and monitor for progression of disease.

The stages of PD are based on the extent of the AL (see 8.11 Dental Charting). Initial assessment of the amounts of plaque and calculus, and the degree of gingival inflammation or bleeding, is a precursory determination only. Complete assessment includes periodontal probing of pockets (areas of AL) combined with evaluation of intraoral radiographs to determine both the extent and pattern of bone loss.

In most cases, teeth are not all at the same level of PD, unless all teeth are very healthy (stage 1) or very diseased (stage 4). There may be a generalized stage 1–2 PD associated with most of the teeth with focal stage 4 PD at a few teeth.

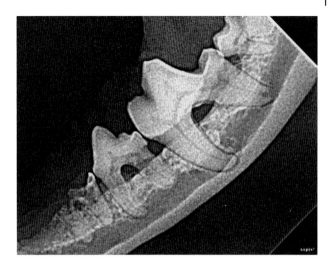

Figure 4.9.2 Horizontal bone loss.

4.9.3 Attachment Loss

If there is loss of the alveolar bone but the gingival height is maintained (minimal gingival loss), there will be a soft tissue PP formed that is deeper than a normal sulcus as the attachment level regresses down the root. If gingiva and bone are lost at the same rate, there will likely be exposed root due to the gingival recession (GR).

In a multirooted tooth, the AL may result in furcation involvement or exposure, assessed by advancing a periodontal probe into the space between roots, under the crown.

- FE1 – furcation 1 involvement; the probe extends less than halfway under the crown.
- FE2 – the probe extends greater than halfway under the crown.
- FE3 – the probe extends completely under the crown, through, and through – from one side out the other.

There can be a combination of GR/root exposure and a PP. The total AL would be the sum of the two measures; for example, PP 3 mm with GR 2 mm would be total AL/level at 5 mm. Horizontal bone loss across several teeth will likely result in either PPs at these teeth or GR with root exposure (Figure 4.9.2). Vertical bone loss at a tooth/root would be found as a deep probing depth straight down a tooth (Figure 4.9.3). The deeper the pocket, the more challenging treatment can be.

4.9.4 Stages of Periodontal Disease [1]

Teeth with stage 1 PD involve only gingivitis. There is no AL although gingival inflammation may result in a slightly deeper sulcus due to swelling and edema. With treatment,

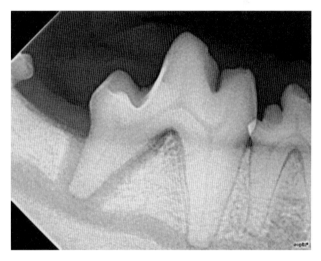

Figure 4.9.3 Vertical bone loss.

the inflammation should subside and the sulcus return to normal depth – this is the only truly reversible stage. Treatment includes complete dental assessment, cleaning, and polishing.

Teeth with stage 2 PD reflects early periodontitis, with up to 25% AL. There is mild to moderate GR with root exposure or moderate PP depth. Treatment includes complete dental assessment, cleaning, and polishing. Closed root planing of pockets up to 5 mm in depth is used to remove calculus, debris, and diseased soft tissue from the root surface and in the sulcus. A local antibiotic gel can be inserted into pockets following root planing/curettage.

Teeth with stage 3 PD involves moderate periodontitis, and 26–50% AL. It is necessary to decide whether to treat or extract, depending on the amount and type of AL. If the tooth is strategic (canine tooth, carnassial), it may be beneficial to perform periodontal therapy to salvage it. If the tooth is less strategic (lower incisor, second molar), extracting it will provide better access to treat an adjacent tooth more effectively.

Patient consideration is also relevant. Periodontal treatment requires additional anesthetic time with more frequent therapy and could still maintain a persistent infection/inflammation. A patient with increased anesthetic or systemic risk may be a better candidate for extraction.

Client concerns and potential compliance issues also need to be considered. Professional periodontal treatment must be followed with meticulous home care and regular retreatments at additional time and costs. Treatment involves complete dental assessment, cleaning, and polishing. Moderate pockets can be managed with closed root planing and placement of an antibiotic gel. For soft tissue pockets deeper than 5 mm, a gingival flap is raised to expose the defect, followed by open root planing with a hand scaler or curette, and suturing the flap closed.

For moderate to deeper pockets with neighboring teeth that are compromised, consider extracting the adjacent teeth to expose the tooth/root to be salvaged. This exposure allows better access for open root planning, debriding excess gingiva and diseased soft tissue (granulation tissue), and then suturing the flap closed. Make sure the remaining tooth is surrounded by healthy attached gingiva if possible. Sometimes the gingival edge will be positioned further apically (lower) on the tooth, potentially exposing some root surface, but the pocket depth will be decreased.

Evaluate for vertical bone loss (see Figure 4.9.3), especially at an important or strategic tooth (canine or carnassial tooth). Extract adjacent, diseased teeth if applicable. There is an option of placing bone graft and membrane to promote healing with bone and even PDL regeneration (guided tissue regeneration), optimally provided by a dental specialist.

Extraction should be considered in some instances. Remove the entire tooth and root if possible, especially if a PDL is visible radiographically. Do not just remove the tooth but manage the soft tissue as well to provide optimal healing. Raise a gingival flap for better exposure and release of tension during closure. Debride extraction sites so all diseased soft tissue and debris are removed. Surgical closure of extraction sites is recommended; be careful to ensure there is no tension along the suture lines.

Teeth with stage 4 PD have greater than 50% AL with extensive bone loss, tooth mobility, and compromised teeth. Treatment involves likely extraction with soft tissue management. If a strategic tooth has just over 50% AL with a specific pattern of AL (vertical bone loss at a root), it may be a candidate for tissue regeneration with advanced treatment attempted by a dental specialist. Furcation involvement increases the risk for the tooth, so the "stage" of PD is elevated (see 8.11 Dental Charting).

- FE1 – "upgrades" the stage to PD2
- FE2 – stage 3 PD
- FE3 – stage 4 PD

EXAMPLES

"M" is a 12-year-old female/spayed toy poodle with extensive PD: heavy plaque and calculus, gingival inflammation and infection and significant periodontal bone loss at many teeth. Overall health is good. M's owner has been concerned about anesthetic risks due to the pet's age but understands that general anesthesia is absolutely necessary for complete dental therapy. Her owner is currently undergoing chemotherapy and further discussion informed her that having less infection and bacteria in M's mouth would be a benefit for the owner as well. With complete evaluation, charting, cleaning, polishing, local, and regional blocks for pain management and constant patient monitoring (she remained stable throughout the procedure), 21 surgical extractions were performed, leaving M with eight teeth (others had been lost previously). Concerns about how she would eat were answered with instructions to feed a softer diet for 10–14 days, along with pain management at home.

While the first night was a little rough for M, by the next day she was eating fairly well, and even better by the next day. At our routine follow-up examination at two weeks, we were thanked profusely and heard how much better M was feeling – more alert and active, and definitely smelling better!

For the great majority of patients with substantial (and even minor) PD, even with systemic issues, the benefits of removing the constant infection, inflammation, and pain absolutely outweigh risks and concerns that can often be minimized with appropriate patient management.

TAKE-AWAYS

- Periodontal disease is a progressive infective, inflammatory disease with potential systemic consequences.

- In most cases, PD is preventable or at least manageable to decrease long-term impact.
- A combination of veterinary examinations, professional care, and home care is the best strategy to provide optimal oral and dental health.
- Complete treatment requires general anesthesia.
- Dental radiographs are essential.

MISCELLANEOUS

4.9.5 Cautions

With severe PD, bone loss can be so extensive that pathological fractures can occur.

Reference

1 American Veterinary Dental College. Stages of Pet Periodontal Disease. https://afd.avdc.org/five-stages-of-pet-periodontal-disease/

Recommended Reading

Eisner ER, Holmstrom SE, Frost Fitch P. *Veterinary Dental Techniques: For the Small Animal Practitioner*, 3 Philadelphia: Saunders, 2004.

Lobprise HB. *Five Minute Veterinary Consult: Clinical Companion – Small Animal Dentistry*, 2 Philadelphia: Wiley Blackwell, 2007.

Lobprise HB, Dodd JR. *Wiggs's Veterinary Dentistry, Principles and Practice*, 2 Philadelphia: Blackwell, 2019.

4.10

Environmental Considerations

Ryane E. Englar, DVM, DABVP (CANINE AND FELINE PRACTICE)

University of Arizona College of Veterinary Medicine, Oro Valley, AZ, USA

BASICS

4.10.1 Summary

Patient health is intimately connected to the environment. As animal health professionals, we often explore and prioritize those internal, patient-specific factors that predispose to, incite, or exacerbate disease. However, the environment also plays a key role in pet health. Environmental considerations are particularly valuable during comprehensive history taking. A patient's access or known exposure to toxins can precipitate disease. A solid understanding of basic pathophysiology facilitates our expedited treatment for presumptive toxicosis and can mean the difference between life and death of the patient. The environment also presents the additional challenge of thermal extremes. Hyperthermia and hypothermia are both possible presentations for companion animals, particularly those who may not be acclimated to either extreme. Furthermore, the environment provides a backdrop to infectious disease, which varies immensely depending upon geographical location. Environmental considerations are essential for the veterinary healthcare team, on whom the burden of diagnosis falls.

4.10.2 Terms Defined

Homeostasis: A "steady state" condition in which the body attempts to maintain itself in spite of external influences, so that core body functions and vital signs remain relatively constant.

Hyperthermia: Sustained elevation of core body temperature beyond that which is considered the normal reference range for the patient.

Hypothermia: Sustained depression of core body temperature below that which is considered the normal reference range for the patient.

Toxicosis: Illness that stems from absorption, ingestion, or inhalation of a toxin.

Toxin: Plant or animal-based poison or venom that causes disease if present at low levels within the body.

MAIN CONCEPTS

4.10.3 Thermal Challenges

The ambient temperature and humidity may challenge our patient's ability to maintain homeostasis. This is particularly true when the individual does not have the opportunity to acclimate to thermal extremes.

4.10.3.1 Heatstroke

Heatstroke is the result of pathological hyperthermia. The body is unable to dissipate heat sufficiently and core body temperature elevates. As the patient's temperature exceeds 40 °C (104 °F), central nervous system (CNS) functions are impaired. The patient may present with varying degrees of abnormal mentation that range from depression to delirium, or even coma. Convulsions may develop. Brain damage may or may not be permanent. Affected patients are often tachycardic. They may develop petechiae or demonstrate other evidence of internal bleeds, such as hematochezia. If hyperthermia is sustained, the patient risks multiorgan shutdown, cellular necrosis, and death.

Patients that are most at risk of heatstroke include those that experience hot, humid environments. Brachycephalic breeds are of particular concern because many have compromised airways. Common brachycephalic breeds include Boston terriers, Boxers, English, and French bulldogs, Pekingese, Shih tzus, and Pugs. These breeds have distinctly foreshortened faces but their associated soft tissue structures are not proportionally reduced. The result is excessive tissue that bulges into the airway lumen, where it may potentially cause obstruction. Airway compromise may be compounded by additional structural defects, including abnormal conchae, everted laryngeal saccules, and stenotic nares.

When dogs are exposed to hot, humid weather, they respond by panting to dissipate heat. Brachycephalic breeds may have difficulty releasing heat because of structurally and functionally abnormal airways (see 3.5 Conformation Extremes and the Veterinary Team). They are more likely to succumb to heatstroke, particularly if they are stressed and/or unable to escape the elements. Obesity also increases their risk for overheating.

Patients benefit most from proactive, as opposed to reactive, veterinary care. Clients need to be educated on how to reduce thermal stress, particularly when patients are overweight or brachycephalic, or both.

At-risk patients should not be confined to outdoor enclosures that lack shade or water. Enclosed environments, such as automobiles, are particularly deadly because the lack of airflow prevents convection cooling. Clients need to be reminded not to lock pets within cars on hot days.

When patients do require prolonged exposure to the heat, such as working dogs or athletes, they should be acclimated to the environment first.

4.10.3.2 Hypothermia

Hypothermia is a common complication of general anesthesia but it also results from prolonged exposure to cold temperatures. Short-coated animals and those at either extreme of age are most susceptible. Initial physiological responses to hypothermia are aimed at retaining heat through piloerection and peripheral vasoconstriction. The patient may also shiver in an attempt to generate heat.

As hypothermia persists and/or worsens, the patient becomes bradycardic, bradypneic, and mentally depressed. Ventricular arrhythmias are common. Ventricular fibrillation may develop, resulting in cardiac arrest.

Hypothermic patients benefit from well-controlled, monitored, active external and internal rewarming. As is true of hyperthermia, hypothermia carries a guarded prognosis, and prevention is the best medicine.

Clients must be educated as to what constitutes an inappropriate environment for patients. Patients should be maintained indoors during periods of extreme cold; if they cannot be, then they must be provided with a means of escaping the elements in an outdoor enclosure, as through a heated doghouse.

4.10.4 Toxin Exposure

In addition to climate and humidity, the outdoor (and indoor) environments provide access to any number of substances, some of which have the potential to be toxic if absorbed (via skin), ingested, or inhaled.

Toxicological emergencies are common events in companion animal practice. Dermal exposure occurs more commonly in cats; oral exposure occurs more commonly in dogs.

4.10.4.1 Nephrotoxins

Several toxins cause acute kidney injury (AKI) in companion animals, including ethylene glycol, lilies (in cats), grapes, and raisins (in dogs).

Ethylene glycol is the active ingredient of antifreeze. When ingested, ethylene glycol is metabolized by the enzyme alcohol dehydrogenase into the following toxic metabolites: glycoaldehyde, glycolic acid, glyoxylic acid, and oxalates. Oxalates bind with circulating calcium to form mineral deposits that occlude renal tubules [1]. This prevents urine formation, and patients present in oliguric-to-anuric renal failure [1]. In addition, patients typically present with changes in mentation that range from depression to stupor. If they are still ambulatory, patients may also present for ataxia.

Lilies within the genera *Lilium* and *Hemerocallis* are also nephrotoxic. These include Asiatic, day, Easter, stargazer, and tiger lilies. The pathophysiology of lily toxicosis is incompletely understood but cats appear to be sensitive to all parts of the plant, including the pollen [2]. Even mere ingestion of water from a vase that contains a lily may result in toxicosis [2]. Affected patients are depressed and may present with hypersalivation, decreased appetite, and vomiting. Swollen, painful kidneys also develop as a result of AKI. Patients will be moderately to severely azotemic. Tubular damage is evident on urinalysis in the form of cylindruria, proteinuria, and glucosuria.

The ingestion of red and white, crushed, and fermented grapes and raisins also induces AKI in some, but not all dogs [3]. The pathophysiology of this toxicosis is incompletely understood but affected patients present in similar fashion to cats that have ingested lilies; gastrointestinal (GI) and renal signs predominate.

4.10.4.2 Cardiac Toxins

Several toxins cause cardiotoxicity among companion animals, including *Taxus* spp. In landscaping, *Taxus* spp. are known as yews. Yew ingestion by livestock and dogs has been reported to cause death due to its cardiotoxic taxine alkaloids. Taxines are maximally concentrated within the plant over the winter months, and dried yew remains toxic for months.

Taxines block sodium and calcium channels within myocytes. This suppresses the contractility of the heart through depression of both sinoatrial (SA) node automaticity and impulse conduction through the atrioventricular (AV) node. In addition, vascular smooth muscle contraction is inhibited, causing arterial vasodilation. If unchecked, this leads to systemic hypotension.

Patients may present with a history of collapse. They are often bradycardic, with characteristic changes on electrocardiogram (ECG) that include absent P wave and/or increased QRS complex duration. Patients may also spontaneously die. Diagnosis may be based on necropsy. Yew fragments may be discovered in the digestive tract or the necropsy may reveal myocarditis, with nonspecific pulmonary edema and congestion.

Lily of the valley, *Convallaria majalis*, also causes cardiotoxicity. Plant material contains cardiac glycosides, which are arrhythmogenic. Affected patients develop bradycardia, which can be significant. They may also develop GI distress and/or seizures. Sudden death is possible.

4.10.4.3 Neurotoxins

Several toxins cause neurotoxicity among companion animals, including heavy metals, such as lead. Paint and paint dust that results from household renovations are primary sources of lead exposure for companion animals but lead may also be found in pipes, solder, putty, caulk, curtain weights, and ceramic glazes. The older the house, the more likely it is to harbor lead-containing components.

Outside the home, companion animals may be exposed to lead through ingestion of bone meal supplements, fishing weights, and automobile batteries.

Lead toxicosis most often affects the nervous system. Nervous system signs are nonspecific but affected patients may present with ataxia, blindness, depression, mydriasis, or convulsions. Ingestion of lead may also impact the GI tract. Affected patients may present with acute abdomen. They are often anorexic and may develop constipation, vomiting, or diarrhea.

4.10.4.4 Carcinogenic Toxins

Several toxins do not cause immediate harm to companion animals but chronic exposure may elevate the risk of other pathologies. For example, malignant lymphoma is a relatively common occurrence in cats. Cats that reside in smoking households are at increased risk for development of lymphoma compared to those that do not [4]. Environmental tobacco smoke (ETS) also increases the risk that oral squamous cell carcinoma (SCC) will develop in cats [5].

4.10.4.5 Other Toxins

Appreciate the diversity of habitats in which our companion animals reside, and recognize that all environments have the potential for toxin exposure. Unusual patient presentations should raise the index of suspicion that toxicosis is possible, and clients should be queried about patient surroundings.

- What does the patient have access to?
- What, if anything, could the patient have gotten into?
- Has anything changed about the patient's indoor and outdoor housing?

Cases involving toxicological exposure often present as emergencies. When these situations present themselves clinically, it is critical that the veterinary team consider the environment as a potential cause, and institute empirical therapy as soon as possible.

4.10.5 Other Reasons to Pet-Proof the Home

Dogs and cats are naturally inquisitive and can get into trouble easily, particularly if they are unsupervised. When pets are introduced into the home, we often hover over them as they explore their new surroundings. However, as they age, they are often increasingly left to their own devices. This is potentially asking for trouble.

Pet-proofing the home is essential to keep pets safe because all ages, not just puppies and kittens, are at risk. Pets typically explore their environments with their mouths, and may be tempted to ingest items, even those that are not intended to be food.

Ingestion of table scraps is likely if garbage is not secured or if used dishes are left in the sink. At best, this provides a source of additional calories for the pet, and may lead to weight gain over time, if food seeking becomes a pattern. At worst, ingestion of people food may precipitate acute gastritis, enteritis, gastroenteritis, colitis, hemorrhagic gastroenteritis (HGE), or pancreatitis, all of which are likely to require medical care.

Vomiting, diarrhea, abdominal pain, and/or anorexia are common presenting complaints. On physical examination, patients are likely to exhibit varying degrees of dehydration. They may exhibit abdominal splinting.

Ingestion of food and nonfood items may lead to foreign body obstruction or even bowel perforation. Corn cobs and peach pits are common sources of obstruction that require exploratory laparotomy. Gastrotomies and enterotomies are commonly performed in clinical practice to alleviate obstruction. Bowel resection with anastomosis may be necessary and depends upon both the duration of the obstruction and the apparent viability of the gut.

Linear foreign bodies present additional challenges to the surgeon. String, cords, fabric, and tape may become caught underneath of the tongue. When swallowed, these items often become lodged at the pylorus. Peristaltic movement of the intestines forces the nontethered end to move forward in the digestive tract. Because one end reminds behind, at the pylorus, the intestines plicate. This often results in extensive intestinal damage and intestinal perforation is likely. When this occurs, septic peritonitis is probable. Multiple enterotomies and/or resections may be required to remove compromised bowel.

To minimize the chance for foreign body ingestion and subsequent obstruction, the following items should be placed out of reach.

- Shoes
- Laundry
- Sewing needles and thread
- Low-lying décor
- Electrical cords
- Telephone wires
- Medications, cosmetics, and lotions
- Garbage and trashbags, particularly those with drawstrings

Other means of pet-proofing include keeping toilet lids in the closed position at all times when the bathroom is not in use, to prevent ingestion of toilet bowl water and/or toilet bowl cleaners. Heating and air ducts should be covered with appropriate registers and/or air vent covers. Likewise, any nooks and crannies should be closed off and/or sealed to prevent pets from escaping into unreachable spaces.

If pets have access to the garage or storage areas, then all chemicals must be confined to pet-proof cabinets or high, out-of-reach shelving. Clients may have childproof cabinets installed to prevent access to cleaners, oils, paints, and poisons, such as rodenticide and ethylene glycol.

Entrance/exit doors should be secured at all times to prevent escape. Doors should be closed cautiously to prevent tails from getting caught as doors slam shut. Tails are not heavily muscled, so any injuries sustained are likely to involve degloving, coccygeal vertebral fractures, and/or compromised blood supply to the tail. When the blood supply is damaged, the tail may become necrotic, necessitating amputation.

Doors within the interior of the house may be used as barriers to limit pet access to rooms that are unsafe. For example, closing the door to a child's bedroom or playroom

is an easy way to limit the pet's exposure to nonfood items that might be ingested. When pets are granted entry to bedrooms, closet doors should be secured to limit exposure to fabric, belts, socks, shoes, and shoelaces.

Baby gates may be effective barriers for small-breed dogs, particularly at entranceways, where dogs may be tempted to bolt outside as people enter and exit from the house.

4.10.6 Exposure to Infectious Diseases

Some environments foster disease. Consider the following three examples.

4.10.6.1 Borreliosis

Borreliosis is a tick-borne disease. Environments that support ticks – *Ixodes scapularis*, *I. pacificus*, and *I. dammini* – reflect higher incidence of disease.

Host response to disease is variable. Lyme disease may be subclinical but it more often presents as acutely debilitating, cyclical, or chronic disease. Dogs and cats may develop nonspecific signs of malaise, including fever, lethargy, and lymphadenopathy, followed by shifting leg lameness. Golden retrievers, Labrador retrievers, and Bernese mountain dogs appear to be predisposed to Lyme nephritis, which is a type of AKI that is often fatal.

4.10.6.2 Leptospirosis

Leptospirosis is another geographically dependent disease. *Leptospira* spp. are shed in the urine of infected animals. Infected urine contaminates the environment and perpetuates the life cycle through the infection of new hosts. For example, infected water exposes dogs that swim in lakes or reservoirs. Exposure to wildlife and, by extension, their urine can also lead to infection. For this reason, both country and city dogs are at risk.

Leptospirosis is more prevalent in regions that experience high levels of rainfall. Outbreaks notoriously follow wet weather. Within North America, the peak season is autumn. *Leptospira* spp. are inactivated by freezing conditions. *Leptospira* spp. are distributed worldwide, and the geographical distribution of leptospirosis within the US is expanding.

Affected patients may present with clinical signs that are suggestive of AKI, hepatic failure, or both.

4.10.6.3 Systemic Fungal Infections

Systemic fungal infections are regional. Patients that live in endemic regions are at increased risk of contracting disease. Patients that reside along the Mississippi, Missouri, and Ohio River valleys are most at risk for contracting blastomycosis. Infection by *Blastomyces dermatitidis* results in fungal pneumonia. Affected dogs may also present with lymphadenopathy or nasal depigmentation, GI, ocular, and/or neurological signs.

Histoplasmosis also concentrates around the Ohio, Missouri, and Mississippi rivers.

Infection in companion animals is thought to occur when patients inadvertently inhale microconidia. The yeast replicates in the lower respiratory tract but infection may spread through blood or lymph. Affected patients may present for fungal pneumonia, cutaneous lesions, behavioral, or vestibular disease.

Coccidioidomycosis, otherwise referred to as valley fever, prefers the arid soils of the southwestern US. When the soil is disrupted by heavy rains, *Coccidioides* sporulates. Inhalation of arthroconidia leads to infection of susceptible hosts. Infection develops within the respiratory tract first. Generalized pneumonia may be severe. Valley fever may also cause infectious pericarditis, lameness, blindness, aberrant behavior, and seizure activity that is caused by CNS involvement.

EXAMPLES

Vulpes is a 5-year-old male castrated Basenji dog that presents for evaluation of acute right thoracic limb lameness. The patient has been lethargic for the past week and his appetite is "off." The patient is resentful of right carpal manipulation but the remainder of the physical examination is unremarkable. A minimum database demonstrates mild hypoalbuminemia and hyperglobulinemia. Thoracic limb radiographs demonstrate a lytic lesion at the distal right radius. Primary bone neoplasia is possible but unlikely, given the age and breed. Because the patient resides in Arizona, a differential diagnosis of coccidioidomycosis (valley fever) is prioritized. Serological testing is performed, and the patient has positive IgM and IgG titers. Long-term treatment with itraconazole is initiated in addition to an analgesic agent. The patient is responsive to therapy.

TAKE-AWAYS

The environment affects patient health.
- History taking is essential to paint a complete picture of the patient's living conditions.
- Indoor and outdoor surroundings may provide a patient with access to one or more toxins.

- Toxicological emergencies are common in companion animal practice and require expedited treatment in the face of many unknowns.
- Environmental considerations include potential exposure to thermal stress as well as to infectious diseases that are endemic to particular geographical zones.

MISCELLANEOUS

4.10.7 Cautions

Toxicological cases are clinically challenging because exposure to a toxic agent is often presumptive, rather than confirmed. In many cases, treatment must be initiated based upon the clinician's high index of suspicion rather than a guarantee of patient exposure. Supportive care, including dermal and GI decontamination, plays a critical role in the triage of such patients. Time is of the essence. These patients require medical intervention before diagnostic evaluation is complete in order to reduce systemic effects of presumptive toxicosis.

Some patients seem compelled to ingest nonfood items over and over again. These patients are said to have pica. Although pica may result from poor nutrition or other underlying medical pathology, it is more often the result of compulsive behavior among our companion animals. These patients do not appear to learn from their past dietary indiscretions and will subject themselves to GI surgery repeatedly. To prevent recurrence, basket muzzles are advised for use in canine patients that demonstrate pica. There is no equivalent for cats with pica but these cases are managed by not allowing cats access to any unsupervised activity with furred or feathered toys.

References

1 Balakrishnan, A. and Drobatz, K.J. (2013). Management of urinary tract emergencies in small animals. *Vet. Clin. North Am. Small Anim. Pract.* 43: 843–867.

2 Fitzgerald, K.T. (2010). Lily toxicity in the cat. *Top. Compan. Anim. Med.* 25: 213–217.

3 Stokes, J.E. and Forrester, S.D. (2004). New and unusual causes of acute renal failure in dogs and cats. *Vet. Clin. North Am. Small Anim. Pract.* 34: 909–922, vi.

4 Bertone, E.R., Snyder, L.A., and Moore, A.S. (2002). Environmental tobacco smoke and risk of malignant lymphoma in pet cats. *Am. J. Epidemiol.* 156: 268–273.

5 Snyder, L.A., Bertone, E.R., Jakowski, R.M. et al. (2004). p53 expression and environmental tobacco smoke exposure in feline oral squamous cell carcinoma. *Vet. Pathol.* 41: 209–214.

Recommended Reading

Greene, C.E. (ed.) (2012). *Infectious Diseases of the Dog and Cat*, 4e. St Louis, MO: Saunders.

Grave, T.W. and Boag, A.K. (2010). Feline toxicological emergencies: when to suspect and what to do. *J. Feline Med. Surg.* 12: 849–860.

Gupta, R.C. (ed.) (2007). *Veterinary Toxicology: Basic and Clinical Principles*, 3e. New York: Elsevier.

Johnson, S.I., McMichael, M., and White, G. (2006). Heatstroke in small animal medicine: a clinical practice review. *J. Vet. Emerg. Crit. Care* 16: 112–119.

4.11

Environmental Enrichment

Ryane E. Englar, DVM, DABVP (CANINE AND FELINE PRACTICE)

College of Veterinary Medicine, University of Arizona, Oro Valley, AZ, USA

BASICS

4.11.1 Summary

Dogs and cats require environmental enrichment. Although their environmental needs change with life stage, dogs and cats benefit from the opportunity to exhibit species-specific behaviors. Unmet needs may result in abnormal behaviors or clinical disease. Indoor-only lifestyles increase lifespan, but potentially sacrifice physical and mental wellness. Indoor/outdoor lifestyles provide stimulation but, increase the risk for trauma or contracting infectious disease.

4.11.2 Terms Defined

Environmental Enrichment: Modifications that improve the quality of one's surroundings.

MAIN CONCEPTS

Companion dogs in most developed countries are integrated into the owner's lifestyle. It is rare to have a strictly outdoor dog, although this may be true of livestock guardian dogs.

The decision to maintain a cat indoors, indoor/outdoor, or strictly outdoors is often made at the time of adoption/purchase. Clients may have preconceived notions about

lifestyles; however, new cat owners may need help exploring which lifestyle best suits the individual patient.

4.11.3 Feline Environmental Needs

A stressful living environment can incite disease. Having a working knowledge of cats as solitary hunters, with keen senses and flexible social systems, facilitates healthy human interactions with cats. Feline communication is largely postural and seeks to avoid conflict. Marking and vocalization are additional cues.

Cats have five environmental needs:

- Safety
- Carefully spaced resources
- Predatory play
- Predictable, positive, social interactions
- Olfaction-friendly surroundings

Indoor-only lifestyles may meet these needs. For example:

- Homes can create vertical space by providing cat trees, shelves, or perches. When cats live with other cats, escape routes are equally important. Cats need to feel that they can get away
- Food, water, scratching, play, rest, and toileting areas should be maintained separately from one other. In multicat households, resources must be multiplied so that each cat has its own
- Prey can be simulated using feathered and furred toys. Cats must be allowed to catch their "prey"
- Cats' preferences for social interactions depend upon genetics and exposure to handling during the socialization period of 2–7 weeks of age. Cats should initiate interactions to establish preferences for physical contact.

Feline body language that demonstrates relaxation and receptivity to handling includes chirruping, head bunting, or the slow blink

- Cats evaluate their surroundings through scent, and "mark" their living space with facial and body rubbing. Strong scents, such as citrus, should be avoided to reduce sensory overload. Synthetic pheromones may be anxiolytic.

Indoor living offers protection from the elements, predators, and automobiles. In addition to preventive medical care, this has the potential to triple the average lifespan from an estimated 4.5 years (in an outdoor cat) to just shy of 15 (in an indoor one) [1].

4.11.4 Complications Associated with Indoor Living for Cats

Indoor living is more sedentary and predictable. The cat no longer hunts to feed itself; it is fed prepared meals, often in excess. Indoor-only cats are commonly obese. Obesity has been linked to the development of osteoarthritis and diabetes mellitus in cats. Barren environments do not allow cats to act out their normal social and predatory behaviors. Cats may develop aberrant behaviors and compulsive disorders, such as feline hyperesthesia syndrome or psychogenic alopecia [2].

Multicat households may lead to resource guarding or competition for prime space. This is intensified if cats are forced to share resources. Territories may develop within a home, through which other cats may not be allowed to pass. This may result in inappropriate elimination.

Stressed cats are more likely to harbor disease. Latent feline herpesvirus (FHV) is reactivated by stress [2]. Stress also is an inciting factor for feline interstitial cystitis (FIC) and inflammatory bowel disease (IBD) [2].

4.11.5 Outdoor Living for Cats

Outdoor living offers the advantage of freedom to roam. Cats may come and go as they please, and hunt. Predation keeps boredom at bay and provides opportunities for mental and physical engagement.

4.11.6 Outdoor Exposure in Dogs

Dogs also benefit from environmental enrichment. Although environmental needs for toy breeds may be met exclusively indoors, it is challenging to provide larger dogs with the appropriate exercise and outlets for play.

Supervised activity on leash and unsupervised access to fenced-in yards are common.

Dogs must be trained to the leash; it is not innate for them to be led. Leash training should be a positive experience for both dog and handler. Positive reinforcement and food rewards are beneficial so that "collar and leash" time is associated with a good experience.

Pups can be acclimated to wearing a collar and leash indoors, before moving outside. Patience is important. The outside world offers sights and smells that are exciting, enticing, and distracting. Dogs may be tempted to pull in the direction that most intrigues them. Handlers will best troubleshoot this by standing like a tree, rather than caving into the knee-jerk reaction to pull the leash in the opposite direction.

If the dog continues to pull, then harnesses that clip at the front end or head halters, such as GentleLeader® headcollars, may be of benefit. Handlers should also be proactive. They should anticipate what may provoke the dog to lunge, redirect the dog's attention using a treat, and/or give the object of interest a wide berth to encourage forward movement.

Harnesses are ideal substitutes for collars for dogs that have medical conditions that involve the neck. For instance, it may be painful for dogs with cervical intervertebral disc disease (IVDD) to have a collar and leash attached to the neck. Dogs with tracheal collapse or any other coughing problem should also avoid neck collars or bandanas in order to prevent pressure from being applied to or over the trachea.

If dogs will be outdoors unsupervised, then it is critical to ensure that they are adequately confined to a safe space. Fenced-in yards are effective, provided that the dog cannot jump over the fences or dig under them. Fences must be routinely surveyed and properly maintained so that gaps in the fence line are repaired before the dog escapes or before the dog catches and/or cuts itself on loose fencing.

Dogs may also wear electronic collars in order to confine them to unfenced yards; however, boundary training is essential so that dogs learn the property line without unnecessary shocking. One should be able to adjust the intensity of electronic collars so that the stimulus is felt, but is not excessive. The downside to the use of electronic collars is that they may instill fear, which is aversive to learning. They also do not reinforce good behavior. Shocks may be delivered by electric fences unintentionally or too often, and dogs may learn to accept the one-time shock of escaping the yard in order to then roam freely. In addition, electric boundaries do not preclude other animals from wandering onto the property and interacting with collar-confined pets. These types of discussions should ideally take place before owners become financially committed to one strategy over another.

Unsupervised dogs should always be provided with fresh water. Shade is an essential escape from thermal extremes, and proper shelter is protective against rain, sleet, wind, and snow (see 4.10 Environmental Considerations).

EXAMPLES

A client recently downsized from a three-bedroom house to a studio apartment. Since the move two weeks ago, she reports that her 5-year-old spayed female Burmese cat has been urinating on the doormat. A medical work-up is unremarkable. The cat has always been indoor-only and the location of the residence precludes a change in lifestyle. You recommend that the client utilize a plug-in pheromone diffuser and provide cat trees or shelving to create vertical space. The house soiling abates.

A client presents her 6-month-old neutered male cat for wellness examination. She expresses concerns about an indoor-only lifestyle, but her residence abuts a busy intersection. She worries about lack of supervision. You recommend that she train him to a harness so that he can be leash-walked.

TAKE-AWAYS

- Indoor, indoor/outdoor, and outdoor lifestyles are choices that our clients make for their pets, with guidance from the veterinary team.
- Regardless of lifestyle choice, cats and dogs have basic environmental needs.
- If environmental needs are not met, then patients may become stressed.
- Stress has the potential to induce aberrant behavior or clinical disease.
- Environmental enrichment is essential to improve the quality of a pet's living space, regardless of its lifestyle.

MISCELLANEOUS

4.11.7 Cautions

Despite the advantages of enrichment that the natural world provides, outdoor living is not without risk. Automobile-related morbidity and mortality are legitimate concerns, particularly in urban environments.

In addition, outdoor resources, such as drinking water, may become contaminated, either by the elements or by

local wildlife. Although the virus is labile, feline leukemia virus (FeLV) is transmitted through saliva and this can occur through the sharing of food and water bowls [3].

Outdoor living also increases the pet's risk of engaging in altercations with other animals. Battle wounds may range from minor scratches, abscesses, and bite wounds to lethal injuries. Even when injuries are medically or surgically manageable, there is the potential for spread of infectious disease. Biting is the primary route of exposure for feline immunodeficiency virus (FIV) [4].

Pets that experience indoor/outdoor lifestyles require year-round protection against ecto- and endoparasites, particularly because they are likely to become reinfested/reinfected. Several of these parasites, including *Toxocara canis* and *T. cati*, are public health concerns because they are zoonotic (see 4.3 Prevention and Control of Infectious Diseases).

Pet overpopulation is a significant problem across the globe. Unneutered roaming pets contribute to this problem.

Wildlife predation by cats is an additional concern by some, but not all of the public.

References

1 Kraft, W. (1998). Geriatrics in canine and feline internal medicine. *Eur. J. Med. Res.* 3: 31–41.
2 Amat, M., Camps, T., and Manteca, X. (2016). Stress in owned cats: behavioural changes and welfare implications. *J. Feline Med. Surg.* 18: 577–586.
3 Lutz, H., Addie, D., Belak, S. et al. (2009). Feline leukaemia. ABCD guidelines on prevention and management. *J. Feline Med. Surg.* 11: 565–574.
4 Hosie, M.J., Addie, D., Belak, S. et al. (2009). Feline immunodeficiency. ABCD guidelines on prevention and management. *J. Feline Med. Surg.* 11: 575–584.

Recommended Reading

Amat, M., Camps, T., and Manteca, X. (2016). Stress in owned cats: behavioural changes and welfare implications. *J. Feline Med. Surg.* 18: 577–586.
Ellis, S.L.H., Rodan, I., Carney, H.C. et al. (2013). AAFP and ISFM feline environmental needs guidelines. *J. Feline Med. Surg.* 15: 219–230.
Levy, J., Crawford, C., Hartmann, K. et al. (2008). American Association of Feline Practitioners' feline retrovirus management guidelines. *J. Feline Med. Surg.* 10: 300–316.
Zoran, D.L. and Buffington, C.A. (2011). Effects of nutrition choices and lifestyle changes on the well-being of cats, a carnivore that has moved indoors. *J. Am. Vet. Med. Assoc.* 239: 596–606.

4.12

Homeowner Insurance Considerations

Tara Harmon, APR

The Cincinnati Insurance Companies, Fairfield, OH, USA

BASICS

4.12.1 Summary

Pet owners face a higher risk of being sued than those who do not own a pet. Even the most well-behaved pet can jump, scratch, bite or even kill. It is not commonly known that pet lawsuits can be paid and defended through homeowner's insurance. This makes the purchase of a homeowner's policy with enough limit of liability particularly important for those who own pets.

4.12.2 Terms Defined

Application: A form that insurance companies collect and use to decide if they want to provide insurance.
Liability: The state of being legally responsible for something.
Personal Property: Movable assets.
Underwriting: The review of a risk with the purpose of approving, declining, and pricing a new insurance policy.

MAIN CONCEPTS

4.12.3 Homeowner's Insurance

A homeowner's insurance policy is a legal contract between an individual and an insurance company. The insurance company agrees to pay for home and liability claims in exchange for payment of premium. Homeowner's insurance contracts are always split into two coverage sections: property and liability. The property section provides financial protection for damages to the home and contents at that property. The liability section provides legal protection for a personal lawsuit brought against the homeowner, household members, and family pets as well as medical payments coverage for third party injuries.

Homeowner's policies provide specific coverage limits for both property and liability. The limit is listed on the declarations page of a home policy and outlines the maximum amount the insurance company will pay for a loss. If there is a claim that exceeds those limits, the homeowner is personally responsible for paying the outstanding balance. For example, if a homeowner with a policy carrying $300 000 in liability coverage is sued for $500 000 after the family beagle bites a small child, the homeowner would be responsible for paying the remaining $200 000 after the insurance company pays their obligated $300 000.

4.12.4 The Application Process

All insurance companies require a completed application before they can quote or issue an insurance policy. Nearly every application inquires if there is a pet kept in the home, and if so, what type of animal and specific breed. There will also be a specific question asking if any pets have ever bitten or caused other injury. Some companies may also ask if the pet is kept in a fully fenced backyard.

So, the insurance quote is only as good as the information included on the initial insurance application. It is extremely important that the application is filled out accurately and with full disclosure. All insurance contracts specifically outline that concealment of information or providing misinformation is considered fraud and will result in declination of claims payment. Insurance fraud is also punishable by law enforcement.

4.12.5 The Underwriting Process

After the application is completed and the insurance agent quotes and sells an insurance policy comes the underwriting process. The purpose of underwriting an insurance policy is to ensure the insurance company fully understands the risk and is collecting accurate premiums. Some insurance companies check reports that disclose prior losses, insurance policies obtained, and members of the household. Others take it further and perform manual online searches of Facebook, Twitter, and other online platforms. Many companies will also visit the home to document the condition of the dwelling as well as confirming pet ownership and fence installation.

Many are unaware that newly issued insurance policies can be canceled by the insurance company after issuance, even if a policy has been paid in full. The cancelation must take place within the initial underwriting period approved by the state or province, which is typically within the first 30–60 days of coverage. A policy is typically canceled in this way if the details included on the initial application do not match the details uncovered during the underwriting process. Common situations for pet owners include undisclosed pets and unacceptable breeds, unsafe conditions such as animal hoarding, or backyard that is not fully fenced.

4.12.6 Dog Breed Exclusions

In the US, dog bites and other pet-related injuries are among the most frequent and severe homeowner claims paid each year. The number of claims and amount paid per claim have increased nearly every year. Many insurance companies have made the decision to withhold from writing homeowner's policies for those who own specific dog breeds because those breeds have generated high claim payouts. Each company's dog exclusion list may vary as each company has differing loss experiences. Some commonly excluded breeds include pit bulls, Staffordshire terriers, Doberman pinschers, and rottweilers.

It is also highly likely that if a pet has bitten once, they will bite again. For that reason, nearly all insurance companies will decline to offer a policy if there was a pet bite within the last five years and the homeowner still owns the pet. Additionally, dog bites to third parties happen more often when a dog escapes from an unfenced yard. For that reason, some underwriters may require a fenced yard to be comfortable offering a policy to a dog owner.

4.12.7 Damages Caused by Pets

Dog bite claims are the most common pet claims paid by insurance companies each year. Over $686 million in liability claims related to dog bites and other dog-related injuries were paid in 2017 [1]. Other less common pet injuries such as dog jumps, cat scratches, horse kicks, and reptile bites can also be covered by homeowner's liability insurance. While these types of injuries are typically less serious, they often result in moderate-sized medical and ambulance bills and occasional lawsuits.

Pets can also cause damage to personal property. If a pet causes damage to its owner's home or personal property, unfortunately there is no coverage available under the homeowner's policy. However, there is coverage for damages to property owned by a third party. For example, if a family pet chews up the carpet in its own home, the homeowner is unable to claim carpet damages through their home insurance. On the other hand, if a dog jumps its owner's fence and chews a patio set in their neighbor's yard, the dog owner's policy would pay for the cost of repair or replacement of the patio set.

4.12.8 Why Every Pet Owner Should Purchase Higher Limits of Liability Insurance

It is extremely important for pet owners to understand the amount of liability insurance they have as well as the stance their insurance company takes on pet ownership. It is extremely common for a homeowner to carry too low a liability limit as well as being unclear if a pet is covered. It is important to consult with an insurance agent or broker to review current coverages and explain policy limits and limitations.

A personal umbrella policy provides an additional layer of liability insurance that sits on top of the underlying limit. Increasing liability limits on the homeowner's policy as well as purchasing an umbrella policy are typically inexpensive and help homeowners stay financially sound in the event of a lawsuit.

Homeowner's insurance policies come in a variety of shapes and sizes, and the amount of liability insurance companies will offer pet owners varies. Many insurance companies limit the amount of liability they will offer, or completely decline to offer coverage to homeowners who own certain dog breeds or other exotic pets. The good news is that there are some insurance companies that do not exclude certain dog breeds, offer higher limits of liability, and a few that may even write a policy after a pet has caused harm. Additionally, there are specialty companies that provide stand-alone dog liability insurance. Pet owners who are unable to purchase a typical homeowner's insurance policy because of a dog breed or other pet they own should consult with an independent insurance agent to see which alternative may provide the best coverage available.

EXAMPLES

Mr and Mrs Smith have just purchased a new home and need homeowner's insurance. They own a 2-year-old Doberman pinscher who is gentle with their family which includes two young children. They contact a local insurance agent who has them fill out an application for insurance. They disclose ownership of their pet as well as confirming their backyard is fenced and that the dog has never caused injury. Unfortunately, their current insurance carrier is unable to offer more than $100 000 in liability insurance due to the dog breed they own. Mr and Mrs Smith understand that this is not enough coverage since they own a dog and contact a different agent who is able to find an insurance company who will offer $500 000 in liability as well as a $1 million umbrella policy. Five years later the family dog jumps on an elderly neighbor during a block party, causing a fall that breaks his hip. Following surgery, the elderly neighbor comes down with an infection which extends his hospital stay for several months. Medical bills exceed $650 000 and are paid by the Smiths' homeowner's insurance company, $500 000 through their liability insurance and the balance through their umbrella coverage.

Ms Thatcher is shopping for a new insurance carrier. She emails a local agent asking for insurance quotes for her home. The agent responds with a list of questions, including if she owns a pet and if so what breed. Ms Thatcher adopted a pitbull a few years ago and understands that the breed may cause an issue when getting insurance. She tells the insurance agent that she does not own any pets. The insurance agent finds her a great home insurance policy with high limits at a low cost. Two weeks after her new policy is issued, an insurance appraiser visits her home and notices the doghouse in her backyard and pitbull bumper sticker on her car. The insurance appraiser notifies the underwriter who cancels her new policy 30 days later. Ms Thatcher scrambles to find another homeowner's policy.

TAKE-AWAYS

- Pet owners face a higher risk of being sued than those who do not own a pet.
- The purchase of a homeowner's policy with enough limit of liability is particularly important for those who own pets.
- It is extremely important that applications for insurance are filled out accurately and with full disclosure.
- Many insurance companies have made the decision to withhold from writing homeowner policies for those who own specific dog breeds because those breeds have generated high claim payouts.
- It is extremely important for pet owners to understand the amount of liability insurance they have as well as the stance their insurance company takes toward pet ownership.

MISCELLANEOUS

4.12.9 Cautions

Homeowner's insurance does not provide coverage for sickness or injury to household pets. Pet health insurance is a separate insurance product and purchase (see 10.16 Pet Health Insurance).

A homeowner cannot file an insurance claim for property damage of their own home or contents caused by a family pet. Because the pet is an extension of the insured, damages would be considered intentional.

Veterinary teams need not be experts in homeowner's insurance, but it is worthwhile for them to be aware of some of these issues as they counsel pet owners on pet-specific care considerations.

Reference

1 Spotlight on: Dog bite liability. Insurance Information Institute. www.iii.org/article/spotlight-on-dog-bite-liability#Dog%20bite%20liability%20and%20homeowners%20insurance

Recommended Reading

Bailey, B. (2018). *The Hammer: Why Dogs Attack Us and How to Prevent It*. Pasadena, CA: Best Seller Publishing.

Wilson, S.L. Dog Bite Statistics (How Likely are You To Get Bit?). www.caninejournal.com/dog-bite-statistics

Section 5

Client Service Considerations

5.1

Pet-Specific Customer Service

Nan Boss, DVM

Best Friends Veterinary Center, Grafton, WI, USA

BASICS

5.1.1 Summary

Customer service in a pet-specific practice setting requires more thought and preparation. Instead of a few choices or protocols, everyone has to be familiar and comfortable with multiple ways to deliver care. It's not enough to be kind, we must also be knowledgeable. This requires planning and training.

5.1.2 Terms Defined

Healthspan: The portion of a pet's life in which it is considered generally healthy, in contradistinction to lifespan which is the quantity of time a pet is alive.

MAIN CONCEPTS

Each patient is unique, just as each client is unique. Flexibility is required if you are to keep many different individual customers happy and meet a variety of their wants and needs. For example, there are three different ways clients prefer to make decisions about their pet's care. Some clients want the veterinary team to tell them what to do. Their question is frequently "What would you do if it were your pet?" Some clients want to discuss information and reach a decision together. The last group wants you to feed them information but make the decisions themselves.

The team needs to communicate differently with these different types of people in order to end up with the client

feeling comfortable with the choices they've made (see 5.10 Discussing Pet-Specific Care). It's also good to be flexible in other ways: with payment plans, with medication administration methods, or with ways you contact the client or follow up. Offer options and let the client decide.

Decisions belong to the client. It is not the job of the veterinary team member to decide what level of care the client wants. The client has the right to make healthcare decisions about their pet. Not offering a certain level of care to a particular customer means the practice has made the decision as to what care the pet receives. In a client-centered practice, the goal is to educate the clients and let them decide.

When developing a pet-specific healthcare plan, the client should be treated like part of the team (see 1.3 Personalized Care Plans). There should be a working relationship with every pet owner to develop the best possible healthcare plan for the pet. More time spent teaching clients about good pet care means better health for the patients and more income for the practice.

How might you present choices and estimates to clients and how will you record their decisions about each?

5.1.3 Getting a Good History

Careful questioning allows the team to determine how best to serve the client and the patient. Getting a good history in a friendly, conversational way will open up a dialogue with a client and engage them in the process of setting up a personalized plan for the pet owner and the pet (see 1.3 Personalized Care Plans). Questions to help open up communication might include "What activities does your dog enjoy?" "What is your cat's favorite game?" "Do you ever travel with your pet?" "What is his favorite snack?" or "How well does she ride in the car?" These sorts of inquiries

Pet-Specific Care for the Veterinary Team, First Edition. Edited by Lowell Ackerman.
© 2021 John Wiley & Sons, Inc. Published 2021 by John Wiley & Sons, Inc.

provide useful information about what needs the pet might have and they also sound caring.

Asking questions and giving clients the chance to talk shows them that we have time to spend with them and gives them a better experience (see 9.2 Asking Good Questions). Talking for a few minutes also gives your exam room technicians the opportunity to dole out treats and schmooze with the patients, or let the cat come out of the carrier on its own – so it improves the pets' experiences as well.

We are all busy and work hard but our clients should perceive that we have time for them and are not just rushing through appointments. Having clients perceive you have time involves the old adage about acting like a swan – looking serene on the surface while paddling like crazy underneath. Having time also involves efficient scheduling, willingness to listen and chat a little, and making sure all your clients' questions and concerns are dealt with.

Templates and forms help the team to ask the right questions and obtain useful information for the programs you are implementing.

5.1.4 Consistency of Care

At the same time that you are working on individualized plans for each pet, you will need to maintain consistency of care (see 9.8 Ensuring Consistency of Care). This means that the same options are offered, explained, and presented well to each client under specific circumstances. A patient or client should never get a greater or lesser level of care because one doctor saw them and not another, or one receptionist spoke with them and not someone else. It's confusing and dismaying to clients when one team member makes one recommendation and another tells them something completely different. Good medical care should be the standard throughout the practice and every team member is part of that.

Practicing high-quality medicine is all about being a better teacher. The only way you can help your patients lead long and healthy lives is to educate their owners. Most of your clients don't have a degree in medicine or behavior. Take the time and make the effort to teach them what they need to know to care for their pets properly.

Using handouts, forms, videos, and other client education tools consistently ensures we are giving the same information to every client (see 5.14 Client Education Materials). Our motto should be: every disease, every medication, every treatment plan, every time. Think of your exam rooms as classrooms. The telephone, the checkout counter, your website, and social media posts are all involved in delivering both customer service and information

to clients. This means the whole team works together. Customer service is not just for the front desk staff!

What educational tools will you need to have for both team members and clients to learn about your pet-specific programs? How will your team deliver useful, actionable information?

5.1.5 Team Training

Team training is essential in this type of practice. In order for clients to receive consistent information from everyone in the practice, team members should have scripts and cue cards for common client interactions, and should all be portraying caring and giving the same advice. This means the veterinary team receives training in communications, including using tone of voice, phrasing, and body language. Each individual team member is trained to handle questions and problems, so the client doesn't have to wait while another person is found to take care of a problem or explain a service offered.

Customers are interested in businesses whose employees are knowledgeable, and who address their needs and treat the client as if they value their business. Have you given your team what they need to shine in your clients' eyes? Very often, the way the business owner treats the team is how the team treats the client.

Pet-specific customer service, like most things in the veterinary hospital, starts with the front desk team. Whether it's a phone call or the greeting when they arrive, the customer service representative (CSR) sets the tone for the entire visit. Don't make the mistake of training your exam room technicians without spending equal time on the front line. If you are working to be a Fear Free™ practice (see 6.6 Fear Free Concepts) or implementing breed-specific medicine, phrases such as "Does your dog pant, yawn or tremble when he visits the vet?" or "We take special care of purebred cats, including DNA testing for early diagnosis of genetic diseases" need to be part of their lexicon. This doesn't happen at a single team meeting or just because you say it should. It takes conscious effort and repetition.

Team members cannot fake being knowledgeable. There is no substitute for team training, continuing education, and staff meetings. The only way your entire team can sound knowledgeable, and be communicating the same messages to clients, is if you have discussed your protocols and recommendations. This means training everyone in the practice to the same high standard, and constantly working to maintain it.

You should have protocols for consistent patient care and customer service and each team member is then trained to those protocols (see 9.4 Standards of Care). Managing the medicine you practice should be rewarding, both financially and emotionally. Being organized gives people the security of knowing exactly what to do, and why.

Much effort may be needed to expand on your vision and mission by creating standards and protocols for everyone to espouse. It isn't enough to simply "tell" your team what they should be doing; you need to explain the hows and whys so that everyone understands the importance of a standard or recommendation. Is your team "in the tell" or "in the know" when they interact with a client?

Here is an example: you want everyone to offer your newly created senior blood panel to every patient when they become a senior (see 11.5 Life Planning by Breed). Why? How will it benefit the patient? What's in it for the team? What's in it for the client? What is your "real" reason for coming up with this new service packet?

First set your goal for your particular business – perhaps it is encouraging senior pets to make regular visits or improving your diagnostic methods to catch disease conditions sooner (see 1.4 Opportunities for Pet-Specific Care). Understand your vision and review your practice management software for your trends. Develop your new service. Now you can go to your team to teach and motivate, armed with information and tools to get them "in the know." Prepare your team for the client visit; how to inform the client, how to create a sense of urgency, how to show the client how this service will improve their pet's healthcare. The client is thinking "What's in it for me?" How will you answer that question? Your team can only become leaders in the exam room if you are able to drive the learning and create the freedom for action.

Your team will be "in the know" and will be able to address the client's needs and concerns because you will have informed them and involved them in the development of this new service. Utilizing team leaders to reinforce the desired behavior will help communicate the message. One attribute of leadership is seeing good things and potential in other people, seeing their passion and helping them grow it. When team members help each other, encourage each other, review each other's charts, and help each other out with talking points and phrases, everyone will benefit.

Communicating your message, the need for senior blood screening in our example, can't be left to chance. You can't assume your team has the same vision for patient care as you do. You can't assume they will discuss the service with a client, much less mention it in passing while they take the rectal temperature.

You also can't assume the client will simply do whatever you say in the exam room, or that every client will respond the same way. Your commitment to your practice's pet-specific care mission must involve building your team up and monitoring for results.

You'll need to take baby steps and break any big project down into small, easily achievable pieces to avoid overwhelming them. Making changes is a step-by-step process. Breed-specific wellness or Fear Free programs are big undertakings that will probably take a year or more to accomplish.

Begin a pet-specific care project with the leaders in your practice, develop team training for each step and involve the team in creating innovative ways to educate each other, as well as the clients. Inform your team about the progress they are making – what doesn't get measured doesn't improve. You can create a sense of urgency for change by simply trying to improve on measurements from one month to the next. A success story about a pet that was diagnosed in the early stages of a condition and how grateful the client was will boost morale and encourage more team participation – so share the stories.

Every practice, regardless of size, can build a pet-specific care team to provide quality care to every patient and a better understanding on the part of every client.

A challenge for the future can be adding new team members when you already have a program up and running. On the one hand, experienced team members will naturally set an example for "how we do things here." On the other hand, one-on-one training tends to emphasize tasks, for example "Here is how to present a wellness plan," but not the *why* behind it. Most people who work in the veterinary profession care deeply about animals. Make sure they know how their work contributes to the mission of increased healthspan for the patients.

A question that correlates well with a patient's overall hospital experience asks whether the nurses and doctors who took care of the patient worked well together as a team. It's vitally important if your client is to maintain a good impression of your hospital that they do not pick up on tension or strife between team members. Respect and professionalism, as well as caring and compassion, should be evident whenever you interact with each other.

5.1.6 Value Statements

The best way to ensure that your team members are giving good presentations is to rehearse and prepare them. Talk about the best ways to say things or to present information, and do some role playing to ensure that they know their stuff. One of the best tools I've found for making this happen is the "value statement."

A value statement is a simple tool we use to communicate with our clients the value of our services both to them and to their pets. It's a sentence or a few sentences that communicate the value of the service or product you are discussing with the client. An example of a value statement would be this sentence: "Wellness plans save you money while keeping Dixie healthy."

Longer scripts are used when offering more complicated things, such as antianxiety medication for an office visit: "Does your dog/cat become anxious or frightened when coming to the veterinarian? We can help to make things better by sending/giving antianxiety medication for you to give Fluffy prior to your visit. This is especially important if she struggles or needs to be muzzled for procedures such as blood draws or nail trims, or if she shows obvious signs of stress when she is here – shivering, cowering, pacing, panting, yawning ... Do you notice any of those things when you come here?" If the answer is yes: "Our comfort kits include antianxiety medication, probiotics to prevent stress-related diarrhea and pheromone products for calming. The kits cost x and we can mail one to you ahead of time."

Value statements increase the perception of our value and also add to the client's perceptions that we care, that we are transparent, and that we are knowledgeable. Value statements can be about what our values are as a practice (what we believe is good care), as well as telling about what goes into a service that makes it costly and why it's worth it to spend money for it. They can be used on the phone or in person.

Value statements provide repetition and reinforcement of the doctors' recommendations. Working together as a team, each person supports the goals of the practice and reinforces the messages we send to clients. Clients may need five or 10 repetitions to remember or purchase something. If the assistant mentions DNA testing, the doctor discusses genetic risks and the receptionist adds a value statement on the client's way out, that's three in one visit!

Getting all our clients and patients the care they deserve is a team effort. It takes a team to get across to the clients the messages you want to send about your hospital, your level of healthcare, and your pride in working there.

EXAMPLES

Here are some examples of using scripts and value statements when serving your customers.

- Always try to add a caring or empathetic statement to your explanation of any service. "I can see that Buddy means a lot to you and you want to take the best possible care of him." "I can see that leaving Heidi here will be hard for you. The doctors and technicians will take very good care of her while she is here." "Having a puppy in the house is so much fun! Let me tell you about our puppy care packages and the vaccination options you have. Which vaccines we recommend will depend on where he will be spending time."

- Precede a price with a value statement. Explain the benefits of the wellness plan, laboratory testing or other service before you tell them the price. Once they hear the fee, most people tune out and don't hear the rest, so talk about value before you mention price.

- If a client questions the cost of an item, you can give a value statement: "Yes, our exam fees are higher than at some other practices. We like to have time to teach you about pet healthcare and we allow the extra time to do that."

- If a client seems hesitant or unsure about something, you can give a value statement: "I can see that you are unsure about whether to have Fluffy DNA tested. It's a bit of an investment, we know, but the results could be life-saving for her."

- If you are offering something new to the client: "Have we talked to you yet about DNA testing for Dixie? Genetic screening for MDR1 allows us to determine if certain medications are safe for her."

- Differentiate yourself from other clinics (see 10.2 The Importance of Practice Differentiation): what do you do better? Every clinic can give a series of puppy vaccinations. Only we are taking the time to "teach you everything you need to know to have a healthy, happy dog, whether you've had many dogs before or this is your first one." "We make sure you are informed about new treatments and improvements in veterinary care every time you come in for a routine exam."

- Always ask if the client has questions or concerns: the whole purpose of the value statements is to make sure the client understands what they will be paying for. Never rush your explanation and be sure you have covered as much as the client seems to want to know. Some clients want to know much more than others. Some will accept anything you offer. Some will hesitate forever and you must be firm in asking for a Yes or No. Be sensitive to clients' body language and questions.

Work with your team to develop scripts and phrases to use with clients. Your scripts should answer the questions "What would your concerns be if you were the client and this was your pet?" "What would you want to know before agreeing to this?" "What fears do you think a client would have about this product?"

TAKE-AWAYS

- Flexibility is required if you are to keep many different individual customers happy and meet a variety of their wants and needs.
- Getting a good history in a friendly, conversational way will open up a dialogue with a client and engage them in the process of setting up a personalized plan for the pet owner and the pet.
- Client education is important in a client-centered and pet-specific practice, and it is an obligation of the entire clinic team to make the visit an educational experience for the client.
- The only way your entire team can sound knowledgeable, and be communicating the same messages to clients, is if you have discussed your protocols and recommendations with them. This means training everyone in the practice to the same high standard, and constantly working to maintain it.
- The best way to ensure that your team members are giving good presentations is to rehearse and prepare them.

MISCELLANEOUS

5.1.7 Cautions

Instituting pet-specific care programs can be more difficult and time-consuming than you think it will be. Being great is hard – if it wasn't, everyone would be great.

Recommended Reading

Boss, N. (2009). *How We Do Things Here: Developing and Teaching Office-Wide Protocols*. Lakewood, CO: AAHA Press.

Boss, N. (2011). *Educating Your Clients From A to Z: What to Say and How to Say It*, 2e. Lakewood, CO: AAHA Press.

Free, F. (2017). *80 Tips to Reduce Your Patients' Fear, Anxiety, and Stress*. Lakewood, CO: AAHA Press.

Lee, F. (2004). *If Disney Ran Your Hospital: 9 1/2 Things You Would Do Differently*. Bozeman, MT: Second River Healthcare Press.

Myers, W.S. (2014). *Become a Client Communication Star DVD*. Lakewood, CO: AAHA Press.

Renfrew, J. (2013). *AAHA's Complete Guide for the Veterinary Client Service Representative*. Lakewood, CO: AAHA Press.

5.2

Meeting Client Needs

Lowell Ackerman, DVM, DACVD, MBA, MPA, CVA, MRCVS

Global Consultant, Author, and Lecturer, MA, USA

 BASICS

5.2.1 Summary

Veterinary teams want to deliver excellent veterinary care, and pet owners want to be the recipients of such care for the benefit of their pets, but separating wants from needs can be difficult, especially when it can be challenging for pet owners to understand what precisely is needed for their pets. Veterinary practices must endeavor to keep their clients satisfied, and that means giving them what they want (and need) most.

5.2.2 Terms Defined

Bedside Manner: Perception of how well a physician relates to a client or patient.

Client: An individual or group who engages in a professional working relationship with a veterinarian or veterinary practice for the delivery of veterinary services.

Customer: Someone who pays for goods or services.

Omnichannel Consumer: A consumer seeking a seamless shopping experience, whether online, through a smart device or telephone, or in a bricks-and-mortar establishment.

Spectrum of Care: The availability and accessibility of veterinary medical care regardless of the socioeconomic status of the pet owner.

 MAIN CONCEPTS

5.2.3 What Do Clients Need?

Clients often have difficulty expressing what they are looking for in a veterinary practice, but assessment of successful practices suggests that those features are known, even if clients cannot enumerate them when asked (see 5.8 The Biology of Marketing).

Most pet owners today are omnichannel consumers and are looking to optimize the value they receive through whichever commercial channels are available to them. Most probably prefer to do business directly with their veterinary hospital, but they are prepared to explore other options if their needs are not being met.

5.2.4 Consistency

Clients can appreciate that medical issues are not black and white and that there is room for medical debate, but they don't want to get mixed messages regarding the healthcare of their pets (see 9.8 Ensuring Consistency of Care). They want the facility to meet their expectations of a hospital, they want the veterinarian to "be a doctor," and they want the staff to act informed and professional.

It is also divisive if clients receive different messages from different members of the healthcare team. Practice protocols should be standardized so that this inconsistency is minimized, as it is confusing for owners and detracts from the trust they place in the practice and its recommendations (see 9.4 Standards of Care).

5.2.4.1 Compassion

Most clients have embraced the human–animal bond (see 2.14 Benefits of the Human–Animal Bond) with their pets, and are visiting the veterinary practice as a reflection of this bond. It is critical that the practice reflects its love of animals in everything that it does, from its logo to its discharge instructions (see 2.15 Promoting the Human–Animal Bond). Although owners want to know that their veterinarian is proficient in his or her trade, they want even more to know that their pets are being cared for by people who clearly understand how important those pets are as family members. For clients, this is reflected in the "bedside manner" of the veterinarian and team, often an overlooked aspect of veterinary training.

Grooming pets before they are discharged, providing give-aways or chew treats, and taking a little extra time with an animal when patience is required (see 6.6 Fear Free Concepts) all speak volumes to clients about the value placed on animals.

Pet owners also perceive the compassion of practices that create completely customized care plans for their pets, recognizing the uniqueness of pets and the need to craft approaches to specifically fit their needs (see 1.3 Personalized Care Plans). Compare the emotional motivators for your best clients (e.g., appreciative that their pet is not afraid to come to clinic, or thankful that their pet's individual needs are being addressed) with other segments and develop messaging that would leverage this appeal to your other clients (see 10.3 Pet-Specific Outreach).

5.2.4.2 Customer Service

Clients want to be loyal to veterinary practices and are often more loyal to us than to other retail businesses. However, they are also consumers and are used to being treated as valued customers by companies with which they do business (see 5.1 Pet-Specific Customer Service). It is important for teams to realize this, because minor lapses in client service can lead to costly losses for veterinary practices.

Much of marketing by companies today is relationship based, in which significant effort is exerted to determine what customers prefer (see 5.13 Improving Client Engagement Through Technology). With pet-specific care, it is often possible to shift customers toward relationships that advance the organization's strategic goals as well. In this case, when clients act in the best interest of their pets, such as with early detection efforts, good preventive medicine, and closing gaps in compliance, the practice and the pet owner both win.

5.2.4.3 Convenience

Today's pet owners are busy individuals, and they routinely pay a premium for convenience. It is important that we make it easy for them to do business with us. There are many practice attributes that clients value, and it is important to consider these. Creating resources that are available online and that the owner has perpetual access to, being available for clients, such as with telehealth (see 2.5 Virtual Care (Telehealth)), and having trained staff who are capable of interacting with clients is a great start.

Today, more than at any time in the past, it is possible to offer convenience by allowing clients to interact with the practice 24 hours a day via online services. There are programs available that allow clients to research their pets' conditions online, book appointments, request prescription refills, and even review an online medical record. Opportunities exist for even more client integration, such as with blockchain applications (see 2.12 Blockchain in Veterinary Medicine). Anything that makes it easier for clients to do business with us is worth evaluating.

5.2.4.4 Competence

Veterinarians may assume that their clients have good reason for realizing they are competent, but in reality, it is very difficult for clients to appreciate the level of skill of any physician. They make judgments based on what they know and feel, and most of this is a subconscious decision (see 5.3 What Clients Expect from the Veterinary Team).

Clients have so little information on which to judge competence that they become excited whenever clues are available to them. Use opportunities to highlight the accomplishments of all professionals and paraprofessionals, such as practice promotional materials, the website, standards of care, customized health plans, and newsletters.

While clients might appreciate an empathetic employee, and empathy is certainly a desirable trait, it is important to realize that sometimes clients can become frustrated by the amount of conflicting information they encounter, and may appreciate individuals who can cut through the clutter and just tell them what they need to know – one who seeks not to solicit more information from the client about what they might like to do, but instead tells them what should be done to get to the fastest and easiest resolution. This can often be effectively communicated through a practice's standards of care (see 9.4 Standards of Care).

5.2.4.5 Cost

Nobody wants to overpay for services, no matter how professional the practice seems. Clients are paying for professional services, but may be interested in buying needed products, or commodities, elsewhere. This is not a lack of loyalty; it is a realization by the client that some products are commodities and without intrinsic value as to where they are purchased, whereas the medical services are value-driven purchases. Veterinary practices should endeavor to learn the same lesson and concentrate on the medical value they can deliver through pet-specific care.

Selling goods, including diets, shampoos, pharmaceuticals, and parasite control products, from a veterinary practice should be a matter of convenience for owners, not a measure of loyalty to the practice, and should be priced accordingly (see 10.15 Putting Price into Perspective). It is important to be an advocate for clients and for practices to understand what they can sell at a premium – professional services.

Still, it is important for practices to understand that not all clients can necessarily afford the level of care that they would prefer (see 2.10 Affordability of Veterinary Services). Thus, it is also necessary to consider the spectrum of care that can be made available to clients in need. There are many strategies available to deal with these situations (see 7.8 Providing Care for Those Unable or Unwilling to Pay; 10.14 Providing Cost-Effective Care for Those in Need; and 2.2 The Role of Incremental Care).

EXAMPLES

Mrs Garcia visited XYZ Veterinary Hospital for an office visit, and learned that her pet had a bacterial folliculitis that would require an antibiotic. The cost of the antibiotic seemed considerable to Mrs Garcia, and she asked if it might be possible to get a prescription for it because she had seen advertisements on television for an online pet pharmacy. She was hoping that she might be able to save some money on the medication. Dr Donaldson became somewhat indignant at the suggestion and proceeded to explain to her that pharmaceutical sales help subsidize surgeries and other services at the hospital, and those prices would have to rise if clients started buying their pharmaceuticals elsewhere. Mrs Garcia thanked him, said she would think about it, and left.

Mrs Garcia was uncomfortable with the discussion, and although she had been a loyal client at XYZ Veterinary Hospital for many years, she decided that she might be more comfortable elsewhere. She visited ABC Veterinary

Hospital and was warmly greeted. Dr Smith reached the same conclusion about the bacterial folliculitis, but thought it would be worthwhile to begin with topical therapy and get a bacterial culture before starting on an antibiotic, to minimize the risk of antimicrobial resistance. She then scheduled a clinical reevaluation to make sure that the treatment did completely clear the infection as anticipated. Mrs Garcia cautiously asked about prescriptions, but this time got a very different response. Dr Smith told her that they could supply any needed medications from the hospital and could either send it to her or have it available for pickup; they also had access to a veterinary online pharmacy if that would be more convenient. In fact, she volunteered to have Nancy, a client service representative, determine the online price so that Mrs Garcia could make an informed decision on what she would prefer. Mrs Garcia was surprised to learn there was so little difference in price between the hospital and the online pharmacy, appreciated the convenience of buying items directly from the hospital, and became a loyal client of ABC Veterinary Hospital.

CAUTIONS

The old saying that the customer is always right is not fundamentally correct. The customer is entitled to courteous, professional, and respectful service; however, it is also true that not all clients are good matches for a practice and not all clients are suitable for a practice. Cultivate the clients who fit the practice's mission, but retention of *all* clients is not a realistic goal.

Veterinary services will constantly be challenged by both veterinary and nonveterinary competitors until practices concentrate on delivering value-added activities rather than just the retail sale of goods and services. Deliver value to clients, and they will deliver at least some degree of loyalty back to the practice.

TAKE-AWAYS

- Clients may have difficulty knowing what they most value in a practice, but they typically know it when they experience it.
- Most pet owners are omnichannel consumers and looking to optimize the value they receive in pet care.
- Clients are more willing to know what you think about their pet's care when they first realize that you care about pets.

- Clients appreciate receiving a consistent message about their pet's care, and this can be facilitated through pet-specific care strategies.
- Clients appreciate both compassion and empathy, and yet sometimes they prefer to just be told what is in the best interest of their pet.

MISCELLANEOUS

Recommended Reading

Ackerman, L.J. (2003). *Management Basics for Veterinarians.* New York: ASJA Press.

Ackerman, L.J. (2020). Giving clients what they want most. In: *Five-Minute Veterinary Practice Management Consult*, 3e, 384–387. Ames, IA: Wiley.

Avery, J., Fournier, S., and Wittenbraker, J. (2014). Unlock the mysteries of your customer relationships. *Harvard Business Review* July/August: 72–81.

Dixon, M., Ponomareff, L., Turner, S., and DeLisi, R. (2017). Kick-ass customer service. *Harvard Business Review* January/February: 110–117.

Magids, S., Zorfas, A., and Leemon, D. (2015). The new science of customer emotions – a better way to drive growth and profitability. *Harvard Business Review* November: 66–76.

5.3

What Clients Expect from the Veterinary Team

Lowell Ackerman, DVM, DACVD, MBA, MPA, CVA, MRCVS

Global Consultant, Author, and Lecturer, MA, USA

 BASICS

5.3.1 Summary

All hospital income is provided by willingly paying clients. Because most consumers are value shoppers, it makes sense to concentrate on providing clients with the value they seek.

Although every client is different, there are some basic rules to providing goods and services that exceed the expectations of our clients. However, to consistently meet expectations, it is first important to appreciate what those expectations are. The next step is to realize that expectations can and should be met by all members of the veterinary team – not just the veterinary professionals.

5.3.2 Terms Defined

Disposable Income: Income remaining after all taxes and mandatory expenses have been deducted that can be spent or saved at one's prerogative.

Omnichannel Consumer: Consumer exposure to information and marketing messages, preferably seamlessly, through a variety of different channels, including bricks-and-mortar stores, the internet, apps, etc.

Risk Management: The identification and assessment of risks and minimization of their impact, such as with insurance or reducing risk factors.

 MAIN CONCEPTS

5.3.3 Determining Expectations

So, what do clients want? There are some expectations regarding clients that can be readily inferred as being standards. All clients will want to be treated fairly and with respect. This should be foundational in all offerings provided. All clients also expect that they will be receiving competent medical care. However, it's actually much more than that. When clients bring in a pet, they expect that the veterinary team will appreciate the pet-specific needs of that pet, given its breed, and specific circumstances as outlined by the client (see 1.2 Providing a Lifetime of Care). Most veterinary teams may struggle with this pet-specific expectation, yet most will admit that it is fair and reasonable for paying clients to expect such expertise. After all, if a client presents a Cavalier King Charles spaniel for evaluation and is paying for that evaluation, is it not reasonable for them to expect that the veterinary team knows breed characteristics and disease susceptibility, and is able to counsel accordingly? If a client travels with their pet, or does specific activities with their pet, or exposes it to other animals at shows, boarding, or grooming, or it has an existing medical issue, it is reasonable for clients to assume that the veterinary team is taking all this into consideration.

To better understand what clients expect, hospitals should have methods in place to actually determine this information directly from clients (see 5.17 Ensuring and Measuring Client Satisfaction). In the most basic method, regularly ask clients if their needs are being met, and if your team is consistently meeting and even exceeding their expectations.

One of the first steps in the process is a risk assessment, which helps the team uncover potential problems proactively (see 1.2 Providing a Lifetime of Care, and 2.7 Risk Assessment). Customer service surveys are critical, especially surveys that allow you to benchmark against others in the industry, with metrics such as the Net Promoter Score (NPS).[1] These surveys are a great way not only to determine if clients are satisfied with your services, but also to ensure that their expectations have been met to such an extent that they would willingly promote you to friends and relatives. It is important to keep in mind, however, that most clients base their satisfaction on impressions (based on appearance, communication, other reviews, etc.) and don't always have reliable criteria on which to base competence. For example, the owner of the Cavalier King Charles spaniel may appear entirely satisfied with their visit until they speak with another owner of the breed who challenges the advice given with a comment such as "What do you mean, the veterinary team didn't talk to you about the risk of heart disease?"

If nationwide surveys are any indication, then most veterinary practices need to reevaluate how well they are doing in the eyes of their clients. In one large study, clients didn't really understand the point of evaluating pets when they appear to be healthy, they found bringing pets to the veterinary hospital stressful, and they also thought veterinary costs were high [1].

From the same study [1], pet owners indicated that they would likely visit the veterinary clinic more if they knew such visits could prevent problems and more expensive treatment later, they were convinced it would help the pet live longer, if each visit was less expensive, and if they really believed the pet needed to be examined as often as recommended.

Pet-specific care answers most of these concerns because it focuses on keeping pets healthy rather than waiting for them to get sick, it takes a proactive approach to prevention and early detection, and it actively engages clients in the health decision-making process (see 1.1 Overview of Pet-Specific Care). While pet-specific care may not lower total costs of care, the value proposition of keeping pets healthy is often an easier discussion to have with clients, since they

are often familiar with the concepts as they apply to human healthcare.

5.3.4 Clear Communication

It is not only important that pet owners receive directions from hospital team members in a clear manner, but consistency of the message is also important, ensuring message integrity from all staff members, the clinic web site, brochures, and other resources that may be provided to the client (see 9.8 – Ensuring Consistency of Care).

Improving communication skills of the veterinary healthcare team is one of the most important things that hospitals can do to help meet client expectations. Obviously, if the intention is to meet and even exceed client expectations, then the first part of the solution is to understand exactly what those client expectations are.

This is best achieved through shared decision making, so the client is intimately engaged in the decision-making process [2]. Clients who are active partners in the care of their pets are more invested in the process, and are also more likely to be compliant with mutually determined recommendations [3].

Although some individuals may have inherently better communications skills than others from the outset, what is clear is that those skills are very trainable and all hospital members can improve their communication skills with appropriate training (see 8.15 Delivering Information to Clients).

5.3.5 Value Delivery and Affordability

Pet owners spend a lot of money on their pets, more with each passing year, and in most cases the money spent is a reflection of the human–animal bond [4] (see 2.14 Benefits of the Human–Animal Bond).

Most consumers are value shoppers and look for the ultimate value in their purchases, rather than merely the price. Whether it is the car they drive, the neighborhood in which they live, or the brand of watch on their wrist, clients want to receive at least as much value as the amount of money they are prepared to pay.

When consumers believe that there are a variety of products or services that are very similar in utility and value, these products or services are regarded as commodities and decisions are then made on the basis of price and convenience. For example, if a veterinarian dispenses a medication when a similar or even identical product is available elsewhere at a much lower price, then even if the client

---

1 Net Promoter, NPS, and Net Promoter Score are trademarks of Satmetrix Systems, Inc., Bain & Company, and Fred Reichheld.

purchases it from the veterinarian, the price differential (if they are aware of it) may cause the client to question the pricing for all services provided at that hospital. Clients will only willingly pay a premium at a veterinary hospital if they perceive they are receiving commensurate value.

Most pet owners today are omnichannel consumers and use many different retail channels (including a variety of online and bricks-and-mortar alternatives) to evaluate products and services and make decisions before they buy. It is natural that they also review their options for veterinary products and services, and clinics should expect this type of client behavior.

Because most pet expenditures are made with disposable income, it is critical that veterinary hospitals detail the amount and type of expenditures that a pet owner might encounter over the life of their pet (see 5.10 Discussing Pet-Specific Care and 2.9 Anticipated Costs of Pet Care). In this way, clients can understand the costs of such care and can plan accordingly, by saving money, buying pet health insurance (see 10.16 Pet Health Insurance), considering payment plans (see 10.17 Payment and Wellness Plans), or other risk management strategies (see 10.18 Financing Veterinary Care) [5].

5.3.6 Advocacy

Clients appreciate that veterinarians run hospitals that need to make money, but they also want to be confident that the recommendations being made are evidence based, in the best interests of their pet, fairly priced, and not motivated by profit. This is best achieved by delivering pet-specific care and creating appropriate standards and protocols within the hospital (see 9.4 Standards of Care) and helping the client to appreciate the needs specific to their pet (see 1.3 Personalized Care Plans).

5.3.7 Confidentiality and Privacy

It is also critical that we do much more for our clients that just deliver medicine. Clients do business with us and trust us with their financial information, and it is important that we safeguard that information. Veterinary clinics can be "hacked" just as any other business, and it is important to safeguard client information (see 7.13 Keeping Client Information Secure). In addition, clients often also trust us with very private information, such as their job status, marital situation, ability to afford services, and much more, and they expect that veterinary hospital staff will keep such information confidential (see 7.6 Privacy and Confidentiality). Accordingly, safeguards should be in

place not only to keep such information private, but to encourage staff not to discuss client matters in nonprivate settings, or even in the form of in-hospital gossip.

TAKE-AWAYS

- Most pet owners are value shoppers and seek value in their expenditures, including expenditures at veterinary hospitals.
- Clients often don't know what they don't know about the care of their specific pet.
- Veterinary teams should be prepared to counsel clients about the specific needs of their pets and help them establish reasonable expectations for the care of their pet.
- If teams make evidence-based recommendations, clients are likely to get confirmation that this is appropriate when those clients engage with other experts, peers, do their own online research, etc.
- Expectations are easier to manage when they are out in the open; encourage clients to share with the team the expectations they have for pet care.

MISCELLANEOUS

5.3.8 Cautions

Each client is an individual, with their own perceptions and expectations. It is not reasonable to assume that any one veterinary practice can meet the needs of all potential clients. The goal should be to practice excellent medicine, deliver uncompromising customer service, and strive to honestly meet the needs of clients, given the practice's mission and vision. In some instances, the needs of individual pet owners might be better met elsewhere. Just as not all consumers shopping for a car are looking for a luxury brand, not all pet owners are necessarily looking for the same level of veterinary care, so meeting expectations is all about first understanding what those expectations are.

References

1 Volk, J.O., Felsted, K.E., Thomas, J.G., and Siren, C.W. (2011). Executive summary of the Bayer veterinary care usage study. *J. Am. Vet. Med. Assoc.* 238 (10): 1275–1282.

2 Cornell, K.K. and Kopcha, M. (2007). Client-veterinarian communication: skills for client-centered dialogue and shared decision making. *Vet. Clin. North Am. Small Anim. Pract.* 37 (1): 37–47.

3 Abood, S.K. (2007). Increasing adherence in practice: making your clients partners in care. *Vet. Clin. North Am. Small Anim. Pract.* 37 (1): 151–164.

4 Lue, T.W., Pantenburg, D.P., and Crawford, P.M. (2008). Impact of the owner–pet and client–veterinarian bond on the care that pets receive. *J. Am. Vet. Med. Assoc.* 232 (4): 531–540.

5 Volk, J.O., Felsted, K.E., Thomas, J.G., and Siren, C.W. (2011). Executive summary of phase 2 of the Bayer veterinary care usage study. *J. Am. Vet. Med. Assoc.* 239 (10): 1311–1316.

Recommended Reading

Aaron, A.P., Kohistrand, M.L., Welborn, L.V., and Curvey, S.T. (2019). Maintaining medical record confidentiality and client privacy in the era of big data: ethical and legal responsibilities. *J. Am. Vet. Med. Assoc.* 255 (3): 282–288.

Ackerman, L.J. (2002). *Business Basics for Veterinarians*. New York: ASJA Press.

Ackerman, L.J. (2003). *Management Basics for Veterinarians*. New York: ASJA Press.

Ackerman, L.J. (2011). *The Genetic Connection: A Guide to Health Problems in Purebred Dogs*, 2e. Lakewood, CO: AAHA Press.

Ackerman, L.J. (2020). What clients expect from their veterinarian. In: *Five-Minute Veterinary Practice Management Consult*, 3e, 250–251. Ames, IA: Wiley.

Ackerman, L.J. (2020). Problem Free Pets: The ultimate guide to pet parenting. Problem Free Publishing (Dermvet).

5.4

The Changing Nature of Pet Owners

Lowell Ackerman, DVM, DACVD, MBA, MPA, CVA, MRCVS

Global Consultant, Author, and Lecturer, MA, USA

BASICS

5.4.1 Summary

Today's pet owner is an informed consumer and, more than at any time in the past, has the ability to acquire pet health information from sources other than the veterinary team. In years past, there would certainly be books on pet care, and members of the "fancy" had access to periodicals targeted to purebred ownership and healthcare. However, now the internet provides ready access to virtually limitless amounts of noncurated information and product sales. That surging volume of available information is not only confusing, but it can adversely affect personal well-being, decision making and productivity, and it can serve as a major interruption in one's day [1].

For veterinarians to compete effectively in such an environment of information overload, they must increasingly rely on value delivery, customer service, and acting as an advocate for pet owners – helping dog and cat owners navigate the confusing path toward optimal pet healthcare.

5.4.2 Terms Defined

Demographics: Description of objective and quantifiable characteristics of an audience or population such as age, marital status, household income, and pet-spending index.

Market Research: Determining attitudes and behaviors of various public segments and their causes in order to plan, implement, and measure activities to influence or change those attitudes and behaviors.

Medicalization: In veterinary medicine, this term has come to represent the percentage of total owned animals that have been seen by a veterinarian at least once in a 12-month period. This is different from the sociological use of the term to describe nonmedical issues that are described in medical terms of prevention, diagnosis, and treatment.

Pet Parent: A term used to designate that the relationship between individuals and their pets in more than just ownership. Such individuals endeavor to do what is best for their pets and seek to maximize the benefits of the human–animal bond for both parties.

Psychographics: Research that attempts to explain behavior by analyzing people's personality traits and values.

MAIN CONCEPTS

Even though the numbers change slightly from year to year, Americans remain a population of pet lovers. In the most recent demographics available, approximately 57% of households in the United States owned a pet and close to two-thirds of those pet-owning households owned two or more pets [2]. This does vary a bit, depending on the survey selected, but it is fairly consistent with the other major survey done that contends that 68% of US households owned a pet, representing approximately 90 million dogs and 94 million cats [3].

5.4.3 Medicalization

Although the US is clearly a country of pet lovers, that affection does not necessarily translate into regular veterinary visits. In addition, there is often a significant discrepancy between veterinary care provided for dogs versus what is done for cats.

Over 60% of pet owners consider their pet a family member, whereas 36% consider them companions, and only 1% consider them property [2]. With those kinds of numbers, one would expect very high levels of medicalization. In this context, medicalization refers to any level of veterinary care that an owned pet receives in a 12-month period, but obviously this does not necessarily represent optimal care.

Close to 75% of pet-owning households took their dogs to the veterinarian at least once a year for routine check-ups and preventive care [2]. From that same study, only 45% of households owning cats had taken them to the veterinarian at least once a year. Feline visits have actually declined 13.5% from the same survey done five years previously, which means that most cats are not receiving the level of veterinary care needed, and the situation seems to be worsening.

One clear determinant of medicalization rates is the human–animal bond (see 2.14 Benefits of the Human–Animal Bond). Although households that owned dogs saw the veterinarian an average of 1.6 times a year, households that saw their dog as a family member had, on average, 2.9 veterinary visits a year, compared with 2.0 visits a year for households considering their dog a companion, and only 1.2 times a year for households considering their dog property [2]. The same benefit seems to hold true for cats. Households that owned cats saw the veterinarian an average of 1.6 times a year, whereas households that saw their cat as a family member had, on average, 1.9 visits a year, compared with 1.2 visits a year for households considering their cat a companion, and only 0.5 visits a year for households considering their cat property. In another study, owners with strong owner–pet bonds took their pets to veterinarians 40% more often than owners with weaker owner–pet bonds [4].

From these studies, it is reasonable to suggest that promotion of the human–animal bond by practices is the best way to improve medicalization of existing patients (see 2.15 Promoting the Human–Animal Bond). Such "pet parents" not only take care of their pets, but often benefit from the interactions themselves (see 5.5 Meeting the Needs of Pet Parents). It is less clear how veterinarians, as a group, can help drive current nonusers of veterinary services to more closely bond with their pets and to seek appropriate veterinary attention.

5.4.4 Demographics and Psychographics

Although the standard family unit of one husband, one wife, and two-plus children has evolved considerably in recent decades, it is less clear that so-called nontraditional families are any less pet friendly, and there is much evidence that total pet numbers and numbers of households owning pets are fairly steady. One thing that seems to be very consistent across all age groups is who is ultimately taking responsibility for pet care. By a resounding 80.7%, the primary pet caretakers are female [2].

The big question on the horizon for veterinary care is the generational differences yet to be observed as the Millennials (those born between 1982 and 1999, although there is not consensus on this range) are now the major generation of pet owners (see 2.6 Generational Considerations). The Millennials, as a cohort, represent about 80 million people in the US, a generation even bigger than the Baby Boomers, and it is not yet known with any certainty what their attitudes will be toward pet ownership and regular veterinary care. However, at present, the Millennials are the predominant pet-owning demographic, and there is at least preliminary evidence to suggest that they take the responsibility seriously and are prepared to spend accordingly [5]. For the generation following the Millennials, sometimes referred to as Generation Z or the iGeneration, time will tell as to how they manage pet ownership, and the generation following them, sometimes referred to as Generation Alpha, are at this moment too young to even guess at their future pet-owning behaviors.

One thing that likely will change regarding the Millennials and Generation Z is how they will want to receive veterinary services. For generations that experienced firsthand the convenience of the internet, smart devices, and social media, will they be content to bring their pets physically to a veterinary office when those pets otherwise seem to be well and not in need of specific services? By the same token, will veterinary offices need to evolve their business models from relying on owners physically bringing a pet to an office, perhaps even considering more telehealth options (see 2.5 Virtual Care (Telehealth))?

Of course, while Millennials tend to get most of the attention, it is important not to lose sight of the next generation, Generation Z, as their needs will not necessarily be identical to those of Millennials. As of 2021, they likely constitute about 20% of the workforce and are very used to convenience. It is possible that iGens will not only want virtual care as an option in healthcare, but might even want veterinary care delivered to their doorstep, or their place of work.

In general, most businesses today do their best to accommodate clients with disabilities. While most veterinary practices have parking spaces available for handicapped clients, most clinics are not necessarily easily accessible for those with mobility-related disabilities. Given that the populations in most developed countries are aging, improving accessibility should be a priority.

5.4.5 Spending

From the most recent statistics available, the US pet industry represents sales of approximately $80 billion per year and of that, only about a quarter is spent on veterinary care [3]. Perhaps more compelling is the fact that although these same surveys indicate that pet spending has grown at a healthy pace, the growth in veterinary spending has been relatively anemic by comparison. This seems to indicate that although pet owners value their pets and spend consistently on them regardless of the economy, veterinary care may not be valued as highly as some other goods and services.

We have already seen that visits to veterinary offices are a direct reflection of the human–animal bond (see 2.14 Benefits of the Human–Animal Bond), but the same is true of expenditures. Dog-owning households that considered dogs to be family members spent 1.6 times more on veterinary expenditures than those that considered their dogs to be companions and 2.3 times more than those that considered their dogs to be property [2]. In the same study, cat-owning households that considered cats to be family members spent 1.7 times more on veterinary expenditures than those that considered their cats to be companions, and 5.1 times more than those that considered their cats to be property.

Veterinary teams have also not done as good a job as needed at educating clients about the need for routine veterinary care (see 1.2 Providing a Lifetime of Care and 5.10 Discussing Pet-Specific Care). Vaccination remains the main reason for pet owners to visit the veterinarian [4] and this can be confusing for owners when vaccination protocols change, or when vaccination becomes available through alternate channels (see 9.11 Vaccination).

Even though there are more cats than dogs, because medicalization rates are higher in dogs than in cats and expenditures per pet are higher in dogs than cats, 68% of total veterinary expenditures are spent on dogs [2]. This represents a challenge, but also a great opportunity to become more feline friendly and to reap the potential benefits of providing needed professional services to cat owners (see 1.5 Feline-Friendly Care and 6.13 Delivering Feline-Friendly Care).

A look at today's pet owners would not be complete without examining their attitudes to the current use of veterinary services. One-third of dog owners and over 40% of cat owners would not take their otherwise healthy pets to the veterinarian if vaccinations were not necessary [4]. This demonstrates that veterinary teams have not done an

acceptable job in detailing the importance of regular veterinary visits and pet-specific care, apart from vaccination.

According to the previously mentioned usage study [6], pet owners would be prepared to take their pets to the veterinarian more often if certain criteria were met. The following are the top four criteria, each followed by the percentage of owners that either completely or somewhat agreed.

- If they knew it would prevent problems and more expensive treatment later (59%).
- If convinced it would help their pet live longer (59%).
- If each visit was less expensive (47%).
- If they really believed their pet needed exams more often (44%).

In addition to all the other factors responsible for driving client visits and appropriate healthcare spending on pets, there is one important aspect that is completely under veterinary control. One of the largest impediments to clients doing the right things for their pets is effective communication about what pet owners should be doing, and making very direct recommendations for action rather than vague suggestions. Clear and thorough communication with the client can ultimately increase compliance by as much as 40% [4].

TAKE-AWAYS

- Pet owners today can be easily distracted by the seemingly limitless amount of information available on the internet. Veterinary practices need to be able to curate resources, so they can be pet specific and relevant for individual pets.
- When it comes to today's pet owners, veterinarians need to convey value in their offerings, take time to educate clients on the immediate and lifelong healthcare needs of pets, and make clear recommendations as to what medical care is appropriate.
- Veterinary practices need to concentrate on providing end-to-end solutions for pet owners, solving their problems, saving them time, providing what is actually needed, and continuously improving the process with the client's total satisfaction in mind.
- It is natural to expect that pet owners will request and even seek out alternate channels of veterinary care that they consider more convenient or cost-effective
- Younger generations of pet owners are likely to have different expectations of the profession from their parents and grandparents

MISCELLANEOUS

5.4.6 Cautions

Along with information overload, we are also seeing global changes in consumer behavior that are reflected in the actions of many customers today. There have been noticeable trends that are likely to affect spending on veterinary care for many years to come. These trends include [7]:

- a demand for simplicity (preference for simpler offerings with the greatest value)
- discretionary thrift (economizing activities, even by affluent consumers)
- the decline of deference (consumers' growing confidence in their own ability to find information and products, and make smart choices, without the need for experts)
- fickle consumption (erratic loyalty, with the belief that there are so many options available that there is no need to settle for what is immediately available).

Businesses that streamline the client experience by providing goods and services that make it easier for customers to buy and use them actually strengthen consumer loyalty, and attract new customers who defect from less user-friendly competitors [8].

References

1 Hemp, P. (2009). Death by information overload. *Harvard Business Review* September: 83–89.

2 American Veterinary Medical Association (2017–2018). *U.S. Pet Ownership & Demographics Sourcebook*. Schaumburg, IL.

3 American Pet Products Association. Pet Industry Market Size and Ownership Statistics. www.americanpetproducts.org/press_industrytrends.asp

4 Lue, T.W., Pantenburg, D.P., and Crawford, P.M. (2008). Impact of the owner–pet and client–veterinarian bond on the care that pets receive. *J. Am. Vet. Med. Assoc.* 232 (4): 531–540.

5 TD Ameritrade. Millennials and their fur babies. https://s1.q4cdn.com/959385532/files/doc_downloads/research/2018/Millennials-and-Their-Fur-Babies.pdf

6 Bayer Healthcare LLC (2011). *Bayer Veterinary Care Usage Study*. Hanover, NJ: Bayer Animal Health.

7 Flatters, P. and Willmott, M. (2009). Understanding the post-recession consumer. *Harvard Business Review* July/August: 106–112.

8 Womack, J.P. and Jones, D.T. (2005). Lean consumption. *Harvard Business Review* March: 59–68.

Recommended Reading

Ackerman, L. (2020). Today's pet owner. In: *Five-Minute Veterinary Practice Management Consult*, 3e, 16–17. Ames, IA: Wiley.

Ackerman, L.J. (2020). Problem Free Pets: The ultimate guide to pet parenting. Problem Free Publishing (Dermvet).

Winkley, E.G., KuKanich, K., Nary, D., and Fakler, J. (2020). Accessibility of veterinary hospitals for clients with mobility-related disabilities. *J. Am. Vet. Med. Assoc.* 256 (3): 333–339.

5.5

Meeting the Needs of Pet Parents

Amanda L. Donnelly, DVM, MBA

ALD Veterinary Consulting, LLC, Nashville, TN, USA

BASICS

5.5.1 Summary

The veterinary profession has consistently focused on the importance of communicating the value of services to pet owners as one of the primary ways to increase client visits, compliance, and retention. The idea has been that if pet owners understand the value of veterinary services and products, they will say "yes" to treatment recommendations.

While conveying the value of veterinary care remains highly relevant, the profession now needs to look at changes in how pet owners value their relationship with veterinary providers. Contemporary business strategy is to evaluate and respond to the needs of a diverse population of pet parents to provide value in all areas they find essential. Veterinary businesses that explore and meet the individual needs of pet parents will be more successful in increasing client loyalty and compliance. Moreover, more pets will get the care they deserve.

5.5.2 Terms Defined

Pet Parent: A term used to designate that the relationship between individuals and their pets in more than just ownership. Such individuals endeavor to do what is best for their pets and seek to maximize the benefits of the human–animal bond for both parties.
Telehealth: Refers to all uses of technology geared to remotely deliver health information or education.
Third-Party Payment: Monetary reimbursement for medical services from someone other than the client/patient.

Holistic Approach: Looks at healthcare for the whole pet, including factors related to exercise, diet, well-being, and the environment rather than just focusing on diagnoses and treatments.

MAIN CONCEPTS

5.5.3 Identify The Needs of Pet Parents

For businesses to consider how to best meet the needs of pet parents, it is critical to look at both the macro view and the micro view. The macro perspective is to think about what pet owners in your community want. This may be somewhat different depending on the demographics of the area (see 5.4 The Changing Nature of Pet Owners). For example, pet parents in a city location with a large population of younger generations may place value on different needs from pet parents in a suburban area with many retirees.

The micro perspective is for teams to identify the specific needs and desires of individual pet parents during each client interaction. While all pet owners appreciate excellent service, they also have unique needs and desires in terms of what they value in the client service experience. For example, one client may value efficiency over all other aspects of service. For this client, employees should keep conversations short and focused. They should update the client on wait times and always set realistic expectations. Another pet owner may tend to be anxious and slow to make decisions. This client needs reassurance and might require that the value of services be explained multiple times.

Pet-Specific Care for the Veterinary Team, First Edition. Edited by Lowell Ackerman.
© 2021 John Wiley & Sons, Inc. Published 2021 by John Wiley & Sons, Inc.

Business strategies and systems need to be put in place aimed at implementing action plans to meet the needs of pet parents. Remember, today's pet owners, particularly younger generations, have a greater desire to stay connected to companies they do business with. Therefore, it is important to consider how to meet the needs of pet parents before, during, and after appointments.

5.5.4 Adopt a Holistic Approach to Pet Healthcare

Surveys have found differences in how pet owners and veterinarians define preventive care. While veterinarians primarily focus on vaccines, spay/neuter, and parasite control for preventive care, increasingly pet owners consider their pet's diet, exercise, play, and emotional well-being as part of preventive care.

Since pets are an integral part of the family, it is vital for veterinary teams to discuss all aspects of the pet's life. Not only will these conversations reveal critical information about the pet's health, this holistic approach reinforces the role of the veterinary team as trusted advisors. The following action steps are examples of how teams can provide value and meet client needs with this holistic approach.

The first is to have clients fill out a health risk assessment survey asking about their pet's lifestyle, exercise, toys, treats, and diet (see 1.2 Providing a Lifetime of Care and 2.7 Risk Assessment). Ideally, this survey would be sent via text/SMS (Short Message Service) or email for clients to complete prior to their appointment. Next, make it a standard to discuss nutrition, obesity management, pain management, and use of supplements as part of every preventive care visit. An educational handout in these topic areas could be sent home with every client. Lastly, give clients a list of trusted websites and other care providers you recommend such as trainers, groomers, and pet sitters.

5.5.5 Enhance Client Education About Quality Medical Care

Providing outstanding client education is paramount for all veterinary teams. Clients want detailed information about medical conditions and preventive care as well as services and products. Be mindful to not assume what clients know. Instead, ask open-ended questions about their knowledge and then tailor client education accordingly.

Teams can build trust and enhance the value of client education by using visual tools and technology to augment verbal messages during every appointment. Examples include brochures, videos, anatomical pictures or models,

and graphs. Be sure to tailor all conversations for care to the client's pet. One way to do this is to reference the breed and the pet's lifestyle when discussing medical conditions and recommendations.

5.5.6 Provide Convenience and Personalized Service

Today's consumers crave convenience. This is why online shopping and home delivery are so popular. Increasingly, technology solutions are available to help meet clients' needs (see 7.9 Using Practice Management Software to Personalize Care). Veterinary hospitals can communicate value and meet the needs of pet parents by using technologies that help pet owners stay connected to the practice, provide customized service, and save time (see 5.13 Improving Client Engagement Through Technology). When considering a technology solution, be sure to evaluate whether it helps the client and helps get the pet the care it deserves. Here is a list of technology solutions desired by pet owners.

- Online scheduling of appointments
- A hospital online pharmacy and home delivery
- SMS/texting for reminders, updates, food or prescription requests, and targeted messages
- Two-way texting with the hospital team
- Completing pet histories and forms before appointments
- Tracking medication usage and pet activity levels
- Social media platforms to post photos, videos, and questions that engage pet owners and create a sense of community
- Video chatting, texting or emailing with a veterinarian in a telehealth approach

5.5.7 Empower Pet Parents

Today's clients want to partner with the veterinary team and be fully empowered to make decisions they feel are best for their family. They want to be an active participant in their pet's care rather than a passive listener to recommendations. Younger generations in particular find value in healthcare providers that ask questions and create dialogue about their pet (see 5.4 The Changing Nature of Pet Owners). Remember, many pet parents have spent time talking to friends or researching on the internet before they visit your practice.

Specific communication skills can be used to form a collaborative relationship that empowers pet parents and helps them see the veterinary team as their trusted advisor.

Open-ended questions help to initiate dialogue rather than just providing educational messages. For example, a veterinarian might ask a client "Tell me what you know about lymphoma in cats?" This approach is more likely to result in a positive outcome than launching into a lecture of what the doctor thinks the client needs to know (see 9.2 Asking Good Questions).

Another communication skill is to use reflective listening statements to invite clients to express what they're thinking or feeling. Examples include statements such as "I sense you're frustrated by Dudley's response to medication" or "It appears you may have some concerns about Roxie's treatment plan."

5.5.8 Focus on Affordability and Cost Savings

Veterinary care can be expensive, and today's consumers are looking for the best value for money spent. Given that pet owners have many choices for pet care services and products, veterinary practices need to have proactive financial discussions with clients (see 5.11 Discussing Finances for Pet-Specific Care).

Make sure your team is trained to present third-party payment plans (see 10.18 Financing Veterinary Care), monthly payment plans (see 10.17 Payment and Wellness Plans), recommended pet health insurance options (see 10.16 Pet Health Insurance) and preventive care plans. Don't be afraid to discuss drug costs. Inform clients of the benefits of in-hospital purchases and the value of promotions or complimentary doses. Offer the convenience of an online store and be willing to write prescriptions when appropriate (see 9.10 Dispensing and Prescribing). Use a mobile app branded to your hospital that includes a client loyalty program. These programs offer added value and can enhance client retention.

EXAMPLES

Mr Brown enjoys bringing his Labrador retriever, Max, to ABC Veterinary Hospital because they offer convenient, personalized service and spend time listening to his needs. Before every appointment, he receives a text/SMS to confirm his appointment and a link to fill out information about Max and his concerns. During the appointment, Max is offered a selection of treats and the veterinarian spends time asking Mr Brown questions about his life with Max. On their last visit, the doctor asked what he knew about joint health. This discussion helped Mr Brown realize Max was having some difficulty with long walks and would benefit from having radiographs as well as a prescription for medication and a joint supplement. As a member of the practice's loyalty program, he was able to use rewards points to save money. After the visit, Mr Brown loved seeing a picture of Max on the hospital's Facebook page.

TAKE-AWAYS

- Veterinary businesses that explore and meet the individual needs of pet parents will be more successful in increasing client loyalty and compliance.
- The human–pet bond is strong. Clients continue to value high-quality care and access to affordable medical services and products.
- Pet owners are interested in a holistic approach to preventive care that includes lifestyle and emotional well-being.
- Today's pet owners have a need for convenience and will choose veterinary healthcare providers that make it easy to do business with them.
- Increasingly, pet parents want to be empowered and involved in decision making for their pet's care.

MISCELLANEOUS

Recommended Reading

Donnelly, A. What's in a story? Today's Veterinary Business. https://todaysveterinarybusiness.com/whats-in-a-story

Donnelly, A. Why Embrace Generation Y? Today's Veterinary Business. https://todaysveterinarybusiness.com/why-embrace-generation-y

Pet Health by the Numbers. 2015 State of Pet Health Report. Today's Veterinary Practice. https://todaysveterinarypractice.com/pet-health-by-the-numbers-3

5.6

Adoption Source Options

Sarah Rumple

Rumpus Writing and Editing LLC, Denver, CO, USA

BASICS

5.6.1 Summary

Getting a new pet is a big deal. When clients ask where they should go to find their next animal companion, the veterinary healthcare team should be prepared to offer advice and a list of trusted and reputable pet adoption sources in the area. The most common pet adoption sources include bricks-and-mortar animal shelters, foster-based pet rescues, breeders, and pet stores. By having a thorough understanding of each, veterinary professionals can help prospective pet owners to support reputable pet adoption sources and make informed decisions.

5.6.2 Terms Defined

No-Kill: A policy that prohibits or severely limits the euthanizing of animals in a shelter.
Backyard Breeder: An amateur animal breeder whose breeding is considered substandard, with little or misguided effort toward ethical, selective breeding.
Puppy Mill: A commercial facility that mass-produces puppies for sale.

MAIN CONCEPTS

When it comes to adopting or purchasing a new pet, the many options – from animal shelters to breeders to pet rescues – can be confusing and overwhelming (see 3.10

Advising Clients on Selecting an Appropriate Pet). A quick internet search can produce thousands of adoptable pets in any given area, but are these pets healthy? Are they coming from reputable organizations? Veterinarians and their teams should be prepared to help prospective pet owners navigate the pet adoption waters. Here's what you should know about some common pet adoption sources so you can offer sound advice to your clients.

5.6.3 Bricks-and-Mortar Animal Shelters

Animal shelters provide places for lost or abandoned animals. Additionally, many shelters provide resources for local pet owners, including low-cost spay/neuter or other veterinary services and educational opportunities for the community. Some animal shelters are municipal agencies, owned by local governments and partially funded by taxpayer dollars, while others are private nonprofit organizations.

Whether shelters are government run or privately owned, most rely heavily on donations from the public to operate. Many shelters will accept any animal, and, because of the high unwanted pet population, animal shelters are often full and are forced to implement humane euthanasia policies to create space for incoming adoptable animals. Other animal shelters have "no-kill" policies and will not euthanize animals for space, regardless of their age, length of time at the facility, or adoptability. Once they reach capacity, these facilities are forced to turn animals away due to space constraints.

Shelters often have relationships with pet supply retailers and will house some of their adoptable animals at these retail stores for periods of time, which can help increase the likelihood of adoption (Table 5.6.1).

Table 5.6.1   Pros and cons of acquiring a pet from an animal shelter

Pros	Cons
Prospective pet owners can see animals available for adoption by simply visiting the bricks-and-mortar facility	The history of many pets in animal shelters is unknown
Many shelters have private spaces where adopters can meet and interact one-on-one with pets they're interested in adopting	Animal shelters are often loud, scary places for pets, and many will be under considerable stress. This can change their behavior and overall demeanor, which affects their adoptability. Once in a less stressful environment, an animal's personality could be entirely different from what it was in the shelter
The pet adoption process is typically faster and easier than adopting through a rescue	Animals may have been relinquished to a shelter for reasons that are not evident at time of adoption
Most pets adopted from animal shelters will be spayed/neutered, dewormed, vaccinated, and microchipped before adoption	Shelters conditions can make it more likely for pets to be exposed to infectious diseases
Adopting from an animal shelter saves a life and opens up a space for another homeless pet	

5.6.3.1 Important Considerations Before Adopting from An Animal Shelter

- What are the animal shelter's standards of care? While potential owners are touring the facility, they should look for signs that animals might not be receiving optimal care. They might even consider signing up as a volunteer before adopting to get a sense of the inner workings of the shelter.
- Are adopters able to spend time alone with potential new pets before committing?
- Can current pets meet the new pet before committing?
- What is the relinquishment policy if an adopted pet doesn't work out?

5.6.4   Foster-Based Pet Rescues

Pet rescues are usually private, nonprofit organizations that are reliant on donations – money, supplies, and volunteer time – from the community to do their work. Rather than investing in bricks-and-mortar spaces to house animals, rescues typically rely on volunteers to foster the animals in their homes until suitable adopters are found (Table 5.6.2).

Rescues sometimes focus on specific species, breeds, or life stages.

Table 5.6.2   Pros and cons of adopting a pet from a pet rescue

Pros	Cons
With the ability to choose a rescue that focuses on a specific species, breed, or life stage, a prospective owner can find the pet desired—whether it's a purebred puppy or a mixed-breed senior pet—without purchasing from a breeder or pet store, yet still saving a life	Adopting can be a considerably lengthy process, including background checks, interviews, and home visits
Foster homes are typically less stressful than shelters, making it easier to see the authentic personalities of pets from the first meeting and enabling pets to maintain regular socialization with humans and other animals in the foster home	Adoption fees can be higher than those charged by animal shelters
Since fosters live with the animals they're caring for, they get a good sense of behavior and habits, and they can convey that information to prospective adopters	Since most rescues are run by volunteers, they can struggle with timely communication and organization. Scheduling times to meet pets with volunteer fosters can be difficult
An adopter will often have multiple opportunities to interact with the animal before the adoption process is finalized	Since rescues are decentralized, there is not a single location to go to consider which pet would be most appropriate
Some rescues partner with animal shelters and focus on animals that are not thriving in the shelter environment. Moving an animal from the stressful environment and into a loving foster home can increase the likelihood of adoption	

5.6.4.1 Important Considerations Before Adopting from a Pet Rescue

- Can a potential adopter tour a foster home or the bricks-and-mortar rescue facility, if applicable? Not all animal rescues are created equal, and some may be hoarding situations or fronts for breeding operations.
- What are the rescue's standards of care?
- Are pets spayed/neutered, dewormed, vaccinated, and microchipped before adoption? Have they received any other necessary medical care?
- What is the relinquishment policy if the pet is not a good fit?

5.6.5 Breeders

Breeders sometimes get a bad rap. After all, why purposely bring animals into the world when there are already so many unwanted pets? While it can be a divisive topic, there are a number of reasons a prospective pet owner might choose to purchase a pet from a breeder, rather than adopting from a shelter or rescue (see 5.9 Dealing with Breeders). When advising your clients, be sure they know the difference between a responsible breeder and a "backyard breeder."

According to the American Kennel Club (www.akc.org), a responsible breeder:

- has spent years researching pedigrees of the breed
- knows the specifics of the breed and the actual line he or she breeds
- knows generations behind the pets he or she is breeding
- will not let a puppy go too young, before the puppy has proper immunizations and socialization
- is willing to talk with and answer the questions of prospective pet owners, whether they've already committed to purchasing an animal or not
- is there for the purchaser and the animal for the pet's entire life, and will take the pet back if something unforeseen happens, regardless of the animal's age
- trains the animals, ensuring they're ready to join their new families when the time is right.

The pros and cons in Table 5.6.3 apply to working with responsible breeders only.

5.6.5.1 Important Considerations Before Purchasing from a Breeder

- Can a prospective pet owner meet the parents of the litter?
- Have health tests been performed on the parents? Does the breeder offer a health guarantee and a contract?

Table 5.6.3 Pros and cons of acquiring a pet from a reputable breeder

Pros	Cons
Owners are able to choose the animal they want and have a better idea of what they're going to get regarding temperament, health, and physical attributes based on the lineage of the animal	Purchasing a purebred animal is much more expensive than adopting from a shelter or a rescue
Animals available from responsible breeders have likely not experienced trauma or abuse	Purebred animals are more likely to be at risk for specific genetic conditions than mixed-breeds
Responsible breeders dedicate years to improving the quality of a particular breed and bringing healthy animals into the world	The process is usually longer than adopting from a shelter or rescue, and reputable breeders are likely to closely scrutinize potential buyers
Medical and behavioral considerations are more predictable, and at least one of the parents is likely accessible	Most reputable breeders only have a few litters a year, and may have a waiting list for those offspring

- How long has the breeder been breeding this particular breed?
- How are animals socialized?
- Are the animals up to date on vaccinations?
- When will the pet be able to go home with the new owner? Responsible breeders should not let a puppy go home with an owner until 8–12 weeks of age.
- Can the new owner contact the breeder at any time after the animal goes home?
- Does the breeder have requirements of prospective owners? Responsible breeders want to ensure their animals are going to good homes.

5.6.6 Pet Stores

If you've ever walked into a pet store, you know how difficult it is to resist those sweet purebred puppy eyes. But, those purebred puppies are often the product of puppy mills, and that means they've experienced abuse, neglect, and misery. According to the Humane Society of the United States (www.humanesociety.org):

- responsible breeders do not sell their puppies to pet stores because they want to meet their buyers in person
- many puppies sold in pet stores come from breeders with one or more animal welfare act violations. United States Department Of Agriculture (USDA) inspection reports have revealed sick and injured dogs who had not been

treated by a veterinarian, underweight dogs, puppies with their feet falling through wire floors, puppies with severe eye deformities, piles of feces, and food contaminated by mold and insects
- pet stores often do not disclose the true origin of their puppies
- puppies sold at pet stores may have serious health or psychological problems.

TAKE-AWAYS

- Veterinarians and their teams should be prepared to help clients make informed decisions and support reputable organizations when considering pet adoption or purchase.
- Bricks-and-mortar animal shelters house homeless pets onsite, usually providing necessary medical care. Potential adopters can meet and visit with pets during the shelter's hours of operation.
- Foster-based pet rescues are typically privately owned nonprofit organizations that rely on volunteers to foster animals in their homes until suitable adopters are found. Some focus on a particular species, breed, or life stage.
- While breeders often get a bad rap, responsible breeders work to improve breed quality and produce healthy animals. They will take the animal back at any time and will provide support for the life of the pet.
- Veterinary professionals should always discourage clients from purchasing animals from pet stores because they are products of puppy mills.

MISCELLANEOUS

Recommended Reading

Newbury, S., Blinn, M.K., Bushby, P. et al. Guidelines for Standards of Care in Animal Shelters. www.sheltervet.org/assets/docs/shelter-standards-oct2011-wforward.pdf

5.7

Preadoption Counseling

Kara M. Burns, MS, MEd, LVT, VTS (Nutrition)

Lafayette, IN, USA

 BASICS

5.7.1 Summary

Pet ownership brings many benefits – physical and emotional. Owning a pet can increase exercise, going outside, and socializing. Regular walking or playing with pets has been shown to decrease blood pressure, cholesterol levels, and triglyceride levels. Through companionship, pets can help manage loneliness and depression. Studies have shown that the bond between people and their pets can increase fitness, lower stress, and bring happiness to their owners.

It is important for potential pet owners to be educated regarding all that pet ownership brings – not only the positive health benefits, but also which pet would be the right fit for the person or family, costs associated with pet ownership, and lifestyle matching between the specific pet and the owner.

 MAIN CONCEPTS

Veterinary healthcare teams are often questioned by prospective pet owners and therefore must be ready to discuss the pros and cons of certain breeds and species, potential costs associated with pet ownership, and which pet is a good fit for that individual potential pet owner (see 3.10 Advising Clients on Selecting an Appropriate Pet).

An animal adoption counselor may be found in veterinary hospitals as well as in shelters. These individuals are specially trained and passionate about making sure pets and families are properly matched. People who work in this role also work with families and potential pet parents to equip and prepare them for any special needs or personality quirks their chosen pets may have, as well as the day-to-day demands and realities of pet ownership. Additionally, if a family already has a pet(s) the healthcare team can advise on how to introduce a new addition to the family, so everyone gets along (see 6.3 Managing Life Changes for Pets)!

Remind the prospective pet owner that they need to ensure the pet they are considering is the correct one for them and the family. Have them do some research regarding the specific breed they are considering [1]. Encourage them to not make a spontaneous decision.

Some questions for prospective pet owners to consider include the following.

- How long will this animal live?
- What does the pet eat?
- How much exercise does the pet need?
- How big will it turn out to be?
- How much will it cost for veterinary care?
- Do I have enough time to properly care for and clean up after the pet?
- What type of habitat does this pet need to be healthy?
- What type of exercise does this pet need?
- Are pets allowed in my house, apartment, or condominium?
- Are there young children, older people, or people with weak immune systems who will care for or be around the pet?

No matter the type of pet, the healthcare team must educate the potential owner about the responsibility for providing regular, life-long veterinary care to keep the pet and the family healthy (see 1.2 Providing a Lifetime of Care). It is important to remind owners that regular veterinary visits are essential to good pet health. Some of the basics in the preadoption discussion should center around how to keep the pet healthy such as:

- proper nutrition
- fresh water
- clean bedding
- plenty of exercise
- vaccinations
- deworming
- flea and tick control

By counseling regarding the pet's health, you are educating the prospective owner on how to keep the entire family healthy (see 2.19 One Health).

Zoonotic disease potential exists and should be discussed. Children under 5 years of age, people with weakened immune systems, and individuals 65 years of age and older are more at risk for diseases spread between animals and people [1]. Pregnant women are also at a higher risk for certain animal-related diseases. Before getting a new pet, keep the following in mind.

- Pet reptiles (turtles, lizards, snakes), amphibians (frogs, toads), or backyard poultry pose a risk of serious illness from harmful germs spread between these animals and family members, especially young children. Proper hygiene in this situation is crucial.
- People with weakened immune systems should take extra precautions when choosing and handling pets.
- Pregnant women should avoid contact with pet rodents to prevent exposure to lymphocytic choriomeningitis virus, which can cause birth defects. It is best to avoid direct contact and have someone else clean the habitat.

5.7.2 Proper Pet Hygiene

When counseling regarding new pets, it is important to educate owners about proper pet hygiene to prevent the spread of germs between pets and people (see 4.3 Prevention and Control of Infectious Diseases). Caution that pets and supplies are best kept out of the kitchen. Cleaning and disinfecting of pet habitats and supplies should be done outside the house when possible. It is prudent to remind them to not clean supplies in the kitchen sink, food preparation areas, or bathroom sink. Proper pet hygiene does not stop inside the house but should also be considered outside the house as well. Remind owners to remove dog feces from the yard and public places by using a bag and disposing of it in proper areas. Dog and cat feces can contain parasites

and germs that may be harmful to other pets and people. Keep children away from areas that might contain dog or cat feces (such as sandboxes at play parks) to prevent them from getting roundworms and hookworms. Clean the cat's litter box daily to lower the chances of exposure to harmful parasites.

Choosing a new pet is not always easy and can be an anxiety-producing process. Potential pet parents who do not take time to learn about the potential pet, breed, or species may find themselves in over their heads with a pet which needs more specialized care than they were ready to provide. Speaking to the veterinary team and adoption counselors can help alleviate that uncertainty and ensure the adoptive pet parents are matched with pets that fit their personalities and lifestyles.

Before clients add a companion animal to their family, offer to help them choose a species and breed that will be a good fit. The veterinary healthcare team and preadoption counselors should be the experts on pets and have a great deal to offer prospective pet owners. Discuss the realistic and unrealistic possibilities that may come with pet ownership. Advise on how to properly socialize and teach/train their pet so the relationship gets off to the best start possible (see 6.9 Preventing Behavior Problems).

EXAMPLES

Joe lives in a high-rise apartment in a big city and works long hours most days. He is contemplating getting a pet and has always heard wonderful things about the Border collie breed but also finds pugs adorable.

The healthcare team at ABC Veterinary Hospital listens to Joe and counsels him on both breeds to help him with a decision on what dog would be a good fit for both Joe and his pet. The Border collie is a high-energy and very intelligent breed. They want to herd as that has been their "job." Depending on gender, they can grow to be 18–22 in. (45–56 cm) and up to 55 lbs. (25 kg). They need lots of activity. The intelligence, athleticism, and trainability of Border collies are perfect for agility training. Having a job to perform, like agility, herding or obedience work, is key to Border happiness [2].

The pug has a very loving personality and can be mischievous. They grow to be approximately 13 in. (33 cm) and 20 lbs (9 kg). They are not a high-activity breed but do need exercise. Pug owners report this breed to be the ideal house dog. Pugs are happy in the city or country, with kids or old folks, as an only pet or in a pack. Pugs do love their food and care must be taken to keep them trim. They do best in moderate climates – not too hot, not too cold – but, with proper care, pugs can be their adorable selves anywhere [3].

Given Joe's current lifestyle, a pug could be a more suitable companion. It is important, though, that Joe is aware that pugs are prone to brachycephalic airway obstruction syndrome (BOAS), and this must be understood and accommodated by any potential pug owner (see 11.3 Heritable Health Conditions – By Disease).

TAKE-AWAYS

- Veterinary healthcare teams must be able to discuss the pros and cons of certain breeds and species, potential costs associated with pet ownership, and which pet is a good fit for a potential pet owner.
- An animal adoption counselor should be specially trained and passionate about making sure pets and families are properly matched.

- The healthcare team must educate the potential owner about the responsibility for providing regular, lifelong veterinary care to keep the pet and the family healthy.
- Counseling regarding the pet's health allows you to educate potential pet owners on how to keep the entire family healthy.
- Potential pet parents who do not take time to learn about the potential pet, breed, or species may find themselves in over their heads with a pet which needs more specialized care than they were ready to provide.

MISCELLANEOUS

References

1 About Pets and People. www.cdc.gov/healthypets/ health-benefits/index.html

2 Border Collie. www.akc.org/dog-breeds/border-collie

3 Pug. www.akc.org/dog-breeds/pug

5.8

The Biology of Marketing

Robert Sanchez

Digital Empathy, San Diego, CA, USA

 BASICS

5.8.1 Summary

One of the most important challenges that a veterinary practice faces is the ability to attract new clients. The internet has caused a fundamental shift in the way that pet owners find their veterinary practices. But while we communicate and learn digitally, we are still looking to satisfy the same psychological needs that we yearned for millennia ago. If the members of a veterinary practice achieve a working understanding of these underlying mechanisms, they can attract more of their ideal clients, build stronger bonds with existing clients, and find more meaning in their work.

5.8.2 Terms Defined

Archetype: A recurrent symbol or motif in literature, art, or mythology.

Buyer Journey: A framework that acknowledges a buyer's progression through a research and decision process ultimately culminating in a purchase.

Meta Description: A snippet of text that summarizes a page's content, used primarily for search engine results purposes.

Sales Funnel: The system or process that companies lead customers through when purchasing a product or service.

Thin Slicing: The ability to find patterns in events based only on "thin slices," or narrow windows, of experience.

 MAIN CONCEPTS

5.8.3 Evolutionary Psychology

As a pet owner looks for a veterinarian, they are consciously asking logical questions. "Who are you, what do you do, and where do you do it?" But the reality is that there is a much older question their mind is subconsciously asking ... "Can I trust you?" Your marketing and communications strategy must be based on the science of relationships – how and why they work. Each member of the team has a potential opportunity, every day, to contribute to an environment where pet owners feel safe, feel trust, and feel comfortable in the relationship.

The biological systems that guide our decision making were developed for an environment that existed tens (or even hundreds) of thousands of years ago. And while we may dress nicer, have better hygiene, and have an incredible and growing body of knowledge that we are privileged to tap into, these same biological systems guide our decision making today.

When we are walking alone in a dark alley, when we are dealing with a mechanic who we feel may have dishonest motives, or when an unwelcomed gaze lingers just a bit too long, it makes us feel wary. Why? Cortisol. When trust is absent, our brain feeds us a dose of this hormone. Cortisol has one job: to make us wary of our environment. To tell us to watch our backs. When we are on a website and something just *feels off*, it's not the website you're feeling. It's cortisol. Your brain is using its early warning system to tell you something is not right, and to be wary of your environment. Chances are, you are unlikely to proceed further with that brand.

This is the lens through which to understand modern consumer behavior. At each successive relationship stage, the prospect will be unconsciously assessing their comfort levels to go a level deeper with you. Your success depends upon your ability to take them through each stage successfully so that you can begin building a real relationship with them inside the practice.

5.8.4 The Sales Funnel

5.8.4.1 Discovery

The first step in the buyer's journey is the search and discovery phase. It occurs when we realize we have a problem, such as needing to find a veterinary practice, and look to solve that problem. It is still common to ask friends for referrals once we have reached this stage, but behavior is quickly shifting to digital research.

Typically, this begins with a Google query, such as "veterinarian near me." The variables that determine the likelihood of progression down your sales funnel are your prominence on the search engine results page, your review score, and your copywriting strategy for your page's title and meta description. Modern pet owners are more likely to diligently compare multiple options now than in the past, making for a more competitive landscape in digital strategies.

5.8.4.2 Consideration

Most of the time spent on the buyer's journey occurs on your veterinary website. Team members who contribute to the website's messaging and strategy have an outsized influence on a practice's success. The initial fraction of a second on your website is disproportionately important. We make decisions about our social relationships quickly – often in a fraction of a second. We're also surprisingly effective at it. This is commonly referred to as "thin slicing." We are so uniquely attuned to this because in our ancestral past this ability was a matter of survival. If the first impression of your website is not warm, modern, and compelling, you will be fighting an uphill neurochemical battle.

Because we are hard-wired to take a small amount of information and extrapolate larger general conclusions about our social groups, it is important that the presentation and quality of your website are very thoughtful. Moreover, you need to be deeply sensitive to the way humans prefer to learn about our world and to communicate – through storytelling.

Your story is not about what you do. Your story is about *what you believe*. And it's about relating how what you do every single day offers proof of you following through on your beliefs. This is how we are wired to build trust. It is when we find a person or social group that shares deeply held values with us that the bonds of trust and community are built. This underlying biology does not change even though the tools we use to connect do change.

These are the real, needle-moving, questions a pet owner is asking on your website. "Do you care about the same things I do? Will you love my pet the way I do? Are you capable of being my pet's caregiver?" You must be thoughtful about the way you present your beliefs, and how they act as your internal motor in everything you do. It may be helpful to learn more about archetypes in branding, such as "the hero" or "the caregiver," to refine your message.

A powerful signal into whether we can or should trust you is whether our community trusts you. Our social group's opinions have a tremendous impact on the way we perceive the world. This is why it can be powerful to strategically place emotional and powerful testimonials throughout your website.

The principle of social proof is exactly why word of mouth has been such an effective driver of business for so many veterinary practices, and it is why online reviews will continue to redefine and shape the landscape of the modern buyer's journey. Many pet owners will not only look at your overall score but will go through the highest-ranking reviews to get a better sense of the scope, depth, and magnitude of the issues raised. It is important to solicit positive reviews on Google and Yelp from your best clients, and to respond empathetically to negative reviews.

5.8.4.3 Action

Once the prospective client feels motivation to act, it is imperative that there is a clear and easy path to action. Humans are wired to balance motivation with energy. All things equal, the harder something is for us to accomplish, the less likely we are to accomplish it. Make sure your website has a "sticky header" so that your phone number follows the user wherever they go. Strategically place multiple calls to action so they are never far from their experience.

If a pet owner progresses down your funnel but does not act, they may still be interested. The timing may just not be right. We live complicated lives, where multiple tasks are on our mind at any one moment. It is smart to adopt similar techniques to the major online retailers (such as Amazon) and utilize retargeting technology.

5.8.5 Cementing the Bond

The initial experience your new client has in your practice is formative for their future decision making. They should be greeted warmly by the front desk staff as soon as they enter. This makes us feel welcome within our new social surroundings and will release positive chemicals (serotonin and oxytocin) in our brain.

Every single member on the team should look at a new client visit as an opportunity to make the pet owner feel like the only person in the room. To show empathy, to project confidence, and to get down on the floor and love their pet like they do.

Once you meet the client in the exam room, shake their hand firmly and look them in the eye. This communicates your interest and trustworthiness. The handshake has been practiced for so long because physical touch is an important way that we reinforce bonds with our social community. It is an important opportunity to begin to shape a strong bond with that client for years to come.

EXAMPLES

ABC Animal Hospital holds a team-wide meeting to incorporate a biological approach to marketing. Jane, a technician responsible for the practice's social media strategy, begins to curate posts that share stories of the team saving lives ad protecting pets. Dr Stevens commissions a redesign of the website from the perspective of storytelling and emotional resonance. The team huddles once every two weeks to talk about how they are making pet owners feel during their visit, and map all the different ways in which they can increase the sense of safety and belonging.

TAKE-AWAYS

- While the channels we use to engage and communicate have changed, we still look for the same biological needs that we always have.
- At our core, humans want the same things: safety, status, belonging, and love. Weave these needs through your marketing and communications, and you will have a significant competitive advantage.
- Start with the website and begin evaluating its efficacy through how well it is speaking to emotions and instincts instead of purely to logic.
- Shift the marketing strategy to be about the common values you share with your clients, and show them how you follow through on those values through social media.
- Train the team regularly on tactics to build stronger bonds with new and existing clients.

MISCELLANEOUS

Recommended Reading

Sinek, S. (2017). *Leaders Eat Last*. New York: Random House.
Damasio, A. (2005). *Descartes' Error*. New York: Random House.

5.9

Dealing with Breeders

Maria Inês Ferreira, DVM, MTB

Veterinarian, Journalist and Author, São Paulo, Brazil

BASICS

5.9.1 Summary

The sharing of information and experiences between veterinarians and breeders has always brought, and still brings, the potential for great benefits, especially for pets. However, this relationship does not always happen to best advantage. Veterinarians and their teams sometimes have preconceptions that breeders think they know everything about the health of the animals they are breeding, being able to solve all problems related to physical and psychological health, and that breeders are not necessarily receptive to the veterinary team's advice. On the other hand, breeders may harbor misconceptions that veterinarians understand little or nothing of the specifics of their breed of interest, and that less than pet-specific insight comes at a high price. Sometimes the veterinary team does not consider breeders to be concerned about animal welfare, being preoccupied more with profit and a mythical breed standard. With this, veterinary and breeder teams can often experience conflict. However, it doesn't need to be this way and all parties benefit from working in a cooperative fashion.

5.9.2 Terms Defined

Breed Clubs: Organization of like-minded individuals concerned about the issues and interest of specific purebreds.

Lineage: Series of generations (ancestors or descendants). Relationship that is established through kinship, of common ancestors, the members of a family, genealogy, race.

Puppy Mill: Indiscriminate breeding facility, where pets are commodities for sale, sometimes with little concern for animal welfare or genetic health. Profitability is typically the primary concern.

MAIN CONCEPTS

5.9.3 Mutual Benefit

Good veterinarians are not only technically capable when it comes to animal care, but they should be up to date on pet-specific care and knowledgeable about the needs of specific pets and their owners (see 1.1 Overview of Pet-Specific Care). On the other hand, good breeders are able to work with a specific breed, knowing its breed-specific issues and concerned with both physical and behavioral health (see 3.10 Advising Clients on Selecting an Appropriate Pet and 5.6 Adoption Source Options). Both veterinarians and breeders are concerned with pet-specific care and the satisfaction of the owners of these animals. But there is still a huge barrier between veterinarians and breeders although both can help and reinforce the benefits for each other.

Veterinarians and breeders can and should work together, cooperate with each other, strengthen positive relationships toward a common goal that is the well-being of pets, and work toward creating healthier pets. Love for animals motivates everyone!

Breeders can sometimes be wary of veterinarians who are not completely informed about the needs of their breed as they themselves tend to be committed to improving their specific breed and doing the best for their animals.

Veterinarians have a lot to learn from breeders as it is almost impossible for them to know details of all breeds of dogs and cats, as well as the sometimes rare disorders to which the breed might be prone. Similarly, breeders may feel at the mercy of the veterinary profession for the medical care their animals require and access to diagnostic tests and medications. Interactions between the two groups can be complicated and challenging, but also provide great opportunities.

5.9.4 Entanglement and Trust

Technique, attention, honesty, and cooperation are key to success in raising healthy animals. Veterinarians are excellent sources of information to pet owners, especially if they are offering a prepurchase service when choosing pets (see 3.10 Advising Clients on Selecting an Appropriate Pet). If veterinarians are knowledgeable about pet-specific care, they can help potential pet owners choose wisely.

When veterinary teams are asked by clients where they might acquire a good representative of a particular breed, teams should know how to indicate a good breeder and for that, they need to work with breeders who are doing the proper screening, preferably under veterinary direction. Even to indicate breeds that may or may not be appropriate for a given client's situation, the veterinary team would be providing an incredibly useful function. To do this effectively, the team needs to understand pet-specific health problems and temperament issues, and ideally how a pet's biological parents could be appropriately screened, and this requires a cooperative working relationship with breeders motivated to do such screening.

Veterinarians should appreciate genetic and behavioral factors relevant for breeds being considered, as well as being able to assess the prospective pet owner for their ability to handle circumstances associated with various breeds (see 11.4 Heritable Health Conditions – By Breed). Good breeders invest time and money in caring for the fruits of their labors, and are a very good source of information on breed-specific issues. That's why most specialists appreciate breeders as great clients, those who will do almost anything for the benefit of their breed. Good breeders are always striving to reach a standard and are extremely involved in the health of their breed. As such, they can be a great resource for the veterinarians who work with them.

Veterinary teams should be well prepared to indicate good breeders to their clients when such requests are made. Otherwise, the practice must be prepared for clients to make such decisions on their own, potentially with disastrous

results. It is not necessary for the veterinarian to endorse any specific breeder, but rather to acknowledge those breeders committed to following appropriate guidelines to do what they can to ensure healthy progeny. That doesn't mean that healthcare problems won't happen, even with a breeder who tries to do everything right, but that steps were taken to mitigate those risks as much as possible.

Good breeders do what they see as necessary to provide a legitimate specimen of the breed bearing not only the physical characteristics but also the expected temperament. They aim for the genetic improvement of the breed to which they are committed, selecting the individuals to reproduce that conform not only to the breed standard but to desirable health goals as well.

Most good breeders provide a written contract with a health guarantee of sorts regarding specific health concerns, allowing time for a prepurchase examination by a veterinarian. In many cases, protective breeders may spend more time screening potential owners of their animals than those prospective pet owners will spend assessing the pet they choose. If medical problems are diagnosed, the breeder may take the puppy or kitten back and provide a refund. There may also be a contractual first option of returning the animal to the breeder in cases when those new pet owners decide they can't keep the pet. In addition, some offspring may be designated as "pet quality" only and not intended for breeding, and there may be a stipulation that such animals be neutered.

Veterinary teams work toward lifelong patient health management, risk assessment, prevention, early detection, and individualized treatment (see 1.2 Providing a Lifetime of Care). In the context of prevention, veterinarians will indicate the best control of parasites, immunizations, adequate nutrition, and hygiene. Genetic testing is often recommended for conditions in the breed for which such testing is available (see 3.4 Predicting and Eliminating Disease Traits). Veterinarians should also be aware of their responsibility to advise breeders to select functionally healthy dogs for breeding. These breeders should practice responsible mating, taking into account genetic predispositions to reduce possible hereditary problems such as hip dysplasia, eye problems, heart problems, etc.

Maintaining good relationships with breeders should be a priority for veterinary teams, along with understanding the specific risks and manifestations of the breed (see 11.4 Heritable Health Conditions – By Breed). At the same time, breeders benefit from following the professional advice of veterinary teams who can provide a balanced perspective on conformation and health concerns. Mutual respect is in the interest of both parties. Such productive relationships will make animals happier, healthier, and better family members.

EXAMPLES

Kate is a female Cavalier King Charles spaniel. Her owner bought her over the internet and the "kennel" said she was 9 weeks old and had already been started on parasite and vaccine control. The owner drove from the airport to the nearest veterinary hospital where the doctors found that Kate was hypoglycemic, dehydrated, and in shock. They estimated the puppy was about 35 days old. She did not come with any documentation of treatments, veterinary care, or any pedigree or registration papers. The owner was desperately worried about the fate of this new little family member, and also had the distinct feeling of being deceived. The veterinary team took care of Kate promptly, managing to reestablish her normal parameters, but directed her new owner to be aware of what is typically recommended when acquiring a pet, the pet-specific care to expect for a Cavalier King Charles spaniel, and what would typically be expected when dealing with a reputable breeder.

TAKE-AWAYS

- Veterinary teams and breeders can and should work together, cooperate with each other, and aim for positive health goals for purebred animals.
- Good breeders are often well informed about the needs of their breed of interest as they tend to be very committed to improving their breed and doing the best for their animals.
- Veterinary teams are excellent sources of information for potential pet owners, including helping them select appropriate pets.

- Veterinary teams and breeders should align around the goal of purebred genetic health. Veterinarians have a lot to learn from breeders about breed-specific issues, and breeders have a lot to learn from veterinary teams about animal health in general.
- Teams of veterinarians and breeders should focus on better understanding the demands and challenges of producing animals with certain characteristics, while keeping healthcare needs in perspective.

MISCELLANEOUS

Recommended Reading

Ackerman, L. (2011). *The Genetic Connection: A Guide to Health Problems in Purebred Dogs*, 2e. Lakewood, CO: AAHA Press.

Ackerman, L. (2019). An introduction to pet-specific care. *EC Veterinary Science* 4 (1): 1–3.

Ackerman, L. (2020). Proactive Pet Parenting: Anticipating pet health problems before they happen. Problem Free Publishing.

American Kennel Club. Finding a "breeder's vet." www.akc.org/expert-advice/news/finding-a-breeders-vet

Canadian Veterinary Medical Association. Dog Breeding – Position Statement. www.canadianveterinarians.net/documents/dog-breeding&prev=search

Humane Society of the United States. How to find a responsible dog breeder. www.humanesociety.org/resources/how-find-responsible-dog-breeder

5.10

Discussing Pet-Specific Care

Lowell Ackerman, DVM, DACVD, MBA, MPA, CVA, MRCVS

Global Consultant, Author, and Lecturer, MA, USA

BASICS

5.10.1 Summary

Although each visit to the veterinary hospital occurs as a discrete encounter, it is actually part of a larger continuum of care that may extend from even before the birth of an individual animal (with preselection counseling, breeding evaluation of the parents, or genetic testing of the sire and dam) to the time of its demise, or even later (see 1.2 Proving a Lifetime of Care). Each episode of veterinary care must therefore be considered as part of an overall strategy for pet-specific care rather than just an isolated event (see 1.1 Overview of Pet-Specific Care).

Very much like purchasing a car or a piece of equipment that comes with a maintenance schedule, creating a personalized schedule of care for individual animals reinforces the concept that there is a plan in place for a lifetime of care, and that it has been created specifically for the needs of a particular pet (see 1.3 Personalized Care Plans).

5.10.2 Terms Defined

Adherence: The extent to which clients administer medications prescribed, including administering the correct dose, timing and use, and completing the prescribed course.

Compliance: The extent to which pets receive a treatment, screening, or procedure in accordance with accepted veterinary healthcare practices. Compliance involves veterinary staff performing and/or recommending treatments, screenings, and procedures, and pet owner follow-through.

Dental Calculus (Tartar): Hardened dental plaque, often caused by the accumulation of minerals from saliva.

Dental Plaque: A biofilm consisting of bacteria, mucus, and food particles that adheres to the surface of teeth.

Epigenetics: The study of heritable changes in genetic expression caused by mechanisms other than those attributable to underlying DNA sequences.

Vaccination: Inoculation with a killed or attenuated microbe with the purpose of preventing disease caused by that microbe.

Zoonosis: Disease that is transmissible between animals and humans.

MAIN CONCEPTS

5.10.3 Genetic Risk Factors

All pets, whether purebred or not, may be predisposed to certain conditions, based on family history or certain genetic (or epigenetic) traits that they carry.

There are now literally hundreds of genetic tests that allow the genotypic determination of physical and disease traits in both dogs (von Willebrand disease, progressive rod-cone degeneration, narcolepsy, etc.) and cats (polycystic kidney disease, spinal muscular atrophy, hypertrophic cardiomyopathy, etc.) (see 3.4 Predicting and Eliminating Disease Traits).

Some of the genetic tests employ actual detection of the disease-causing variant (mutation) and therefore are very predictive for risk, whereas others detect genetic markers that may be associated with increased or decreased risk of disease. Superimposed on the actual genotype are a variety of environmental factors that impact disease or trait expression. There are many more conditions that rely on phenotypic testing, such as hip dysplasia, diabetes mellitus, and atopic dermatitis (see 3.11 Integrating Genotypic and Phenotypic Testing).

The environment can also affect expression of traits, and certain environmental "shocks" can leave imprints on the genetic material in eggs and sperm, which can be passed on to future generations (so-called epigenetics). Epigenetic marks can switch genes on or off, affecting disease risk, and can be passed on to offspring.

It is important that veterinary teams feel comfortable with genetic testing and its opportunities and challenges related to preventive healthcare, or the profession might find itself lagging behind. Because most genetic testing can be performed with a cheek swab, testing is not restricted to veterinary professionals and in many areas, the majority of genetic testing is being performed by nonveterinarians. Veterinarians have not been early adopters of genetic testing and may be less informed on developments than some owners and breeders. This trend must be reversed if veterinary teams want to remain in the vanguard of preventive care and early detection for dogs and cats. At the current time, there are hundreds of genetic tests currently available to identify conditions [1], and yet most of that testing is being requested by nonveterinarians.

5.10.4 Lifestyle Management

Veterinarians must be cognizant of many factors that can affect pet health and educate pet owners as to how best to prevent problems.

Some issues can be attributable to geography, including the prevalence of various conditions and toxins (e.g., blastomycosis, risk of rattlesnake bite, risk of heatstroke or frostbite, etc.).

Pets can also be at increased risk based on exposure to other animals (such as at a boarding facility, groomer, or even within the veterinary hospital) or environments (e.g., drinking from or swimming in ponds, walking in wooded areas, access to disease vectors, etc.), travel outside the home area to another area in which a condition is enzootic, or through owner indiscretion (accidental ingestion of chocolate by pet, sandbox not covered to prevent fecal contamination, yard debris not cleared, which serves as point of entry for ticks, etc.).

It is important that veterinary teams use a consistent risk assessment protocol to help determine risk factors that might not be evident on physical examination (see 2.7 Risk Assessment).

Veterinary teams must counsel owners on both medical and lifestyle issues if the goal is to prevent healthcare issues from occurring, and make recommendations that are relevant for the needs of each pet and owner (see 1.3 Personalized Care Plans).

When it comes to medications to be administered for either prevention or management, it is important to consider compliance and adherence (see 9.17 Improving Compliance and Adherence with Pet-Specific Care) challenges and to favor routes of administration that make it convenient for clients to follow veterinary directions precisely.

5.10.5 Life Stage Management

Although pets need personalized and individualized care throughout their lives, breaking down requirements by life stages is often useful in discussions with owners (see 4.1 Canine and Feline Life Stages).

Because not all animals reach the same life stages by the same age, life stages may be designated on the basis of certain characteristics, albeit arbitrarily (see 11.05 Life Planning By Breed). Proposed life stage guidelines have been proposed for both dogs [2] and cats [3]. Separate senior guidelines have been proposed for both dogs and cats as well [4].

Risk factors, environment, behavior, nutrition, parasite control, vaccination, dental care, zoonotic disease control, safety, and reproductive health should be addressed regularly with pet owners throughout a pet's life.

5.10.6 Parasite Control

Parasite control is not only an important element in preventive care for pets, but is also a critical public health issue with potential legal liability for underestimating its significance.

Many common forms of fecal testing used in veterinary offices have relatively low sensitivity, especially when samples tested are not fresh, so standard fecal testing alone may not fully predict parasite burdens and thus may not ultimately protect the public from parasites spread in pet feces.

Integrated parasite control should be considered, evaluating the best combination of products to provide control for both internal and external parasites. Because many parasite control products are available over the counter and without a prescription, veterinarians must be aware of all products being used in pets, whether prescribed or not. Control protocols should target local parasite prevalence and take into account individual lifestyle characteristics that might increase or decrease risk. In addition, teams should make recommendations for products that take compliance issues into consideration.

The Companion Animal Parasite Council (www. capcvet.org) provides guidelines for parasite control in North America, and advice for mitigating risk of zoonotic transmission of disease. Recommendations include year-round control of internal and external parasites in dogs and cats, routine testing and deworming, and minimizing the risk of humans contacting animal feces and disease vectors (see 4.5 Prevention and Control of Parasites).

Public health is everyone's concern and clients should understand their role in protecting everyone in the community (see 2.19 One Health). Those clients that choose not to follow the hospital's recommendations for parasite control should be informed of their potential liability, and the hospital should consider the use of a signed waiver in these instances. Preventing the spread of parasites within a community is everyone's responsibility.

5.10.7 Vaccination

Vaccinations have been important in controlling a variety of diseases in the dog and cat population, including fatal zoonotic diseases such as rabies.

There are many considerations to be made in creating a vaccination schedule for a hospital, including government mandates, local disease prevalence, safety of the vaccine, efficacy of the vaccine to prevent disease, duration of immunity, any risks posed by the vaccine itself, and any animal-specific issues to be considered (including age, state of health, concurrent problems, etc.).

In general, vaccines are divided into core products that should be used on all animals serviced by the hospital and noncore vaccines that are used based on appropriate risk assessment (see 9.11 Vaccination).

In general, vaccines are to be avoided in animals less than 6 weeks of age, where interference with maternally derived protection would be anticipated.

Most vaccines are given as an initial series every 2–4 weeks as indicated on label recommendations and then periodically as needed. For some agents, a titer can be used to determine relative protection whereas for others, there will be reliance on a sensible vaccination schedule.

Guidelines have been developed for both canine vaccination [5] and feline vaccination [6] within North America, as well as global recommendations, but all rely on veterinary judgment because not all generalizations can be supported by currently available scientific studies.

5.10.8 Oral Care

Despite the fact that dental care is needed in dogs and cats as much as it is in humans, most pets do not receive the level of oral care required.

Because preventive care is often not sufficient, dogs, and cats commonly develop periodontal disease in which dental

plaque adheres to the teeth, and bacteria within the plaque irritate the gum tissue and may even result in infection of the underlying bone. By 3 years of age, most dogs and cats have some evidence of periodontal disease (see 4.9 Periodontal disease).

Although owners are often most concerned with offensive breath odor or unsightly calculus (tartar), it is actually the progressive nature of periodontal disease that poses the most risk for pets.

Periodic dental cleaning should be performed by veterinary teams and general anesthesia is required. Scaling the teeth without anesthesia is not recommended by most dental professionals.

In between dental prophylactic procedures in which cleaning and polishing are performed, home care is extremely important. This might include regular brushing with pet-specific toothbrushes and toothpastes (dentifrices), oral rinses with specially formulated antiseptics such as chlorhexidine, and diets and chews specifically created for this purpose.

5.10.9 Discussion

The goal of pet-specific care is to provide healthcare advice that is relevant for the individual pet, and the emphasis is to prevent problems whenever possible, to embrace early detection so problems can be dealt with when there are the most options available, and finally to provide treatment or intervention according to evidence-based principles.

Pet-specific care cannot be delivered in a vacuum. It requires client engagement, and it is best to start that engagement during puppy and kitten visits when the veterinary hospital team can serve as advocates of pet care from the earliest possible opportunity.

To accomplish pet-specific care, hospital teams need to be capable of soliciting information from the pet owner, either by standardized questionnaire or direct inquiry, as a typical history collected during an office visit may not uncover all needed information on which to base recommendations. Pet owners also need to be aware of why compliance is so important to the care of their pets, and what will be expected of them in the personalized medicine process.

The message needs to be conveyed to pet owners that the veterinary hospital team has the expertise to be a resource for quality of life issues for pets, and to attempt to guide the process of keeping the pet as healthy and happy as possible, for as long as possible.

Early detection is an important part of pet-specific care, and pet owners need to understand the importance of such surveillance systems (see 4.7 Embracing Early Detection). Such early detection includes not only things like parasite testing and routine laboratory profiles, but potentially also genetic screening, orthopedic screening, geriatric screening, etc.

While many pet owners have heard of the tremendous medical breakthroughs that have been made in genomic medicine, and that there are many genetic tests available for use in dogs and cats, it is important to convey that genetic testing is an important aspect of pet-specific care, but not sufficient on its own to answer all questions about risk, so a more balanced approach of genetic and nongenetic screening is indicated (see 3.11 Integrating Genotypic and Phenotypic Testing).

In many hospitals, it is the veterinary team (especially nurses and client service representatives) that drives pet-specific care programs, including initiating questionnaires, discussions with pet owners, collecting samples, and maintaining contact to ensure compliance. Accordingly, it is imperative that staff be appropriately trained to accomplish these tasks.

In conversations with pet owners, it is also important to communicate that such pet-specific care may frontload some expenses, even though prevention tends to save money over treatment in the long run. Such conversations should take place during puppy and kitten visits, so it is possible there will need to be some financial discussions as well (see 5.11 Discussing Finances for Pet-Specific Care). This is important so the clients can be fully aware of when such care should be initiated, and how much it is likely to cost. This is also the ideal time for pet owners to consider whether pet health insurance will help mitigate such risks and better allow them to follow hospital recommendations (see 10.16 Pet Health Insurance).

EXAMPLES

Example 1

Mrs Green arrived at ABC Veterinary Hospital with her new 8-week-old Coton de Tulear puppy, Pierre, and she was interested in commencing a lifetime of sensible healthcare for her new family member.

The doctors at the hospital did not have much familiarity with the breed (the receptionists and technicians had originally debated whether it was a bichon frisé, Havanese, or poodle), so before engaging the client in any healthcare discussions, they first did some research on the subject [1].

In addition to their regular discussions of vaccination, nutrition, training, and parasite control, they informed the owner that the breed actually had a few health concerns, and that it would be worth performing genetic testing to determine any potential risk for canine multifocal retinop-

athy (I and II), neonatal cerebellar ataxia, primary hyperoxaluria-1, and von Willebrand disease.

Pierre had an uneventful physical examination, other than finding a mild umbilical hernia that would be repaired at time of neutering, and appeared to be in good health. The doctor laid out plans with the owner for how they were going to keep Pierre healthy over the breed's potentially long lifespan, in a step-by-step approach, starting with the immediate pediatric needs. The doctor assured Mrs Green that even though it might seem a bit daunting initially, ABC Veterinary Hospital would be there every step of the way to help guide them through the process.

Example 2

Rocky Goodwin is a young Doberman pinscher and his owners are interested in him living a long and healthy life. Following his examination, it was concluded that Rocky was a healthy pup, and a personalized health profile was recommended to help him remain that way. Mrs Goodwin seemed fixated on one of the risk factors that had been identified for his breed – cardiomyopathy – and was particularly anxious as her father recently died of congestive heart failure. The opportunity was taken to learn more about this experience, including her remorse that the diagnosis hadn't been made earlier in her father's situation, when more could have been done.

The veterinary team was empathetic with her concerns and suggested that although the risks cannot be eliminated with Rocky, the team would be committed to early identification of problems, should they exist. The first step would be to perform genetic tests for the risk of cardiomyopathy, as a positive result would indicate that Rocky is more likely than other Dobermans to be at risk, but it would still not be a foregone conclusion that Rocky would develop the heart disease; a negative result means less likelihood, but the risk still does not drop to zero. It was explained that cardiomyopathy is an adult-onset disease, and although perhaps most commonly first detected around 5–6 years of age in affected animals, it can be quite variable and even diagnosed as early as 1 year of age in some dogs.

Based on the information provided, Mrs Goodwin agreed that the genetic tests made sense as a first step (along with the other genetic tests that are part of the recommended panel, including von Willebrand disease, narcolepsy, and malignant hyperthermia) and she indicated she would also appreciate learning more about these conditions at home if there were resources that could be provided. Given the facts presented, a lifelong healthcare plan would be created for Rocky that would take into consideration all his determined risk factors, not only for genetic diseases but also for environmental and lifestyle risks.

Although Mrs Goodwin was understandably concerned that her healthy new family member could possibly develop a devastating disease later in life, she appreciated being apprised so early in the process, being provided with so much supporting information, and having such a credible action plan already in place. Mrs Goodwin was committed to her role as Rocky's "parent" and was also prepared to investigate pet health insurance (see 10.16 Pet Health Insurance) and other mechanisms for being able to afford Rocky's care. Before leaving the hospital, she once again indicated her appreciation for such customized care and asked if it would be acceptable if she recommended the hospital to her family and friends.

TAKE-AWAYS

- With pet-specific care, it is important to concentrate on discussing how our actions help keep pets healthy, rather than waiting for pets to get sick before we intervene.
- Client engagement is improved when they can see "the big picture" of how pet care will be implemented over a pet's anticipated lifespan, not just on a visit-by-visit basis.
- Be aware that most of the resources needed to provide pet-specific care are already available. It's just a matter of assembling things into an easy-to-explain format.
- Most of the communication that takes place regarding pet-specific care involves the nonveterinary hospital team, so make sure they are appropriately trained and fully conversant with the topics of interest.
- Pet-specific care works best when it is started with young puppies and kittens, when pet owners can not only see the interventions that will take place over time but can also prepare for how they are going to pay for them.

MISCELLANEOUS

5.10.10 Cautions

When discussing lifelong care with pet owners, it is impossible to anticipate all problems that might potentially occur, and the intention is also not to alarm the owner unnecessarily; attention is typically focused on risks that pose the most concern and for which prevention or successful management might be attained.

References

1 Ackerman, L. (2011). *The Genetic Connection*, 2e. Lakewood, CO: AAHA Press.

2 Creevy, K.E., Grady, J., Little, S.E. et al. (2019). 2019 AAHA Canine Life Stage Guidelines. *J. Am. Anim. Hosp. Assoc.* 55: 267–290.

3 Hoyumpa Vogt, A., Rodan, I., Brown, M. et al. (2010). AAFP-AAHA Feline Life Stage Guidelines. *J. Am. Anim. Hosp. Assoc.* 46: 70–85.

4 Epstein, M., Kuehn, N., Landsberg, G. et al. (2005). AAHA senior care guidelines for dogs and cats. *J. Am. Anim. Hosp. Assoc.* 41: 81–91.

5 Ford, R., Larson, L.J., McClure, K.D., et al. (2017). AAHA Canine Vaccination Guidelines. www.aaha.org/guidelines/canine_vaccination_guidelines.aspx

6 Scherk, M., Ford, R.B., Gaskell, R.M. et al. (2013). 2013 AAFP Feline Vaccination Advisory Panel Report. *J. Fel. Med. Surg.* 15: 785–808.

Recommended Reading

Ackerman, L.J. (2011). *The Genetic Connection: A Guide to Health Problems in Purebred Dogs*, 2e. Lakewood, CO: AAHA Press.

Ackerman, L.J. (2020). Discussing pet-specific care. In: *Five-Minute Veterinary Practice Management Consult*, 3e, 344–347. Ames, IA: Wiley.

Ackerman, LJ. (2020). Problem Free Pets: The ultimate guide to pet parenting. Problem Free Publishing (Dermvet).

Ackerman, L. (2020). The new e-commerce: E-commerce is more than just selling products online. *AAHA Trends*; 36(11): 51–54.

American Animal Hospital Association-American Veterinary Medical Association (2011). 2011 AAHA/AVMA Preventive Healthcare Guidelines. *J. Am. Vet. Med. Assoc.* 239 (5): 625–629.

Lacroix, C.A. (2007). Discussing parasite control and zoonosis liability. In: *Blackwell's Five-Minute Veterinary Practice Management Consult* (ed. L. Ackerman), 112–113. Oxford: Blackwell Publishing.

Partners for Healthy Pets. www.partnersforhealthypets.org

Shaw, J.R. (2019). Evaluation of communication skills training programs at north American veterinary medical training institutions. *J. Am. Vet. Med. Assoc.* 255 (6): 722–733.

5.11

Discussing Finances for Pet-Specific Care

Brandon Hess, CVPM, CCFP

VetSupport Inc., Cincinnati, OH, USA

 BASICS

5.11.1 Summary

Finances in general can be an uncomfortable topic for discussion. When emotions and the life of an animal are involved, it is even more challenging. When finances are not discussed effectively, clients tend to have complaints or, even worse, social media rampages. Effectively communicating finances takes practice, but prevents sticker shock and complaints and helps retain valuable relationships.

5.11.2 Terms Defined

Care Plan: An alternative term for "estimate" that sounds more personalized.

Paraverbal Communication: The pitch, tone, inflection, and pace of a communication. Often referred to as: "It's not what you said, it's *how* you said it." The "how" is the paraverbal.

Pareto Principle: The concept that 80% of outcomes come from 20% of causes. For example, 80% of revenues come from 20% of clients.

Perceived Value: What someone feels they have gotten in return (not always financial) in return for money they have paid.

Return on Investment (ROI): What financial return is seen from investing in something.

Sticker Shock: Surprise on receiving a bill due to lack of communication and not being prepared for the amount.

 MAIN CONCEPTS

5.11.3 The Challenge

One of the most challenging things within veterinary medicine is discussing fees. In fact, a study showed that thousands of veterinary professionals found "discussing or disputing fees" as a top three stressor [1] (Table 5.11.1). It is not unusual for clients to put veterinarians, or support staff, in an uncomfortable situation. There are many types of challenging financial conversations.

- Client doesn't have money, but the patient is treatable.
- Client has the money, but won't spend it.
- Client is willing to put themselves into a difficult financial situation to treat.

Since every client has a different, at times unknown financial situation, each situation poses different challenges. There are, however, consistent things that should be taken into consideration.

- *Time and place*: What conversation are you having, and who is around? When a financial conversation occurs in front of others, the chance of it escalating increases. Along with public conversation comes potential embarrassment and defensiveness.
- *Condition of patient*: The more critical the patient is, the more caution should be exercised when discussing finances.
- *Client history with practice*. Loyal and long-term clients tend to be more understanding at times, but also may expect special treatment. "I've paid for a few of these exam rooms" is not an uncommon thing to hear from clients like these.

Table 5.11.1 Top stressors in veterinary practice [1]

Veterinarians	Veterinary support staff
Difficult or noncompliant clients	Difficult or noncompliant client
Not enough time	Problems with co-workers
Discussing or disputing fees	Not enough time

Source: Modified from Figley and Roop [1].

5.11.4 Client Expectations

The expectations that clients have of veterinary professionals has substantially increased over the last 10 years, and will continue to do so. More and more focus is being put on the full experience that the client has, rather than just the medicine (see 5.3 What Clients Expect From the Veterinary Team). You could have the best doctors, surgeons, or technicians in your area but none of that will matter if the client has a negative experience. This negative experience could be as small as not effectively communicating what the final invoice will be.

5.11.5 Education and Training

There are two different mindsets on what staff should be trained on. One approach is the "product" approach, where staff are trained on the ins-and-outs of a product so that they can better sell it to a client. The other is the "soft skill" approach. The idea behind this is that if the team is taught how to be effective communicators; they will be able to deliver solutions and increase compliance. In fact, Shawn Achor, who is a Harvard-trained psychologist, provides the following statistic in his TED talk titled "The Happy Secret to Better Work" [2].

Your brain at positive is 31% more productive and 37% more successful at sales, than at negative, neutral or stressed. Doctors are 19% more accurate at coming up with diagnoses with their brains at positive, than at negative, neutral or stressed.

The ROI that can be expected from focusing on soft skill-based training is not only increased sales (topline revenue), but also decreased expenses. By investing in training such as effective communication, conflict resolution, confident recommendations, etc., staff turnover rates can be decreased. With a decrease in staff turnover rates comes a decrease in payroll, due to less demand for training, recruiting, and onboarding. Within education and training, there are some key areas that should be focused on: verbiage, empathy, and consistency.

Verbiage training is about what, how, and when to say things. When a financial conversation occurs at the wrong time, it can easily escalate a situation. In the same way, if attention is not paid to the nonverbal and paraverbal aspects of communication, a disconnect can occur between the intent and perception of that conversation. Imagine driving down the road and being cut off by another car. Our first instinct is that person intentionally cut us off. However, if we take a step back and try to give the other the benefit of the doubt, that is an empathetic reaction. In this example, other reasons that we could think of include: they didn't see us, they were in a hurry due to an emergency or they just got off a long shift and weren't paying attention. While it does not decrease the danger of cutting someone off, practicing empathy decreases the likelihood that a situation will escalate.

In short, *empathy* is figuratively being able to put yourself in someone else's shoes. With clients, co-workers, or even personal interactions, practicing empathy is essential for effective communication, especially with finances. A video that drives this topic home for the veterinary field can be found on YouTube titled "Empathy in Veterinary Practices," or on the Veteos Facebook page [3].

Lastly, *consistency* is something clients look for and need. Consistency allows for the communication of the same message in the same way, but also increases the value of that message. When finances are communicated at the same points of a visit, in a similar way, it is easier for a client to receive and also shows the client the value of that message. For instance, when the value of a fecal test is communicated on a reminder card, by confirmation phone call, triage team member and then the doctor, the chance of compliance increases substantially. Consistency in wording is important too. There are some forbidden phrases that should be avoided, or alternative phrasing considered. As an exercise, have the staff brainstorm alternatives to the phrases in Table 5.11.2.

Table 5.11.2 Alternative wording for phrases that should be avoided in practice

Forbidden phrase	Alternative wording
Estimate	Care plan or treatment plan
We can't do payment plans	What we can offer is _____
I'm sorry it's so expensive	We understand that pet care can be pricey. Can I review the charges with you?
The total for your visit today is ____	Itemize services/products and then state total

EXAMPLES

Mrs Smith, a long-time client of ABC Veterinary Hospital, called the clinic during a packed day of appointments. She informed the front desk team member that her dog Fluffy was having breathing problems and she would like to bring him in immediately. The front desk staff member sensitively informed Mrs Smith that they would be more than happy to see Fluffy and just wanted to make sure she knew there would be an emergency fee. When Mrs Smith came in, a technician immediately took Fluffy to the back to triage her. The front desk team roomed Mrs Smith and kept her updated on what was going on with her pet. After the doctor examined Fluffy and discussed the plan with Mrs Smith, the doctor informed Mrs Smith that a technician would be in to discuss the care plan with her. The technician came in minutes later with a printed, personalized care plan for Fluffy. The care plan contained an anticipated care total, which had a low and high range for care. The care plan was signed by Mrs Smith, and she was given a copy. Mrs Smith provided a deposit for hospitalized care and left Fluffy to be treated by the clinic. If the clinic needed to go outside the agreed price range, they would call Mrs Smith to inform her.

TAKE-AWAYS

- Client expectations will continue to grow as they experience different veterinary and nonveterinary services.
- Education and practice are essential to effective financial communication.
- Clients want consistency, and to be told about finances throughout the visit so they are not surprised when they check out.
- Empathy is a valuable soft skill which gives you an appreciation for what someone else is going through or is wanting. It's essential when discussing finances or handling a financial complaint.
- Avoid terms such as "estimate" with clients. It does not communicate "individualized care" and it sounds optional.

MISCELLANEOUS

References

1 Figley, C.R. and Roop, R.G. (2006). *Compassion Fatigue in the Animal Care Community*. Washington, DC: Humane Society Press.

2 Achor, S. TEDx Talk: The Happy Secret to Better Work. www.youtube.com/watch?v=fLJsdqxnZb0

3 Veteos Facebook Page. Veterinary Empathy: Real People, Real Stories. www.facebook.com/veteos/videos/398305467598205

5.12

Discussing Anesthetic Risk

Tamara Grubb, DVM, PhD, DACVAA

Washington State University, Pullman, WA, USA

BASICS

5.12.1 Summary

Anesthesia for a pet can be very frightening for the pet owner, and this is an understandable reaction since there is some inherent risk of complications during anesthesia. Ensuring that the veterinary hospital team is committed to practicing safe anesthesia, and communicating this commitment to the client, is the most effective way to alleviate the pet owner's anesthetic fears. Although a brief statement of the safety commitment may suffice to alleviate most pet owners' concerns, taking the time to discuss these protocols and procedures in depth may occasionally be necessary. Anticipating frequently asked questions and having prepared, standardized answers is the most effective and efficient way for the entire veterinary team to address anesthetic risk concerns.

MAIN CONCEPTS

5.12.2 Decreasing Anesthetic Risk

The mere thought of a beloved pet undergoing anesthesia can be incredibly frightening for the pet owner. When checking on a pet following a procedure requiring anesthesia, "Did my pet survive anesthesia?" is often the first question asked by the owner – even before "How did the procedure go?" Pet owners are rightfully, but sometimes exaggeratedly, concerned about their pet's safety during anesthesia. As occurs in humans, there is a small inherent risk of anesthesia-related complications, or even death, in healthy animal patients, and the risk increases in unhealthy patients. However, the risk can be minimized by appropriate stabilization prior to anesthesia and with diligent monitoring and support during anesthesia (see 9.13 Preanesthetic Considerations).

The most effective means of alleviating pet owner fear of anesthesia-related risk is steadfast commitment to practicing the safest anesthesia possible and communication of that commitment to the pet owner. The practice should follow these guidelines to decrease anesthetic risk.

- Adhere to the latest safety recommendations for veterinary anesthesia. Safety guidelines are available from a variety of organizations, such as the American Animal Hospital Association (AAHA).
- Assign a nurse trained in anesthesia and pain management to each patient. The training should be both in-house and through anesthesia-specific continuing education. In some instances, nurses could specialize in anesthesia through the National Association of Veterinary Technicians in America (http://navta.net) or an equivalent group in the nurse's country of practice.
- Tailor the anesthetic and analgesic protocol, including drugs, monitoring, and support, for each patient after a thorough evaluation of the patient's health status.
- Ensure that the patient's needs are addressed and that a plan is in place for all four phases of anesthesia: preanesthesia, induction, maintenance, and recovery.

Pet-Specific Care for the Veterinary Team, First Edition. Edited by Lowell Ackerman.
© 2021 John Wiley & Sons, Inc. Published 2021 by John Wiley & Sons, Inc.

5.12.3 Client Communication Regarding Anesthesia and Anesthetic Risk for their Pet

Although a brief statement on the practice's commitment to safe anesthesia is often enough to alleviate pet owner concerns, a more thorough description of the practice's anesthetic procedures and detailed answers to questions may be necessary in some instances. Fear of anesthesia can be the reason that owners choose to cancel a much-needed procedure for their pet. The job of the veterinarian and veterinary nurse is to alleviate those fears by taking the time – occasionally quite a bit of time – to fully answer all the pet owner's questions and to explain the process of anesthesia in your hospital. Insufficient time with the pet owner, dismissive answers, and apparent lack of knowledge of the anesthetic process will do nothing to alleviate, and actually may worsen, the client's fears of anesthesia for their pet.

Both the veterinarian and veterinary nurse play a role in discussion of anesthesia with the pet owner. The veterinarian should discuss anesthetic risk with the owner and answer any medical questions. The owner's comfort with anesthesia is often enhanced if they can also speak with the specific nurse in charge of their pet's anesthesia and the nurse can go into a more detailed description of the anesthetic process.

Below are some frequently asked questions and answer examples regarding risk of anesthesia. By anticipating questions and having standardized answers, the entire veterinary team can present a strong and consistent message regarding the hospital's dedication to decreasing anesthetic risk in their patients. Of course, some questions are patient specific and, along with the standardized answers, veterinarians and veterinary nurses should be ready to provide answers individualized to any given patient. The pet owner needs to know that the team cares and that their pet is important to the team.

5.12.4 Frequently Asked Questions

I don't understand why my pet needs anesthesia. Why is anesthesia necessary for some procedures, like dentistry, that do not require anesthesia in humans?
Example answer: Because our pets don't understand that a procedure that might be uncomfortable is being done to improve their health, they can become extremely frightened and uncooperative, or even aggressive, during the procedure. They are also more likely to experience pain, which can add to

the fear. By using anesthesia, we keep the patient calm and pain free during the procedure. The fact that the pet isn't moving is also beneficial since we can do a better, more thorough job with the dental procedure (or other procedure).

Is there a risk of complications or death with general anesthesia?
Example answer: Like most medical procedures, there is a slight risk that anesthesia could make your pet worse or even cause death. We know that this can be a very scary process for pet owners and at our animal clinic we do everything we can to decrease anesthetic risk and to keep your pet as safe as possible. We adhere to the latest anesthetic safety guidelines, use the same anesthetic drugs that are used in humans, and utilize patient support like intravenous (IV) fluids, pain control, patient warming, and advanced patient monitoring. In addition, our nurses have received training in anesthesia from our doctors and attend continuing education courses. Your pet will have a nurse dedicated to monitoring the pet's vital signs throughout the entire anesthetic period and into the recovery period. If you would like more detail, we are happy to discuss each step of the anesthetic procedure with you.

What is the risk that my pet will die?
Example answer: The risk is very low. The reported risk of death in healthy pets is about one in 2000 (0.05%) in dogs and about 1 in 1000 in cats (0.11%) [1]. The risk is slightly greater in unhealthy pets, but we will make sure that your pet is as healthy as possible before we anesthetize him/her.

I'm sorry, I am very nervous about anesthesia. Please describe the anesthetic process in more depth.
Example answer: After we have done a physical exam and completed all the diagnostic tests, we will choose drugs and drug dosages specific for your pet. First, your pet will receive a sedation drug and a pain-relieving drug. This will allow your pet to be calm and comfortable as the process starts. Then a catheter will be placed in your pet's vein for administration of further drugs and IV fluids. Your pet will be receiving oxygen and will be placed on a warm blanket during the catheterization. Next, a drug to make the pet go to sleep will be injected into the catheter and a tube will be placed in your pet's windpipe (trachea) as soon as it is asleep. Anesthetic gases, that will keep your pet asleep, and oxygen will be administered through the tube. At this point, we will be using physiological monitors to assess your pet's blood pressure, heart rhythm, breathing, oxygen level, and body temperature. We will also be administering more pain medication if necessary. I (or "a nurse" if the

answer is from a doctor) will be watching your pet the entire time and will be documenting all this information on the anesthetic record. When the procedure is finished, the anesthetic gases will be turned off, but your pet will still be breathing oxygen for several minutes. The tube in the windpipe will be removed when your pet starts swallowing. We will still be watching your pet and keeping it warm and we will administer more pain drugs when your pet needs them. When we are comfortable that your pet is fully awake, we will call you and let you know that everything went fine. (An approximate time that the owner can expect a call could be added to the conversation.)

What can I do to decrease the anesthetic risk for my pet?
Example answer: The doctors and staff at our animal clinic will discuss the anesthetic procedure with you and you should be prepared to provide the doctors and staff with a complete history of your pet's health, including medications that the pet might be on that were not prescribed by the doctors at our clinic. Be sure to tell us if your pet is on over-the-counter drugs like aspirin or on any kind of herbal supplement. The doctors may also recommend diagnostic tests like blood work, x-rays ("radiographs"), ultrasound, or other tests. The information provided in the history and by the diagnostic tests will allow the doctors and staff to tailor the anesthetic protocol to your pet's specific needs, which improves the safety of anesthesia for your pet. You should be sure to ask any questions that you have – we want you to be very comfortable with our care of your pet during anesthesia.

Is my pet too sick to be anesthetized?
Sometimes, unfortunately, the answer is, "Your pet is too sick NOT to be anesthetized" when patients present with conditions that require emergency surgery. A patient with a gastric dilation/volvulus (GDV) or "bloat" is an example. In this situation, the risk of anesthesia is likely no more or less than the risk of the procedure, which is necessary to save the patient's life. The fact that the anesthesia is not avoidable should be communicated to the pet owner, while also emphasizing that the hospital practices anesthesia that is as safe as possible, even in critical patients. In all situations other than dire emergencies, the patient should be stabilized prior to anesthesia to decrease the risk of anesthesia-related complications. Stabilization can decrease the risk of anesthetic death by 3–6 times [1]. Stabilization can mean short-term treatment in urgent situations, like administering IV fluids and analgesic drugs overnight to a cat with a traumatic orthopedic injury (e.g., a fractured bone) in anticipation of surgery to repair the

injury after the cat is stable. Stabilization can also mean long-term treatment, like sending a dog with newly diagnosed cardiac disease home with appropriate medication for several weeks before an elective dental procedure (see 9.13 Preanesthetic Considerations). Regardless of whether short-term or long-term treatment is required, once the patient is stabilized, the answer could be as follows.
Example answer: Your pet has responded well to the treatment and we have minimized the risk of anesthesia as much as we possibly can. At this point, the risk of not doing the procedure is greater than the risk of anesthesia. (An example of this scenario is a patient who isn't eating because of dental pain and needs to be anesthetized for a dental procedure. Not doing the procedure would mean that the pet still won't eat.) We will take very good care of your pet.

Is my pet too old to be anesthetized? I have been told that he/she is too old.
Age is not a disease but as patients age, their response to anesthetic drugs and their need for physiological support during anesthesia do change. In general, aged patients require lower anesthetic drug dosages, closer monitoring and more aggressive physiological support than healthy middle-aged patients. Aged patients are also more likely to have concurrent disease and the specific disease might increase anesthetic risk. In all patients a thorough physical exam and routine lab testing (e.g., complete blood count [CBC] and/or serum chemistry) should be performed prior to anesthesia. In aged patients, the exam and testing may need to be expanded to include tests like diagnostic imaging (e.g., ultrasound or thoracic radiographs), electrocardiogram (ECG) and specific blood tests such as those for liver, kidney, or thyroid function. See 9.13 Preanesthetic Considerations for more information. If conditions are found that require stabilization, refer to the process described in the previous section prior to anesthetizing the patient.
Example answer for healthy and/or stable geriatric pets: We routinely anesthetize older patients at our animal hospital and are prepared to give them the extra care that they might need. Your pet needs this procedure and the benefit of the procedure for your pet outweighs any small risk of anesthesia.

Is my pet too young to be anesthetized?
Unless the patient needs emergency surgery, anesthesia should be delayed until the pet is at least 12–16 weeks old. This allows neonatal physiological processes to mature. If the pet needs anesthesia at a younger age, the answer to this question will be similar to the previous answers, emphasizing the clinic's commitment to safe anesthesia and attentive care of their pet.

My breeder (or the internet) said that my dog breed is "sensitive" to anesthesia. Do you know how to safely anesthetize this breed?

Although well-meaning, these comments are often not medically based and can actually compromise care if the owner is adamant that the pet be anesthetized by methods other than those that are utilized in your clinic. You should always adhere to the protocols that you are most familiar with and that have been proven safe in your experience. There are very few true breed-related sensitivities but there are certainly breed-associated risks due to breed-related conditions or diseases (e.g., brachycephalics) (see 3.15 Breed-Related Anesthetic Considerations). In most instances, an answer like this is appropriate.

Example answer: We anesthetize patients of all breeds at this hospital and take excellent care of all of them. Your pet will be carefully watched, and a nurse will be with him/her for the entire anesthetic period.

Who will be taking care of my pet during anesthesia?

The veterinarian should assure the client that doctors oversee every component of anesthesia but that a veterinary nurse will be the direct caregiver for their pet during anesthesia. The doctor can introduce the nurse for a conversation that might be similar to:

Example answer: Hi Mrs Kat. I am the veterinary nurse in charge of your pet's anesthesia today. I will work with the doctor as he/she designs an anesthetic protocol specific for your pet. I will help to anesthetize your pet and will be with your pet, watching it throughout the entire procedure and in recovery until it is awake and comfortable. Don't worry about your pet while it is here. I will take very good care of him/her and will call you just as soon as he/she is awake

Is anesthesia for animals the same as anesthesia for humans?

Example answer: It is very similar. We use the same anesthetic drugs and monitoring techniques that are used in human medicine, but we include specific care that is needed for animals, like your dog (or cat). Just like in human medicine, in veterinary medicine we first use sedatives to make sure that your pet is calm, and then we induce sleep using drugs injected into the veins. For short procedures, this may be all that is necessary, but for longer procedures we use inhaled anesthetic drugs delivered through a special tube ("endotracheal tube") in your pet's airway (or 'trachea). For support, just as in humans, we use oxygen, IV fluids, anesthetic monitoring, patient warming, and pain control to make sure that anesthesia is as safe, and that your pet is as comfortable as possible.

What should I anticipate following my pet's anesthesia? Will he/she be OK? Is there anything special I need to do or anything that I should watch for?

Pet care should be discussed not only for postanesthesia but also postsurgical requirements. Since pet owners are generally nervous when picking up their pets after a surgical procedure and often more focused on the pet than on the doctor or nurse, written instructions that describe what to watch for and guidelines of when to call the clinic with concerns should be provided for the pet owner to take home.

Example anesthesia-specific answer: Most animals tolerate anesthesia very well, especially when the anesthetic protocol is tailored to your pet's needs, like we do at our animal clinic. Animals generally wake up rapidly and are ready to return home with you by the end of the day (or whenever you determine). Your pet may still be a little sleepy the night of the procedure and may not want to eat a large meal. We recommend keeping your pet quiet and allowing it to sleep. Offer it a small meal of something it really likes to eat. If your pet is still sleepy or not wanting to eat the following day, it might be normal depending on the procedure, but please give us a call so that we can discuss your pet's care.

Is there anything else that you can do to ensure the safety of my pet? I am really afraid to do this.

If the owner continues to be exceedingly concerned, or if the patient does indeed have risks that you are more concerned about than usual, consider consulting with or referring to a board-certified anesthesiologist, who may be at a university or specialty practice. Depending on your area, anesthesiologists may also be available to come to your practice. Anesthesiologists can be found through the American or European Colleges of Veterinary Anesthesia and Analgesia (ACVAA or ECVAA, respectively) or other organizations depending on your country. Patient referral can be specifically for anesthesia – not just for the surgical, dental, or medical procedure. An example is referral of patients with severe cardiac disease for anesthesia for a routine dental procedure. Although the dental procedure is routine, the anesthesia for that patient will likely include advanced monitoring and support and a dedicated anesthesiologist.

TAKE-AWAYS

- Anesthesia can be very frightening for pet owners. This is an understandable reaction but can result in a needed procedure not being scheduled for their pet if fears of anesthetic risk are not alleviated through effective client communication. Take the time to listen and to answer questions.
- The veterinary team (veterinarians, veterinary nurses, etc.) must be committed to safe anesthesia for every pet and should be prepared to discuss that commitment and the anesthetic process with pet owners.
- Patients should be stabilized prior to anesthesia so that the veterinary team can assure the client that, at this point, the benefit of the procedure for the pet outweighs the anesthetic risk.
- Prepared answers to frequently asked questions and written discharge instructions allow the clinic to provide a strong and consistent message regarding their approach to decreasing anesthetic risk for pets.
- If the client continues to be exceedingly concerned or if the pet is indeed at high risk for anesthesia complications, consider recommending a consult with or referral to a board-certified anesthesiologist.

MISCELLANEOUS

Reference

1 Brodbelt, D.C., Blissitt, K.J., Hammond, R.A. et al. (2008). The risk of death: the confidential enquiry into perioperative small animal fatalities. *Vet. Anaesth. Analg.* 35 (5): 365–373.

Recommended Reading

American College of Veterinary Anesthesia and Analgesia (ACVAA). www.acvaa.org/Owners

American Veterinary Medical Association (AVMA). www.avma.org/resources/pet-owners/petcare/when-your-pet-needs-anesthesia

Bednarski, R., Grimm, K., Harvey, R. et al. (2011). American animal hospital association. AAHA anesthesia guidelines for dogs and cats. *J. Am. Anim. Hosp. Assoc.* 47 (6): 377–385.

Grubb, T., Sager, J., Gaynor, J.S. et al. (2020). AAHA anesthesia and monitoring guidelines for dogs and cats. *J. Am. Anim. Hosp. Assoc.* 56: 59–82.

5.13

Improving Client Engagement Through Technology

Caitlin DeWilde, BS, DVM

The Social DVM, LLC, Webster Groves, MO, USA

BASICS

5.13.1 Summary

Technology, utilized in multiple formats, can help a veterinary practice better engage with existing and potential clients, educate pet owners, create a loyal clientele base, and even improve clinical outcomes. While initial adoption and utilization of the latest technological advances can seem daunting, meeting growing client desires and expectations for communication and engagement can be rewarding for all involved.

5.13.2 Terms Defined

Engagement: The ongoing interaction between a practice and a customer.

Telehealth: All uses of technology geared to remotely deliver health information or education.

Telemedicine: The use of medical information exchanged from one site to another via electronic communications regarding a patient's clinical health status.

MAIN CONCEPTS

5.13.3 The Need

Today's pet owners, particularly the millennial generation of pet owners, now the largest pet-owning segment of the population [1], have created a demand for improved

technology as part of their pet's healthcare. Pet owners are utilizing technology at touchpoints throughout the veterinary experience – everything from online research of review sites and social media when selecting a veterinarian, to visiting a practice's website to check hours and scheduling an appointment, to requesting records via email, app, or portal access, and utilizing texts and emails for notification of results and next steps.

By providing access and information where and how pet owners are looking, veterinary practices can increase appointments, revenue, compliance, and loyalty.

5.13.4 Opportunities

5.13.4.1 Social Media

Pet owners, particularly millennial pet owners, are more likely to be active on social media (see 5.4 The Changing Nature of Pet Owners). More than 15% of millennial pet owners will consult social media when looking for pet information [1], and a leading economic study has identified consistent social media use as one of the top four predictors of practice sustainability and success [2]. With billions of daily users, Facebook currently offers the largest base of existing and prospective clientele. Additional platforms such as Instagram and Twitter can be considered based on individual practice demographics, and there will be doubtless many other options going forward.

Social media presents the ultimate opportunity for veterinarians to literally and figuratively engage with their clientele on a daily basis, instead of the once- or twice-yearly in-person visits (see 7.5 Connecting with Clients Through Social Media). In addition to sharing social media-friendly pet articles and photos, practices have the opportunity to share trusted resources, client education materials, and more personalized content that differentiates the practice from its competition and allows clients to become more bonded to the staff of the practice. In addition, based on the practice's staff resources and online offerings, social media can present yet another opportunity for online booking, highly targeted yet low-expense advertising, and online messaging.

5.13.4.2 Apps and Push Notifications

At the time of this writing, over 80% of Americans owned a smartphone [3], and mobile apps are now ubiquitous, allowing the user to do everything from order groceries to arranging a ride share to managing their finances, and, now, their pet's healthcare. The average user spends more than four hours each day in nonvoice use of their smartphone, and 90% of that time in apps [4]. For many, but not all clientele, a veterinary-specific mobile app can improve client engagement, communication, and pet health. A recent study demonstrated that 86% of pet owners would like instant access to their pet's medical records through a mobile app [5], yet just 3% of practices in 2018 were utilizing this technology [1]. See Table 5.13.1 for a full comparison of client app and phone communication preferences.

Push notifications, or communications sent via an individual app, may have a higher read rate – up to four times more likely to be read than email. Because they can be turned on or off by a client, they also offer pet owners the most control over when and how they'd like to receive information.

Current market offerings allow veterinary practices to send mobile notifications of upcoming services due, patient updates, area pet health alerts, and test results. Others give pet owner access to patient records, appointment and prescription refill requests, messaging with the practice, and the opportunity to earn loyalty rewards. Medical journaling between veterinary teams and pet owners, along with remote patient monitor integration (e.g.,

with pet wearables), is also emerging features (see 2.5 Virtual Care (Telehealth)).

5.13.4.3 Digital Client Communications

Texting clients can be an economical and efficient way to engage with them. Texting (SMS) is widely adopted by today's population with some studies showing use as high as 97% of Americans. In addition, text messages are often read and responded to within three minutes, compared to 90 minutes for email messaging [6]. Veterinary practices can utilize texting for a variety of client interactions, including:

- appointment reminders and confirmations
- hospitalized patient updates
- boarding patient updates and photos
- dosing/medication reminders
- routine diagnostic test results
- health alerts/area outbreaks
- emergency practice closings.

Email communications are also helpful when it comes to providing clients more accessible information, and many users still prefer email communications to direct mail. Answering client emails can create a helpful dialogue preferred by many pet owners, as nearly 24% of millennial pet owners currently email questions to veterinary practices [1], and nearly 80% of pet owners would like to consult with their veterinarian via email [7].

Email may present additional, yet still affordable, methods of client engagement when a less immediate approach is preferred, including:

- appointment reminders and confirmations
- postvisit surveys and online review links
- promotion of new services and products
- sharing relevant health topic information, e.g., emailing owners a specific list of resources on a particular disease topic.

Table 5.13.1 Comparing client app and phone communication preferences

	Like app better than phone	Like app equal to phone	Like app less than phone	Don't use/Don't know
Make appointments	78 (50.3%)	53 (34.2%)	19 (12.3%)	5 (3.2%)
Order medication	62 (40.0%)	47 (30.3%)	20 (12.9%)	26 (16.8%)
Order pet food	52 (33.5%)	36 (23.2%)	22 (14.2%)	45 (29.0%)
Checking clinic hours	104 (67.1%)	34 (21.9%)	9 (5.8%)	8 (5.2%)
Looking for vet info	89 (57.4%)	35 (22.6%)	10 (6.5%)	21 (13.5%)
Accessing pet medical record	85 (54.8%)	42 (27.1%)	8 (5.2%)	20 (12.9%)

Source: Santi Kogan [5].

5.13.4.4 Website Offerings

Having a mobile-friendly website is essential, and now prioritized by leading search engines. Since 94% of US users access information on a smartphone [8], having a mobile-responsive website with multiple client-friendly features can make meeting client demands a reality.

5.13.4.4.1 Client Portals

Allowing clients to access important information like vaccine records to share with boarding, training, and grooming facilities can improve customer satisfaction and decrease calls to the front desk. In emergency or referral situations when clients seek outside veterinary care, medical record access can limit frustrations and improve patient care. Portals can also provide areas for owners to request appointments and prescription refills, and send secure messages to their pet's care team. In 2018, just 28% of practices offered a client portal [1].

5.13.4.4.2 Online Scheduling

Real-time appointment scheduling online is a solution to frustrations of both pet owners and practice staff. Clients can book an appointment online, at their convenience, even if your office is closed. Receptionists are freed up for more tasks when they spend less time on the phone discussing various scheduling options with clients, which takes eight minutes on average for each appointment.

In our human healthcare counterpart world, 66% of US health systems will offer online self-scheduling and 64% of patients will book appointments digitally by the end of 2019 [9]. In addition, recent human healthcare research suggests that nearly 40% of appointments are booked when businesses are closed [10]. Why would veterinary appointments be any different? In 2018, just 45% of practices offered online scheduling [1], indicating significant room for improvement to meet this client need. Client engagement and satisfaction, along with practice revenue, improve when clients are able to book appointments promptly, and receive online confirmation and/or reminders through your service or their own digital calendars.

5.13.4.4.3 Pet Health Information

Cat and dog owners alike indicated that a practice's offering a list of online resources for accessing reliable pet health information was one of their top five preferred services. Less than half of practices were found to offer client education resources on their website as of 2018 [1]. Providing clients the information they want, in the location that they are seeking it can improve client satisfaction, engagement, and, best of all, pet owner education. In addition, online pet health information, articles, and blogs can also bolster search engine rankings and serve as a source of social media content.

5.13.4.4.4 Online Store

In today's era of outside pharmacy use, having easy access to a trusted resource for online shopping for prescriptions, diets, and parasite preventives in the same place as other pet health information can be beneficial to both clients and veterinary teams. A 2018 study identified that dog owners in particular viewed having an option for online purchasing and home delivery as one of the top five most desired veterinary practice offerings, yet just 14% of clinics offered an online store [1].

5.13.4.5 Patient Update Notifications

A recent study assessing pet owner preferences on being updated on the status of their hospitalized pets indicated that the majority preferred to be updated every 4–6 hours (Table 5.13.2) [11]. In addition, when asked how they preferred to receive these updates, phone call and text were the top two responses (42% and 38%, respectively; see Table 5.13.2) [11]. This and other aspects of this study demonstrate that owners prefer updates more frequently than practices are currently delivering, and that preferred communication modalities are being underutilized. Offering these more frequent and varied communications can be time consuming and challenging for some practices but services such as texting and app push notifications may provide a more economical and time/cost-efficient option when compared to phone calls.

Table 5.13.2 Client preferences for patient update frequency

	Number	Percent
Hourly	86	8.4
Every 2–3 h	278	27.2
Every 4–6 h	358	35.0
Every 8 h	145	14.2
Every 12 h	96	9.4
Every 24 h	40	3.9
I would not want updates	3	0.3
Other	16	1.6

Most of the "other" responses wanted updates if something changed or there was something to report.

Source: Kogan et al. [7].

Table 5.13.3   Client device preferences for receiving patient updates

	Ranked 1	Ranked 2	Ranked 3	Ranked 4	Ranked 5
Phone call, cell/home	430 (42.0%)	242 (23.7%)	185 (18.1%)	111 (10.9%)	55 (5.4%)
Text	390 (38.1%)	307 (30.0%)	218 (21.3%)	88 (8.6%)	20 (2.0)
Phone at work	91 (8.9%)	202 (19.7%)	159 (15.5%)	261 (25.5%)	310 (30.3%)
Video	64 (6.3%)	74 (7.2%)	141 (13.8%)	235 (23.0%)	509 (49.8%)
Email	48 (4.7%)	198 (19.4%)	320 (31.3%)	328 (32.1%)	129 (12.6%)

Source: Kogan et al. [7].

5.13.5   Reputation Management

Online reviews are the new word of mouth, with 90% of customers visiting a business's online review rankings before selecting them [1]. The more reviews a business has, the more trustworthy it is deemed. While negative online reviews can certainly be a source of headache and heartache for the veterinary professional, few are working hard to elicit the feedback of their loyal and supportive clientele. Engaging with clients to encourage them to share experiences and reviews can minimize the impact of negative online reputation comments and reviews if and when they occur. In addition, valuable insight into your customers' experiences can be gained and utilized to improve future visits.

By sharing visual reminders of online reviews in person and online, creating clickable direct links to online review sites, sharing positive reviews on practice websites and social media channels, embedding review links in digital communications and sending postvisit survey and feedback requests, practices can engage with their clients and improve their overall customer service and online reputation.

5.13.6   Telemedicine

Perhaps the newest and most rapidly growing method of client engagement is via a veterinary practice's telemedicine and telehealth offerings. Mirroring trends in human healthcare, pet owners are increasingly interested in communicating with their veterinary team via text, email, and video (see 2.5 Virtual Care (Telehealth)).

According to a recent study, a practice's offerings of online texting or chat services was rated by pet owners in the top two most preferred offerings – #1 for dog owners and #2 for cat owners. Further, cat owners identified online video health consultations as one of the top five most desirable services a veterinary practice could offer [1].

As of this writing, many states are in the process of developing updated Practice Act language to determine legal and professional guidance on the use of telehealth. The American Veterinary Medical Association (AVMA)'s current position statement is that veterinary telemedicine should only be conducted within an existing veterinarian–client–patient relationship (VCPR).

Current industry offerings will allow practices to utilize video and chat telemedicine for a variety of client appointments, particularly those for recheck examinations and instances where the owner has difficulty transporting the pet to the practice.

5.13.7   Remote Patient Monitoring

Wearable pet devices such as activity trackers and glucose monitors can provide large amounts of data for both the pet owner and the veterinarian, while limiting the time that the pet must remain in the hospital (see 2.5 Virtual Care (Telehealth)). Combined with remote patient monitoring software, veterinarians can implement programs for:

- weight management
- arthritis/mobility assessment
- glucose monitoring
- atopy and pruritus scoring
- medication administration compliance.

Owners can become more engaged and have increased dialogue with the veterinary team using these ongoing monitoring approaches.

 TAKE-AWAYS

- Pet owners increasingly rely on technology to connect with their veterinary team via websites, social media, and apps.
- Practices can increase engagement by increasing communications via text messaging, emails, and push notifications.

- Hospitals should continue to provide interesting and relevant educational content on their websites and social channels where pet owners are looking for information.
- Consider early adoption of emerging technologies like telemedicine and remote patient monitoring.
- Connect with clients and reinforce your messaging by providing information and accessibility to your team in multiple digital touchpoints online.

MISCELLANEOUS

References

1 Pet Owner Paths Study. (2018). National Pet Owners Survey.

2 Volk, J.O., Felsted, K.E., Thomas, J.G., and Siren, C.W. (2011). Executive summary of phase 2 of the Bayer veterinary care usage study. *Journal of the American Veterinary Medical Association* 239 (10): 1311–1316.

3 Pew Research Center. Mobile Fact Sheet. https://www.pewinternet.org/fact-sheet/mobile

4 Santi, S. You Need a Mobile App for your Veterinary Hospital but Not for the Reasons You Think. https://vet2pet.com/2017/07/you-need-a-mobile-app-for-your-veterinary-hospital-but-not-for-the-reasons-you-think/

5 Santi S, Kogan L. Vet2Pet and Colorado State University Release Pet Owner's Perceptions and Use of Veterinary Mobile Applications Study? https://vet2pet.com/2017/02/vet2pet-and-colorado-state-university-release-pet-owners-perceptions-and-use-of-veterinary-mobile-applications-study

6 Patterson Veterinary. 10 Stats that Will 100% Convince You To Start Texting Your Clients. https://www.pattersonvet.com/vet/blog/10-stats-that-will-100-convince-you-to-start-texting-your-clients

7 Kogan, L., Shoenfeld, R., and Santi, S. (2019). Medical updates and appointment confirmations: pet owners' perceptions of current practices and preferences. *Frontiers in Veterinary Science* 6: 80.

8 Google. Be Mobile Friendly Overview. https://developers.google.com/search/mobile-sites

9 Accenture. Patient Engagement: Digital self-scheduling set to explode in healthcare over the next five years. www.accenture.com/t20170412t073547z__w__/us-en/_acnmedia/pdf-6/accenture-patient-engagement-digital-self-scheduling-explode.pdf

10 Truman, B. The Benefits of Online Appointment Booking. www.americanveterinarian.com/journals/amvet/2018/october2018/the-benefits-of-online-appointment-booking

11 Kogan, L., Schoenfeld-Tacher, R., Simon, A.A., and Viera, A.R. (2010). The internet and pet health information: perceptions and behaviors of pet owners and veterinarians. *Internet Journal of Veterinary Medicine* 8 (1).

Recommended Reading

Frankel, C. Top 5 Ways to Leverage Client Smartphones to Enhance Care. www.cliniciansbrief.com/article/top-5-ways-leverage-client-smartphones-enhance-care

5.14

Client Education Materials

Peter Alberti, BSBA

Inulogica, Northborough, MA, USA

BASICS

5.14.1   Summary

Educating clients is a vital, yet often difficult accomplishment. In the realm of pet-specific care, the opportunity exists to engage pet owners more easily by tailoring client education directly to the patient. A deliberate effort to offer recommendations in a consumable, actionable, and relatable form can make concepts contextually relevant for the pet owner and improve overall effectiveness of the education process.

MAIN CONCEPTS

Since pet-specific care involves the entire veterinary team, along with pet owners and other stakeholders, it is vital that everyone is aligned with the overall goals for each pet as well as the protocols and procedures involved. Educating clients and encouraging compliance have always been challenging in animal health. Consumerism and social media have further complicated the matter. Adding terminology and concepts pertaining to pet-specific care that are likely to be highly technical and complicated for pet owners to comprehend only adds another burden to an already difficult task.

One client education challenge inherent to pet-specific care is also an opportunity – the guidance must be unique to a particular pet. More sophisticated decision making will be required to determine what education is needed, at what time, and how best to communicate it to a client.

Making these decisions collaboratively will certainly be challenging. However, education tailored to a specific pet is much more contextually relevant to the pet owner than generic pet health education content, and therefore is likely to be more readily accepted by the client. This should facilitate better, more informed decision making.

Three elements should be considered when selecting client education materials for pet-specific care.

- Relevance – selecting materials that are appropriate.
- Distribution – identifying effective method(s) and times to reach clients.
- Confirmation – ensuring clients understand what they are being told and are compliant with the guidance given.

5.14.2   Relevance

The bottom line is that recommendations will be most effective if the client can understand and relate to the guidance being offered. There are a number of strategies that can be employed to accomplish this.

Use patient medical records as the basis for selecting materials and explain the reasoning for providing the material as it relates to the pet (see 7.9 Using Practice Management Software to Personalize Care). It may not be readily apparent to an owner why certain materials pertain to their pet's situation. It may be easier for a client to grasp a health concept if it is presented in context with the pet. Avoid distributing industry-supplied materials purely for the sake of convenience. Ensure they are truly relevant to the pet's needs.

When discussing recommendations, identify areas of specific client friction for which supporting material could lower barriers. When you provide supplementary resources that the client can use to learn more about your recommendation, you are helping to ensure the client understands the association to the pet-specific guidance. Clients can get off track easily, especially when they do not understand something well.

Most adults are reticent to ask questions if they think it will make them appear unintelligent. Also, different people learn in different ways. Therefore, leveraging multiple sources of educational material can help to make the adult learner feel more comfortable. Having said this, do not overwhelm clients with numerous materials just because they are available. Introduce materials with a clear explanation about why they are relevant to the pet and ask which one(s) resonate best. Give the client sufficient time to digest the content and formulate questions. Prompt them to relate their questions to their own pet.

Ensure the entire veterinary team provides consistent messaging as it relates to the pet (see 9.8 Ensuring Consistency of Care). This is likely to require new protocols/approvals, as well as training, for the practice. Help the team resist the temptation to talk about complex pet-specific concepts which, although relevant and exciting in a medical context, won't help the pet owner understand what's going on.

5.14.3 Distribution

People are always busy. They have become less and less capable of consuming large amounts of information, especially when it is complicated. To ensure pet-specific educational content is effective, consider employing some of the following strategies.

Whenever possible, send materials to clients ahead of time to give them an opportunity to review and understand them. If you do this, provide an outlet for them to ask questions or request more information if they need it.

Consider providing content in small doses. If there is a series of content available, send one part, allow the client to confirm understanding, and then send the next one. Doing this while maintaining the context of the client's specific pet will help keep the pet owner engaged and creates a *customer journey* to follow (see 5.8 The Biology of Marketing). It also allows you to identify if there are any breakdowns in understanding or compliance around a given topic.

Using multiple channels to send content can be helpful as well. Enabling clients to access email, websites, internet search terms, brochures, and other resources will help differentiate content and keep the interest of the audience by virtue of having different learning experiences (see 5.13 Improving Client Engagement Through Technology). Having said this, ascertain the client's preferred channels so you do not risk a missed opportunity if a client dislikes or rejects a particular medium.

Verifying that the educational resources you recommend are current is a priority. This applies particularly to digital assets, but also to printed materials. Reviewing materials together with clients and specifying them in context with pet-specific care are two excellent ways to actively perform this validation.

5.14.4 Confirmation

Ensuring the client clearly understands pet-specific guidance is the job of the veterinary team. Ideally, specific and measurable actions can be taken by the pet owner which can be monitored and evaluated by the clinical team. This will help ensure the pet-specific education is effective.

It can be easy to assume the client will review educational materials when they are offered. This is not a safe assumption. There are many reasons why pet owners do not read educational materials, including lack of time, lack of understanding about the content itself, misunderstanding your expectations about what to review, and losing the materials, among others. Establish methods to confirm the client reviews the material, such as the following.

- Ensure the client understands why the material is relevant to his/her pet.
- Confirm the client knows how to follow advice/take action based on the materials.
- Establish a means for the client to ask questions and interact with your team.
- Help the client devise pet-specific strategies, goals or measurements that align with the educational content.
- Since a good deal of pet-specific care focuses on prevention and early detection, whenever possible try to help the client establish a degree of excitement about the goals and actions that will make his/her pet healthier. Leverage this during future interactions by referring to it and relating it to the educational content to reinforce compliance.

EXAMPLES

Mrs Jones has a dog named Sparky who has been diagnosed with a certain form of cancer. Multiple teams will be involved in Sparky's care. Mrs Jones needs to be informed about diagnostics, therapies, risks, financial considerations, follow-up care, and many other topics. The primary care veterinarian determines that Mrs Jones is technically savvy and uses online resources frequently.

It is also demonstrated that she is not particularly organized and tends to forget things and lose items. It becomes apparent that digital education materials are likely to be most productive for Mrs Jones.

The primary care veterinarian creates an education program that includes the following.

- Emailing one document or website link at a time to Mrs Jones.
- When applicable, copies of the emails will be provided to specialists or other veterinary team members with directions, so Mrs Jones knows who to contact with questions.
- Before sending a new email, the primary care veterinarian asks Mrs Jones to confirm her understanding of the previous materials that were sent. If applicable, Mrs Jones is asked to answer a question, complete a task or perform some other action confirming her understanding.
- Included at the bottom of each email is a history showing previous education materials sent, the action(s) taken, and any other notes. This helps Mrs Jones and the team maintain context for current activities and review history if/as needed.
- Whenever possible, specific notes, images, or other assets from the medical records are included in the emails and are referenced specifically, correlated to the education materials being sent. When this is not possible, a follow-up discussion is initiated to help Mrs Jones relate what she learned to Sparky's specific case.

By following this process, Mrs Jones is not overwhelmed with information, she can participate productively with Sparky's care, and the veterinary teams can monitor her participation and understanding about what needs to be done.

TAKE-AWAYS

- Client education materials in a pet-specific care context must be meaningful and understandable for clients.
- Client education is inherently difficult. Adding pet-specific concepts can potentially make it appear more complicated. Strategies must be employed to ensure effectiveness.
- The entire staff must be aligned on how to educate clients.
- Educational content should be current and relevant.
- Clients are likely to need guidance and oversight to make effective use of educational materials.

MISCELLANEOUS

5.14.5 Cautions

The potential exists for veterinary teams to talk in very technical terms about pet-specific concepts. Care must be taken to ensure pet owners understand what is being discussed.

Recommended Reading

Pritchard, D.E., Moeckel, F., Villa, M.S. et al. (2017). Strategies for integrating personalized medicine into healthcare practice. *Per. Med.* 14: 141–152.

5.15

Client Appointment Scheduling

Kurt A. Oster, MS, SPHR, SHRM-SCP

Bay State Veterinary Emergency and Specialty Services, Swansea, MA, USA

 BASICS

5.15.1 Summary

Management of the practice scheduling system and client appointments is a major driver of client satisfaction and practice profitability. Unfortunately, automation breeds apathy and few veterinary practices proactively manage their scheduling system with the same oversight that was commonplace with paper-based scheduling systems.

5.15.2 Terms Defined

10-Minute Flex: Scheduling system that allows the user to determine the appropriate amount of time for the appointment based on the number of 10-minute blocks that are combined. Therefore, an appointment could be 10, 20, 30, or 40 minutes, as needed.

Anybody: Generic term used by many practices to identify a client that scheduled an appointment but did not request a specific doctor. Therefore, "anybody" can see this client.

Bonding Philosophy: There are two primary bonding philosophies in multidoctor practices. The first is to bind clients to the practice. The second bonds the client to a specific doctor.

Bonding Rate: A measure of the client bond with a specific doctor, calculated as the percentage of appointments with a doctor in which that doctor was specifically requested.

Fill Rate: Percentage of available appointment slots that were scheduled during a specific period of time. If, for example, a doctor is seeing 15-minute appointments from 8.30 a.m. to 10.00 a.m., there are 10 available appointment slots. If six of these slots are scheduled, the fill rate for this appointment block is 60%.

Forward Booking: This is the process of scheduling a client's next visit to the practice before they leave so a client always knows when they need to return, instead of waiting or receiving a reminder notification.

Patient Recovery: In multipet households, the staff always checks the status of all pets during each transition to ensure that no pets in the family are past due to receive and recommended care.

Request: Generic term used by many practices to indicate that a client has requested a specific doctor when scheduling an appointment.

Straight 15s: Historically the most common scheduling system. The staff would schedule a steady stream of appointments at 15-minute intervals (e.g., 8.00, 8.15, 8.30, etc.). Currently, it is estimated that 10–15% of companion animal practices still use this system.

Straight 20s: A popular expansion of the straight 15s approach. Appointments were scheduled at 20-minute intervals (e.g., 8.00, 8.20, 8.40, etc.). Currently, it is estimated that approximately 40% of companion animal practices use this system.

Straight 30s: A popular time-scheduling option in very competitive markets and perhaps the schedule of choice for new practices trying to bond clientele. It is estimated that less than 5% of companion animal practices use this system.

MAIN CONCEPTS

Typically, each client/patient encounter has a fixed number of tasks. Examples could include introducing yourself to the client, eliciting the client's chief complaint, taking an appropriate history, performing a physical exam, formulating a treatment plan, performing necessary treatments, answering client questions, preparing for future encounters, documenting the encounter, and assisting with any billing or follow-up procedures.

Time/motion studies indicate that the majority of veterinarians can complete the above tasks in approximately 12 minutes. In a straight 15-minute appointment system, this leaves three minutes of quality client education time (unless other care is sacrificed). Given that the average companion animal visits the veterinarian two or fewer times per year, this gives the veterinarian six minutes or less each year to educate the client on all healthcare issues and/or needs relevant to their pet. Most veterinarians find this amount of time woefully inadequate.

Implementation of a standard 20-minute appointment system increases a veterinarian's quality education time per encounter from three to eight minutes. These five additional minutes represent a more than 250% increase in the amount of time a veterinarian has to educate and bond with her clients. Although a veterinarian will only be able to see three patients per hour (instead of four), productivity per visit typically increases so dramatically that productivity per hour is greater with fewer patient encounters. Decreased client volume has multiple benefits. It also decreases stress on support staff, increases doctor time with the client and improves a practice's on-time performance (significant drivers of client satisfaction).

Utilizing 30-minute appointments is rarely an effective strategy in the general practice setting. Most veterinarians are unable to fill the additional 10 minutes with quality client communication and education. Therefore, clients perceive these longer appointments to be inefficient and poor customer service. Veterinarians rarely increase their productivity enough so that two patient visits per hour can be as profitable on a per-hour basis as three visits per hour.

The 10-minute flex system allows the staff to capitalize on the advantages of each of the systems described above without being locked into one specific time block. Ten-minute flex scheduling starts by breaking your appointment book into 10-minute slots. The number of slots utilized for each patient encounter depends on the needs of the client, patient, and/or veterinarian (or all three). In a typical practice, a 10-minute appointment could be a suture removal or a simple recheck exam. A 20-minute appointment could be the majority of routine appointments or more complex rechecks, and 30-minute appointments can be for two pets that belong to the same client, more involved procedures (second opinions, for example), or new client visits.

On-time performance is a key component of all customer service programs. By providing staff with the flexibility to schedule visits for the precise amount of time the staff will need to complete all necessary services and communication, 10-minute flex scheduling can dramatically improve a practice's on-time performance.

Practices should calculate the fill rate for each doctor, each quarter, as described above. The results should be entered into a table similar to the one below.

Time	Monday	Tuesday	Wednesday	Thursday	Friday	Saturday
Morning	120%	80%	70%	60%	Off	120%
Afternoon	70%	40%	40%	50%	Off	Off
Evening	Off	Off	96%	Off	Off	Off

In a typical general practice, about 70% of the appointment schedule is routine preventive healthcare driven by the reminder system. Driving even a 5% increase in reminder compliance can help a practice reap huge dividends. Practices can often achieve this increase (or more) by changing from a monthly to a weekly reminder protocol. Instead of sending out a first reminder for next month, a second reminder for last month and a third reminder for two months overdue, the practice changes to two weeks out for first reminders, two weeks past due for second reminders, then six weeks past due for third reminders. This simple change in protocol increases the practice's reminder compliance rate dramatically and provides the added benefit of evenly distributing work across the entire month instead of the practice being busy early in the month and slow near the end of the month until the next wave of cards goes out.

Another simple yet effective technique for driving compliance and fill rate is patient recovery. Patient recovery is the process by which the team ensures that all members of a multipet household are up to date. If a client receives a reminder alert and calls to schedule an appointment for Fluffy, the receptionist should check the reminder status of the other pets in the household. If Rusty is past due, they should recommend bringing Rusty in at the same time so they can both be brought current. If unsuccessful when scheduling Fluffy, the staff has a second opportunity to schedule Rusty during Fluffy's checkout process.

Once the appointment book is full, the team will want to ensure that all the clients actually arrive for their visit. Missed appointments are missed opportunities for production that are lost forever. Therefore, many practice management software programs now have features built into their appointment book to track the reason for a missed appointment and flag habitual offenders.

Confirming appointments two days in advance can dramatically decrease missed appointment rates. Some software systems are able to send email, telephone, and/or text (SMS) confirmations to clients to help improve compliance. Confirming one day in advance rarely allows clients to alter their schedule if they have forgotten about their appointment. However, confirming appointments two days in advance allows clients an opportunity to alter their schedule, or notify you of the cancelation far enough in advance that you can fill the open slot. Contacting missed appointments and rescheduling them will dramatically improve client compliance, patient care, and practice profitability.

Internet portal systems and client apps allow clients to request and/or confirm their appointments online. These systems offer clients 24-hour convenience for negligible monthly cost.

EXAMPLES

Last year, Dr Smith had a receptionist calculate her appointment fill rate for the last three months. Overall, her average fill rate was 71%. She had her staff initiate a patient recovery program and they began confirming all appointments at least two days in advance. She measured her fill rate each quarter and one year later it had risen to 94%. This represented an addition of a little over four additional appointments in her schedule each day. The result was over $100 000 in additional practice revenue of which she received additional wages of over $20 000.

TAKE-AWAYS

- Select a scheduling system that supports your practice style and philosophy that supports the correct amount of time for each visitor to ensure patient care, customer service, and efficient use of practice resources.
- Train each team member on the value of having a full appointment schedule.

- Measure and monitor your reminder return rates. A practice should achieve at least 45% compliance from a first reminder with a goal of 85% within three reminder cycles.
- A patient recovery program and an effective appointment confirmation program can be put in place at virtually no cost. It just requires some simple customer service and communication training.
- Practice automation can be your friend. Utilize your management software and ancillary software products to customize and automate as much of your confirmation process as possible. Extend your appointment book out 18 months to support forward booking and consider a practice app if you don't already have one.

MISCELLANEOUS

5.15.3 Cautions

During the transition to a new scheduling system, staff members will inevitably make mistakes. Teamwork and communication can minimize the impact of these errors on the clients as well as on the staff. Typically, it takes 2–4 weeks for most practice staff to transition smoothly and efficiently to 10-minute flex scheduling. Once introduced to a 10-minute flex scheduling system, rarely does a practice choose to revert back to its previous scheduling system.

Patient recovery and forward booking programs initially create additional work for reception teams. Offering training (including role playing) and small rewards or incentives for hitting targets will go a long way in driving staff compliance.

Recommended Reading

Ackerman, L.J. (2002). *Business Basics for Veterinarians*. New York: ASJA Press.

Judah, V. (2012). *Veterinary Office Procedures*, 2e. Clifton Park: Delmar.

Oster, K. (2020). Client appointment scheduling. In: *Five-Minute Veterinary Practice Management Consult*, 3e (ed. L. Ackerman), 288–289. Wiley.

Smith, C. (2009). *Client Satisfaction Pays*. Lakewood, CO: AAHA Press.

5.16

Maintaining Client Contact Between Appointments

Robert Sanchez

Digital Empathy, San Diego, CA, USA

BASICS

The ability to think critically from the customer's perspective is a significant competitive advantage. Because while you may feel that you sell quality veterinary medicine, that is not what people buy. Everyone, everywhere, buys something because of one simple reason: *doing so makes us feel a certain way*.

The ability to do this within your veterinary practice is paramount. However, with modern digital tools, we can begin to extend the walls of our communication and create stronger bonds with clients even when they aren't directly in front of us. Our industry's commodity is trust and when you build a deep relationship filled with trust and insightful advice, it solves many problems and creates a brighter future for your practice, your team, and your community.

5.16.1 Terms Defined

Brand: The conscious and unconscious feelings and attitudes that consumers have about a business.
Brand Equity: The value of a brand.
Churn: The percentage of customers who cease their patronage of a given service.
Customer Success: The business methodology of ensuring customers achieve their desired outcomes while using your product or service.
Ideal Customer Profile: A description of the customers that are a perfect fit for your services.

MAIN CONCEPTS

Often times, a practice will have a disjointed strategy in maintaining engagement with pet owners between visits. That is a mistake, as there should be a very purposeful strategy around improving sentiments toward the practice across as wide a network as possible, and improving the success of pet owners in having happier and healthier relationships with their pets.

5.16.2 Branding

If you can't make me feel, it's hard to make me act. The most important piece of brand equity that your veterinary practice owns is the way that its community and customers feel about the practice. The ability to build, strengthen, and nurture relationships is likely the best predictor of success for a veterinary practice.

Trust is the foundation of any relationship. Your practice should, at all levels, have well-defined and delineated strategies to build trust with customers and prospects at every potential touch point. Trust does not emerge from logical calculations. It is much closer to an instinct. In our ancestral past, early humans had to quickly discern who would have our backs when there were threats. That is why we are constantly, and unconsciously, sizing up our social surroundings in order to determine our level of comfort with a person or social group.

Modern consumer attitudes about pets have shifted significantly in the last generation. Owners now think of their pets as more like family members than commodities to be maintained and replaced when necessary. This is the attitude you must tap into – the love that we all have for animals, the passion that lives within that space, and the celebration of the bond that exists between humans and animals (see 2.14 Benefits of the Human–Animal Bond).

We learn about the world through narrative and story. We are hungry for stories with characters who face a compelling situation and who share our values (see 5.8 The Biology of Marketing). The backbone of your relationship-building strategy should be a celebration of people and animals doing amazing things for each other. The majority of this should be unique content that happens within everyday practice.

It is important to begin cataloguing this so that your community can share the successes that your team experiences on a consistent basis. Share these incredible stories consistently and widely. The work that veterinary professionals do every day is powerful and meaningful, and it changes lives. This is the steady drumbeat that will build brand equity with your clients and community between visits. The best channels through which to market these stories are social media (specifically Facebook and Instagram), and email marketing.

Another trust-building strategy is to revel in transparency. Humans crave connection, and we want to get to know you. Find someone on the team who is a talented writer, or outsource to a professional, and start putting together staff and event profiles. When there is something unexpected about a team member, for example a technician who is a local jazz performer, that should be celebrated. When you put on an event or have a charitable cause, speak to the underling *why* of the event.

5.16.3 Customer Success

A pet owner longs to be their pet's hero. They are not looking for another hero. They need a guide. Someone to help them walk the path that helps them live happier and healthier lives together.

Customer success is a business methodology that shapes strategy around ensuring that customers achieve their desired outcomes. It was developed by executives at the popular customer relationship management company Salesforce, after the company began to experience high churn from disengaged and confused customers. After implementing customer success, their churn plummeted. And while a veterinary practice faces different obstacles from a software company, the lessons can be broadly applied to any kind of patron-based relationship. The idea is to make your relationship with them as valuable for them as possible on an ongoing basis (see 5.1 Pet-Specific Customer Service).

The foundation of a sound customer success strategy is education. There are significant education gaps within the veterinary industry that must be addressed, such as feline visits and dental care, that are largely due to ineffective or nonexistent education strategies. Digital media gives us the platform to create a scalable and valuable education strategy between visits (see 5.13 Improving Client Engagement Through Technology).

The best place to start is by strategizing with your team on the most important topics that face compliance gaps. Then, begin putting together a content calendar to raise and celebrate awareness of these topics. An example content calendar looks like this.

Month	Emphasis
January	Internal parasites
February	Dental health
March	Obesity awareness
April	Puppy and kitten care
May	Flea and tick prevention
June	Breed-specific health issues
July	Feline health
August	Nutrition
September	Senior care
October	Pain management
November	Training
December	Holiday hazards

As an industry, we must begin to adopt a broader view of how we can make successful pet owners. Pet owners are hungry to learn about how to better care for their pet's health issues, but there are also important education gaps in nutrition, behavior, lifestyle, and other aspects of the human–animal bond. The entire team is a well-spring of insight, as they see the compliance gaps first hand and can help craft and execute on a concerted strategy.

Once you have created a content calendar, the next step is to begin writing articles and curating social content to effectively market the education. Aim for two blog posts a month, with a post a week that chronicles a "success story" of an owner acting as a hero to a pet to overcome the given obstacle. Blogs can also be sent out as a newsletter via your practice management software or a third-party email marketing solution.

Also consider utilizing digital platforms for real-time events that bring together your community, such as Facebook Live. Market the event ahead of time on social media so that pet owners know that they can submit their questions on your post, and that the top questions will be answered during the event.

Many clients may find value in automated reminders for their pet's healthcare and visits. You can integrate the "awareness topics" into a reminder system – whether it is through your practice management software or a third-party solution, such as a smartphone app. Reminder systems add the value of individualization – you can automate the system to remind pet owners about upcoming checkups, lapses in vaccinations, and more. Text and app-based reminders tend to have higher compliance rates, especially among younger clientele.

EXAMPLES

ABC Animal Hospital holds a team-wide meeting in order to build a system for categorizing success stories that happen in the practice and assign leadership roles within this system. Jan, a technician, is responsible for taking photos of memorable moments. Susan, a customer service representative with a knack for writing, is responsible for typing a one-paragraph summary of the event that happened (such as Milo's rescue). And Rick, a veterinary assistant who also manages the practice's Facebook account, is responsible for scheduling these posts, monitoring activity, and responding accordingly.

Dr Jessica, an associate (employed) veterinarian, begins to curate topics for a content calendar based on the team's feedback of the most common questions and compliance issues that they see within the practice. She finds an outside writer with experience in the industry and a talent for storytelling to translate these ideas into well-developed blog posts, approximately 500–1000 words in length. And Rick works with Dr Jessica to curate weekly posts and success stories around the given topic for that particular month.

TAKE-AWAYS

- Few practices think deeply about how to build relationships with clients outside the walls of the practice. With

digital tools, consistently building brand equity simply requires strategy and execution.

- Trust is the currency of our business. We trust people and organizations with whom we share deeply held values. Think about those values and celebrate them on social media and through direct marketing such as email.
- Be authentic during your digital communications. When you are supporting a charitable cause or when a team member has a unique skill or passion, celebrate that. Humans yearn for genuine connection and feeling like we are seeing behind the curtain grows the bond we feel with you.
- Begin to adopt a customer success strategy instead of merely customer service. Be proactive about educating pet owners between visits about different health, behavior, nutrition, and lifestyle topics that have important compliance issues.
- Involve the entire team in this strategy. Every person on the team has a unique vantage point about where the most meaningful moments in the practice occur, and where the most important education opportunities exist.

MISCELLANEOUS

5.16.4 Cautions

In order to chronicle client-based stories across social media, you will first need their permission (see 7.6 Privacy and Confidentiality). Consider adding an opt-in for this in your new client intake forms. Also, to avoid voiding their consent, pictures of the visit must be taken from a practice-owned camera, not an employee-owned camera.

Recommended Reading

Garcia, E. Instant success with Instagram. https://ericgarciafl. com/instant-success-with-instagram

Sinek, S. How great leaders inspire action. TED Talks. www. ted.com/talks/simon_sinek_how_great_leaders_inspire_ action?language=en

Weinstein, P. Reach out and touch someone. Today's Veterinary Business. https://mydigitalpublication.com/pub lication/?m=60566&i=597090&p=30

5.17

Ensuring and Measuring Client Satisfaction

Caitlin DeWilde, BS, DVM

The Social DVM, LLC, Webster Groves, MO, USA

 BASICS

5.17.1 Summary

As veterinary professionals, we would love to measure the success of our careers and businesses in the wagging tails and friendly nuzzles of our patients. However, it is essential that we instead rely on the feedback given by our ultimate client, our patient's human owners. Ensuring and measuring client satisfaction allows our practices to best address and respond to concerns, reward successes, tailor future decisions, and ultimately provide better patient care and clinical outcomes.

 MAIN CONCEPTS

5.17.2 The Need

In order for veterinary practices to be successful and profitable, client satisfaction must be high. A satisfied customer will be a loyal customer, leading to repeat patient visits, higher acceptance of proposed services and products, increased spending at the practice, and referral of additional clients and pets.

To build an army of these loyal clients, practices must first ensure that their clients are satisfied. Second, tools to elicit, measure, and respond to client feedback must be implemented.

Many practices are quick to assume that a booked schedule or the absence of negative online reviews means that their customers are satisfied. Without any quantitative data to confirm that assumption, however, practices leave themselves open to missed opportunities. These include giving practices an avenue to address concerns, providing disgruntled clients a private "offline" space to share their feedback, reaffirming the strengths of the practice and team, identifying new client services and revenue streams, and overall suggestions for continual improvement.

5.17.3 Ensuring Client Satisfaction in a Pet-Specific Care Practice

Practices with a pet-specific care emphasis often offer a communication-based and team-based healthcare approach. In many ways, the very nature of this approach lends itself to naturally eliciting client feedback due to the frequency of communication. Increased feedback means more opportunities to meet, and hopefully exceed, client expectations.

The key to meeting those client expectations and ensuring satisfaction is to clearly demonstrate the value of the care and services provided.

Clients often subconsciously "calculate" value at the time of a veterinary transaction. This is the value of what they expected, plus the additional value they weren't expecting (value-add) but experienced, divided by the total costs (which includes both financial and nonfinancial costs). In short, it is the value add (such as pet-specific care) that drives a premium price over a commodity price for most consumers.

Fortunately, pet-specific care models give veterinary professionals many opportunities to impact these equation variables. In particular, the "service delivered" and the "service expected" can be affected by multiple team members within a client's cycle of care.

Improve your "services delivered" experience by addressing four key areas of the client experience: (i) preappointment (ii) during appointment, (iii) postappointment, and (iv) nonappointment.

Preappointment service delivery focuses on the process of making the appointment. Clients making appointments over the phone or in person should have the full attention of the receptionist, who is cordial and friendly. Avoid placing callers on hold, and if unavoidable, offer to call them back or set up an appointment via email or text. After the appointment is made, confirm via phone call, email, or text (ideally having asked the client's preference for how they prefer to receive their communications). Confirm at the time of making the appointment and again as a reminder the day of the appointment. Same-day reminders should also include any reminders for additional needs and be specific, for example "Please remember Fluffy should be fasted for two hours for her bloodwork sample" or "Please bring a fecal sample less than one hour old for Fido's intestinal parasite screening." This helps eliminate additional trips and client frustration.

At the time of the appointment, greet the client (and pet!) by name. If the clients must wait, direct them to the best area of the reception for their pet (e.g., avoid placing a cat next to a pacing dog). Address the pet's comforts first, such as a pheromone-infused towel to cover the cat carrier or a bowl of water for the dog. Client comforts can be addressed with water, coffee and reading material, and perhaps even WIFi. Make sure the reception area is cleaned throughout the day, and each exam room is clean before the client and pet are placed. Staff members should have regular training and assessment on communication skills and bedside manner to ensure they are providing friendly and compassionate care to both clients and pets.

In addition to discussing and offering quality medical care for their pet, it's important to communicate the costs of these and give the owner time to make decisions. Ideally, provide estimates in written form (or visible on a digital device) and discuss them with owners prior to performing diagnostics and treatments. One- to two-page medical summary reports, written in lay terms, sent home at the time of the visit can provide clarity, reinforce veterinarian recommendations and help owners communicate information with family members at home. If not readily available, offer to email this to the owner after they've returned home. Prior to concluding the visit and leaving the exam room, the veterinarian asks the owner for any final questions or concerns.

After the appointment, reach out to the owner within 24–48 hours (or sooner as the clinical course dictates) after nonwellness visits to check on the pet and address any new issues and client questions. Preventive care visits should also receive follow-up contact, along with supporting information that corresponds to the veterinarian's preventive health recommendations (e.g., instructions for the next annual visit, preventive dental care, nutrition/supplement recommendations, screening tests, etc.). Diagnostic test results should be communicated and discussed, and if possible, clients should be provided a copy for their records through a pet portal, or via email or traditional mail. After all medical issues have been addressed, clients should receive a postvisit survey or other opportunity to share feedback. Practice-specific feedback surveys and online review links should be clickable/embedded within any email or text communications to make it as easy as possible to respond.

As an ongoing relationship between a practice and a client progresses, the practice must continue to add value (nonappointments). In order to compete with internet services and other local clinics, practices must continue to establish themselves as the ultimate resource for all things related to their pet's care (see 5.16 Maintaining Client Contact Between Appointments). Key ways to achieve this are to meet client needs for educational information (e.g., via blogs, newsletters, social media articles, infographics, and videos), provide value in related pet services such as grooming, day care and training, and hold pet-friendly and client-friendly events (such as kitten socialization and puppy training classes, weight management weigh-ins, etc.). Reward owners who are loyal to your practice with perks and prizes such as discounted services or products, nominal gifts and recognition of their pet's care. Determine your loyal clientele by running client referral source reports, use a veterinary-specific loyalty app, and survey online review sites for feedback. Above all, thank these clients for their support and continue demonstrating the value you bring to them and their pet.

The other variable of the value equation, "service expected," is an accumulation of perceptions, some of which may be beyond the control of the veterinary team (e.g., when a client's perception is based solely on the word of mouth of an outside individual). However, it may also be impacted by past experiences, biases, and the expectations your practice and staff communicate before their visit. Clearly, veterinary professionals have the largest ability to impact the latter.

"Service expected" can be best met by clearly establishing and setting expectations from a client-facing viewpoint. From the very beginning, the mission, values, and culture the practice offers should be clear – in person and online. The practice's services provided and business information (hours, location, payment options) should be readily accessible. Team members should be trained and regularly assessed for their ability to provide information and answers to client questions and concerns throughout a veterinary visit or touchpoint (e.g., call or online contact). When these items are clear, the "services expected" will be most closely aligned with the "services delivered."

As many new client appointments come after an online search, ensure that your practice is readily represented (see 5.13 Improving Client Engagement Through Technology). The practice website should be mobile device friendly and load quickly (check this with several free online speed test tools). In addition, the practice accounts should be claimed and information should be regularly updated on Google Business, Yelp, Nextdoor, and Facebook. Optional platforms like Twitter, Instagram, Linkedin, and others can be considered based on client demographics. All platforms should contain consistent information, messaging, and brand elements (e.g., logo, colors, messaging, and style) to increase recognition. Information new clients are most likely to be searching for (hours, address, product/service availability) [1] should be prominently displayed.

Emotional marketing techniques should be implemented whenever possible – avoid stock photos and instead focus on imagery that shows the staff interacting with pets, happy pets of all species and ages and in general, photos that convey the true culture of the practice (see 5.8 The Biology of Marketing).

Finally, communication should be emphasized throughout the client cycle. Team members should not only be educated on what information to provide clients, but also how to provide it. Understanding that clients have different communication and learning styles is key to delivering the information in the best way. Be prepared to present the information to owners in person and remotely, in a variety of formats from email to blog to specific website to social media. The "New School" pet owner often wants to get their information from their veterinarian, but may also need longer to research, likes to have additional online resources, and is influenced by data-backed facts.

Value, and in turn client satisfaction, will be high when clients are happy with the "services delivered" and the "services expected" components of the above equation. Assessing "how high" requires implementing data-quantifying tools within the practice.

5.17.4 Measuring Client Satisfaction

Just as veterinary professionals rely on statistically validated, evidence-based data for clinical diagnostics and treatments, calculating client satisfaction should also involve quantifiable information. Measuring client satisfaction regularly has been identified as a significant opportunity to increase veterinary visits [1].

There are many methods and tools to consider based on your practice's needs and capabilities, ranging from a single-question Net Promoter Score questionnaire to a multi-question survey to a simple monitoring of online reviews. Choose a measurement tool that works for your practice based on your technological capabilities, the practice's goals and, most importantly, the practice's ability and commitment to analyzing and acting on client responses.

The most common tool to utilize is a postvisit client survey. Several veterinary industry companies offer this service as an email or web-based link, and some may integrate with existing practice management software (PMS) for an automated solution. Simple options include using a free online service such as http://surveymonkey.com to craft a survey and create a link that can be shared with clients via email, website, or social media.

Before implementing any client satisfaction measuring tools, be sure that a process exists (and has been tested) to collect, notify the practice of responses, and store the data.

The exact questions that should be included in the survey will vary based on the specific practice offerings, goals, and objectives. Members of certain veterinary industry organizations may have access to an existing survey and/or implementation service as a member benefit. These surveys often come with the benefit of being created with field-tested questions as well as having answer benchmarks for comparison.

Sample questions for a client satisfaction questionnaire
From your visit today, how would you rate:

The amount of attention the veterinarian gave to your pet

How well the veterinarian understood the reason for your visit

Your sense of the vet's confidence interacting with you and your pet

How well the veterinarian involved you in the entire appointment

The veterinarian's examination of your pet

How well the veterinarian explained treatments and procedures

How well you understood the costs today

How well the veterinarian involved you in decisions

The veterinarian's discussion of options with you

The veterinarian's discussion of the cost with you

The interest the veterinarian expressed in your opinion

The amount of information you received from the veterinarian

How well the veterinarian addressed all of your concerns

The veterinarian's recognition of the role this pet has in your life

The amount of time the veterinarian spent with you and your pet

Your likelihood to recommend this veterinarian to others

Providing clients with short, simple questions will increase the likelihood of responses. Avoid long sentences or multiple topics per question. Do not limit responses with multiple choice-only questions. Include blank space for clients to add their own additional thoughts and feedback, if they choose.

Encourage your clients to participate in your survey. Emphasize the direct benefits, such as how it will benefit their pet's well-being. Let them know that their input will help shape improvements and future service in the practice. Consumer research indicates response rates can increase by as much as 15% by offering even a nominal incentive, such as a discount off their next visit or a small service (e.g., a free nail trim) [2].

Consider including a final question to ask if the reviewer can be contacted for further input or clarification, and how they would like to be contacted. After a survey has been completed/submitted, thank the client for their response and reiterate the importance of their candor and feedback.

Analysis of client satisfaction feedback is crucial to identify and repair discrepancies, to celebrate successes, and to dictate next steps. Make analysis and response of any client feedback a priority and a regular task. A key staff member or management team should have a policy in place for when and how client feedback is handled. For instance, if a client survey returns with negative feedback, a manager should call them within three business days. All responses are summarized and discussed at each monthly management meeting.

Regularly schedule time at the management and entire staff levels to ensure that all members of the team have received the feedback as well as the steps taken to correct or improve based on this feedback. Keep a running log of feedback over time in order to ensure an upward, or at least steady, trend of client satisfaction.

Pair this quantifiable client feedback data with new client referral numbers, online review numbers and rankings, and client retention data to create a comprehensive picture of practice success.

EXAMPLES

Jane searches for local feline practitioners for her cat Maxine after they move to the area. Finding ABC Veterinary Hospital's website showcasing their accreditation as a cat-friendly hospital and having convenient evening hours, Jane also sees that they have numerous five-star reviews on Facebook and Yelp. She uses their online pet portal to schedule an appointment and receives a confirmation email immediately. The day of the appointment, Jane receives a text message reminder. When she arrives at ABC Veterinary Hospital, she is greeted promptly by a friendly receptionist and then given a feline pheromone-infused towel to place over Maxine's carrier as they wait in the cat-only side of the lobby. Jane and Maxine are quickly escorted to the cat-only exam room, where Jane answers patient history questions asked by the technician. The veterinarian enters the room and after greeting both Jane and Maxine, does a thorough exam and recommends vaccines based on Maxine's indoor/outdoor lifestyle, and a bloodwork panel to screen for relevant diseases. The technician presents Jane with an estimate for these services prior to the veterinarian administering the vaccines or the technician drawing the blood, which she approves.

After completing these services, the veterinarian asks Jane if she has any other questions, which she does not. The veterinarian explains that she will email Jane within 72 hours with the bloodwork results, and before Jane leaves she gives her a summary of her medical exam as well as a pamphlet about a recommended diet for senior pets.

The next day, Jane receives the email with the bloodwork attached and a note from the veterinarian explaining that everything looked good. The following day, Jane received a five-question quick email survey, which she completed, giving five stars! She received a thank you email confirming her survey submission and links to the practice social media accounts. She continues to follow the practice on social media for the latest news in cat health and the occasional cute pet photo!

TAKE-AWAYS

- Clients calculate their satisfaction and value of a veterinary visit based on financial and nonfinancial costs, services delivered, and services expected.
- Meet and exceed client expectations by clearly communicating the practice's culture, values, services, and key business info (e.g., hours, payment options, etc.) long before their first appointment.
- Pet owners, particularly "New School" pet owners, prefer multiple digital touchpoints for information gathering and practice communication.
- Client satisfaction surveys should be concise and direct. Consider offering a nominal incentive for participation.
- Client feedback should be taken regularly and analyzed as soon as possible in order to best respond. Trend these results over time and correlate with patient visits, referral source reports, and overall profitability to ensure you are meeting your customers' needs.

MISCELLANEOUS

References

1 Volk, J.O., Felsted, K.E., Thomas, J.G., and Siren, C.W. (2011). Executive summary of phase 2 of the Bayer veterinary care usage study. *J. Am. Vet. Med. Assoc.* 239 (10): 1311–1316.

2 Understanding consumers' local search behavior. www.thinkwithgoogle.com/advertising-channels/search/how-advertisers-can-extend-their-relevance-with-search-download

Recommended Reading

American Animal Hospital Association. Client Satisfaction Survey. www.aaha.org/professional/membership/client_satisfaction_survey.aspx

Coe, J., Adams, C., Eva, K. et al. (2010). Development and validation of an instrument for measuring appointment-specific client satisfaction in companion-animal practice. *Prev. Vet. Med.* 93 (2): 201–210.

The Opportunity Survey Tool. www.partnersforhealthypets.org/opportunity_login.aspx

Volk, J.O., Felsted, K.E., Thomas, J.G., and Siren, C.W. (2011). Executive summary of phase 2 of the Bayer veterinary care usage study. *J. Am. Vet. Med. Assoc.* 239 (10): 1311–1316.

5.18

Lifetime Support – Pet Trusts and Wills

Lowell Ackerman, DVM, DACVD, MBA, MPA, CVA, MRCVS

Global Consultant, Author, and Lecturer, MA, USA

 BASICS

5.18.1 Summary

Pet-specific care implies a philosophy of caring for pets across their entire lifespans. So, as pets are treated more and more like family members, it is only natural that pet owners will want to plan for the eventuality when they may no longer be able to provide the care needed for those family members. This is not only the case for long-lived animals, or even for older pet owners, but anyone can find themselves in a situation (accident, infirmity, debilitating illness, natural disaster, terrorist event, etc.) when they are unable to properly care for their pets and need assistance in this regard, either while still alive or following death.

Despite the aging of the US population, the recognition of the human–animal bond as an important connection between people and their pets (see 2.14 Benefits of the Human–Animal Bond), and a continuous trend for increased spending on our pets, most pet owners do not consider what might happen to their pets if they die, are displaced, or become even partially disabled. In perhaps too many instances, these pets do not receive the continued care their owners would have wanted, and may end up relinquished to a shelter or even euthanized.

Even if there are individuals willing to care for a decedent's pet(s), if there is not a will or trust that mentions the pet and the owner's intentions for its care, then there may be legal quandaries over who is allowed to take the animal and how to deal with pet-related expenses.

Wills and trusts are methods for individuals to make their wishes known regarding their pets. However, pets cannot directly be left property, including money, following their owner's death, so a human intermediary is required.

A will can transfer assets following a death, but it cannot dictate ongoing supervision. A trust, on the other hand, can outline the continued care of pets, name new caregivers, provide funding for pet care, and empower the trustee, who has a legal duty of carrying out the wishes of the settlor. Accordingly, most attorneys recommend trusts for pets rather than just including a pet in a will.

An additional estate instrument that is sometimes used for similar purposes is known as a pet protection agreement. This is actually a layperson's document that can be used to help ensure the well-being of pets after a pet owner's death or disability. It does not have the legal weight of a trust or a will, but it is a low-cost alternative that can be completed without the assistance of an attorney.

5.18.2 Terms Defined

Beneficiary: The individual who benefits from a trust agreement.

Decedent: A person who has died.

Executor: A person or entity appointed by a testator to carry out the terms of their will.

Grantor: An individual who transfers or conveys ownership.

Probate: The court process by which a will is proved valid or invalid.

Responsibility: The duty to perform or complete an assigned task.

Settlor: A person who has created a trust. Also known as a trustor or grantor.

Testator: A person who has made a will.

Pet-Specific Care for the Veterinary Team, First Edition. Edited by Lowell Ackerman.
© 2021 John Wiley & Sons, Inc. Published 2021 by John Wiley & Sons, Inc.

Trust: A relationship whereby property is held by one individual for the benefit of another.

Trustee: The individual or organization who receives the settlor's property for the benefit of the beneficiaries.

Will: Also known as a testament, the legal declaration by which a person names one or more persons to manage aspects of the estate after the testator's death.

 MAIN CONCEPTS

5.18.3 Wills

A will is a legal declaration by a testator in which an individual or individuals are named to manage an estate and transfer property after death. In the strictest historical sense, wills refer to real estate property whereas testaments refer to personal property, but today everything is included under the so-called last will and testament.

Pet owners can include their pets as provisions in their wills, but there are several reasons why this might not be the optimal solution. Wills can take weeks or months to be executed, might have to go through probate, and can be contested by others. When pets are transferred in a will, they are conveyed as any other type of property and the testator can specify what they hope for in terms of pet care, and even provide support in the form of monetary assets for this purpose, but the beneficiary is under no obligation to act as the grantor intended.

Although a will may allow a pet to be transferred to someone else following the owner's death, it is important to realize that this may not be helpful if the owner remains alive but is unable to provide adequate care and would just benefit from some assistance in caring for their pet(s). The will is strictly an instrument for transferring property after the testator's death.

It is for this reason, and many others, that trusts are often considered better options for pet owners but if that is not possible, the will does offer the prospect for the pet owner to make their wishes known regarding the transfer of ownership of any pets.

5.18.4 Trusts

A trust is a legal agreement that provides for the care of a pet in the event of an owner's disability or death. The owner does not need to be incapacitated for the trust to take effect, as long as the pet owner is deemed unable to manage their pet's care.

With the adoption of a new provision for the Uniform Trust Act of 2000, many states allowed laws that permitted the creation of pet trusts. Although not universally available in all states, pet trust laws have been enacted in almost all states and the District of Columbia [1].

Pet trust laws do vary on a state-by-state basis, so pet owners should enlist an attorney skilled in estate planning in their state of residence. Because there may be some states in which a pet trust is not valid and others where enforcement is discretionary, trusts need to be reviewed whenever moving to another state.

Some states allow a trust to provide for an animal for its entire life, whereas others may be limited to 21 years, so it is important to know the law in any particular state of residence.

Typically, the trust is written for the trustee to hold property (including money) "in trust" for the settlor's pet(s), and it can take effect during their lifetime or after their death. The trustee can then make payments to a designated caregiver, as provided in the trust. Trust funds are not subject to probate, the terms of the trust are not part of the public record, and there are no funding delays once the trust has been triggered by a specified situation.

The instructions in a pet trust can be very specific, so pet owners can feel confident that the trust is likely enforceable by law and that their wishes regarding their pets will be respected. Such instructions might include the frequency of veterinary visits, favorite foods to be fed, grooming requirements, and even the mode of burial or cremation after the pet's death. The pet's anticipated standard of living should be well documented within the trust.

Pet owners should not be secretive with friends and family members about their intentions for their pets. They should especially discuss such arrangements with anticipated caregivers to ensure that such individuals are willing and prepared for the task proposed. Without this agreement, it will likely be left up to the trustee to find an appropriate individual or organization to provide such services.

When the pet dies and there is still money left in the trust, the assets are distributed to a second beneficiary, such as an individual, a charitable foundation, or a corporation. The trust can also be written to cover offspring of the pet beneficiary.

In preparing a trust, it is important to select trustees who will be responsible for following the directions specified, and the caregivers who will ultimately be providing the day-to-day care requested. Because both trustees and caregivers are susceptible to the same fates as the rest of us, thought should be given also to successor trustees and caregivers who would be next in line should first choices no longer be able to provide the services requested. Secondary beneficiaries are also named, in the event that assets remain in the trust after the beneficiary pets have died.

TAKE-AWAYS

- If pet owners do not create a trust or will, they should consider what will likely happen to their pets in the case of death or disability. Other options exist, including life trusts, pet protection agreements, or private arrangements with friends, family members, or charitable pet-related organizations or shelters. Not having any plan can create a hardship not only for any pets involved but also for those who are ultimately left with making decisions related to those pets.
- Because pets cannot legally hold title to property in the United States, they also cannot be direct beneficiaries of a will or trust. Therefore, individuals or other legal entities must fulfill the intermediary role, with pets being the eventual beneficiaries of the instrument.
- Veterinary teams can assist pet owners in the creation of a pet trust by providing them with a personalized pet profile for pet-specific care that would enable them to estimate the costs of medical care over the pet's anticipated lifespan. To that end, they would also need to add reasonable costs for feeding, grooming, and miscellaneous other expenses that would be relevant to a particular pet. It is also important for the pet owner to consider the assets necessary to adequately cover the administration of the trust, including trustee fees, attorney consultation, and other such expenses.
- It is possible to create a trust for each individual pet to be cared for, but an alternative is to create one trust meant to serve all pets that would be owned during a pet owner's lifetime.
- Situations change, including moving to a state with different pet trust laws or enforcement, changes in relationships with would-be trustees and caregivers, and changes in number or types of pets that might alter the circumstances in a pet trust. Whenever such changes occur, it is important to revisit the trust and consider whether amendments are warranted.

MISCELLANEOUS

5.18.5 Cautions

Whenever money is involved, fraud can also exist, so care should be taken to ensure that the pet can be accurately identified. Suitable permanent forms of identification include microchipping and archived DNA samples from which identification can be confirmed. Photos and veterinary documentation of identifiable markings also help with identifying pet beneficiaries.

There are significant differences between states in pet trust laws, including how long they can remain in effect, how much can be left for a pet beneficiary, and how enforceable a pet trust might be, so trusts should only be created after consultation with an experienced estate attorney, with expertise in the likely state of residence of the pet and caregiver.

Abbreviation

DNA   Deoxyribonucleic acid

Reference

1 American Society for the Prevention of Cruelty to Animals. Pet Trust Primer. www.aspca.org/pet-care/pet-planning/pet-trust-primer

Recommended Reading

Ackerman, L. (2020). Pet trusts & wills. In: *Five-Minute Veterinary Practice Management Consult*, 3e (ed. L. Ackerman), 852–853. Ames, IA: Wiley.

American Bar Association (2013). *The American Bar Association Guide to Wills and Estates: Everything you Need to Know about Wills, Estates, Trusts, and Taxes*, 4e. New York: Random House Reference.

Congalton, D. and Alexander, C. (2002). *When Your Pet Outlives You: Protecting Animal Companions After You Die*. Troutdale, OR: NewSage Press.

Dekker, J. (2016). *Planning for Pets: Trusts, Leash Laws and More*. Briarcliff Manor, NY: Parker Press.

Hirschfeld, R. Ensure your pet's future: estate planning for owners and their animal companions. www.animallaw.info/sites/default/files/arus9marqeldersadvisor155.pdf

Hirschfeld, R. (2010). *Petriarch: The Complete Guide to Financial and Legal Planning for a Pet's Continued Care*. New York: AICPA.

Hoyt, P.R. (2009). *All My Children Wear Fur Coats: How to Leave a Legacy for Your Pet*, 2e. Oklahoma City, OK: Legacy Planning Partners.

Kass, R.E. (2011). *Who Will Care When You're Not There? Estate Planning for Pet Owners*. Detroit, MI: Carob Tree Press.

Lacroix, C.A. (2007). Pet trusts and wills. In: *Blackwell's Five-Minute Veterinary Practice Management Consult* (ed. L. Ackerman), 476–477. Ames, IA: Wiley Blackwell.

Section 6

Pet-Specific Considerations

6.1

Normal Development Stages of Dogs and Cats

Jacqui Ley, BVSc (Hons), PhD, DECAWBM, FANZCVS (Veterinary Behaviour)

Melbourne Veterinary Specialist Centre, Glen Waverley, Victoria, Australia

 BASICS

6.1.1 Summary

As our most popular companion animals, dogs and cats are often lumped together for their management and general care. There are many similarities in the developmental stages of dogs and cats but there are also important differences, particularly in the early weeks of life. Knowing what is normal for dogs and cats at different stages of their lives means all staff at the veterinary clinic can provide sensible and scientifically sound advice to owners about managing their pets.

6.1.2 Terms Defined

Adolescence: The period between puberty and social maturity.
Juvenile: Young, immature, looking like the adult except in size and reproductive ability.
Juvenile Period: The time after the socialization period and before puberty.
Puberty: Period in development characterized by the onset of reproductive system activity.
Sensitive Period: Times in the development of young where the brain is more sensitive to environmental stimuli.

 MAIN CONCEPTS

There are major differences in the development of dogs and cats that reflect differences in their evolution and domestic history. Dogs have been domesticated much longer than cats. The role of the cat in ancient times was to clear vermin from food stores. The animals they hunted were small, active at night, and numerous. The cat was largely left on its own to get the job done. In contrast, dogs developed from scavengers of garbage to a settlement early warning system and a helper on hunts. The jobs of the dog then diverged further into the many jobs we know only by the historic names of the dogs. Cats just kept doing what cats do best and no great changes occurred until they became pet cats and mutations leading to varied appearance became desirable.

The developmental stages of the dog and cat can be summarized as neonate, transitional, socialization, juvenile, adolescent, adult, and geriatric (Table 6.1.1). This represents one of many different potential models for life stages in dogs and cats (see also 4.1 Canine and Feline Life Stages).

6.1.2.1 Neonatal Stage

Puppies and kittens are born after approximately nine weeks gestation. Both species are born deaf, blind, and unable to walk although they can crawl along using their forelimbs. They have strong rooting reflexes when touched

Table 6.1.1 Developmental stages in dogs and cats

Life stage	Dogs	Cats	Characterized by
Neonatal	0–14 days	0–7 days	Deaf, blind, limited mobility
Transitional	14–21 days	7–14 days	Ears and eyes open, standing, and walking
Socialization	21 days to 12 weeks	14 days to 7 weeks	Interaction with conspecifics and the environment; adult body language may be seen
Juvenile	12 weeks to 12–18 months	7 weeks to 6–12 months	Ends with onset of puberty. Puberty is characterized by the activation of the reproductive systems
Adolescence	12–24 months	6–12 months to 36–48 months	Increasing independence, increase in impulsive behavior, time of learning, exploring
Adult	12–24 months to 8–12 years	36–48 months to 10 years	Period of stability, seeking territory, mates, raising young
Geriatric	8–12+ years	10+ years	Decline in sensory abilities, strength, immunity, cognitive abilities

on the nose and lips. This helps them find their mother's nipples when suckling. Both species require external stimulation to defecate and urinate. Neither species can regulate their temperature at this stage of life.

6.1.2.2 Transitional Stage

During this roughly week-long stage, the eyes and ear canals of the puppies and kittens open. They can start to gather more information from their environment. Their muscles and coordination improve so they start being able to stand on all fours and to walk.

Table 6.1.1 shows that kittens go through this stage sooner than puppies. Kittens are ready to leave the nest at about week 3. However, they need handling from week 2 to have them become more comfortable with being handled as adult cats. As many feral or semiferal kittens are not seen until after week 3, this has important implications as to whether they can adapt to be an owned cat which is handled by humans.

6.1.2.3 Socialization Period

This is a time of great learning for puppies and kittens. During this phase of development, puppies and kittens are able to fully interact with their environment and conspecifics. They learn what is safe and beneficial to interact with, they learn how to interact and how to respond to others. During this time they are flexible in their learning and can learn to accept animals of other species [1, 2]. Important differences between cats and dogs can be seen through this sensitive period. Kittens show a rise in play with other kittens which peaks around 16 weeks before declining in favor of object-directed play as the kittens get ready to hunt for themselves [3]. Puppies show conspecific play throughout

this period. Owners are often upset and embarrassed by their puppy's sexual play. "Humping" may be seen and is generally normal behavior. The puppy can be gently distracted to another, socially acceptable activity.

In the canine world, the socialization period has reached almost mythic importance. A lack of socialization is blamed for many behavior problems and is offered as an explanation for mental illness in the dog. Some puppies are subjected to extreme socialization programs to prevent undersocialization. The puppy is exposed to as many things from a checklist as possible. But overdoing the socialization may be as problematic as undersocializing.

Socialization is about learning that the world is complex but manageable. The youngster learns some general rules by which they can organize their environment (i.e., listening for certain sounds made by people helps avoid negative consequences and also helps get food treats). What has been found to be most important through this period is that the young animal is supported and reassured in its exploration by its primary caregiver. This is what helps them develop resilience and the ability to cope with adversity.

Socialization is not about experiencing everything that the dog may encounter across its whole life before it is 12 weeks old. Too much exposure may lead to a puppy that is tired and overwhelmed and unable to regulate its emotional state. The learning experience that the puppy may receive is that meeting people and being in new places is overwhelming. They may carry this over into adulthood and learn to be avoidant of new environments and new people and/or other animals.

The best advice that new puppy owners can be given is that the puppy needs reassurance and support as it explores. They should act as the puppy's secure base. It must explore at its own pace with plenty of opportunities to retreat if needed. The puppy should also be protected against people wanting to pat it when it gets tired. Puppies need to sleep to recharge and to let their brains make the changes needed for learning to occur.

Again, compared with puppies, kittens spend less time in this stage of development, completing it by week 7 [4]. Kittens have passed through the socialization period by the time they are old enough to be adopted. Breeders need to be exposing kittens to normal household activities and noises and frequently handling the kittens well before they are old enough to be adopted to maximize their opportunity to become comfortable with a varied environment.

If feral or wild kittens are found, they need to be gently exposed to people and home environments [1]. Ideally, this should be done after they have formed a secure attachment to a person or another cat. This individual then acts as the secure base from which the kittens can explore.

6.1.2.4 Juvenile Stage and Puberty

The juvenile stage is one of continued physical, mental, and emotional growth for the puppy and kitten. There is increasing independence and it can be a rough time for owners. Often their compliant baby animal seems intent on having its own way. Owners need to know that this will occur and to be prepared for this change. Having plenty of activities for the pet is very important. Toys, food-dispensing items, regular exercise, play, and manners training can all help the pet's journey through the juvenile stage to pass with only minor problems. Kittens especially become completely independent and may go missing if let outside. Encourage owners to let their kitten explore outside before they feed it so that it is motivated to come inside.

This stage finishes with the onset of puberty. During this stage, the reproductive systems of the body start to function [5]. In dogs, puberty is generally considered to occur between 6 and 12 months of age although the size of the dog affects the onset of puberty, with small breeds starting at about 6 months and giant breeds starting at 18 months [5]. Bitches are considered to have entered puberty when they show their first proestrus and male dogs are in puberty when they can be induced to ejaculate. Cats are more variable, with the age of onset of puberty in kittens being as young as 3.5 months although it is more usually at 5–9 months [4].

Puberty is an important period of brain development, with the changes eventually leading to the cautious adult brain. But throughout adolescence, regardless of species, there is an increase in risk-taking behavior, sensation seeking, and impulsive behavior [6]. In companion animals, this may result in them exploring their environments more and damaging items they may have previously ignored. They may also be more defiant and inclined to be demanding. This behavior must not be met with aggression by the owner. Dogs may be pushy at the dog park and some, if not supervised, can become obnoxious.

Generally, the best advice for clients with cats and dogs going through puberty is to set clear household rules, be supportive but not a pushover, provide opportunities for exploration, and for the pet to physically challenge themselves. Provide opportunities for exercise. Male cats can be especially frustrating at this time of their lives and need lots to do if they are confined. Be prepared for the odd tantrum and stand firm against it.

6.1.2.5 Social Maturation

This is when the baby animal becomes an adult and has adult responses to stimuli. For example, a young dog may stand up to an older dog pushing it around. It is during this stage of development that many mental illnesses first appear or a pet with a mental health problem may change strategies from hiding and running to fighting back or even being offensively aggressive as a form of defense. Multipet households may go through a period of unrest as a youngster takes an adult position in the social group. This should not be taken to mean that there is a rearranging of hierarchies but rather that the new adult animal may not respond like a youngster, which may upset some routines. Normal animals will sort this out with minimal fuss but if the problem continues or there are injuries to pets due to fighting then a mental health issue may be present in one or more pets. A behavior consultation involving all pets may be needed.

Clients should be specifically asked about problem behaviors at their pet's first adult health check and vaccination.

6.1.2.6 Geriatric

Veterinary and aging experts are divided as to when cats and dogs become old and geriatric. The exact timing may vary with species, breed, and/or size of the animal (giant breeds seem to become aged quickly compared with smaller breeds). Differences in the physiology of aged small, medium, and giant breeds has been found as they age, although all three sizes showed an age-related decline in overall metabolism [7].

As pets become elderly, there may be age-related declines in vision, hearing, sense of smell and taste, and a reduction of muscle strength and stamina. The pet may have pain related to chronic problems such as arthritis.

Owners need to be asked about how elderly pets are coping. Some owners believe that their pets are just slowing due to age, but the pet may have chronic health problems that are reducing their abilities to function fully.

Advice for owners at this stage may involve helping owners care for their elderly pets by making adjustments for mobility, reduced exercise tolerance, loss of hearing or vision, reduced appetite and also cognitive decline syndrome. Some owners may not be prepared to hear that their pet is aging and needs some adjustment to its lifestyle. All staff members should be supportive and give owners time to adjust and ask questions.

EXAMPLES

A client contacts the clinic concerned that her elderly dog is growling at her 6-month-old puppy when the older dog used to play with and tolerate the puppy's behavior. The staff member taking the call ascertains that the older dog is a healthy 10-year-old Jack Russell terrier mix and the puppy is a Labrador retriever. The staff member explains that it is likely that now that the puppy is in the juvenile stage, its play is more boisterous and it is less likely to listen to the older dog. The older dog has to be more assertive to make the puppy listen. The best approach is to monitor play and for the owner to interrupt before the puppy gets too rough. The older dog may like something to shelter under (a chair or small table) so it can play from a protected space. The owner is also asked to separate the dogs so the older dog can have a break from the puppy. The staff member also tells the owner that if these strategies do not help settle things down, she is welcome to contact the clinic to discuss the problem in greater detail. At a two-week follow-up, the client reports that the dogs are more settled now that she has implemented the suggestions.

A client brings her 18-month-old domestic shorthair cat to the clinic for his annual examination and vaccinations. She mentions when asked that the cat is waking family members early in the morning by climbing on beds, patting faces, and vocalizing. He is also jumping on window ledges, cupboards, shelves, and knocking items off them. The clinical examination shows that the cat is in very good health. The veterinarian takes a behavior history using a questionnaire and no other behavior problems are identified. A diagnosis of being a normal, young male cat is made. The veterinarian discusses the motivation for the behaviors the cat is showing and that it is normal for cats to explore their environment and to be active early in the morning. Strategies are discussed such as providing more opportunities for the cat to explore his environment through hiding food-dispensing toys for him to find during the day, the owner is encouraged to play with the cat when she comes home from work, toys can be left for the cat at night time so he has something to do in the early morning. Providing high spaces or allowing the cat to access some high areas is also encouraged. Lastly, an outside enclosure is recommended to give the cat more space to explore. A two-week follow-up is booked, at which the owner reports that the food toys have really helped, as has giving the cat access to some shelves. She is not playing with her cat when she gets home and an outdoor enclosure is not possible. The improvement is enough for the owner to be happy.

TAKE-AWAYS

- During the socialization period, puppies and kittens need to be exposed to the world while being supported, reassured, and protected. This support is what is most important in helping a young animal develop resilience.
- Kittens pass through the developmental stages at earlier ages than puppies and often spend less time in each stage. So, when adopted, kittens are in their juvenile stage and entering puberty while puppies are only about halfway through their socialization phase. Kitten socialization must start earlier than puppy socialization.
- The juvenile or adolescence stage of life is tough for everyone, including pet parents. Clients need information to let them know that increased activity, exploration, and independence are all normal. Opportunities to exercise and socialize, more activities at home and positive reinforcement training can all help owners negotiate this time.
- Social maturity is a time when some pets will show a mental illness such as an anxiety disorder. Clients need to be asked about any problem behavior at the first adult vaccination of their pet. Being proactive in asking about behavior problems helps uncover owner concerns and allows clinic staff to provide support and help.
- Older age affects individual dogs and cats differently. Some may need more help with chronic conditions and age-related declines in sensory abilities. Advice needs to be tailored to the limitations of the patient, not given as blanket advice for dogs or cats of a certain age.

MISCELLANEOUS

References

1 Casey, R.A. and Bradshaw, J.W.S. (2008). The effects of additional socialisation for kittens in a rescue centre on their behaviour and suitability as a pet. *Applied Animal Behaviour Science* 114 (1–2): 196–205.

2 Kuo, Z.Y. (1938). Further study of the behavior of the cat toward the rat. *Journal of Comparative Psychology* 25 (1): 1–8.

3 Bateson, P. and Barrett, P. (1978). The Development of Play in Cats. *Behaviour* 66 (1–2): 106.

4 Beaver, B.V. (2003). *Feline Behaviour: A Guide for Veterinarians*, 2e. St Louis, MO: Saunders.

5 Gobello, C. (2014). Prepubertal and pubertal canine reproductive studies: conflicting aspects. *Reproduction in Domestic Animals* 49: 70–73.

6 Laviola, G., Macri, S., Morley-Fletcher, S., and Adriani, W. (2003). Risk-taking behavior in adolescent mice: psychobiological determinants and early epigenetic influence. *Neuroscience & Biobehavioral Reviews* 27 (1–2): 19–31.

7 Speakman, J.R., van Acker, A., and Harper, E.J. (2003). Age-related changes in the metabolism and body composition of three dog breeds and their relationship to life expectancy. *Aging Cell* 2 (5): 265–275.

6.2

How Animals Learn

Alicea Howell, LVT, VTS (Behavior), KPA, CTP

Barks and Rec, Traverse City, MI, USA

BASICS

6.2.1 Summary

Why do animals do what they do? Answering this question is a complex topic but one deep rooted in the understanding of learning theory. It's critical that anyone interacting and training an animal of any species has a fundamental understanding of classical conditioning, operant conditioning, counterconditioning, and desensitization. Learning theory can be applied to modifying behavior in or out of the veterinary hospital.

6.2.2 Terms Defined

Classical Conditioning: Also known as pavlovian or respondent conditioning, this describes the pairing of a neutral stimulus with an unconditioned stimulus; through repeated pairing, the neutral stimulus becomes a conditioned stimulus and elicits a conditioned response.

Classical Counterconditioning (CCC): Changing the emotional or physiological response of an animal.

Conditioned Response: After classical conditioning has taken place, it is the response to a conditioned stimulus. It is also the response of an organism after learning has occurred.

Conditioned Stimulus: After classical conditioning has taken place, it is the stimulus that creates the conditioned response.

Desensitization (DS): The decrease of an emotional response to a stimulus after gradual exposure.

Learning: The process by which a behavior is acquired, omitted, or changed as a result of experience.

Negative Punishment: Subtraction of a pleasurable stimulus to decrease the likelihood of an animal performing a behavior again.

Negative Reinforcement: Subtraction of an aversive stimulus to increase the likelihood the animal will perform a behavior again.

Neutral Stimulus: Anything that has an effect on behavior before conditioning occurs.

Operant Conditioning: Also called Skinnerian conditioning or instrumental conditioning, this is a method of learning through trial and error that creates associations between behavior and consequence.

Operant Counterconditioning (OCC): Also called response substitution, this is a form of behavior modification performed by changing the animal's behavioral response from an unwanted behavior to a desired behavior in response to the same stimulus.

Positive Reinforcement: Addition of a pleasurable stimulus to increase the likelihood the animal will perform a behavior again.

Punishment: Addition of an aversive stimulus to decrease the likelihood an animal will perform a behavior again.

Unconditioned Stimulus: Anything that elicits a reaction from an animal without prior conditioning.

MAIN CONCEPTS

Learning is the process by which a behavior is acquired, omitted, or changed as a result of experience [1]. Without an understanding of learning theory, we cannot understand the reason animals perform undesired behavior or how to get them to perform a desired one. This chapter will discuss classical conditioning, operant conditioning, counterconditioning, and desensitization.

6.2.3 Classical Conditioning

Classical conditioning, also referred to as pavlovian conditioning, was discovered by Ivan Pavlov, a Russian physiologist. Classical conditioning is about associations between stimulus and emotion, physiological, or secretion response [2]. There are many examples of classical conditioning in the veterinary hospital, such as white coat syndrome. After many pairings of people wearing white being linked to painful vaccinations, blood draws, and scary procedures, the white coat all by itself elicits a fearful emotional response. Many cats run and hide when they see a carrier, dogs run from nail trimmers, and some patients gag at just the site of a syringe filled with anything.

There are three phases to classical conditioning. Before conditioning, there is a neutral stimulus (syringe) and neutral response (no interest). The second phase, called the conditioning phase, is where a repeated pairing occurs with an unconditioned stimulus (bitter medicine) and an unconditioned response (gagging). After repeated pairings of the syringe (neutral stimulus) containing the bitter medication (unconditioned stimulus) that causes the gagging (unconditioned response), the syringe becomes a conditioned stimulus causing a conditioned response (the gag reflex).

6.2.4 Operant Conditioning

Operant conditioning, also called Skinnerian conditionomg. was first described by John B. Watson and B. F. Skinner. Operant conditioning is based on cause and effect learning. Unlike classical conditioning, which is learning by association, operant conditioning is learning based on consequences. These consequences fall into four categories: positive reinforcement, negative reinforcement, positive punishment, and negative punishment [3].

Reinforcement is anything applied to or removed from the learner to increase the likelihood the behavior will happen again. Punishment is anything applied or taken from the learner to decrease the likelihood the behavior will happen again. Positive reinforcement training is adding something the learner desires to increase the likelihood the behavior will happen again. Negative reinforcement is the subtraction of something the learner does not desire to

increase the likelihood the behavior will happen again. Then there is positive punishment which is adding something the learner does not desire to decrease the likelihood the behavior will happen. Lastly, negative punishment is removal of something the learner desires to decrease the likelihood the behavior will happen again.

These are the foundations of any training program and are used in conjunction with each other. For instance, when using positive reinforcement to teach a sit, you give a treat, toy, praise, or petting to the dog once he is seated. The dog learns to sit for good things. However, whatever he was doing before, whether it was jumping or just standing, was negatively punished and was decreasing. Notice that using the positive punishment/negative reinforcement concepts relies on adding something that the animal will work for to avoid things that lead to an increase in fear, anxiety, stress, and even aggression [4].

6.2.5 Counterconditioning

6.2.5.1 Classical Counterconditioning (CCC)

Counterconditioning is the process of changing an existing classically conditioned response (emotion, reflex, secretion), and replacing it with a new response to the same stimulus [5]. By pairing a previously feared stimulus with something we know causes the desired emotional response, we can change the fear response to a happier one. Common tools used during CCC include high-value treats, toys, pleasurable forms of touching, and happy verbal praise. CCC is a useful tool in the treatment of fearful animals in and outside the veterinary hospital.

Classical counterconditioning is the change of an emotional response – it is not dependent on the animal's behavior. The goal is simply to form good associations with something that was previously feared. In the exam room, every touch can predict something wonderful like a favorite treat. When the touch predicts the treat for enough repetitions, the animal should begin to anticipate something pleasurable associated with touching. If the animal is nervous about touching, the touch should be broken down into smaller segments (desensitization), and progress should be made at the animal's comfortable pace. DS and CCC to veterinary procedures will be described in depth using numerous examples.

6.2.5.2 Operant Counterconditioning (OCC)

Operant counterconditioning is teaching the animal to perform a desired behavior in the presence of a previously important stimulus [5]. Some trainers call this differential reinforcement of an alternative behavior (DRA) or differential reinforcement of incompatible behavior (DRI), while others call it OCC or response substitution. By teaching the desired behavior, we can make it easy for an animal to cooperate with treatments. Teaching an incompatible behavior means the desired behavior could physically not be performed when the undesired behavior is being performed. An easy example of this is teaching a dog to sit for greeting. Currently, a jumping dog understands that to elicit attention from the owner, he must jump up in response to his owner's presence (stimulus). To teach him an incompatible behavior, "Sit" is usually used. You can't jump while sitting. The stimulus of a new human is operantly counterconditioned by every human waiting for the dog to naturally sit or respond to a sit cue to receive any attention from the person. After many repetitions, the new human becomes a stimulus that means sit.

A good example in the veterinary setting is teaching a dog to offer his paw for nail trims. A dog who usually pulls his paw back when we try to trim a nail can be taught to stand and offer a paw. Standing and offering a paw is incompatible with pulling the paw away. Of course, this behavior needs more than just counterconditioning; something that has a history of being bad needs desensitization at the same time.

6.2.5.3 Desensitization (DS)

Desensitization is a process where a stimulus is presented repeatedly in a controlled and gradual fashion [6]. DS is a useful behavior modification tool and is used in conjunction with counterconditioning to change an animal's emotional and behavioral responses to stimuli. Unfortunately, this tool is often misused, and the animal is rushed into steps of training it is not ready for. In systematic DS, the stimulus is separated into steps and the trainer should evaluate what aspect of the stimulus is least fearful and organize the different aspects from least to most feared by the learner. In order to set up a good DS plan, you need to start at the first stressor, which for some patients will be entering the exam room. The animal should become comfortable at one level before moving to the next.

EXAMPLES

Most dogs and cats are afraid of nail trims but it is an achievable behavior to train. The training plan would have elements of positive reinforcement (food for correct responses) and negative punishment (withholding food for

incorrect responses). The training plan would require a nonstressful starting point so as part of the DS plan, we would need to identify when the stress occurs and start there. For our example, it is the sight of the nail trimmers. The steps of the desensitization and counterconditioning plan would look something like this.

- Presence of nail trimmer = treats change emotional response (DS/CCC)
- Presence of nail trimmers in human hand = treats (DS/CCC)
- In absence of nail trimmers teach paw target to hand for a treat (DS/CCC/OCC)
- In presence of nail trimmers teach paw target to hand for a treat (DS/CCC/OCC)
- In absence of nail trimmers teach dog to accept touching on nail (DS/CCC/OCC)
- Inpresence of nail trimmers teach dog to accept touching on nail (DS/CCC/OCC)
- By inching slowly, bring nail trimmers closer to nail reinforcing each calm approximation (DS/CCC/OCC)
- Touch nail trimmer to nail (DS/CCC/OCC)
- Trimmer around one nail (DS/CCC/OCC)
- Small amount of pressure to nail with trimmer (DS/CCC/OCC)
- Successfully through all above steps with no fear and anxiety, and a willing paw target to your hand and trim one nail (DS/CCC/OCC)

Keep in mind that every step is repeated multiple times until the animal is having fun performing the behavior *before* moving to the next small step and each repetition is paired with food or something else the animal will work for.

TAKE-AWAYS

- Classical conditioning is a physiological or emotional response after repeated pairing of two stimuli.
- Positive reinforcement is the training method of choice that has fewer side effects of creating fear, anxiety, and stress.
- Positive punishment-based training can result in fear, anxiety, and aggression.
- When changing an emotional response, counterconditioning, desensitization, and positive reinforcement are all working together.
- Successful systematic desensitization occurs only when the animal's triggers are identified and the behavior is broken down into small approximations.

MISCELLANEOUS

6.2.6 Cautions

When training any animal, take necessary safety precautions. If the animal has a history of aggression or if the procedure is painful, desensitization and counterconditioning the animal to wear a cage muzzle or enter a restraint cage may be needed. Furthermore, the use of positive punishment and adverse training has been linked to an increase in aggression.

References

1 Leuscher, A. (2003). *DOGS! Course in Behavior Modification*. West Lafayette, IN: Purdue University.
2 Chance, P. (2008). *Learning and Behavior*, 6e. Boston, MA: Wadsworth Cengage/Learning.
3 Howell, A. and Feryercilde, M. (2018). *Cooperative Veterinary Care*. Ames, IA: Wiley.
4 Herron, M., Shofer, F., and Reisner, I. (2009). Survey of the use and outcome of confrontational and non-confrontational training methods in client-owned dogs showing undesired behaviors. *Applied Animal Behaviour Science* 117 (1–2): 47–54.
5 Yin, S. (2009). *Low Stress Handling, Restraint and Behavior Modification of Dogs & Cats*. Davis, CA: Cattle Dog Publishing.
6 Shaw, K. and Martin, D. (2015). *Canine and Feline Behavior for Veterinary Technicians and Nurses*. Ames, IA: Wiley.

Recommended Reading

Pryor, K. (1999). *Don't Shoot the Dog: The New Art of Teaching and Training*. New York: Bantam Books.
Ramirez, K. (1999). *Animal Training: Successful Animal Management through Positive Reinforcement*. Chicago: Shedd Aquarium Society.
Skinner, B.F. (1945). The operational analysis of psychological terms. *Psychological Review* 52 (5): 270–277.

6.3

Managing Life Changes with Pets

Jacqui Ley, BVSc (Hons), PhD, DECAWBM, FANZCVS (Veterinary Behaviour)

Melbourne Veterinary Specialist Centre, Glen Waverley, Victoria, Australia

BASICS

6.3.1 Summary

Pets are part of the lives of many people. Many families have pets so children can learn about life, empathy, and responsibility. Many young adults get a pet as part of growing up and for many young couples, a pet is a way to test out the idea of sharing the WORK and benefits of looking after someone together. For families whose children have grown up, a pet is a companion and may act as a conduit for communication with other people. Human lives may change considerably during the life of a pet but often these life changes are not managed well for pets, resulting in a break-down of the human–animal bond (HAB). Attention to how life stage changes may affect a pet means changes in management of the pet can be implemented to minimize disruption.

6.3.2 Terms Defined

Human–Animal Bond: A mutually beneficial and dynamic relationship between people and animals that is influenced by behaviors that are essential to the health and well-being of both.

MAIN CONCEPTS

Human lives can change considerably, resulting in reorganization of households, routines, and who lives where. Modern living means that people can expect to have several jobs and move home several times. They may also have more than one partner, co-parent and have blended families. All this change is hard for humans to manage and some pets may also struggle to adjust. Helping owners with advice about managing their pets may reduce stress for the owner as well as the pet.

In general, if changes to the pet's life are coming, the earlier adjustments are made the easier it is for everyone to cope. Often, pets are not given enough time to adapt and their stress adds to their owner's stress. Animals may need weeks to months to adapt to changes

6.3.3 Moving House

A frequent stress for families is moving to a new house and this is a high-risk time for pets to be lost or injured. Visiting the new property with the pet before the move helps them start to familiarize themselves with the house.

Boarding pets during the moving period keeps them in a safe place until they can be moved to the new property. This is a service veterinary clinics may be able to offer.

Alternatively, pets can be left in a familiar room and moved last of all.

Encourage the owner to set up a space for the pet in the new home that has familiar furniture, bedding, water bowls, and food and toilet facilities. Feliway®, Feliway Multi/Feliway Friend (for cats) and Adaptil® (for dogs) diffusers or sprays may help and should be on for 24 hours or sprayed around before the pet is introduced to the new home.

Pets and owners will be stressed so extra vigilance about gates, doors, and keeping pets on leashes when outside can all reduce accidents.

Similarly, updating microchipping details and tags with cell/mobile numbers can help maintain current contact information.

6.3.4 Introducing New Partners

For many pet owners, introducing a new partner to their pet can be stressful. The acceptance of both parties is important. Owners can help make the introductions and future management problem free (almost).

Introduce the new partner to the pet gradually. Owners need to discuss their pet's likes and dislikes to prevent misunderstandings and lay the groundwork for the new partner being around the pet.

The new partner should not be too familiar when introduced to the pet. Many animals are cautious about meeting new people. Cats and smaller animals may be avoidant until they are comfortable with the new partner. Let them approach in their own time and dictate the development of the pet–new partner relationship. Acceptance can be encouraged by including the new partner in activities the pet enjoys.

Pets may have changes to their sleeping arrangements. Making these changes and maintaining them when the partner is not present helps the pet to accept the new sleeping plan.

6.3.5 Melding Pet Families

Many couples have pets when they meet. Combining pet families to create one, hopefully, happy family can be stressful. Planning helps reduce stress. If one partner is moving in with their pets, the new animals are being forced to invade the territories of the incumbent animals. If both families are moving into new property, all the pets are disrupted. Regardless of the species, planning for separate housing and possibly complete separation for a while is important. Cats especially need their own areas to retire to and are best introduced by having a timesharing arrangement for the main living areas. If one cat or family of cats is out, the other family of cats is confined, and vice versa. By sharing the space at separate times, the cats become aware of each other without encountering each other and fighting. This pattern mimics how cats interact with other cats naturally. As they become comfortable, feeding and other pleasurable activities can be introduced in the area at the same time but at opposite ends of the room.

Set aside regular time with the pet(s) to maintain the bond with them. Creating a routine that provides this is essential to help pets relax and adjust to new routines.

6.3.6 Babies and Children

Pets and interactions with animals are good for the development of children but are not without risk of injury [1]. Preparation minimizes risks to the child and pet.

Make changes to household routine early in the pregnancy. If pets will be excluded from some areas or moved outside, then the sooner this happens the more likely they will accept the change by the time the baby arrives. Pet barriers are very helpful for restricting pets but allowing them to still be inside.

If a pet is used to a quiet household then introducing baby noises on a high-quality audio device may help them adjust. Play the recording when the pet is eating or playing to help them become used to it. The owner can carry a baby doll or rolled-up towel to acclimate the pet to them having something in their arms. The owner and pet can practice trained cues such as the pet going to their mat or bed while the owner carries the "baby." Pets may need to be taught to stay away when the owner is nursing. Referral to a positive reinforcement trainer to help the owner and pet learn safe skills may be needed.

6.3.6.1 Mobile Baby

Mobile babies can frighten pets. Babies are attracted to pets [2] and once crawling may focus on the pet and head toward it. From the animal's point of view, this is very aggressive behavior, and some may react by trying to escape or by being aggressive back. The pet and the baby need protection from each other. Child or toddler barriers can be installed to control where the pet goes in the home and pets can be put outside or in another room while the child is playing or on the floor. Tying the dog up is not safe as it does not prevent the child approaching the animal which is restricted in its ability to retreat.

Many owners have unrealistic expectations of their pets when around their children. The advice from everyone in the veterinary clinic should reiterate that dogs and cats have limited reasoning abilities and that they cannot understand the intentions of a baby or young child. Similarly, the babies and young children cannot understand the warning signals of a dog or a cat and so avoid injury. Adults *must* protect both child and pet through direct supervision (which may mean one adult for the baby and one for the pet) or by providing safe places for each (see 8.12 Preventing Animal-Related Injuries).

6.3.6.2 Children

Children gain a lot from interactions with pets. Helping them be safe around their pets is very important. Dog bite statistics show that the group of children most at risk for bites is 5-year-old boys [3]. This age group is also more likely to be bitten on the face due to their height.

Children must be actively supervised around the family pet. Parents and other adults can encourage and model appropriate ways to interact with pets.

Growling is the dog's early warning system; it is their way of asking for more space. A dog that growls should be acknowledged and protected with the space it needs.

Children who visit their friend's home can be hard for pets to accept. Visiting children may not realize that the way they interact with their pets at home may not be tolerated by other pets. Dog bite data shows that many children are bitten by dogs that they know but with whom they dog not necessarily live.

Most parents do not inherently have a good understanding of the factors that increase the risk of bites to children [4]. Veterinary clinics can help educate parents and children about how to interact with their pets and other animals they may encounter. Puppy and kitten classes are good places to start talking about this with parents, grandparents, and anyone with children in their lives. Veterinary staff can also advise parents and talk with children about what pets like at clinic visits. Newsletters, clinic websites, clinic blogs, clinic open days and visiting preschools, kindergartens, and schools are all other ways in which the message can be discussed and demonstrated.

6.3.7 Co-parenting

Some couples co-parent their pet after their relationship has broken down. The pet may live between two houses with different routines. Many adjust to this. Sticking to routines for feeding, exercise, and sleeping helps the pet.

Management of the pet does not have to be the same at each house but must be sensitive to the pet's needs. Cats are territorial and do not like to leave their territory so co-parenting between two properties is less likely to work.

Encourage owners to be clear as to who the clinic should address mail, email, and phone calls to for efficient care for the pet. This also applies to consent for treatment and who will be covering any bills, decisions about treatment, and end of life decisions.

6.3.8 Leaving/Death/Family Breakdown

When a family member leaves the home, it can be disrupting for pets, especially if they were close to the individual. Their distress can be upsetting for the owner and remind them of the loss of that person. Clinic staff can help owners by being supportive. Simple advice can be that the owner reassures the pet while also instituting changes in the routine that may help the animal adjust to the new household organization. Walking at different times and engaging in play may all help. Leaving a blanket, chair or cushion with the missing person's scent for the pet to sit on may also help them adjust to the person being gone.

From a psychological view, it is not clear if animals grieve but they can show loss of energy, no interest in play or other activities, and loss of appetite. This can be a normal response to a loss and should pass in a few weeks. If it continues for more than a few weeks, depression must be considered. The pet may need treatment for this and may need referral to a behavior specialist.

EXAMPLES

Scout is a 7-year-old, neutered male Australian cattle dog. He was brought into the clinic as he had bitten a visiting 6-year-old boy on the leg. The child had required stitches. Scout's owners were very upset and were considering euthanizing Scout. His owner reported that he had never bitten before and was gentle and well behaved in lots of situations. Their son and the visiting boy had been playing a rowdy game of basketball and their son had fallen, and the other boy had fallen on top of him. Scout had rushed in and bitten the visiting boy, tearing his pants and bruising his leg.

The veterinarian explained that Scout was probably excited by the boys' rowdy game and had been upset by the boys falling over. Scout had inhibited his bite as evidenced by the lack of serious injury to the boy. Managing the situation in the future so that Scout was separated while the children played would prevent this from happening again. The owner took Scout home to think about this information. The clinic followed up a week or so later and the owner told them that they had installed a gate on their verandah that allowed them to keep Scout locked in when the children were playing basketball. The owner was very grateful for the advice.

Bosley's male owner had died after a long illness and after a month, Bosley, a 5-year-old male domestic longhair cat, was quiet, not playing with his toy mouse and hiding away. Bosley's female owner was worried about him. His veterinarian examined Bosley and found him to be in good health. She discussed how Bosley's owner could support Bosley and encourage him to move around and play by introducing some new food-dispensing toys, changing his feeding routine and also playing with him like his male owner had played. Bosley's owner changed the routine a little at home but left a blanket her husband had used on his favorite chair for Bosley to use. She reported that Bosley spent time sitting there but was starting to move around and investigate his new feeding toys and was starting to engage in some play with her.

TAKE-AWAYS

- Life changes for people and for pets. Preparing pets for changes as early as possible helps them adjust before the stress of the actual change.
- When changes happen, give the pet(s) time to adjust – this may take many weeks longer than owners think.
- Children and dogs need supervision and more supervision and even more supervision by adults.
- Pets need their own space in the house where they can retire for rest. Their need to rest or take time out *must* be respected.

MISCELLANEOUS

6.3.9 Cautions

Veterinarians must document advice given to owners of dogs that bite or show aggressive behavior. The advice must emphasize the risk and the duty of care of the owner to control the dog at home and in public. Referral to a behavior specialist is highly recommended.

Owners may be very distressed after the loss of a family member. If an owner is upset and reaching out to clinic staff, the owner may need gentle referral to a grief and loss counselor for help.

References

1 Esposito, L., Mccune, S., Griffin, J., and Maholmes, V. (2011). Directions in human–animal interaction research: child development, health, and therapeutic interventions. *Child Development Perspectives* 5 (3): 205–211.

2 Kidd, A.H. and Kidd, R.M. (1987). Reactions of infants and toddlers to live and toy animals. *Psychological Reports* 61: 455–464.

3 Ozanne-Smith, J., Ashby, K., and Stathakis, V.Z. (2001). Dog bite and injury prevention – analysis, critical review, and research agenda. *Injury Prevention* 7 (4): 321–326.

4 Reisner, I.R. and Shofer, F.S. (2008). Effects of gender and parental status on knowledge and attitudes of dog owners regarding dog aggression toward children. *Journal of the American Veterinary Medical Association* 233 (9): 1412–1419.

Recommended Reading

Kirkham, L. (2012). *Tell Your Dog You're Pregnant*. London: Little Creatures Publishing.

Pellar, C. (2013). *Living with Kids and Dogs … Without Losing Your Mind: A Parent's Guide to Controlling the Chaos*, vol. 2. Woodbridge, VA: Dream Dog Productions.

6.4

Creating a Pet-Specific User's Manual

Peter Weinstein, DVM, MBA

PAW Consulting, Irvine, CA, USA

 ## BASICS

6.4.1 Summary

When someone purchases a new car, they expect to receive an owner's manual and have directions for all the maintenance the vehicle is anticipated to need over time. Pets certainly are not cars, but like cars, there is a routine maintenance schedule that pets can benefit from to increase their longevity and prevent problems from occurring. And, unlike cars, you can take a pet home with little to no experience in raising or housing or feeding or maintaining or caring for a pet and most significantly, there is no agreed-upon "maintenance" schedule for pets found in the world of the internet.

It is the role of the veterinary practice to be the expert on the maintenance of the pet from womb to tomb. Thus, it behooves veterinary practices to have consistent and mandated standards of care for wellness that outline, initially, a puppy/kitten wellness program, and then a year-by-year maintenance schedule that not only includes wellness needs but other pet-specific or age-related diagnostic and preventive care. For a pet owner to know when their pet's "tune-up" is needed is a first step to transparent and compliant care.

 ## MAIN CONCEPTS

6.4.2 What is a User's Manual for Pets?

Since some pet owners may never have had a pet before, they could have little if any knowledge or understanding of what it entails to be a responsible and caring pet owner. It is more than just the food and exercise and love that is routinely provided with minimal knowledge or understanding. Both your practice and your clients will benefit from a step-by-step guide and support information that has been written and approved by your team (see 1.3 Personalized Care Plans). A user's manual (also known as a personalized care plan) can be more than just a schedule. It can answer all of the more frequently asked questions about puppy care and kitten care and outline the needed wellcare parameters required by your community and your practice. But a user's manual doesn't stop there – it clearly outlines pet care through the pet's entire life up to the end of life discussion (Table 6.4.1). This is a road map to keeping a pet happy, healthy, protected and cared for from birth until the rainbow bridge is reached.

A user's manual must be easy to read and broken up into sections that reflect the growth and development of the pet similar to your automobile's care reflecting mileage.

Table 6.4.1 Example of a grid for ABC Animal Hospital, whose standard of care includes annual visits for wellness care

	6–9 weeks	9–12 weeks	12–16 weeks	>16 weeks	6 months	1 year	2 years	3 years	4 years	5 years	6 years	7 years	8 years	9 years	10 years	11 years	12 years	13 years
Physical exam	X	X	X	X		X	X	X	XX	XX	XX	XX	XXX	XXX	XXX	XXXX	XXXX	XXXX
DHPP	X	X	X	X		X			X			X			X			X
Rabies				X		X			X			X			X			X
Bordetella	X	X	X	X		X	X	X	X	X	X	X	X	X	X	X	X	X
Leptospirosis		R	R	R		R	R	R	R	R	R	R	R	R	R	R	R	R
Lyme		R	R	R		R	R	R	R	R	R	R	R	R	R	R	R	R
Intestinal parasite exam	X	X	X	X		X	X	X	X	X	X	X	X	X	X	X	X	X
Oral deworming	X	X	X	X														
Heartworm testing[a]						X	X	X	X	X	X	X	X	X	X	X	X	X
Heartworm preventive[b]	X	X	X	X		X	X	X	X	X	X	X	X	X	X	X	X	X
Flea/tick preventive[c]	X	X	X	X	X	X	X	X	X	X	X	X	X	X	X	X	X	X
Spay/neuter[d]					X or	X												
Microchip					X													
Wellness panel[e]					X	X	X	X	X	X	X	X	X	X	X	X	X	X
Breed-specific discussion[f]					X	X	X	X	X	X	X	X	X	X	X	X	X	X
Breed-specific testing[g]					X	X	X	X	X	X	X	X	X	X	X	X	X	X

X = Frequency per year.

R = Regionally specific.

[a] Heartworm testing, based upon American Heartworm Society Guidelines.

[b] Heartworm preventive, based upon American Heartworm Society Guidelines and regional risk assessment.

[c] Flea/tick preventive, based upon regional risk assessment.

[d] Spay/neuter – based upon discussion with the veterinarian and breed and size, the most appropriate time for surgery will be determined.

[e] Wellness panel – based upon age, history, and risk factors, more or less testing may be recommended.

[f] Breed-specific discussion – age- and breed-related conditions will be discussed.

[g] Breed-specific testing – based upon age and breed, specific diagnostic tests will be recommended.

Additionally, the manual should have sections for the more common nonveterinary pet care needs where questions might arise – nutrition, grooming, behavior, insurance, etc. Any services that your practice offers should be highlighted. And any services that your practice does not provide should include recommended sources for that service (think referral marketing here).

6.4.3 Getting Started

Before you can create a user's manual, you must get 100% agreement and commitment from the veterinary staff and hospital team as to the standards of care you have for wellness from puppyhood through development, middle age, and eventually geriatrics.

Think about what you want to have as a protocol for:

- full examination
- vaccinations – include both core and regionally specific risks
- intestinal parasite examination
- deworming
- heartworm preventive
- flea/tick control
- neutering/desexing procedures
- microchips
- laboratory testing
- other basic wellcare parameters that you believe in
- regionally specific risk factors, such as heartworm, Lyme, leptospirosis, etc.

Starting at 1 year of age, what do you expect wellness to look like annually? With these protocols in mind, what are your expectations for compliance on an annual basis? With the wellness parameters annualized, integrate breed-specific discussions, testing, and monitoring into an annual grid.

And finally, consider other preventive testing, procedures, etc. that you believe should be included.

Remember, all doctors and staff should have acceptance of the year-by-year patient needs. And with this user's manual, you have now created a perfect staff training and discussion tool as well as a consistent, predictable, and reliable series of standards.

6.4.4 Putting Together the User's Manual

With the foundation built, you can create your user's manual.

1) Create a cover with the pet's picture taken at their most recent visit and entitled: [PET'S NAME] MANUAL FOR CURRENT AND FUTURE HEALTHCARE.

2) Create a grid reflecting puppy or kitten minimum wellness standards of care that take the pet through its spay/neuter surgery to include vaccinations, deworming, flea/tick control, heartworm, and other needs specific to your community. Don't forget to include breed-specific needs as well.

3) Create a grid with a year-by-year set of minimum wellness and preventive standards and breed-specific needs for care for pets from post desexing surgery until a year deemed geriatric (based upon size and breed in many cases).

4) Create a grid with year-by-year set of minimum wellness and preventive standards and breed-specific needs for care for geriatric pets.

5) For each line item or need identified in the grid, there needs to be concomitant discussion on what the item is and why it is needed. This can be included in each section after the grid and is a perfect way to give your clients homework after their visit. For example: DHPP is a vaccination to prevent four diseases: distemper, hepatitis, parainfluenza, and parvovirus. In puppies, it is given every 3–4 weeks until they are 16 weeks of age or older to ensure that their immune system has been provided with sufficient time to mature and develop the ability to protect the puppy.

6) Put this all together in a notebook or disk or online resource customized for the pet and pet owner and linked to reminders and recalls with associated checklists to measure compliance.

7) Present this on day one of your relationship as the pet's user's manual

You have now given your clients a huge bonus for their first visit and something for them to talk about with their friends and family. And you have told them exactly what to expect for every basic wellness or preventive visit for the rest of their pet's life. Barring any unforeseen emergencies or breed-specific problems (and you've told them about those as well), they have a road map to keep their pet happy and healthy for a long time.

6.4.4.1 Frequently Asked Questions

It has been asked, do you give this all at once or should you provide different sections with each regular visit? Clients rarely remember to bring their user's manual with them and most pets don't have a filing system for pet documents. It is suggested to give them the entire manual at once and provide any updates on a visit or via email so as to keep the list of resources or updated information fresh and to keep you front of mind with your clients.

Estimates for costs can be included but must include a statement that these costs are current as of the date of printing and are subject to change to reflect the costs of delivering care, or something similar.

Consider rewards for completing the checklist for care.

6.4.4.2 Oh My Gosh

This seems daunting in its scope but you are already doing something like this, you just haven't documented it. Recognize that clients only absorb about 20% of what is told to them in the exam room and even less if they are stressed. Additionally, people learn and absorb differently – by combining auditory training (exam room conversation), visual training (exam room demonstrations; reading) and kinesthetic training (things to do at home), you can amplify your effectiveness in client compliance and patient care.

For overachievers, you can create video content to support much of the above. And although not as readily customizable, it may appeal to a whole new generation of pet owners.

Recognize that 80% of the manual is redundant from pet to pet within a species. The customization comes with pet-specific details and age-related details (which fit with breed specifics). With the completion of a generic template for cats, small dog breeds, medium dog breeds, large dog breeds, and giant dog breeds, you are 80% complete. The real benefit of computers is the ability to integrate the pet's name, breed, and breed-specific information very easily (see 10.7 Breed-Specific Marketing).

6.4.5 Real Benefit

This manual could be a great marketing tool as well. Expect clients to be overjoyed to have all of the answers for their pet's care in one resource. Imagine the dog park, pet store, social media conversation, etc. that clients will drive with this amazing added value.

Compliance is an area of great frustration in practice (see 9.17 Improving Compliance and Adherence with Pet-Specific Care). In many cases, compliance comes up short because of the lack of transparency and the ultimate surprise that occurs from visit to visit. The manual defines upfront the standards of care that the practice expects and delivers upon. There should be no surprises from visit to visit if the practice uses the user's manual to provide clear expectation.

Before each visit, you can let your clients know to review their user's manual. Additionally, you can forward book future visits based upon the checklists for future needs. Send the checklists and expectations to the client as a reminder a week or two before the visit. Explain what to expect. Tell them to be ready with questions they may have. Set expectations ahead of time and compliance is more likely to be adhered to.

A great benefit of the manual is that it allows you to set the standard of care that your practice wants to offer (see 9.4 Standards of Care). Way too often, we try to accommodate to the needs of all pet owners in a community. It is very challenging and extremely frustrating, especially with healthy animals, to go from exam room to exam room negotiating care. Your manual can be used to define which clients your practice wants to see and lets clients know ahead of time what their expectations are.

And the other major benefit is consistency (see 9.8 Ensuring Consistency of Care). In a multidoctor practice, there is no room for different doctors to have different wellness plans and standards of care. This creates chaos and confusion for the doctors, staff, and clients. By creating different standards, you allow clients to choose the standard that they want rather than the optimal standard for the pet. By creating consistent standards, you make it much easier for the client service team, technician team, and exam room team to communicate a uniform message to clients. Consistency sends a strong message to clients. And if clients receive a consistent and transparent message, the level of trust that they have in the practice will grow. And trust is what can make you stand out to the clients and subsequently the community.

EXAMPLES

The samples below may or may not reflect your standards of care. They are strictly provided as an example for you to think about when creating your own templates.

Table of Contents

6.4.5.1 Puppy to Nine Months User's Manual Action Items

We expect three or four wellness visits up to and including the spay or neuter procedure.

At each visit you can expect:

	6–9 weeks	9–12 weeks	12–16 weeks	>16 weeks	16–36 weeks
Doctor's exam	X	X	X	X	X
DHPP	X	X	X	X	
Bordetella	X	X	X	X	
Rabies				X	
Deworming	X	X	X	X	
Heartworm preventive	X	X	X	X	
Fecal examination	X		X		
Genetic screening			X		
Microchip					X
Spay/neuter					X
Breed specific-orthopedic screening					X

One to seven years user's manual action items for a golden retriever, ncluding wellness, behavioral, preventive care and breed-specific needs

	1–2 years	2–3 years	3–4 years	4–5 years	5–6 years	6–7 years
DVM examinations	XX	XX	XX	XX	XX	XX
DHPP	X			X		
Bordetella	X	X	X	X	X	X
Rabies	X			X		
Heartworm test	X	X	X	X	X	X
Heartworm preventive	X	X	X	X	X	X
Flea and tick preventive	X	X	X	X	X	X
Intestinal parasite examination	X	X	X	X	X	X
Screening lab test – blood	X	X	X	X	X	X
Screening lab test – urine	X	X	X	X	X	X
Breed-specific screening	Hip and elbow radiographs				Add thyroid	Add thyroid

NOTE: Each X = frequency.

Seven years and above user's manual action items for a golden retriever, including wellness, behavioral, preventive care and breed-specific needs

	7–8 years	8–9 years	9–10 years	10–11 years	11–12 years	12–13 years
DVM examinations	XXX	XXX	XXX	XXX	XXX	XXX
DHPP	X			X		
Bordetella	X	X	X	X	X	X
Rabies	X			X		
Heartworm test	X	X	X	X	X	X
Heartworm preventive	X	X	X	X	X	X
Flea and tick preventive	X	X	X	X	X	X
Intestinal parasite examination	X	X	X	X	X	X
Screening lab test – blood	X	X	X	X	X	X
Screening lab test – urine	X	X	X	X	X	X
Breed-specific screening	Add thyroid	Add thyroid	Add thyroid	Add thyroid	Add thyroid	Add thyroid

Note: Each X = frequency.

6.4.5.2 Sample Information Sheet

5.8 Your pet's medical needs as a seven year old.

Goldie is now 7 years old. That is almost 50 years old in people years!!

As Goldie progresses into "middle age" we want to maintain the same wellness parameters that we have done in the past but also increase our levels of surveillance for age-related changes as well as some of the specific breed-related changes.

From a breed-specific standpoint, here are our concerns during her seventh year.

- Hypothyroidism
- Progressive retinal atrophy
- Cataracts
- Cancer
- Arthritis

There are other conditions that middle-aged golden retrievers may present with and we will discuss those if there is evidence of those conditions based upon our discussions with you and our physical examination findings.

Here is our checklist for Goldie's veterinary care during her seventh year.

- Wellness Visit
  - Full examination
  - Update all relevant vaccinations
  - Check for intestinal parasites (stool sample)
  - Check for heartworm disease (blood test)
  - Refill heartworm preventive
  - Refill flea and tick preventive
- Senior and Breed-Specific Visit
  - Full examination
  - Full blood chemistry and complete blood count (blood sample)
  - Full urinalysis (urine sample)
  - Discussion on breed specific risks for Goldie
    - Hypothyroidism
    - Progressive retinal atrophy
    - Arthritis
    - Cataracts
    - Cancer
  - Testing for breed-specific risks for Goldie
    - Thyroid level (blood test)
    - Thorough eye exam and vision testing (cataracts and progressive retinal atrophy)
    - Thorough joint manipulation for pain (arthritis)
    - Radiographs of joints (x-rays) (arthritis)
    - Thorough palpation of lymph nodes and abdomen (cancer)
    - Radiographs of chest and/or abdomen for cancer
    - Ultrasound of abdomen for cancer
- Discussions:
  - Nutrition
  - Exercise
  - What to look for over the next year
  - What to expect at the next visit

For additional information about today's visit, please review the relevant chapters in the user manual including but not limited to:

- Chapter 1 Goldie is a Golden Retriever (for breed-specific information)
- Chapter 2 Nutrition (for age-related dietary modifications)
- Chapter 5 Teenage to Middle Age (for exercise and other aging related information)

Should you have any questions, before or after your visit, our email hotline for clients is breedspecific@ouranimalhospital.com

TAKE-AWAYS

To enhance compliance, be transparent and explain wellness and responsible pet ownership needs on day one of your relationship with the pet.

- Consistent standards, adhered to by all doctors, are essential to client and pet compliance and enhance staff understanding of patient care.
- Pet owners want to know what to expect from visit to visit and a user's manual not only delineates this but can help owners to predict and budget for future costs.
- By including wellness, preventive, behavior and breed-specific discussions in one manual, a pet owner has resources created by a veterinarian and specific to their practice and can mitigate the need to go to Dr Google for information.
- A customized user's manual indicates to the client that their pet is not just a number but a member of your practice's family.

MISCELLANEOUS

Recommended Reading

AAFP vaccination. https://catvets.com/guidelines/practice-guidelines/feline-vaccination-guidelines

AAHA vaccination. www.aaha.org/guidelines/canine_vaccination_guidelines.aspx

AAHA dental guidelines. www.aaha.org/guidelines/dental_guidelines/default.aspx

American Heartworm Society. www.heartwormsociety.org/veterinary-resources/american-heartworm-society-guidelines

Canine life stage guidelines. www.aaha.org/public_documents/professional/guidelines/canine_life_stage_guidelines.pdf

End of life guidelines. www.aaha.org/professional/resources/end_of_life_care_guidelines.aspx

Feline Life stage guidelines. www.aaha.org/professional/resources/feline_life_stage.aspx

www.partnersforhealthypets.org

Preventive healthcare guidelines. www.aaha.org/public_documents/professional/guidelines/aaha-avma_preventivehealthcareguidelines.pdf

6.5

Opportunities and Challenges of Providing Services for Low-Income Clients

David Haworth, DVM, PhD

Vidium Animal Health, Phoenix, AZ, USA

BASICS

6.5.1 Summary

Veterinary healthcare is not free but pets are considered family members or companions by most owners, consistently across all income levels, and not every family can afford care. All owners want to be responsible pet parents, but in too many cases cannot find care options with what they are able to spend, but they want to spend something. This discrepancy between what is offered and what can be paid creates a potentially very large unsatisfied market for providing some kind of care for low-income owners.

Providing care options across the cost spectrum, recognizing that responsible care (on the part of the owner and veterinary team) is not defined by what can be afforded, and acknowledging as a reality that some treatable diseases must go untreated are keys to providing care for pets in low-income communities.

6.5.2 Terms Defined

Incremental Care: A philosophy of providing medical options along the cost spectrum for owners, as opposed to only offering the very best (and usually most expensive) option.

Low-Income: Typically living at between 100% and 200% of the federal poverty threshold.

Poverty: Living with an income below an amount determined to provide a basic standard of living.

Standard of Care: An agreed-upon minimum care protocol for a given medical condition. This protocol may or may not take cost of care into consideration.

Subsidized Care: Programs in which all or part of the cost of veterinary care is paid by an entity other than the pet's owner.

MAIN CONCEPTS

A significant proportion of the population live at or below the poverty threshold during any given year. Many times, that number is categorized as "low-income" and the majority of the population has lived in poverty for at least one year of their lives. Pet ownership rates are consistent across all income levels and, thanks in part to the relatively long lives of our pets, this means that there is a very high likelihood that pets will be a bonded part of families experiencing a temporary or permanent state of low-income or poverty. For a large percentage of those bonded families, veterinary care is unavailable or not affordable (see 2.10 Affordability of Veterinary Services). This is due to several contributing factors, but regardless of the reasons, it represents a very large potential market for veterinary services.

Since the early 1970s, veterinary practices have focused, rightly, on maximizing revenues and demonstrating high value to the pet owner. Like all small businesses, location is a key component in client selection and therefore the logical location of any new veterinary practice has been in the highest income community available. While reasonable, this has resulted in large "veterinary care deserts," where populations do not have access to veterinary clinics within a reasonable distance. This effect is compounded by the fact that most public transport systems do not allow non-service animals to use their services. Even those families that are highly motivated to seek care may be logistically prevented from accessing it.

In addition, veterinary medical education has focused increasingly on specialized care, deemphasizing routine or wellness care in favor of advanced diagnostics and procedures that are unaffordable for many pet owners. As a result, veterinarians, especially recent graduates, often only consider "gold standard" options to diagnose or treat a condition, offering other options only if forced to by the client. All too often, this results in an unsatisfactory outcome for the client (who feels guilty they cannot afford to follow the veterinary team's recommendations), the veterinary team (who know there were "better" options that the client couldn't or wouldn't afford), and the pets themselves.

An alternative, termed "incremental care" (see 2.2 The Role of Incremental Care), involves a philosophy of offering – without judgment – options of care along the cost spectrum. Incremental care, as opposed to gold standard therapy, can be offered in individual appointments within any practice, or can be the basis for new business models (see 10.14 Providing Cost-Effective Care for Those in Need). Practices that serve low-income communities can be financially successful by offering every client treatment options priced with appropriate margins, but with at least some at more affordable prices. While this sometimes sacrifices higher success rates, newer, more effective drugs and more sophisticated diagnostics, some care is unquestionably better for pets than no care (see 7.8 Providing Care for Those Unable or Unwilling to Pay). Because many diseases and conditions cannot be treated incrementally – there are simply no low-cost options – humane euthanasia must always be considered and offered nonjudgmentally in those cases where no other affordable option exists.

In order to seize the opportunity available in low-income communities, several other considerations should be taken into account beyond the philosophy of incremental care. Among these are menu-driven services, transparency in pricing, clear communication, and strict cost containment. Menu-driven services simply means that clinics cannot offer everything to everyone and remain efficient. Low-income communities routinely deal with service providers that offer limited services and veterinary care does not need to be any different. Vaccinations, parasite control, limited wound or infection care and quasi-grooming procedures (anal sac expression, nail trimming, etc.) are not only important parts of pet care but can be done efficiently and for low cost. Complicated medical or surgical work-ups might not be possible. Clear communication of costs is critical, likely through a combination of posted prices for common procedures and stated or written estimates during the decision-making process. Clients without a lot of money are still willing to spend money on their pets, but

this amount may need to be strictly constrained, and it is likely that any surprise expenses will be refused. Additionally, if an owner is made to feel they are anything less than a good pet parent because they cannot afford more expensive care, there is a high likelihood that they will not seek out care the next time, which would be catastrophic for the pet as well as representing lost revenues to the profession.

Clearly, cost containment is critical to success when providing veterinary services to low-income families in order to maximize the potential for acceptance of recommendations and to create a viable business. Since the two largest costs in most practices are payroll and overheads, minimizing location costs not only makes a significant impact but also allows payroll costs to be optimized, since offering services to low-income communities should not include a vow of poverty on the part of veterinary teams. One less expensive option is a mobile clinic that allows for scheduled rotations along an established route of parking lots and corners. Importantly, this is not a mobile clinic that travels to patients by appointment, but instead locates in communities and lets clients come to them. Another option to explore is free or subsidized real estate from a municipality or community members. Storefront offices, even if only occupied on a periodic (but consistent) schedule, are frequently donated by cities or real estate developers trying to attract other businesses into an area.

Lastly, there is a large and growing set of grants available from philanthropic organizations that subsidize pet care costs for low-income families. Each granting program is unique but in general program goals should be clearly defined, the community problem that is being addressed articulated, and contingency plans described in case assumptions are not met. Often grantors require that the recipient is designated a not-for-profit organization, but clinics can either qualify for this status themselves or they can partner with an established nonprofit which would receive the grant and contract with the clinic to provide services. In cases of extreme poverty, for instance those families that are experiencing homelessness, subsidized care may be the only option available.

Veterinary care is an essential part of pet ownership but all too many communities do not have access to that care because of geographic, financial, or other logistic barriers. Not only does this mean that a large number of pets routinely go without healthcare, it also means that there is a significant market need that goes unmet. Billions of dollars are not coming into veterinary practices because this segment is being largely ignored. There are, however, viable practice models that will allow the need to be met and the practices to thrive.

TAKE-AWAYS

- The bond between a family and their pet is not defined by their income level, with consistently strong feelings across all income levels.
- In some ways, the positive benefits of a pet may be more extreme in low-income families than those with higher income.
- Low-income families want to be responsible pet owners, and understand they need to provide veterinary care for their pets.
- In order to provide that care, service providers must be willing to engage in compassionate communication, offer options across the cost spectrum (i.e., incremental care), and accept that some "treatable" conditions will have to remain untreated.
- There is a very large unmet need and therefore significant opportunities for veterinary clinics in servicing low-income communities.

MISCELLANEOUS

6.5.3 Cautions

Veterinary licensing boards are struggling with the concepts of "standards of care" and incremental care. Familiarize yourself with the current understandings in your jurisdiction before offering clients options that may be considered below standard.

Recommended Reading

Blackwell, M.J. Access to veterinary care, barriers, current practices, and public policy. *Access to Veterinary Care Coalition* https://avcc.utk.edu/avcc-report.pdf.

6.6

Fear Free® Concepts

Marty Becker, DVM

Fear Free, LLC, Denver, CO, USA

 BASICS

A major barrier to pets receiving veterinary care is the fear, anxiety, and stress (FAS) they suffer when visiting the veterinary hospital. From being placed in a carrier, to the car ride, to the smells and sounds outside the clinic, to the waiting room, to the exam room, and then back home again, the entire experience ranges from bewildering to outright terrifying for many pets. This in turn makes the client reluctant to bring their pet in for anything but the most serious of illnesses or injuries. It also creates stress in the veterinary team members who, having entered the profession because of a love of animals, find themselves feared. To keep pets in our practices in an era of competition from internet sites and pet store pseudo-experts, decreasing FAS for pets, pet owners, and the practice team is both the right thing and the smart thing to do.

6.6.1 Terms Defined

Anxiety: A diffuse generalized feeling of apprehension, unease, and/or nervousness regarding an imminent event, uncertain outcome, or danger.

Classical Counterconditioning: Changing a patient's conditioned emotional response (CER) to a perceived stimulus from an unpleasant emotion to a pleasant emotion.

Conditioning: A reaction to an event modified by learning or experience.

Considerate Approach: A specific form of interaction between the veterinary team and the patient designed to minimize the negative emotional responses that may arise during patient care.

Distraction Techniques: Utilizing things the individual pet finds desirable, such as treats, brushing, toys, petting, etc. to focus their attention away from a perceived negative experience and alleviate FAS.

Fear: An aversive emotional state involving physical and psychological responses to a stimulus that is perceived as a threat or danger.

Gentle Control: Handling method that allows the veterinary team to comfortably and safely position patients for veterinary care without causing FAS.

Stress: Physiological changes experienced when the animal's emotional state is disrupted by an aversive trigger or event. The response exists along a spectrum from mild to extreme stress, which is called distress.

Tonic Immobility: A state of motionlessness caused by fear or a sense of being overwhelmed with stimulus to the point of freezing.

Touch Gradient: Initiating and maintaining continual physical contact and gradually increasing intensity when administering treatments that involve contact with the body such as injections, nail trimming, and others.

Victory Visits: A veterinary hospital visit designed to reinforce the idea that the veterinary clinic is somewhere good things happen rather than one where treatments or procedures are performed.

 MAIN CONCEPTS

When trying to understand why a pet's emotional experience at the veterinarian is such a barrier to veterinary care, consider these statistics from the Bayer Veterinary Usage Study [1].

Pet-Specific Care for the Veterinary Team, First Edition. Edited by Lowell Ackerman.
© 2021 John Wiley & Sons, Inc. Published 2021 by John Wiley & Sons, Inc.

- Fifty-eight percent of cat owners and 38% of dog owners report their pet hates going to the vet.
- Thirty-eight percent of cat owners and 26% of dog owners say just the thought of taking their pet to the vet stresses them out.
- Twenty-eight percent of cat owners and 22% of dog owners say they'd go to the vet more often if it wasn't so stressful for them or their pet.
- Twenty-six percent of cat owners and 19% of dog owners say they'd go to the vet more often if their pet didn't dislike it so much.

It might help to think of a pet as a 1-year-old child who doesn't know why a procedure benefits him or her, and can't anticipate the relief of pain even if it's moments away. Pet owners, seeing the obvious stress in their pets during veterinary visits, feel like they are hurting their pets by trying to help them.

Who wants to intentionally hurt someone you love, especially a dependent being like a beloved family pet? That's one of the major reasons an increasing number of pet owners have relied on the internet for a diagnosis and treatment plan, have sought a treatment for many common medical problems such as allergies, periodontal disease, or anal sac impaction from a Facebook group or pet store employee. Pet parents think visiting the veterinarian for preventive care or treatment simply isn't worth the hurt to the pet or the hassle for them. It's all too easy for them to believe the hype and try a new food or the supplement of the moment.

The harm this causes to the veterinary professional is certainly felt in the pocketbook, but that's not the real bottom line. We entered the veterinary profession to help animals. We have a high degree of empathy for our patients, and want only to keep them healthy and well. Instead, we spend our days restraining pets while they are dragged resisting from their carriers, held down to get blood drawn, or wrestled onto the procedure table. We all have patients who come happily to us, but we have also stopped thinking it's unusual how many of them hide from us.

For years, board-certified veterinary behaviorists have been preaching to the profession about the need to look not only at the physical well-being of pets but at their emotional well-being as well. Most veterinary healthcare professionals routinely saw the signs of FAS, but thought of it as collateral damage of practice. The best response, we reasoned, was to just "get 'er done" and let the pet go home.

But what is the cost of all this on *our* stress levels? How hard is it for us to work in that environment, day in and day out? How does this impact high levels of burnout, and an increased risk of depression and suicide, in our profession?

Fear Free is based on the belief that veterinary practice can be a positive experience for the patient, the client, and the veterinary team if attention is paid to the FAS of the pets in our care (see 6.8 Managing Routine Procedures to Minimize Problems). The training and certification courses were developed by veterinary behaviorists to demonstrate how to remove or reduce our patients' FAS triggers or treat them if they arise.

6.6.2 Getting Started with Fear Free Visits

The good news is that embracing Fear Free doesn't require major remodeling of our hospitals. All we have to remodel are our own habitual behaviors, including increasing awareness of the signs and consequences of FAS. Nor does adopting this way of practice take too much time. In fact, the average Fear Free exam only takes 29 seconds longer to perform than a non-Fear Free exam, and it's estimated the hard costs of a Fear Free visit are 50 cents to $1.00 per visit, mostly for pheromones, treats, and nutraceuticals.

It's relatively easy to get started with providing Fear Free veterinary visits. The first and most important step is to learn to recognize the signs of FAS, and to take them seriously. Those include biting, clawing, yawning, lip licking, salivating, shivering, panting, hiding, fidgeting, freezing, and escape attempts. A dog who appears to be "napping" on the exam room floor may really be in a state of tonic immobility, as can the cat who appears to be "sleeping" in the hospital cage. These high-stress states look restful, but are very difficult for the patient to experience and can interfere with both accurate diagnostic test results and healing.

6.6.3 The Pet's Perspective

Walk through your practice. Look at it through a pet's eyes, maybe a particularly difficult patient of yours. Sit in your practice's reception/waiting area, and ask if it's reasonable to expect different species, strange pets, and unfamiliar people to be happy and calm together, especially when many of the pets are in pain, most are in distress, and almost all can't wait to leave the premises.

Ask yourself what you can do to reduce the FAS triggered by the waiting area. While some modifications can be made to improve them, such as separating cats and dogs, many progressive practices instead usher client and patient immediately into exam rooms for check-in or have clients leave their pets in their vehicles, come inside to check in, and then go back outside to wait with their pets until it's their turn to be seen.

Now, take a deep breath. What do you smell? Our patients have senses of olfaction that far outstrip ours, so the mingled aroma of feces, anal sac secretions, urine, and bleach or other harsh chemicals is even more overpowering to them than to us. In fact, those strong smells can be aversive and may cause a temporary loss of the sense of smell that can be as disorienting to a pet as a loss of sight or hearing.

Pets will also be affected by something we can't smell: pheromones. Pheromones are chemicals emitted by an animal which are detected by animals of the *same* species. These chemical signals of emotion can be positive to a nursing kitten blissfully at her mother's nipple, but fear and stress also leave their chemical signature in the environment and our patients can detect them. They're like a big neon sign saying, "Danger within!"

Fortunately, there are powerful yet sensory-friendly cleaners available, such as those utilizing accelerated hydrogen peroxide. Feces can be picked up immediately and disposed of in airtight containers; same for anal sac secretions. Vertical surfaces both inside and outside the practice can be cleaned several times per day and then spritzed with positive cat or dog pheromones. Common items used in examinations such as stethoscopes, otoscopes including the battery pack, muzzles, and nail trimmers can be cleaned with accelerated hydrogen peroxide cleaners and then wiped over with pheromone wipes.

6.6.4 Fear Free Takes a Team

Now that you've taken a pet's eye-nose-and-ear view of your practice, move on to the front desk. Watch your customer representative check in a few clients. What's the experience like? Is it calm? Does the staff member interact with the pet? Is there an opportunity for the pet's FAS to be noticed and dealt with? Are treats available and offered? Is the pet owner asked about the pet's FAS, to help guide the pet to the best waiting option for that patient? Are there notes in the pet's file that can keep their FAS at a low level?

This is a component of Fear Free that can be surprising to some veterinary professionals, but it's as important for the client and your front desk team to be on board with Fear Free as it is for the veterinarian. And there's an important nonhuman piece of the puzzle, too: your records. Each pet should have an emotional medical record (EMR) the same way it has a record of procedures given, diagnoses, and prescribed treatment.

The basis of the EMR is the previsit questionnaire (PVQ), which every new client should be asked to complete. Along with basic information about the pet and a medical history, questions about the pet's behavior, fears, favorite treats, and other emotional information should be included.

By consulting the EMR, FAS triggers and escalation of fear states can be avoided. That's why the EMR should be referenced and updated at every visit. It should be consulted when the client calls to schedule the appointment, to ensure any preparation, such as previsit pharmaceuticals (PVPs), is handled.

The PVQ and EMR are also opportunities to remind the client how best to transport the pet to the hospital. A pet owner can't bring in a wild feline or terrified canine and expect us to wave a treat under the pet's nose and achieve a magical state of calm. Rather, the pet owner must start preparing for a veterinary visit a week ahead of time by:

- getting (or better yet, keeping) the carrier out so the pet doesn't only associate it with negative experiences. give the pet treats in the carrier, spray it with pheromones, or put soft bedding or food inside
- keeping the pheromones flowing on the day of the visit, from carrier to car
- preheating or precooling the car so the same temperature is maintained from home to vehicle to clinic
- covering the carrier on three sides to reduce visual stimuli, and making sure the carrier is secured and placed on a surface that is level, not slanted
- not baby talking or chattering with the pet in the car, but instead playing calming music
- having the pet come in hungry. Unless it is medically contraindicated, which is rare, the pet owner on the direction of veterinarian should reduce the pet's food or even eliminate a meal before the veterinary visit, in order to increase the value of treats during the visit.

Owners should also be educated about the value of the "victory visit." This is a structured service offered by a qualified team member. It could be a preventive service or an intervention for existing FAS associated with the veterinary hospital. Victory visits might be set up as short private sessions. To maximize efficiency, you might schedule them during a block of time each week. For example, every Tuesday from noon to 2 pm a victory visit is available every 15 minutes. Or you may have a team member offer a group class after hours that focuses on preparing patients for veterinary visits. The focus is not just on making the environment a good place but also acclimating the pet to gentle control and veterinary equipment. If utilized as an intervention service for pets with high FAS scores, trust and positive associations can take several repeated visits to establish.

6.6.5 Examining the Exam

Walk from the reception area to the exam room. Close the door and sit there. What do you hear, see, smell? Is it comfortable? Is it cool or warm enough? Are there places for a cat to get up high? Is there enough floor space for a large dog, or one unable or unwilling to get on the exam table, to be examined? Are the lights bright and glaring? Is it an environment that will reduce or escalate a pet's FAS?

Look for simple changes you can make, like dimming the lights and adding calming music and pheromones. Have all team members learn to lower their voices and maintain a calm atmosphere in the hospital. The goal of time spent in the exam room is to give the pet a chance to relax, not escalate into an even greater state of anxiety.

Think about where the exam takes place. In the bad old days, each pet was hoisted up onto the table or lifted on a hydraulic lift that rocked like the horse ride outside a grocery store. Now, besides food rewards, pets are given choices of where they're to be examined including on a yoga mat on the floor, in the bottom half of the carrier, on an easily sanitized cat tree, in the owner's lap, or up on the table on a warm, nonskid surface.

One of the tenets of Fear Free is that we "put the 'treat' into 'treatment'." That means laying in a supply of highly palatable treats, from soft treats such as squeeze cheese and peanut butter to baby food, whipped cream, deli meats, fish flakes, tuna, and other high-value foods. Give them liberally, and use techniques such as smearing cheese or peanut butter on a cabinet door to distract the pet from an injection or other potentially uncomfortable procedure.

Distraction can also be accomplished by utilizing anything the individual pet finds desirable, including brushing, toys, or petting. The point is to get their attention off the unpleasant situation.

Some specific Fear Free exam room techniques involve changing how you approach each pet, how you handle them, how you achieve positional compliance, and how you respond to a pet whose FAS escalates during the exam.

- *Gentle control.* Most of us were taught restraint in veterinary school, where the goal was always to protect the practice team. Now with Fear Free we embrace low-stress handling and gentle control. The goals are still positional compliance and ensuring safety but we also look after the pet's physical and emotional wellbeing. No more cats being stretched out, or dogs being held down by veterinary nurses.
- *Considerate approach.* Considerate approach encompasses the interaction between the veterinary team and the patient. It requires keeping the pet's emotional well-being in mind and noting how the pet responds to the sensory inputs of the physical environment, the client, and the veterinary team, and any procedures being performed.
- *Touch gradient.* Instead of touching the patient sporadically or intermittently, once you establish contact with your patient maintain it with at least one hand while slowing and gently moving between areas of the patient's body. Sporadic touch can result in a startle response, which may lead to FAS. Begin your touch in a nonsensitive area and maintain contact with your hands as you gently slide toward other areas of the pet's body. Touch gradient also includes acclimating a patient to an increasing level of touch intensity associated with veterinary procedures while continuously measuring the patient's acceptance and comfort.
- *If you can't abate, medicate.* The dozens of boarded veterinary behaviorists and veterinary anesthesiologists who developed and continue to advise Fear Free have several mantras when it comes to reducing FAS including (i) sedate early and often, (ii) think of sedation as a first option rather than a last resort, and (iii) just give medication a chance.

Like animals in severe respiratory distress, animals in a state of high emotional arousal are also in distress. This means you must address those patients' needs immediately. Ignoring emotional harm in the interests of "getting 'er done" will negatively impact the practice's financial health, violate the trust of the client, damage the well-being of the veterinary team, and violate our oath as veterinarians to promote animal health and welfare and relieve animal suffering.

EXAMPLES

A senior greyhound named Lily suffered very severe FAS during veterinary visits all her life. She developed kidney disease and required regular monitoring of her blood pressure. Her blood pressure readings were extremely high when they were taken at the hospital, but when the Fear Free Certified technician offered to take her blood pressure in the owner's car, the readings were normal.

A mixed-breed dog named Copper experienced FAS so bad that her owner had not taken her for veterinary care for several years. After an emergency room visit, she had to see a general practice veterinarian for follow-up. The veterinarian she chose was Fear Free Certified, and he immediately offered to examine and treat her dog in the outdoor garden area at the side of the hospital. By the end of the visit, the dog was happy and relaxed.

Jax, an 11-year-old cat who had not been to the veterinarian since the age of 3, needed to see a specialist. At the time of the initial appointment, the specialty practice solicited information for the pet's EMR, and suggested obtaining PVPs from Jax's primary veterinarian before the initial visit. Once Jax arrived, they put a pheromone-drenched warm towel over the carrier and brought him directly to the exam room. It was the first time Jax was not highly stressed and fearful during an appointment, and also the first time he didn't hide under the bed once he got home.

TAKE-AWAYS

- Veterinarians and all veterinary practice team members need to be familiar with the signs of FAS in pets.
- Emotional health and well-being need to be diagnosed, and treated to the same extent as physical health and well-being.
- Fear Free practice does not involve a large investment of time or money. Most of what we need to remodel is our habits and mindset, not our hospitals.
- Fear Free can provide a competitive advantage to a veterinarian or practice over internet resources, pet store employees, and social media.
- Fear Free practice can free veterinarians and team members from sources of stress in our own professional lives, including having our patients fear us, resistance to treatment from patient and client, and the effects of negative client experiences.

MISCELLANEOUS

Reference

1 Volk, J.O., Felsted, K.E., Thomas, J.G., and Siren, C.W. (2011). Executive summary of the Bayer veterinary care usage study. *Journal of the American Veterinary Medical Association* 10: 1275–1282.

Recommended Reading

Becker, M., Becker, M., Sung, W., and Radosta, L. (2018). *From Fearful to Fear Free: A Positive Program to Free Your Dog from Anxiety*. Deerfield Beach, FL: HCI.

Horwitz, D. and Horwitz, D. (2018). *Blackwell's Five-Minute Veterinary Consult Clinical Companion*. Hoboken, NJ: Wiley.

Howell, A. and Feyrecilde, M. (2018). *Cooperative Veterinary Care*. Newark, NJ: Wiley.

Landsberg, G.M., Hunthausen, W.L., and Ackerman, L. (2013). *Behavior Problems of the Dog and Cat*, 3e. Edinburgh: Saunders/Elsevier.

Overall, K.L. (2013). *Manual of Clinical Behavioral Medicine for Dogs and Cats*. St Louis, MO: Elsevier.

Yin, S.A. (2009). *Low Stress Handling, Restraint and Behavior Modification of Dogs & Cats: Techniques for Developing Patients Who Love Their Visits*. Davis, CA: CattleDog Publishing.

6.7

Cooperative Care

Alicea Howell, LVT, VTS (Behavior), KPA, CTP

Barks and Rec, Traverse City, MI, USA

 BASICS

6.7.1 Summary

Visiting the veterinary clinic is a stressful time for both clients and patients. If there is a struggle, clients are less likely to keep their dogs and cats up to date on preventive care. Adopting a pet-specific approach to handling will allow all patients to receive the care they need. Cooperative veterinary care training is at the very center of pet-specific handling.

6.7.2 Terms Defined

Aggression: Behavior intended to harm, or at least threaten to harm, another.

Antecedent: Anything that happens before the target behavior, such as a cue or a trigger. Antecedents can be environmental, a gesture, sound, smell, person, etc.

Approximation: A step toward the desired behavior.

Consent: Giving permission for something to happen. In animal training, it is a behavior that has been taught to allow the trainer to touch or perform a procedure on the animal.

Cooperative Care: The animal either gives consent by performing a behavior or is easily distracted by food during veterinary procedures.

Consequences: Anything that happens immediately after the target behavior. The process by which these consequences influence behavior is called operant conditioning.

Desensitization: The decrease of an emotional response to a stimulus after gradual exposure.

Positive Reinforcement: Addition of a pleasurable stimulus to increase the likelihood the animal will perform a behavior again.

Shaping: Teaching a new behavior through selectively reinforcing small criteria toward the desired behavior.

 MAIN CONCEPTS

A domestic animal, like a cat or dog, has no reason to defend itself through aggression if it does not feel threatened. Most will choose to flee rather than fight. An animal that is in control of what is happening during a training session does not feel his safety is in jeopardy and if he does, he can simply walk away. Not only do they begin to feel safe, but they also learn how to turn on good things and turn off the bad things. Furthermore, through the use of positive reinforcement, counterconditioning, and desensitization, we can condition the "bad stuff" to be "good stuff."

Cooperative care training is focused on husbandry tasks the patient will need to comply with for its healthcare (see 6.8 Managing Routine Procedures to Minimize Problems). A cooperative approach means that the learner and the trainer are working together. In order to know when an animal is ready to have a medical procedure performed, it is necessary to have consent. How do you receive consent from an animal that doesn't speak English? It's easy – through a consent behavior that is previously taught. Consent behaviors are "I'm ready" behaviors. Cooperative care training relies on consent work but also requires the animal have some foundation skills as well.

Pet-Specific Care for the Veterinary Team, First Edition. Edited by Lowell Ackerman.
© 2021 John Wiley & Sons, Inc. Published 2021 by John Wiley & Sons, Inc.

6.7.3 Foundation Skills for New Learners

No matter what cooperative behavior you are teaching any animal, they will need a foundation in learning and a few beginner skills. Most dogs will have a nice sit you can use to your advantage, but most animals have no idea how to learn and what it feels like to have true positive reinforcement training (see 6.2 How Animals Learn). These skills can be taught in a group training session for more behaviorally normal dogs or one on one with dogs with behavior problems or other species that would become nervous in a group class.

6.7.4 Teaching Consent

Consent implies giving permission for something to happen. In animal training, it is a behavior that has been taught to allow the trainer to touch or perform a procedure on the animal [1]. In order to teach consent, the animal must have a way to communicate that he is "ready to go" or is "not ready." Teaching a consent behavior is the first step in true cooperative care. Any behavior that is salient to the learner and the teacher will work.

Training a consent behavior is all about building a history of reinforcement for this behavior. Stationing or a chin rest is a good start for my consent behaviors because they are typically new to the learner and therefore have no history of bad stuff. The station becomes a place of reinforcement and training.

Pets learn that getting down off the station (often a low table) means the training stops. So, in other words, all the scary stuff stops but all the good stuff (treats, attention) also stop. It is up to the trainer (and deliverer of reinforcement) to make sure the good stuff far outweighs the bad, break the behavior into small workable chunks, and keep the promise to the animal that they are in control.

6.7.5 Teaching Targets

Targeting is a useful skill making it easy to move an animal into position without tugging or coaxing. It can also teach new learners to place a body part into a needed position. When working on movement, most dogs and cats can be taught to touch their nose to your hand for a click and treat. Then start to move the placement of your hand a few inches away, making them lean into it to touch it. Once the nose to hand target is understood, they can come from one, two, three, even 50 ft away to touch your hand. Placing your hand above a table can prompt the animal to step up onto the platform to reach and touch your hand.

Teaching a body part to target can teach them to offer a limb or paw when needed. Target sticks or other targets are available at training stores online.

6.7.6 Responding to Cue

In cooperative care, oftentimes cues will be objects like the table, target, syringe, etc. However, get used to naming everything you do so then animal knows what to expect and can decide to stay on the consent table or move away. Naming body parts or procedures will build consistency in the interactions with the trainee.

6.7.7 Training Process

When you start counterconditioning a fearful dog to enjoy nails trims, it will not happen in one session. Most likely it will take many sessions, especially if the dog has been overrestrained or injured in the past and has learned to be fearful. When teaching complex new behavior such as non-restraint venipuncture, vaccines, or exam, it will be critical to break these large behaviors into small approximations. Cooperative care behavior will require shaping, bridging, counterconditioning, and desensitization. Understanding these training concepts is the key to any good trainer.

Shaping is breaking a complex behavior into pieces and training them in successive approximations toward the end behavior [2]. For example, for the stationing behavior, the best way to teach it is through shaping. It's unlikely the animal will just leap onto the table – you will have to teach them to step all four paws up onto the platform. To achieve this behavior easily, we will use a bridge, also known as an event marker. The clicker is my bridge of choice. The clicker means "you are correct, here comes your food" (in shaping plans, it's a click and treat – C/T); the lack of C/T means "incorrect, please try again or try what you're doing harder." For the clicker to be used as an effective bridge, it needs to mark the exact moment the behavior is occurring and then the trainer can follow it with food. A shaping plan for "go to station" might look something like this.

- Animal looks at platform C/T
- Animal walks toward platform C/T
- Animal touches platform with nose or paw C/T
- Animal raises foot on to or next to platform C/T
- Animal places one foot onto platform C/T
- Animal places front two feet onto platform C/T
- Animal steps up with back feet, placing all four on platform C/T

Each of the steps will need multiple repetitions before moving onto the next but don't wait too long to progress or the animal will think that they have it and are done. If at any step the learner fails more than three times in a row, go back a step and reinforce that behavior again. Once the animal immediately gets up onto the platform, the next step would be to cue behavior the animal already knows, like sit, down, paw, etc. This teaches the learner that the station is a place of training and reinforcement.

6.7.8   Husbandry Behavior

Now that the learner has a consent behavio,r you can start counterconditioning and desensitization to the procedure (see 6.02 How Animals Learn). If it's a painful medical procedure like a blood draw or injection, consider the rule of 100 times trained for every real procedure [3]. Practice each step 100 times before moving to the next and once the entire behavior is ready, practice it 100 times for every time the actual painful procedure will be performed.

6.7.9   What to Do with Wrong Choices

The hardest part for new trainers is understanding the importance of what to do when the animal performs an undesirable behavior. During the shaping process, sometimes the animal will get down off the table, squirm or with newer trainers the animal might show small signs of anxiety or aggression. Hopefully, the worst behavior you get is the animal getting down off the training platform (exam table). However, no matter what "bad" behavior that animal shows, it's important to ignore it, NEVER punish it, but make notes on it. Good training notes or mental notes will let you know when you are progressing too quickly through the shaping/desensitization process. If the animal shows signs of stress or removes itself from training in a session, you're asking too much of it, so go back a few steps and progress more gradually.

EXAMPLES

Coco is a 1-year-old Australian shepherd who is aggressive when touched by veterinary staff. Due to her age, she now needs booster vaccines and a heartworm check. Coco learned to station on a platform for food reinforcement during her first visit. After repeated stationing for food reinforcement, she was slowly introduced to touch, first on her side, then shoulder and slowly progressing to wrist, then paw. If at any time Coco became nervous, she simply removed herself from the stationing platform to signal she wasn't ready for the next step. As the behaviors became more complex, new consent behaviors emerged. For example, after lifting her paw multiple times, she began to offer her paw to the trainer. Once she began lifting and offering her paw, that became the new consent behavior for paw work. If she got down off the platform or stopped performing other consent behaviors, the trainer would reduce the training plan to the previously successful step and repeat multiple times before moving forward again. After multiple training sessions, staff were able to complete a physical and vaccinations without Coco leaving the station.

TAKE-AWAYS

- Cooperative veterinary care starts with teaching a consent behavior the animal can use to communicate readiness to participate.
- Husbandry behavior should be trained through positive reinforcement.
- Complex behaviors need a lot of repetition, especially if the animal has a history of bad experiences with performing them.
- Break large behaviors into small steps to make both trainer and learner successful.
- Using an event marker like a clicker is an easy way to capture the moment the animal performs the behavior correctly.

MISCELLANEOUS

6.7.10   Cautions

When working with aggression that is hard to predict or when performing painful procedures, use protective contact training. This training can be performed by teaching the animal to press a body part against a gate for injection or offering a leg through a gate for venipuncture. Teaching aggressive dogs to accept wearing a cage muzzle and take treats through the bars is another valuable safety measure.

References

1 Howell, A. and Feryercilde, M. (2018). *Cooperative Veterinary Care*. Hoboken: Wiley.

2 Pryor, K. (1999). *Don't Shoot the Dog: The New Art of Teaching and Training*. New York: Bantam Books.

3 Ramirez, K. (1999). *Animal Training: Successful Animal Management Through Positive Reinforcement*. Chicago, IL: Shedd Aquarium Society.

Herron, M., Shofer, F., and Reisner, I. (2009). Survey of the use and outcome of confrontational and non-confrontational training methods in client-owned dogs showing undesired behaviors. *Applied Animal Behaviour Science* 117 (1–2): 47–54.

Shaw, J. and Martin, D. (2015). *Canine and Feline Behavior for Veterinary Technicians and Nurses*. Ames, IA: Wiley.

Yin, S. (2009). *Low Stress Handling, Restraint and Behavior Modification of Dogs and Cats*. Davis, CA: CattleDog Publishing.

Recommended Reading

Chance, P. (2008). *Learning and Behavior*, 6e. Boston, MA: Wadsworth Cengage/Learning.

6.8

Managing Routine Procedures to Minimize Problems

Jacqui Ley, BVSc (Hons), PhD, DECAWBM, FANZCVS (Veterinary Behaviour)

Melbourne Veterinary Specialist Centre, Glen Waverley, Victoria, Australia

 ## BASICS

6.8.1 Summary

Veterinary clinics are generally not places where dogs and cats feel comfortable. Many interactions and routine procedures can be made more animal friendly with simple changes. The way staff interact with the animals is important, as is preparing the pet for the visit to the veterinary clinic. The clinical examination should be pleasant for the patient. Vaccinations can be given in such a way as to reduce pain and routine procedures can be practiced, making them familiar for the pet. Cooperative care is a model from zoos and marine parks that encourages training of the animals to facilitate their own examination and healthcare which is becoming more familiar to veterinary clinics seeing companion animals (see 6.7 Cooperative Care).

6.8.2 Terms Defined

Cooperative Care: System of management teaching, using positive reinforcement and animal behaviors that make examination and treatment easier.

Human-Animal Bond (HAB): A mutually beneficial and dynamic relationship between people and animals that is influenced by behaviors that are essential to the health and well-being of both.

 ## MAIN CONCEPTS

Creating a clinic that focuses on the animal's and client's experience has benefits for the animals, staff, and clients. If owners feel their pets are not comfortable at the veterinary clinic, they may delay bringing their pet in for a consultation [1]. It is relatively easy to make small adjustments for patient well-being in procedures such as the clinical examination, vaccination, ear examination, blood collection, and catheter placement.

Stressed and anxious pets display their distress differently. Animals may use aggressive behavior, struggle, or repeatedly jump up seeking reassurance. But don't forget that a quiet, still, and nonresisting pet may still be very stressed.

Veterinary clinics must not forget the experience of the animal within their services. New clinics should be designed to be quiet, and to allow separation of species. Existing clinics can make small, effective changes.

- Keep the clinic quiet and calm. Noise levels have been shown to increase stress levels in dogs [2]. Use noise-absorbing materials and soft-close features on drawers and cupboards where possible. Keep background music and televisions down low, playing calming music (for people and animals) and keeping voices calm.
- High-pitched voices add to animal stress. Encourage all staff to keep their voices calm, soothing, and low pitched when handling animals.

Pet-Specific Care for the Veterinary Team, First Edition. Edited by Lowell Ackerman.
© 2021 John Wiley & Sons, Inc. Published 2021 by John Wiley & Sons, Inc.

- Offer highly palatable treats to help animals feel more relaxed. If treats are not taken or taken then dropped, stop offering as the pet is too stressed.

6.8.2.1 The Clinical Examination

When pets are calm, clinical examination findings are more accurate. Stressed dogs and cats have higher heart rates and respiratory rates, panting prevents auscultation of the heart and lungs, dilated pupils make eye examinations difficult, and tense muscles make examination of the musculoskeletal system difficult. Bloodwork may be altered from normal baseline. It is good medical practice to make the examination calm to reduce patient stress.

- For some pets, the trip to the clinic is very stressful. Cats especially do not like leaving their home territory. Nonsedating previsit medication can help reduce stress and make the whole visit easier to tolerate [3]. Trial medication to find the best fit with the patient.
- Encourage owners to familiarize their cat or dog to the carrier and mode of transport. Many animals are more comfortable in familiar carriers. There are several that open from the top allowing easy access to the animal while it stays in the carrier.
- Let the pet explore the room or just sit in their carrier for a while before starting.
- Handling of the pet has been shown to increase behavioral signs of stress [2]. Minimize this by keeping the clinical examination smooth and gentle. The routine should start at the head – meet the pet before launching into examining it! Avoid any nonemergency activities until there is some rapport with the pet.
- Give the pet breaks – a chance to move away or step back during the examination. This allows the pet to reduce its stress level and prevent problems. Encourage the owner to reassure their pet.
- If the pet responds, intersperse the examination with just patting the pet. It may help them relax. Owners like to see that veterinarians and staff like pets – especially their pet!
- Use treats during the examination. Eating helps lower stress levels and helps change a negative experience into something that was worth going through to get the "good stuff."
- Show the pet any equipment that will be used. Letting them briefly sniff it helps with acceptance of the equipment.
- Work where you and the pet are comfortable. Some pets are calmer on the floor, or on their owner's lap or even on your lap.

6.8.2.2 The Vaccination

- Some vaccines are better given cold, others are less painful if given at body temperature. Check with the vaccination manufacturer.
- Use minimal restraint – many pets will stay still if they are offered a treat to lick at (peanut butter or similar sticky treats) while they are vaccinated.
- Use a new needle on the syringe for delivering the vaccine. Numb the skin's nociceptors by pinching before injecting.
- Be prepared to distract the pet if the vaccine stings a little after it is given. Rubbing the area firmly and offering treats can help them forget the sting.

6.8.2.3 Ear Examination

- Use a quiet area. If the animal moves during the examination, the otoscope may hurt the ear canal.
- If the ears are obviously sore, swollen, or discharging, examination under sedation with pain relief may be more appropriate.
- Let the animal see and smell the otoscope before attempting the examination.
- Warm the cone in your hand – this is important if the cones are metal but can also help with plastic cones.
- Reward the pet after the exam is finished.

6.8.2.4 Blood Collection

- Prepare all the equipment needed in a calm and quiet area.
- Use minimal restraint to keep the animal still. Most animals are calmer with less restraint.
- Do not tap the head to "distract" the pet. This is most likely seen as threatening and may cause the animal to freeze rather than sit quietly. Use food treats or stroking to help distract the patient. If the owner is calm, having them stay nearby and in contact with their pet may help the animal settle.
- Use quiet, low-pitched voices.
- Short breaks between clipping, cleaning, and taking the blood allows the animal a rest. Step back and reduce restraint to give the animal space.
- New needles are less painful.
- Some owners may be interested in training their pets to hold a suitable position for medical procedures.
- Aggressive cats may need to be restrained using a towel to minimize the risk of injury to staff.

6.8.2.5 Catheter Placement

- Use a calm and quiet room or area.
- All conversation should be in calm, low-pitched voices
- Use enough restraint to keep the animal still.
- Consider using a rear leg vein if a pet is worried about handling around its front legs.
- Use treats or frozen stock for the pet to lick to divert their attention.
- Clipping and applying a lidocaine (lignocaine) gel for a few minutes may help make introducing the catheter less stressful for the pet.
- Take breaks between parts of the preparation to give the pet a chance to relax.
- Use a new catheter if the vein is missed and withdrawn from the skin. Catheter tips get damaged as they go through the skin, increasing discomfort.
- If a vein is difficult to get, take a break; repeated attempts with the pet restrained increase its stress.

EXAMPLES

Slate is an aggressive 74 kg Great Dane with a severe head tilt and trouble walking from otitis media. A catheter is needed for general anesthesia. Slate is left in the consulting room with his owner until it is time for his procedure. He is given a subcutaneous sedative to help relax him. Peanut butter is offered through his basket muzzle and he is cuddled by his owner as his saphenous vein is prepared for a catheter. Everyone around Slate uses calm, soothing tones as he is gently restrained while his leg is catheterized. He doesn't growl and his general anesthetic induction is smooth and his anesthetic and procedure go well. He is recovered in the consulting room with his owner and he is calm when he wakes.

TAKE-AWAYS

- Veterinary clinics can be frightening for animals. Owner perceptions of how their animals feel at the clinic may cause them to delay presenting their pet to the clinic.

- Many routine procedures can be made more animal friendly with simple, low, or no cost changes
- Talking in low-pitched and quiet tones is calming and helps animals settle.
- Treats, treats, and more treats! Have a variety and offer them.
- Use minimal restraint when holding pets for procedures. Many pets struggle less and are more compliant when held with less restraint.

MISCELLANEOUS

6.8.2.6 Cautions

Safety of staff and owners is important. If a pet is aggressive or very anxious, sedation is preferable for the animal's well-being and safety of staff.

References

1 Volk, J.O., Thomas, J., Colleran, E., and Siren, C. (2014). Executive summary of phase 3 of the Bayer veterinary care usage study. *Journal of the American Veterinary Medical Association* 244 (7): 799–802.
2 Stellato, A.C., Hoffman, H., Gowland, S., and Dewey, C. (2019). Effect of high levels of background noise on dog responses to a routine physical examination in a veterinary setting. *Applied Animal Behaviour Science* 214: 64–71.
3 van Haaften, K.A., Eichstadt Forsythe, L., Stelow, E., and Bain, M. (2017). Effects of a single preappointment dose of gabapentin on signs of stress in cats during transportation and veterinary examination. *Journal of the American Veterinary Medical Association* 251: 1175–1181.

Recommended Reading

Howell, A. and Feyrecilde, M. (2018). *Co-operative Veterinary Care*. Wiley.
Jones, D. A., (2018) Co-operative care: Seven Steps to Stress-Free Husbandry

6.9

Preventing Behavior Problems

Kymberley C. McLeod, DVM

Conundrum Consulting, Toronto, Ontario, Canada

BASICS

6.9.1 Summary

Behavioral problems are, sadly, both very common in pets and incredibly frustrating for owners. As a group, they are the number one reason for animal relinquishment and euthanasia over a lifetime, far outpacing medical issues. Early introduction of positive training techniques establishes a positive rapport between pet and owner, builds and strengthens the human–animal bond, and offsets or prevents future behavioral problems.

Behavioral screening and counseling are essential components of every veterinary visit. Providing client education on the benefits of preventing negative behaviors and opportunities to learn and practice beneficial training techniques encourages a positive long-term relationship with the clinic and healthcare team. Demonstration and utilization of low-stress handling techniques in clinic can be an effective way to increase client loyalty, and further strengthen the bond between the pet, the owner and the practice, for greater economic and welfare gains long term.

6.9.2 Terms Defined

Anxiety: Anticipation of a negative event with no clear threat currently present.

Behavioral Counseling: The systematic approach to discovering, diagnosing, and treating behavioral issues, encouraging better client compliance and success.

Desensitization: Gradual exposure to a stressor with positive reinforcement of calm behaviors.

Five Freedoms: Internationally recognized and accepted standards of care detailing the need for freedom from hunger/thirst, discomfort, fear/distress, pain/injury/disease, and the freedom to express normal behavior.

Positive Reinforcement: Rewarding a pet for a desired behavior in order to increase the frequency of that behavior.

Punishment: The removal or addition of something in order to attempt to decrease a behavior (positive punishment = yelling, leash corrections, physical reprimands; negative punishment = removing something desired, e.g., attention or food).

MAIN CONCEPTS

The client's understanding of the importance of preventive healthcare is most easily influenced during early pet ownership. Veterinary visits are the ideal time for members of the healthcare team to check in with owners on current behavioral health and help solve problems where needed. When prevention is not successful, relinquishment to shelters or euthanasia may occur.

The veterinary profession is called to uphold the welfare needs of the animals in its care. One way to quantify and evaluate an individual patient's welfare status is by utilizing the Five Freedoms. Not all "normal" behavior is desirable or understood by owners. However, animals should be able to satisfy their needs to vocalize, socialize, scratch, dig, play, and hide. Early education of owners about the potential harm that surgical alteration can have on future behavioral patterns may help them understand why procedures such as ear cropping, tail docking, declawing, and debarking are not recommended.

Pet-Specific Care for the Veterinary Team, First Edition. Edited by Lowell Ackerman.
© 2021 John Wiley & Sons, Inc. Published 2021 by John Wiley & Sons, Inc.

Owners should be encouraged to offset and prevent boredom in their mainly indoor companion animals. Proper crate selection and crate training instruction, and help with choosing and fitting proper head/body control harnesses should be discussed with every new client. Assistance selecting appropriate toys (chase, tug, chew, and enrichment type), pet-safe outdoor runs ("cattios" for indoor cats), sensory items (pheromone sprays, food puzzles/mazes, catnip), and interactive technology encourage better environments for indoor pets. Counsel clients to recognize signs of anxiety or stress early, and introduce the anxiety-reducing tools that are available (compression vests, pheromones, etc.). Discuss litterbox hygiene and product selection, and effective stain/odor products. Finally, consider utilizing technology-friendly ways to disseminate ideas for better client uptake.

We must address training techniques that have negative welfare impacts. The inappropriate use of force, domination, or punishment techniques can increase fear, anxiety or stress for the pet. It can also be helpful to research and personally interview local trainers to find local options you can refer clients to. If there is a board-certified behaviorist available, discuss this as a potential early intervention strategy for animals showing issues.

A team approach is best for behavioral counseling, allowing the hospital to maximize the team's comfort level and education. Client-facing staff members can assist with intake exams/questionnaires, demonstrating products (such as head collars) and their appropriate use, and providing follow-up literature for the rest of the family, while behavioral counseling and diagnostic/therapeutic plans may be best addressed by doctors. Offer preadoption consultations to discuss temperament, activity level, mental and physical health needs, and suitability to a client's lifestyle (see 3.10 Advising Clients on Selecting an Appropriate Pet). Also pertinent are common medical concerns for the breed, and any genetic testing recommended (see 3.4 Predicting and Eliminating Disease Traits).

There are many advantages to beginning appropriate behavioral learning as early as possible for companion animals. In dogs, the socialization and learning period occurs between 3 and 12 weeks of age. Cats have a tighter window, between 3 and 7 weeks of age. During this time, appropriate social behavior, both with other animals as well as with humans, is cemented (see 6.1 Normal Development Stages of Dogs and Cats). Additionally, acclimatization to situational stressors occurs most readily during this time.

Relinquishment for behavioral reasons peaks between 6 and 24 months of age. Maximizing juvenile vaccine appointments to promote preventive behavioral and life skills training is highly recommended. The importance of appropriate socialization opportunities should be stressed. Assist owners with habituation techniques for children,

loud noises, kennels, cars, etc. Basic obedience and life skills training (such as daily tooth brushing, nail trimming, and grooming) allow animals to accept these procedures more readily in the future, increasing the likelihood of regular preventive care (see 6.8 Managing Routine Procedures to Minimize Problems). Owners who report that their animal appears stressed by the very act of visiting the veterinary hospital are less likely to comply with regular wellness or preventive care visits.

Since the human–animal bond is a dynamic relationship, activities that help to establish a positive bond early in life maximize the benefits for both the animal and its human family (see 2.15 Promoting the Human–Animal Bond). Both negative behaviors themselves and the anticipation of those behaviors occurring break the bond, leading to less investment in the animal's overall health and wellness. Conversely, owners who report a strong bond with their animal are less likely to relinquish or euthanize their pet even in the face of severe behavioral concerns (see 2.14 Benefits of the Human–Animal Bond).

One of the common ways to positively influence the bond between the pet and owner is to encourage age-appropriate socialization and obedience training. Training techniques that positively reinforce desired behaviors rather than punishing negative behaviors have been shown to be more successful and welfare-centric (see 6.2 How Animals Learn). Beyond basic commands, the aim for companion animals is to graduate with positive emotional wellness. Our companion animals need to handle being alone in any situation, to behave in a friendly, safe and appropriate manner, and to adjust to change in a healthy way (see 6.3 Managing Life Changes for Pets). Habituation to loud noises, children, veterinary visits, and basic handling of sensitive body parts is also an essential skill. All pets need to learn appropriate housebreaking skills and show normal vocalization patterns.

Actively preventing pets from being in situations where they may perform undesired behaviors is far more successful than punishment after the fact. Since inappropriate elimination is one of the most common reasons for choosing euthanasia/relinquishment, stressing at each visit the importance of appropriate elimination training and hygiene will help clients to understand how important prevention is.

The human–animal bond is a strong driver of the level of healthcare a pet receives. Discussing the human benefits of a strong human–animal bond (such as decreased cardiopulmonary disease), as well as for the pet, increases the likelihood that clients will invest more time and money in the healthcare of that pet (see 2.14 Benefits of the Human–Animal Bond). Additionally, they are more likely to retain the pet for a longer time and be more compliant pet owners who value preventive care. Attracting clients that invest more, for longer, and in more areas leads to a financial gain for the practice that is ethically sourced and may lead to better client satisfaction and retention numbers.

Finally, it is important to acknowledge the contribution healthcare team providers can make to behavior in the clinic. Animals who exhibit behaviors clients attribute to stress or agitation, or for whom veterinary visits seem significantly traumatic, are less likely to seek out preventive care than clients whose animals appear relaxed and comfortable at the veterinarian (see 6.8 Managing Routine Procedures to Minimize Problems). When patient visits decrease, both the welfare of the pet and the economic health of the practice suffer. Reducing the fear, anxiety, and stress provoked by veterinary visits must be a top priority for clinics (see 6.6 Fear Free Concepts). Low-stress techniques start the moment a pet is bound for the clinic and should be encouraged until the moment the pet returns to the safety of their home environment. Educating the entire healthcare team on the value of lowering stress in our patients and practicing these handling techniques until they become second nature are essential to better patient welfare during the veterinary visit.

EXAMPLES

Daisy is an 8-year-old Yorkshire terrier, and is the third Yorkie her family has owned. Due to behavioral issues with her predecessors, her parents were quite receptive to the suggestion that they work with Daisy's breeder to choose a puppy with the personality type they desired. Thorough socialization and obedience training in puppyhood turned into a desire to try something more exciting with Daisy. Surprisingly, agility was a great fit, and her family attribute her brave outgoing personality to her early socialization, training, and exposure to novel experiences in puppyhood.

TAKE-AWAYS

- Prioritizing positive behavioral health and the prevention of behavioral problems are essential to building and nurturing the human–animal bond.
- Early socialization, positive training techniques, and environmental enrichment are key to maximizing companion animal welfare.
- Behavioral screening and counseling should be part of all veterinary exams.
- Low-stress handling techniques encourage positive behaviors during veterinary visits.
- A strong human–animal bond with their pets leads to better, more satisfied clients, who contribute more significantly to ethical financial growth for the hospital.

MISCELLANEOUS

Recommended Reading

Ackerman, L., Landsberg, G., and Hunthausen, W. (1996). *Cat Behavior and Training. Veterinary Advice for Owners.* Neptune, NJ: TFH Publications.

Ackerman, L., Landsberg, G., and Hunthausen, W. (1996). *Dog Behavior and Training. Veterinary Advice for Owners.* Neptune, NJ: TFH Publications.

Landsberg, G., Hunthausen, W., and Ackerman, L. (2013). *Behavior Problems of the Dog and Cat.* St Louis: Saunders-Elsevier.

Webster, J. (2016). Animal welfare: freedoms, dominions and "A Life Worth Living.". *Animals* 6 (6): 35.

Yin, S. (2009). *Low Stress Handling, Restraint and Behavior Modification of Dogs and Cats: Techniques for Patients Who Love Their Visits.* Davis, CA: CattleDog Publishing.

6.10

Behavior Problems – Advice

Jacqui Ley, BVSc (Hons), PhD, DECAWBM, FANZCVS (Veterinary Behaviour)

Melbourne Veterinary Specialist Centre, Glen Waverley, Victoria, Australia

BASICS

6.10.1 Summary

The recognition of behavior problems and mental health in animals is growing among the veterinary industry. Not many professional organizations include the normal behavior of the species being managed as part of their training. The result is that many veterinarians, technicians, and nurses are not completely comfortable in providing advice to clients to help them manage their pet's behavior. In the worst cases, the advice that is given may actually be misinformation! But good, scientifically based information is available. Normal species-specific behavior needs to be taught to all staff. Then staff need to know how to recognize and ask about problem behaviors. Once the behavior the owner has concerns about is identified as normal or a sign of mental illness, safe and practical advice can be given.

6.10.2 Terms Defined

Anxiety: A negative emotional state that may be triggered by uncertainty. It is a normal emotion and usually transient.

Anxiety Disorder: A persistent state of negative emotional state without identifiable trigger or stimulus. Interferes with the individual's daily life and causes significant distress.

Cognitive Dissonance: Mental discomfort experienced when an individual's beliefs or expectations clash with new information perceived by the individual.

Fear: A negative emotional state brought on by the threat of pain, danger or harm. It is triggered by an identifiable stimulus.

Mental Health: An individual's condition with regard to their emotional, cognitive psychological well-being.

Mental Illness: Condition which causes serious disorder in an individual's behavior, emotions or thinking.

Problem Behavior: Any behavior by a pet that the owner considers to be undesirable. The behavior may or may not be normal for the species.

Stress: Internal or external factors that move the animal from a physiological state of homeostasis.

Veterinary Psychiatry: The arm of veterinary medicine that diagnoses and treats mental health disorders in animals.

MAIN CONCEPTS

Undesirable behavior in our pets is a challenge for all owners and can spill over into other areas of the animal's life, making it hard for professionals to handle the animal. But not all undesirable behavior is a sign of a mental health problem. Some behavior that is normal and appropriate for animals at certain ages and stages of development is not desirable to owners. The difficulty can be working out the motivation for the behavior – normal or ill health?

6.10.3 Normal Behavior

The normal behavior of species generally seen at the veterinary clinic should be common knowledge for all staff. It is normal for dogs to bark, growl, and bite as well as mark things and destroy items they find. It is normal for cats to scratch vertical and horizontal surfaces, be active at dawn and dusk, vocalize, hide, kill small animals, and spray. Helping owners accept and manage these behaviors helps preserve the human–animal bond and keep pets in their families (see 6.1 Normal Development Stages of Dogs and Cats).

6.10.4 Mental Illness

Mental illnesses in companion animals and other species kept in farms, laboratories, zoological collections, marine parks, and aquaria are recognized by veterinary behavior specialists. Recognition by general practitioners and other professionals working with companion animals and by owners tends to be poor but it is improving with increasing education. Mental illnesses occur due to imbalances within the brain's biochemistry. It is not clear if the initial problem is caused by an internal defect in brain function or external factors such as early environments or cognitive dissonance. It is likely that it is a combination of both groups of factors.

As the mental illnesses that are recognized in animals can affect their responses to real and perceived threats, recognizing mental health problems, encouraging treatment, and adapting clinic procedures to minimize stressors for animals are all important for animal and human welfare and safety. Affected animals may experience greater fear, anxiety, and stress when visiting the clinic (even when well) and when handled. Painful procedures may hurt them more; they may be more difficult to anesthetize and managing anesthesia and analgesia may be more complex [1]. All these factors can have significant effects on how the animals approach the veterinary clinic and staff. Some patients will be difficult and dangerous to handle. Recognizing when a patient has a mental illness is important for their welfare and, in some cases, for owner and staff safety.

The types of mental health problems diagnosed in patients include anxiety disorders that may present as aggression directed at familiar people and/or animals, aggression directed toward unfamiliar people and/or animals, separation anxiety and distress, marking and house soiling, phobias, and Generalized Anxiety Disorder (GAD). Obsessive compulsive disorders (OCD) and cognitive decline syndrome (CDS) may also be seen. Depression is also recognized but rarely presented. Developmental disorders of young animals are also becoming recognized.

6.10.5 Recognition of Mental Illnesses May Be Hampered by Several Factors

The behavior displayed may not necessarily be odd or unusual. Some mental illnesses, such as OCD, may cause the animal to present with abnormal behavior such as repetitive spinning, tail chasing, trancing, eating (pica), grooming, pacing, or swaying, for example. The behavior is obviously abnormal and the motivation to perform the behavior may be causing distress and preventing the animal from undertaking normal social and self-care activities.

But these presentations are not common. Most problem behaviors present as normal behavior such as seeking attention, avoiding social contact, aggression, protecting resources or toileting in inappropriate places and marking behavior. It is important to recognize that problem behavior is due to a mental illness when the behavior is out of context or extreme in its intensity and/or its frequency. So a dog may be aggressive and lunge and bark when it sees an unfamiliar dog on the street – the aggression is not needed if the other dog is not being aggressive. A cat may spray urine on furniture around the house, on curtains, on any new or moved item – the urine spraying is extreme in its frequency. A puppy may be excessively active and not appear to be learning typical cues such as its name, to sit and where to toilet normally. Its behavior is abnormal with regard to the context for the activity, its frequency, and intensity.

Misinformation about normal behavior of many companion animals and how problem behavior should be addressed is widespread. Many people cling to the notion that dogs have a dominance hierarchy and unwanted behavior is related to the dog trying to dominate the owner. Therefore, unwanted behavior should be addressed by being tougher and more assertive, so the dog perceives the owner to be dominant. This ignores the true situation and can exacerbate anxiety for the affected dog. Sometimes the sources of the misinformation are trusted by owners. They may choose to follow the advice even when the animal is suffering due to the "advice." This means that clients may not hear the information presented to them by staff. Staff need to be supported in providing correct advice but also helped to understand that some clients will not accept the advice, which can be disheartening for staff members. Some clients will start to listen if they hear the same message several times so staff should always provide the correct advice.

Having all staff familiar with the normal behavior of the species the clinic sees frequently helps them answer questions for clients and raise concerns about the behavior of patients.

Staff may hold incorrect views as to what is normal behavior for the species they handle, even if they are experienced with that species. This may affect how they handle animals and approach problem behavior. To address this takes a whole-clinic approach. All team members need to be aware of patient mental health and be empowered to open conversations with clients and know how to address questions about pet behavior. Awareness of how animals may perceive and react to our handling efforts encourages sympathetic and empathetic handling and management for routine care.

Staff and clients may hold different views about mental illness. Some people do not believe that animals have mental lives and that they can be affected by mental illness. Supporting staff to understand why some people will ask for advice but then reject it can help them manage their own feelings and look after their own mental health.

6.10.6   Safe Advice

The advice given by all staff members must first do no harm to people or animals and keep everyone (the owners, the public, other animals, and the affected pet) safe. Sometimes the simplest and most obvious advice is the best for an animal with a behavior problem. If a pet does not like an activity, shows signs of distress, is avoidant or aggressive when approached or taken to a place then, if it is not necessary for everyday survival, the animal doesn't have to take part. For example, if a dog is aggressive at the local dog park, not taking it there is a sensible, safe and welfare-friendly thing to do. Alternative activities could be explored such as playing at home or walking on the street or even going to a different park. A cat that is aggressive to other cats in the household can be given their own space that the other cats cannot access.

Many owners need advice as to how to manage normal behaviors in their pet. Many owners are surprised at how active normal young pets can be. More exercise may be the answer but many pets need more at-home activities as they spend considerable time alone in the home. Safe items can be left for pets to play with (and destroy), food can be hidden in toys that reward interaction by dispensing the food and the toys can be hidden. Feeding can be moved from a bowl to toys or even spread on the ground so the animal has to work to get its food. This encourages normal foraging and exploratory behavior.

More time spent on training can help pets and their owners learn to interact. Trainers suggested must be positive reinforcement trainers because this training method will do no harm to the animal. The training may be for manners but can also be tricks and other fun activities or for sports.

If the issue is more than a training problem, lack of stimulation and exercise or just misunderstanding normal behavior, then a consultation with a veterinarian may be needed. Mental illness must be diagnosed after the collection of a detailed history, clinical examination, and observation of the animal. Medical causes for changes in behavior must be ruled out. Suitable behavior medications coupled with a behavior modification plan and environmental management can successfully treat straightforward behavior problems. Storm fears and phobias are a common example of problems that require medication to help the patient manage.

Sometimes it is not possible to treat behavior problems in clinic. Referral to a board certified or recognized specialist in veterinary behavioral medicine is best. If one is not located near the clinic, many specialists offer consultations by phone or over the internet and can be accessible to clients in remote areas. However, immediate advice to help the client should also keep the patient, owner, other people, and other animals safe.

Follow-up with the owner is very important to check that things are improving and if they are not, to see what else can be done to help.

 EXAMPLES

A client telephones the clinic worried about the aggressive behavior her male Australian terrier shows whenever he sees another dog. She has been advised to take her dog up close to other dogs and correct him harshly when he growls at the other dogs. She has tried this and her dog's behavior is worsening.

Being aggressive toward others who are not being threatening is a commonly misunderstood behavior. The dog is not being dominant. Rather, the aggressive behavior is out of context and extreme in its intensity for the situation (walking down the street and seeing an unfamiliar dog walking calmly with its owner).

The owner's Australian terrier requires a medical examination to rule out health problems and then referral to a veterinary behaviorist for diagnosis and treatment. In the meantime, the owner was advised to actively avoid other dogs when out walking. Pushing her dog close to other dogs makes him feel more anxious and gives him more chances to practice his aggressive behavior. Avoidance allows him to be calm and to feel safe.

The owner followed this advice and also had a phone consultation with a veterinary behaviorist who recommended specific exercises and medication. When her practice followed up a month later, the client was happy with her understanding of her dog's problem and his progress.

A couple brought their pair of Burmese cats in for their annual health check-up and vaccinations. The owners mentioned that one of the cats was urinating and defecating on the bed in the spare room. They were very upset about this behavior and were considering rehoming the cat. The cat was found to be healthy and bloods and urinalysis were normal. The technician ran the owners through a questionnaire about cat toileting and found that the owners provided their cats with two litter trays side by side in the laundry. The litter brand was the same and there had been no recent changes. The trays were scooped daily and cleaned every few weeks with hot water and disinfectant. The soiling cat was noticed to always use the litter trays as soon as they were cleaned. The two cats were reported to get along well – they were seen to sleep curled up together and to groom each other. The veterinarian tentatively diagnosed a house-soiling problem due to poor litter tray management and a substrate preference for the bed. The owners were asked to provide at least 1–2 more trays in different parts of the house and to completely empty and clean the trays every time they were soiled. They were also asked to clean the bedding using an enzymatic cleaner, and to keep the door to the spare room shut or consider installing a self-closer on it. A two-week follow-up was booked. At two weeks, things had improved (there was one urination on the bed when the door was left open). The owners were very happy and were no longer thinking of rehoming their cat.

TAKE-AWAYS

- Behavior problems may be normal behavior that owners do not understand or like or they can be caused by mental illness.
- A good history is needed to define the problem behavior and the situations when it occurs.
- Mental illness is recognized by assessing the context, intensity, and frequency of the problem behavior.
- It may take the owner time to accept the information, especially if it challenges their beliefs about how pets should behave or their views on mental health.
- Any advice given should first keep the pet, owner, and other people and animals safe. Referral for treatment may be necessary.

MISCELLANEOUS

6.10.7 Cautions

Before attempting to treat mental health problems in patients, veterinarians should have training in veterinary behavioral medicine.

Reference

1 Väisänen, M.A.M., Valros, A., Hakaoja, E. et al. (2005). Pre-operative stress in dogs; a preliminary investigation of behavior and heart rate variability in healthy hospitalized dogs. *Veterinary Anaesthesia and Analgesia* 32 (3): 158–167.

Recommended Reading

Beaver, B.V. (2003). *Feline Behavior: A Guide for Veterinarians*, 2e. St Louis, MO: Saunders.

Howell, A. and Feyrecilde, M. (2018). *Co-operative Veterinary Care*. Ames, IA: Wiley Blackwell.

Landsberg, G., Hunthausen, W., and Ackerman, L. (2012). *Handbook of Behavior Problems of the Dog and Cat*, 3e. Edinburgh: Elsevier Saunders.

www.dogwelfarecampaign.org

6.11

Treating Animals with Behavior Problems

Kymberley C. McLeod, DVM

Conundrum Consulting, Toronto, Ontario, Canada

BASICS

6.11.1 Summary

Behavioral counseling, whether for undesirable or abnormal behaviors, begins with a thorough history, physical exam, and diagnostic testing. Once the medical and/or primarily behavioral causes for the problem have been diagnosed, treatment can ensue with appropriate therapy. Therapeutic options may include owner education, environmental modification, behavioral modification, neuropharmacology, nutritional intervention, and/or auxiliary products. Educating the client about the causes and therapeutic plan is the key to owner compliance, and therapeutic consistency is key for success. Where possible, seek advanced education to further develop knowledge in behavioral medicine. Consider referral for complicated cases.

6.11.2 Terms Defined

Abnormal Behaviors: Behaviors rooted in abnormal anxiety stress or fear, such as compulsive disorders/picas, thunder phobias, separation anxiety.

Anxiety: Anticipation of a negative event with no clear threat currently present.

Behavioral Counseling: The systematic approach to discovering, diagnosing, and treating behavioral issues, encouraging better client compliance and success.

Desensitization: Gradual exposure to a stressor with positive reinforcement of calm behaviors.

Neuropharmacology: Utilizing substances to influence the nervous system and behavior.

Positive Reinforcement: Rewarding a pet for a desired behavior in order to increase the frequency of that behavior.

Punishment: The removal or addition of something in order to attempt to decrease a behavior (positive punishment = yelling, leash corrections, physical reprimands; negative punishment = removing something desired, e.g., attention or food).

Whale Eye: A body language signal where the dog shows the whites of its eyes. This is a warning signal of anxiety and, potentially, aggression.

MAIN CONCEPTS

When assisting clients who are experiencing behavioral issues with their pets, remember problem behaviors can include both undesirable and truly abnormal behaviors. Differentiating between the two is important for both client education and therapeutic pathways.

Thorough behavioral consultations include both a medical and behavioral history, physical exam, and, if applicable, diagnostic testing (bloodwork, urinalysis, advanced imaging, skin scraping, cytology, etc.). Bloodwork and urinalysis may assist in determining appropriate medications. Information about the family and housing situation, the pet itself, and all aspects of the problem behavior should be gathered at this time. Questionnaires provided to the client prior to the appointment and videos of the behavior can be especially useful.

Pet-Specific Care for the Veterinary Team, First Edition. Edited by Lowell Ackerman.
© 2021 John Wiley & Sons, Inc. Published 2021 by John Wiley & Sons, Inc.

As with any other consultation, the history, exam, and diagnostic findings will lead to a series of differential diagnoses, some primarily behavioral, others medical. Only after medical causes have been ruled out can a primary behavioral concern be determined. Remember that health and behavior are intimately linked. Stress and pain can also present as primary behavioral issues, so drug trials and stress management techniques may be warranted, even in the face of "normal" medical work-ups.

Behavioral therapy may include owner education, environmental modification, behavioral modification, neuropharmacology, nutritional intervention, and/or auxiliary products. First, uncover what your client understands about the behavioral issues the pet is facing, and what knowledge gaps need to be closed. Explore underlying assumptions as to cause and prognosis, as well as what the owner can achieve therapeutically. Highly engaged, motivated clients are far more likely to get a successful resolution than those who aren't. Client behavioral education is a major driver of compliance (see 9.17 Improving Compliance and Adherence with Pet-Specific Care). Be patient, be thorough, be kind, and be empathetic to the situation. Clients who feel they are part of the team to decide what they can and can't do in their home situation will be more likely to continue with recommendations.

Coach the client to identify potential triggers for the behavior where possible. By avoiding these triggers, they may be able to reduce the frequency of the undesired behavior. For example, dogs who struggle with aggression in their own homes can benefit from creation of a "safe zone" without triggers – the dog's own crate, a closet or separate room, etc. The safe zone allows the dog to avoid its own triggers, and many animals will do this on their own (e.g., bury under blankets during a thunderstorm or hide under the bed when strangers are in the house). Also, care should be taken to discuss with owners any additional contribution, positive or negative, other animals and/or people may be making to the negative behaviors in the home environment.

Environment enrichment is key to reducing boredom-related negative behaviors (see 4.11 – Environmental Enrichment). Utilizing stimulating activities like food puzzles, hunting games, pheromones or essential oils can all increase an animal's sense of enjoyment of the home. Areas to escape, climb, dig, run, and play are important aspects of the pet's environment. From an animal welfare point of view, environmental enrichment also helps to satisfy an animal's need to perform normal species-specific behaviors daily.

Reward-based training can be considered enrichment too! Pets can be motivated to perform positive behaviors more often when they recognize something positive will follow (see 6.10 Behavior Problems – Advice). Mark desired behaviors immediately as they're performed with an audio cue as well as an immediate reward the pet desires. Punishment-based training (positive or negative punishment) rarely targets the cause of the problem, but simply leads to the animal avoiding the behavioral "symptom." Artificially muting the symptoms may lead to escalation, as the instigating stressor or trigger is still present. Food doesn't have to be the only reinforcing reward – some pets may be motivated by a few moments of play with a desired toy, affectionate verbal encouragement, or grooming/petting.

Exercise can also be a good addition to behavioral modification options. Natural endorphin release occurs with exercise, leading to increased relaxation and decreased stress and anxiety. Exercise can be a source of daily enrichment, as it can increase exposure to new sights/smells/interactions. However, it must be appropriate in its time length, intensity, and location. Increasing exercise length or intensity too quickly may increase stress and anxiety for the pet. Also realize that for undesirable behaviors, or those that are boredom related, enrichment and exercise can be a wonderful outlet for excessive energy. However, for those with abnormal or compulsive behaviors, remember panic and anxiety result from increased stimulation of the hypothalamic–pituitary–adrenal axis. Conditions such as separation anxiety are rarely caused by unmet exercise or enrichment needs.

Nutritional supplements and pharmacological options should be considered when anxiety and fear are components of the issue. There are both fast-acting and slow-acting options. In general, prescription medications will create positive change more quickly than supplements by nature. Consider how acute the pet's needs are. Ethically, always treat with the fastest acting appropriate option to start, as anxiety and panic are detrimental to both brain function and systemic health. Knowing that many clients will prefer "natural" supplements to prescription options, advocate for early diagnosis and therapy so these options can still be used.

Products that help to reduce stimulus may be very helpful for anxiety. Deep pressure compression vests, hoods to decrease visual stimuli, white noise machines, and species-specific music/video channels can all help assist with anxiety management.

Predicting the success of a treatment plan can be complex. However, early intervention for a problem that is easily identified, and where the stimulus is controllable, has a better prognosis. Consistency is key to the success of any behavioral intervention. Client education to increase compliance and motivation will improve the chances of success. Reevaluate the treatment plan when possible, adjust where necessary, and continue to encourage client compliance.

Lastly, never hesitate to ask for help when dealing with clients requesting behavioral consultation and therapy. Whether due to lack of knowledge, skills, staff time or the financial investment needed to do behavioral work, know your limits. If seeing complicated behavior cases is interfering with seeing primary care patients from the hospital, consider referring. Partnering with a board-certified behavioral specialist, a veterinarian with significant additional training and interest in behavior (or who has a practice limited to behavior), or a qualified trainer can all be reasonable decisions. Also consider referral if psychoactive drugs may be necessary. However, behavioral consultation and therapy can be an amazing economic driver for clinics who value and charge for them appropriately, are motivated to create programs that are client friendly, and utilize a team approach to delivery.

EXAMPLES

Boomer, an 18-month-old collie, began yawning and showing "whale eye" when strollers approached. He had previously been very confident around new people and experiences. The owner had no idea what caused the change but recognized the behaviors as signs of anxiety or fear. They reached out for advice to the veterinary hospital where Boomer's puppy socialization classes had been held. A thorough exam showed no physical reason for Boomer's behavior. The trainer began reward-based desensitization training, working on distinct skills to keep focus on the owner, and rewarding relaxed and calm behaviors. By allowing Boomer to choose whether he wished to approach the stroller, and rewarding positive behaviors, he was finally able to conquer his fear of the large scary buggies and realize that the small humans inside sometimes had treats for him too.

TAKE-AWAYS

- Whether undesired or abnormal, all behavior patterns that negatively affect the bond between pet and owner should be addressed.
- Thorough behavioral counseling requires a full history, physical exam, discussion of environment, diagnosis, therapeutic plan, and follow-up to ensure compliance.
- A multifocal approach to therapy with a highly motivated client tends to be most successful.
- Ethically, always treat with the fastest acting appropriate option to start, as anxiety and panic are detrimental to both brain function and systemic health.
- Don't hesitate to refer early when an issue requires more time, skill, or pharmacological knowledge than you currently have.

MISCELLANEOUS

Recommended Reading

Ackerman, L., Landsberg, G., and Hunthausen, W. (1996). *Cat Behavior and Training. Veterinary Advice for Owners.* Neptune, NJ: TFH Publications.

Ackerman, L., Landsberg, G., and Hunthausen, W. (1996). *Dog Behavior and Training. Veterinary Advice for Owners.* Neptune, NJ: TFH Publications.

Hammerle, M., Horst, C., Levine, E. et al. (2015). AAHA canine and feline behavior management guidelines. *J. Am. Anim. Hosp. Assoc.* 51: 205–221.

Landsberg, G., Hunthausen, W., and Ackerman, L. (2013). *Behavior Problems of the Dog and Cat.* St Louis, MO: Saunders-Elsevier.

Overall, K.L. (2013). *Manual of Clinical Behavioral Medicine for Dogs and Cats.* St Louis, MO: Elsevier Mosby.

6.12

New Puppy/Kitten Considerations

Ryane E. Englar, DVM, DABVP (Canine and Feline Practice)

College of Veterinary Medicine, University of Arizona, Oro Valley, AZ, USA

BASICS

6.12.1 Summary

New puppies and kittens are welcome additions to veterinary practice because they represent new life as well as the opportunity to forge lifelong veterinarian–client–patient relationships (VCPRs). The initial visit sets the tone for subsequent consultations and facilitates conversations about pet-specific care. It may be tempting to default to a cookie-cutter approach that outlines the same medical plan for every new patient that enters the consultation room. However, there is no universal recipe for puppy or kitten wellness. Companion animal healthcare must be tailored to the patient (pet-specific care), keeping in mind the individual's needs and risk factors. Key considerations for every new puppy and kitten include, but are not limited to, breed-related predispositions to disease, behavior, diet, parasite control, and vaccination protocol.

MAIN CONCEPTS

6.12.2 Tailoring Care to the Individual

There is no set script for the new puppy/kitten visit. Each consultation is an opportunity to develop a unique VCPR and to address pet-specific care. To provide this level of care, veterinarians must cover the following areas.

- Breed
- Behavior
- Diet
- Reproductive health
- Parasite control
- Vaccinations

Veterinarians also need to appreciate the client's perspective: what are their expectations for the patient, including its anticipated function (companion vs show animal vs breeding stock vs other) and lifestyle?

6.12.3 Breed-Specific Considerations

With dozens of feline and several hundred canine breeds, there is immense variety in morphology and genetics among companion animals. Veterinarians should actively research unfamiliar breeds because they may possess unusual characteristics that are considered "normal," including vital signs that fall outside the "normal" reference ranges (see 4.8 Pet-Specific Relevance of Reference Intervals).

Clients should be informed of breed predispositions to disease (see 11.4 Heritable Health Conditions – By Breed). More than two-thirds of dog breeds have one or more genetic disorder [1]. Collies, for instance, are predisposed to choroidal hypoplasia (collie eye anomaly) and many other conditions. Puppies can be examined for morphological changes as early as 6–8 weeks of age, and genetic testing can detect risk by as early as one day of age [2].

Awareness is key to successful management of disease, if not prevention. Recognizing the prevalence and genetics of disease may also help veterinarians work with breeders concerning appropriate testing and examination of prospective studs, bitches, queens, and toms so that diseases are less likely to be inherited by offspring.

6.12.4 Behavior Considerations

Behavioral issues may initially seem minor but a patient's behavior as it matures determines whether the pet is a suitable companion. Many are surrendered to shelters because of unacceptable behaviors that are incompatible with owners' expectations [3].

Canine separation anxiety, reactivity, and aggressiveness are potential triggers for relinquishment. Aggressive and/or destructive tendencies need to be addressed early and consistently [4].

Puppy socialization to conspecifics, people, sounds, inanimate objects, and tasks, such as nail trimming, can also facilitate a successful transition into the home environment [4].

Inappropriate elimination is a common reason for feline relinquishment. Clients may require education on litterbox etiquette in terms of substrate type, cleaning frequency, box size, and style [5]. In addition, clients need to recognize that predatory behavior is normal in kittens, but that acceptable outlets for play are necessary to avoid play biting that may led to relinquishment in adulthood [5].

6.12.5 Dietary Considerations

Commercial diets should meet Association of American Feed Control Officials (AAFCO) or other regulatory standards; however, there is a vast range of acceptable feeds for dogs and cats in canned, semi-moist, and dry formulations. Diets tend to overestimate daily intake if fed according to label. To prevent inappropriate weight gain, discuss individual needs relative to life stage, activity level, and sterilization status [5]. Needs can be further refined based upon body condition score (BCS).

Home made diets are increasingly popular and can be nutritionally complete [5]. However, proper education is essential to avoid nutrient deficiencies. Without supplementation, cats that are fed vegetarian diets may develop taurine-deficient retinopathy or dilated cardiomyopathy (DCM).

Consult available nutritional assessment guidelines as needed to individualize patient plans.

6.12.6 Reproductive Health

Pet overpopulation and overcrowding in shelters are two concerns that have historically been addressed through surgical sterilization (see 4.2 Gender-Related Considerations).

Ovariohysterectomy, ovariectomy, and orchiectomy are popular elective sterilization surgeries that may reduce undesirable hormone-associated behaviors, such as roaming (see 2.18 Population Control). These procedures are also associated with health benefits, such as reduction of mammary neoplasia in females; however, they may increase the risk for development of other diseases. For instance, pediatric gonadectomy may influence a patient's predisposition to orthopedic disease [6, 7]. This association is particularly concerning to clients of large- and giant-breed puppies, who may wish to postpone sterilization surgery until skeletal growth is complete.

Transparent dialogue concerning risk–benefit analysis and client expectations is essential for appropriate patient planning in the context of what is best for the individual.

6.12.7 Dental Prophylaxis

All dogs and cats benefit from some degree of at-home dental care [5]. Few ever receive it. Both puppies and kittens can be acclimated to tooth brushing and cursory inspections of the mouth by the client, which allow for early detection of dental disease before it becomes systemic (see 4.9 Periodontal Disease). Oral care chews and treats may be beneficial when client or patient compliance fails but they are a poor substitute for brushing [5].

Small-breed dogs are more likely to retain deciduous teeth than their large-breed counterparts [4]. Small-breed puppies should be watched closely for eruption of permanent dentition so that, if necessary, dental corrections can be paired with sterilization surgery to avoid multiple anesthetic events [4].

6.12.8 Parasite Control

Ecto- and endoparasites are vectors for disease, some of which are public health concerns given their potential for zoonosis (see 2.19 One Health). The Companion Animal Parasite Council (CAPC) provides guidelines on how to screen for and ultimately prevent infestation and infection [4, 5]. However, individuals may be at greater risk for contracting disease depending upon lifestyle, geographical state of residence, and travel [5]. For example, kittens that will maintain some degree of outdoor living are likely to be exposed to *Taenia taeniaeformis*, a tapeworm that is contracted when cats hunt and ingest infected mice. Fecal screening is an essential way to protect patient and client health.

Risk factors should be discussed in the consultation room, particularly if immunocompromised individuals reside in the home (see 4.5 Prevention and Control of Parasites).

6.12.9 Vaccine Considerations

Core vaccinations are recommended, if not required by municipality, and often include FVRCP (for kittens), DA2PP (for puppies), and rabies virus (for both, in enzootic areas) [4, 5]. American Animal Hospital Association (AAHA), American Association of Feline Practitioners (AAFP), and World Small Animal Veterinary Association (WSAVA) vaccination guidelines are available to establish evidence-based protocols for developing protective, acquired immunity [4, 5, 8]. However, the veterinarian's experience as well as the individual patient's needs and risk factors determine how many vaccines should be administered at once (see 4.3 Prevention and Control of Infectious Diseases).

Additional noncore (elective) vaccinations may or may not be necessary, depending upon the patient's anticipated lifestyle and exposure to conspecifics (see 9.11 Vaccination).

Some vaccinations, such as those protective against *Bordetella bronchiseptica,* may be formulated for different routes of administration: oral, intranasal, or injectable. These products require the clinician to consider which option offers the most protection to the patient while still allowing the patient to meet client expectations concerning performance. For instance, working dogs rely heavily upon scent to perform their function. These patients would least benefit from an intranasal vaccination, which could interfere with their ability to perform.

EXAMPLES

A 6-month-old female bloodhound puppy presents for ovariohysterectomy. Her blood pressure is measured as part of her preoperative exam. You recall that hounds consistently have blood pressures that register 10–20 mmHg higher than in mixed-breeds [9].

A 5-month-old male Labrador retriever puppy presents for unilateral blepharospasm and corneal edema after roughhousing with a kitten. There is a curvilinear sliver of fluorescein uptake at the central cornea. The client reports that this patient is in training to be a Seeing Eye dog. Aggressive treatment for corneal ulceration is initiated to preserve this patient's vision.

TAKE-AWAYS

- There is no one-size-fits-all approach to the care of a veterinary patient, particularly puppies and kittens.

- Beginning with the initial wellness visit, all consultations and associated veterinary care should be tailored to the patient.
- Although many puppies and kittens share certain care recommendations, such as core vaccinations, their individual needs can and will vary based upon lifestyle, geography, exposure to conspecifics, and travel plans.
- Areas to explore with new puppies and kittens include, but are not limited to, breed, behavior, diet, parasite control, reproductive health, and vaccination protocol
- Pet-specific care strengthens the VCPR by matching patient needs with client expectations.

MISCELLANEOUS

6.12.10 Cautions

Pet-specific care requires an initial investment of time to take a thorough history, elicit the client's perspective, and individualize recommendations. This investment may not be considered economical or efficient by some practice managers but the veterinarian should resist the urge to abbreviate the initial new puppy/kitten visit. There is not one script for care that fits everyone, and clients do not appreciate an assembly line approach to veterinary practice. Clients are also more likely to comply when recommendations are crafted to fit the patient instead of the other way around.

References

1 Ackerman, L. (2011). *Genetic Connection: A Guide to Health Problems in Purebred Dogs*, 2e. Lakewood, CO: AAHA Press.

2 Gough, A., Thomas, A., and O'Neill, D. (2018). *Breed Predispositions to Disease in Dogs and Cats*, 3e. Hoboken, NJ: Wiley.

3 Scarlett, J.M., Salman, M.D., New, J.G. Jr. et al. (1999). Reasons for relinquishment of companion animals in U.S. animal shelters: selected health and personal issues. *J. Appl. Anim. Welf. Sci.* 2: 41–57.

4 Bartges, J., Boynton, B., Vogt, A.H. et al. (2012). AAHA canine life stage guidelines. *J. Am. Anim. Hosp. Assoc.* 48: 1–11.

5 Vogt, A.H., Rodan, I., Brown, M. et al. (2010). AAFP-AAHA feline life stage guidelines. *J. Am. Anim. Hosp. Assoc.* 46: 70–85.

6 Kustritz, M.V.R. (2007). Determining the optimal age for gonadectomy of dogs and cats. *J. Am. Vet. Med. Assoc.* 231: 1665–1675.

7 Reichler, I.M. (2009). Gonadectomy in cats and dogs: a review of risks and benefits. *Reprod. Domest. Anim.* 44 (Suppl. 2): 29–35.

8 Day, M.J., Horzinek, M.C., Schultz, R.D. et al. (2016). WSAVA guidelines for the vaccination of dogs and cats. *J. Small Anim. Pract.* 57: 4–8.

9 Acierno, M.J., Brown, S., Coleman, A.E. et al. (2018). ACVIM consensus statement: guidelines for the identification, evaluation, and management of systemic hypertension in dogs and cats. *J. Vet. Intern. Med.* 32: 1803–1822.

Recommended Reading

Bartges, J., Boynton, B., Vogt, A.H. et al. (2012). AAHA canine life stage guidelines. *J. Am. Anim. Hosp. Assoc.* 48 (1): 1–11.

Day, M.J., Horzinek, M.C., Schultz, R.D. et al. (2016). Guidelines for the vaccination of dogs and cats. *J. Small Anim. Pract.* 57: E1–E45.

Gough, A., Thomas, A., and O'Neill, D. (2018). *Breed Predispositions to Disease in Dogs and Cats*, 3e. Hoboken, NJ: Wiley.

Scherk, M.A., Ford, R.B., Gaskell, R.M. et al. (2013). 2013 AAFP feline vaccination advisory panel report. *J. Feline Med. Surg.* 15: 785–808.

Vogt, A.H., Rodan, I., Brown, M. et al. (2010). AAFP-AAHA feline life stage guidelines. *J. Am. Anim. Hosp. Assoc.* 46: 70–85.

6.13

Delivering Feline-Friendly Care

Kim Kendall, BVSc, MANZCVS (Cat Medicine and Animal Behaviour)

Feline-Friendly Care, Roseville, NSW, Australia

BASICS

6.13.1 Summary

Many people enjoy the company of their cats but may not understand what cats need. For many veterinary clinics, managing the fractious feline patient while not upsetting the owner is a delicate balance. By paying attention to the species-specific needs of cats, making some clinic changes and educating owners about managing their cat, clinics can expect to have more consultations that have calmer cats and happier cat people.

6.13.2 Terms Defined

Cat-Friendly Practices: Veterinary clinics where attention to the process of transporting, attending to the examination, testing and treatment of clients' cats has been planned and orchestrated to minimize distress to feline patients.

Fear-Free Homes and Clinics: A broad group of recommendations that encompass the environment and husbandry of pets in the home and in the veterinary clinic. The concepts are based on the view of the pets rather than the human participants and are designed to improve the welfare of pets in all places.

Feline-Friendly Care (FFC): Quiet, calm, controlled cat care, respecting the individual cat's preferences and health parameters. FFC also involves the use of in-home and outpatient management of the most important feline diseases and disabilities.

Hypercarnivore: This term refers to specialized digestion and metabolism requiring elements only available from animal (meat) sources. Shared with dolphins, spiders, ferrets, owls, and alligators.

MAIN CONCEPTS

6.13.3 The Ecology of the Cat

Cats and humans began co-habiting about 10 000 years ago, when cats were thought to have moved closer to human habitats to take advantage of animals exploiting grain stores. Cats are considered hypercarnivores by ecologists and have an essential requirement for meat. They are remarkable hunters, employing an ambush strategy to snatch unwary prey. Their claws are strong, their teeth are efficient daggers, and their athleticism is remarkable. The little domestic cat has the added problem that, while out hunting, they may become prey and be eaten or injured themselves.

Of the limited number of species of animals that have undergone the process of domestication, cats have probably had the least intervention by humans. Cats demonstrated that they were capable of surviving without much input by humans; mate selection and breeding were not controlled by humans and cats were left to do the useful vermin control without much interference.

Now domestic cats live as companion animals and can be very good at this role. They are often recommended for busy people who live in high-density housing as cats are quiet and do not need external exercise and can be left on their own for long workdays. However, while this does meet many of their needs (social contact after hunting alone could be considered to be mimicked by people going to work/school and coming home), they express their bonds with others differently from what people expect, resulting in misunderstandings such as sprayed urine, hiding cats, and scratched humans.

There is a lot that can be done to improve how people (owners and the healthcare team) interact with cats. Owners will need guidance and encouragement.

6.13.3.1 The Keys to Cat Health – Physical, Mental, and Social Health

All cats benefit if their owners understand more about cats in general and their cat in particular. The information needs to be reinforced by all the healthcare team at every visit. It requires them to do a minimum of training and will help them provide the best care they can for the cat. It also needs to be reinforced that this applies in sickness as well as in health.

6.13.3.2 Feeding

All cats are fascinated by food. As hypercarnivores, they have to be fussy, as their digestive tract is short. In addition, their vitamin, fatty acid, and amino acid requirements are specific, and a reduced capacity to detoxify components of plants (e.g., aspirin) means the cat is easily poisoned. The feline habit of licking their coats to cleanliness also makes them susceptible to ingesting air-borne intoxicants – including lead from paint, polychlorinated biphenyls (PCBs), pollens from lilies, grease from diesel, inorganic pesticides blown in on the wind – the list is as long as your imagination.

There is a huge amount of information and pseudoinformation available on feeding a cat. As a rule, recommend feeding the best-quality food an owner can afford. Because of the vagueness with which some pet food manufacturers are allowed to label their products, the wording they use should be checked carefully.

If the cat can catch rats or mice or has outdoor access, then they will balance their needs themselves. Interestingly, insects, mollusks, honeybees, and spiders have a very high level of taurine in them, which may explain the hunting habits of young cats especially, since cats have an irreducible metabolic requirement for taurine.

Cats can be vegans or vegetarians, and can be fed raw diets, but the supplementation required is more complex than most owners will cope with.

An easier way to the "best" recipe for cats is to look for a complete and balanced diet off the shelf, from a reputable manufacturer, and supplement it with a "little of what the cat likes."

Hunting is at the core of what it is to be a cat. It is pleasurable for a cat, releasing dopamine in the brain. Food presentation and play parameters that mimic hunting (without anyone getting hurt) are essential substitutes for the cat which does not go outside. Reductions in wildlife capture for those cats which do go outside to hunt and forage can be achieved using brightly colored collar attachments (e.g., http://birdsbesafe.com) and flashing light attachments (LED collars) and by controlling the time cats go out.

6.13.3.3 Parasite Control

Why worry about parasites? Because they carry disease, create irritation, and some are zoonotic to humans. It will be necessary to devise a parasite control program that deals with both internal and external parasites (see 4.5 Prevention and Control of Parasites).

6.13.3.4 Clean Toilet

Only 25% of cat owners even notice house soiling with urine [1], but once they do, 50% seek veterinary advice – the others either ignore it or relinquish the cat, so spraying (sometimes colloquially referred to as pee-mail) is a big deal.

It is generally accepted that confined cats need a clean, private toilet. However, few owners are aware that kittens at 3 weeks old start – independently of their mother – to scratch up dirt and other diggable or sand-like material, in a secluded place, to create a hole to eliminate in and then cover over. This behavior is purely instinctive and appears nonselective in young cats.

What the adult cat wants to eliminate in or on, though, is learned and individual. This means that if a cat is not using a litter tray, the owner needs to assess why. As a rule of thumb in decoding the message: if the urine (or feces) is near the tray, then the location is OK, but the litter substrate is unsuitable (dirty, wrong type, tray too small), and the solution is to get another tray or clean it more regularly, make the substrate deeper or a different type. If the urine is under a window or near a door to the outside, then something outside (most likely another cat) is the problem and no amount of litter trays will solve the problem. The cat is likely marking the boundaries of its territory.

Eliminating away from the tray is always a message, never a mistake, and the owner and veterinary team have to work together to decode the message and fix the problem (see 6.11 Treating Animals with Behavior Problems). No cat ever changed voluntarily – the environment has to change so the cat can cope and then the litter tray will become the preferred elimination site again.

6.13.4 Transport – The Biggest Barrier to Feline Healthcare?

Kittens can be trained surprisingly easily. They are expecting instructions from their mothers and siblings and are much more easily influenced than an adult cat.

The cat carrier is a signal for many cats that they will soon be undergoing an unpleasant experience, which starts with being confined, may include transport by car or other vehicles and result in them being out of their territory and, worse, maybe in another cat's territory. The noise, smell, and instability of the carrier during transport all add to the unpleasant experience for the cat. No wonder some cats vomit, urinate, and defecate on their way to the veterinary practice, but it need not be that way.

Training a kitten to go into a carrier is as simple as (gently) picking them up and putting them in a suitable carrier, then helping them out again, repeated three or four times a day for the first few days. The carrier becomes "no big deal." Turning the carrier into a "safe place" and bed works even better, and there is nothing wrong with bribing a cat to go into the carrier.

For the cat that needs to be transported with no time for training, there are some tips to help the owner make their veterinary visit on time. A cat will observe its owner very closely and will pretty much always know when they plan to take the cat out of the house. Owners can have the carrier ready in another room, then use a pillowcase to scoop the cat up (head first into the open end of the pillowcase). The end can be tied off (yes, the cat can breathe – you've noticed they breathe under duvets) and then load the cat carefully into the carrier and release the tie. The pillowcase can then absorb any elimination products. There are a number of other methods demonstrated on the internet. Check a few out and consider showing them to clients when they bring their cat in. However, the preferred method is always to train appropriately from the start, and avoid causes of fear, anxiety, and stress.

6.13.5 Mental and Social Health – Starts Young and Is Critical for Future Behavior and Adaptability

Cats are known to be very adept at making associations. This is just learning – and cats have to be good at it as they will not often get a second chance to evade a predator or find some prey. Owners rarely take the time to teach their cats behaviors that are beneficial to cat and owner, but it is time well spent. An early start is recommended as this helps the kitten develop good habits for a lifetime.

There are several critical stages of growth in cats – much of it, up to the age of 16 weeks, is preprogrammed and all healthy kittens go through them (see 6.1 Normal Development Stages of Dogs and Cats). Humans are particularly enamored of the "object play" of kittens 8–10 weeks old (when patting and chasing small objects occur), but not so keen on the "social play" of 12–16 weeks old (when hunting and biting all-comers occur). For both of these periods, the kitten is honing their coordination and muscle strength for hunting, and their social, defense, and fighting skills for later in life. The first stage is "cute," the second commonly labeled as "feline terrorist" or other tag. If you can explain to the owner the reasons for this developmental drive, and how to redirect the more painful play strategies, there will be a happier and healthier relationship between owner and cat. The advice basically revolves around setting aside enough time each day to play with the kittens – and playing their kind of game. Pounce and kill small furry toys (never hands and feet). Adult cats also need at least 2×20 minutes of pounce-and-play daily, especially if they are confined.

There is a wealth of information on how to feed and maintain the health of kittens without mothers (aka fostering orphan kittens). However, the problems associated with future mental and social health that occur with hand-rearing any species – while well researched and well known among behaviorists and zookeepers – remain unaddressed and unacknowledged among the kitten nursery and fostering community. A kitten raised in isolation from other cats and kittens will have long-term negative effects to their behavioral stability and sociability. Social isolation affects all the kittens raised alone or even in pairs, if they have only human contact, and no input from socially stable adult cats.

Everyone needs their mother, and kittens do best if raised with a sociable female until 12–14 weeks old. At the very least, kittens should be kept in litters or groups of between three and six kittens to develop in a more flexible social environment. You can assure novice owners that two kittens, raised together from 10 weeks old, will almost certainly remain feline friends for their lifetime. About 5% of pairs will fall out, but some of these pairs can have their bond restored.

If the owner plans to keep the cat indoors for its whole life, a second feline (not canine, rabbit or human) may be beneficial for that cat's long-term mental and social health. An indoor-only cat is obviously much safer, will live longer and be physically healthier than cats who go outside. However, it is effectively in solitary confinement, and this is known to disturb even adult humans. The easy solution is get two kittens, under 6 months old, keep them indoors with a scratching post (furniture damage is another source of irritation for owners), and provide suitable toys and foraging opportunities. The kittens will play hunting games with each other, instead of human toes and hands, and will learn manners from each other, in cat language.

Kittens can easily be trained to (i) hold still while their nails are clipped – gently play with their toes and learn to extend the nail from the sheath, (ii) swallow a pill – pretend a piece of chicken is a pill and just pop it down the back of their throat, and (iii) have their coat ruffled which may reduce the tendency to bite when their back is petted. Practicing these skills will set most cats up to be more cooperative at the times when they need husbandry and medical procedures performed (see 6.8 Managing Routine Procedures to Minimize Problems).

Cats will typically warn before they bite, but owners have to know the warning signs. Most cats do not enjoy having their tummy rubbed or being stroked near the base of the tail. Almost all cats like being rubbed around their checks and above the eyes in the oily areas where they naturally rub objects and other cats.

Adult cats can be trained – but actually they spend more time training their owners. The feline brain has very little prefrontal cortex, which means they react quickly, without much inhibition ("executive function"). Again, very useful for a small, solo hunter which is also hunted. It also means that cats do not have a concept of "other" (that we know of). Like toddlers, they think you already know what they are thinking and that, very definitely, they are the center of the universe.

How many cats is the right number for owners to have? It actually depends on the cats, rather than the humans! Important factors to consider are the amount of living space (including vertical space), the number and distribution of resources available and whether the cats have the choice and opportunity to remove themselves from situations in which they do not want to participate. Cats tend to use a time-share arrangement for accessing resources when confined. When there is insufficient space and resources (remember cats do not wait their turn for litter trays) then there may be conflict. Sometimes cats will just move out and find another owner. But if they are confined, they cannot do this and must find other ways of coping, which often leads to problem behaviors.

6.13.5.1 Sampling Methods in a Feline-Friendly Fashion

Cats are always more cooperative with their owner around. FFC aims to keep the owner safe and the cat calm, so allowing the owner to be present during the sampling procedure is recommended in most situations. Cats can generally be gently restrained and positioned to get urine and blood samples (e.g., "low-stress handling" and Fear Free® techniques).

Urine is very useful for providing information about the health of a cat. Cystocentesis is a relatively easy procedure that generally gives high-yield results. However, should a cat not have sufficient urine for cystocentesis, there are other methods of sampling such as free catch samples using nonabsorbent materials.

It is also possible to test urine from the bottom of the carrier (although it cannot be cultured), and any blood should be discounted if the cat has fleas. The urine specific gravity (USG), glucose, pH, and protein levels are accurate enough to use. If the urine has been absorbed (into paper litter, a paper or cloth towel), then rehydrating the sample with a few drops of water and pressing a dipstick onto the surface will show whether there is glucose or blood in the urine. These are two very useful pieces of information for veterinarians and owners alike.

Collecting *blood* requires some preparation before the cat is even taken from its carrier. Have all materials ready and use a small needle and syringe. Avoid alcohol on the skin prepuncture, and handle the specimen gently to prevent hemolysis. A great deal can be done with small samples if prepared carefully and put in microtubes.

Sample for blood glucose from the ear vein, using a glucometer, rather than trying to get extra for a sodium fluoride/potassium oxalate (NaF/Kox) tube. The sample will be accurate if the cat has not been sitting around stressed for an hour or been permitted to "paddle." Muscle activity accompanied by distress raises the blood glucose in nondiabetic cats.

Consider whether analysis is going to change your recommendation before attempting to get a *feces* sample!

In general, avoid uncomfortable procedures where possible. Taking a core temperature should be done with a digital thermometer for accuracy. It is only relevant for a cat which is not eating or very lethargic – including times when a cat's body temperature drops so low it stops moving.

EXAMPLES

6.13.6 Fractious Cats

A clinic is seeing a large number of cats that are difficult to handle in the consultation room and in hospital. The clinic decides to implement a cat owner education program after several serious bites to staff members. They develop some information boards about species-specific behavior, discuss and demonstrate carrier training, tableting, nail trimming, and handling cats with clients. They offer a kitten kindergarten program for new owners which covers these topics. They implement cat-friendly handling and previsit anxiolytic medications. They have pheromone diffusers on in the clinic. Staff members practice handling techniques and sedation protocols for very distressed and aggressive cats.

A review 12 months later shows that staff members have not been injured beyond scratches and clients feel better about bringing their cats to the clinic.

TAKE-AWAYS

- Train early to make husbandry procedures nonconfrontational.
- Think of the mental and social health of kittens, not just their medical health, as this sets them up to be lifelong companions.
- Work with the natural behaviors of cats rather than against them.
- Teach cats that the carrier is a safe place.
- Be prepared with all equipment before getting the cat out of the carrier – the best tests are done on unstressed felines.

- Encourage owners to provide sufficient resources distributed in the area available for their cats to help reduce conflicts.

MISCELLANEOUS

6.13.7 Cautions

Every cat is representative, but no cat is average. Each must be assessed individually, and a custom-made approach designed and implemented. Cat body language is subtle, and most messages are defensive and distance increasing.

Any cat can put you in hospital. Be respectful of their armory – they only use it for defense, essentially to preserve life, and that perspective matters. You will be warned beforehand so know your cat signals!

Reference

1 Data from 2013 survey by Cats Protection. www.cats.org.uk/wolverhampton/news/behaviour-survey

6.14

Pain Prevention, Management, and Conditioning

Robin Downing, DVM, MS, DAAPM, DACVSMR, CVPP, CCRP

The Downing Center for Animal Pain Management, Windsor, CO, USA

BASICS

6.14.1 Summary

Pet owners fear pain and suffering for their beloved animal family members. By partnering with and educating clients, veterinary healthcare team members can help to prevent pain in young healthy patients, and to better manage pet pain once it is present. Leveraging nutrition, controlled exercise and conditioning, as well as physical and pharmacological medicine means happier (and healthier) patients.

6.14.2 Terms Defined

Acupuncture: A form of medical treatment in which thin needles are inserted into the body at very specific locations in order to exert a neuromodulatory effect.

Cannabidiol (CBD): A compound found in the flower of the cannabis plant. CBD is nonintoxicating and has been investigated for use in pets for seizure control and pain management.

Central Sensitization: A condition within the nervous system in which there is the development and maintenance of a chronic pain state. This is sometimes referred to as *wind-up* and reflects a state of abnormal nervous system reactivity.

Chiropractic: A form of medical treatment that relies on the restoration of normal movement throughout the musculoskeletal system, especially in the spine, by way of small-amplitude, high-velocity adjustments.

Maladaptive Pain: A chronic pain state in which the pain is out of proportion to tissue damage and that persists long after tissues have healed. This is "pain as disease."

Medical Massage: The application of specific massage techniques to a specific issue the patient is showing.

Multimodal Pain Management: A balanced approach to pain management using more than one treatment at once to deliver a synergistic effect that is superior to monotherapy.

Nutraceutical: A nutritional supplement that behaves like a drug without being a pharmaceutical agent.

Nutrogenomics: The study of the effects of nutrition on the expression of genes on the DNA, and focuses on how specific nutrients may affect health.

Physiotherapy: Physiotherapy (also referred to as physical therapy) involves the use of physical medicine techniques and modalities (such as therapeutic laser, neuromuscular electrical stimulation, etc.) to restore mobility and function.

Therapeutic Exercise: Physical activities that are used to restore function and build physical strength, balance, and endurance.

MAIN CONCEPTS

6.14.3 Introduction

The human–animal bond is a powerful force (see 2.14 Benefits of the Human–Animal Bond). With advances in disease and parasite prevention, pets are now living longer and better than ever. Advancing age is often accompanied by health concerns like the development of osteoarthritis (OA) and its attendant inflammation and pain (see 8.20 Team Strategies for Arthritis). Pet owners want their beloved animal family members to live as long as possible, and they are rightly concerned about the potential for pain to undermine their pets' quality of life. Our clients fear that their pets will suffer, and they want the veterinary healthcare team's help and guidance to prevent that suffering from happening.

The good news for pets and pet owners is that there are excellent strategies for preventing pain before it happens, and for managing inflammation and pain once degenerative changes occur in the body.

6.14.4 Pain Prevention Strategy #1: Keep Them Lean

The rise of overweight and obese pets has paralleled that in humans (see 6.15 Approaching Obesity on a Pet-Specific Basis). Across cultures, food is equated with love. As a consequence, many pets grow too quickly as puppies and kittens which results in more fat cells in the body, setting the stage for a lifelong battle of the bulge. The single most important pain prevention strategy the veterinary team can adopt is to partner with pet owners to help them keep their cats and dogs lean from the very beginning.

Many pet owners have been misinformed about feeding their puppies or kittens. They often think that young animals need an endless supply of food in order to grow properly. This is an unfortunate myth as it leads to higher numbers of fat cells in the body, resulting in juvenile-onset obesity, an increased risk for degenerative diseases like OA and cancer, shortened life expectancy, and compromised life quality (see 8.25 Team Strategies for Weight Management). Pet owners want the veterinary team to partner with them for the benefit of their pets. Our partnership should start at the beginning of the pet's life with the recommendation of a specific nutrient profile and a specific portion per day divided into a specific number of meals – generally 2–3 meals per day.

Create the expectation that managing nutrition and portions will be a lifelong process. Nutritional needs change over time as the pet's body changes. Allow your clients to know that they can rely on you to provide evidence-based nutritional advice that will help maximize the health of their pet throughout the pet's lifetime (see 9.15 Nutritional Counseling). Of course, keeping your patients lean with appropriate nutrition means keeping up your own knowledge on the topic. Fortunately, continuing education options abound!

What about pets who come to us already overweight and obese? All is not lost. The clinical nutritional science of nutrogenomics has revealed that there are genes on the DNA associated with obesity, and a different set of genes is associated with lean body composition. Further, we now know that we can alter the expression of those genes through specific combinations of nutrients – upregulating the "lean" genes and downregulating the "fat" genes. This allows the pet's body to burn fat selectively as its primary energy source, preserving muscle. Thus, a specific nutritional recommendation alongside specific portion recommendations is critical to success.

Don't forget about snacks. Pet owners want to – and will – provide snacks for their dogs and cats. A reasonable recommendation for easy-to-use snacks includes air-popped popcorn and water-based vegetables like green beans, broccoli, and cauliflower. Be aware of vegetables with high starch or sugar content like yams or carrots. Also, be mindful of any mineral concentration that may occur in some vegetables, for instance calcium, which could negatively affect pets with a metabolic tendency toward urocystolith formation.

A critical key to success in helping a pet achieve a lean body composition is client engagement and persistence (see 6.15 Approaching Obesity on a Pet-Specific Basis, and 8.25 Team Strategies for Weight Management). Physique remodeling takes time and will only succeed if the healthcare team creates realistic expectations for the timeline involved, and remains in partnership with the client throughout the process.

On the human side of weight loss, one reason for the success of programs like Weight Watchers® (now WW) is accountability – regular weigh-ins and evaluation of consumed food. Consider an accountability program for your practice. Such a program works like this.

- The pet is identified as overweight or obese.
- A nutrient profile and portion are prescribed.
- An approved snack list is provided.
- An appointment is set for every 4–5 weeks for a no-charge weigh-in for the pet.
- At the weigh-in the profile and portion are reviewed, confirmed, and adjusted if needed.
- The next weigh-in is then set.

This kind of program provides regular opportunities to celebrate success and to fine tune feeding if needed. It provides incentive and rewards the owner for their diligence and attention to detail. Further, it celebrates the human–animal bond, and reinforces the client's relationship with the practice and healthcare team. Finally, it enhances job satisfaction for the veterinary team and allows for the cultivation of one-on-one relationships with clients and their pets. Overall pet healthcare delivery is enhanced. Regular weigh-ins provide the team with the opportunity to ask "Is there anything else you need today?" allowing the client to bring up any health concerns that could prompt a follow-up appointment. In this scenario, everyone wins!

Once an appropriate body composition is achieved, a specific maintenance nutrient profile and portion can be prescribed, and the need for ongoing vigilance is communicated to the client. This strategy lays a strong foundation for lifelong care of the pet by enhancing the owner's understanding of the profound impact something so routine – like daily feeding – can have on their beloved animal companion's health, wellness, and longevity.

6.14.5 Pain Prevention Strategy #2: Keep Them Active

An important key to pet pain prevention and keeping pets lean is to keep them active. Calories burned must exceed calories ingested. Pet owners may not appreciate or understand the positive impact of regular exercise on their pet's health, wellness, and longevity. The veterinary team can and should play a role in guiding pet owners about appropriate activity for particular dogs and cats.

For instance, growing puppies whose growth plates are open and generating new bone should not have the regular rhythmic concussion on those growth plates that occurs with running at a steady pace for long periods. It is better for young growing puppies to have a varied pace, so walking with short bursts of running or playing is more appropriate. Swimming, once they know how, is another great way for puppies to be active and burn calories.

Adult dogs who have a normal body composition score and do not have any joint issues like OA can benefit from many different types of activity. Walks, runs with their owners, off-leash play like chasing a ball or a hunting dummy, and swimming make for lots of fun and build cardiovascular fitness.

Old age is not a disease so old dogs do not, by definition, need to be retired from regular activity. Regular walks provide ongoing benefit. A dog who has enjoyed running and swimming its entire life can continue to participate in those activities until any painful conditions emerge. As their bodies change with age, it is likely that OA will develop at some point in one or another joint. This is the time in a dog's life when a partnership with the veterinary healthcare team becomes especially important. When issues like OA emerge, it is critical that pain be identified early so that appropriate pain relief, joint support, and activity modification can be implemented. Dogs are very willing to mask their discomfort and push on, even though to do so may result in injury or harm to their bodies.

Our job as healthcare providers is to advocate on behalf of beings who cannot advocate for themselves. Identifying pain and its source (whenever possible), relieving that pain, and modifying activities as needed are all a part of that advocacy (see 2.16 Pain and Pain Management). Dog owners often mistake changes in their dogs' stamina or interest in being active as "just getting old." This is a myth that we are obligated to dispel. Partnership with clients for the benefit of our patients provides the opportunity for such myth busting.

What about cats? Cats need to be active as well, although our approach will be quite different from that with dogs. Cats are instinctive hunters and leading an indoor lifestyle, while the safest option, can turn them into bored couch potatoes. There are many excellent (and easy) ways to provide environmental enrichment that can keep cats mentally stimulated and physically active. The American Association of Feline Practitioners is one source for ideas about how to play with cats:

https://catfriendly.com/cat-care-at-home/playing-with-your-cat

Cats can learn to walk with a harness and leash, so don't rule that out as an exercise option. Interactive toys, interactive feeders, and interactive treat dispensers are all ways to engage a cat in various activities. Providing vertical climbing options and placing food at various levels uses the cat's climbing and hunting drives to our (and their) advantage.

Cats who stop "going vertical" are sending a signal that they are painful – a signal we must not ignore. Remember to ask about a cat's activities during regular examinations in order to identify changes that may signal pain and require intervention.

6.14.6 Pain Prevention Strategy #3: Keep Them Strong

Alongside appropriate nutrition and regular exercise, getting strong and staying strong can help prevent pain in pets. Therapeutic exercises can target specific parts of the body to facilitate good movement and function. Strength-building activities can include simple functional exercises like the following.

- Sit-to-stand – have the dog sit, then stand up in place; repeat for up to 10 repetitions per set, three sets per session, 1–2 sessions per day
- Backward walking – This skill must be taught. Work up to 20 steps, first on a level surface, then backward up an incline, then backward down a decline.
- Serpentine walking – walk along a curb with two to three steps in the street, then two to three steps on the curb; repeat for two to three blocks.

- Diagonal walking – walk up a hill at an angle, then down at an angle; change directions in order to put the both sides of the body toward the uphill side.
- Dancing – hold the dog up so that it is standing on its rear legs and step forward three to four steps, then step backward three to four steps; repeat for two to three cycles.
- Slow walking up steps and down steps – the goal here is to have the dog use each leg one at a time while stepping up and then stepping down.
- Air mattress walking – a partially inflated air mattress creates an unstable surface that focuses effort on core strength, balance, and proprioception.
- Sand/beach walking/running – aand creates an unstable surface that focuses effort on core strength, balance, and proprioception.
- Walking in shallow water – the effort to move forward against the surface tension of shallow water works both limb extensors and core muscles.

Additional therapeutic exercise options are given in the resources in the Recommended Reading list.

As for cats, climbing and scratching activities are useful for strength building and maintenance.

6.14.7 Once Pain Is Present

Once pain and inflammation from OA are present, an appropriate multimodal pain management strategy must be designed and implemented in order to break the pain cycle, and allow the pet to engage in regular activities (see 8.20 Team Strategies for Arthritis).

Multimodal pain management typically utilizes one or more pharmaceuticals, an appropriate joint support nutrient profile, joint support nutritional supplements, and physical medicine (see 2.16 Pain and Pain Management). Nonsteroidal antiinflammatory drugs (NSAIDs) form the cornerstone of relieving chronic pain. A metabolic profile should be in place to set a baseline in case a patient experiences an adverse event from the medication. Some individuals will demonstrate sensitivity to an NSAID – generally gastrointestinal sensitivity. Should that occur, consider offering a different NSAID; sensitivity to one does not necessarily mean sensitivity to them all. That said, should an individual experience an adverse reaction to two different NSAIDs, they should not receive NSAIDs.

Complementing the NSAID, gabapentin exerts its effects on the dorsal horn of the spinal cord to modulate the pain experience. Gabapentin remains an important part of managing chronic maladaptive pain in humans, and has demonstrated its utility for chronic maladaptive pain in dogs

and cats. In addition, amantadine, an NMDA receptor antagonist, can also complement the effects of NSAIDs.

When choosing joint support nutrition and nutraceuticals, it is important to review the most current data and clinical studies to ensure that patients are receiving products whose use is grounded in evidence. One emerging pain management strategy utilizes hemp-derived CBD. Initial studies demonstrate efficacy for chronic maladaptive pain. It is important to utilize products whose contents have been verified by independent analysis, as well as products that have been assessed for efficacy and safety in the target species.

Physical medicine and physiotherapy relies on the use of modalities (for instance, therapeutic laser, electrical stimulation, targeted pulsed electromagnetic field therapy), as well as hands-on techniques often referred to as "manual therapy." Physical medicine options that may be chosen for chronically painful pets include:

- medical acupuncture
- chiropractic
- medical massage
- physiotherapy.

EXAMPLES

Sage was a 9-year-old spayed female golden retriever whose owner was considering euthanasia due to Sage's declining quality of life. The owner reported that Sage could barely walk across the living room of the home, and she had difficulty rising from a down position. Sage no longer sought out interactions with the human family members. She was morbidly obese at 40 kg (her ideal body weight was 25 kg) and pain was detected along her back, over her rostral thorax, and in the hip flexors. Diagnostics revealed hypothyroidism and thyroid replacement hormone was prescribed. A nutrient profile that leveraged the principles of nutrogenomics was prescribed in order to upregulate Sage's metabolism. A multimodal pain management plan including a NSAID, gabapentin, a therapeutic dose of EPA, and a joint support nutraceutical was put in place.

A regimen of controlled, timed walks for calorie expenditure and cardiac conditioning, as well as therapeutic exercises for strength building, was initiated. Exercise was expanded as Sage's abilities increased. Within eight months, Sage had achieved an ideal composition and was enthusiastically capable of walking 3–5 miles per day with her owner. Gradually the NSAID and gabapentin were reduced and ultimately discontinued.

TAKE-AWAYS

- Overweight and obesity are much easier to prevent than to reverse.
- Chronic maladaptive pain is easier to prevent than to manage.
- Conditioning for lifelong health, wellness, and activity is best begun early in a pet's life.
- Cats should not be exempted from our conditioning and pain prevention protocols.
- Pet owners want our help and guidance to allow their animal companions to live as long and as well as possible.

MISCELLANEOUS

6.14.8 Cautions

Normalizing body composition is not a "quick fix." Nor is it a "one size fits all" proposition. It is important to consider the whole patient, all of its particular medical issues and any quirks, as well as the environment and lifestyle of the home and family. We must ask questions in order to better understand the patient and family, but we must be sure to *listen* carefully so as not to jump to erroneous conclusions that could potentially undermine our success. We must create reasonable expectations about the outcomes we seek when working with a particular pet, and we must be ready to adjust our plan for a pet as needed, based on the progress that pet makes.

These same caveats apply as we work either to prevent pain or to reverse it once it is present. Each pet is an individual, and as such deserves our attention to the details of its life, family, environment, and activities of daily living. By taking the time to pay attention to the details, we can forge a rewarding and long-lasting relationship with both pet and pet parent.

Abbreviations

DNA   Deoxyribonucleic acid
EPA   Eicosapentaenoic acid
NMDA N-methyl-D-aspartate

Recommended Reading

Bockstahler, B., Levine, D., and Millis, D. (2004). *Essential Facts of Physiotherapy in Dogs and Cats*. Babenhausen, Germany: BE VetVerlag.

Gaynor, J. and Muir, W. (2015). *Handbook of Veterinary Pain Management*, 3e. Philadelphia, PA: Mosby.

Goldberg, M.E. and Tomlinson, J.E. (2017). *Physical Rehabilitation for Veterinary Technicians and Nurses*. Hoboken, NJ: Wiley Blackwell.

Millis, D. and Levine, D. (2014). *Canine Rehabilitation and Physical Therapy*, 2e. Philadelphia, PA: Saunders.

Zink, C. and van Dyke, J.B. (2018). *Canine Sports Medicine and Rehabilitation*, 2e. Hoboken, NJ: Wiley Blackwell.

6.15

Approaching Obesity on a Pet-Specific Basis

Ernie Ward, DVM, CVFT (Certified Veterinary Food Therapist)

Association for Pet Obesity Prevention, Ocean Isle Beach, NC, USA

BASICS

6.15.1   Summary

Obesity in dogs and cats is one of the most common diseases encountered in small animal veterinary practice, affecting approximately 20–40% of all pets. Weight-related co-morbidities such as diabetes, osteoarthritis, organ impairment, and many forms of cancer are increasingly common. The recognition, diagnosis, and treatment require the veterinary team to focus on the individual patient's needs, develop a comprehensive communication strategy, and offer sustainable treatment options.

6.15.2   Terms Defined

Body Condition Score (BCS):   A one to nine whole-integer scale used to describe a pet's morphological status and provide an estimate of body fat.

Muscle Condition Score (MCS):   Assessment of a patient's muscle mass graded as normal, mild, moderate, or severe muscle loss.

Narrative Nutritional History Taking: Using narrative veterinary medicine techniques to obtain a more accurate nutritional and lifestyle history.

Narrative Veterinary Medicine: Clinical communication technique utilizing open-ending questions to facilitate more open, thorough, truthful, and sensitive medical conversations.

Obesity: 30% above ideal body weight, equivalent to 8–9/9 using the preferred nine-point BCS system.

Patient-First Language: Communication technique that emphasizes the pet patient first, not the disease or medical condition, in order to decrease bias and judgment by veterinary professionals.

Resting Energy Requirements (RER):   An estimate based on metabolic body size of daily energy needed to sustain essential bodily functions.

MAIN CONCEPTS

Obesity or excess weight in dogs and cats is one of the most commonly diagnosed medical disorders in general veterinary practice. In the United States, an estimated 56% of dogs and 60% of cats are classified as overweight or obese [1], in the United Kingdom 46% of dogs, 34% of cats and 30% rabbits [2], and global estimates of overweight or obese pets range from 22% to 44% [3]. Veterinarians report that pet obesity is one of their primary health and welfare concerns for animals, with 98% of US veterinary professionals considering pet obesity "a significant problem" [4] and 60% of UK veterinarians saying, "obesity is the biggest health and welfare concern for UK pets" [5]. There is increasing evidence that obesity is beginning to affect dogs and cats in emerging countries, particularly Brazil and China [6]. Obesity is also reported to be increasing in growing animals, with studies documenting 21% of dogs overweight by 6 months of age [7].

In 2018, 25 of the world's largest and mosst respected veterinary organizations declared their support for the "Global Pet Obesity Initiative Position Statement," creating a standardized definition of obesity in dogs and cats, universal BCS, and "for the veterinary profession formally to recognize canine and feline obesity as a disease" [8]. Despite increasing prevalence rates, global awareness campaigns, and advances in treatments, many pet owners fail to recognize the risks of pet obesity and veterinarians struggle to accurately diagnose, effectively communicate with pet owners, and successfully treat pets with obesity.

6.15.3   Health Effects of Obesity

Small animal obesity has a multitude of contributors and causes, including overfeeding, inadequate physical activity, genetics, concurrent diseases (i.e., acromegaly, hyperadrenocorticism, osteoarthritis, heart, or respiratory disorders), hormonal imbalances, certain medications, microbiome alterations, potential environmental metabolic disruptors (i.e., bisphenol-A), and more. To effectively diagnose and treat obesity in dogs and cats, veterinary teams must eliminate other causal factors and use a combination of therapeutic approaches.

Diagnosing and treating a pet with obesity is important to preserve or improve well-being and quality of life. Obesity in dogs and cats can reduce life expectancy by 2–2.5 years [9] and negatively impact quality of life [10], and is associated with a wide variety of co-morbidities [11, 12]. Obesity contributes to metabolic derangements (including diabetes), can cause significant functional impairment (most notably respiratory, cardiovascular, and renal function) [13, 14], and is costly for pet owners [15]. Excess weight can exacerbate osteoarthritis and associated pain and debilitation [16] and is associated with many forms of cancer [17]. Overweight cats are more likely to be diagnosed with lower urinary tract disease, diabetes mellitus, respiratory disease, skin disorders, locomotor disease, and trauma [18].

Obesity has been shown to adversely affect a pet's quality of life [19]. Dogs with obesity that lose as little as 6% of their body weight experience a significant increase in overall enjoyment and quality of life, according to their owners. Mobility, activity levels, and human interaction all improve after successful weight reduction, often within 12 weeks of beginning a weight loss program.

6.15.4   Challenges to the Diagnosis and Treatment of Obesity

Many veterinary professionals struggle to educate and convince clients to begin or sustain a weight loss program for their pets. Veterinarians may lack communication training or educational tools to effectively implement change [20, 21]. Many veterinary clinics have few standardized medical or communication protocols, increasing the likelihood for inconsistent patient care and incomplete client service. In addition, many veterinarians report they are hesitant to discuss obesity with pet owners due to lack of time, concerns about compensation for their efforts, and doubts about effective treatments. Veterinary teams need to present a consistent, pet-specific approach to effectively treat pet obesity and overcome these clinical challenges (see 8.15 Delivering Information to Clients).

Many veterinarians are also apprehensive to inform a pet owner their dog or cat is obese [22]. Veterinarians fear a diagnosis of obesity will offend, upset, anger, or even cause the client to leave the practice. This hypothetical outcome can cause professional anxiety and discomfort, and may lead to avoidance of the topic [23]. Most people, including veterinary healthcare providers, often choose to ignore issues that make them uncomfortable or which they view as controversial. Despite these concerns, surveys show the majority of US pet owners appreciate a veterinarian's recognition of their pet's weight status and value their nutritional advice [1].

Veterinary teams may also become pessimistic when a pet owner ignores their nutritional advice or if a patient fails to successfully lose weight. This may lead veterinary teams to become discouraged, preventing them from addressing obesity and nutritional issues in the future. Obesity in dogs and cats is a complex, challenging, and emotionally charged topic for both pet owners and veterinary professionals. By recognizing the sensitivity of the topic and creating thoughtful communication tactics, veterinarians can more efficiently and effectively address the disease. Diagnosing and treating obesity is our professional responsibility, and we should approach it as any other serious disease. We must create effective communication and treatment strategies, involve our staff, and actively engage our clients to successfully resolve obesity.

6.15.5   Recognition of Overweight and Obesity

The first step in diagnosing obesity is to weigh the pet and perform a BCS (Figures 6.15.1 and 6.15.2). A MCS [24] is a helpful adjunct to body weight and BCS to more accurately assess a patient's physical status and categorization. We recommend using the universal 1–9 BCS scale using whole-integers validated by the World Small Animal Veterinary Association (WSAVA). In general terms, a BCS of 1–3 is "under ideal weight," 4–5 is "ideal," 6–9 "over ideal."

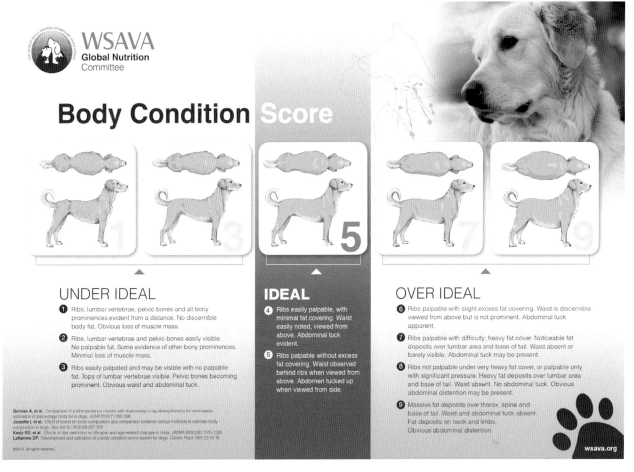

Figure 6.15.1 Canine body condition score. *Source:* Courtesy of the World Small Animal Veterinary Association. https://wsava.org/wp-content/uploads/2020/05/WSAVA-Global-Nutrition-Toolkit-English.pdf.

The Association for Pet Obesity Prevention's Global Pet Obesity Initiative Position Statement makes the following measurement recommendations and definition of obesity [8].

Our recommendation is that the term *obesity* be defined as 30% above ideal bodyweight. While excess bodyweight (overweight and obesity) represents a continuum and any cut-point for onset of disease is somewhat arbitrary (see below), this definition correlates with the determination of obesity in humans using the standard metrics such as body mass index (BMI) and abdominal circumference. It is also consistent and broadly supported by veterinary studies where there are associations with various co-morbid diseases, functional impairment, and decreased quality of life. The most practical clinical measure of adiposity is body condition score (BCS, see below), and 30% above ideal weight is equivalent to 8/9 using the preferred nine-point system.

However, defining obesity on the basis of "above ideal weight," rather than on the basis of condition score, is preferable because it enables veterinarians to use other strategies to identify the onset of obesity precisely in addition to definition by BCS. For example, if a veterinary practice recommends routine bodyweight and BCS assessment throughout life, and such practices formally identify and record the "healthy adult weight" of a dog or cat (i.e., an early-adult life bodyweight where BCS is ideal), weight gain could then be accurately quantified as a percentage change from the healthy adult weight, enabling the onset of obesity to be accurately determined.

Another key data point in identifying weight trends and obesity is comparing the pet's last known weight with the current measurement. Many dogs and cats will have a seemingly insignificant increase that clearly represents a long-term trend. By recognizing increase in bodyweight

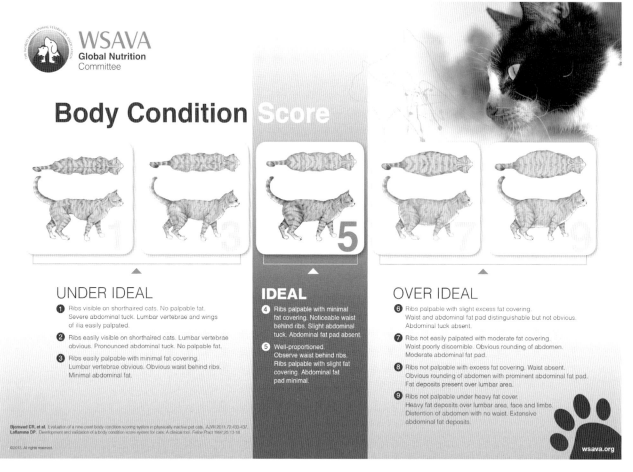

Figure 6.15.2 Feline body condition score. *Source:* Courtesy of the World Small Animal Veterinary Association. https://wsava.org/wp-content/uploads/2020/05/WSAVA-Global-Nutrition-Toolkit-English.pdf.

and adiposity early, interventions will be more successful and require less dramatic efforts. We recommend adding to each pet's physical exam report the last weight and BCS compared with current findings. This simple dataset can alert veterinarians to a possible emerging problem and establish that changes in diet, exercise, lifestyle, or additional diagnostic tests may be necessary.

6.15.6 Patient-First Language

The concept of weight bias and personal bias has been well documented in human medical literature [25]. "Fat shaming" is now recognized as a key barrier to treatment and successful outcomes in treating human obesity [26]. The American Medical Association (AMA) encourages physicians to use a "person-first language" approach to obesity [27]. We recommend a similar "patient-first language" strategy when discussing pet obesity. The terms "dog with obesity" or "cat with obesity" indicate to pet owners that

obesity is a disease and that medical and lifestyle interventions are required. When a pet is described as an "obese cat," this implies the cat (or the owner) is to blame for the condition and activates neurolinguistic pathways that dismiss the severity of the condition and a client's desire or ability to successfully change the pet's condition. In the same way, a veterinary professional would articulate "a dog with cancer" or "your dog has cancer," instead of "a cancer dog"; we advise using more compassionate and solutions-oriented patient-first language when discussing obesity with clients.

It is important that veterinary staff avoid using words such as "fat," "heavy," "chubby," "plump," or other derogatory terms. It is also essential that staff members do not passively diminish the importance of obesity by making statements such as "He's not that fat. I've seen worse" or "Most pets need to lose a little weight." Minimizing the potential severity of excess body fat in a patient undermines future weight loss counseling. The goal of the communication process is to gather information, not make a diagnosis or pronounce judgment. Veterinary teams should strive to create a clinic culture that understands and values preventive care, especially diet, lifestyle, and body condition, and seeks ways to enhance compassionate communication to support medical recommendations.

6.15.7 Narrative Nutritional History

The next step in diagnosing and treating obesity is to obtain a nutritional history. Consistency in communication and standards of care are needed for success in veterinary practice, especially weight-related disorders. Veterinarians should train their teams to communicate about a pet's diet, lifestyle, and quality of life with clients in a clear, medically sound, and methodical manner. Feeding and weight loss recommendations should be integrated into routine vaccination and wellness visits, puppy and kitten appointments, and sick pet examinations. Standards of care exist that encourage every veterinary team to evaluate a patient's nutrition as a "fifth vital sign" [28].

One of the most effective methods for inquiring about a pet's current diet and activity involves asking open-ended questions during an examination (see 9.2 Asking Good Questions). Open-ended questions allow a client to provide additional information, and foster collaborative decision making. Some veterinarians fear asking an open-ended question will lead the client to provide excessive or extraneous information or take too much time. In practice, this is rarely the case. In fact, the quality and veracity of closed-ended questions such as "What type of dog food are you feeding?" may lead to inaccurate data. For example, a pet owner may be reluctant to truthfully give the pet food brand they purchase for fear of being judged by the veterinary team. Others may underreport feeding volumes, omit treating behaviors, or fail to include when they share "human foods."

Narrative veterinary medicine or narrative nutritional history are terms we use to describe using open-ended medical history questions to facilitate story telling by a client. These conversations are more natural for clients and give veterinary team members the opportunity to elicit and investigate subtle client behaviors and activities.

Obtaining a medical history using narrative veterinary medicine as a conversational structure only takes a few minutes, and the veterinary team member is able get a more accurate assessment of the patient's diet, activity, and lifestyle in an inviting and nonjudgmental format. The general steps of a narrative nutritional history are as follows.

1) *Conversation invitation* – a broad, open-ended question that encourages a conversation.

2) *Pivot and acquiring trust* – many clients are accustomed to closed-ended, "yes or no" medical inquires, and the team member may need to gain the client's trust in order to obtain thorough and truthful answers.

3) *Active listening* – a key element of narrative veterinary medicine is attentive listening and allowing the conversation to progress naturally, rather than a team member simply recording dictation and not forging a personal connection.

4) *Elaboration* – as the narrative progresses, the team member can ask for clarification or elaboration on medically salient points.

6.15.8 Treating Obesity and Excess Body Fat

The foundation of obesity treatment in dogs and cats remains caloric restriction and increased caloric expenditure through physical activity (see 8.25 Team Strategies for Weight Management). Once a diagnosis of obesity is made, the next step is to rule out any underlying causal or contributing conditions. The presence of hypothyroidism, hyperadrenocorticism, acromegaly, diabetes, hypertension, masses, and conditions that lead to decreased physical activities such as cardiac and respiratory diseases, osteoarthritis, and neuromuscular diseases needs to be evaluated.

An individualized weight loss program is needed for each pet. Careful consideration of the client's personal food philosophy, lifestyle, ability to pay, and interest along with meeting the pet's nutritional needs are crucial for successful outcomes. The role of food rewards, treats, and shared eating habits (i.e., offering "people foods" at mealtimes) must be addressed and viable options offered (i.e., baby carrots as treats or offering plain vegetables from the owner's plate instead of starches and animal products).

Begin by estimating the pet's current caloric intake and reduce this amount by 20–25% [29, 30]. Reweigh the pet in two weeks, and adjust caloric intake as needed. Ideal weight loss rates between 0.5–1.5% bodyweight/week should be your initial clinical goal. For dogs, this may be 3–5% bodyweight loss per month; for cats, an ideal weight loss of 1–3% (approximately 0.5 lb per month for an average-sized cat) is realistic. During the first three months, rapid weight loss is often achieved, followed by plateauing as metabolic adaptations occur. It is important to reweigh the pet every 2–4 weeks during the first 3–6 months of weight loss.

If a pet fails to lose weight or plateaus, you may need to adjust caloric intake or dietary formulation. Before adjusting diet, be certain the client is compliant. In general terms, you may begin caloric restriction at 1.2–1.4 times RER for canines,and 1.0 RER for felines [29]. You may decrease further based on the pet's weight loss results and rate of loss. We do not recommend restricting calories less than 80% to 70% RER for any dog or cat. If you reduce below 70% RER, you risk creating nutritional imbalances.

To calculate an approximate RER for a dog or cat in kilocalories per day:

$70 \times$ [(ideal weight in kg)]^3/4 or $70 \times$ [(ideal weight in kg) to the 3/4 power]

or

$30 \times$ (body weight in kilograms) + 70 (not to be used for very small or very large dogs)

If you reduce daily caloric intake to 70% RER of starting caloric intake and fail to observe weight loss within the first 90 days, you may need to change dietary formulation. If you started with a higher protein/higher fiber formulation, try a lower protein/higher fiber (or different fiber composition) diet. Sometimes a slight alteration in the ingredient or macronutrient profile can trigger metabolic change. We recommend making these changes at 1–3-month intervals. After 90 days, if the pet does not experience appreciable weight loss, change your treatment. Monitoring and adjusting daily caloric intake, diet formulation, and physical activity becomes increasingly important as you continue the weight loss program. Many pets will reach an ideal weight within a few months, only to relapse due to poor owner adherence or metabolic adaptations.

6.15.9 Physical Activity

In general, dogs need 20–30 minutes of walking or other aerobic activity per day. Cats benefit from three or more 3–5-minute intense play periods. Here are some additional methods to encourage physical activity in pets.

- Walk the dog at a brisk walk pace (12–18 minutes per mile) on a short leash (four-foot leash ideal for most dogs).
- Use food puzzles for all feedings to slow feeding rates and enrich the feeding experience. Owners often perceive a dog as "hungry" if they witness the dog rapidly consuming all its food. Slow feeders may discourage overfeeding in this manner. Consider automated pet food dispensers.
- Play "find the food" – move the food bowl upstairs or downstairs or to different parts of the house to require the pet to walk to its food bowl. Moving the feeding location also provides additional environmental enrichment.

- Use feather dusters, flashlights, paper bags or balls, remote-controlled and sound-activated toys, anything the pet finds interesting to physically interact with or chase. Try to engage your dog or cat in stimulating play at least twice a day.
- Have the client play with their pet if it begs for food. Many dogs substitute food for attention and affection; train the client to teach their dog that playtime replaces mealtime.
- When a dog begs for food, take it outside. This environmental distraction and interaction may be enough to make the dog forget its desire for food.
- Feed small meals frequently, especially a last feeding before bedtime or "midnight snack" for dogs and cats prone to wake the client up during the night or early morning.
- If a dog or cat begs for food at an empty bowl, add a low-calorie vegetable treat, a few kibbles, or small dollop of canned food.
- Feed dogs healthy treat substitutes such as baby carrots, broccoli, zucchini, cucumber, celery, and asparagus.
- Offer fresh water instead of food. Many dogs and cats love fresh water, so try filling up the water bowl instead of the food bowl when a pet is begging at the feeding station.

EXAMPLES

Here is an example of narrative veterinary medicine used to obtain a diet and physical activity history. In this example, the client was invited to tell her pet's story, revealing several key interventional opportunities in the process. This technique yields considerably more information in a friendlier, more engaging process than closed-ended questioning.

6.15.10 Conversation Invitation

During the initial conversation invitation, the veterinary team member uses an open-ended question focused on the primary objective, in this case to determine the client's feeding habits, and the pet's lifestyle, environment, and physical activities.

Veterinary team member (VTM):   "Describe for me a typical day in Buster's life."

Client (C):   "Oh, I don't know, nothing unusual, Buster just has a normal dog's life!"

6.15.11   Pivot and Acquiring Trust

Many clients are uncertain how to answer an open-ended question at first, often because a medical professional has never spoken with them in this manner. You may need to earn the client's trust by sharing your care and compassion for the pet and asking a slightly more specific or tangential question, known as a communication "pivot."

VTM: "I think Buster is not only 'normal,' but a very special   with a fantastic family. OK, for starters, what's the first thing Buster does when he gets up each morning?"

C: "Well, I get up around 6.00 a.m., and the first thing I do is let Buster out to go potty."

VTM: "Do you take him for a walk then?"

C: "Heavens no! That's much too early and I haven't had my coffee! I let him out and he usually does his business and comes right back inside. While he's out, I usually pour his food."

6.15.12   Active Listening

It is imperative in narrative veterinary medicine to actively listen to the client's responses in order to refine their answers. In this example, the client mentions "pour his food," indicating imprecise feeding behavior and increasing the likelihood of overfeeding. The veterinary team member has the opportunity to discover the client's actual feeding practices within the client's story telling in a nonjudgmental manner.

VTM: "What kind of food? Do you use a measuring cup?"

C: "Right now I'm using XYZ Dog Brand because my groomer recommended it for his coat. I fill the bowl about half full (indicates size bowl)."

Even though the client didn't report an exact food volume, the veterinary team member has determined the client does not measure the pet's food portions and the brand. An approximate feeding volume can be made, or the client can be asked to measure the food at the next meal. If the pet is diagnosed with obesity, the veterinarian can advise measuring or weighing feeding as a viable treatment option.

6.15.13   Elaboration

One of the biggest challenges in obtaining an accurate nutritional history is uncovering the number of treats and food rewards given. Clients are often reluctant to share each daily treating occasion for fear of judgment. Most pet owners understand that excessive treating is potentially unhealthy, and don't want to risk being viewed as providing improper care. In order to uncover hidden treating habits, the veterinary team must allow the client to elaborate and spontaneously share their daily routine in a nonthreatening way.

VTM: "Thanks. What's next for Buster?"

C: "Well, I get everyone out of the house and then I leave for work. I let Buster out again before I leave, and I usually give him an ABC Dog Cookie when I leave to tide him over until I come back at lunch to let him out."

VTM: "When you get home, what does Buster do?"

C: "I let him out again, and then I give him a 123 Doggie Treat if he's been a good boy. He always is!"

VTM: "And then he stays in until you get home from work?"

C: "Yes, as soon as I get from work we go straight for a walk. He starts twirling as soon as he sees me grab the leash!"

VTM: "How long do you walk him usually?"

C: "Oh, a good 15–20 minutes."

VTM: "And dinner?"

C: "Yes, I give him the same as in the morning. Although I have to admit, I usually give him a little something as soon as I get home. He must be a little hungry after being alone all day."

VTM: "What about after dinner? Does he go outside or anything else?"

C: "Sure, I let him go potty a few minutes after he's done eating, and he stays out a good 10–15 minutes. My husband will also give a cookie after dinner when we sit down to watch television."

What this narrative nutritional history teaches us.

- The client feeds a specific brand twice daily.
- Doesn't precisely measure food.
- Gives at least two brands of treats.
- Give treats at least 4–5 times a day.
- Minimal exercise/physical activity.

Your team now has the opportunity to make more precise treatment recommendations based on more accurate information than traditional closed-ended question-and-answer experiences. This technique also improves the veterinary professional–client relationship and creates a framework for authentic, meaningful conversations to occur.

TAKE-AWAYS

- Obesity in dogs and cats continues to be a significant health disorder, causing disease, reduced life expectancy, and decreased quality of life.

- The diagnosis and successful treatment of obesity continue to challenge veterinary healthcare professionals. Training and utilizing all members of the veterinary care team can improve the recognition of obesity and outcomes.
- Successful weight loss programs include assessing a client's needs, abilities, and goals integrated within an individualized, multimodal therapeutic approach.
- Patient-first language can help overcome veterinary bias and encourage dialogue and obesity treatment.
- Narrative veterinary medicine and narrative nutritional history taking can be a highly effective communication strategy for veterinary professionals.

MISCELLANEOUS

References

1 2018 Pet Obesity Survey Results – US Pet Obesity Rates Plateau and Nutritional Confusion Growshttps://petobesityprevention.org/2018

2 PAW Report. (2018). PDSA Animal Wellbeing. www.pdsa.org.suk/media/4371/paw-2018-full-web-ready.pdf

3 Sandøe, P., Palmer, C., Corr, S. et al. (2014). Canine and feline obesity: a one health perspective. *Vet. Rec.* 175 (24): 610–616.

4 2016 Pet Obesity Survey Results – US Pet Obesity Expands, Owners Disagree with Veterinarians on Nutritional Issues. https://petobesityprevention.org/2016

5 Pet obesity epidemic is top welfare concern for vets. www.bva.co.uk/news-campaigns-and-policy/newsroom/news-releases/pet-obesity-epidemic-is-top-welfare-concern-for-vets

6 Mao, J., Xia, Z., Chen, J., and Yu, J. (2013). Prevalence and risk factors for canine obesity surveyed in veterinary practices in Beijing, China. *Prev. Vet. Med.* 112: 438–442.

7 German, A.J., Woods, G.R.T., Holden, S.L. et al. (2018). Dangerous trends in pet obesity. *Vet. Rec.* 182: 25.

8 The Global Pet Obesity Initiative Position Statement. Ward E, German AJ, Churchill JA. https://static1.squarespace.com/static/597c71d3e58c621d06830e3f/t/5da311c5519bf62664dac512/1570968005938/Global+pet+obesity+initiative+position+statement.pdf

9 Kealy, R.D., Lawler, D.F., Ballam, J.M. et al. (2002). Effects of diet restriction on life span and age related changes in dogs. *J. Am. Vet. Med. Assoc.* 220: 1315–1320.

10 German, A.J., Holden, S.L., Wiseman-Orr, M.L. et al. (2012). Quality of life is reduced in obese dogs but improves after successful weight loss. *Vet. J.* 192: 428–434.

11 Lund, E.M., Armstrong, P.J., Kirk, C.A. et al. (2005). Prevalence and risk factors for obesity in adult cats from private US veterinary practices. *Intern. J. Appl. Res. Vet. Med.* 3: 88–96.

12 Lund, E.M., Armstrong, P.J., Kirk, C.A. et al. (2006). Prevalence and risk factors for obesity in adult dogs from private US veterinary practices. *Int. J. Appl. Res. Vet. Med.* 4: 177–186.

13 Mosing, M., German, A.J., Holden, S.L. et al. (2013). Oxygenation and ventilation characteristics in obese sedated dogs before and after weight loss: a clinical trial. *Vet. J.* 198: 367–371.

14 Tropf, M., Nelson, O.L., Lee, P.M., and Weng, H.Y. (2017). Cardiac and metabolic variables in obese dogs. *J. Vet. Intern. Med.* 31: 1000–1007.

15 Bomberg, E., Birch, L., Endenburg, E. et al. (2017). The financial costs, behaviour and psychology of obesity: a one health analysis. *J. Comp. Pathol.* 156: 310–325.

16 Pettitt, R.A. and German, A.J. (2015). Investigation and management of canine osteoarthritis. *In Practice* 37: 1–8.

17 Pérez Alenza, D., Rutteman, G.R., Peña, L. et al. (1998). Relation between habitual diet and canine mammary tumors in a case-control study. *J. Vet. Intern. Med.* 12 (3): 132–139.

18 Öhlund, M., Palmgren, M., and Holst, B.S. (2018). Overweight in adult cats: a cross-sectional study. *Acta Vet. Scand.* 60 (1): 5.

19 German, A.J., Holden, S.L., Wiseman-Orr, M. et al. (2012). Quality of life is reduced in obese dogs but improves after successful weight loss. *Vet. J.* 192: 428–434.

20 National Research Council (2013). *Workforce Needs in Veterinary Medicine*, 99–101. Washington, DC: National Academies Press.

21 CABI (2012). *Veterinary Practice Management*, 63–66. Bristol: University of Bristol.

22 Ward, E. Trone Brand Energy. Association for Pet Obesity Prevention proprietary research. Reprinted by permission. 2014.

23 Strategies to Overcome and Prevent Obesity Alliance. Why Weight? A Guide to Discussing Obesity and Health with Your Patients. www.waterloowellingtondiabetes.ca/userContent/documents/Professional-Resources/STOP-Provider-Discussion-Tool.pdf

24 World Small Animal Veterinary Association. Muscle Condition Score, Dogs: https://wsava.org/wp-content/uploads/2020/01/Body-Condition-Score-Dog.pdf. Cats:

https://wsava.org/wp-content/uploads/2020/01/
Cat-Body-Condition-Scoring-2017.pdf

25 Tomiyama, A.J., Carr, D., Granberg, E.M. et al. (2018).
How and why weight stigma drives the obesity 'epidemic'
and harms health. *BMC Med.* 16 (1): 123.

26 Phelan, S.M., Burgess, D.J., Yeazel, M.W. et al. (2015). Impact
of weight bias and stigma on quality of care and outcomes
for patients with obesity. *Obes. Rev.* 16 (4): 319–326.

27 2017 American Medical Association Annual Meeting
Resolutions, no 402. Person-First Language for Obesity.

www.ama-assn.org/sites/ama-assn.org/files/corp/
media-browser/public/hod/a17-resolutions.pdf

28 WSAVA. Nutrition – The Fifth Vital Sign. www.vin.com/
apputil/content/defaultadv1.aspx?pId=11349&
catId=34755

29 Brooks, D., Churchill, J., Fein, K. et al. (2014). 2014
AAHA weight management guidelines for dogs and cats.
J. Am. Anim. Hosp. Assoc. 50 (1): 1–11.

30 Perea, S. (2010). What's the take-home? Nutrition.
ClinBrief 8: 63–65.

6.16

Assessing Blood Pressure as an Early Indicator of Disease

Ryane E. Englar, DVM, DABVP (Canine and Feline Practice)

College of Veterinary Medicine, University of Arizona, Oro Valley, AZ, USA

BASICS

6.16.1 Summary

Vital signs are patient-specific measurements used in both clinical practice and triage to assess the status of an individual's whole-body health. Historically, pulse rate, respiratory rate, and temperature have been the standard three vital signs documented in the veterinary medical record. However, blood pressure (BP) has recently been recognized as a fourth vital sign because of its impact on a patient's essential body functions. In small animal practice, systemic hypertension is increasingly diagnosed as canine and feline patients live longer and, as seniors, often face concurrent diagnoses of chronic renal, metabolic, and endocrine disease. Systemic hypertension in dogs and cats is most often secondary to one or more of these disease processes. Therefore, tracking changes in BP at each veterinary visit is prudent so as to diagnose disease early and initiate medical management before significant target organ damage (TOD) occurs.

6.16.2 Terms Defined

Blood Pressure (BP): The force of blood moving through the arteries as produced by myocardial contractility, represented most typically in medicine as two numbers: the first number represents systolic pressure and it occurs immediately after the heart contracts; the second number represents diastolic pressure and it is the lowest number that is seen throughout the cardiac cycle.

Systemic Hypertension: A condition characterized by a persistent increase in BP within systemic vessels, that is,

those that carry blood from the heart to the rest of the body, with the exception of the lungs.

Target Organs: Those organs that are exceedingly sensitive to systemic hypertension and will develop pathology if systemic hypertension is unchecked; these include the central nervous system (CNS), cardiovascular system, kidneys, and eyes.

MAIN CONCEPTS

6.16.3 Measuring BP in the Dog and Cat

Direct BP measurement involves placing an arterial line in the patient [1]. This line attaches to a transducer, which connects to an oscilloscope. Systolic BP (SBP), diastolic BP, and mean arterial pressure (MAP) are measured continuously [2].

Direct BP measurement is accurate, but impractical outside the intensive care unit (ICU) [1, 3, 4]. Placing an arterial line requires skill and is not without risk [2].

Indirect BP measurement, using Doppler or oscillometric monitoring, is more practical [1]. Doppler requires a cuff and crystal-containing probe to detect arterial blood flow [2]. The cuff is placed over the radial or coccygeal artery [2]. When inflated, the cuff occludes blood flow. As the cuff deflates, arterial blood flow is reestablished [2]. This change in blood flow is detected by the probe, which transmits an audible signal [2].

Oscillometric monitoring also requires a cuff. Changes in cuff inflation allow arterial pulse oscillations to be detected electronically and conveyed to a screen for viewing [2].

Doppler measurements correlate with direct BP measurements better than oscillometric devices [2, 5, 6]. However, validation of both approaches has been challenging [1].

6.16.4 Normal BP in the Dog and Cat

The 2018 American College of Veterinary Internal Medicine (ACVIM) guidelines summarize BP readings for dogs and cats as reported in the current veterinary literature. Canine SBP ranges from 131 ($\pm$20) to 154 ($\pm$31) mmHg, and feline SBP ranges from 111 ($\pm$4) to 160 ($\pm$12) mmHg [1].

Aging in cats and dogs may increase BP by 1–3 mmHg per year [1, 6–10].

Hounds consistently have BP that is 10–20 mmHg higher than mixed-breeds [1, 7].

6.16.5 Causes of Secondary Hypertension in the Dog and Cat

Systemic hypertension may be primary (essential) or secondary. Primary hypertension represents most of the caseload in people with high BP, but it is not as commonly seen in veterinary patients.

Hypertension in dogs and cats is more often secondary to [1, 4, 11–16]:

- chronic kidney disease (CKD)
- hyperadrenocorticism (Cushing's disease)
- hyperthyroidism
- pheochromocytoma
- primary hyperaldosteronism (Conn's syndrome)
- prescription drugs
- erythropoietin
- phenylpropanolamine.

6.16.6 Adverse Effects of Persistent Systemic Hypertension

Systemic hypertension injures tissues, particularly the CNS, heart, kidneys, and eyes [1]. TOD includes the following pathologies [1, 3, 6].

- Neurological
  - Altered mentation and behavior
  - Seizure activity
- Cardiovascular pathology
  - Left ventricular hypertrophy
  - Systolic murmur and/or gallop rhythm
  - Congestive heart failure (CHF)

- Ocular
  - Blindness
  - Hyphema
  - Retinal detachment
- Renal
  - Microalbuminuria
  - Proteinuria
  - Azotemia

When SBP exceeds 180 mmHg, patients are at extreme risk for TOD [1].

6.16.7 Screening for Systemic Hypertension

The current standard of care dictates that BP should be assessed in [1, 17]:

- middle-aged to older cats
- dogs with hyperadrenocorticism
- patients that are about to start treatment with prescription drugs that elevate BP
- patients with historical data that could be consistent with TOD, such as apparent blindness
- patients with abnormal physical exam findings that are consistent with TOD, such as retinal detachment(s)
- patients that are undergoing anesthetic procedures.

However, it pays to be proactive and screen for hypertension in patients before there is systemic or concurrent disease. Healthcare is in the process of evolving from diagnosing and managing disease to identifying risk factors present in patients before they actually develop and are clinical for disease.

Routine BP screening among apparently healthy patients is key to establishing their baselines so that deviations from the norm can be noted and evaluated in light of trends.

Being proactive about BP measurements allows the veterinary team to identify subclinical, prehypertensive patients before TOD has occurred.

How often to screen heathy patients and at what age to begin screening remain to be determined.

 EXAMPLES

Smudge is a 9-year old male castrated Tonkinese cat that presents for annual wellness examination. The client reports that he has "slowed down" and is unusually cautious with his movements. Physical examination discloses a Grade 3/6 systolic murmur and bilateral mydriasis. Fundoscopic examination confirms bilateral retinal detachment. TOD is suspected and BP measurement is advised. SBP obtained through Doppler is 185 mmHg. A case work-up confirms renal disease. Antihypertensive therapy will not resolve the detached retinas but it may slow progression of renal disease.

TAKE-AWAYS

- BP is a reflection of whole-body health.
- Secondary hypertension is common in companion animal practice.
- Screening for hypertension is important to patient wellness; being proactive catches disease early.
- Systemic hypertension is associated with TOD.
- Early recognition of systemic hypertension allows the clinician to initiate treatment before TOD is irreversible.

MISCELLANEOUS

6.16.8 Cautions

Measurement of BP is an imperfect science. Interpretation of BP may be complicated by the following factors [1, 2, 18].

- Breed
- Temperament
- Patient positioning
- Operator's skill
- Cuff size
- Cuff placement

An additional complication of BP measurement is that not all elevations in BP reflect persistent systemic hypertension. There is also a condition called situational hypertension, sometimes called "white coat syndrome" [1, 6]. In white coat syndrome, the stress associated with a clinical setting activates the sympathetic nervous system in some but not all patients. Although transient, the resultant hypertension may still damage target organs [19–22].

Cats are particularly sensitive to white coat syndrome [6, 11]. This may make it challenging to know when to treat feline hypertension as "real." If SBP readings exceed 180 mmHg, then situational hypertension is unlikely; however, white coat syndrome makes it difficult

to know how to approach a clinical case in which SBP is in the gray zone.

Abbreviation

mmHg   millimeters of mercury

References

1 Acierno, M.J., Brown, S., Coleman, A.E. et al. (2018). ACVIM consensus statement: guidelines for the identification, evaluation, and management of systemic hypertension in dogs and cats. *J. Vet. Intern. Med.* 32: 1803–1822.

2 Scislowicz, O.D. Blood Pressure Measurement. Veterinary Team Brief 2018: 23–27.

3 Henik, R.A. (1997). Diagnosis and treatment of feline systemic hypertension. *Comp. Cont. Educ. Pract.* 19: 163–179.

4 Acierno M. Diagnosing and treating hypertension. http://veterinarycalendar.dvm360.com/diagnosing-and-treating-hypertension-proceedings-0

5 Haberman, C.E., Morgan, J.D., Kang, C.W. et al. (2004). Evaluation of doppler ultrasonic and oscillometric methods of indirect blood pressure measurement in cats. *Int J. Appl. Res. Vet. Med.* 2: 279–289.

6 Taylor, S.S., Sparkes, A.H., Briscoe, K. et al. (2017). ISFM consensus guidelines on the diagnosis and management of hypertension in cats. *J. Feline. Med. Surg.* 19: 288–303.

7 Bodey, A.R. and Michell, A.R. (1996). Epidemiological study of blood pressure in domestic dogs. *J. Small. Anim. Pract.* 37: 116–125.

8 Bright, J.M. and Dentino, M. (2002). Indirect arterial blood pressure measurement in nonsedated Irish wolfhounds: reference values for the breed. *J. Am. Anim. Hosp. Assoc.* 38: 521–526.

9 Meurs, K.M., Miller, M.W., Slater, M.R. et al. (2000). Arterial blood pressure measurement in a population of healthy geriatric dogs. *J. Am. Anim. Hosp. Assoc.* 36: 497–500.

10 Remillard, R.L., Ross, J.N., and Eddy, J.B. (1991). Variance of indirect blood pressure measurements and prevalence of hypertension in clinically normal dogs. *Am. J. Vet. Res.* 52: 561–565.

11 Jepson, R.E. (2011). Feline systemic hypertension: classification and pathogenesis. *J. Feline. Med. Surg.* 13: 25–34.

12 Brown, S.A. and Henik, R.A. (1998). Diagnosis and treatment of systemic hypertension. *Vet. Clin. North Am. Small Anim. Pract.* 28: 1481–1494, ix.

13 Reusch, C.E., Schellenberg, S., and Wenger, M. (2010). Endocrine hypertension in small animals. *Vet. Clin. North Am. Small Anim. Pract.* 40: 335–352.

14 Syme, H. (2011). Hypertension in small animal kidney disease. *Vet. Clin. North Am. Small Anim. Pract.* 41: 63–89.

15 Watson, N., Murray, J.K., Fonfara, S. et al. (2018). Clinicopathological features and comorbidities of cats with mild, moderate or severe hyperthyroidism: a radioiodine referral population. *J. Feline Med. Surg.* 20: 1130–1137.

16 Hoffman, J.M., Lourenco, B.N., Promislow, D.E.L. et al. (2018). Canine hyperadrenocorticism associations with signalment, selected comorbidities and mortality within north American veterinary teaching hospitals. *J. Small Anim. Pract.* 59: 681–690.

17 Stepien, R.L. (2011). Feline systemic hypertension: diagnosis and management. *J. Feline Med. Surg.* 13: 35–43.

18 Dixon-Jimenez A, Rapoport G, Brown SA. Systemic hypertension in dogs and cats. https://todaysveterinary practice.com/systemic-hypertension-in-dogs-cats/

19 Verdecchia, P., Schillaci, G., Borgioni, C. et al. (1995). White coat hypertension and white coat effect – similarities and differences. *Am. J. Hypertens.* 8: 790–798.

20 Ogedegbe, G. (2008). White-coat effect: unraveling its mechanisms. *Am. J. Hypertens.* 21: 135–135.

21 Cardillo, C., Defelice, F., Campia, U. et al. (1993). Psychophysiological reactivity and cardiac end-organ changes in white coat hypertension. *Hypertension* 21: 836–844.

22 Palmer, B.F. (2001). Impaired renal autoregulation: implications for the genesis of hypertension and hypertension-induced renal injury. *Am. J. Med Sci* 321: 388–400.

Recommended Reading

Acierno, M.J., Brown, S., Coleman, A.E. et al. (2018). AVCIM consensus statement: guidelines for the identification, evaluation, and management of systemic hypertension in dogs and cats. *J. Vet. Intern. Med.* 32: 1803–1822.

Taylor, S.S., Sparkes, A.H., Briscoe, K. et al. (2017). ISFM consensus guidelines on the diagnosis and management of hypertension in cats. *J. Feline Med. and Surg.* 19: 288–303.

6.17

Senior Care

Heidi B. Lobprise, DVM, DAVDC

Main Street Veterinary Hospital and Dental Clinic, Flower Mound, TX, USA

BASICS

6.17.1 Summary

With advances in veterinary medicine, we are seeing more pets advancing in age. This "graying" of our patient population provides both opportunities and challenges as we strive to provide them with optimal care throughout their life stages. While "age is not a disease," there will always be a decrease in older patients' ability to respond to stresses and handle a decrease in organ function and capacity. With "healthy aging" these changes can be minimized, but dogs and cats can develop myriad problems, often multiple co-existing problems (co-morbidities), and it is often up to the primary care practitioner and their team to manage these patients.

6.17.2 Terms Defined

Aging: The progressive changes after maturity with a decrease in organ functional ability and the depletion of physiological reserves

Geriatric: A pet's life stage defined when the pet has reached its expected life span and beyond.

Life Stage: A segment of a life span defined not just by a set of years, but also by characteristics.

Relative Age: The age in "people years" that corresponds to a dog's or cat's age

Senior: Life stage defined as the fourth quartile of a pet's expected life span (from 75% to 100% of its life span).

MAIN CONCEPTS

Aging has been described as the progressive changes that occur after the maturity of an individual. There is a decrease in organ functional ability and depletion of physiological reserves, and therefore recovery from illness or dysfunction is more challenging than when young. Oxidative changes and telomere shortening have been identified as hallmarks of aging, and the impact of inflammation on the aging process is being closely studied. It is important to manage these alterations in our patients as subtle fluctuations may not be noticed early on, and without intervention, changes can progress to significant disease that will be more challenging to handle.

When we look at our patients' life spans, we should also consider evaluating the "healthspan" or quality of life (QOL). As pet patients deteriorate, the human–animal bond can suffer as well, and this can lead to abandonment or even euthanasia (see 6.20 Quality of Life and End of Life Issues).

To define what is "senior," we must first realize that determining the relative age of a veterinary patient is not as simple as multiplying their biological age by a factor of 7 (see 11.05 Life Planning by Breed). Contrary to common perceptions, not all pets are senior at 7 years of age, and some are senior before the age of 7. The designation "senior" can be applied to a pet that has reached 75% of its life expectancy, with maturity reached at 50% of the life span and a pet that has outlasted its life expectancy considered geriatric. This can be easy to compute if you know the life expectancy of the pet, or a breed life expectancy, but challenging in other instances (see 1.2 Providing a Lifetime of Care). That being said, the most current version of the AAHA Canine Life Stage Guidelines has eliminated the category "geriatric" altogether (see 4.1 Canine and Feline Life Stages). According to the AAFP, cats are easier to categorize, becoming senior at 11 years of age and geriatric at 15 years of age.

In dogs, it is known that giant- and large-breed animals age more quickly than smaller breeds, making it more complicated. You can use relative age charts that have been developed based on bodyweight, to account for the small dog–large dog variance to get an estimation of relative age and life stage. But what about pets adopted as adults, as their age is an estimate and they may be older than assumed? Extrapolated from a commonly used relative age chart, we can estimate that small dogs under 20 lb (9 kg) become senior at about 9 years of age, and geriatric at 14 years of age; medium-sized dogs (21–50 lb, 9.5–23 kg) become senior at 8 years of age and geriatric at 13 years of age; large dogs (51–90 lb, 24–40 kg) reach senior at 7 years of age and geriatric at 12 years of age, while giant-breed dogs (over 90 lbs, 40 kg) hit that senior status as early as 6 years of age and are geriatric at 9 years of age.

We use these categories of determining the life stage to help us guide the care that is recommended for these groups. If we start with a lifetime of optimal care and screening, transitioning to a senior level of care should be a smooth continuum from youth to geriatric. As you discuss life stages and care with the pet owner, they anticipate the differences as their pet ages, so don't just start the information about senior care when their pet reaches that stage.

So, what should a senior care program look like? Most programs will increase the frequency of comprehensive physical examinations to twice yearly if not already being done, including blood pressure measurement, body condition scoring, and muscle condition scoring (lean body mass [LBM]). This will likely include a full diagnostic panel (chemistry, electrolytes, thyroid panel, urinalysis, hemogram). It has been shown that routine screening in healthy animals can reveal early changes that have not yet manifested in detectable symptoms or signs [1, 2], and early detection can positively impact management of the disease. Many senior and geriatric pets will have multiple issues and these co-morbidities will require coordination of therapies. In fact, the best geriatric "specialists" are general practitioners who have to integrate all the body systems in their evaluations, diagnostics, and management.

In managing these patients, collate and track any changes that may occur. Look for early changes and trends within the normal range of diagnostic parameters that may indicate where the "high normal" values may soon become abnormal (e.g., creatinine creep and evaluating SDMA). Be sure to communicate the importance of senior care to the owners. If you correlate senior pet care with human aging milestones such as recommendations for testing as we age (PSA, mammogram, colonoscopy), owners can understand that changes occur more rapidly in our pets and work with us to support optimal wellness in aging. There are also many conditions that humans and animals may share, such as weight control, osteoarthritis, diabetes, and cognitive issues.

6.17.3 Nutrition and Body Condition

An important aspect of senior care involves monitoring body condition and providing nutritional consultation. In most pets, base metabolism rate (BMR) decreases with age, yet with older cats (11 yrs+), BMR can increase. Assessing the body condition score (BCS) is commonly done, is easy to record and there are good scales for assessment (see 6.15 Approaching Obesity on a Pet-Specific Basis). Owners can be taught to palpate spine and ribs, and to take sequential photos of face, side view, skyline view. Some seniors may benefit from a slightly higher BCS around 6, especially those with chronic heart or renal disease, as the reserves of body mass can be beneficial during periods of stress.

With decreased activity levels, though, weight gain can lead to obesity, which can influence other factors, including an increased risk of osteoarthritis and diabetes (see 6.15 Approaching Obesity on a Pet-Specific Basis). Overweight dogs have shorter lives, so making dietary adjustments, including restricting treats, can help maintain a healthy weight (see 8.25 Team Strategies for Weight Management). Encourage the owner to provide exercise and environmental enrichment that can help both physical and mental health. Be sure to set intermediate weight loss goals as a percentage of bodyweight and celebrate milestone goals that are met.

Weight loss can be even more critical in senior and geriatric pets, especially with cats. Determine why a pet might not be eating well, possibly due to nausea, dental disease, or even cognitive issues. If the pet is eating but still losing weight, evaluate gastrointestinal or other systemic issues such as hyperthyroidism. Distinguish whether the weight loss is due to loss of fat or loss of muscle (see LBM or muscle condition scoring below). Loss of weight in older cats is often an indication of the presence of a chronic disease and can be used as a predictor of mortality. As inappetence can exacerbate other conditions such as hepatic lipidosis and decrease recovery, appetite stimulants can be helpful, or feeding tubes may be necessary.

Lean body mass or muscle condition score (MCS) may be more critical to assess than BCS, as healthy muscle plays a role in endocrine function, not just movement and skeletal support. Aging pets may show signs of sarcopenia as normal aging changes that are anticipated. Here, fat slowly replaces muscle tissue, but this can be minimized with feeding good-quality proteins and regular exercise. Senior and geriatric cats may require additional protein if no renal issues are present. In contrast, cachexia or excessive loss of muscle mass is often due to an advanced disease state. The patient may have excessive fat with minimal weight changes and seem obese, but still have significant LBM loss. Once lost, muscle levels can be very difficult to revert to normal.

Determining the appropriate diet for any individual senior pet can be quite challenging. While there are minimums set for growing and adult pets, there are no particular recommendations for senior diets. In commercially available "senior" diets, there are huge variations in diet components. There will also be huge variations in individual need, with specific requirements for certain disease processes. Generally speaking, diets with higher digestibility, higher quality proteins (at increased levels for some patients), antioxidants and caloric adjustment seem to have desirable qualities that could benefit most seniors. Patients with chronic kidney disease (CKD) may need restricted protein and phosphorus, and sodium may be restricted for patients with chronic heart failure. Gastrointestinal issues in pets may benefit from antigen-restricted or hydrolyzed protein diets, or low-fat formulations for pancreatitis patients.

6.17.4 Pain in Senior Pets

Osteoarthritis and other painful conditions are common in older dogs and cats, but they will often hide their pain until it is advanced (see 8.20 Team Strategies for Arthritis, and 6.14 Pain Prevention, Management and Conditioning). Owners may think that their decreased activity and slowing down is due to age, but that is not always the case. Dogs may be reluctant to climb stairs or jump onto favorite places, or they may have decreased exercise tolerance (assess cardiopulmonary health as well). If they aren't going through the doggie door and are now house soiling, both pain levels and cognition need to be evaluated. Cats may be less active with less jumping, and either grooming less or excessively grooming around a painful joint or area. If they aren't able to get into a little box with high sides, they may go outside the box.

 Managing the pain for any pet with issues can benefit from a multimodal approach, selecting the appropriate medication and supplements while adding in complementary pain management modalities (see 2.16 Pain and Pain Management). If there is a positive response to medication, then there was definitely an analgesic deficiency! With seniors, don't forget to manage the environment as well, by covering slick floors with stable rugs or runners or using toe grips for dogs. Assist them getting onto furniture or perches with steps or ramps, and the occasional helping hand. Adjust the doggie door to be more comfortable to get through or take them out more often. For cats, get litter boxes with lower sides and place floor covers around them. Provide any level of activity and environmental enrichment that they can tolerate to help maintain flexibility and muscular stability (see 4.11 Environmental Enrichment).

6.17.5 Senior Behavioral Issues

Cognitive decline (dementia) is common in aging dogs and cats, and their QOL can be greatly impacted (see 6.19 Problem Aging). If signs are detected early in the process, management can help keep the changes minimized and help pet owners adjust accordingly.

The DISHAA acronym can help you evaluate behavioral decline in pets by looking for these early signs. D – for disorientation; pets don't recognize family members, seem to get lost easily, may stare blankly, and are less reactive to common stimuli. Signs of decreased interaction (I) may manifest as decreased affection, being hesitant to approach, and showing increased irritability and anxiety with owners, visitors, and other animals. When the sleep/wake cycle is disrupted (S), the day/night sleeping cycle may be reversed and they may pace or be restless at night, or have increased vocalization at night, especially cats. House soiling (H) may be one of the more frustrating signs of decline and is often due to deficits in learning and memory. They may eliminate in the house or don't ask to be let out, and they may also show a decreased response to previously learned behaviors. The first A stands for activity, referring to decreased purposeful activity, such as aimless wandering or repetitive behaviors such as circling. The second A, anxiety, has been more recently added to the DISHAA acronym. As the pet ages, there can be increased stress with otherwise innocuous stimuli (sounds, sights), as well as increased separation anxiety or anxiety with new situations.

A practitioner arrives at a cognitive decline diagnosis often after ruling out any medical issues that could be contributing to the signs. If there is polyuria/polydipsia due to any other disease, this could be exacerbating issues with house soiling. Osteoarthritis can prevent a cat from using its litter box or a dog from using the doggie door, also resulting in soiling. Chronic disease may contribute to decreased activity, increased sleep, and lethargy. Hearing and sight loss can contribute to irritability and lack of recognition. These issues may exist concurrently with cognitive dysfunction or exacerbate it. Early assessment and detection can allow you to start with medications, diets, and supplements that can help decrease the impact of cognitive dysfunction, but a slow decline will likely continue. Be sure to reassess QOL on a regular basis, as the decline can be rapid in some pets.

6.17.6 Senior Dental Care

Older pets have a higher incidence of dental disease, primarily because the teeth and periodontal tissues have been there longer to accumulate problems (see 4.9 Periodontal Disease). In addition, small dogs have a higher incidence of periodontal disease compared to larger dogs, with more crowded teeth and less alveolar bone. Since small dogs tend to live longer than larger dogs, small, older dogs are often in need of dental care. The infection and inflammation that accompany oral and dental disease can have a significant negative impact on the systemic health of the pet.

With few exceptions, managing the patient to minimize their anesthetic risks will greatly benefit the patient once the dental disease is cleared (see 5.12 Discussing Anesthetic Risk). Appropriate preoperative diagnostics will help identify any underlying systemic disease, and if the disease is minimal to mild, the dental procedure can be scheduled. If there is moderate disease detected, the patient can be treated to stabilize them sufficiently for the anesthetic procedure. Animals with severe systemic disease that cannot be easily controlled may be less optimal as patients. Anesthetic and analgesic protocols can be tailored to the patient by decreasing the amount of preanesthetic agents used and the amount of induction agent, if possible. Keeping the procedure as short as possible will benefit the patient, as will minimizing the depth of anesthesia. Providing adequate pain management before, during, and after procedure will not only make the animal more comfortable but can also help to decrease the extent of general anesthetic gas needed to maintain a stable depth of anesthesia.

With most seniors, it is no longer recommended to withhold water for extended periods of time; they can usually have water available until they leave home for the appointment. It has been shown that it can be beneficial to feed a small meal up to four hours before the procedure. Bringing a blanket or toy from home can help decrease stress and anxiety.

For specific disease conditions, other considerations are made. In diabetes mellitus patients, it is critical to have a healthy mouth, as dental disease and diabetes are often co-morbidities. These patients can have a small meal early in the morning with a half dose of insulin. Glucose levels should be checked several times, such as before, during, and after the procedure; if levels are low, supplementation is given. The goal is to return the patient to normal meals and insulin as soon as possible.

Mitral insufficiency and heart disease can be very common in senior pets, so additional preoperative assessment is recommended. There should be an assessment of ProBNP and thoracic radiographs at a minimum, adding in echocardiography if these show any abnormalities. With more advanced cases, a full cardiology consultation is recommended to coordinate anesthetic protocols. Once the patient is deemed stable enough for the procedure, a decision can be made whether preoperative antibiotics are necessary. If there is sufficient infection in the oral cavity, minimizing the bacteremia during the procedure may be of benefit. The patient should be stabilized with medication prior to the anesthetic event for mild sedation and pain management. Preoxygenate the pet if it can be done with minimal stress and handling. The intravenous fluids should be decreased by half to one-third of the typical rate, while monitoring cardiac and pulmonary function closely. All efforts should be made to minimize surgery time and depth of anesthesia, and maintain body temperature.

Patients with preexisting renal disease will often benefit from intravenous fluids given prior to the anesthetic event. Intraoperative fluid rates can be increased with monitoring for any pulmonary issues and postoperative urine production. If nausea is an issue with pets with gastrointestinal issues, an antiemetic can be administered perioperatively, and medication dispensed for postoperative use. Consider an appetite stimulant if needed and make dietary recommendations (soft food post surgery) with minimal changes (moisten dry food instead of making an abrupt change to canned food), especially if the patient is on a prescription diet.

Continue the dental care with a follow-up call the day after the procedure to make sure the patient is recovering sufficiently. Schedule a two-week recheck to assess tissue healing and start an appropriate home care program.

6.17.7 Senior Care Program

In order to maximize the level of care your senior patients can receive, the first step is identifying which patients fit this category. It is fairly straightforward to identify patients prior to each visit, and if additional senior-level care is not being requested, make recommendations appropriate for that pet. Trying to identify entire groups of senior and geriatric pets is not as simple, as "Senior at Seven" is not applicable to many patients. It would take a formula using weight and actual age to categorize these groups.

6.17.8 Pet Owner Advocates

As in human medicine, a patient's care can be enhanced if they have an advocate that can monitor their care and health parameters. Educate the pet owner to be more aware of small changes that can herald the beginning of health issues. Encourage them to keep a "health diary" where they can keep records of veterinary visits and diagnostic results. They can also monitor BCS images on a quarterly basis and record water consumption, dietary changes, and elimination habits, if unusual. They can take pictures of any masses with a familiar object for size comparison to make a tumor map that can be used to detect any changes in a suspicious area. Any other subtle changes, from behavioral problems to activity levels, can also be noted.

Environment enrichment has been shown to benefit both the physical and mental health of individuals – human and animal alike. Having regular, stimulating interaction with their pet, including exercise that can be structured to their abilities and limitations, can even improve the human–companion animal bond. Using food toys and games that encourage foraging techniques can help slow down the meal while providing a task to complete.

The aging of our pets and patients shouldn't be faced with dread, but we should celebrate the milestones as we help these individuals have a good healthspan. Have a space on your website, Facebook page or bulletin board in your office to recognize when pets reach their senior or geriatric life stages. Make this visible to other pet parents, who may want to compare their pets to others. In this act of celebrating, consider the process of aging as an "upgrade," with elite status for each life stage. Mature patients can be "awarded" silver elite status, seniors get gold elite status and geriatric pets can have platinum elite status bestowed upon them!

When you share these success stories, you can tell when routine diagnostics helped to identify a disease early in its progression, allowing for optimal management. Despite an owner's concerns about anesthesia for their pet, let them share how extensive dental extractions made a big difference in how their pet now feels. Communicate how a lifetime of prevention, wellness care, and weight management can result in a patient living beyond their expected life span – from puppy or kitten life stages to geriatric and beyond. In addition to this, encourage people to adopt a senior dog or cat to allow them to live out their remaining years with optimal care.

EXAMPLES

Mrs V adopted an adult shih tzu cross when her elderly Japanese chin passed away. Opal was estimated to be 3–4 years of age and in good general health but needed good dental care. Preoperative diagnostics were unremarkable except for moderately high blood pressure readings and an SDMA reading of 14 (high normal). Not unusual for a small breed dog, several teeth required extraction due to crowding and bone loss. However, the pulp canals of the teeth seemed very narrow, an indication that Opal was actually quite a bit older than 3–4 years. Given the likelihood that Opal was approximately 9–10 years of age and considered senior, the owner agreed with recommendations to further pursue diagnostics on a more regular basis (blood pressure every three months – it has remained stable – and bloodwork and urinalysis every six months). With her dental disease under control, Opal became more active and playful, so even though she is a senior, we expect many years of good health to come.

TAKE-AWAYS

- Many changes in senior and geriatric pets may be subtle or attributed to aging, but if associated with disease and addressed early in the progression, optimal care can be provided.
- The relative age of a dog or cat is not simply "times 7"; there are good resources for determining the life stage of a pet – from mature to senior to geriatric.
- Body condition scoring should be paired with muscle condition scoring to evaluate the LBM of a pet.
- "Senior" diets have no guidelines for recommendations and can vary greatly. The veterinary team should evaluate each individual to make appropriate diet choices.
- Good dental care can be provided to almost any senior pet.

MISCELLANEOUS

Abbreviations

AAHA	American Animal Hospital Association
ProBNP	Pro B-type natriuretic peptide
PSA	Prostate-specific antigen
SDMA	Symmetric dimethylarginine

References

1 Paepe, D., Verjans, G., Duchateau, L. et al. (2013). Routine health screening: findings in apparently healthy middle-aged and old cats. *J. Feline. Med. Surg.* 15 (1): 819.

2 Willems, A., Paepe, D., Marynissen, S. et al. (2017). Results of screening of apparently healthy senior and geriatric dogs. *J. Vet. Intern. Med.* 31 (1): 81–92.

Recommended Reading

AAHA. Canine Lifestage Guidelines. www.aaha.org/aaha-guidelines/life-stage-canine-2019/life-stage-canine-2019

AAHA. Senior Care Guidelines. www.aaha.org/globalassets/02-guidelines/senior-care/senior-care-guidelines

Cognitive dysfunction syndrome evaluation tool (DISHAA). www.purinainstitute.com/sites/g/files/auxxlc381/files/2018-08/DISHAA.pdf

Gardner, M. and McVety, D. (2017). *Treatment and Care of the Geriatric Veterinary Patient*. Hoboken, NJ: Wiley.

International Cat Care. Life Stages. https://icatcare.org/advice/life-stages

Vogt, A.H., Rodan, I., Brown, M. et al. (2010). AAFP-AAHA feline life stage guidelines. *J. Fel. Med. Surg.* 12: 43–54.

WSAVA. Nutrition Guidelines Toolkit. www.wsava.org/nutrition-toolkit

6.18

Aging Gracefully

Jacqui Ley, BVSc (Hons), PhD, DECAWBM, FANZCVS (Veterinary Behaviour)

Melbourne Veterinary Specialist Centre, Glen Waverley, Victoria, Australia

BASICS

6.18.1 Summary

Helping pets age well is an important part of veterinary care. With pets living longer, veterinary teams juggle more health problems and owners need good practical advice as to how to help their pets as their abilities decline. Simple tips can help owners make adjustments to their pet's environment to encourage movement and mental activity – important for aging gracefully.

6.18.2 Terms Defined

Aging: A complex set of biological changes occurring in older individuals that result in a progressive reduction of the ability to maintain homeostasis when exposed to internal physiological and external environmental stresses.
Cognitive Skills/Abilities: Brain-related skills such as memory, learning, and reasoning that are needed for most tasks.
Geriatric: Relating to elderly individuals.
Metabolism: The physical and biochemical processes that make or use energy in the body.

MAIN CONCEPTS

Getting older results in declines in sensory, physical, and cognitive abilities [1, 2]. These changes are all seen in companion animals and need to be discussed with owners to

help them meet the needs of their pet. Many owners fail to notice signs of illness in their older pets but do notice changes such as that the pet sleeps more, is stiff, has loss of hearing, loss of sight, and is slowing down [3].

6.18.3 Aging

There are several changes seen in the body as it ages. Weight loss and change in body composition are seen in older dogs and cats [4, 5]. Higher body condition scores (BCS) have been linked with longer survival rates when faced with serious health problems such as neoplasia [5] or cardiac insufficiency [6].

Owners frequently report noticing changes in sensory abilities. Age-related decline in hearing and changes in the histology of the inner ear have been demonstrated in dogs [7] and are suspected in cats. Visual deficits such as cataracts also occur. Nuclear (lenticular) sclerosis causing clouding of the pupil is commonly seen but does not appear to affect vision [8].

Old dogs have been found to have atrophy of the olfactory epithelium [9] and probably suffer reduction in their sense of smell, an important sense for navigation, social interaction, and appetite stimulation.

6.18.4 Helping Pets Age Gracefully

Owners can be given advice and help to give their older pets a good quality of life and to have a pet that is active and engaging.

Start discussions about managing old age when a pet is still young (see 6.17 Senior Care). Different breeds and individuals age at different rates. In breeds with known predispositions for heart disease, neoplasia, renal disease, etc., implement screening programs for detection and introduction of management strategies early.

Body weight and BCS should be assessed and recorded across the pet's life. Decreases in BCS below healthy need to be investigated.

Early management of chronic disease such as orthopedic conditions helps keep the animal as independently mobile as possible. Diet, dietary supplements, weight management, and specific exercise programs designed by a physiotherapist all may help. As the animal ages, the nature of the management program can be adjusted to include pain-relieving medications and treatments such as ice and heat packs.

Exercise often needs to be adjusted gradually. Shorter exercise more frequently keeps joints that may stiffen up moving without overtaxing them. Changes from chasing a ball or Frisbee to walking may be needed. Swimming and exercise in water are supportive of joints while providing resistance for muscles, making it good exercise for older pets.

Small changes help older pets navigate safely.

Steps, ramps, and nonslip carpet runners can all help a pet move around its home without falling. Owners may require advice as to how to lift and/or support their pet safely when navigating stairs. Harnesses are available that make it easier to lift larger dogs. A pet stroller/buggy/pram allows the owner to take the pet out with them and provides a comfortable place to rest when the pet needs. Being outside provides important mental stimulation for many older pets.

Providing padding on beds, heating pads, moving older animals inside to sleep at night also help with joints that get stiff. Jackets can also help keep pets warm when previously they may have been more tolerant of cold. Some animals will need help with grooming. Cats with arthritis often cannot groom thoroughly. Clipping longer haired animals may also help with the management of their coats.

Keeping the layout of the house the same helps pets with vision deficits. If changes are made, the pet will need to be guided until they learn the new layout. Night lights and motion-operated lights can help a pet with reduced vision navigate at night time or in dark parts of the house. Specific odors such as a perfume or essential oil sprayed onto furniture or doors and sounds can help the pet navigate.

It is easy to startle pets with hearing loss and can cause bites to people or other pets. If a loss of hearing is suspected or diagnosed, the client needs to understand that the animal will sleep more deeply and may startle if awoken suddenly. Clapping or calling the pet may not be enough to awaken the animal but often stamping on the ground is effective. A remote-activated vibrating collar may be helpful for getting their attention safely.

For loss of smell, heating up food and applying highly odiferous and palatable toppings can encourage older pets to eat. Offering smaller meals more frequently may also help.

Older pets still need mental stimulation even if they cannot undertake exercise. Teaching new tricks, introducing new toys, especially puzzle toys, can help keep an older pet mentally active. Scent work training can be a great activity for older pets to learn as it engages their minds, can be done slowly taking physical abilities into account and is fun!

Some older pets need protection from younger pets in the home. The younger pets may be too boisterous and knock the older pet over. Some younger pets are intolerant of mistakes made by the older pet such as failing to see them or hear them. Providing some time apart and supervision is often needed.

Attention to pain is very important. Many dogs and some cats have low-grade chronic pain that is hard to detect but should be suspected if a pet is quieter than usual or irritable. Sometimes an antiinflammatory trial is needed to identify pain. If the pet improves then longer term medical management can be used along with therapies such physiotherapy and massage.

Lastly, clients need to listen to their pet. Many older animals develop strong likes and dislikes – it is part of their charm.

EXAMPLES

A client reports that her older vizsla is lagging on his daily runs with her. On clinical examination, the veterinarian finds that the dog has significant loss of range of motion in his hindlegs, loss of muscle mass and overall a reduction in BCS based on the dog's records. The client also reports that the dog has trouble changing position. Radiographs of the dog's hindlegs and back show significant changes associated with arthritis of the hips, sacroiliac, and other vertebral joints. A plan involving pain relief, joint supportive supplements, and an exercise program designed by a physiotherapist attached to the clinic is implemented. The owner is advised not to run her dog but to walk him twice a day for shorter periods. Swimming is also recommended. After a month the dog is reassessed. He shows an increase in his BCS, has slightly improved range of motion in his hip joints, is reported to be happier, and able to settle in the evening.

A client presents her mother's 10-year-old domestic shorthair cat because it has significant matting of its coat all down its back. The cat is found to have fleas, is thin, and resists palpation of its back. Due to cost constraints, it is not possible further work up the cat. The mats are clipped off and it is treated for fleas. As the veterinarian is suspicious that the cat has a painful back and cannot groom, a nurse/technician is asked to demonstrate some grooming tools and discuss some changes to help the cat's mobility. The client takes a suitable comb and reports back that her mother can groom the cat and keep its coat healthy. She has raised the cat's food and water bowls slightly off the ground and provided some steps to help the cat move around. The cat is eating better and has been moving around the house more.

TAKE-AWAYS

- Many treatable health problems are dismissed by owners as just old age.
- Older animals may need changes to their environment, exercise, and diet to help them stay active and well.
- Start discussing older age in pets with owners when pets are young. Be proactive with preventive healthcare for chronic conditions.
- Keep older minds active with new training, toys, and experiences. It's the "use it or lose it" idea!
- Listen to the pet for their likes and dislikes, and for changes in their ability to cope.

MISCELLANEOUS

References

1 Goldston, R.T. (1995). Introduction and overview of geriatrics. In: *Geriatrics and Gerontology of the Dog and Cat* (eds. R.T. Goldston and J.D. Hoskins), 1–8. Philadelphia, PA: WB Saunders.

2 Reed, D.M., Foley, D., White, L. et al. (1998). Predictors of healthy aging in men with high life expectancies. *American Journal of Public Health* 88 (10): 1463–1468.

3 Davies, M. (2012). Geriatric screening in first opinion practice – results from 45 dogs. *Journal of Small Animal Practice* 53 (9): 507–513.

4 Speakman, J.R., van Acker, A., and Harper, E.J. (2003). Age-related changes in the metabolism and body composition of three dog breeds and their relationship to life expectancy. *Aging Cell* 2 (5): 265–275.

5 Laflamme, D.P. (2016). Sarcopenia and weight loss in the geriatric cat. In: *August's Consultations in Feline Internal Medicine* (ed. S.E. Little), 951. St Louis, MO: Elsevier.

6 Slupe, J.L., Freeman, L.M., and Rush, J.E. (2008). Association of body weight and body condition with survival in dogs with heart failure. *Journal of Veterinary Internal Medicine* 22 (3): 561–565.

7 Shimada, A., Ebisu, M., Morita, T. et al. (1998). Age-related changes in the cochlea and cochlear nuclei of dogs. *Journal of Veterinary Medical Science* 60 (1): 41–48.

8 Bellows, J., Colitz, C., Daristotle, L. et al. (2014). Common physical and functional changes associated with aging in dogs. *Journal of the American Veterinary Medical Association* 246 (1): 67–75.

9 Hirai, T., Kojima, S., Shimada, A. et al. (1996). Age-related changes in the olfactory system of dogs. *Neuropathology and Applied Neurobiology* 22 (6): 531–539.

Recommended Reading

Boneham-Webster, S. (2007). *Senior Cats*. Neptune, NJ: TFH Publications.

Dodman, N. (ed.) (2012). *Good Old Dog: Expert Advice for Keeping Your Aging Dog Happy, Healthy, and Comfortable*. Boston, MA: Mariner Books.

Hoskins, J.D. (2003). *Geriatrics and Gerontology of the Dog and Cat*, 2e. St Louis, MO: Saunders.

6.19

Problem Aging

Jacqui Ley, BVSc (Hons), PhD, DECAWBM, FANZCVS (Veterinary Behaviour)

Melbourne Veterinary Specialist Centre, Glen Waverley, Victoria, Australia

BASICS

6.19.1 Summary

It is common for animals well into their teens to be presented to companion animal practices. Aging in companion animals mostly parallels aging in people with the expected decline in sensory abilities along with more complicated medical problems. The brain also suffers from age-related change which shows as a loss of cognitive ability.

In some animals the degree of cognitive decline is greater than expected and is the result of abnormal processes in the brain. The pet gets lost, loses learned responses, wakes at night and is generally anxious and irritable, all of which is difficult for owners. Treatment to help slow the changes and management of the pet's environment can help owners navigate this challenging time.

6.19.2 Terms Defined

Aging: A complex set of biological changes occurring in older individuals that result in a progressive reduction of the ability to maintain homeostasis when exposed to internal physiological and external environmental stresses.
Cognitive Decline: Normal age-related reduction in memory, learning, and reasoning skills.
Cognitive Impairment: Problems with concentration, making decisions, learning, and memory that affect the individual's everyday life.

Cognitive Skills/Abilities: Brain-related skills such as memory, learning, and reasoning that are needed for most tasks.
Monoamine Neurotransmitters: Noradrenaline/norepinephrine, dopamine, and serotonin.

MAIN CONCEPTS

It is expected that as pets age, they will experience some cognitive decline as their brains become less efficient, similar to the situation in humans [1]. Some pets show cognitive impairment and their behavior is challenging for owners to manage. Cognitive decline is due to normal aging, while cognitive impairment is a loss of learned responses and other cognitive skills due to damage to the brain. In elderly dogs and cats, it leads to cognitive decline syndrome (CDS). CDS parallels dementia and Alzheimer's disease (AD) in humans [2].

Animals affected by CDS show a variety of signs. They tend to be remembered by the mnemonic Disorientation, Interactions, Sleep/wake cycles, Housetraining, Anxiety, Activity (DISHAA) (Table 6.19.1).

In humans, tests of memory and recall are used to assess the cognition domains such as learning, episodic memory, and working memory [3]. Laboratory tests with aged dogs and cats show that deficits in complex learning can be seen in some elderly animals. Tests that require the animals to learn a rule then learn the reverse of that rule (reversal learning) or to retain information (delayed nonmatching

Table 6.19.1 DISHAA explained

Explanation
D Disorientation – the pet gets lost in the house or yard, seems confused, not recognizing familiar people or other pets
I Interactions – altered interactions, often reduced, possibly irritable
S Sleep/wake cycle changes – night time waking is often what prompts owners to contact the clinic
H House training loss. Loss of other learned responses
A Anxiety – may appear for the first time or worsen
A Activity – altered, may be increased or decreased

test) reliably separate elderly animals into unimpaired and impaired groups [2].

The onset of CDS is insidious and many pet owners do not notice the small changes in the pet. At present, it is not possible to measure the onset of CDS in pets. AD in humans is thought to have a significant preclinical onset and the same is probably true of CDS in pets.

6.19.3 Causes

There are several theories as to what causes CDS. Some animals have the changes in the brain associated with AD in humans and it is thought that it may be the same disease process occurring [2].

Low levels of a group of neurotransmitters called the monoamine neurotransmitters (serotonin, dopamine, and noradrenaline/norepinephrine) are theorized as a cause of CDS. Monoamine neurotransmitters are important for learning, memory retrieval, and responding to stimuli. When levels become too low, there is a concurrent loss of functioning in the brain. Some patients respond to medications that increase the amount of these neurotransmitters.

Another theory is that the mechanisms in the brain that clean up free radicals are failing, resulting in oxidative injury to individual neurons. Some patients respond to medication to increase blood flow to the brain and diets that result in fewer free radicals being generated.

6.19.4 Presentation and Diagnosis

Cognitive decline syndrome must be considered on the differential diagnostic list when owners present an elderly pet with a history of being irritable, showing signs of being anxious or having fears or phobias, losing toilet training and other learned behaviors and seeming confused. Owners most commonly complain of altered social interactions,

increased sleeping during the day and nighttime restlessness and vocalizing in dogs and cats [4].

Many of these signs overlap signs of other medical conditions. House soiling may occur due to pain from arthritis and other musculoskeletal conditions preventing pets getting up to go out to the toilet. Illness that alters urine output or toileting routines may also result in house soiling. Ruleouts include diabetes, hyperadrenocorticism (Cushing's disease), renal insufficiency, bladder stones, and intestinal disease. Heart disease, syncope, deafness, and blindness may all cause a pet to be vague and not respond to cues.

Diagnosis is made by ruling out medical causes for the problems reported by owners. It has been demonstrated that veterinary teams need to be proactive in asking owners of older pets if there are any behaviors concerning them [5]. A checklist questionnaire is an efficient way of screening for problems [4].

6.19.5 Treatment

Treatment of CDS aims to improve clinical signs and slow progression of the disease to improve the welfare of the pet and owner and delay the onset of dementia. Treatment may include environmental enrichment, diets, supplements, and medication. A combination of treatments often gives the best results.

6.19.5.1 Environmental Enrichment

Individuals with CDS are still able to learn and interact (see 4.11 Environmental Enrichment). Studies in humans and animal species have shown repeatedly that physical and mental exercise helps relieve some of the symptoms of AD in humans and CDS in animals [6]. Providing favorite activities and games that suit the pet's physical abilities helps slow their decline. Activities may include walks, time outside in the garden, training for sports or just for fun, swimming or even just introducing new toys or food-dispensing toys and helping the pet find hidden treats.

Daily routine is also very important for helping pets manage as it provides structure and reliability to the day and helps pets orientate themselves. Memory is complex and multilayered and while the pet may be having a vague moment, they may still respond to cues for their daily routine.

6.19.5.2 Diets

There are some helpful commercial diets that are well supported by efficacy research. All are high in antioxidants and a variety of compounds, such as medium-chain fatty acids

Table 6.19.2 Commercially available diets, supplements, and medications

Treatment type	Treatment	Active ingredients
Diet	Hills B/D	Antioxidants, fatty acids, dl-alpha-lipoic acid and L-carnitine
	Purina Pro Bright Minds/ Optiage	Medium-chain triglycerides which supply ketone bodies as a possible alternative energy source for neurons
	Royal Canin Mature Consult (Canine and Feline)	Phosphatidylserine, antioxidants, L-tryptophan
Supplements	Senilife (Ceva Animal Health)	Phosphotidylserine, *Gingko biloba*, vitamin E, resveratrol, vitamin B6
	Neutricks (Neutricks)	Apoaequoin, a calcium-buffering protein derived from jellyfish
	Akatvait (Vet plus Ltd)	Phosphatidylserine, omega-3 fatty acids, vitamins E and C, alpha-lipoic acid (not in feline product), coenzyme Q and selenium
	Novafit (Virbac Animal Health)	S-adenosylmethione – helps preserve cell membrane fluidity, receptor function and regulate neurotransmitter levels and increase glutathione production
Medication	Selegiline	MAOB inhibitor
	Propentofylline	Increases microcirculation, improving oxygenation of the brain and removing free radicals

found to be useful for brains as alternative sources of energy. Examples of these diets that have been shown to help relieve some of the signs of CDS in dogs and cats are Hills Pet Nutrition Prescription Diet B/d, Purina Proplan Bright Minds (North America) or Optiage (UK) and Royal Canin Canine Mature Consult and Feline Mature Consult. Table 6.19.2 summarizes some commercially available diets.

6.19.5.3 Medications

Medication aims to improve functioning of the individual nerve cells. Suitable medications may be protective and supportive of biochemical pathways inside the cells or in the synapses.

Selegiline is a monoamine oxidase B inhibitor (MAOB-I). Monoamine oxidase is the enzyme that breaks down monoamine neurotransmitters which are important for learning and memory and many other functions in the brain. Selegiline results in higher levels of these neurotransmitters and helps improve functioning. It is licensed for dogs in North America and has also been effective in cats. Some animals respond within a few weeks while others may take two months before showing improvement [6].

Propentofylline is licensed for use in dogs in some parts of Europe and Australia. It increases microcirculation in the brain and periphery with the net result of providing more blood and therefore more oxygen to the brain. Laboratory tests have shown variable results for its effects [6].

6.19.5.4 Medications to Avoid

Medications that have anticholinergic effects may worsen the signs of CDS, sometimes permanently, and should be avoided where possible. Examples of anticholinergic medications are atropine, amitriptyline, clomipramine, and diphenhydramine (Benadryl®).

EXAMPLES

Frosty, a 13-year-old, neutered female Siberian husky, was presented by her owners due to house soiling and nighttime waking. Her clinical examination found that she was thin with reduced range of motion in her hips and a painful back. She seemed confused and was nonresponsive to being called by the veterinarian or her owners. She was diagnosed with arthritis and CDS. Treatment for her CDS included a therapeutic diet and propentofylline. She was also treated for her arthritis and her owners put down nonslip matting, provided her with a night light and started physiotherapy. A revisit two weeks later showed that Frosty was able to get up and go to the toilet unaided and the house soiling had stopped. The nighttime waking was improving and Frosty was noticeably more alert and interactive.

TAKE-AWAYS

- CDS is an insidious disease that probably has a long preclinical time before signs of cognitive decline are detectable.
- The signs associated with CDS are covered by the mnemonic DISHAA.
- Asking owners specifically about changes in an elderly pet's behavior is essential for early identification and monitoring of behavioral signs for establishing a diagnosis and monitoring treatment success.
- Diagnosis may be difficult due to other overlapping medical conditions that may mask signs of CDS.
- Treatment may include prescription diets, supplements, medication, and environmental management.

MISCELLANEOUS

References

1 Goldston, R.T. (1995). Introduction and overview of geriatrics. In: *Geriatrics and Gerontology of the Dog and Cat* (eds. R.T. Goldston and J.D. Hoskins), 1–8. Philadelphia, PA: WB Saunders.

2 Landsberg, G.M., Nichol, J., and Araujo, J.A. (2012). Cognitive dysfunction syndrome: a disease of canine and feline brain aging. *Vet. Clin. North Am. Small Anim. Pract.* 42: 749–768.

3 Dubois, B., Feldman, H., Jacova, C. et al. (2014). Advancing research diagnostic criteria for Alzheimer's disease: the IWG-2 criteria. *Lancet Neurology* 13 (6): 614–629.

4 Landsberg, G.M. and Malamed, R. (2017). Clinical picture of canine and feline cognitive impairment. In: *Canine and Feline Dementia* (eds. G.M. Landsberg, A. Maďari and N. Žilka), 1–12. Cham: Springer.

5 Landsberg, G.M. and Araujo, J.A. (2005). Behavior problems in geriatric pets. *Vet. Clin. North Am. Small Anim. Pract.* 35: 675–698.

6 Denenberg, S. and Landsberg, G.M. (2017). Current pharmacological and non-pharmacological approaches for therapy of feline and canine dementia. In: *Canine and Feline Dementia* (eds. G.M. Landsberg, A. Maďari and N. Žilka), 129–144. Cham: Springer.

Recommended Reading

Landsberg, G.M., Maďari, A., and Žilka, N. (eds.) (2017). *Canine and Feline Dementia*. Cham.: Springer.

6.20

Quality of Life and End of Life Issues

Mary Craig, DVM, MBA, CHPV

Gentle Goodbye Veterinary Hospice and At-home Euthanasia, Stamford, CT, USA

 BASICS

6.20.1 Summary

Quality of life (QOL) is a term we use to describe the qualitative, less clinically measurable components of a pet's condition. While there is broad agreement that our goal is to avoid suffering for our pets at end of life, because our nonverbal patients communicate through sometimes subtle signs and behaviors, caregivers can miss these signals if they aren't aware or attentive to them.

Helping clients to understand how to read their pet's behavior to determine their quality of life can not only facilitate conversations about whether it is time to consider euthanasia, but it can also prompt treatment discussions about pain management or other palliative care.

6.20.2 Terms Defined

Co-morbidities: More than one disease or condition occurring at the same time, often complicating treatments and responses.

Multimodal Pain Management: An approach to pain that considers the source of the pain as well as the mechanism of action of available drug choices, often combining several drugs at lower doses.

Palliative Care: Treatment which supports or improves the patient's QOL by relieving suffering. This term can be used when treating curable or chronic conditions, as well as during end of life care.

QOL: The total well-being of an individual animal, taking into account the physical, social, and emotional components of the animal's life.

QOL Assessment: The assessment a caregiver makes about how well or poorly an animal is doing, considering the totality of an animal's feelings, experiences, and preferences, as demonstrated by the animal.

Suffering: An unpleasant or painful experience, feeling, emotion, or sensation, which may be acute or chronic in nature. Suffering is an umbrella term that covers the range of negative subjective experiences, including (but not limited to) physical and emotional pain and distress, which may be experienced by humans and by animals.

 MAIN CONCEPTS

6.20.3 Why Do Caregivers Need to Understand Quality of Life?

Clients will say they don't want their pet to suffer or be in pain, but what does that really mean? Suffering is a difficult concept to quantify, and pain can present in a number of ways (see 8.13 Team Approach to Pain Management). Especially in the face of co-morbidities, it's the overarching quality of life that's more important and more measurable. Most veterinary professionals intuitively understand what "quality of life" is but may have difficulty articulating it to clients.

Furthermore, it's nearly impossible for us to accurately assess a pet's QOL in a practice setting. Except in the most extreme cases, the behavior a pet displays in an exam room or waiting area can markedly camouflage behaviors they may show at home. It can be a disservice to the pet and caregiver for veterinary personnel to make a judgment about a pet's QOL based on a few minutes' observation outside the home.

Therefore, it is important that we educate and equip caregivers to be able to evaluate their pet's comfort level at home. A subjective and educated observer who sees the pet in their normal environment, throughout the day and night, will detect behavior that reflects true QOL and indications of suffering. This understanding will allow them to ask for support, additional diagnostics or treatment, and often eventually euthanasia.

6.20.4 What is Quality of Life?

Certainly, the absence of pain is important (see 2.16 Pain and Pain Management), but other feelings contribute to what we consider suffering. When asked, many caregivers say they don't want their pet to be in pain but in fact, the factors affecting their pet's QOL go well beyond the absence of pain.

There are a number of published QOL scales, and most include similar components (Table 6.20.1). Find one that you feel comfortable discussing with clients. As a pet reaches the end of life, it is often helpful to ask clients to rate their pet's QOL on a daily basis to help them think more objectively about it.

With an effective ongoing QOL assessment in place, clients may also be more likely to reach out when the QOL slips to seek further hospice or palliative care. We often expect that multimodal pain management may be required

(see 6.14 Pain Prevention, Management and Conditioning), but without ongoing QOL communication with caregivers, we may miss the opportunity to increase therapeutics as the disease progresses. A quick QOL status check can signal the need for a deeper discussion.

Another advantage of monitoring QOL with a daily diary is the ability of family members to assess individually and then compare notes. Often a family member who is at work all day may not be seeing what others are. Children in the family may be less experienced in pet care, but still profoundly invested in the life of the pet. Helping everyone to see and hear what a pet is communicating can be critical as a family considers euthanasia and deals with grief at the end of life.

6.20.5 Quality of Death

Among caregivers facing the end of their pets' lives, it is an almost universal hope that "she goes peacefully in her sleep." The reality is that this rarely happens without a long drawn out period of *poor* QOL and it's often not peaceful at all. While hospice-supported natural death can be accomplished, it can be very time intensive and expensive (see 9.18 Hospice and Palliative Care). For most clients, that's not what they want.

An important part of a caregiver's education at their pet's end of life is understanding what this specific death might look like if they delay euthanasia too long. It need not be a dramatic guilt trip, but a gentle discussion of what is likely to occur as the disease(s) progresses is important. Renal failure is a very different death from cardiac failure. Armed with this information, caregivers are much better equipped

Table 6.20.1 Typical components considered in a quality of life (QOL) assessment

Mobility	Depending on the disease process, mobility issues can reflect a level of discomfort, strength or cognitive acuity. The ability to move also impacts a pet's sense of autonomy and the loss of mobility often causes frustration, anxiety, and an unsettling sense of vulnerability
Nutrition	Unwillingness to eat can reflect nausea, pain or other uncomfortable sensations. That said, as humans approach natural death, the appetite diminishes or ceases altogether
Hydration	Especially important in diseases that affect kidney function, hydration can have a significant effect on the way a pet feels. Dehydration and the build-up of toxins can be uncomfortable
Interaction/attitude	Any changes in behavior can signal quality of life concerns. Hiding, disengaging, or altered interactions with other pets may be because of discomfort, anxiety or both
Elimination	Normal urination and/or defecation are important health issues, but as important to consider is where the elimination is occurring. Pets' toileting habits are instinctual and long-standing behaviors that when abandoned often indicate pain, dementia, anxiety or other forms of suffering
Favorite things	Whether it's seeking out a sunny spot or barking at the mailman, when pets no longer take pleasure in the things they used to enjoy, they are signaling a decreased QOL
Disease-specific parameters	Many diseases have specific indicators that require education and monitoring. Caregivers can monitor a resting respiratory rate in patients with diseases that could affect a pet's ability to breath. Mucous membrane color and capillary refill rate can be useful monitors in bleeding or cardiovascular diseases. Helping owners understand one or two disease-specific parameters can be valuable

to decide when it's the right time. This is much more valuable than telling a caregiver "You'll know when it's time."

Choosing to end the life of a pet is the most difficult decision a caregiver has to make, and it is a decision that they have to live with, so it's important that it be their decision and that we support them in it.

EXAMPLES

Malcolm was a 15-year-old neutered male beagle who lived with a family of four, including two teenaged girls. He had developed arthritis a few years ago, particularly in his knees and spine. He was receiving several different medications in escalating doses for his arthritis pain that kept him comfortable, relatively active and happy to be with his family. With instruction from their hospice veterinarian, his caregivers were monitoring his QOL with a daily diary. For Malcolm, the parameters that were most predictive of how he was feeling included mobility, interactions, and elimination. On days he was uncomfortable, he would have difficulty getting up, would pace before finally lying down, and would defecate inside even after going outside to urinate. The family used the diary to help know when it was time to discuss increased pain management with their veterinarian. Each time the score ticked down for more than a few days, they would consult with their veterinarian about a dose change or additional drug. After more than two years of monitoring and managing his pain, Malcolm started to refuse even people food, and resisted taking pills. The family decided together that his QOL score had dipped to a point where euthanasia was the humane choice. They made an appointment for a house call the next day and said goodbye to Malcolm all together outside under his favorite tree.

TAKE-AWAYS

- QOL goes beyond just the absence of pain.
- Veterinary practices should adopt a QOL scale they are comfortable with and teach caregivers how to use it.
- An educated client is better able to judge when QOL is poor.
- Understanding what their pet's specific disease will look like as death approaches can help a caregiver make the difficult decision to euthanize.
- A daily diary is often the best way to be objective as caregivers assess and align on QOL.
- Euthanasia can be a gentle death, but it is such a difficult decision to make through which we need to support caregivers.

MISCELLANEOUS

Recommended Reading

Gaynor, J. and Muir, W. (2008). *Handbook of Veterinary Pain Management*, 2e. St Louis, MO: Elsevier.

Pope, G. (2015. https://archangelink.com/). *The BrightHaven Guide to Animal Hospice*. Archangel Ink.

Shanan, A., Shearer, T., and Pierce, J. (2017). *Hospice and Palliative Care for Companion Animals: Principles and Practice*. Ames, IA: Wiley-Blackwell.

Shearer, T. (2011). Palliative medicine and hospice care. *Veterinary Clinics of North America: Small Animal Practice* 41 (3).

Section 7

Hospital Considerations

7.1

Creating a Client-Centered Hospital

Amanda L. Donnelly, DVM, MBA

ALD Veterinary Consulting, LLC, Nashville, TN, USA

BASICS

7.1.1 Summary

Historically, veterinary practices have been doctor centered. Hospital operations, protocols, and communications have centered on doctors because they provide medical care for pets. Traditionally, veterinarians have taken a paternalistic approach when educating clients and giving them recommendations. Gradually, there has been a movement away from this approach to one focused on client needs. Research has shown that with a client-centered approach to communications and pet care, hospitals can achieve better patient outcomes and greater pet owner satisfaction.

7.1.2 Terms Defined

Client Engagement: The communication connection and relationship between a client and the veterinary business.
Forward Booking: Scheduling the patient's next appointment.

MAIN CONCEPTS

7.1.3 The Value of Being a Client-Centered Hospital

Being a client-centered hospital is somewhat different from being a service-oriented hospital. The goal of providing excellent client service is to make clients happy and build client loyalty (see 5.1 Pet-Specific Customer Service). This goal is embraced by client-centered hospitals as well but the concept of putting the client at the center of the business is based on the premise of getting more pets the care they need. Client-centered hospitals understand that the needs and preferences of clients must be met for pets to receive optimal care. Client-centered teams strive to enhance client engagement, build trust, and develop partnerships with clients so they are part of the decision-making process for their pet's healthcare.

7.1.4 Creating a Client-Centered Culture

Being a client-centered hospital doesn't mean following the motto "the client is always right." Rather, it is about ensuring the team knows that a primary business goal is to always make sure clients feel cared about. One way to accomplish this goal is for teams to convey a desire to help clients at all times.

Conveying a desire to help involves letting clients know the team wants to do whatever it can to make a visit to the hospital easy, efficient, and enjoyable. It is beneficial to create dialogue with team members about being client focused rather than task oriented. Employees who focus on building relationships, rather than just completing transactions, will enhance client engagement and build client loyalty.

Conveying a desire to help goes beyond the basics such as saying, "We'll get you in an exam room as soon as possible." Because clients expect those cordial statements, they don't bond pet owners to a practice. On the other hand, team members who say or do something unexpected will impress clients. For example, rather than asking "Do you need help carrying everything?" (or, worse yet, not offering help), a client-focused employee will come from behind the front desk carrying the client's products and say, "Let me help you out to your car."

7.1.5 Focus on Enhancing Client Engagement

Client engagement is about making authentic, emotional connections with pet owners. When clients are emotionally bonded to the veterinary team, they tell friends and co-workers "I wouldn't dream of going anyplace else with my little Sophie."

To connect emotionally with clients, teams can use specific communication skills to provide personalized service and build rapport with clients (see 8.15 Delivering Information to Clients). A simple yet often overlooked way to do this is to use the name of the client and the name of the pet when speaking with pet owners. Using someone's name shows respect and conveys you know who they are – they aren't just a number in your day. Likewise, people love to hear their pet's name. Service appears customized when a client hears "How is Sophie doing?" rather than "How is she doing?"

Giving compliments is another easy way to enhance client engagement. One of the best compliments is to praise clients for how well they take care of their pet. Pet owners can be commended on their efforts to get their pet to lose weight or for being consistent with heartworm and flea control products. Praise reinforces a position on patient advocacy and lets pet parents know they're doing a good job (see 5.5 Meeting the Needs of Pet Parents).

Client-centered teams also use communication skills to build trust and form partnerships with pet owners (see 5.1 Pet-Specific Customer Service). Today's pet owners want to be empowered and participate in making decisions for their pet (see 5.2 Meeting Client Needs). Specifically, teams can ask open-ended questions to elicit information from clients that allows the team to provide tailored service and personalized care for a pet owner (see 5.3 What Clients Expect from the Veterinary Team). Here are examples of excellent open-ended questions that engage pet owners.

- What is important to you for Chloe's nutrition?
- Tell me what you know about arthritis in senior dogs.
- Tell me what you know about diabetes in cats.
- What concerns do you have about Oliver's treatment?
- How are you feeling about Sadie's prognosis?

Clients may experience anxiety, sadness, or frustration while at the hospital. A common response to upset clients is silence because team members aren't sure what to say. In these instances, it's best to respond with kind and reassuring words which can create lasting impressions for clients. For example, a client may be grumpy because they are exhausted after being up all night with a sick pet. A trained team member might say, "So Charlie kept you up all night. I can see how tired you are. That must have been so frustrating."

7.1.6 Team Approach to Care

In client-centered hospitals, teams work together to meet the needs of pet owners and create an exceptional client service experience. To promote effective teamwork, it's critical to designate job roles. Just telling your team "everyone help and work together" doesn't work well to achieve consistency of service. Individual team members need to be accountable for completing specific job tasks (see 8.3 The Importance of Accountability in Pet-Specific Care). Implement systems so everyone knows their job roles and assignments for each day. Examples include having a designated veterinary nurse who will answer questions for the front office team and making daily assignments for which team member will provide assistance to the client service team during their busy lunch break.

7.1.7 Implement Client-Focused Systems and Standards

Practices need systems and standards to ensure pet owners have a positive client experience every time they visit the hospital. Additionally, protocols should be implemented that cater to clients' needs. To create a client-centered hospital, be sure to view protocols from the client's perspective. For example, many practices have a policy that prescription refill requests will take 24–48 hours to fill. This seems like a reasonable policy because it favors the hospital. But does it meet the needs of clients who routinely can pick up medications from a human pharmacy within a few hours?

Be sure to think about client interactions that take place before, during, and after visits to the hospital. For example, evaluate the system you use to remind clients when their pets are due for preventive care. Consider if the system is effective by looking at it from the client perspective. Are you still using paper postcards generated in-house or heavy card stock postcards with color pictures that are tailored for the pet owner? Are you sending text reminders and using a practice app to help clients book appointments?

Two systems that should be examined at all veterinary hospitals are the patient admission and discharge processes.

To ensure these client interactions go smoothly, consider what protocols you may need to put in place. This could include advising clients via text (SMS) before their appointments that the check-in process will take 10–15 minutes. Or perhaps you need to create a checklist for team members to use during admissions so they can efficiently gather correct information from the client, such as their best contact number (see 2.4 Checklists in Veterinary Medicine).

Client-centered hospitals are increasingly moving to exam room discharge processes. Once clients have seen the doctor and/or leave the exam room, they don't like to wait to check out. Joining a line at the front desk can be aggravating, especially if the pet owner is juggling kids, bags of food or medication, and a rowdy or scared pet. Checking clients out while they are still in the exam room can create a much nicer experience for pet owners. Exam room checkout also allows privacy for a client who might need to discuss finances or other sensitive topics.

Exam room check-out also makes it easier to do forward booking. Team members aren't distracted so they can focus on communicating the value of the next appointment. Likewise, the pet owner is in a more comfortable position to hear the message and think about their schedule. Ideally, forward booking should be done before collecting money for services.

EXAMPLES

After moving to a new city, Emily asked her colleague, Jack, if he could recommend a veterinary hospital. Jack told her she must go to ABC Pet Hospital because of how they cater to his needs and partner with him to provide the best care for his beagle, Sam. He explained that on his last visit, he was anxious because Sam was vomiting. The staff were empathetic and reassured him they would take care of Sam. The certified veterinary technician asked a series of questions about Sam's diet, daily routine, and medical history. She praised Jack for being such a good pet parent and bringing Sam in before he became dehydrated. The doctor reviewed the laboratory tests, which showed no

serious abnormalities. Jack particularly likes this doctor because she always asks questions about his concerns and what he knows about veterinary conditions rather than just telling him what to do. Sam was sent home on a bland diet and medication. Jack was able to check out and schedule his next appointment in the exam room.

TAKE-AWAYS

- Being a client-centered hospital means focusing on clients' needs and wants with a goal of guiding them to provide optimal care for their pets.
- The value of being a client-centered hospital is that more pets will get the care they deserve.
- Client-centered hospitals develop a culture dedicated to helping pet owners at all times and creating an exceptional client experience.
- Teams at client-centered hospitals focus on enhancing client engagement to build trust and form strong relationships with pet owners.
- Client-centered hospitals implement systems and standards to ensure the consistent delivery of customized pet care and high levels of client service.

MISCELLANEOUS

Recommended Reading

Berry, L. and Seltman, K. (2008). *Management Lessons from the Mayo Clinic*. New York: McGraw-Hill.

Fleming, J. and Asplund, J. (2007). *Human Sigma: Managing the Employee–Customer Encounter*. Washington, DC: Gallup Press.

Gerber, M. and Weinstein, P. (2015). *The E Myth Veterinarian*. New York: Prodigy Business Books.

Hsieh, T. (2013). *Delivering Happiness: A Path to Profits, Passion, and Purpose*. New York: Grand Central Publishing.

7.2

Managing the Pet-Specific Workplace

Lowell Ackerman, DVM, DACVD, MBA, MPA, CVA, MRCVS

Global Consultant, Author, and Lecturer, MA, USA

 BASICS

7.2.1 Summary

Workplace management is about balancing the needs of those receiving care through the hospital with those providing the care. Building the support infrastructure into the practice business model is essential for this purpose and can make the difference between the business strategically driving outcomes and or the outcomes driving the business.

Most veterinary teams are trained to deal with healthcare issues and are not necessarily trained in how to manage the business aspects of the workplace, but a hospital cannot survive and thrive without both aspects being managed effectively.

7.2.2 Terms Defined

Cross-Selling: Encouraging a buyer to purchase related or complementary products or services.

Economy of Scale: The reduction in cost per unit that results when operational efficiencies allow increased production. Thus, there is an increase in savings because as production increases, the cost of producing each additional unit decreases.

Economy of Scope: The reduction in costs of operations when a company enters two or more markets where the operations in one market can be used to make operations in another market more efficient.

Holacracy: A flat organizational structure in which authority and decision making are controlled by self-organizing teams rather than by a management hierarchy.

Open-Book Management: The premise that employers should share with employees the measures of the practice's business success so that employees better understand the efforts that impact that success.

Profit Center: A section of a practice that can be assessed in terms of its revenues and expenses (e.g., surgery, imaging, laboratory, etc.).

Upselling: Encouraging a buyer to purchase a higher level of items or services.

Workstream: The step-by-step process by which tasks are completed by teams working within the hospital.

 MAIN CONCEPTS

7.2.3 Attitudinal Differences

It is important to realize that operating a for-profit veterinary hospital is done with the intention that the business should be profitable. In most cases, there are not governmental or charitable organizations supporting the care of animals in these facilities, so they need to be profitable to survive and fairly compensate all concerned, as well as provide the services that pet owners crave. Still, veterinary teams often appreciate that the public believes there must be some charitable component to the business, and teams are often asked to subsidize or discount care, which partly explains the relatively low salaries not only of veterinarians but also of the other positions employed by the hospital (see 2.11 Discounting in Veterinary Practice). Most pet owners are not aware of how expensive it is to operate a veterinary hospital, and it is not their duty to know, but owners of such businesses are keenly aware that payroll, overhead, and materials can be difficult or impossible to

Pet-Specific Care for the Veterinary Team, First Edition. Edited by Lowell Ackerman.
© 2021 John Wiley & Sons, Inc. Published 2021 by John Wiley & Sons, Inc.

manage without adequate and consistent revenue generation. It is also difficult for most pet owners to appreciate how often veterinary hospitals are approached for such financial support or accommodation.

Partially associated with this attitude is the misconception that clients do not want to spend money for veterinary care. Frankly, nobody wants to spend money on things if they don't have to. There is abundant evidence that pet owners spend more money on their pets with every passing year, although it is clear that the growth in spending on veterinary care may be much less. This implies that clients might not be recognizing the value in the veterinary care offered, rather than indicating reluctance of clients to provide their pets with appropriate veterinary care.

The main impediment to growth in veterinary spending is likely a failure on the part of the veterinary profession to communicate effectively with clients about the importance of following recommendations, and perhaps the value of services being offered [1]. Improving communication skills is the most effective way to increase revenue generation in veterinary hospitals, which is critical if the current business model is to survive (see 5.10 Discussing Pet-Specific Care).

7.2.4 Business Model Differences

The current business model for veterinary practices in the United States is one of many small primary care hospitals serving communities. Most of these practices have relatively few full-time-equivalent veterinarians and limited opportunities to grow substantially, other than by mergers and acquisitions. Regarding acquisitions, in many countries more and more practices are becoming corporate owned. Since most of the practices being acquired tend to be larger, this can have an outsized impact on client visits. So, while corporate-owned practices may still be in the minority, if the trend continues, they might still represent the majority of actual client visits.

Each veterinary hospital has essentially the same types of services to offer, and the same types of equipment. Accordingly, there are relatively few opportunities to improve economies of scale and/or scope, which makes it difficult to be more competitive in pricing while assuring profitability.

Because of high fixed overhead costs and the necessity of providing some services that might not be profitable, hospitals sometimes engage in pricing that might make little sense from a profit center perspective (see 10.13 Approach to Pricing).

Staff are often confused by veterinary pricing schemes, and if they are not certain where the value is delivered, then they are likely to be less than convincing when communicating that message to clients. Partially because of the confusion with the veterinary business model, there is often a dichotomy between the goals of practice owners and managers, who are seeking to assure adequate revenue generation, and associate (employed) veterinarians and nonveterinary staff who are often most concerned with meeting the needs of clients while saving them money. It is true that there are clients who may not be able to afford recommended services, but it is challenging for individual veterinary practices which may already be struggling financially to serve the role of community benefactor when it comes to the provision of veterinary services (see 6.5 Opportunities and Challenges of Providing Services for Low-Income Families and 7.8 Providing Care for Those Unable or Unwilling to Pay). It's unrealistic to expect that individual small businesses can take on this burden themselves, and yet many practices try to do what they can.

7.2.5 Pet-Specific Considerations

In the traditional veterinary workplace model, the emphasis is on getting clients into appointments and then augmenting with add-ons to basic care, such as needed diagnostic tests, procedures, and dispensed items (parasite control, laboratory testing, dental cleaning, etc.). This menu-driven model of basic services and then à la carte recommendations can work, but the process makes it difficult for clients to foresee expenses, and staff are often uncomfortable with the process and the reaction of clients to expenses they were not anticipating. The goal of pet-specific care is transparency, so in most instances there should not be any surprises about what services are to be recommended, and what the costs will be.

With pet-specific care, the focus from the start is on investing in prevention and early detection, and clients have the opportunity to better appreciate the costs involved with procedures and testing recognized from the very earliest office visits. Staff can then be better coaches and educators without a need to appear to be "cross-selling" or "upselling" products and services, and clients are better consumers because they are not surprised by recommendations when they come in for office visits. For example, all veterinary teams want pets to receive comprehensive parasite control to protect pets and their families, and this is true whether clients come in for a basic examination and receive "add-on" parasite testing and appropriate medications, or if the recommendation is understood from the start on what is involved with keeping pets parasite free.

To begin to embed pet-specific care into the practice workstream, teams need to first appreciate the "big picture" of what is being attempted – focusing on keeping pets healthy rather than waiting for them to become ill before we begin intervention (see 1.1 Overview of Pet-Specific Care). As teams start to grapple with some of the ways of accomplishing this, it quickly becomes evident that there are many aspects of practice that need to change to achieve the kinds of outcomes that are desirable. The team needs to determine which pets are at risk for different issues (see 1.2 Providing a Lifetime of Care). They need to understand how effective the hospital currently is in terms of desired outcomes (see 9.17 Improving Compliance and Adherence with Pet-Specific Care). They need to appreciate challenges regarding the affordability of veterinary practice (see 2.10 Affordability of Veterinary Services), and they need to appreciate some of the tools that can help make the situation more manageable, such as pet health insurance (see 10.16 Pet Health Insurance).

Veterinary teams implementing pet-specific care also need to appreciate one other thing – that pet-specific care is not for everyone. While all pet owners should aspire to the virtues of pet-specific care, not all will. Since this is a relatively new concept for most pet owners, and is different from the old model that pet care just requires some vaccinations and periodic visits to the veterinary clinic, expect that in any rollout there will not be universal acceptance of these new concepts and offerings.

As team members work to improve practice models of better understanding the needs of specific owners and pets, it is also worthwhile to consider which clients would be most receptive to the message of pet-specific care (see 10.4 Client and Patient Segmentation) and then design outreach for those clients (see 10.3 Pet-Specific Outreach). In most cases, the initial outreach for this new model of care would be to owners of puppies and kittens who can be introduced to the new concepts without previous bias, and to the market segment often referred to as pet parents (see 5.4 The Changing Nature of Pet Owners and 5.5 Meeting the Needs of Pet Parents). This would typically account for about 20% of practice patients, but they are the population most likely to be receptive to these new concepts.

It might initially seem questionable to put so much effort into such a small segment of the hospital population, but it's important to recall that according to the Pareto Principle, it is typically 20% of such endeavors that contribute to 80% of outcomes (see 10.2 The Importance of Practice Differentiation). So, rather than the team trying to launch pet-specific care and discussing it with all clients (where 80% will probably not be interested in being early adopters), it is best to focus on those most responsive to the messaging, where uptake is more likely to occur.

During the initial rollout, it is also worth limiting the offer to those most interested because there are bound to be fixes needed, as is common with all new programs (see 7.3

Leading the Change Towards Pet-Specific Care). However, once the program is working well with those core clients, it is much easier for the team to use their positive experience to then offer the system to other clients. It is also likely that clients who are happy with the pet-specific care offering will share their appreciation with friends and family, so the team may encounter clients who ask about pet-specific care even if it is not directly offered to them.

7.2.6 Generational Differences

It is natural for there to be attitudinal differences among generations in the workplace, but the current veterinary business model often makes it difficult to reconcile some of these differences within veterinary hospitals.

Currently, most veterinary hospitals in the US are owned by the Baby Boomer and Generation X generations, but most young veterinary team members are Generation Y (Millennials), and they already account for more than half the employees in most practices. While most attention is focused on Millennials, it is important not to forget about Generation Z (iGeneration) individuals in the marketplace (see 2.6 Generational Considerations). For this cohort, there was never a time in their lives that the internet did not exist and there is an expectation of convenience associated with their purchasing power.

Millennials tend to set high standards for themselves, but in return they expect their work to be fulfilling, and they have hopes that they will receive mentorship, clear career path advice, ongoing training and education, and a workplace that blends well with the rest of their life [2]. Gen Z appears to be more entrepreneurial, may have experienced more hardships growing up in a recession, and may be more money focused than Millennials.

Millennials currently represent the largest population of pet owners as well as veterinarians, but there are concerns that today's veterinarians do not appear to be that interested in practice ownership and those changes are very apparent. In 2006, 53% of veterinarians surveyed aspired to veterinary practice ownership, but by 2016, that number had dropped to 30% [3].

Currently, the majority of pet owners in the US are Millennials, so the veterinary workplace needs to change to meet the needs of this demographic.

7.2.7 Gender Differences

It is an inescapable fact that there is a major demographic shift in the veterinary profession as far as gender is concerned. In most US veterinary schools, over 70% of the classes are female, with some schools approaching 90%. Although men used to predominate in the profession, that is no longer the case and the current population of licensed veterinarians is close to parity between the sexes, but females will predominate in the years ahead if current student ratios persist.

Regarding practice ownership, nearly 60% of practice owners are male, whereas almost three-quarters of associate (employed) veterinarians are female [4]. The salaries of female veterinarians seem to lag those of males but males typically work longer hours, so it is difficult to interpret such pay discrepancies.

To date, it is unclear what effect this demographic shift in the profession will have. At present, it does not seem to affect practice ownership as males were actually less likely than females to aspire to practice ownership [3].

In the United States, new graduate veterinarians are more likely to be female, veterinary technicians/nurses are more likely to be female, and receptionists are more likely to be female, so whatever changes come with the female predilection for the profession are likely to be magnified in the years ahead.

7.2.8 Open-Book Management

The premise of open-book management is that organizational business information shared with employees not only helps them to do their jobs better, but helps them understand their role in the company and the company's ultimate success.

It is important to realize that open-book management does not require business owners to share sensitive financial data with staff. In most instances, the information presented may be productivity ratios or key performance indicators (e.g., percentage of dog and cat patients with pet health insurance policies) that allow employees to see how their overall efforts are reflected, positively or negatively, in the company's performance. For example, if the company's target is to keep nonveterinary wages below x% of total revenue, it is easy for everyone in the hospital to check if things are on target if they have access to this statistic. If the goal is for the clinic to cultivate a certain percentage of clients who have year-round integrated parasite control for their pets, then readily sharing this metric on an ongoing basis is the best way for staff to determine whether objectives are being met.

When employees understand the metrics of business success for the hospital, it is easier for them to appreciate how altering their performance to move those numbers in the needed direction can improve outcomes for all concerned (see 7.10 Analytics and Informatics).

Because pet-specific care involves so many different potential data points, this information must be easily available to teams. In fact, there are often so many different metrics that need to be tracked that dashboards may actually be customized to the need of individual teams, so they are not overwhelmed by the different aspects being measured (see 10.12 Dashboards and Key Performance Indicators).

7.2.9 Change Management

The care of pets is changing profoundly, especially with the introduction of pet-specific care, and the ability of veterinary hospitals to change along with it will ultimately determine the success or failure of many veterinary hospitals (see 7.3 Leading the Change Towards Pet-Specific Care).

For many years, practices have been perhaps overreliant on revenues from product sales, which allowed them to undercharge for professional services while keeping overall profitability stable. With the advent of the internet, and many products entering the retail channel, it has been challenging for veterinary hospitals to consider pricing their products competitively now that the marketplace is much more transparent. This poses a concern for the current business model because veterinary owners are now going to have to be much more aware of individual profit centers and be prepared to price their professional services much higher than they have done previously, because profitability from retail sales is likely to be much lower (see 10.15 Putting Price into Perspective).

In addition to pricing issues, veterinary practices will need to be more responsive to the needs of pet owners. This includes taking a lifelong perspective on healthcare needs, rather than concentrating on individual transactions (see 1.2 Providing a Lifetime of Care). In the end, this is better for pets, clients, and practices.

To be effective, all employees will need to be aligned around the common hospital mission and will need to effectively charge clients for the value they receive (see 8.4 Alignment – The Key to Implementing Pet-Specific Care). This is made easier in the case of pet-specific care, where the emphasis is on keeping pets healthy rather than waiting for them to get sick before veterinary intervention occurs. With a focus on prevention, early detection, and closing compliance gaps, veterinary teams have many more opportunities to add value to the pet care equation, and there are many more ways to charge appropriately for the expertise of the veterinary team.

Telehealth options are also likely to be more important to the veterinary business model as veterinary teams seek to provide services requested by clients (see 2.5 Virtual Care (Telehealth)). This is much easier to accommodate within a pet-specific care model, where clients are already more receptive to the concept of lifelong care rather than periodic transactional care.

New business models are being contemplated in some sectors, including self-management models like holacracy. While on the surface, it might appear that such systems lack structure, in reality the teams are the structure, the teams govern themselves, and leadership tends to be distributed among roles rather than individuals [5]. There are a variety of such self-management terms (e.g., podularity, circle, cabal, etc.) and some are bound to take root in the veterinary workplace.

7.2.10 Work–Life Balance

Everyone functions better with appropriate work–life balance, but this can be difficult in veterinary practices where profitability is a concern.

Some of the issues are generational in nature, yet they can't be ignored. Members of the Baby Boomer generation who started many of the veterinary practices currently in existence were used to working long hours with few niceties, and there might be some resentment of Millennials and Gen Zers who might not share the same motivations. On the other hand, we are at a crisis point with new graduates who value work–life balance, but have relatively meager starting salaries given the student debt they likely need to service [6].

Despite this issue and the fact that there is no shortage of veterinary clinicians, veterinary schools have actually increased the number of graduating students, and new veterinary schools are under consideration, creating additional concern for the future of the profession [7].

The salary concerns don't end there and many veterinary paraprofessionals and receptionists do not make enough money for them to be able to regard their job as a career that would allow them to own a home and make a living in their work position. Improved revenue generation with pet-specific care should mean there is adequate practice income to ensure that all employees are properly compensated for the value they provide to clients and the practice.

In reality, it is not "life" and "work" that need balance as much as the tasks that we enjoy doing versus those that cause us anxiety. As much as possible, strategic planning can help make changes to increase tasks that we enjoy and minimize those that cause us angst.

7.2.11 Regulatory Compliance

Although veterinary medicine in many respects is a "mom-and-pop" industry, hospitals still need to be accountable for many aspects of practice.

Product dispensing and administration is the largest revenue center in most veterinary hospitals, but is tightly governed in the US by a variety of laws, principally the Food and Drug Administration (FDA) for prescription drugs, the Environmental Protection Agency (EPA) for over-the-counter medications such as many flea and tick control products, and the US Department of Agriculture (USDA) for pet foods. Hospital employees are protected under many different laws that regulate pay, conditions, and permitted work hours. The workplace itself warrants safety precautions, most regulated in the US by the Occupational Safety and Health Administration (OSHA).

Operating a business contrary to any of the regulations cited is not only improper and can lead to fines and other punishments, but also undermines the sanctity of the workplace for all who work and do business there.

TAKE-AWAYS

- There are many different aspects that make workplace management challenging for veterinary hospitals.
- Delivering pet-specific care differs from the traditional transaction-based model of healthcare, and veterinary teams need to be appropriately trained.
- Pet-specific care isn't for everyone. Hospital teams need to appreciate which clients are likely to be most receptive to the messaging.
- Early adopters of pet-specific care are more likely to be new pet owners and pet parents.
- Pet-specific care is often embraced by hospital teams because the idea of helping clients keep their pets healthy is one of the main driving forces for why they went into veterinary care in the first place.

MISCELLANEOUS

7.2.12 Cautions

While prevention and early detection save clients money because preventing problems typically costs less than treating problems, keeping pets healthy can cost owners more than traditional care because of improved surveillance, closing compliance gaps, and providing better care (oral care, nutrition, weight management, pain management, etc.).

References

1 Lue, T.W., Pantenburg, D.P., and Crawford, P.M. (2008). Impact of the owner-pet and client-veterinarian bond on the care that pets receive. *J. Am. Vet. Med. Assoc.* 232 (4): 531–540.

2 Meister, J.C. and Willyerd, K. (2010). Mentoring Millennials: delivering the feedback gen Y craves is easier than you think. *Harv. Bus. Rev.* May: 68–72.

3 DVM360. State of the Profession: Checking in on veterinarians' practice ownership plans. www.dvm360.com/view/state-profession-checking-veterinarians-practice-ownership-plans

4 American Animal Hospital Association (2018). *Compensation and Benefits*, 10e. Lakewood, CO: AAHA Press.

5 Bernstein, E., Bunch, J., Canner, N., and Lee, M. (2016). Beyond the holacracy hype. *Harv. Bus. Rev.* July–August: 38–47.

6 Shepherd, A.J. and Pikel, L. (2013). Employment of female and male graduates of US veterinary medical colleges, 2013. *J. Am. Vet. Med. Assoc.* 243 (8): 1122–1126.

7 National Research Council (2012). *Workforce Needs in Veterinary Medicine*. Washington, DC: National Academies Press.

Recommended Reading

Ackerman, L.J. (2020). Workplace management. In: *Five-Minute Veterinary Practice Management Consult*, 3e (ed. L. Ackerman), 92–95. Ames, IA: Wiley.

Ackerman, L.J. (2003). *Management Basics for Veterinarians*. New York: ASJA Press.

Groysberg, B., Lee, J., Price, J., and Cheng, J.Y.-J. (2018). The leader's guide to corporate culture. *Harv. Bus. Rev.* January–February: 44–52.

Lee, T.H. (2010). Turning doctors into leaders. *Harv. Bus. Rev.* April: 50–58.

Meindl, A.G., Roth, I.G., and Gonzalez, S.E. (2019). Never apologize for wanting to be "just" a general practitioner. *J. Am. Vet. Med. Assoc.* 255 (8): 891–893.

Society for Human Resource Management. www.shrm.org

Vande Griek, O.H., Clark, M.A., Witte, T.K. et al. (2018). Development of a taxonomy of practice-related stressors experienced by veterinarians in the United States. *J. Am. Vet. Med. Assoc.* 252: 227–233.

7.3

Leading the Change Towards Pet-Specific Care

Randy Hall

4th Gear Consulting, Huntersville, NC, USA

BASICS

7.3.1 Summary

Leading any change in your practice can be difficult. By definition, we want ourselves and others to do something different in the future than they have in the past and that is often quite the challenge. We tend to think that getting others to change is difficult but even getting ourselves to change can feel like an uphill battle. All we have to do is look at the incredibly low success rate of New Year's resolutions to understand just how tough individual change can be.

Many of us approach change with the expectation that we will simply explain the changes to others, and they will understand and then behave differently. That all we really require for change as humans is information. But despite many of us having that expectation, nothing could be further from the truth.

MAIN CONCEPTS

Change follows a process that is predictable and can be executed successfully on a consistent basis, but it's not intuitive or generally practiced due to our expectations of how change *should* happen.

As you are thinking about moving to pet-specific care, there will be myriad behavioral changes that are needed for the humans in your practice and even the clients. The process that you use to make all of this change happen in your practice is critical to executing pet-specific care effectively and without multiple failed attempts.

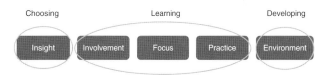

7.3.2 Insight

Change first begins in the human brain with an insight about something that could be, should be or needs to be different. Just the occurrence of insight creates the possibility of human change. We have all experienced this when we get a thought like "I should do that differently next time" or "That might be a really good idea" or "Pet-specific care is something we really need to embrace." Once that insight happens, we release neurotransmitters that can create a path to *how* we might actually accomplish the shift in behavior, new skill or process or other lasting change. So, the first component of change is insight.

7.3.3 Involvement

The next component of human change is involvement. For instance, one might have the insight to eat healthier, but then nothing actually changes. Obviously, in that case, no lasting change happens. We have thousands of insights weekly that result in absolutely no change. They are necessary for change but by themselves, insights do not create change. One of the challenges in leading change is that we will hear insights from others, verbalized as intentions, that we believe actually create change when they only

Pet-Specific Care for the Veterinary Team, First Edition. Edited by Lowell Ackerman.
© 2021 John Wiley & Sons, Inc. Published 2021 by John Wiley & Sons, Inc.

create the possibility of change. If we have an employee who frequently shows up late and we have a conversation with them and they say "I will be better about getting to work on time," we think that we have created a change simply because we have created the intention to change. The intention, no matter how well intended it is, does not equal any change. It is just the verbalization of an insight, which means the precursor for change is present.

Involvement happens when we interact with all the circumstances and challenges surrounding the change. Involvement is where we build mental maps that help us understand the way through the change, the actions we will need to take, the habits we will need to shift, the thoughts we will have to reconsider, the process we might have to use or the plan we will have to create. If we wanted to embrace pet-specific care, for example, we would need to involve ourselves with the different conversations with clients, the different processes in the practice, the different interactions between functions, the different educational materials we might create and multiple other small shifts or changes that would have occur for us to successfully execute the change. Every change that lasts has this mental map created for how the change will be executed before it is successful. We simply cannot execute a change without working through in our minds the way to execute the change.

It is during this process that the first level of resistance can occur. Our inner thoughts surrounding the challenges associated with change will immediately surface during this process. If we want to eat healthier, we might think about how to prepare food differently for the week. That might create a mental map of new shopping habits or cooking processes. We often, as we explore those new ways of behaving, conceive of reasons why the change simply won't work. "I don't have the time to cook everything" or "There's no way I could do all that food preparation every week with my schedule." Or with pet-specific care, we might feel like "The clients will never buy into this" or "This feels like too much trouble to execute" or "My team will never get on board with all of this extra work." Involvement is where early resistance shows up in our brain, and also a critical part of any lasting change. It's where intention meets reality and no intention that hasn't been tested against reality has ever resulted in lasting change.

Sometimes, as leaders in a practice, we resist this involvement phase of change because it's where opposition shows up initially. People find all kinds of reasons why it won't work due to their internal conversations. As leaders, we seek to get "buy-in" by telling people why it's good for them. But buy-in only happens when we internally think that it might work, and that only happens when we work through all the reasons why it might not work.

Involvement is messy and difficult and sometimes feels counterproductive and yet no change happens without it.

We learned to walk, talk, ride a bike and drive a car using it. As much as we wish we could just tell people to do something and they would find a way through it, change does not happen that way for humans. We need to confront our thoughts about why it won't work and then explore ways that it might work. We need to weigh the benefits of the change against the effort required to produce and sustain it. When we have done that, and, through involvement, found a path that might work and a reason to make it work, we are ready for the next step – focus.

7.3.4 Focus

Focus is the act of putting energy and more thought into the path through the change that we think might work. For example, if we decide to implement pet-specific care in our practice and we believe that if we do have a good conversation with our clients about it, they will embrace it and it will set us apart as a practice, then we need to figure out what that conversation will sound like. We will need to focus on the details of the words and the order of them so that we can execute the change.

Without focus, all of that involvement can go to waste. If we believe through our involvement with the change that "Clients probably will think it's a good thing" and then go to have a conversation with a client about it, without thinking more about the words we will use and the details of the client conversation, we will meet the second level of resistance – this is harder than we thought. The first level of resistance to change is the belief that it won't work. The second level is when we believe that it might work, but then find it to be more difficult than we expected.

This is where focus can save us. If we were to think through the exact conversation we might have with our clients, including sentences like "We are embracing pet-specific care because we know every animal has different genetics and leads a different lifestyle from every other animal and we believe that our best care means learning about your pet and taking all of that into account as we partner with you to give them their best possible life," we now have a plan that has a level of detail in it that is possible to execute against. That's something we can actually say, not just an idea that if we say the right things it might work. That only arises through focus on the actionable details associated with the change.

One rule of thumb is that if we can't now practice something, then we have not focused on it enough. If you watch a child learn to walk, taking those first few steps and the moments before they try, that's true focus. We need to focus on the details of the actions associated with any change before we can do the next step – practice.

7.3.5 Practice

After we focus well enough to have a completely defined set of actions, then we have to create a neural pathway that will help us execute that set of actions. That happens when we practice, and only when we practice. We have never executed any set of actions repetitively without creating a neural pathway that guides those actions. Our neural pathway for brushing our teeth, for example, is very well formed. Our neural pathway for saying the sentence we think the clients might embrace is not developed at all. As leaders in a practice, we sometimes think that because we conceive of the sentence, we or anyone else should be able to execute it immediately, either because they heard it or because they were told to. But actions don't happen that way. Telling a child to brush their teeth for the first time, despite the fact that they have made many previous motions with their hands for all kinds of other things, does not work for helping them change. Only practice does. And practice with support works even better as we coach them through the brushing process and give them feedback as they learn.

Often when we are leading change in a practice, we simply tell people what to do differently and then get back to work. In this way, we set change up for complete failure because we have not practiced any of the new patterns, behaviors, words or processes. When we do not practice, we can expect people to fail with incredible frequency even with tasks that they had good intentions around and wanted to execute. As a further example, without going back and reading our sentence above, try to deliver it well right now as if a client were right in front of you. Even if you really want to, you will struggle with making that happen. And having a real client in front of you will add much more difficulty to something that has never been practiced. We don't have a neural pathway for that set of words yet. Now if you were to practice it 20 times, you would immediately be better after maybe 10 minutes of practice. Change follows a pretty clear pattern in humans but if we understand it and support each of the components of change, we greatly increase our chances of leading a successful change in our practice, no matter what it is.

7.3.6 Environment

The last component of sustainable change is environment. This means that people need to be surrounded with the right environment in order for change to be successful in most cases. There are certainly cases of highly driven or motivated individuals who executed significant changes in environments that did not help them at all and in fact were part of their biggest challenge. But those cases are far more about the individual or the specific change than they are

representative of a model for successful change. People can, and do, overcome incredible odds to make personal changes happen but why, as a leader of a practice or team that was trying to change, would we count on all of our people doing that?

Our best option is to create an environment around our team that supports lasting change so that we can smooth the path for them so that change happens more quickly and easily and they can focus on clients and pets more than they do the change. That means building an environment where people are allowed to make mistakes to learn, are coached and supported as they learn, and where there is dedicated time for involvement and practice. In the work world, we often spend all our time doing the work and there is no dedicated time for improvement and practice. We do not get good, much less great, at anything that we do not spend enough time working on, outside the actual "during work" execution. By definition, all the things that we did well yesterday we should be pretty good at today. But also by definition, we cannot expect anything to be better or different from yesterday without working through the steps of change associated with it.

Change happens when we build a world where it can and where we do the things that consistently support people as they work through the changes for themselves. Some practices very effectively use team meetings or daily "huddles" to work on new behaviors or improved performance. These become safe places to fail, learn, and grow where people are encouraged to try new things and make mistakes. We all make mistakes every day and we aren't good at anything that we didn't mess up at initially. As humans, we are simply bad at things before we are good at them and the act of being bad at them is actually part of how we get better. I refer you back to the child learning to walk, or even a first surgery or a first catheter placement or a first client check-in. People who aren't in a great environment for learning will decide that learning is too difficult and opt for just staying at their current level of competency, because improvement only comes with failure and mistakes and support and if those things are not OK in this hospital, then learning will not be OK either.

EXAMPLES

ABC Animal Hospital wants to implement pet-specific care and they are walking through the components of change in order to do that. They use questions to create insight for the team first by having a meeting that openly discusses pet-specific care, why it might be better, why it might help clients and/or patients, why it might create a higher level of care, and how it might set the practice apart from others in the area.

They then have a second meeting that involves everyone on what would have to happen, as a team, to execute it well. They ask questions like "What will the challenges be? What will need to be different? What new habits or processes will we need to adopt to be good at this?" The team is encouraged to brainstorm and discuss and share thoughts that would help everyone build mental maps for how this change might look and feel.

Then they break into smaller groups to work through the focus needed to explore the details of the new actions. Maybe they will need to define a new check-in process, a new way to take a patient history, a new conversation with clients during an office visit, a new set of diagnostic tools or a new set of educational tools.

The practice then uses meetings to practice all the new behaviors or actions associated with the change. They role-play the check-in process and the patient history. They take turns practicing and perfecting their introduction to pet-specific care that they would share with clients.

Regular practice and improvement time are dedicated in the practice to help people learn and improve. They spend five minutes every morning before they open for the team to walk through the new behaviors and take turns practicing them as they get ready for the day. They spend a few minutes at the end of each shift talking about what worked and where they still have opportunities for improvement.

TAKE-AWAYS

- Lasting, sustainable change follows a predictable pattern in humans consisting of five components: insight, involvement, focus, practice, environment.
- As leaders, we can follow a set of steps that will help changes happen quickly and effectively.
- Telling people to change is generally ineffective at actually helping them to change.
- We can force short-term change using our role or our authority, but sustainable change only happens when people work through the process for themselves in a supportive environment.
- Resistance is part of any change and we cannot eliminate it. We need to work through it and use it to find ways in which the change can work.

7.4

Getting Informed Consent

Betsy Choder, JD, MS

VetCounsel LLC, Crown Pointe Parkway, Atlanta, GA, USA

BASICS

7.4.1 Summary

There are numerous laws, regulations, and ethics that are triggered when providing veterinary medical care to animals, especially depending upon the particular facts and circumstances. By law, animals are characterized as "property" and, accordingly, an animal's owner/guardian must provide some type of consent before veterinary treatment can be rendered. Clients' expectations (sometimes unrealistic expectations) of veterinary medical services can be the source of significant misunderstandings, potentially resulting in lawsuits, internet shaming, or veterinary board complaints. Even though practitioners might believe they provided clear communications to the client, the client might not have heard, nor listened, nor understood what was being stated. It is important to minimize misunderstandings and complaints from clients – while maximizing communications and viable defenses against such claims – by using *informed* consents from clients regarding veterinary medical treatment of their animals.

MAIN CONCEPTS

7.4.2 "Informed Consent" Versus "Owner's Consent"

In veterinary medicine, the doctrine of informed consent is quite different from human medicine. Three differentiating factors include (i) consent for treatment can only be provided by the patient's owner/guardian, (ii) being informed about costs is an integral part of the client's/owner's consent, and (iii) the patient does not have legally recognized "rights of consent." Accordingly, in 2007, the American Veterinary Medical Association (AVMA) chose to replace the term "informed consent" with "owners' consent" for all AVMA references. The AVMA stated, in part, "[t]he public is best served when veterinarians provide sufficient information in a form and manner that enables owners or their authorized agents to make appropriate decisions when choosing the veterinary care needed for their animals."

For the purposes of this topic, the term "informed consent" will be used synonymously for "owner's consent" or "authorized agent's consent."

7.4.3 "Consent" Comes in Different Forms – Direct, Implied, Verbal or Written

Consent for treatment can be made by nodding or by physically presenting an animal to a veterinary facility (such as emergency situations or appointments for annual examinations). This type of consent, referred to as "implied consent," is very common. The most significant problem associated with implied consent is being able to define what exactly the client was granting.

Implied consents can be enforceable to a limited extent under limited circumstances. For example, an "emergency exception" usually exists – while trying to stabilize any animal in a life-threatening situation, it is impractical to wait until a formal written informed consent from the owner is obtained.

TIP: For unforeseen emergency treatment care of animals, consider training clinical personnel to obtain signed consents from the client/owner, when possible, while stabilizing treatment is being rendered – including client's choice for poststabilization treatment options such as resuscitation and cost range estimates.

7.4.4 All "Consents" are Not the Same

With limited exceptions, asking a client to sign a generic statement simply giving "permission to perform" a treatment on an animal – without any other materially related information – can be problematic, especially if an outcome occurs that was neither discussed nor expected by the client. A veterinarian should be able to minimize the potential for miscommunications and misunderstandings within the veterinarian–client–patient relationship (VCPR) by providing sufficient information from which a client can decide to accept or deny the course of treatment for their animals. This type of communication, whether verbal or written, is known as "informed consent."

7.4.5 What is Required for "Informed Consent"?

The information presented to an owner/guardian for consent of treatment on an animal should include:

- the diagnoses (or description of the animal-patient's medical status) and general treatment available (including probability of success and risks involved)
- alternative treatments available (including probability of success and risks involved for each treatment mentioned)
- the prognosis or risks of rendering no medical treatment
- risks involved for each treatment option (including specifying the potential for death, physical impairments, stroke, allergic reactions, and other known general risks)
- potential prognosis of recovery for each treatment option
- written estimated costs for each of the treatment options, including for the "no treatment" option.

A "one type fits all" consent form should not be used for every situation. The standard of care applicable to different situations will vary, depending upon degrees of risk for the animal's survival and continuing good health.

Depending on the facts and circumstances, an owner's/guardian's informed consent could also include:

- choice of resuscitation or no resuscitation (in case of emergency or during surgery/anesthesia/treatment)

- provisions when overnight care of the animal is necessary (such as extra costs involved or whether client needs to make other arrangements if a veterinarian is not available)
- whether "cosmetic" procedures are requested by the client while the animal is sedated (such as claw burring, dewclaw removal, and other treatments)
- maximum limit of fees, if any, that client is willing to spend (especially in case of problems encountered during treatment)
- information required by state regulations (such as name of attending veterinarian or surgical location)
- additional expenses, if applicable, in case of death (burial/cremation, necropsy)
- essential home care instructions for animal's recovery (TIP: In situations where failure of the client to follow the doctor's advice could result in significant harm to the animal, consider having the client sign a copy of the potential risks, warning signs and other take-home instructions)
- veterinarian's "no guarantee of outcome." Veterinary medicine is not an exact science and is dependent upon many factors such as severity of medical issue, age and health of animal, type of treatment being provided, owner's compliance with home care, and more.

TIP: If client opts to refuse certain provisions or recommendations of veterinary care, such as choosing no resuscitation in case of emergency or during treatment, request that they provide signature of their refusal either on the consent form or directly into the medical record to help avoid future misunderstandings.

7.4.6 Not all Consents are Legally Enforceable

When drafting consent-for-treatment documents, the wording of the form should be easily understood by any reasonable person with average intelligence. Consider the following "traps."

- *Client's condition and circumstances.* Minors, those unable to understand English and those impaired by alcohol/drugs are legally incapable of providing "consent" to an agreement.
- *Missing essential terms.* The information within a consent form should reflect at least the minimum requirements defined in the jurisdiction's statutes or regulations.
- *Use of ambiguous, vague or medical terminology.* Avoid using medical terms (i.e., enucleation, ovariohysterectomy) that an average person might not understand. For example, consider using, as applicable:

– "teeth cleaning and possible teeth removal/loss" instead of the word "dental"
– "potential risks may include inflammation, infection, permanent physical impairment or death" instead of generic "many risks and adverse reactions are possible."

Even though obtaining an owner's written consent before rendering treatment on their animals might minimize the potential for misunderstandings, the most effective method is to ensure that the clients are part of the decision-making process. Applicable laws differ regarding requirements of veterinary informed consent, yet a practitioner can minimize the potential for disgruntled, upset clients by taking the time to educate and answer their questions, especially on treatment options, benefits, risks, and costs. Consider consulting with an attorney knowledgeable in the field of veterinary medicine to assist with drafting an informed consent form.

TAKE-AWAYS

- Ensure a veterinarian's presence when obaining client consent. Avoid the possibility of a client being able to claim that consent was given only through interactions with a receptionist or assistant, neither of whom are able, by law, to provide prognoses or diagnoses of animals' medical issues in response to owner's questions.
- Waivers/release from liability are not consents for treatment. Waivers are not always enforceable nor recommended – such as in circumstances of gross negligence, intentional acts, wanton conduct or fraud by the practitioner. In many instances, courts will not enforce waivers if perceived as (i) being "forced" on a client and/or (ii) the veterinarian's higher level of knowledge regarding the risks of medical issues created "unequal bargaining power" for the client.
- Not necessary to list all possible outcomes. If the probability of a potential risk happening is very low, consider whether mentioning it would really be a significant factor. Use reasonableness as your guide rather than writing a medical compendium of everything possible.
- Failing to follow consented treatment can be problematic. Aside from raising ethical issues, a veterinarian's failure to follow the client's consent for treatment – such as failing to euthanize (or to resuscitate) as requested or performing a necropsy without informing client – could also result in criminal and/or civil legal action.

- Avoid client's "transfer of responsibility." A practitioner should be cautious when clients make special requests such as "Money is no object. . .whatever it costs to save his life – do it!" or "I obviously have no choice. . .I have to trust you" or "What would you tell your brother/sister to do in this case?" Consider responding to clients in the same manner as if these statements were not made, with professionalism and courteousness. Ethically and legally, it is the client's decision alone whether to accept or decline treatment on their animals after having been informed of the potential treatments, outcomes, risks, benefits, and costs.

MISCELLANEOUS

7.4.7   Cautions – Do Statutory Requirements Open Doors to Public Lawsuits?

Several states have enacted mandatory informed consent statutes as part of their veterinary practice acts. This has created tension among veterinarians, animal owners, animal law experts, and animal rights groups as to the issue of whether the statutory requirement of informed consent raises the bar on the "property" status of animals – when no such informed consent is required for other types of property treatment such as car repairs, home/furniture remodeling or landscape maintenance.

7.4.8   Disclaimer

This discussion incorporates references to laws and organizations solely in the USA. Other countries might have similar laws and organizations applying to this subject matter. However, this discussion is not intended as legal advice nor to establish an attorney–client relationship – it is for generic educational purposes only.

Recommended Reading

JAVMA News. (2007). "Informed consent" versus "owner consent." www.avma.org/News/JAVMANews/Pages/071215d.aspx

7.5

Connecting with Clients Through Social Media

Caitlin DeWilde, BS, DVM

The Social DVM, LLC, Webster Groves, MO, USA

BASICS

7.5.1   Summary

Social media offers veterinary practices a variety of ways to connect with their clients. Posting photos, videos, infographics, and articles on social media channels can help bond existing clientele to the practice, educate pet owners, and help catch the eye of potential clients. In addition, features like targeted advertising, advanced online messaging, call-to-action (CTA) buttons, online scheduling, and social media reviews can all be utilized to help build a practice's business both online and in practice.

Recent studies demonstrate the pet owner's increasing desire for more online information, social media activity and practice accessibility, with more than 15% of pet owners using social media to find information about their pet [1].

7.5.2   Terms Defined

Call-to-Action Button: A CTA button directs your page visitors to do something specific, like visit your website, call your practice or book an appointment.

Facebook Boost: Boosted posts are ads you create from posts on your Facebook page. Boosting a post may help you get more people to react, share, and comment on it. You may also reach new people who are likely interested in your page or business but don't currently follow you.

Facebook Pixel: The Facebook Pixel is an analytics tool that allows you to measure the effectiveness of your advertising by understanding the actions people take on your website.

Instagram Stories: Instagram feature that lets users post photos and videos that vanish after 24 hours.

MAIN CONCEPTS

7.5.2.1   The Need

Pet owners, particularly millennial pet owners, are more likely to be active on social media than the general population [1]. More than 15% of millennial pet owners will consult social media when looking for pet information [1], and a leading veterinary economic study has identified consistent social media use as one of the top four predictors of practice sustainability and success [2]. With billions of daily users, Facebook offers the largest base of existing and prospective clientele. Additional platforms such as Instagram, YouTube, and Twitter can be considered based on individual practice demographics, and new platforms are bound to be developed.

Social media presents the ultimate opportunity for veterinarians to literally and figuratively engage with their clientele on a daily basis, instead of the once- or twice-yearly in-person visits. In addition to sharing social media-friendly pet articles and photos, practices have the opportunity to share trusted resources, client education materials, and more personalized content that differentiates the practice from its competition and allows clients to become more bonded to the staff of the practice (see 5.13 Improving Client Engagement Through Technology). In addition, based on the practice's staff resources and online offerings, social media can present yet another opportunity for online booking, highly targeted yet low-cost advertising, and online messaging.

7.5.3 Platforms

7.5.3.1 Facebook

Facebook is the most commonly used social media platform, both for general users and for the veterinary industry. Boasting nearly 1.8 billion daily active users [3], the platform is used by about 70% of veterinary practices [1]. Photos, videos, and links can be shared easily, and Facebook offers specific business page features, including CTA buttons, targeted advertising, reviews and recommendations, user insights, and client messaging.

7.5.3.2 Instagram

Instagram is rapidly growing among users in the general population and in the veterinary community. There are more than 1 billion daily users sharing photos and videos via traditional posts, 15-second Instagram "stories" that are visible for just 24 hours, or long form video up to 10 minutes on Instagram TV (IGTV). Ninety percent of the platform's users follow business pages [4], so despite a more "informal" vibe, businesses and brands have significant opportunity to connect with their clients. Veterinary practices can take advantage of specific business account features including CTA buttons, targeted advertising, user insights, and client messaging.

7.5.3.3 Other Platforms

Lesser utilized platforms in the veterinary industry include Twitter, YouTube, LinkedIn, Snapchat, and Pinterest. These platforms also offer business support but veterinary usage is less common. Based on specific practice demographics, however, these platforms may still be of value if a practice's clientele is using them frequently. Surveying owners regularly about their preferred platforms to communicate with the practice may help assess the need, if any, for these platforms.

7.5.4 Strategies to Connect

7.5.4.1 Providing Valuable Content

Over 70% of veterinary clients report using the internet to search for pet health information [5], but 41% of veterinary practices provide no educational resources online [1]. A list of online resources with reliable pet care information was identified by "New School" pet owners as one of the top five preferred offerings from veterinary practices [1]. Similarly, this need echoes the findings of the Bayer Veterinary Care Usage Study, in which 65% of cat owners

Table 7.5.1 Examples of marketing content

Shared content examples	Promotional content examples	Personalized content examples
Educational articles from AVMA, AAHA and other trusted sources	Service highlight (e.g., spotlight practice's offering of laser therapy)	Pet health original blog from practice website
Community events	Special offers and discounts (e.g., parasite preventive rebates)	Get to know your team: biography features
Locally relevant pet news	Book Now post	Photos of patients with staff

reported that their veterinary team could provide better educational material to help them understand their pet's health needs [2].

Social media presents an opportunity for veterinarians to provide educational content in a medium where pet owners are already spending a large amount of their time. Veterinary practices can present educational information via links, photos, infographics, or, for the highest engagement, video.

Traditional social media marketing best practices recommend following a rule of thirds when it comes to diversifying content: one-third shared content, one-third promotional content, and one-third personalized content (Table 7.5.1). The latter may be even more important in the veterinary industry, where connection with the veterinary team and facility can reassure pet owners, create stronger bonds, and differentiate the practice from local competition.

Regularly sharing content of value and interest to pet owners can help increase the bond between the practice and client, as well as establish the practice as a source of online information.

7.5.4.2 Video

Video content gives your clientele a look at the "real people" behind the medicine and patient care at your practice – something no one else can replicate. Mobile video usage has increased by nearly 10 million daily viewing minutes in the last two years [6]. Better yet, memory and understanding are increased, with viewers retaining 95% of a message after watching it through video, as opposed to just 10% when reading the same message in text form [7]. Facebook's algorithm prioritizes video and Instagram video watch time is also increasing.

Table 7.5.2 Example of video length on different platforms

Platform	Type of video	Length
Facebook	Video	Up to 240 minutes max; at least 3 minutes recommended
	Live video	Recommended: 10 minutes minimum, up to 4 hours
	Story	1–120 seconds
Instagram	Post	3–60 seconds
	Story	15 seconds per story
	IGTV episode	15 seconds to 10 minutes
YouTube	Video	Up to 15 minutes long, longer if verified

In veterinary practice, creating video gives team members the chance to share interesting, engaging content with clients and let them get to know the team and facility. In addition to creating another digital touchpoint form of educational content, video also presents a content medium that can easily be repurposed and reused. For instance, when a video is recorded, the file can be submitted for transcription, creating a text file that can be repurposed into a blog post.

Whenever possible, videos should be captioned. Facebook provides a free automatic caption generator when uploading files to the platform, although the punctuation and spelling can be inaccurate. Submitting the file to an online service is very affordable and more effective, often generating the required SubRip (.srt) file type cost-effectively and within a few hours. Up to 85% of video on social media is watched without sound [8], so adding captions (which will automatically appear if sound is not turned on) will increase both watch time and understanding of the material (see Table 7.5.2 for video lengths on different platforms).

7.5.4.2.1 Example Video Prompts

- Tour of the hospital.
- Tour of a specific room, e.g., the cat-only exam room, recovery areas.
- DIY: how to trim nails, how to clean ears, how to brush teeth.
- Microchipping demonstration.
- Examination (repeat with different life stages).
- Explain an accreditation received (AAHA, Fear Free, Cat Friendly).
- Five facts: Dr Smith.
- Dog go-pro tour!
- Share a success story!

7.5.4.3 Targeted Advertising

Social media presents arguably the best and most affordable type of advertising in the modern world. Practices can cost-effectively target existing and potential clientele based on their age, education, interests, demographics, even previous interest in dogs or cats. Advertisements, boosts, and promoted posts can be created in just minutes, and parameters adjusted in real time. Analytic information about engagement, reach, and clicks is readily available, and in some cases, overwhelming in its sheer size (see 10.6 Target Marketing and Targeted Client Outreach).

Unfortunately, social media platforms have become a pay-to-play world in which some form of ad spend is almost essential to seeing the quality and quantity of success businesses had in the platform's early days. That said, with such a low cost and ability to set up in just a few minutes, even from a mobile device, paid advertising is a very efficient use of a practice's time and money.

Facebook offers two forms of advertising: Facebook ads and Facebook boosts, while Instagram offers "promoted posts." Ads can be seen in the platform's normal feed, in Stories, Messenger, Facebook Marketplace or Audience Networks (other websites and apps). Regardless of the type or placement, these paid and targeted advertisements can be created with photos, links, videos, slideshows, and more.

Advertising objective types can also vary, anything from brand awareness to booked appointments to video views. Each objective type will have different options for ad media and placement. Based on your practice's goal, you may choose a specific ad type to help refine targeting and improve your return on investment.

Using customer data you already have on hand (such as email lists, website visitors, previous ad engagers), practices can create custom audiences. Custom audiences make it easy for a practice to reconnect with people who have already shown an interest.

Additionally, these custom audiences can be used to create "lookalike" audiences in which other social media users who match many of the characteristics of the original group are collected, providing a useful source of potential clients for a practice to target.

Examples of effective social media advertising include the following.

- Boosting a post showing off a practice's new cat-friendly exam room, targeting cat owners within a 5-mile (8-km) radius of the practice.
- Creating a "Book Now" ad for new puppy owners, targeted to adults within a 5-mile (8-km) radius who have liked the local shelter's Facebook page.
- Using a Facebook Pixel to retarget website visitors with a special "book now" or "get offer" ad.

- Boosting a post with a "Learn More" button, linked to a blog on the practice website about top reasons for more frequent geriatric pet exams, targeted to a custom audience created from existing client email addresses.

7.5.4.4 Messaging

As mobile device use continues to grow, pet owner (and general consumer) expectations of business accessibility also increase. Many find the asynchronous nature of messaging appealing, since responses can come quickly but the conversation and information can be exchanged at both parties' convenience. Messaging also offers businesses an opportunity for more personal, conversational interactions and streamlined interactions with the ability to provide easy access to information and conversions, especially in terms of appointment booking and online shopping.

7.5.4.4.1 Facebook Messenger

Nearly 1.3 billion people use Facebook Messenger alone [9]. Among those who use the platform to communicate with businesses, the majority say being able to message a business makes them "feel more confident about the brand" [9]. In the veterinary-specific industry, the Merck Pet Owner Paths study identified that among "New School" pet owners (millennial generation and younger), having the ability to communicate online was a key desired feature when choosing a practice [1]. Further, 24% of "New School" pet owners email or submit questions on clinic websites or Facebook pages, compared to just 4% of traditional pet owners [1].

Compared to other platforms, Facebook Messenger offers some significant advantages and features for business profiles.

- Personalized Messenger greetings.
  - Create a greeting that people will see the first time they open a conversation with you on Messenger.
  - Example: Hi Caitlin! We look forward to helping you and your pets. If you need immediate assistance, please call our office at (555) 555–5555.
- Away messages
  - When away messages are on, your page is away and sends away messages. You can manually make your page away in Inbox or schedule times for your page to be away each week.
  - You can customize your message to let people know how long you'll be away and when you'll respond.
  - Example: "Hi Caitlin! We are closed right now. If you have a medical emergency, please call Veterinary Emergency Services at (555) 555-5555. If you have a nonurgent issue, please respond and we'll get back to you within 1 business day."
- Instant replies (e.g., where to contact if a medical emergency).

  - Respond to the first message someone sends your page.
  - You can customize your message to say hello, give them more information about your page or let them know when to expect a response.
  - Example: "Hi Caitlin! We look forward to helping you and your pets. You can expect a response to your message within 24 business hours, but if you need more immediate assistance, please give us a call at (555) 555-5555."
- FAQ automated responses.
  - Contact information.
    o Customize your message to include additional contact information.
  - Location.
    o Respond to a message asking about the location of your business. You can customize your message to include additional information about your location, such as options for parking or public transport.
  - Hours.
    o Respond to a message asking about your business hours. You can customize your message to include additional information, such as upcoming holiday hours.
  - Page recommended and page not recommended.
    o Send a message after someone publicly shares that they recommend your page. You can customize your message to thank them, send an offer or start a conversation. If not recommended, you can customize the message to learn more about the customer's experience.
  - Job application received.
    o Respond to someone who applied for a job you posted. You can customize your message to thank them for their interest or let them know when to expect a response.
- Subscription messaging (allowing pages to send nonpromotional content on a recurring basis through the Messenger platform).
- Integration with Facebook posts and practice website chat plugin.
- Online booking (via appointment booking interface in the Messenger Platform API) and appointment reminders.
- Advertising opportunities.

For those practices that do not wish to use messaging, this feature can also be disabled.

7.5.4.4.2 Instagram Direct

Instagram also allows for easy communication via business messaging, and nearly 150 million users connect with businesses each month [10]. A third of these conversations begin with an Instagram story [10].

While Instagram does not offer as many automated messenger features, common questions can be answered with customizable "Quick Replies," available in your practice's account settings.

7.5.4.5 Social Media Reviews

Gain the trust of existing and potential clients with online reviews and recommendations via Facebook. Ninety percent of "New School" pet owners and 40% of traditional pet owners will research a practice's online reputation before selecting a practice [11]. According to Facebook, nearly one-third of the platform's users are utilizing business reviews and recommendations [12]. Facebook "Reviews" have recently evolved into "Recommendations" on Facebook, and practices can choose whether or not to allow these reviews to be visible on your page. Clients can now easily indicate a simple "yes" or "no" instead of a star ranking if they recommend your business. They can also elaborate with tags, text, and photos.

While managing online reviews has traditionally been a source of stress for many veterinary professionals, reviews can help bolster our reputation and provide valuable client feedback, both negative and positive.

Efforts should be made to respond to most reviews and recommendations. Thanking a customer for a positive review may strengthen the relationship, demonstrate your commitment to your clientele to others reading, and encourage more positive reviews. Negative reviews should be handled on a case-by-case basis, but in many cases, responded to without defensiveness and following the AVMA's recommendation of being (i) compassionate, (ii) confident, and (iii) competent. In some cases, best practice may be to first call the owner or alternatively, respond to the online review and offer direction for the reviewer to call the office to discuss further, thereby directing the conversation offline.

While Facebook is the only true social media platform that offers online reviews, additional platforms such as Google Business and Yelp offer the ability to directly share reviews onto a Facebook page account. This can also help improve the visibility of a practice's positive reviews and encourage additional feedback and reputation building.

7.5.4.6 Call-to-Action Buttons

Call-to-action buttons, available on Facebook and Instagram business accounts, provide clickable links to key information and conversion opportunities. This gives pet owners a quick and direct way to contact you, book an appointment, get directions, and more without having to leave the platform.

Facebook offers a single CTA button on a business page just below the cover photo, and practices can choose to allow visitors to:

- Book Now
- Contact Us (link to website contact page)
- Send Facebook Message
- Call Now
- Send Email
- Sign Up
- Watch Video
- Learn More
- Shop Now
- See Offers
- Use App.

Instagram offers the ability to provide multiple CTA buttons, accessible in your practice's profile. These include:

- Email
- Phone
- Directions
- Booking.

Ultimately, regular and effective use of CTA buttons can increase a practice's social media return on investment by driving clients to their objective (e.g., contact, booking, or website visits).

7.5.4.7 Online Scheduling

The average appointment made over the phone takes eight minutes to schedule [13]. Using online scheduling options on social media CTA buttons or paid social advertisements, practices can improve client satisfaction, accessibility, and ultimately patient appointment numbers. Both Facebook and Instagram will allow for direct appointment booking using their free appointment tools, or integration with third-party programs. Facebook in particular can offer a customized menu of services, availability views, sync with Google calendars and automated appointment reminders via the Messenger platform or text messages.

For practices not wishing to use social media booking, "Book Now" CTA buttons on a practice page or boosted posts/ads can simply be directed to the "Contact" or "Request Appointment" page on their website.

Online scheduling is essential, even if a real-time scheduling service is available. One survey found that nearly 70% of millennial pet owners (the largest pet-owning population) [14] preferred to book online. Another survey found that 50% of appointments were made after business hours, and 17% of appointments made with an online booking tool were from new clients. However, only an estimated 25–45% [11, 15] of practices offer this function.

Practices can easily take advantage of this opportunity to reduce staff time, improve client appointment numbers, and be more accessible to their clients.

7.5.5 Strategies to Connect with More Clients

Growing your social media following can help increase your local reach and strengthen your brand awareness. Consider the following strategies to ensure your clientele, new and existing, know how to connect.

- Include social media links on website, email signature, and digital communications.
- Include social media channels as referral sources on client registration paperwork.
- Ask new clients if their pet has their own social media account, and tag their photos if so!
- Have visible reminders of social media channels in the practice and on print materials (e.g., window decals, "Follow Us" signs, social icons on business cards, letterheads, and brochures, etc.).
- Respond to social media comments, messages, visitor posts, reviews, and check-ins to foster communication.

TAKE-AWAYS

- Pet owners increasingly rely on technology to connect with their veterinary team via websites, social media, and apps.
- Veterinary teams can and should use a variety of digital touchpoints to communicate with pet owners, including photos, videos (ideally captioned), and articles.
- Social media messaging can provide an affordable and simple way to communicate with clients, and business page tools can simplify responses to decrease workload.
- Targeted advertising can help practices ensure that their social media content is seen by pet owners in their geographic region.
- Online reviews and comments can help build a practice's reputation and social proof. Respond to negative reviews with the three C's: compassion, confidence, competence.

MISCELLANEOUS

7.5.6 Cautions

Use of social media platforms can open a practice up to cyberbullying and negative reviews. While this is rare, the effects can be extraordinarily stressful. Visit www.avma. org/onlinereputation for helpful resources.

If using online messaging, develop a social media protocol so all your team are aware of how you intend to monitor and/or record conversations held with clients in order to keep accurate medical records and boost the veterinary–client–patient relationship (VCPR).

Abbreviations

AAHA American Animal Hospital Association
AVMA American Veterinary Medical Association

References

1 Up Your Website Game. Merck Pet Owner Paths. https://merckpetownerpaths.com/action-steps/step-10/
2 Executive summary of the Bayer veterinary care usage study. https://avmajournals.avma.org/doi/full/10.2460/javma.238.10.1275
3 Facebook Reports Second Quarter 2020 Results. https://investor.fb.com/investor-news/press-release-details/2020/Facebook-Reports-Second-Quarter-2020-Results/default.aspx
4 Instagram Business. https://business.instagram.com/
5 The Internet and Pet Health Information: Perceptions and Behaviors of Pet Owners and Veterinarians. http://ispub.com/IJVM/8/1/12921
6 50 Visual Content Marketing Statistics You Should Know in 2020. https://blog.hubspot.com/marketing/visual-content-marketing-strategy
7 27 Video Stats for 2017. www.insivia.com/27-video-stats-2017/
8 85 percent of Facebook video is watched without sound. https://digiday.com/media/silent-world-facebook-video/.
9 Facebook Messenger for Business. www.facebook.com/business/marketing/messenger
10 Why messaging businesses is the new normal. www.facebook.com/business/news/insights/why-messaging-businesses-is-the-new-normal
11 Pet Health Overview – Merck Veterinary Manual. www.merckvetmanual.com/resourcespages/pet-health-overview
12 Recommendations: Build Reputation Locals Trust. www.facebook.com/business/recommendations
13 Assessing Online Scheduling as an Emerging Trend in Physician Appointments. https://partners.healthgrades.com/blog/assessing-online-scheduling-as-an-emerging-trend-in-physician-appointments
14 How can pet clinics please millennials? https://mma.prnewswire.com/media/973536/Weave_infographic_millennial_pet_owners.pdf

15 How online booking can boost practice revenue. https://softwareservices.covetrus.com/global/client-solutions/how-online-booking-can-boost-practice-revenue/

Recommended Reading

Pet Owner Paths Study: 2018 National Pet Owners Survey. file:///C:/Users/Owner/Downloads/merck_petownerpaths_whitepages%20(2).pdf

Frankel, C. Top 5 Ways to Leverage Client Smartphones to Enhance Care. www.cliniciansbrief.com/article/top-5-ways-leverage-client-smartphones-enhance-care

Establish your reputation with recommendations. Facebook blog. www.facebook.com/business/recommendations?ref=fbb_blog#

Online reputation management and cyberbullying. www.avma.org/PracticeManagement/Administration/reputation/Pages/default.aspx

7.6

Privacy and Confidentiality

Betsy Choder, JD, MS

VetCounsel LLC, Crown Pointe Parkway, Atlanta, GA, USA

BASICS

7.6.1 Summary

Veterinary medical practices are facing many of the same increasing challenges as other business operations in trying to deter access to, and exposure of, confidential and proprietary information. With technological and electronic advances, news headlines are filled with stories related to the hacking or exposure of confidential information ranging from retail store chains, hospitals, insurance companies, governmental offices, online service providers, and even consumer credit companies. This invasion of people's/business's confidential information is usually gained through unauthorized access into various electronic systems, through personal scams or due to careless security management practices.

It is important that veterinary practices explore methods and reasons for ensuring the confidentiality of proprietary business information as well as protecting uniquely identifiable information of private individuals and businesses.

MAIN CONCEPTS

7.6.2 Balancing Interests

In business settings, the needs of an employer's legitimate business interests must be balanced with the rights of employees and clients. This can be very challenging.

Employers must understand the importance of maintaining the confidentiality of employee and client information (such as Social Security numbers, email, or telephone contact information, workplace injury reports, background checks, workplace investigation findings) while also preserving confidentiality of business information that is not available to nonmanagement employees or the public (such as financial and other proprietary data).

Typically, limitations against the release of business information considered to be "confidential" are used in two situations: (i) relative to employment, usually through use of restrictive covenants in workplace policies and contracts, and (ii) the sale of a business, usually through the use of nondisclosure agreements. Employers should seek the assistance of legal counsel in efforts to draft contracts or policies related to confidentiality and privacy issues in the workplace, to assist in providing parameters for training staff or conducting workplace investigations, to identify what types of information are considered "proprietary" or "confidential," how to avoid the unauthorized release of "private" or "confidential" information, and defining the circumstances and types of confidential/proprietary information that can be released on a limited, need-to-know basis.

7.6.3 Privacy, Confidentiality, and the Law

Protecting proprietary and confidential interests relies upon legal, ethical, and moral foundations. Protecting privacy rights and confidentiality of information should be a business's priority without a time limit – whether during employment, after business hours, and even after employment has ended. As our society becomes more dependent upon electronics and the advancement of technology, our laws governing the collection and use of private information also evolve. In the United States, the Supreme Court has held that many of the Constitutional amendments (such as the First, Third, Fourth, Fifth, Fourteenth Amendments) provide the basic protection for many individuals' privacy. Yet, there are also federal and state laws that carve out exceptions and limitations of an individual's expectation of privacy. Knowing the applicable federal or state laws is essential before requiring employees to sign confidentiality agreements, before performing criminal background checks or workplace investigations, and even before video surveillance at the workplace.

7.6.3.1 Individuals' Right to Privacy and Confidentiality

Depending upon the particular facts, the applicable state's laws, the type of information and how it is transmitted (such as the internet, social media, newspapers, or to persons within the workplace), courts might yield different outcomes on privacy/confidentiality issues. Some of the laws protecting privacy and confidentiality of individuals and businesses, that are most likely applicable to your workplace, include the following.

- *Health Insurance Portability and Accountability Act of 1996 (*HIPAA*)*: Under federal law, employees in the US have the legal right to keep their medical and health information private – not to be divulged to other employees. The US Department of Health and Human Services (HHS) has established that employers that handle, store, and/or transmit personal health information – "protected health information" – must abide by the privacy requirements of the HIPAA of 1996. Accordingly, veterinary practice employers should take steps to ensure that protections are in place to safeguard the confidentiality of an employee's health/medical information – accessible only by a few key employees who need to know such information.
- *Legal protection of veterinary medical records and clients' information*: Respecting the privacy of clients in a veterinary practice is essential to building trusting relationships – both professionally and personally (see 7.13 Keeping Client Information Secure). Oftentimes clients provide information to veterinary businesses that they might not want other people to know – such as an unregistered phone number, residential address which should not be divulged to the public, or credit card information on account – all of which the client considers personal or private.

Many states have laws that provide protection of information contained in a veterinarian's record – including the client's information – as being confidential or private. These laws usually require that clients provide written consents before a veterinary medical record can be released. Yet limited exceptions for release of medical records without the client's written consent are also permitted – such as when a veterinarian receives a court order, a subpoena from an established civil or criminal proceeding, or a State Board's investigation for the medical record. Before releasing any information about an animal-patient or client, check your local laws or contact an attorney in your area to define the applicable requirements.

TIP: Unscrupulous callers might falsely claim to be boarding facilities, veterinary clinics or groomers requesting information about an animal when, in reality, they are seeking information about the client/owner. Train personnel to refrain from giving client information over the phone or sending records by fax/electronic transmission to other veterinary, boarding, or grooming facilities without the client's prior express written consent or, if applicable, obtaining a client's verbal consent.

- *Identity theft*: Federal and state laws provide penalties for those committing identity theft or impersonating individuals and businesses. These laws carry heavy penalties, including felony charges, incarceration, and fines. Yet, the primary problem is identifying the theft or impersonator. A veterinary business owner might potentially be considered as enabling crimes associated with identity theft, under particular circumstances – such as allowing the following acts at the workplace: (i) publishing photos and names in public view – such as lobby, website, social media – of animals boarding at facility "during owners' vacation" (potentially enabling burglary or theft to occur at client's home); (ii) leaving employees' tax forms or personal documents easily accessible on a desk or any unlocked location (potentially enabling fraudulent use of personally identifiable information, social security number and date of birth); (iii) discussing employee's medical information to staff members without the employee's knowledge or consent (exposing employee's right to privacy of health status), or (iv) placing documents in the trash without shredding (enabling others to gain information that could potentially be used for any unlawful activities).

The identity of your business can also be "stolen" for unlawful purposes. Keep financial information and credit cards secured. Unscrupulous people might use electronic signatures saved in your computers for obtaining controlled drugs or use passwords to divert funds from business bank accounts, or potentially use a business's credit card information (or access to a business credit card) to purchase electronics and office equipment to be delivered to another address.

- *The Fair Credit Reporting Act* contains strict regulations and processes that employers must follow when conducting postemployment criminal and consumer background checks on employees. Be sure to adhere to those provisions – such as proper documentation and obtaining the employee's consent prior to seeking the information.
- *Civil privacy laws*: Many states have laws defining protections for a person's reasonable expectation of privacy – including criminal/civil penalties related to a business's intrusion of solitude (such as expected privacy in a bathroom or locker room area), to appropriation (such as posting a client's or employee's face/pet for the benefit/marketing of the business without the client's/employee's consent) or false light (such as using social media postings to distort the truth or to mislead). Business owners should take proactive measures by implementing and maintaining workplace policies to ensure any employee's reasonable expectations of privacy are not violated.
- *The Electronic Communications Privacy Act (*ECPA*)* places limitations on an employer's right to monitor phone calls and emails at the workplace – unless the employee knows and consents to it. The ECPA also provides protection for an employee's voicemail messages at work – an employer may not listen to, delete, or prevent access to an employee's voicemail messages. Consult with an attorney to draft legally enforceable policies that allows the employer to monitor phone calls, emails, and social media use on business equipment for legitimate business reasons and business protections.

TAKE-AWAYS

- Draft an identity theft protection policy and train staff on the confidentiality of clients' personal information, employees' personal information, and proprietary business information.
- Ensure the privacy of employees' health information to avoid violations of the HIPAA by (i) maintaining medical/health-related reports in a separate folder/separate area from other personnel files, preferably in a locked cabinet, and (ii) avoiding discussing reasons for an employee's medically related absence with other members of the workforce, unless there is an overriding legitimate business reason for doing so.
- Draft workplace policies limiting employees' use of business computer and telephone systems. Prohibit employees from reading/opening emails from unknown senders on business computers (potentially providing a gateway for malware through a "fake" email message that enables hacking, loss, or shutdown of the entire business's stored data and information).
- Minimize theft of the business's financial information by having "two-layer confirmation" for electronic withdrawals of business funds from financial institutions (notifications by text to owner's cellphone or personal email before withdrawal transactions can be made) and change business passcodes often (sharing only with those who need to know).
- Draft workplace policies that prohibit disclosure of employee's/client's personal information by phone to nonemployees without the express prior consent of the protected individual, and refrain from uploading or posting photos of pets or people without the owner's/person's consent.

MISCELLANEOUS

7.6.4 Cautions

Maintaining confidentiality and privacy in a workplace can be extremely challenging for employers, especially in this age of electronic and technological advances. Veterinary practice owners and employers should contact an attorney for assistance to comply with laws that help protect the privacy and confidentiality of individuals and the business.

Recommended Reading

Choder, B. (2020). Identity theft prevention programs at the workplace. In: *Five-Minute Veterinary Practice Management Consult*, 3e (ed. L.J. Ackerman), 818–821. Ames, IA: Wiley.

7.7

Puppy and Kitten Classes

Jacqui Ley, BVSc (Hons), PhD, DECAWBM, FANZCVS (Veterinary Behaviour)

Melbourne Veterinary Specialist Centre, Glen Waverley, Victoria, Australia

BASICS

7.7.1 Summary

Puppy classes and kitten classes are invaluable services that can be offered by a clinic to their community – if they are done well. A class for owners of new puppies and kittens can help clients understand their pet and guide their development, can advise them on the routine healthcare for their pet and encourage their comfort in seeking help from the clinic. The classes are an opportunity for puppies and kittens to become familiar with and be comfortable attending the clinic. Well-trained staff can watch for health and behavior concerns so they can be addressed sooner. All clinic staff need to support a puppy or kitten class for it to be a success.

7.7.2 Terms Defined

Kitten: Young cat aged 8–16 weeks.
Puppy: Young dog aged 8–16 weeks.

MAIN CONCEPTS

The benefits of providing a well structured puppy or kitten class to clients are many; for the pets themselves, for clients and their families, for staff members, for the business and for clinic's community. The puppies and kittens are given a safe environment for socializing. Puppies can play with other puppies while supervised to encourage appropriate behavior and puppies and kittens can meet a variety of people who may not be part of their everyday life. The animals are also becoming familiar with the clinic and the staff and are building positive associations with them which can help with ongoing healthcare [1].

During the classes, the owners are also becoming comfortable with the clinic and staff. The class is a safe place to ask questions about health, development, and behavior which aids in developing realistic expectations which helps retention in the home [2]. Clients can be educated about how to handle their puppies and kittens and practice this under the guidance of trained staff. It is also a good time to provide further information about healthcare and vaccination, parasite control, diet, dental care, and grooming as well as discussing routine reproductive control. Common problems such as toilet training and mouthing can be discussed as a group, allowing owners to clarify any points.

Puppy classes are typically run by a veterinary nurse or technician, sometimes with a local dog trainer. Kitten classes are generally run by a veterinary nurse or technician. Running the classes gives staff members the opportunity to develop organization and communication skills and establish relationships with clients and their pets which lead to an increase in job satisfaction.

The clinic also benefits as better educated clients who understand their pets and are comfortable seeking advice from the clinic are likely to stay with the clinic for the life of that pet and others. Being able to provide care for pets as their health needs change over their lives also adds to staff job satisfaction and the success of the clinic.

The community overall benefits from good puppy and kitten classes being offered at local veterinary clinics. More pets are retained in their homes, reducing the number of dogs and cats abandoned or relinquished to shelters. The

Pet-Specific Care for the Veterinary Team, First Edition. Edited by Lowell Ackerman.
© 2021 John Wiley & Sons, Inc. Published 2021 by John Wiley & Sons, Inc.

owners are more likely to be aware of their responsibilities as pet owners and to comply with local laws. Puppy classes have long-term positive effects for puppies, with participants displaying less aggression to unfamiliar people [3].

7.7.3 Resources Needed

All clinics can run a puppy or kitten class if resources are allocated for this. The class needs a suitable area. The space will dictate how many people and pets can be in a class. Small spaces may mean multiple classes are run rather than just one larger space. The space may be the waiting area, a dedicated room or even a large consulting room for a very small class. A good class can be provided for just one or two pets.

The person delivering the class needs to be trained. These classes are not just play times but important points of contact for clients. Staff should know the normal behavior of the species as well as healthcare for that species (see 6.1 Normal Development Stages of Dogs and Cats). They must understand how animals learn. Staff also need to be excellent communicators who enjoy speaking with clients about their new pet. If outside experts are brought in (local dog trainers, local groomers), they should be vetted to ensure that their values align with the veterinary clinic. Positive reinforcement trainers are strongly recommended.

Puppy and kitten classes need dedicated time. The staff members involved need time to prepare for the class and to deliver the class without interruption. A correct level of staffing is also needed to make sure the class runs smoothly. Extra staff members to help with unruly or upset pets and to help with clean-ups are very helpful.

7.7.4 Structure

7.7.4.1 Puppy Classes

There appear to be two main ways of structuring puppy classes. The most popular is a set number of classes, between four and six, delivered once a week. The first class is an information night and puppies are left at home. The rules of the class are explained so that clients know what to do and how to manage their puppies. The next 3–5 weeks of classes cover basic manners such as sit, down/drop, recalls, stay, give/drop it, and beginning walking on a lead. Health-related topics include diet and feeding, oral care, parasite control, vaccination programs, and general healthcare, including how to check the puppy for health problems. Handling and examination of the puppy's feet, ears, skin, under the tail and mouth can be practiced

along with calming and soothing the puppy. Pilling can be practiced using treats. Care of the different types of coats and grooming can be discussed and demonstrated. Problem behaviors such as crying at night, mouthing and biting, jumping, and toilet training are all discussed. Socialization exercises may include supervised playtime between two and three puppies, navigating obstacles such as small barriers or a children's play tunnel, and engaging with people dressed in unusual clothes (dress-ups for the participants).

Working on the manners exercise for the week and some socialization time is interspersed with short information sessions. While listening, owners practice calming their puppies. Generally, the last class is a fun "graduation" class.

The other system of organizing classes is a rolling class that puppy owners can join at any time. The classes are repeated in sequence and puppies graduate when they have attended all classes.

7.7.4.2 Kitten Classes

Kitten classes are different from puppy classes. Species differences and the developmental stage of the kittens mean that some things undertaken in puppy classes are not suitable for kitten classes. Topics covered include feline healthcare, dietary recommendations, oral care, coat care, parasite prevention, vaccination schedules, litter box management, and general healthcare. Pilling is an important skill for kitten owners to learn and for kittens to learn to tolerate. Owners can be shown appropriate and safe toys for their kitten and give them a trial run to see what their kitten likes. The kittens can be socialized to unfamiliar people. Traveling to and from the clinic also helps the kittens to become familiar with their carrier.

EXAMPLES

Sunnyside Veterinary Clinic start offering puppy classes to their community. The class is 90 minutes once a week for five weeks. The first week is puppy free and each subsequent week involves periods of supervised play, short training sessions learning a new exercise each week, and information for clients about dog care and management. The classes are a success and a year in, the clinic is seeing more new puppy clients and is retaining clients beyond the first year, resulting in greater income for the practice. A second staff member is being trained to participate in puppy classes to broaden her skill set and allow the clinic to offer classes year round.

TAKE-AWAYS

- Puppy and kitten classes can be invaluable services for a clinic to offer their community if they are well resourced and delivered by trained staff.
- Puppy and kitten classes can aid retention of new clients to the practice beyond the first year.
- They are an excellent way to deliver healthcare messages to clients in a safe environment designed to encourage questions and conversation.
- Puppies and kittens who attend the classes become familiar with the clinic, which reduces their stress levels at subsequent visits.
- Staff who are supported in delivering puppy and kitten classes broaden their skills and report greater job satisfaction.

MISCELLANEOUS

7.7.5 Cautions

Areas used for puppy and kitten classes must be thoroughly cleaned to prevent transmission of infectious diseases. Staff must practice infection control to prevent transmitting diseases from hospitalized pets to the participating pets (see 4.4 Preventing Infectious Diseases in the Small Animal Veterinary Hospital). The type and level of control needed may vary by region.

References

1 Overall, K.L. (1997). *Clinical Behavioural Medicine for Small Animals*. St Louis, MO: Mosby.

2 Duxbury, M.M., Jackson, J., Line, S., Anderson, R. Evaluation of association between retention in the home and attendance at puppy socialization classes. *Journal of the American Veterinary Medical Association*, 2003. 223: 61–66.

3 Casey, R., Loftus, B., Bolster, C. et al. Human directed aggression in domestic dogs (Canis familiaris): occurrence in different contexts and risk factors. *Applied Animal Behaviour Science*, 2014. 152: 52–63.

7.8

Providing Care for Those Unable or Unwilling to Pay

Ryane E. Englar, DVM, DABVP (Canine and Feline Practice)

University of Arizona College of Veterinary Medicine, Oro Valley, AZ, USA

BASICS

7.8.1 Summary

Veterinary healthcare providers are obligated by the Veterinarian's Oath to act as stewards of the animal kingdom. This ethical agreement requires veterinarians to prioritize patient welfare and the prevention of disease above all other external influences, including finances. On paper, these tasks seem self-explanatory and clear-cut but in reality, clinical cases are rarely so black and white. Patients more often present in shades of gray that threaten the provider's understanding of how to provide gold standard medicine, particularly in cases in which patient outcomes are almost entirely dependent upon cost. How to provide care for those who are unable or unwilling to pay presents the provider with an ethical dilemma. How do we uphold our oath to the profession while balancing the limitations of care that comes with a price tag? Viable options include tailoring the minimum database to suit the immediate needs of the patient, staging the diagnosis, payment plans, and in some cases, euthanasia of the patient in spite of a treatable condition.

7.8.2 Terms Defined

Gold Standard: That which is considered the best available diagnostic test, treatment plan, or other benchmark that is available to manage patient care.

Minimum Database: A set of diagnostic tests that is recommended to be performed on every patient to provide the clinician with sufficient data to either confirm a diagnosis or narrow down the possibilities of what may be ailing the patient.

Payment Plan: A contractual agreement for paying off outstanding debt, in which the borrower pays back a set amount of money at scheduled intervals, typically monthly.

MAIN CONCEPTS

7.8.3 Prioritizing Patient Care

When new graduates gain admittance to the profession of veterinary medicine, they take an oath to use their knowledge and skills to advance animal health and welfare [1]. In addition, veterinarians are expected to practice medicine in a matter that is consistent with the Principles of Veterinary Medical Ethics (PVME), a code of conduct that is under the purview of the American Veterinary Medical Association (AVMA) [2]. This code maintains that veterinarians are ethically obligated to place the needs of the patient above financial interests.

The need to prioritize patient care comes naturally to healthcare providers but balancing this need against the cost of care does not. Veterinarians are trained to offer gold standard care for every patient. This standard of care, in combination with the minimum database, helps the practitioner to diagnose with the greatest accuracy. Stress can occur when veterinary teams feel they are being asked to compromise on this standard (see 8.17 Dealing with Compromise Fatigue).

In a world of ideals, the gold standard is always possible. However, as scientific advances revolutionize the number of diagnostic tests available to our patients, is the gold standard always feasible? What happens when the price of diagnosis and/or treatment exceeds the client's ability or willingness to afford the gold standard?

7.8.4 The Cost of Care

As diagnostic testing and treatment options expand, so too does the cost of care. Each test expands the arsenal of what healthcare providers can test for, and each test gives the clinician a better understanding of the patient's individual circumstances. However, each test is associated with a cost. This raises an important question: "Are we pricing people out of owning pets?" [3]

Today's pet owners are concerned about the monetary aspects of veterinary care (see 2.10 Affordability of Veterinary Services). They expect cost of care to take a backseat to patient care [4–6]. However, pet owners are also price-conscious [7]. They want veterinarians to be upfront about costs and to initiate discussions about cost early on in the consultation [4, 8]. They need to be prepared for what bills to expect, particularly since the majority of pet owners in the US and Canada do not subscribe to pet health insurance (PHI) [5, 8–10]. Clients frequently experience sticker shock and they may not understand the value of the services provided [4, 7, 11–14]. It is up to the veterinarian to justify each line item on an estimate [15].

7.8.5 Options for Financing Care

In order for veterinary practices to survive, they must receive payment for services rendered. Options for financing care include the following [16–18]:

- Establishing wellness plans within individual veterinary practices (see 10.17 Payment and Wellness Plans).
- Tailoring the minimum database to the patient to, in effect staging the diagnosis (see 2.2 The Role of Incremental Care).
- Offering in-house payment plans (see 10.17 Payment and Wellness Plans).
- Accepting third-party payments (see 10.18 Financing Veterinary Care).
- Promoting PHI (see 10.16 Pet Health Insurance).
- Establishing a charity fund.
- Considering euthanasia as a realistic treatment option.
- Refusing clients, when the patient is not in critical condition.

7.8.6 The Role of Communication

Regardless of how financing is achieved, it is important that the veterinary team communicate effectively (see 8.15 Delivering Information to Clients). Clients may feel self-conscious about what they can and cannot afford, and veterinarians may feel defensive about clients who question costs [4, 8]. Both emotions detract from patient care. It is important to address these emotions when they arise and maintain the examination room as a safe zone, free from judgment. Financial limitations do not reflect lack of care on the part of either the veterinarian or the client (see 5.11 Discussing Finances for Pet-Specific Care).

EXAMPLES

Purrkinje, an 8-year-old, spayed female Siamese cat, presents with a two-day history of stranguria (straining to urinate) and hematuria (blood in the urine). Physical examination confirms pain on palpation of the urinary bladder; the remainder of the examination is unremarkable. A urinary tract infection (UTI) is suspected but to be complete, a minimum database is recommended: complete blood count (CBC), chemistry panel, urinalysis (UA) with culture, thyroxine (T4), and abdominal radiography. Cost of care is discussed with the client, who is unable to afford the recommended approach. A cost–benefit analysis (CBA) determines that the best approach for Purrkinje's care is to stage diagnostic testing, beginning with a UA and urine culture. No uroliths are apparent during ultrasound-guided cystocentesis. UA is positive for *Escherichia coli*, and antibiotic therapy is initiated based upon culture and susceptibility. The patient responds well to treatment, clinical signs abate, and the UTI resolves.

TAKE-AWAYS

- Cost of veterinary care is rising as scientific advancements increase the diagnostic and therapeutic tools available to healthcare providers.
- Although veterinarians are required by their professional oath to prioritize the need of the patient over the cost of care, clinical cases often become a balancing act between what the patient needs and what the client can afford.
- Veterinarians need to prepare clients for anticipated expenses and explain the value of care.

- Practices need to look beyond traditional methods of payment and implement financing strategies that assist clients with patient care expenses.
- Wellness plans and third-party payment are viable tools that help clients afford care now.

MISCELLANEOUS

7.8.7 Cautions

Financing solutions for the cost of care are imperfect at best. Not all clients will qualify for third-party payment plans, and even if the practice itself is willing to offer a payment system, there is no guarantee that the client will pay.

Problems also arise when discussions about cost are not upfront. Written estimates can facilitate finance-based conversations but they are infrequently referenced [4, 5]. Clinicians may be faced with a client that says "do everything," only to have the client balk at the bill after the fact [4]. Blind faith that a client will follow through on promises to pay is not an ideal strategy for running a business.

Not all clients who refuse care do so because of finances. Some do not prioritize pet care. This can incite discord between the client and veterinary team. Provided that the client is not engaging in neglect or animal cruelty, we must accept that not all clients see value in investing in optimal healthcare. In these situations, it is important to avoid rash judgments about client character. Instead, center conversations on common ground: what can we agree to do for the pet now to facilitate healthcare? The client may decline care today, but be open to discussion in the future. If clients and veterinary teams cannot respect each other's approach to care in a way that is mutually agreeable, the client should be directed to seek care elsewhere.

References

1 Veterinarian's Oath. www.avma.org/KB/Policies/Pages/veterinarians-oath.aspx
2 Principles of veterinary medical ethics of the AVMA. www.avma.org/KB/Policies/Pages/Principles-of-Veterinary-Medical-Ethics-of-the-AVMA.aspx
3 DVM360. Is the gold standard the old standard? http://veterinarymedicine.dvm360.com/gold-standard-old-standard
4 Coe, J.B., Adams, C.L., and Bonnett, B.N. (2007). A focus group study of veterinarians' and pet owners' perceptions of the monetary aspects of veterinary care. *Journal of the American Veterinary Medical Association* 231: 1510–1518.
5 Coe, J.B., Adams, C.L., and Bonnett, B.N. (2009). Prevalence and nature of cost discussions during clinical appointments in companion animal practice. *Journal of the American Veterinary Medical Association* 234: 1418–1424.
6 Kipperman, B.S., Kass, P.H., and Rishniw, M. (2017). Factors that influence small animal veterinarians' opinions and actions regarding cost of care and effects of economic limitations on patient care and outcome and professional career satisfaction and burnout. *Journal of the American Veterinary Medical Association* 250: 785–794.
7 Lue, T.W., Pantenburg, D.P., and Crawford, P.A. (2008). Impact of the owner-pet and client-veterinarian bond on the care that pets receive. *Journal of the American Veterinary Medical Association* 232: 531–540.
8 Brockman, B.K., Taylor, V.A., and Brockman, C.M. (2008). The price of unconditional love: consumer decision making for high-dollar veterinary care. *Journal of Business Research* 61: 397–405.
9 Brown, J.P. and Silverman, J.D. (1999). The current and future market for veterinarians and veterinary medical services in the United States. *Journal of the American Veterinary Medical Association* 215: 161–183.
10 (2001). *Paws and Claws: A Syndicated Study on Canadian Pet Ownership*. Toronto, Canada: Ipsos Reid.
11 Volk, J.O., Felsted, K.E., Thomas, J.G. et al. (2011). Executive summary of the Bayer veterinary care usage study. *Journal of the American Veterinary Medical Association* 238: 1275–1282.
12 Volk, J.O., Felsted, K.E., Thomas, J.G. et al. (2011). Executive summary of phase 2 of the Bayer veterinary care usage study. *Journal of the American Veterinary Medical Association* 239: 1311–1316.
13 Volk, J.O., Thomas, J.G., Colleran, E.J. et al. (2014). Executive summary of phase 3 of the Bayer veterinary care usage study. *Journal of the American Veterinary Medical Association* 244: 799–802.
14 DeHaven, W.R. (2014). Are we really doing enough to provide the best veterinary care for our pets? *Journal of the American Veterinary Medical Association* 244: 1017–1018.
15 Arman, K. (2015). What can't be taught. *Canadian Veterinary Journal* 56: 197–198.
16 Kondrup, S.V., Anhoj, K.P., Rodsgaard-Rosenbeck, C. et al. (2016). Veterinarian's dilemma: a study of how Danish small animal practitioners handle financially limited clients. *Veterinary Record* 179: 596.
17 Kinnison, T. (2016). When veterinary teams are faced with clients who can't afford to pay. *Veterinary Record* 179: 594–595.

18 Durrance, D. and Lagoni, M.S. (1999). I can't pay for treatment. *Veterinary Economics*: 64–66.

Recommended Reading

Coe, J.B., Adams, C.L., and Bonnett, B.N. (2007). A focus group study of veterinarians' and pet owners' perceptions of the monetary aspects of veterinary care. *Journal of the American Veterinary Medical Association* 231 (10): 1510–1518.

Coe, J.B., Adams, C.L., and Bonnett, B.N. (2009). Prevalence and nature of cost discussions during clinical appointments in companion animal practice. *Journal of the American Veterinary Medical Association* 234 (11): 1418–1424.

7.9

Using Practice Management Software to Personalize Care

Peter Alberti, BSBA

Inulogica, Northborough, MA, USA

BASICS

7.9.1 Summary

Implementing pet-specific care can be much easier and more effective when medical goals are supported by data and information. Practice management software (PMS), also known as a pet information management system or "PIMS," facilitates the process of storing, retrieving, and using the data and information. Aligning the use of the PIMS with your practice's pet-specific care initiatives is no different than setting it up for traditional diagnostic and preventive care purposes. It simply requires some planning and execution.

7.9.2 Terms Defined

Electronic Health Record (EHR): A comprehensive report of a patient's overall health. It may or may not include EMRs from one or more practices and is intended to be shared among authorized providers, staff, and other users.

Electronic Medical Record (EMR): The specific notes, codes, diagnoses, prognoses, prescriptions, and other data that specifically relate to a patient's medical history within a practice. It may be a standalone record or may be incorporated into a PIMS record. It is typically not shared outside the practice.

PIMS: The software used by the practice to record appointments, notes, prescriptions, vaccines, reminders, invoices, and more. Also known as PMS.

Wearables: Electronic devices that are worn by a person or animal that gather, store, and share data. For pets, these often include collars or tags that have sensors.

MAIN CONCEPTS

7.9.3 Planning

Early detection is a key principle of pet-specific care (see 4.7 Embracing Early Detection). Once a few conditions have been identified on which to focus, you can use the PIMS to identify patients who meet risk criteria for these conditions. Whether it is species/breed, age, gender, weight/composition, vaccine history, or any other criteria, you can create profiles and segments to devise care plans and measure outcomes. You can then use your PIMS to track which clients are most aligned to the practice goals, and which ones might be receptive to creating a care plan.

By combining historical data with new data sets created through deliberate coding and analysis, your PIMS system will help you substantiate your commitment to ongoing care. Your team and your clients can have more productive conversations when a specific plan and data-driven results drive the discussions.

7.9.4 Encoding and Integrating Data

Once you have identified care plan protocols for pet-specific care it is time to evaluate – and possibly update – the way you work with your PIMS.

Cleaning up data is an excellent first step. Over time, data can become stale or inconsistent. Ensure all data values that are relevant to your care plan protocols are complete and accurate. For example, if your protocol will profile patients based on age, ensure the age value exists for all patients in the database. Evaluate how the age is specified. Is it calculated by the PIMS based on the pet's birthday? If so, you also need to check the birthday values to ensure they are complete and accurate. Or is the age entered manually by your staff? If so, it's very likely it doesn't get updated every year, so you'll need to get them updated and ensure they are updated regularly.

One the PIMS data are verified and ready, ensure your practice team is aware of your policies about encoding data. Explain why it's necessary to enter data a certain way, what the impact is of failing to do so, and ideally give each team member an intrinsic reason to want to comply with your standards. Also, create a process to verify that the encoding is being done properly. Create audits or checks and balances that ensure the data are clean on a day-to-day basis. The more accurate the data are, the better the outcomes will be since the PIMS outputs will become a pivotal tool for creating, monitoring, and reviewing care plans with clients.

Many PIMS systems can store or integrate data from external sources such as diagnostic equipment, laboratory results, wearables, mobile apps, client communication systems, and more. When devising a plan for pet-specific care, consider what opportunities beyond your own clinic data could be helpful. For example, if the pet's weight is a factor in a care plan, you can easily weigh the pet at the appointment and use this data point in your discussions with the client. However, if you make it easy for the client to record and report the pet's weight at home, along with deploying an exercise monitoring device that regularly records the patient's activity level, you now have a far better data set with which to do analysis and make recommendations (see 2.5 Virtual Care (Telehealth)).

7.9.5 Sharing Results

There are a few stakeholders who can benefit from the data and information your PIMS makes available with pet-specific care.

Your own healthcare teams are the obvious beneficiaries. Your staff and clients should use the PIMS results regularly as part of the care plan process. Ideally, every aspect of a patient's care plan will be made easily available whenever it is productive throughout the year. Some PIMS systems integrate with client portals to make results available online or through mobile apps. Automated reminders and monitoring/alerts can help the teams remain focused.

Integrations that allow other members of a patient's care team (e.g., groomers, dog walkers, pet sitters, etc.) to participate are ideal. Bidirectional sharing and communication among these participants help create a holistic EHR, a shared repository of pet health data that can help everyone work toward common goals for a pet. Selected portions of your practice's EMR can be shared at your discretion to contribute to the EHR. The more you and the client make available to others, the better the entire care team can help the pet.

Surveillance networks are being developed that will seek to leverage PIMS data. These programs will not only benefit from receiving your PIMS data, should you choose to allow it, but could also become a valuable data set for your own planning. By aggregating certain data sets, surveillance networks identify trends and patterns that can help you make decisions. This information may or may not be something you can produce with your own, limited data sets. Additionally, surveillance networks may provide you with insights and concepts you may otherwise not have considered. Finally, they are doing a great deal of work on your behalf, saving you time.

Your client is, of course, the ultimate stakeholder on the care team. A key success factor for care plans is client adoption and compliance. Your PIMS data give you the opportunity to craft a story with your client that is powerful since it is evidence based. Leveraging the PIMS for planning, monitoring, and outcomes sharing will help clients feel they are in control of their pet's journey, which in turn is likely to result in better compliance (see 9.17 Improving Compliance and Adherence with Pet-Specific Care). Making it easy for clients to access appropriate PIMS information and helping them to receive it in a timely manner will improve results.

 TAKE-AWAYS

- PIMS, when properly configured, is a valuable tool to make pet-specific care feasible and effective.
- Align PIMS with the practice's protocols and standards of care. Avoid creating protocols based on software features.
- Leverage as many sources of data as are available. Don't limit yourself to your own data.
- Incrementally add and improve pet-specific care capabilities over time to ensure staff acceptance, accuracy, and return on investment.

- Use the PIMS to showcase outcomes as well as to share information across multiple teams.

MISCELLANEOUS

7.9.6 Cautions

When leveraging PIMS results in client-facing conversations, ensure they are consumable by a pet owner. The potential exists for discussions to be very technically detailed which could have a negative impact on client adoption. If a pet owner does not clearly understand and agree with a care plan, compliance is likely to be low.

There are myriad opportunities to improve a patient's care through pet-specific care, and they are exciting (see 1.3 Personalized Care Plans). Don't "boil the ocean" and try to deploy every possible care plan all at once. Just because your PIMS system enables you to do something doesn't mean you should. Staff acceptance and adoption of your processes, along with accuracy and true return on investment, will be reduced if you try to do too much at once. Determine which care plan elements have the highest impact and are most likely to succeed and start with those. Once your team enjoys a few successes with pet-specific care, they will be more receptive to making other changes in the future.

Some PIMS systems are extremely feature-rich. One common trap is to leverage software capabilities just because they are available. It can be helpful to learn what the system can do, be inspired by ideas it offers, and implement best practices, as long as ultimately you only enable features that produce measurable results and support your goals. Do not create protocols in your practice based on software capabilities. Use the software's capabilities to implement your chosen protocols.

7.10

Analytics and Informatics

Peter Alberti, BSBA

Inulogica, Northborough, MA, USA

BASICS

7.10.1 Summary

Analytics and informatics are two discrete disciplines which are integral to making veterinary data productive for multiple stakeholders including doctors and staff, practices, suppliers, researchers/academics, and the animal health industry as a whole.

7.10.2 Terms Defined

Analytics: Techniques and processes used to enhance productivity through data analysis.
Informatics: The process of using data to improve health and the delivery of healthcare services.
Interoperability: The ability for data or information to be consumed by disparate systems or processes.

MAIN CONCEPTS

7.10.3 The Difference Between Analytics and Informatics

There is no formal distinction between analytics and informatics, but they are technically quite different. Analytics may be considered as the discovery, interpretation, and communication of meaningful patterns in data, whereas informatics deals more with the practice of information processing.

The simplest way to distinguish the two is to understand the ultimate outputs derived from each. Analytics, a function performed largely by data analysts, produces charts, graphs, tables, and other information organized to support a decision of some sort. Informaticists identify what decisions need to be made, how data should be organized and articulated as information, and how information could (or should) be interpreted.

While analytics nearly always involves some sort of data and very often requires use of technology, informatics does not always imply the use of either of these. Human interaction, human interface, processes, and systems are often key contributors to the work of an informaticist.

7.10.4 The Opportunity: Analytics and Informatics for Pet-Specific Care

A core concept in pet-specific care is evidence-based medicine (see 2.1 Evidence-Based Veterinary Medicine and Personal Bias). This inherently lends itself to analytics and informatics at multiple levels. On a per-patient basis, there are many dimensions to work with. Take each of those dimensions to a per-breed, per-species, per-practice, or per-region level and there are countless ways to identify trends.

Data points associated with early detection of conditions, reactions, diseases, etc. will be defined and redefined on an almost continuous basis. Computational analysis of the relationships between each of the entities involved will not only accelerate early detection, it will likely help identify components that could not have been considered by manual analysis.

7.10.5 Interoperability

A key challenge that limits advances in analytics and informatics in any field, but particularly in healthcare, is the availability of compatible data. In both academic and commercial realms, the fundamental need to protect intellectual property often offsets the benefit of collaboration and data sharing. This driver, coupled with market-driven demand for fast-paced innovation, has resulted in an abundance of incompatible data sets.

In the context of pet-specific care, interoperability is even more challenging. The very nature of "personalizing" medicine requires very detailed and specific data points. The pace of innovation and the very large scope of opportunity drive the creation of an incredible amount of data and information. Enabling productive use of disparate data sets and information realms requires willing collaboration and disciplined approaches.

Veterinary practices can help to encourage and improve interoperability by:

- training teams to create and follow standards of care for data entry
- embracing and capitalizing on the opportunities that exist with data sharing
- challenging suppliers to adhere to standards that enable the exchange of data which benefits the practice and its patients
- actively identifying and implementing uses of data within the practice and then sharing aggregate results within the animal health industry so everyone benefits.

7.10.6 Privacy, Security, and Ethics

Inherent in any digital system is concern over appropriate use of data and information. Analytics and informatics both have unique considerations that transcend basic notions of data security (see 7.13 Keeping Client Information Secure). Privacy is defined here as the appropriate availability of data and information. Security is more aligned to the protection of data within digital systems. Ethics revolves around appropriate uses of data and information by stakeholders who are entitled to use it (see 7.6 Privacy and Confidentiality).

Although human health data are aggressively protected by regulation, animal health data are generally not. However, the personally identifiable information of pet owners that often accompanies pet health records remains well protected by law. As such, systems built to accommodate analytics and informatics must be developed to adhere to the regulations. Clients remain unclear or uninformed about these matters and typically expect that their information, and that of their pets, will be safeguarded.

Regardless of the extent of regulatory requirements, animal health data are regarded as valuable property and are consequently restricted by many veterinary practices. While this is justifiable on some level, it is problematic at the same time. Veterinary practices who refuse to allow their data to be included in the universe of analytics and informatics services and programs are, more than ever, restricting their ability to modernize their practices, tap into the potential of the data to make animals healthier, and remain competitive in their markets. Unfortunately, intentional and unintentional misappropriation of practice data by third parties has created a great sense of fear in some practice decision makers. The resolution to this is finding a balance between reasonable care to protect data and unreasonable stashing of the data.

The myriad implementations of analytics and informatics, and the ease with which powerful outputs can be created, creates new ethical concerns. A veterinarian's oath is to strive to promote animal health and welfare. Under certain pressures (economic, client-driven, etc.) veterinary teams could be compelled to misuse available information. For example, the sale of identifiable pet health data without permission from clients could be intriguing to a practice struggling financially. Leveraging aggregated data to unduly influence a pet parent when it is not truly in the best interest of the patient could potentially occur under certain circumstances.

Although the privacy, security, and ethics considerations described here are not necessarily unique to pet-specific care, they can be more impactful when the "personalized" aspects of pet-specific data are involved. Legal and regulatory considerations are becoming more prevalent. The increasing correlation of human health with animal health and the coupling of research and commercial data from both of these realms have resulted in added scrutiny by government agencies.

EXAMPLES

1) A new heartworm preventive becomes available. From a medical perspective, it is more likely to be effective in pets with specific characteristics. The practice can identify the best candidates for the drug by querying the practice data and making recommendations to clients based ib the characteristics of the particular patient. The practice can then initiate a deliberate plan

to test the effectiveness and confirm the correlation to specific pets.

2) Practices join forces in a defined geographical region to share data about a disease of concern. They agree to code instances of the disease in a consistent manner. When their data are combined and analyzed they are able to identify trends across multiple dimensions. The disease is more prevalent in urban than rural areas. It is also more common in pets who are not overweight. Further investigation reveals that dog walking with professional dog walkers may be an associated factor, even if a causal relationship is not immediately evident. This could help direct further epidemiological investigation. Practice teams in urban areas can now work to identify clients who use professional dog walkers and alert them to the issue and what is currently known about it, through whatever means are appropriate.

TAKE-AWAYS

- Analytics and informatics are two distinct disciplines that play a major role in animal health.
- Opportunities abound to leverage analytics and informatics to continuously improve animal health, particularly for pet-specific care scenarios.
- Care must be taken to ensure data and information are only available to those who need them, but also that they are not kept inappropriately hidden away.
- Proper use of data and information is vital.
- Analytics and informatics concepts are not limited to business and technical professionals. Clinical staff can, and should, play a major role in endorsing and using analytics and informatics in the practice.

MISCELLANEOUS

7.10.7 Cautions

An abundance of data and information can easily lead to misuse. While deliberate abuse by clinical staff seems generally unlikely, generating and accessing information just because it is available can be distracting and sometimes even misleading. Care should be taken to ensure information is accurate and productive.

Since data and information in the realm of pet-specific care are particularly focused on a team approach, ensuring consistency and clarity across all stakeholders will produce better results. If team members code records differently, review results in an inconsistent manner, or interpret reports without a framework, pet-specific care can easily become "staff-specific care." Information systems should create alignment across teams (see 8.4 Alignment – The Key to Implementing Pet-Specific Care).

Recommended Reading

Ethical issues for today's veterinarian in the digital age. www.veterinarypracticenews.com/ ethical-issues-for-todays-veterinarian-in-the-digital-age

Electronic Health Records in Veterinary Medicine. www.embs.org/pulse/articles/ electronic-health-records-veterinary-medicine/

Leveraging EHR Interoperability For Transitions of Care. https://vynamic.com/insights/ leveraging-ehr-interoperability-for-transitions-of-care

Veterinary Informatics. https://sbmi.uth.edu/blog/mar-15/03182015.htm

7.11

Client Safety

Saya Press, BVSc, MS, DACVECC

The Veterinary Specialty Hospital of San Diego, Sorrento Valley, San Diego, CA, USA

 BASICS

7.11.1 Summary

Client safety is of the utmost importance in all areas of veterinary medicine – not just the veterinary clinic or hospital, but also in the home and community. Particularly in novel situations, it becomes the veterinary professionals' duty to educate and guide clients in ways that ensure their ongoing safety, especially when their pet may be in pain or stressed. Client safety encompasses an understanding of animal psychology and awareness of how the environment may impact this, as well as an appreciation of special circumstances, such as administration of medications, zoonotic diseases, and emergency situations, among others.

7.11.2 Terms Defined

Cytotoxic Waste: Waste associated with cytotoxic drugs (often chemotherapeutics) that is toxic to cells.
Fecal–Oral Transmission: Transmission that occurs due to ingestion of organisms from another animal's feces.
Genotoxic Waste: Waste that may have the potential to damage genetic information, typically derived from drugs used in chemotherapy or radiation oncology.

 MAIN CONCEPTS

7.11.3 The Veterinary Hospital

Fortunately for most hospitals, client safety concerns extend only as far as the waiting and exam rooms, as it is not generally standard practice to allow clients in treatment areas for more than a brief visit of their hospitalized pet.

It is important for veterinary staff to remember that animals may be more anxious at a veterinary clinic, or may be in pain, which may result in behaviors the client is not expecting. This may result in clients being injured as they attempt to intervene, especially if they are restraining their pet for examination (see 8.12 Preventing Animal-Related Injuries). Veterinary staff should be aware of the potential for owners to misinterpret or be surprised by their animals' different behavior and should communicate this possibility early, as well as educating clients on signs of anxiety when possible.

Safest practice is that clients are not permitted to restrain their pet for the physical examination, especially parts that the animal may find distasteful (such as rectal temperatures, ear inspections or examination of painful areas). Trained veterinary personnel should be available to assist the veterinarian when needed. Practices should note that they may be liable for expenses related to any injury sustained on their premises, even if it is by the client's own dog.

Pet-Specific Care for the Veterinary Team, First Edition. Edited by Lowell Ackerman.
© 2021 John Wiley & Sons, Inc. Published 2021 by John Wiley & Sons, Inc.

For hospitals that permit visits with hospitalized pets, it is recommended that these visits are directly supervised by veterinary staff. Any sharps, heavy equipment or potentially toxic medications should be removed from the patient's environment while owners are visiting. Thorough counseling of owners on appropriate personal protective equipment prior to a visit should be performed for any animal on chemotherapeutic medications requiring isolated disposal of waste, or any patient with a zoonotic disease.

Owners should never be permitted in any part of the practice with active radiation, including x-ray rooms, computed tomography (CT) or fluoroscopy when in use, and can never be allowed to restrain their own pet for these procedures. In such situations, appropriate chemical restraint should be employed if needed.

7.11.4 Emergency Situations

Undoubtedly, all veterinarians and veterinary hospitals will, at some point, treat an emergency patient. This may range from trauma to collapse to toxin ingestion and everything in between. Many of these situations have the potential to put owners at risk of injury as they try to help their pet or transport them to the hospital. Pets which are not normally aggressive but have been injured may be in pain and more likely to bite or scratch their owners. Owners should be cautioned about this possibility if they are trying to move their injured pet post trauma. Large dogs who have collapsed and thus are "dead weight" may cause back or neck injury to owners (and staff) attempting to lift them.

Snake bites and animal attacks present another situation whereby owners may get hurt attempting to help their pet. Veterinary staff should advise owners not to attempt to pick up any snakes or spiders (including those they believe to be dead) to minimize any chance of the owner getting bitten. Depending on geographic region, the risk of rabies or other zoonotic disease from feral or wild animals may need to be communicated to the owner, and they should be discouraged from approaching any feral or wild animal.

Animals that are entangled and/or caught in wire or rope may be particularly fractious and painful. If there is concern, owners may be advised to muzzle their dog prior to cutting it free. The same recommendation can be given to owners attempting to transport any animal in pain, as long as the animal is not in respiratory distress and is safe to be muzzled. Ideally, the owners should have access to a basket muzzle rather than cloth muzzle, as the former allows easier respiratory effort. If the above criteria are not satisfied, a towel or comparable blanket may be used loosely around the animal's neck as a way to restrain and control its head, as long as no pressure is put on the airway.

An owner witnessing their pet having a seizure may be tempted to take measures to prevent it biting its own tongue. This should be discouraged, and nothing should be placed in the animal's mouth as it is likely to result in inadvertent biting of the owner.

7.11.5 Medications

Many animals will require oral medications at home at some point. Ideally, a patient willingly takes their medications in a small treat. However, if a sufficiently high-value disguise cannot be found, transdermal or long-acting injectable preparations may be sought. Additionally, compounding pharmacies may be able to flavor medications to increase palatability. If these options are unavailable or are cost-prohibitive, some animals may require pilling. Teaching clients to pill their animal requires demonstration by veterinary staff. If clients are still unable to do this, a piller (or pill gun) may be useful and reduce risk of injury.

Some medications may have the potential to harm owners, including but not limited to chemotherapeutics. Gloves should be dispensed with all medications that carry such risks. Table 7.11.1 provides a list of some (nonchemotherapeutic) medications that have the potential for adverse effect when handled. A complete list of all such medications is lengthy; the reader should consult pharmacology textbooks or dispensing guidelines for information on medications not listed here.

Patients being treated with chemotherapeutic medications may excrete these drugs in their urine or feces, resulting in cytotoxic or genotoxic waste. Ideally, patients should remain hospitalized until their feces and/or urine are no longer of concern; however, if this is not feasible, gloves should be sent home with the client, to be used for 72 hours following administration of therapy. Patients should not urinate or defecate in high-traffic areas or where children may play.

7.11.6 Zoonotic Diseases

A zoonotic disease is one that can be transmitted from animal to human. A full list of these conditions is beyond the scope of this topic, but the more common or infamous ones include toxoplasmosis, leptospirosis, dermatophytosis (ringworm), *Giardia*, *Salmonella*, Lyme disease, *Campylobacter*, *Cryptosporidium*, some intestinal worms, and rabies. Specific recommendations given to avoid human exposure depend on the route of spread, the infectious potential of the pathogen, and the immune status of the client (see 4.3 Prevention and Control of Infectious Diseases).

Table 7.11.1 Examples of nonchemotherapeutic medications that may have the potential to harm owners [1]

Medication	Route of injury	Potential toxicity in people	Recommendations for client safety
Chloramphenicol	Accidental exposure – residue on hands, inhaled particles (if tablet broken or crushed)	Aplastic anemia	Gloves should be worn when handling Thorough hand washing after dosing
Misoprostol		May induce miscarriage in pregnant women, or asthma attack in susceptible individuals	Gloves when handling, thorough hand washing after dosing Pregnant women and asthmatics should avoid touching this medication
Nitroglycerin	Transdermal due to inadvertent contact	Hypotension, headaches, rash locally	Gloves when applying, and do not pet animal where medication was applied
Fentanyl patch	Transdermal absorption, either unintentionally during placement or removal, or intentional abuse	Sedation, dysphoria, respiratory, or CNS depression, rashes at contact site	The author recommends placement be performed in a veterinary clinic, removal with gloves only. Disposal by flushing down the toilet
Injectable medications	Needlestick injury	Variable depending on drug; infection if the needle is "dirty"	Clear education on appropriate infection technique and disposal Offer clients to return needles to clinic for disposal

Parasites or bacteria that spread by the fecal–oral route (*Salmonella*, *Campylobacter*, toxoplasmosis, intestinal worms) rely on good preventive care (including regular anthelminthic treatment) when appropriate and strict hygiene while handling fecal material. Due to the increased risk for fetal transmission, pregnant women are advised against cleaning cat litter trays, especially cats fed raw meat, or indoor/outdoor cats which hunt. *Leptospira* is shed in the urine, so clients should be advised to avoid contact with their pets' urine, and when handling infected (or suspect) animals' urine or soiled areas, appropriate protective equipment should be used (gloves), and hands should be thoroughly washed.

Rabies is rare in many parts of the world but continued vaccination is paramount in protecting the pet population and thus our clients. Owners should be advised to avoid any contact with a suspected rabid animal, and should seek immediate medical attention if they are bitten.

EXAMPLES

Oliver, a 2-year-old male castrated Labradoodle, presented following ingestion of a toxic amount of a nonsteroidal antiinflammatory drug. Due to financial constraints, the owners chose outpatient care with gastric protectants, subcutaneous fluid, and misoprostol. The veterinary team communicated clearly to the owners the risks of misoprostol and provided gloves to be used when administering the medication. The owners received a detailed demonstration

of how to administer subcutaneous fluids and were instructed to put used needles inside a closed container and return this to ABC Veterinary Hospital for disposal of sharps at the recheck appointment.

TAKE-AWAYS

- Client safety can be managed through good communication of risks and concerns.
- It is the responsibility of the veterinary team to ensure clients remain safe while on the premises.
- Clients may need to be made aware that when their animal is hurt, they may be more likely to bite, scratch, or injure them.
- Clients must be well educated on the risks of various medications and the risks associated with different routes of administration (transdermal, subcutaneous).
- Zoonotic diseases represent special cases that require education about route of spread and populations at risk.

MISCELLANEOUS

Reference

1 Plumb, D.C. (2018). *Plumb's Veterinary Drug Handbook*, 9e. Stockholm: PharmaVet Inc.

7.12

Patient Safety

Helen Ballantyne, PG Dip, BSc (Hons), RN, RVN

Cambridge University Hospitals NHS Foundation Trust, Cambridge, UK

BASICS

7.12.1 Summary

Patient safety within the veterinary environment is threatened by the increasing complexity of healthcare combined with emerging disease profiles, financial pressures, and pharmaceutical resistance.

Maintaining patient safety is essential to prevent animals coming to harm during veterinary treatment. It is the responsibility of all members of the multidisciplinary team as adverse events are not restricted to animals undergoing clinical procedures.

An open, no-blame culture of patient safety should be cultivated whereby unexpected outcomes and near-misses are embraced as learning opportunities so steps can be taken to prevent similar events happening again.

7.12.2 Terms Defined

Adverse Event: When patients come to harm as a result of their veterinary treatment journey.

Human Factors: The organizational, individual, and environmental characteristics that influence behaviors that can impact patient safety.

Near-Miss: A situation where an adverse event nearly happened but was prevented.

Patient Safety Incident: An umbrella term for an episode of failed or substandard healthcare that causes or has the potential to cause an adverse event.

Polypharmacy: The simultaneous use of multiple drugs in an individual patient.

Root Cause Analysis: A systemic approach to establishing the fundamental cause or causes of a problem.

MAIN CONCEPTS

Huge advances in veterinary healthcare have been accompanied by an increasing complexity of care. In a model that echoes human-centered healthcare, companion animals are living longer, often with multiple chronic conditions requiring ongoing treatment. This can result in complicated treatment plans, polypharmacy, and multiple goals of care. In addition to this increase in patient acuity, emerging disease profiles, resistance to pharmaceuticals, and increasing financial pressures add a further dimension of complexity. Each of these factors is a threat to the safety of patients within the healthcare environment as clinicians need to find new ways of working with increasingly restricted resources.

Human-centered healthcare began to prioritize patient safety after worldwide research demonstrated that patient safety incidents were on the rise. A patient safety incident is an umbrella term for an episode of failed or substandard healthcare that causes or has the potential to cause harm. When patients come to harm as a result of their healthcare treatment, it is an adverse event. While all healthcare procedures have some inherent risk, such risks are known and discussed openly with owners as part of the process of obtaining informed consent (see 7.4 Getting Informed

Consent). In contrast, adverse events are unexpected and unintended. Examples of adverse events include medication errors, hospital-acquired infections, diagnostic errors, and failure to rescue deteriorating patients. If a situation in clinical practice has led to circumstances where an adverse event nearly happened but was prevented, this is termed a near-miss.

The veterinary profession is starting to learn lessons from their human medicine counterparts and implement patient safety practices and precautions. The aim of all patient safety measures is to prevent adverse events during the provision of healthcare. The pursuit of patient safety is complex, with no single tool or philosophy guaranteeing success. In contrast, there is a requirement for a collaborative approach combining specific patient safety tools with a working culture that supports patient safety as a priority.

7.12.3 Creating a Patient Safety Culture

Prioritizing a philosophy of patient safety is probably one of the most important measures a veterinary healthcare team can implement to keep animals safe in the clinical environment. It is also probably one of the biggest challenges a team may encounter as it requires a significant paradigm shift in attitudes and culture.

7.12.4 The Multidisciplinary Team

The first shift in attitude is the assumption that patient safety is the responsibility of frontline clinical staff; patient safety incidents are not restricted to clinical errors (see 8.14 Appropriate Handling of Medical Errors). Unintended harm may come to a patient waiting in reception before they have seen a member of the clinical team. Consider a cat that enters the practice in the arms of its owner; it is vulnerable to harm from the other patients waiting to see the veterinarian. A patient safety approach would be for the receptionist to offer the owner a carrier for their pet, or alternatively find a safer place for the cat to wait. All members of staff need to be fully committed to patient safety no matter what their remit and responsibility may be.

7.12.5 Support, Report, and Learn

The second major shift in culture is the need for patient safety incidents and unexpected clinical outcomes to be reported within a no blame culture. There needs to be a support, report, and learn approach. Traditionally, adverse events in healthcare have been addressed by establishing the cause and effect of the action or actions of an individual or group. This approach concentrates on the behavior and characteristics of the person or people associated with the error and apportions blame accordingly. Efforts to address the problem are targeted at the people involved and focus on individual reprimands and retraining.

There are several problems with this blaming method of addressing patient safety incidents. Primarily, it is an approach based on a flawed assumption. Adverse events in healthcare rarely arise purely from individual recklessness or ignorance, but are more likely to occur from basic flaws in the way the healthcare system is organized and delivered. Therefore, it is inappropriate to apportion blame to members of the team. Instead, in a process known as the systems model, operational and organizational procedures are examined instead.

As a basic example, consider a patient who requires blood glucose monitoring at 30-minute intervals. The nurse/technician in charge of the patient realizes the glucometer he is trained to use is not available; it is being used elsewhere. As he is not appropriately dressed for the operating room, he is unable to enter the surgical wing of the hospital to retrieve the equipment. He finds an alternative glucometer but realizes that there are substrates missing and he is unsure how to use it. Meanwhile, the animal has missed two blood tests and is suffering from hypoglycemia.

Under the traditional model, a blaming method, when the omission of blood tests was discovered, the nurse in charge of the patient would be blamed for the animal developing potentially life-threatening hypoglycemia. He would likely be reprimanded by the senior clinician for neglecting the patient and sent on a diabetes awareness course to refresh his knowledge of the condition.

Examining the same situation from a systems model provides an alternative point of view. The nurse knew and understood the importance of monitoring the blood glucose level. There is no evidence that he omitted the procedure through ignorance or malevolence, he was spending time seeking out the necessary equipment. The questions that should be asked are directed to the organizational systems. Why were clinical staff not aware that the glucometer was going to be needed for a prolonged period of time in the operating room? Why were staff not trained how to use the back-up glucometer? Why is the back-up glucometer not adequately maintained so that it can be used when required? Is the number of glucometers currently available to staff in the hospital sufficient? Putting measures in place to address each of these questions would prevent the incident happening again.

Another problem with apportioning blame to patient safety incidents is that it promotes a culture of secrecy and fear. This may be to the detriment of any animal involved if staff feel unable to report problems and attempt to manage the situation independently. Treatment to offset the effects of the incident may be delayed, insufficient or absent if staff feel too frightened to seek assistance.

Finally, the fear and secrecy often linked with the blame model prevents the opportunity to learn from patient safety incidents as staff involved feel ashamed and fearful. Consider the glucometer case, in which sharing the details of the case would facilitate learning. Perhaps other members of the team would examine their own skill set and realize that they have also not received training on the back-up glucometer. Training could be performed for the whole team, potentially preventing the same situation happening again.

Robust leadership is essential to shift the paradigm of blame. Leaders must adjust their own attitudes and assumptions and embrace adverse events, unexpected outcomes and near-misses as learning opportunities. They need to demonstrate to the entire multidisciplinary team that patient safety incidents can be reported within a no blame culture.

On a practical level, the provision of incident report templates can facilitate robust data collection. Digital methods, with online submission of information, are probably the most effective way of obtaining the necessary facts but the key point is that all staff need to be able to access the reporting system.

7.12.6 Patient Safety Investigations

As well as facilitating and supporting the reporting of patient safety incidents, team leaders need to demonstrate that they are able to perform thorough impartial, no blame investigations. A systematic approach should be instigated; often a root cause analysis is appropriate. This is a logical step-by-step approach to unraveling complex incidents. Understanding what happened, how it happened, and why it happened are key to developing recommendations and changes to practice that can prevent the situation occurring again.

7.12.7 Embracing Client Complaints

Embracing client complaints is another paradigm shift that will support patient safety. Traditionally, client complaints have been viewed as negative, but just as with adverse events and unexpected outcomes, they should be approached as learning opportunities. Ignoring complaints or failing to investigate them properly may result in failure to identify weaknesses in care processes. The clients of a veterinary team should be considered as secondary team members and their input valued as such.

7.12.8 Speaking Out

There are further paradigms within veterinary healthcare teams that must be challenged to support patient safety. Not only must staff be supported to report patient safety incidents, but they also need to be empowered to challenge each other on patient safety regardless of levels of expertise, seniority, and management. Staff need to be taught to respect and listen to such challenges and treat them seriously. There are valuable lessons to be learnt from cases in human-centered healthcare, of adverse events that might have been prevented if junior members of the team had been listened to or had the courage to speak out.

Leaders need to deconstruct traditional hierarchical structures within the veterinary healthcare team and eliminate any practice that supports deference or subordination. As an example, veterinary nurses/technicians have historically worked under the direction of veterinarians with little to no autonomy; this can lead to feelings of deference and submission to the veterinarian which could limit open and honest conversation regarding mistakes.

7.12.9 Near-Misses

It has been said that near-misses are "the gold dust of patient safety." Such incidents provide a highly valuable substrate for learning. Near-misses will happen daily within a complex environment such as veterinary healthcare. Examples include discovering incorrectly labeled medication, faulty equipment or patients without identification collars. Each of these examples could result in catastrophic incidents – poisoning, injury, and mistaken surgery respectively. Learning from errors with the potential to harm before actual harm occurs means causal factors can be identified and corrected. An emphasis on reporting near-misses supports a culture of continuous improvement, and requires supportive leadership and protected time to exploit the full benefit.

7.12.10 Shared Learning

Human-centered healthcare has learned valuable lessons on safety from other complex and risky industries. The aviation, nuclear power, and oil industries have all been labeled as high-reliability organizations. They consistently avoid adverse events despite operating in highly complex and dangerous conditions with high levels of inherent risk. A key part of their success has been attributed to the acceptance and application of human factors and more recently human-centered healthcare has begun to utilize this emerging science to support patient safety.

Human factors are the organizational, individual, environmental, and job characteristics that influence behavior in ways that can impact safety. One of the foundational principles is an open acknowledgment that errors can and will occur. This acknowledgment is crucial and should not be looked upon as a defeat, but more as the acceptance of humanity and fallibility. It acknowledges that humans are in fact human and may be the most substantial sources of risk. It encourages the application of ergonomics to prevent error, the consideration of workplace design and environmental factors that may support safety and prevent accidents and errors.

One of the most basic examples of the application of human factors in healthcare is the strategic positioning of emergency equipment. Such essential and important tools are kept in consistent, high-profile locations to support easy access in times of stress.

The use of checklists, now widely used in human healthcare and increasingly in the veterinary profession, is a prime example of a tool used to address human factors (see 2.4 Checklists in Veterinary Medicine). Checklists are used in aviation to support complex routine processes. Their use makes allowances for the understanding that the more complex a procedure becomes, the higher the likelihood of error associated with it. Checklists are also used by pilots in times of emergency. In this instance, checklists prevent the omission of crucial interventions due to stress-induced memory lapses. They also prevent another recognized reaction to stress – fixation. This is when people repeatedly continue to take the normal or expected course of action, even when it is not working. Within veterinary healthcare, repeated unsuccessful venipuncture could be an example of fixation. Animals will quickly become agitated at multiple uncomfortable attempts to collect blood samples. As their agitation escalates, so other methods of restraint and blood collection should be attempted. If the staff member continues the same method over and over again, it is less likely that the blood sample will be successfully collected, and staff may be in danger of harm from a highly agitated animal. The fixation behavior could be addressed by a predetermined decision to only make two attempts at venipuncture before trying an alternative method.

Primarily, the science of human factors acknowledges that it is far simpler to change the situation, the environment, and/or the equipment than the ingrained behaviors and reactions of human beings.

7.12.11 Pet-Specific Care

Another valuable tool to support patient safety is the acknowledgment and identification of the wide variation in patients, even between those animals of the same species, the same breed, or those presenting for the same routine procedure. Thorough assessment, identification, and comprehension of the animal's normal baseline will support the application of individualized care, promoting safer care (see 3.14 Pet-Specific Relevance of Reference Intervals). As a basic example, knowing that an animal will only eat a dry diet is essential to support adequate postoperative nutrition. Making an assumption that they will eat the same wet food as the other patients could result in a compromise in patient safety as the patient's nutritional needs will not be met. Furthermore, observation of the patient's apparent anorexia could result in inappropriate escalation of treatment – assisted feeding, for example. Treating each patient as an individual is key to providing appropriate and safe veterinary care.

7.12.12 Think Big

Patient safety must never be considered a finite activity; it is a continuum and measures must be put in place to constantly assess and evaluate existing patient safety strategies. Healthcare is always evolving and as patients change from needing acute reactive care to chronic complex care, so the aims of patient safety should also evolve. Improving patient safety should incorporate the safety of those patients undergoing care outside the hospital environment through comprehensive support and education of owners via a mutually respectful therapeutic relationship. In addition, there are advocates within human healthcare suggesting that patient safety may be improved by developing and implementing strategies to improve population health. Surely the same might be applied to veterinary healthcare. As increasing numbers of pets suffer from obesity, so their susceptibility to associated co-morbidities increases (see 6.15 Approaching Obesity on a Pet-Specific Basis). Might this be an example of a broader patient safety incident which the veterinary team has a duty of care to try and address?

EXAMPLES

On a busy Monday morning at a small animal veterinary practice, a staff member from the local cat shelter has brought in four black kittens for neutering. Consent is taken for the procedures and the sexes of the litter checked, whereby it is established there are three males and a female. The kittens are then settled into the hospital ward.

According to practice protocol, the female neutering is planned as the first procedure. The female kitten is anesthetized and prepared for surgery. While the nurse is clipping the patient, it is noticed that the kitten is in fact a male. The veterinary surgeon is alerted, who confirms the observation and the appropriate surgery is performed which is uneventful. The kitten suffers no ill effects apart from the loss of fur due to his inappropriate and unnecessary clip.

While no harm was done, this is an extremely valuable learning opportunity. The potential for causing harm is very high as an animal was presented for an incorrect surgical procedure. The nurse involved speaks to the nursing team leader and together they do a root cause analysis on the case, taking the time to speak to all members of the team working that day. Several observations were made.

- None of the kittens had identification collars.
- When supplies were checked, it was established that there were no ID collars in the practice for the admitting nurse to use.
- The nurse selecting the relevant kitten for surgery was a new member of staff and therefore didn't know that when litters of kittens are admitted in this way, identification collars should have been applied.
- The sex of the kitten was not checked again before he was anesthetized.
- It was established that the operating clinician was about to check the sex of the kitten, but they were called away by a colleague who needed some advice. The procedure then continued on the surgeon's return without the final presurgical check.
- The colleague only asked the operating veterinarian for help, interrupting the preoperative procedure because the phone in their room wasn't working and so they couldn't access help from anybody else. They were forced to break the accepted convention of not interrupting the operating team.

As a result of this near-miss and the associated root cause analysis, it is clear that the incident occurred as a result of multiple breakdowns in practice systems and protocols.

This near-miss was centered on the potential for performing incorrect surgery, but the benefit of analyzing such an event is that other near-misses can be identified and addressed. In this case, the fact that the phone didn't work in one of the rooms could have been a serious staff safety compromise. Should a member of staff fall ill or be trapped in that room with an angry client or patient, they would have had no means of communication. Equally,

patient safety may have been compromised; should an animal have suffered a cardiac arrest, the potential for delay in getting help to them could have severely compromised the outcome.

Several action points were instigated as a result. First, it was decided that there would be a new protocol and all animals admitted to the hospital would have identification collars placed on them in the presence of their owner, during the initial admission consultation. Second, the broken phone was mended and a system of weekly checks on the entire phone system was put in place and assigned to the hospital maintenance team. Third, a new protocol for reporting broken equipment was put in place that made it easier for action to be taken. Finally, the case was presented to the entire team during a staff meeting and the associated planned changes explained and discussed.

TAKE-AWAYS

- Advances in veterinary healthcare have led to increasing complexity of care which can have a detrimental impact on patient safety.
- Patient safety is the responsibility of every member of the multidisciplinary team; adverse events are not restricted to clinical situations.
- Adverse events, unexpected outcomes, and near-misses should all be embraced as valuable learning opportunities.
- A work culture that promotes patient safety should hold an open acknowledgment that human error is inevitable; such errors should be addressed with a no blame attitude.
- Acknowledgment and identification of variation between patients is a key step toward keeping patients safe.

MISCELLANEOUS

Recommended Reading

Ballantyne, H. (2019). Basic concepts of patient safety – exploring the terminology. *Veterinary Practice Today* 7 (2): 16–18.
Clinical Human Factors Group. (2017). What are clinical human factors? https://chfg.org/what-are-clinical-human-factors

NHS Improvement. (2018). Patient Safety. https://improvement.nhs.uk/improvement-hub/patient-safety

Yu, A., Flott, K., Chainani, N., Fontana, G., Darzi, A. Patient Safety 2030. London: NIHR Imperial Patient Safety Translational Research Centre, 2016. www.imperial.ac.uk/media/imperial-college/institute-of-global-health-innovation/centre-for-health-policy/Patient-Safety-2030-Report-VFinal.pdf

McCaughan, D. and Kaufman, G. (2013). Patient safety: threats and solutions. *Nursing Standard* 27 (44): 48–55.

7.13

Keeping Client Information Secure

Peter Alberti, BSBA

Inulogica, Northborough, MA, USA

BASICS

7.13.1 Summary

Implementation of pet-specific care inherently involves storage and retrieval of data and information, whether paper-based, digital, or both. Protecting client personal data is not only a best practice, in many places it is required by law. It is therefore important to define "confidential" information, assess existing systems and processes that store or use the information, and make improvements as necessary.

7.13.2 Terms Defined

Confidential Information: Information intended to be kept secret and not disclosed to others.
Personally Identifiable Information (PII):   Any information that can be used to identify an individual. Regulatory definitions vary by location, including what information requires protection.

MAIN CONCEPTS

7.13.3 Defining "Confidential" Information

Personally identifiable information, often called "PII," is any single piece of data or collection of data that enables identification of an individual. While regulatory requirements are usually specific about what data comprise PII, in places where regulations are not in place the determination is often subject to interpretation. It is well known that PII should be kept secure, but PII is not the only type of data that should be kept confidential.

Pet medical records, the confidentiality of which may or may not be protected by law, should be secured as well (see 7.6 Privacy and Confidentiality). Pet owners, like all consumers, are becoming increasingly sensitive to data privacy issues. Some perceive they are entitled to protection similar to laws that protect human health information, even when this is not the case. From a client satisfaction perspective, and to protect the reputation of your practice, it is strongly recommended that the medical record be kept confidential.

As pet-specific care advances, a pet's medical and other record(s) and the pet owner's own PII will become more tightly coupled. Personalized approaches to care will inevitably involve consumer behavioral science as well as medical facets. As such, the medical record itself can ultimately become a component of client-specific PII, and must therefore be protected.

7.13.4 The Importance of Keeping Information Secure

In the past, a simple paper-based or computer-based file was appropriate for record keeping. The information generally never left the practice unless it was in the hands of the pet owner. The value of the information was fundamentally limited.

Modern pet care typically involves numerous stakeholders which could include multiple veterinary professionals, online services and home delivery services, suppliers offering direct-to-consumer engagement, third-party

Pet-Specific Care for the Veterinary Team, First Edition. Edited by Lowell Ackerman.
© 2021 John Wiley & Sons, Inc. Published 2021 by John Wiley & Sons, Inc.

support services for veterinary practices, and more. The only way all these parties can properly and accurately support a pet's needs is to share data. Consequently, the systems to store, share, and use the information have become robust, which in turn increases the value of the data.

The value of the data is well known to many who have ties to your practice. Disgruntled employees, unhappy clients, competitors, and professional data hackers are all sources of penetration and misuse. No business is "too small" to be a productive source of a data breach.

7.13.5 How Data Breaches Can Occur

In the digital age, a great deal of attention is given to large-scale database breaches and nefarious computer hackers. Often overlooked are the smaller and less sophisticated sources of confidential data, yet they are just as important when seeking to protect client information.

Paper-based data sources are frequently overlooked. This includes faxes, intake, or other forms, contest entries, and any other places where a client or staff member writes down client information.

On the digital side, a challenging "landmine" to avoid is email. When an email is transmitted, it almost always travels in unencrypted form. This means anyone with access to the data as it is sent across the internet can read the email, including any attachments. Sending forms or requesting personal information through email is very insecure and should be avoided.

Wi-Fi networks have become commonplace. Many practices use consumer-grade equipment, typically self-installed and configured. Some offer guest access for clients and others do not. No matter how it is implemented, Wi-Fi networks connected to practice computer systems must be protected in multiple ways. Simply requiring a Wi-Fi password is no longer sufficient. Although the likelihood of a professional hacker arriving onsite to steal data is unlikely, it's not impossible and is easily circumvented with a few basic steps.

Many new digital capabilities have emerged to help veterinary practices operate. From customer communications to diagnostics equipment to practice consulting and reporting services, data are being shared with outside vendors at a rapid rate. These integrations are typically well intentioned and are deployed carefully. Ultimately, however, the responsibility lies with the practice to ensure client data are protected, and this includes third-party access and use of the data.

7.13.5.1 Best Practices

There are many best practices for keeping client and patient information secure.

- Conduct an analysis of your existing data/information. Identify what should be kept confidential and prepare formal documentation that outlines what is expected. Include a process to identify new types of data/information that should be added to the documentation.
- Create a formal process for handling each type of confidential information, including business impact of a breach and, where appropriate, disciplinary measures that could be taken if processes are not followed. Place emphasis on less obvious breach sources such as paper-based or email data.
- Train staff regularly about the importance of securing confidential data and how your practice handles this. Regular updates to the training will help ensure the team always has this top of mind.
- Periodically conduct audits to ensure processes are being followed. Include in-house audits but also consider having an outside source involved.
- Direct clients to communicate with your practice in specific ways that explicitly protect their confidential information. For example, many clients will be unaware that sending a credit card number by email is insecure. It is appropriate to tell them "Please call our office with your credit card number and *do not* send it by email since email is not secure."
- Disallow practice staff from using personal devices (laptops, mobile devices, etc.) for business use since such devices may be vulnerable to attacks. If personal devices are required, it is appropriate to insist that they be inoculated with business-class security software and subject to audits.
- Ensure all business digital systems have updated security software (e.g., antivirus, internet protection, email scanning, etc.).
- If third-party services can access your data, ensure their privacy policies and data protection processes appropriately protect your practice's interests and that they are compliant with any applicable regulatory requirements for your location.
- Prepare for a breach. Have a communication plan, a recovery plan, and appropriate levels of insurance and legal representation.

EXAMPLES

ABC Veterinary Hospital decide to actively protect their data. They hire an outside data security expert to perform an audit. Based on the results of the audit, they make a few changes.

Their most important change is to focus on the staff. They develop a simple but powerful training program to train staff on the importance of data protection. They also create a few processes that isolate certain PII to a limited number of places, and they limit which staff members can access this information. For example, address, phone number, email, and other information provided on a paper-based form are only handled by front office staff. The information is entered into the practice management software and is then shredded. One practice owner is identified as the primary point of contact in the event of a breach, with one other practice owner as the back-up.

The data security firm is then hired to install protection and monitoring systems for all computers and networks. A monthly report is sent to the practice indicating risk areas that were protected, updates that were made, and potential breach concerns, if any. The practice assigns a staff member to actively review the reports and take action if necessary.

Finally, the practice creates a breach plan that describes how the practice will communicate with clients, who at the practice will handle communications, and how the rest of the staff should respond if asked about the breach.

TAKE-AWAYS

- It has become more important than ever to concern yourself with protecting client privacy because of the way data and information are used.

- Knowing what must be secured is vital. There may or may not be regulatory requirements. Maintain vigilance.
- Establish procedures, processes, and expectations.
- Regularly train staff and conduct audits.
- Be prepared for a breach and know how to handle one if it happens.

MISCELLANEOUS

7.13.6 Cautions

Data breaches happen, even to businesses which have no reason to believe they are susceptible. It is not necessary for a professional hacker to manually target a particular business or specific computer. Automated software programs (often called "bots") scan for vulnerabilities in data networks and find systems to penetrate. Do not make the mistake of believing your practice is impervious to data breaches.

Because of this, it is extremely important to create a data breach plan ahead of time. Think about what information you store, how it could be breached, and what actions you would take if a breach occurs. Actions should include an immediate communication plan with your local authorities and your clients, as well as a protocol for staff. For example, your team should know what to say and what not to say about the breach. Waiting until a breach occurs before creating a plan will likely result in problematic actions and outcomes.

7.14

Premise Disinfection

Kara M. Burns, MS, MEd, LVT, VTS (Nutrition)

Lafayette, IN, USA

BASICS

7.14.1 Summary

Pathogens are microorganisms that cause disease. Different classes of pathogens vary in their resistance to destruction by chemical methods. In veterinary hospitals, microbial control is best accomplished with sanitation, disinfection, and sterilization. Oftentimes, sanitation and disinfection create acceptable levels of microbial control.

Disinfection is crucial to prevent the spread of infectious disease, especially in the veterinary hospital [1]. However, proper sanitation can be confusing. It is imperative for veterinary teams to use proper sanitization products, so the hospital is not at risk of an outbreak.

Information on disinfectants for specific animal disease agents can be obtained from regulatory animal health agencies. Disinfectants utilized in veterinary hospitals should bear the approval statement of the Environmental Protection Agency in the USA or a similar agency in other countries. Be sure that all members of the veterinary team understand and follow the label instructions.

7.14.2 Terms Defined

Antiseptic: Agent capable of preventing infection through the inhibition of growth of infectious agents.
Asepsis: A state where no living organisms are present.
Cleaning: Physical removal of microbial contaminants.
Disinfection: Using physical or chemical approaches to ensure the destruction of pathogens from nonliving objects.
Pathogens: Microorganisms that cause disease.

Sanitization: Reducing microbial populations to safe levels.
Sterilization: The eradication of all life from an object, or complete microbial control.

MAIN CONCEPTS

Disinfection of the entire veterinary hospital is crucial to keeping disease under control (see 4.4 Preventing Infectious Diseases in the Small Animal Veterinary Hospital). Ensure your hospital has cleaning and disinfection protocols. These protocols should not only be written down, but should be in the employee manual in every hospital, as well as posted where all members of the team can review them. A "one and done" approach to protocol review is never a good standard of care (see 9.4 Standards of Care).

Veterinary team members should also review the protocol itself. How long ago was the protocol instituted? Is the protocol current? Are the steps leading to proper disinfection? Which type of disinfectant is being used? Ensure the team is using the correct disinfectant and using it properly. Improper disinfectants or improper mixing of disinfectants may not be beneficial and may even harm patients and people in the hospital. Remember, cleaning is not the same as disinfecting.

A three-step process is recommended to truly sanitize a surface [1].

1) Mechanical removal of organic material such as feces, urine, blood, respiratory secretions, etc.
2) The surface must be thoroughly cleaned with soap/general cleaner, rinsed, and dried. Once the surface is clean

Pet-Specific Care for the Veterinary Team, First Edition. Edited by Lowell Ackerman.
© 2021 John Wiley & Sons, Inc. Published 2021 by John Wiley & Sons, Inc.

and dry, apply the disinfectant, which must be allowed to sit for the required contact time as directed by the disinfectant manufacturer.

3) Using a damp cloth, rinse away the disinfectant and dry the area well.

The veterinary team must remember that not all disinfectants are equal. Therefore, we must carefully read the label to ensure understanding of the specific product's uses and dilution instructions. Some products both clean and disinfect – these are great for routine cleaning and disinfection. However, there are products that disinfect only. This means the surface/area must be cleaned first. In these cases, the surface must be cleaned with a detergent and then rinsed and dried before applying the disinfectant. One example of this is bleach. Bleach disinfects only, so the veterinary team must clean the surface with a detergent first, before rinsing, drying, and applying the disinfectant. If the surface is not cleaned first, bleach will not be efficacious in killing pathogens.

It makes sense that different parts of the clinic will require different levels of cleaning and disinfection. Obviously, there will be more specific protocols for isolation, infectious disease areas, surgical suites, etc., than for doctor's offices, reception, and computer workstations.

When cleaning, it is prudent to start with areas that are exposed to healthy animals. Next would be areas with ill animals, leaving the isolation area for last. Remember to have the team avoid cross-contamination; different cleaning equipment should be used in each area.

When it comes to cleaning and disinfecting, the entire area must be cleaned and disinfected – from ceiling to floor and everything in between. Have the healthcare team ensure that only what is needed in that specific area is actually there. If it does not need to be there – get rid of it! This will decrease the cleaning and sanitizing time and decrease the risk of infection.

Ensure that the hospital's sanitization protocols are effective and easy to understand and execute. The healthcare team must be trained on disinfection protocols, and whatever supplies the team needs should be provided without question.

As cleaning and disinfecting protocols become part of a veterinary hospital's culture, the healthcare team will be more confident when admitting and treating patients, including those with infectious diseases, while minimizing the risk of exposure to other patients, the healthcare team, and pet owners.

The AAHA Infection Control, Prevention, and Biosecurity Guidelines recommend appointing a practice "champion" to take primary responsibility for implementing cleaning and disinfection protocols and ensuring

compliance by every member of the veterinary team [2]. The champion's focus should be to:

1) limit pathogen introduction, exposure, transmission, and infection within the hospital population
2) evaluate the effectiveness of infection control practices at controlling disease.

EXAMPLES

Post protocols in highly visible (to veterinary teams) areas.

Ensure the duties associated with cleaning and disinfecting are provided on checklists and put a team member (practice manager, head credentialed technician) in charge of ensuring that the cleaning and sanitizing duties are checked off.

Ask team members for their feedback about the hospital's disinfection protocols. Oftentimes, it is small changes that make compliance with protocols much easier.

Have the practice manager ask the various team members to demonstrate how they clean an exam room or disinfect an area after a sick animal has been in the clinic. Discuss with each employee.

Keep the protocol easy and straightforward.

TAKE-AWAYS

- Disinfection, sanitization, and cleaning remove most microorganisms.
- Disinfection of the entire veterinary hospital is central to keeping disease under control.
- Ensure your hospital has cleaning and disinfection protocols.
- The entire area must be cleaned and disinfected – from ceiling to floor and everything in between.
- Remember the three-step process of true disinfection.

MISCELLANEOUS

7.14.3 Cautions

Beware of products that disinfect only. This means the surface/area must be cleaned first. In these cases, the surface must be cleaned with a detergent and then rinsed and dried before applying the disinfectant.

References

1 Brown, J. Disinfection protocols: a clean start. Veterinary Practice News. 2018). www.veterinarypracticenews.com/disinfection-protocols-a-clean-start/

2 Stull, J.W., Bjorvik, E., Bub, J. et al. (2018). AAHA infection control, prevention, and biosecurity guidelines. *J. Am. Anim. Hosp. Assoc.* 54 (6): 297–326.

Recommended Reading

American Animal Hospital Association. 2018 AAHA Infection Control, Prevention, and Biosecurity Guidelines. www.aaha.org/aaha-guidelines/infection-control-configuration/aaha-infection-control-prevention-and-biosecurity-guidelines/

American Animal Hospital Association. Sample environmental cleaning and disinfection protocol. www.aaha.org/aaha-guidelines/infection-control-configuration/protocols/cleaning-and-disinfection2/

Section 8

Hospital Team Considerations

8.1

Delivering Pet-Specific Care as a Team

Jason C. Nicholas, BVETMED (Hons)

Independent Consultant, Author and Speaker, Co-founder, Preventive Vet, Portland, OR, USA

 BASICS

8.1.1 Summary

Once pet-specific care (PSC) has been considered for a practice and clients are "on board" with the philosophy, it is important to consider how the veterinary team can best deliver this level of care and embed the concepts in the practice workstream.

Each member of the hospital team has a role – or rather, several roles – to play in the successful delivery of excellent PSC. Utilizing and engaging the whole hospital team won't just increase efficiency and provide a better healthcare experience for your clients and patients, it will also lead to a more empowered, engaged, and happier team.

8.1.2 Terms Defined

Care Team: The veterinarian(s), technicians, assistants, and customer service representatives (CSRs) who regularly and consistently care for and interact with a particular patient and client.

Forward Booking: The practice of scheduling a patient's future visits and procedures prior to them leaving the practice for the current visit.

 MAIN CONCEPTS

8.1.3 Get the Team on the Same Page

Make discussions about the hospital's PSC approach a regular part of "all-team" meetings. Encourage questions from team members and see if there are any specific cases or patients that team members wish to discuss or learn more about. This is also an opportunity to discuss and align on the pet health insurance providers you and your team are going to recommend (see 10.16 Pet Health Insurance), determine which genetic testing products you'll recommend and use (see 3.4 Predicting and Eliminating Disease Traits), and periodically review and evaluate your patient workflows and protocols to ensure that they're working as well as they can for everybody.

Pro tip: Use regular doctors' meetings to review and discuss the current body of evidence that will help to guide and determine the hospital's diagnostic and treatment protocols for specific conditions (see 9.4 Standards of Care and 9.6 Care Pathways).

8.1.4 Schedule for Success

Forward booking of upcoming visits, exams, and procedures isn't just better for your practice, it's also better for your clients. Like us, our clients often lead very busy lives, attempting to balance work, relationships, childcare, and everything else on top of pet care. Without forward booking, you're putting the onus on your clients to remember to call in and schedule at a later date (which all too often doesn't happen). Or you're putting additional work on your CSRs to do otherwise avoidable reminder communications (calls, texts, emails, etc.). Forward booking improves your team's ability to deliver successful PSC. After all, providing care (whether pet-specific or otherwise) depends on your clients actually booking and showing up for appointments and procedures, which they are more likely to do with forward booking.

Pro tip: The PSC approach also makes forward booking easier, as the care plan is laid out in advance and reviewed at each visit, so your client and your team know when the next visit(s) should be scheduled (see 1.3 Personalized Care Plans).

When possible and practical during appointment booking, try to keep the same "care team" (both veterinarian and technician/nurse) assigned to a particular patient. This helps to establish and build stronger bonds between the client/pet and the hospital team. Having dedicated care teams also helps those members of the care team become more intimately aware of and involved in the details of a particular patient's health, environment, and overall care.

When blood, urine, genetic and other diagnostic tests are anticipated at a wellness visit, aim to schedule a paraprofessional visit for those tests a week or so in advance of the pet's scheduled wellness appointment. Similarly, health risk assessment questionnaires should also be completed in advance of the visit (see 1.2 Providing a Lifetime of Care, and 2.7 Risk Assessment). Doing so gets the results back in enough time to be evaluated by the team *prior* to the wellness exam, so that they can discuss those results, along with any changes they may necessitate in the patient's care plan, with the client at the time of their pet's wellness visit. These face-to-face conversations help improve efficiency (e.g., avoiding "telephone tag" to discuss results) and allow for better client communication and comprehension.

8.1.5 Focus on the Care Plan

The "rooming" process provides the perfect opportunity for the technician/nurse on a pet's care team to review with the client the aspects of their pet's care plan that are anticipated for that visit and to ask the client if they have any questions about the diagnostics, treatments, or other anticipated aspects of their pet's visit.

Pro tip: Because new historical data, physical exam findings, and other factors may necessitate a change in the care recommendations for the visit, it is important for the technician to use the word "anticipated" (or similar) when referring to the recommendations on the care plan for the visit. This helps to avoid causing client confusion or disappointment should the recommendations need to be altered by the doctor after they have talked with the client and examined the patient.

Following each visit, and as part of their record writing, the doctor should make any updates to the care plan and recommendations that are warranted by the information, exam findings, and other data that they have obtained at that visit (see 9.1 Medical Record Entries). They should then email that updated care plan to the client, along with (brief) explanations for any recommended changes to the care plan going forward.

Pro tip: In that email, invite the client to either email back with any questions they have or (more ideal) call the practice to schedule a time for a phone call or virtual care visit (see 2.5 Virtual Care (Telehealth)) to discuss any questions or concerns they may have. Scheduling such interactions can make them more efficient and informative, as both parties can be better prepared, and scheduling also helps avoid "phone tag" and missed connections.

EXAMPLES

Henrietta, a 13-year-old tortoiseshell cat, was due for her semiannual wellness visit. As was done the year before, she was prebooked into the schedule for this visit, and Henrietta's mom brought her in for a technician visit the week prior to her wellness exam so that blood and urine samples could be obtained and submitted to the reference laboratory. Her results, which came back in plenty of time for her veterinarian to evaluate prior to her wellness visit, were suggestive of early chronic renal failure (CRF). At the veterinarian's request, the CSR extended the scheduled time for Henrietta's upcoming scheduled wellness visit to accommodate the time they would need to further discuss and answer Henrietta's owner's questions about CRF in cats and the additional diagnostics that would be recommended on the day. Thankfully, Henrietta did not have hypertension and she happily took to the prescribed renal formula diet at this early stage of her disease. Her mom felt well prepared for what may lie ahead, as she was able to have all her questions answered by her veterinarian in an unrushed, face-to-face fashion during Henrietta's visit.

Danielle, the nurse/technician at ABC Animal Clinic who was assigned to now 5-year-old Australian cattle dog Dundee's care team during his initial puppy visits, knew that something was "off" with Dundee the moment he came in for his annual wellness visit. Dundee, normally eager to see Danielle and the rest of the team at ABC, shied away and got stiff as Danielle extended her hand to give him his favorite scratches behind his ear. She asked his owners if he had been more head-shy at home. They said that they hadn't really noticed but now that she mentioned it, they did think that he'd been a little less eager for scratches on his head and even a little more quiet in general. While discussing Dundee's care plan with the doctor prior to the exam, Danielle mentioned the change she noticed and this new piece of history. During the examination, it was discovered that Dundee was exhibiting signs of neck pain and had repeatable decreased range of motion in his neck. The recommendation for starting pain medications and dropping off the following morning for sedated neck radiographs was added to Dundee's care plan and accepted by the clients. A presumptive diagnosis of possible cervical disc extrusion was made on radiographs the following day. Given the lack of neurological deficits and a positive response to pain medications, it was decided to try conservative therapy of crate rest and continued pain management (as well as switching from a neck collar to a front-clip body harness). Dundee's personality had returned to normal by the end of the crate rest period and the presumptive cervical disc problem was added to his master problem list. His owners were counseled on continued precautions to take and signs to watch for which would indicate that further diagnostics or an emergency trip to the local specialty hospital would be necessary.

TAKE-AWAYS

- Engaging the entire hospital team, and having them "on the same page," is important for delivering PSC as efficiently as possible. Incorporating discussions and Q&As about PSC into your regular hospital team meetings can help keep everyone engaged and on the right track.
- Scheduling correctly – in terms of the time and team allotted to each visit, as well as the number and types of visits themselves – is central to the ability of your team to best deliver PSC.
- Forward booking of appointments, procedures, and other visits is an easy and effective way to increase the likelihood that your clients will actually show up for the care that their pets need and benefit from. It also happens to be an easy way to increase practice revenues.
- When appropriate, obtaining samples for diagnostic testing prior to a patient's scheduled wellness visits can help to improve care, efficiency, and client engagement with the PSC approach.
- A patient's "care plan" is the roadmap for their particular health and well-being journey, but it is not set in stone. Refer to it often and update it as needed, and don't forget to send and discuss the updated care plan with your client.

MISCELLANEOUS

Recommended Reading

Partners for Healthy Pets. Forward booking tools. www. partnersforhealthypets.org/forward_booking.aspx

8.2

Developing Staff Competencies

Lowell Ackerman, DVM, DACVD, MBA, MPA, CVA, MRCVS

Global Consultant, Author, and Lecturer, MA, USA

 BASICS

8.2.1 Summary

Working in a veterinary practice presents some personal growth challenges for employees, because in many cases the organizational chart is relatively flat and there are not many opportunities for advancement. However, with the implementation of pet-specific care, there are actually many opportunities for the individual advancement of staff within certain disciplines and niches.

For career advancement, an employed veterinarian may have an opportunity to become a partner or even buy the practice from the owner, but once paraprofessional and administrative staff reach a supervisory position, they have typically advanced as far as they can. Some customer service representatives and technicians/nurses might advance to management positions, and practice ownership is possible for some, but such a career path is not assured.

To keep the very best employees, and for them to remain challenged and motivated, staff development must be part of the practice's core strategies. Pet-specific care allows specific competencies to be developed which can lead to career fulfillment regardless of the career ladders available in a particular practice.

8.2.2 Terms Defined

Individual Development Plan (IDP): A staff member's individual plan for self-development that is approved by a manager to ensure it is aligned with the organization's goals.
Presenteeism: Workers being on the job but not fully productive.

 MAIN CONCEPTS

The financial realities for most veterinary practices are that they tend to pay employees less than comparable businesses, and often provide fewer benefits. In many cases, we try to rationalize this as a requirement of working with animals, as though working in a veterinary practice requires a charitable component from its employees, even if we then want the staff to be motivated to help ensure that the financial needs of the practice can be attained.

All employees deserve to be paid wages and benefits commensurate with their skills and working in a veterinary clinic is no exception. However, because there is limited room for vertical advancement in most veterinary practices, additional attention should be paid to career development of employees, especially for potential horizontal advancement.

There is one other feature of staff development that is worthy of reflection. Staff who develop skills and leave the practice to take more advanced positions elsewhere should be viewed as successes, not failures, especially if there are no appropriate opportunities for them within the practice. In too many instances, practices look at such career advancement as abandonment or disloyalty, rather than considering the bigger picture of our employees having their own lives and goals and that career development of these employees can definitely be a win–win situation for both the individual and the practice.

Superimposed on this career development process is that some staff turnover is natural and inevitable for a practice A practice that has been in existence for a prolonged period of time and still has all the same employees is not necessarily a model of an ideal workplace.

8.2.3   Pet-Specific Opportunities

Pet-specific care focuses heavily on prevention, early detection, evidence-based treatment and attention to closing compliance gaps, and practices need systems in place so that implementation is as close to seamless as possible. This involves strategies for the development of clinic resources, staff training, internal dissemination of information and strategies, and messaging to clients.

When professional and paraprofessional staff develop specific subject competencies, it is important that strategies be developed for how practice resources should be leveraged to achieve specific outcomes, how all the staff will be trained so that implementation happens practice-wide and can be delivered to all appropriate clients, and some method to determine client uptake and satisfaction with the offerings.

Examples of subject competencies might include:

- genetic testing
- pet health insurance
- pet identification/microchipping
- integrated parasite control
- antimicrobial stewardship
- oral care
- weight management
- diet and nutrition
- senior care
- premise disinfection
- privacy and security of client information.

In most cases, subject competencies are going to be developed by veterinary and paraprofessional staff as a result of strategic planning exercises, interested individuals will take "ownership" of the projects, and ad hoc committees of representative staff stakeholders will determine the resources needed and the potential challenges to be overcome to ensure success. During this development phase, it is worth introducing the topic to appropriate clients and gauging their interest as well as any concerns they may have that could interfere with a successful rollout.

Developing appropriate systems and messaging plans is critical, because with most pet-specific topics, much of the actual implementation is done by nonveterinary team members. Thus, when it comes to a subject such as pet health insurance, if the program is properly implemented, most of the client conversations on the topic will happen with front office staff and technicians, and will not be a distraction to veterinary time with clients.

Because most veterinary team members do not have access to much in the way of vertical career advancement, it is important to recognize the commitment and leadership development they display with subject competencies.

A staff member who shows interest in a subject like genetic testing should be given the opportunity to explore what is available in the marketplace and report back to a team meeting about the pros and cons of such an offering. The management team can then do a more involved assessment of the value proposition and if it seems to correspond well with the hospital mission and strategy, the staff member can be authorized to form a group (typically including at least one veterinarian, one technician/nurse, and one receptionist) to determine what would be necessary for successful implementation and rollout.

It is important to realize that when staff members step forward to take responsibility for such projects, they may need some coaching for leadership skills and the communication skills necessary to explain all parts of the program to the staff prior to implementation. Their "ownership" of the task and their attempt to create value should be recognized and rewarded at employee reviews, even if the project does not materialize as ultimately successful for the practice. Not every project considered will be successful, but having staff willing to do the work to explore potential opportunities is something to be recognized and celebrated.

The staff member who becomes a subject matter expert will be given the opportunity to be recognized as such within the practice, to oversee implementation, and collect information on outcomes to share at team meetings (see 8.6 Nursing Leadership). With appropriate assistance and oversight, they can even engage in problem solving if uptake is not as robust as first anticipated, which is not unusual. The original ad hoc group can usually provide useful feedback on why the program is not being implemented as originally planned and the management team can help redeploy the initiative, as needed, to achieve better results.

A useful lesson for such subject leaders to learn is that to be successful, most new processes need to be embedded in the current practice workstream or staff quickly resort to old habits (see 7.3 Leading the Change Towards Pet-Specific Care). The challenge is to make new efforts "sticky" so that they become an automatic part of how office visits are conducted. For example, with genetic testing, the initial rollout might include flagging all puppy and kitten visits for the front office team to discuss such postnatal screening in advance of office visits (and even send owners a brochure or weblink in advance of the visit), to remind them of such testing when they present for the visit, and then for the technician/nurse to inquire if they have any questions before they collect a sample for testing.

For the most part, subject competencies are straightforward, but it is not always possible to know what offerings will be best received by clients. In addition, some staff members might propose developing competencies which might initially seem to only indirectly benefit the practice.

Realizing that when staff show initiative, they are demonstrating their desire to better themselves (and hopefully the practice), it is always worthwhile to listen to the whole proposal and offer constructive feedback. Sometimes providing a submission form with questions to be answered can help staff think through the entire process, including how the concept might benefit the pet, the client, and the practice.

8.2.4 Goal Setting

Most employees are hired for a specific job, with a specific job description, and little thought about other strengths they might have that could be important to the practice.

It is therefore worthwhile to explore strengths (and weaknesses) of employees in a standardized setting and to determine where personal development can coincide with strategic needs of the practice.

The first step is often determining an employee's aspirations, by asking such questions as "What do you see yourself doing five years from now?" If a receptionist sees herself as a receptionist five years hence, then it is clear that she should hone her skills in customer service and communication. If an employed veterinarian sees herself in an ownership role, then it might be worth cultivating skills in practice management and mentoring her in those duties within the hospital.

8.2.5 Performance Management

While many veterinary practices tend to have informal and often infrequent employee evaluations, timely feedback is an important component of goal achievement.

Annual reviews have many limitations, including holding people accountable for past behavior and not necessarily emphasizing current performance and mentoring others in the practice, both critical to long-term success. To better support employee development, many organizations are dropping or changing their annual review systems in favor of giving people less formal but more frequent feedback that follows the natural work cycle [1].

When managing staff performance, it is also important to be aware of subtle issues, such as presenteeism – employees being present but, for one reason or another, not being fully engaged or functional on the job. It has been estimated that this can cut productivity by one-third or more and can actually be far more expensive to a business than other health-related costs [2]. Some common causes of presenteeism include migraine, arthritis, allergies, depression, lower back pain and many other common maladies that allow employees to come to work but not necessarily on a fully productive basis.

Motivation is another important concept in performance management. It will probably not surprise many business owners but if employees are not self-motivated, it is extremely difficult if not impossible to motivate them. The job of management is to create an environment in which self-motivated employees have the support they need to achieve their goals. Interestingly, even so-called "problem employees" may show evidence of motivation in other aspects of their lives. If these individuals are going to remain as valuable members of the organization, it will be necessary to find their locus of energy and leverage it to achieve needed goals [3]. Otherwise, it is exceedingly unlikely that they can be motivated to do what you are already paying them to do (but that they are not currently doing). Going round and round on the same issues is not to anyone's advantage.

8.2.6 Core Competencies

Every veterinary practice should have a mission and those values should be captured in certain core competencies that are expected of employees. Although some core competencies will be hospital-wide, others may be specific to individual positions, such as veterinarians, nurses/technicians/assistants, receptionists/customer service representatives, and managers.

Core competencies are important in staff development, because they can be tiered (e.g., beginner, intermediate, expert, etc.) and considered in terms of reward-based compensation.

Core competencies can be vague, but the actions and outcomes derived from them should actually be as specific as possible. Examples of core competencies might include:

- customer focus
- technical skills
- accountability
- change management
- mentoring
- teamwork
- leadership
- business skills
- self-awareness.

8.2.7 Individual Development Plans (IDP)

Individual developments plans are documents created by employees with the input of their managers which help define specific goals towards which the employee would like to strive over a set period of time, typically one year.

Although the plan itself is meant to support the initiatives of the employee, it is the manager's responsibility to ensure that the actual goals are aligned with the visions of the practice, so that it becomes a win–win scenario. For example, an employee might like the practice to provide time off and financial support for getting a pilot's license, but unless this can be substantially aligned with the needs of the practice, then this would be an unsuitable goal for an IDP. On the other hand, enrolling in a certificate course in human resources might be entirely appropriate for a receptionist or technician with aspirations of progressing into a management role.

The IDP is an agreement between the organization and the employee and both must be involved in its creation. Although the employee will be responsible for their part of the IDP, the manager will need to ensure that the practice supports the initiative, in time allowed and/or with financial support.

8.2.8 70/20/10

A learning and development model known as 70/20/10 was introduced by Lombardo and Eichinger [4] some years ago, and different versions are often used in allotting resources for IDPs.

The basic premise of the model is that about 70% of learning within an organization should come from on-the-job training, 20% from coaching and mentoring, and 10% from actual courses, lectures, and formal training.

It is important to realize that there is nothing magical about the 70/20/10 rule and it is just an approximation. There is no empirical evidence that this ratio is optimal or that the three components are independent of one another, and the model prioritizes on-the-job training, which can be extremely variable in quality from hospital to hospital. The ratio is just a starting point for discussions and can be customized for each individual circumstance.

8.2.9 Career Ladders

As already mentioned, the organizational charts of most veterinary practices are relatively flat and in very small hospitals, all positions might report to one individual – the owner.

As practices increase in size, more positions become available as managers and supervisors are needed to maintain alignment and this creates opportunities for new and existing employees (see 8.4 Alignment – The Key to Implementing Pet-Specific Care).

As many veterinarians have learned the hard way, it is not always possible to promote existing successful employees to new roles and assume they will be similarly competent. Accordingly, core competencies can be extremely useful in determining the skills needed for each job description.

 EXAMPLES

Karen is a certified veterinary technician who has been working for ABC Veterinary Hospital for five years. She is the most technically gifted employee in the practice and the only technician in the practice who knows how to determine blood pressure with the hospital's Doppler unit. This has been a great source of pride for her, as whenever a blood pressure reading is required, the other technicians need to call Karen. However, Karen has been reluctant to teach any of the other technicians this skill and this has been a source of tension within the practice. The owner has announced that within a year, there will likely be a need to hire one or two more technicians, and he will be considering a technician supervisor at that time for the hospital. Karen has expressed interest in the new position and considers herself a prime candidate because of her excellent technical skills.

The hospital owner and manager, in anticipation of the growth of the practice, have decided that they should develop core competencies for the hospital positions and IDPs for all the employees, and specify which skills need demonstrated mastery before promotions can be made.

In meeting with Karen for her quarterly review, the manager assures her that her technical competencies are excellent, but that the supervisor role requires expert competency in mentoring and teamwork, which are currently not her strengths. An IDP is created and as part of that Karen is tasked with creating a skills program for technicians in which she will teach several skills, such as blood pressure determination, placing jugular catheters, and dental charting, and then will supervise those technicians as they teach those skills to the others in the practice. The process is able to channel Karen's strengths into important progress for the technical workforce within the practice. Karen's new expertise in mentoring earns her the promotion to supervisor when that position becomes available.

TAKE-AWAYS

- Because of the structure of most veterinary practices, there are relatively few opportunities for career advancement.
- Despite the lack of structured advancement, with pet-specific care, there are many opportunities for niche advancement and specialization.
- Staff who feel empowered and competent are better able to engage clients and advance pet care initiatives.
- Staff should be encouraged to develop competencies needed by the practice.
- It is important that there are processes in place for staff to share their expertise with others in the practice.

MISCELLANEOUS

8.2.10 Cautions

Veterinary practices being what they are – small businesses – they are not always able to create challenging new positions to which employees can aspire. Even in these cases, it is possible to ascertain the potential strengths of employees and channel appropriate skills into outcomes that are to everyone's benefit.

References

1 Capelli, P. and Travis, A. (2016). The performance management revolution. *Harvard Business Review* October: 58–67.

2 Hemp, P. (2004). Presenteeism: at work – but out of it. *Harvard Business Review* October: 49–58.

3 Nicholson, N. (2003). How to motivate your problem people. *Harvard Business Review* January: 57–65.

4 Lombardo, M.M. and Eichinger, R.W. (1996). *The Career Architect Development Planner*. MN: Lominger.

Recommended Reading

Ackerman, L.J. (2002). *Business Basics for Veterinarians*. New York: ASJA Press.

Ackerman, L.J. (2003). *Management Basics for Veterinarians*. New York: ASJA Press.

Ackerman, L.J. (2020). Staff development. In: *Five-Minute Veterinary Practice Management Consult*, 3e (ed. L. Ackerman), 202–203. Wiley.

Fernandez-Araoz, C., Groysberg, B., and Nohria, N. (2009). The definitive guide to recruiting in good times and bad. *Harvard Business Review* May: 74–84.

McCord, P. (2018). How to hire – chances are you're doing it all wrong. *Harvard Business Review* January: 90–97.

8.3

The Importance of Accountability in Pet-Specific Care

Lowell Ackerman, DVM, DACVD, MBA, MPA, CVA, MRCVS

Global Consultant, Author, and Lecturer, MA, USA

BASICS

8.3.1 Summary

Accountability is a critical attribute in the functioning of a veterinary hospital. Although it might at first appear that it is the doctors who are responsible for the perception created by a practice, careful review of experiences both positive and negative shows that all staff – doctors, technicians/ nurses, receptionists and managers – have an important role to play in how the practice is perceived by the world outside the walls of the clinic.

Regardless of the quality of a surgical procedure and the prowess of the surgeon, what is the perception of the public if an animal is released with fecal matter in its fur or incomplete discharge instructions, or is checked out by bickering front office staff? In most organizations it was long ago appreciated that to deliver quality care and excellent client service, everyone within the organization must realize their critical roles and endeavor to deliver on the practice's mission and vision. When that does not occur, the medical care may be second to none but customers will still flock to other alternatives . . . and there are always alternatives.

For a hospital to function at its best, especially when delivering pet-specific care, every employee must not only be accountable for their own duties but also deliver on implied promises to all stakeholders regarding the mission and vision of the practice. Without accepting "ownership" of all responsibilities in this regard, a practice will need to rely on only its medical skills. With competition for veterinary services increasing regularly, and with the very high cost of delivering those services, being second best can be a costly demotion.

8.3.2 Terms Defined

Accountability: The obligation to be responsible and to act in the best interest of the organization and its mission.
On-Boarding: The process of helping new employees become productive more quickly by providing them with documentation and training related to practice culture, vision, policies, protocols, and expectations.
Responsibility: The duty to perform or complete an assigned task.

MAIN CONCEPTS

Client service experts understand that there are many experiences that clients can have with a practice, and these exposures are sometimes referred to as "moments of truth" [1]. In many cases, these moments of truth may have little to do with the medical care actually being delivered and everything to do with how the clients *feel* they were treated or valued by the practice and its staff.

Consider the previous examples, such as when a pet is discharged in an unclean condition. What does it say about the level of care delivered by the practice, even if the surgery went flawlessly? What impression does the client get when responding to their telephone calls is considered an imposition? What about the situation when the team seems unaware of the well-documented breed-specific attributes of a patient? All of these seemingly insignificant "moments of truth" can easily add up to a bad experience, even when all medical services are delivered with excellence.

Although it is easy to brush off the rants of a single client, in veterinary practice this can have a decidedly bad cascading effect. Happy clients tell a few of their friends about a good experience, but unhappy clients share their displeasure with many more. Clients will only accept so many negative stories before they consider their other options (see 5.2 Meeting Client Needs).

It's impossible to guard against all negative experiences, but staff who are empowered and accountable are much less likely to create scenarios that get blown out of proportion and can usually easily document their good-faith efforts to make things right. That's really all that anyone can hope for (see 5.1 Pet-Specific Customer Service).

It's important to avoid artificial boundaries within the practice so that the practice identity, vision, and mission won't become clouded. There might be distinctions between departments, issues between shifts, tension between front-office and back-office staff, and many other instances in which personal accountability is lost or camouflaged. This must not be allowed to fester or it can have long-time deleterious consequences on practice success.

To some extent, personal accountability tends to lapse in any organization in which anonymity is possible. So, the challenge with veterinary hospitals is to make accountability a scalable attribute. People voluntarily must maintain their accountability even as staff numbers grow, and everyone must tie their collective success on each other stepping up to always do the right thing, and then to be prepared to ask what else they can do to keep things moving in the right direction (see 8.1 Delivering Pet-Specific Care as a Team).

This notion of always asking "What else can I do?" is the foundation of the Oz Principle [2], based loosely on the premise that the characters of the book and movie (Wizard of Oz) spent their time looking for a wizard to fix their problems, when all along they had the power to make those things happen themselves. It's a simple but powerful premise and the Oz Principle challenges each employee to "See it, own it, solve it, and do it."

One thing that needs to consistently happen is to unite staff in the pursuit of practice excellence by codifying the vision and mission of the practice, at least its intent. It helps immensely if this intent can be summed up in a short phrase that every employee can identify with and respond accordingly. In the Oz Principle, that catchphrase reflected whether behaviors were *above the line* (desirable for the given organization) or *below the line* (undesirable for the given organization). For veterinary practices, it is best if this catchphrase is customized into something meaningful to the employees, because they will be expected to live and work to those ideals.

Accountability is important for the organization in general because without it, bad leaders drive out good staff and it is very easy for even high-producing teams to be reduced to mediocrity. In a very short period of time, such mediocrity can become institutionalized and paralyze the organization from achieving strategic goals.

If accountability is not a practice directive, staff become preoccupied with tasks and job descriptions (to which they can still be accountable), rather than "big picture" strategies. The easiest way to determine this is to ask employees to describe their purpose in the clinic.

If a receptionist is asked about his or her purpose, and responds that it is to answer telephones, make appointments, and collect money from clients, they are clearly missing the real intent – to be the client-facing representation of the practice and all its values, to create a welcoming environment into which clients can bring their pets, and to help pet owners understand how the recommendations of the practice are in their best interests and those of their pet. Clearly, a properly motivated receptionist (client service representative) is much more than just someone to answer telephones, book appointments, and refile medical records. They must realize that even if tasked to answer the telephone and perform office duties, their primary responsibility, and that of everyone else working in the clinic, is to engage clients in a friendly and professional manner, strive to create positive "moments of truth" for pet owners, and to be a champion of the practice's approach to pet healthcare and the value provided.

EXAMPLES

Suzanne is a nurse at ABC Animal Hospital, and during lunch, she overhears some of the other nurses complaining about a newly hired veterinary nurse who doesn't seem to be keeping the medical records at a level dictated by the practice's standard of care. Suzanne joins her colleagues in the discussion, reminding them that the clinic's motto is "We strive to be our best – every day" and that being *our best* means mentoring one another so everyone achieves and surpasses the practice's standard of care.

A meeting of all the nurses was convened to discuss standards of care regarding medical record entries. In the discussions that ensued, Heather, the new nurse, admitted that what was being discussed was different from what she was used to in her previous practice. In a nonthreatening manner, the other nurses assured her that there were many different ways that medical entries could be made, but at this hospital, for the good of all pets being treated, the nurses decided to unite around best practices and codify certain practices to avoid confusion. Several nurses shared anecdotes from other practices where they had worked in which inconsistencies could have ended up harming the patient (including the use of nonstandard abbreviations, and weights for dosing sometimes reported in kilograms and sometimes reported in pounds). Because all nurses needed to rely on one another to ensure pet health, several nurse duties benefited from standardization, including medical record entries.

One fact that came to light in the discussions was that when the standards of care were first proposed, there were only three nurses in the practice and so the standardization was really just a verbal directive, shared among the existing nurses. Since that time, several more nurses and assistants had been hired and there was no official document that actually captured those standards of care for the on-boarding of new employees, which is why Heather just assumed that what she was doing (and was doing successfully at her previous practice) was acceptable.

Suzanne asked Heather if she would help her codify the standards of care around medical record entry into an actual document that could be shared with all the technical staff. Heather agreed, and two other nurses also expressed an interest in participating. The goal was to codify the standard into a document within four weeks, ratify the document with all the nurses, get endorsement from the veterinary director and practice administrator, and then present the new standards at the next full employee meeting. The document would then be part of the on-boarding training for all professionals and paraprofessionals. Heather volunteered to be the official mentor for these standards as new nurses joined the practice.

TAKE-AWAYS

- Clients judge a practice not just on its medical merits, but on how comfortable they feel with interactions involving all staff members.
- To effectively deliver pet-specific care, staff members must act in a complementary manner to help assure optimal outcomes.
- For accountability to be successful, team members must be empowered to do the right thing, and support the efforts of others to do what is needed.
- Accountability is not an excuse to scapegoat employees for the actions of others, but to foster the collective responsibility of achieving what needs to be achieved.
- Accountability only works within a practice if leadership creates an appropriate vision, and supports team members to always do the right thing.

MISCELLANEOUS

8.3.3 Cautions

Employees should not be expected to be accountable for tasks beyond their appropriate job description. For example, a surgical nurse can be accountable for tracking the use and recovery of surgical sponges in a procedure and for keeping the surgeon informed of the count, but cannot be held responsible for the surgeon's activities during the procedure.

Veterinarians are often hesitant about empowering employees, for fear that they will overstep their authority or discount goods and services to clients, but there is no evidence to support such fears. In actuality, empowering staff while making them accountable is one of the best ways of ensuring that they share the same practice vision, goals, and objectives as the owners of the practice. Alignment and accountability are in everyone's best interests (see 8.4 Alignment – The Key to Implementing Pet-Specific Care).

References

1 Carlzon, J. (1989). *Moments of Truth*. New York: HarperBusiness.

2 Connors, R., Smith, T., and Hickman, C. (2004). *The OZ Principle – Getting Results Through Individual and Organizational Accountability*. New York: Penguin Books.

Recommended Reading

Ackerman, L. (2003). *Management Basics for Veterinarians*. New York: ASJA Press.

Ackerman, L. (2020). Accountability. In: *Five-Minute Veterinary Practice Management Consult*, 3e (ed. L. Ackerman), 106–107. Ames, IA: Wiley.

Blanchard, K., Carew, D., and Parisi-Carew, E. (2000). *The One Minute Manger® Builds High Performing Teams*. New York: HarperCollins.

Connors, R. and Smith, T. (2012). *Change the Culture, Change the Game*. New York: Portfolio Trade.

Ricks, T.E. (2012). What ever happened to accountability? *Harvard Business Review* October: 93–100.

8.4

Alignment – The Key to Implementing Pet-Specific Care

Lowell Ackerman, DVM, DACVD, MBA, MPA, CVA, MRCVS

Global Consultant, Author, and Lecturer, MA, USA

BASICS

8.4.1 Summary

Running an efficient and effective veterinary hospital doesn't happen by accident. It takes all staff members working collectively to achieve hospital goals.

Alignment is critical for a variety of reasons, not the least of which is that without alignment, it is impossible to deliver on a unified mission and vision to pet owners. Also, in most veterinary hospitals, profit margins are so tight that there is no room for misalignment – salaries and jobs are at risk.

8.4.2 Terms Defined

Goodhart's Law: The observation that when a metric becomes a target for control, it often stops being a good measure.

MAIN CONCEPTS

Perceptions sometimes differ between staff members and management about the direction in which the hospital needs to go, but hospital goals are only achieved when attention is paid to the following factors:

- consumer value
- customer satisfaction
- hospital profitability and sustainability
- staff development
- standards of care
- consistency of care
- appropriate resource allocation.

Every hospital has its own reasons to harness alignment, and yet hospital goals are not difficult to enumerate. Most hospitals would be happy enough if all staff members united around a few common themes, such as:

- to have all hospital staff identify with and exemplify the spirit of the hospital mission
- to deliver consistent high-quality care to all clients, regardless of the experience or expertise of individual staff members
- to have hospital staff concerned with the business success of the practice, as well as desirable medical outcomes
- for all staff members to be accountable for the success of the practice, regardless of their positions.

As simple as these goals might appear, it is rare to find hospitals that appropriately achieve them with any consistency. To consistently achieve alignment, hospitals need to develop and prioritize the following.

- Leadership
- Differentiation
- Shared goals and expectations
- Accountability
- Strategic planning

Most veterinary owners are "reluctant leaders." They like the concept of "being the boss" but not necessarily the actual leading. Accordingly, many veterinary hospitals do not have established reporting structures, and care becomes inconsistent when there is not a senior "champion" for ensuring a level of care is delivered for every client visit (see 7.3 Leading the Change Towards Pet-Specific Care). When there is a lack of clear leadership, the typical result is that the hospital relies on gimmicks (such as production or bonuses) to motivate employees to do what they are supposed to be doing.

If staff are to believe that their practice is different from the others in the area, then differentiation becomes an important concept to embrace (see 10.2 The Importance of Practice Differentiation). The hospital must first define and then celebrate these distinctions, realizing that the differentiated practice may not be ideal for every client. In the real world, consumers have lots of choices, such as the type of car they drive, the type of restaurants they prefer, where they shop for clothes, etc., and it is quite possible that the newly differentiated practice might be a better fit for some clients, but not necessarily for all of them. However the practice is differentiated, it will be important to be able to measure and illustrate the value that the practice offers its clients. To fully embrace this concept, it is important to understand the "core" market sought by the practice, and not to panic when clients who don't want that type of practice seek a better fit elsewhere. If hospitals don't provide this differentiation, then clients are likely to differentiate themselves, and they most often do this based on price.

To have a well-defined hospital vision and mission is fine, but to reflect this to staff and clients requires the practice to have shared goals and expectations. To make this work, staff need to appreciate that it's not just about the medicine – it's about the total client experience and clients receiving value for their money spent. It's not just about individual excellent doctors, technicians, and receptionists – it's about individuals functioning as a team to deliver excellent care and ensuring that things don't fall through the cracks (see 8.1 Delivering Pet-Specific Care as a Team). It's also not just about meeting client needs – it's about delivering care in a way that meets hospital goals as well (see 5.2 Meeting Client Needs). Like any successful business exchange, there needs to be a commitment to the concept of "win–win."

Accountability is a critical attribute in the functioning of a veterinary hospital (see 8.3 The Importance of Accountability in Pet-Specific Care). While it might at first appear that it is the doctors who are responsible for the perception created by a practice, careful review of experiences both positive and negative show that all staff – doctors, technicians/nurses, receptionists, and managers – all have an important role to play in how the practice is perceived by the world outside the walls of the clinic.

For a hospital to function at its best, every employee must not only be accountable for their own duties but deliver on implied promises to all stakeholders regarding the mission and vision of the practice. Without accepting "ownership" of all responsibilities in this regard, a practice will need to rely on only its medical skills. With competition for veterinary services increasing regularly,

and with the very high cost of delivering those services, being second best can be a costly demotion.

One aspect of trying to drive alignment around common directives is the need to contend with a rule of thumb referred to as Goodhart's Law. Named after a prominent economist, Goodhart's Law refers to the observation that when a metric becomes a target for control, it often stops being a good measure. For example, if there is a directive to reduce accounts receivable, this can often be achieved by harsh means, but after that, measuring accounts receivable will do little to assess how effectively policies are promoting optimal cash flow. It is important to consider how our directives might actually have unintended consequences, and manage the process, and the alignment of our teams accordingly.

8.4.3 Strategic Planning

As was mentioned from the very start, running an efficient and effective veterinary hospital doesn't happen by accident – it takes planning. The fundamental design of a strategic planning initiative is to deliver exceptional medical care and client service in a team-based fashion, pay staff appropriately for the value they deliver, pay employee veterinarians appropriately for the value delivered (and owners a fair return on investment), and then charge clients appropriately for the value they receive. In some cases, this might mean adding services, in others it might mean changing the way services are delivered, and in other cases it might suggest discontinuing services that cannot be delivered profitably (or those for which clients aren't prepared to pay).

In a well-designed strategic plan, there is a division of duty between the management team (the trained practice management consultant, owners, and hospital manager/administrator) and the hospital staff who will be implementing the changes.

Once a core group of actionable missions has been created, the value of which is evident to all stakeholders, then specific plans for implementation should involve staff. In many cases, teams are the most effective way to ensure the success of the process. In many ways, this is more like acting as the captain of a ship rather than the dictator of a small empire. Management determines the destination for the voyage, and the staff explore options for the best way to get there, acting on smaller tactical pieces of the strategy.

In any strategic action plan, it is important to regularly determine whether the plan is still on target, whether the stakeholders are all happy with the program, and whether the target is still desirable. Strategic plans are fluid and flexible, and some plans may not be able to be successfully implemented. The most important aspect is to be responsive to the needs of clients and to alter programs accordingly.

TAKE-AWAYS

- Pet-specific care relies on the successful interaction and collaboration of *all* hospital team members.
- Individual team members must be accountable not only for their duties, but for the final outcomes desired.
- Alignment begins with effective leadership.
- Hospital team members must understand the "big picture" of what the practice is trying to achieve, and their role in delivering desired outcomes.
- Including team members in strategic planning efforts, and sharing metrics that allow them to see the impact of their actions, help assure alignment around best practices.

MISCELLANEOUS

Recommended Reading

Ackerman, L. (2020). *Five-Minute Veterinary Practice Management Consult*, 3e. Ames, IA: Wiley.

Buckingham, M. and Goodall, A. (2015). Reinventing performance management. *Harv. Bus. Rev.* 93 (4): 40–50.

Connors, R., Smith, T., and Hickman, C. (2004). *The OZ Principle – Getting Results Through Individual and Organizational Accountability*. New York: Penguin Books.

Detert, J.R. and Burris, E.R. (2016). Can your employees really speak freely? *Harv. Bus. Rev.* January: 81–87.

Fowler, S. (2014). *Why Motivating People Doesn't Work. . .and What Does*. Oakland, CA: Berrett-Koehler Publishers.

Kerr, J.M. (2014). *The Executive Checklist. A Guide for Setting Direction and Managing Change*. Basingstoke: Palgrave Macmillan.

Koch, R. (2013). *The 80/20 Manager: The Secret to Working Less and Achieving More*. London: Little, Brown.

Moore, I.C., Coe, J.B., Adams, C.L. et al. (2014). The role of veterinary team effectiveness in job satisfaction and burnout in companion animal veterinary clinics. *J. Am. Vet. Med. Assoc.* 245 (5): 513–524.

Ricks, T.E. (2012). What ever happened to accountability? *Harv. Bus. Rev.* October: 93–100.

Shapiro, S.M. (2011). *Best Practices Are Stupid*. London: Portfolio/Penguin.

Trout, J. and Rivkin, S. (2008). *Differentiate or Die*, 2e. Ames, IA: Wiley.

8.5

How Important Is Emotional Intelligence?

Lowell Ackerman, DVM, DACVD, MBA, MPA, CVA, MRCVS

Global Consultant, Author, and Lecturer, MA, USA

 BASICS

8.5.1 Summary

Emotional Intelligence (EI), also referred to as Emotional Quotient (EQ), has become a popular topic but its roots can be traced back over 100 years. Many claims have been made for EI but there is still some controversy over the validity of some of these claims.

EI is important in the workplace, but its relationship to actual intelligence has been disputed. Various definitions have been proposed for EI and various models exist. If you are going to implement pet-specific care initiatives in your practice, how much attention needs to be paid to EI?

8.5.2 Terms Defined

Emotional Intelligence: The capacity to perceive, assess, and positively influence one's own and other people's emotions.

Empathy: The ability to appreciate the feelings of others.

Motivation: The desire to accomplish things for the sake of achievement.

Self-Awareness: The ability to know one's emotions, strengths, and weaknesses and their impact on others.

Self-Regulation: The ability to control or redirect one's disruptive emotions and adapt to changing circumstances.

Social Skills: The ability to manage relationships and direct others in a desired direction.

Stakeholder: Anyone who is impacted by, or impacts, an organization's actions, products, or services.

 MAIN CONCEPTS

8.5.3 Models

Emotional Intelligence is a common buzzword in practice management, but it is important that the concept be viewed in context. There is substantial disagreement among experts as to what EI is and how it is best measured, and there are often conflicting reports on its predictive ability. However, even with these issues, the topic remains important.

The mixed model of EI, introduced by Daniel Goleman [1], focuses on the skills and competencies that drive leadership performance. These skills are: Self-Awareness, Self-Regulation, Social Skills, Empathy, and Motivation.

There are several tests for the mixed model, including the Emotional Competency Inventory (ECI), the Emotional and Social Competency Inventory (ESCI), and the Emotional Intelligence Appraisal (EIA); 360° assessments are also considered measures of this mixed model.

The ability-based model suggests that emotions are important and help individuals make sense of social environments. The four types of abilities recognized in this model are: perceiving emotions, using emotions, understanding emotions, and managing emotions.

The most common measure of the ability-based model is the Mayer-Salovey-Caruso Emotional Intelligence Test (MSCEIT), which has some similarity to ability-based IQ tests; these generate a total score as well as scores in each of the four branches of this model.

The Trait EI model concerns one's self-perceptions of emotional abilities. In many ways it considers EI to be a personality trait rather than a cognitive ability. There are many self-tests for Trait EI, including the Trait Emotional

Intelligence Questionnaire (TEIQue), the EQ-I, the Schutte EI model, and the Swinburne University Emotional Intelligence Test (SUEIT)

8.5.4 Concerns

It is important to realize that although most researchers appreciate EI as a recognizable attribute, there are still many questions as to what is being measured. Does EI actually reflect a form of intelligence, and is it actually predictive of social and leadership success within an organization? Is EI an important attribute when hiring team members to help implement pet-specific care in a practice? This type of debate will continue to rage but it is likely that EI reflects more on social skills than intelligence.

Possibly more concerning is that validation studies have not really found EI to be predictive of important outcomes, such as academic and work success [2]. One other concern about these self-report tests is that they are actually measuring the test-taker's perception of what would be a good response, rather than measuring some intrinsic ability.

8.5.5 Recommendations for Veterinary Practices

Although academicians will continue to debate the merits and constraints of EI, veterinary practices are most interested in forming functional hospital teams that can deliver both exceptional medical care and customer service and those attributes are critical for the successful implementation of pet-specific care (see 8.1 Delivering Pet-Specific Care as a Team).

In this regard, whether EI is a form of intelligence or a skill is not as relevant as employees being aligned with the hospital mission, their commitment to functioning as part of a larger team, their ability to communicate effectively with clients and each other, and their willingness to be accountable in their role within the hospital (see 8.3 The Importance of Accountability in Pet-Specific Care).

For most veterinary practices, the primary method of assessing EI will likely be to increase self-awareness with the use of self-tests (such as EIA from Emotional Intelligence 2.0), or 360° evaluations which look at the interactions of individuals with other stakeholders.

The EIA (www.talentsmart.com) has four parts, based upon the connection of what one sees and does with oneself and with others. The answers to the self-test provide an overall EI score along with personal competence (and contributing scores for self-awareness and self-management) and a score for social competence (and contributing scores for social awareness and relationship management).

8.5.6 360° Feedback

Also known as multirater feedback, 360° evaluations include feedback from subordinates, peers, and supervisors, as well as a self-assessment. In some cases it can also include other stakeholders, including specialists accepting referrals, clients, vendors, and anyone else who might provide useful feedback to an individual to help them grow as a professional.

The feedback is not meant to be punitive, but rather to provide the individual with useful information about how they are perceived by others, so that they can plan their personal development for future success (see 8.2 Developing Staff Competencies).

The accuracy of such an assessment is somewhat affected by the length of time the rater has known the individual being evaluated, with the most legitimate ratings being for those who have known the individual for 1–3 years. 360° evaluations are valuable, but need to be used cautiously as a measure of performance, because there can be weak correlation between such assessments and performance appraisals done by supervisors because they are measuring different attributes.

EXAMPLES

Dr Amelia Gold has been an employed veterinarian for three years at ABC Veterinary Hospital and has expressed some interest in becoming a partner. The owners of the practice have decided that a 360° evaluation may help Dr Gold in her personal development and identify strengths and areas that might need further attention.

The practice contracted with a consultant to facilitate the testing and that consultant suggested that some of the competencies to evaluate might include customer focus, technical skills, business acumen, communication, integrity, team building, motivating others, and managing workload.

To conduct the evaluation, Dr Gold and the practice owners jointly selected representative receptionists, nurses, other doctors at the practice, the owners, and the itinerant radiologist and surgeon who visit the practice to work on specific cases, to participate in the process, with the only criterion being that all raters had personally worked with Dr Gold and been familiar with her work for at least one year.

The consultant sent an email with rater links to Dr Gold and the others so they could complete the assessments online. Each of the participants was assigned a code of self, boss, peer, nonveterinarian, or other, and afterward the consultant prepared a report with the rating scores for

Dr Gold's self-appraisal, the average from all responses, and the responses for each of the participant groups.

Dr Gold was pleased that her overall assessment was quite positive, with particular strengths in technical skills, integrity, and customer focus. It was illuminating that there was an apparent discrepancy between her self-rating for business acumen and the owners' ratings, and they proposed that as part of an individual development plan (see 8.2 Developing Staff Competencies), they would involve Dr Gold in more of the management aspects of the practice. Part of her duties in the plan will be to be aware of key performance indicators and how they are impacted by the actions of the hospital team under Dr Gold's direction. If she does wish to pursue becoming a partner in the hospital, this will be an important aspect of her development.

TAKE-AWAYS

- Emotional intelligence is a common buzzword in practice management but somewhat controversial in what it measures and how applicable that is to workplace success.
- Emotional intelligence is likely not as relevant as employees being aligned with the hospital mission, their commitment to functioning as part of a larger team, their ability to communicate effectively with clients and each other, and their willingness to be accountable in their role within the hospital.
- The results of EI tests can be "gamed" by employees who know how to answer questions that determine EI scores.
- It's important to keep in perspective that few validated studies support the notion that standardized EI tests can predict workplace success.
- For many veterinary practices, a 360° evaluation will provide a more functional measure of how well employees perform within a healthcare team. Such tests are one, but only one, indicator of employee self-awareness.

MISCELLANEOUS

8.5.7 Cautions

There are significant limitations to EI tests, and the concepts are really meant to be used to foster self-awareness and positive interactions between team members. While the general perception of EI is very positive, there are some cautions worth considering.

- As individuals develop their emotional skills, it is also possible that they could enhance some abilities to manipulate others, even if unintentionally. If those individuals have self-serving motives, EI can influence others in a negative way.
- Individuals who are good at controlling their emotions may also become good at hiding their true feelings and motivations.
- An emotional "pitch" may motivate people to act against their best interests, and even against the best interests of the clinic.
- By perceiving what others feel, we are also capable of using those feelings to influence or compel their actions.
- Emotional Intelligence is not consistently correlated with job performance unless jobs actually require attention to emotions (e.g., customer service). In certain task-based jobs, enhancing EI can actually be a hindrance to improving performance.

References

1 Goleman, D. (2005). *Emotional Intelligence: Why it Can Matter More than IQ*. New York: Bantam Books.

2 Landy, F.J. (2005). Some historical and scientific issues related to research on emotional intelligence. *Journal of Organizational Behavior* 26: 411–424.

Recommended Reading

Ackerman, L. (2020). Emotional Intelligence. In: *Five-Minute Veterinary Practice Management Consult*, 3e (ed. L. Ackerman), 128–129. Ames, IA: Wiley.

Bradberry, T. and Greaves, J. (2009). *Emotional Intelligence 2.0*. San Diego, CA: TalentSmart.

Chamorro-Premuzic, T. (2017). Could your personality derail your career? *Harvard Business Review* September–October: 138–141.

Cornwall, M. (2012). *Go Suck a Lemon: Strategies for Improving your Emotional Intelligence*. CreateSpace.

Detert, J.R. and Burris, E.R. (2016). Can your employees really speak freely? *Harvard Business Review* January–February: 81–87.

Goleman, D. (2011). *The Brain and Emotional Intelligence. New Insights*. Florence, MA: More than Sound.

Grant, A. The Dark Side of Emotional Intelligence. (2014). www.theatlantic.com/health/archive/2014/01/the-dark-side-of-emotional-intelligence/282720

8.6

Nursing Leadership

Helen Ballantyne, PG Dip, BSc (Hons), RN, RVN

Cambridge University Hospitals NHS Foundation Trust, Cambridge, UK

BASICS

8.6.1 Summary

Effective nursing leadership is associated with a culture of high-quality care and continuous improvement. It is a challenging role, demanding an ability to blend and adapt leadership styles depending on the situation at hand. Traditionally, there was an assumption that certain people were born with the necessary characteristics to make them good leaders. Now it is accepted that leadership skills can be learned and developed.

The increasing complexity of veterinary healthcare makes it difficult for one member of staff to lead alone. The ability and willingness to delegate and share leadership responsibilities is a valuable skill that can streamline a leader's workload and empower employees, raising levels of job satisfaction and motivation.

8.6.2 Terms Defined

Autocratic Leadership: A style of leadership whereby one person has sole influence on a group of people within an organization.

Democratic Leadership: A style of leadership that encourages opinion and input from everyone involved within an organization.

Leadership: The ability to influence a group of people to behave in a particular way to achieve a shared goal.

Link Nurse: A member of the nursing team who takes on extra responsibility to develop their knowledge and skills in a particular area of nursing care with the aim of sharing their learning with their colleagues.

Management: The responsibility for the administration of an organization.

Transactional Leadership: A style of leadership that involves offering a reward for the adherence to instructions.

Transformational Leadership: A style of leadership that influences people to decide to adhere to instructions.

MAIN CONCEPTS

Leadership behaviors are intrinsic to nursing. At the beginning of a nursing career lessons are taught about the delegation of tasks, the responsibility to share knowledge with others and the need to advocate on behalf of patients.

As qualified nurses, leadership behaviors continue through adherence to professional codes of conduct that outline responsibilities toward patients, colleagues, and the general public. It is these behaviors that lead nurses to be held as both professional and social role models. The requirement every nurse has to ensure their knowledge and skills are up to date is a fundamental leadership behavior, for nurses must be self-aware and self-critical and seek out the relevant training to facilitate their professional development.

Despite these daily intrinsic leadership behaviors which are demonstrated across all levels of nursing, leadership is still often perceived as only something senior nurses with formal leadership roles are responsible for. There is a belief that it is something that is done by senior staff to their juniors.

Some of this misperception stems from a confusion between management and leadership. These terms are regularly used interchangeably but are very different and require different approaches and skill sets. Nursing managers are primarily task orientated, performing practical tasks. They are usually responsible for the delivery of quality clinical care and accountable for any unexpected outcomes. Their actions are usually short term with a single focus and may include budgeting, staff planning, and the monitoring and delegation of work streams.

Leadership is different in that it primarily focuses on workplace culture in line with organizational strategy and vision (see 7.2 Managing the Pet-Specific Workplace). It involves motivating others to be part of a shared vision to achieve a shared goal, and to design and support the ongoing strategy of the organization. Leadership is transformative – while management may tell staff how to behave, leadership aims to change behaviors for the long term, influencing people to behave and work in a particular way. It is associated with high-quality nursing care and a culture of continuous improvement.

Consider the introduction of a new brand of anthelminthic prophylaxis. A nursing manager would likely be responsible for ordering in the stock and organizing the date and time of training sessions to teach staff about the product. Nursing leadership would concentrate on consistent open communication about the change in practice, educating staff members as to the goals of the new treatments (see 7.3 Leading the Change Towards Pet-Specific Care). There should be explanations as to why the change is happening and how it fits into the organizational strategy and vision – for example, explaining that the new treatment has better clinical evidence associated with it, is cost-effective, and is easier to administer to the animals. Employees are much more likely to adhere to a change in work practice when they understand why it is needed and the benefits of its implementation.

Veterinary healthcare is complex, and a large busy veterinary environment can be described as a volatile, uncertain, complex, and ambiguous (VUCA) environment. A term originally used by the military, VUCA is now being used to highlight some of the challenges experienced in rapidly changing environments. While not every day will present such challenges, it cannot be denied that most veterinary healthcare professionals are never quite sure what their day will have in store for them, or how it will affect them personally and professionally. In the face of such challenges, effective leadership behaviors are essential to support staff to perform their role to the best of their ability.

There are two main styles of leadership associated with nursing. Transactional leadership is essentially the exchange of rewards in return for behavioral compliance. Staff who adhere to instructions receive benefits, in the form of remuneration, status or respect and praise. Returning to the new anthelminthic product example, a transactional approach would focus solely on promoting the fact that every time a staff member achieves a compliance target, they will receive a bonus in their wages.

In contrast, transformational leadership is a form of influence. Staff are empowered and motivated to behave in particular ways, adhering to and being part of the organizational vision and strategy of the organization. In this case, leading the change of product would focus on education of employees, ensuring that they understand how the product works and how they can explain it to clients. It will provide them with the tools to encourage the use of the product, knowing that using that particular product is part of the ongoing vision of the organization.

Transactional leadership is a style which is primarily task based and functional and possibly the style of leadership that is nearest to management. It is usually autocratic and leaves little room for negotiation or consultation with employees. As such, staff members can report feeling relatively stress free, as they have a leader who is so involved with every aspect of their work that individual staff members feel little to no responsibility for their actions. However, the leader may be extremely stressed and anxious as they feel they need to supervise every employee. This is a poor leadership cycle as the more anxious a transactional-based leader becomes, the more detail they want to know about actions within the organization. This can create a culture where staff do not feel respected or trusted. They may disengage, leading to more pressure on the sole leader.

The critical problem with this approach is consideration of what happens when the leader is not present within the organization. Often, staff are unable to perform, paralyzed by the fear of not being able to check their actions. They stagnate and stall, not wanting to make decisions potentially affecting clinical outcomes. Businesses may see a dip in turnover while key leaders are away, again due to staff feeling fearful and unable to think for themselves. It is this phenomenon that leads to this form of leadership also being known as the "hero" approach. Often, once the leader has returned, normal service is resumed and staff are reassured by their presence. While this might gratify the individual leader, it is an alarming prospect in the long term, leaving a veterinary business extremely vulnerable both clinically and economically.

An alternative approach to transactional leadership is the more democratic transformational leadership. In this "servant" approach, the leader is often seen to be working for the staff rather than the other way around. This style concentrates on empowering staff, encouraging them to develop their strengths and specialist interests. It also generates a culture of continuous improvement as staff members are encouraged to reflect and evaluate their practice and make suggestions as they learn from formal training and experiences. It often leads to individuals or small groups within the team taking on extra responsibilities or research projects as part of the wider organizational vision and strategy.

For example, consider a veterinary practice which has a long-term aim of providing mobile veterinary services to a remote community. A transformational leader may notice that two of the nursing team are interested in wound management, a discipline that is expected to form a key part of a mobile service. The nurses are invited to attend advanced training on wound management, the long-term goal is shared with them and they are able to engage on a wider level with the organization. Transformational leadership such as this can improve job satisfaction, reduce sickness, and increase loyalty to the organization.

The transformation approach relies heavily on open and honest communication, which at times can be difficult, particularly when dealing with commercially sensitive information. Emotional responses can interfere with business approaches. Consider a practice that has recorded disappointing financial outcomes. These outcomes may not be serious, may be entirely predictable and safe within the financial constraints of the business, but require some input to improve them (see 7.2 Managing the Pet-Specific Workplace). Sharing financial information within an appropriate context can be challenging as there is the danger that a primitive, fearful response may be stimulated by conversations regarding financial pressures. There may be assumptions that staff are to be laid off, resulting in mistrust, anxiety, and increasing absenteeism and presentism. In addition, the democratic open approach of transformational leadership can be a barrier to effective working as it can be difficult to make rapid decisions when every member of a large team requires consultation.

In fact, it is a combination of both styles of leadership that can support staff to deal with a VUCA environment. Transactional leadership can address the complexity of the healthcare environment by trusting expert experience and opinion so decisions can be made quickly. Autocratic methods of leadership can help leaders address the volatile element of the healthcare environment with a task-based approach responding to rapidly changing situations. To look at a basic example, consider a cardiac arrest; the democratic division of tasks would waste valuable time. In fact, a transactional leader, taking charge and allocating areas of responsibility, could save time and save a life.

The shared vision and organizational loyalty created by the democratic transformational leadership can assist staff to cope with the uncertain and ambiguous nature of healthcare. A culture of staff empowerment is created so that individuals feel able to adapt their ways of working,

make suggestions, and share responsibility. It will support the ability of staff to adapt in the face of rapid change and potentially offer protection of their mental well-being as they deal with a difficult environment.

Nurses in formal leadership roles need to blend their styles of leadership and offer a combination of autonomy and empowerment. A further step to optimize leadership, as previously mentioned, is to encourage leadership behaviors in all staff members, not just those with a formal leadership role.

Within human-centered nursing, there is a model of leadership empowerment known as link nursing. The link nurse is an individual member of a nursing team who volunteers to take a proactive role in developing knowledge, skills, and professional networks in a specific area of nursing care. This has benefits across the team as the link nurse makes a commitment to ensure they stay up to date with the most contemporary and evidence-based information on their subject and crucially, shares their learning with the rest of the team (see 8.2 Developing Staff Competencies). A common example is a link nurse role for diabetes. A link nurse is able to support their colleagues with treatment plans, and will have professional networks on which to call should further help be required. This model can optimize patient care and improve the knowledge base of a team.

There are also benefits to the individual through their exposure to senior staff network who may act as mentors, offering unique support and learning opportunities. Each of these skills and experiences can support nurses as they develop leadership skills to progress their career trajectory. In addition, the team benefits from having an engaged member who is keen to share their positive experiences. The feeling of empowerment from having a designated area of responsibility can be strong and lead to high-level clinical care as staff are encouraged to constantly evaluate and improve the care they give.

Supporting leadership behaviors in junior members of staff also has the benefit of supporting the long-term planning of staffing. Members of the team who have been exposed to leadership experiences are more likely to be effective leaders in the future. The link nurse role is not the only model of shared leadership that may be applied. Encouraging staff members to take responsibility for clinical audit, or for leading changes in practice or for gathering client feedback are all valuable experiences that can benefit both staff member and organization. Furthermore, a culture of leadership doesn't need to extend to big projects with sole responsibility. Positive leadership behaviors should be encouraged on a day-to-day basis. Examples include robust detailed handovers, prioritizing a holistic nursing approach, the fair and democratic organization of coffee breaks or encouraging colleagues to speak up at meetings. If all staff are supported to perform these day-to-day tasks, it can lead to a strong leadership culture where staff work together to achieve shared goals.

There are also benefits to nurses in formal leadership roles if they are able to delegate areas of responsibility effectively. To some extent, it can lighten their burden of work, although there will always be work associated with delegation to ensure staff feel supported and not overwhelmed by additional responsibilities. Delegation can ease the complexity of leadership. In VUCA environments, it is simply unrealistic for leaders to have detailed knowledge of every area of work. Nursing leaders need to be able to demonstrate humility, and rely on others to gather information, to weigh options and present balanced, relevant opinions to facilitate high-level decision making.

There has been a movement away from the belief that leaders are born, to the acceptance that leadership skills can be taught and learned. Much has been written about the skills required for effective leadership in both nursing and the general domain. There are multiple lists available that outline characteristics and talents that are deemed useful or even essential for leaders to display.

Within the context of nursing, the ability to be able to reflect and self-evaluate is one of the most important skills. The ability to take time, think things through and crucially adapt behaviors and approaches as required are the foundations of sound leadership. Such behaviors are particularly relevant for leadership within the complex and rapidly evolving nursing environment. They are also the foundations of other critical skills, including emotional intelligence (see 8.5 How Important is Emotional Intelligence?) and the ability to develop high trust relationships.

 EXAMPLES

Great Mates was a large veterinary hospital in the UK with a nursing team consisting of 10 qualified and registered nurses and five nursing assistants all managed by a head nurse who was responsible for the management and support of the entire nursing team. The head nurse had a very formal leadership style, keeping tight control on all clinical protocols, retaining the only set of keys to storage cupboards, and making all the decisions that affect the nursing team, from daily tea break timings to recruitment.

Several of the registered and qualified veterinary nurses had been at Great Mates Hospital for many years and were experienced and highly skilled. Many of them struggled with the head nurse's approach, particularly when her large workload had an impact on her ability to make decisions that might easily be delegated to others.

When a new veterinarian arrived at the clinic, keen to initiate laparoscopic surgical techniques, some of the nurses were pleased and excited to be part of a new way of working. They were looking forward to learning different skills and supporting a more modern approach to surgery. When all the relevant equipment arrived, the head nurse took charge and explained she was going to be the only nurse in the practice who would learn about the new techniques and once she had written all the relevant standard operating protocols, she would teach all the other nurses what to do.

The head nurse went on a course to learn about laparoscopic surgery and began working with the surgeon to use the new equipment. However, the head nurse also had other priorities, including the annual appraisal of staff members, a change in therapeutic diet provider, and organization of a upcoming client evening.

Quickly, she was unable to continue to participate in the laparoscopic surgery. However, as she had not shared any of her newly acquired knowledge, there was nobody else to step into her place. The veterinarian in question was very quickly frustrated that they could not continue to practice their new skill. The owners of the hospital were angry that highly expensive equipment was sitting idle in operating rooms, collecting dust. One of the most experienced nurses became demoralized and resigned when she learned that this new and interesting project would not be shared among the team, having sought out a new and more challenging role in a surgical referral center.

The practice manager raised the issue with the head nurse and an action plan was made. Volunteers were sought to attend the course on laparoscopic surgery, and both veterinarians and veterinary nurses were included, with the aim being to ensure as many people as possible began to familiarize themselves with the new technique. In-house training sessions were organized with the entire team so knowledge could be shared.

Several benefits were observed. The head nurse was able to concentrate on the review of the new therapeutic diet provider which ensured there was little overlap of superfluous stock levels. Members of the nursing team were motivated and enthused by the new way of working, with one nurse using the laparoscopic surgical cases as a basis for a research project as part of her postgraduate training. More veterinarians got involved with the new techniques, so more animals benefited from the minimally invasive surgeries. The hospital administrator quickly noticed a return on the investment which pleased the hospital owners.

The head nurse was so pleased with this approach to the project that she expanded the idea and asked for volunteers to organize the upcoming client evening. A nurse with a particular interest in media offered to help and designed a new and exciting client evening that resulted in the highest ever attendance at a client evening and local press coverage promoting the hospital.

The head nurse embraced this new style of leadership and continued to delegate projects, offering ongoing support and supervision but handing over the day-to-day responsibility to others. This had a positive impact on her work–life balance due to a lighter workload. The nursing team demonstrated high levels of motivation and enthusiasm for work as each developed their own areas of interest and responsibility. Monthly team meetings allowed the dissemination of new information and ideas, contributing to robust clinical governance and effective team working. The head nurse continued to monitor and support the nurses to ensure that they were not becoming overwhelmed by their extra responsibilities and the new style of working meant that if someone did need a break, others were equally informed so could help out at short notice.

TAKE-AWAYS

- Leadership behaviors are intrinsic to the process of nursing and are not restricted to those with formal leadership roles.

- Effective leadership has the potential to optimize clinical care and support a culture of continuous improvement.
- Good leaders are not always born with the relevant characteristics required for leadership; leadership skills can be learned, practiced, and developed.
- The ability to reflect and self-evaluate is one of the most crucial skills for nursing leaders.
- Sharing leadership responsibilities with other members of staff who have relevant areas of interest and ability can support effective information gathering so leaders can make appropriate and well-informed decisions. It may also empower employees, leading to higher levels of job satisfaction and motivation.

MISCELLANEOUS

Recommended Reading

Ballantyne, H. (2019). Leadership for veterinary nurses: the theory. *Veterinary Nursing Journal* 34: 69–71.

Ballantyne, H. (2019). Leadership for veterinary nurses: the practice. *Veterinary Nursing Journal* 34: 108–110.

Hartley, J. and Benington, J. (2010). *Leadership for Healthcare*. Bristol: Policy Press.

Henwood, S. (2014). *Practical Leadership in Nursing and Healthcare*. Boca Raton, FL: CRC Press.

8.7

Nursing Care Plans

Helen Ballantyne, PG Dip, BSc (Hons), RN, RVN

Cambridge University Hospitals NHS Foundation Trust, Cambridge, UK

BASICS

8.7.1 Summary

Nursing care plans are the written records of nursing care intended for a patient. They are unique to each animal and are created as a result of a comprehensive assessment where both actual and potential problems are assessed.

They can support holistic approaches, pet-specific care, continuity of care, and clinical governance. Additionally, they can be useful educational tools for newly qualified nurses or experienced nurses dealing with unusual cases.

8.7.2 Terms Defined

Assessment: The gathering of data about a patient.

Care Planning: The process of recognizing an animal's problems and making decisions about clinical interventions to assist in addressing them.

Clinical Governance: The process of checking that care being given is to the highest possible standard, usually compared to contemporary evidence-based practice and or previously agreed practice benchmarks

Holistic Care: Also known as the "whole patient approach." It involves the assessment of an animal incorporating their physical and behavioral needs, as well as the needs of their owner, with the aim of addressing existing health problems and preventing future problems.

Medical Model of Nursing: An approach to nursing whereby only the signs and symptoms that are presenting are treated, usually linked to a specific diagnosis.

Nursing Care Plans: The written record of the care planning process.

Nursing Process: A systematic approach to nursing comprising a four-stage cycle of assessment, planning, implementation, and evaluation.

Objective Data: Data obtained by performing procedures that result in measurements that can usually be compared to an expected value, e.g., body temperature, blood pressure.

Patient-Centered Care: Human-centered healthcare concept that strives to ensure all decisions are made with the involvement of the patient and their chosen support network.

Subjective Data: Data obtained through qualitative descriptive reports from an owner or healthcare professional after assessing an animal, e.g., coat condition or level of pain.

Therapeutic Relationship: A series of interactions between nurse and owner that supports the clinical treatment of an animal.

MAIN CONCEPTS

A nursing care plan is a document outlining intended treatments for patients under the care of a veterinary nurse. It is formed as a result of the care planning process which involves a thorough patient assessment and development of nursing care goals.

Historically, nursing was based on a medical model. Interventions were very much reactive, a task carried out in response to a particular disease or set of clinical signs. Anecdotes from human-centered nursing outline stories of lists of patients needing particular treatments. One nurse would be responsible for one intervention on any one shift. Therefore, a nurse might go around the ward, changing all the patients' dressings, while another helped with hygiene and cleanliness, while another took blood samples.

Such a transactional pattern of work left very little room for individualized care and therefore it prevented the recognition of patient-specific patterns, for example a nonhealing wound in a patient who also had a poor appetite.

During the 1960s, leaders in human-centered nursing instigated discussions about the definition of nursing. This led to an awareness of the need for individualized, patient-specific care, as nurses began to recognize and develop their own skill sets that optimized the medical treatment of patients. Providing care that was specific to the needs of one individual avoided patients receiving unnecessary treatments and supported improved clinical outcomes as adjuvants to medical treatment were given due time and attention. Nurses began to think in a holistic way, considering the whole patient rather than simply the disease or symptoms in front of them. A basic example in veterinary nursing would be the suturing of a wound without consideration of the animal's ability to access the wound and quickly and effortlessly remove the stitches.

More recently, this individualized approach has been extended throughout human-centered nursing to a concept of patient-centered care, defined by the UK Royal College of Nursing as "care that puts people at the center, involves patients, service users, their families and their careers in decisions and helps them to make informed choices about their treatment and care."

It may be speculated that healthcare professionals who work with animals will already take an individualized pet-specific approach to each of their patients and plan care accordingly. Logistically, veterinary nurses are far more likely to be caring for a ward containing a variety of species, with each requiring a different approach and different medication, as well as having variable physiological parameters.

Working with animals requires an implicit ability to prioritize and plan. Animals cannot be asked to "sit still" or be reassured with "this won't hurt." An inappropriate approach, poor handling technique or poor prioritization of interventions could lead to animals becoming hostile and aggressive.

Implicit care planning may come naturally to veterinary nurses, but there are several advantages to explicitly planning patient care and creating a detailed nursing care plan. Taking the time to plan the care of an animal can improve clinical outcomes, through the implementation of individualized, pet-specific care. By assessing a patient as an individual, actual healthcare problems can be addressed and potential problems can also be taken into account, so a more proactive approach is facilitated. Short-term health may be restored and long-term health promoted. In addition to the patient's needs, the assessment should also include the needs of the owner who will have their own thoughts and opinions about their animals' health which need to be taken into account.

One of the most useful tools in planning nursing care is the nursing process. This is a cyclical, continuous process of assessment, planning, implementation, and evaluation.

8.7.3 Assessment

Assessment is primarily the gathering of data about a patient. Both subjective and objective data are valuable within this process. Subjective data may be described as qualitative information and are often drawn from the owners' thoughts and opinions. Examples include levels of pain, vocalization, or swelling. Objective data are generally quantitative, involving a numerical measurement that can be compared to an expected normal level, for example, body temperature, electrolyte levels or respiratory rate. There are many tools available to structure the process of assessment. Human-centered nursing often uses Roper, Logan, and Tierney's list of activities of daily living [1] as a prompt to ensure all areas of the patients' health and well-being have been assessed. There are other tools associated with different areas of nursing such as intensive care or operating rooms. All these tools are equally applicable to veterinary patients.

Once the data have been collected, nurses need to consider three elements to establish conclusions about the needs of their patient. First, they need to consider the actual health problems the patient is presenting with, second they need to think holistically and consider the potential problems the animal may have and finally, they need to consider all the information within the context of the animal's normal health and husbandry.

So, for example, consider a cat who has had a collision with a car and now has a fractured jaw. The actual problem is the fracture which needs further examination, imaging, and perhaps surgery. The potential problem is that this patient may struggle to eat, especially when this is considered in the context of the animal's normal husbandry – this cat only eats dry food. Taking the time to consider in advance can support positive clinical outcomes. It may be more advantageous to the cat to place a feeding tube for assisted feeding at the time the fracture is repaired, rather than learn at a later date that the cat is going to struggle to eat and so require a second anesthetic to place a feeding tube.

8.7.4 Planning

Planning the nursing care of a patient is a two-stage process. First, goals of care should be set. This involves thinking through the ideal outcome for the patient and working with the owner to support the treatment. All goals should be set within the specific, measured, achievable, realistic, and timed (SMART) principles. Consider the nutritional needs of an animal; a goal to "improve food intake" is lacking detail to support its application and has no means of measurement to establish if it is being achieved. The same goal approached with SMART principles would be specific and measurable – feed 250 g dog food three times a day; it will be achievable, as the animal has previously eaten this amount; and realistic as while the animal is in hospital, three meals can be delivered. Finally, it can be timed as an endpoint can be marked for reassessment, for example feed 250 g dog food three times a day for three days and then repeat blood tests and weight of patient.

Patient goals need to be planned with the support and consent of pet owners. Taking the time to plan goals of care and discuss them with owners supports the development of a therapeutic relationship. Defined as a "series of interactions between the veterinary nurse and the owner of the animal that support effective patient care," a therapeutic relationship can be the key to essential adherence to home treatment regimens and therapy. Owners who know, understand, and, crucially, agree that an animal needs a particular medication are far more likely to administer it (see 9.17 Improving Compliance and Adherence with Pet-Specific Care). Furthermore, setting the foundations of open and detailed communication can support other elements of the care planning process such as financial planning and follow-up consultations.

Common barriers to therapeutic relationships include nurses making assumptions and not approaching the patient and owner as individuals. If an animal has a condition that requires long-term medication, the nurse might assume that the obvious decision is to agree to that long-term commitment. The owner may feel differently, as time pressures, stress for the animal and financial implications will all affect their decision-making process, and nurses need to be able to accept the owner's decision without judgment.

The second part of the planning process is preparation. This is a broad task that ranges from preparation of the physical environment and associated equipment to mental preparation where nurses evaluate their own skill sets and associated confidence to ensure that the relevant tasks are within their scope of practice. Such planning steps can allow nurses to seek further support if they need it, perform safety checks on equipment, and potentially optimize patient safety. It also allows the nurse to individualize the procedure for the patient. A nervous animal may need a quiet, dimly lit room, with minimal personnel. A boisterous happy dog may need toys and many hands to distract him.

8.7.5 Implementation

The implementation stage of the nursing process is the action of caring, by whichever intervention is required, be that basic nursing care, supporting diagnostics or surgery. It is the action, the doing stage of the process.

8.7.6 Evaluation

The evaluation stage is key to the nursing process and supports the continuum of care (see 9.7 Continuum of Care and Convergence Schedules). The evaluation is simply a question as to whether the care intervention has achieved the planned goal. So, has the care helped the patient? There may be several answers to this question, each leading to the same action – reassessment and development of a new plan of care. If the intervention has helped the patient, then the next step is to reassess their status and perhaps set care goals related to their discharge from hospital. If the care intervention has not helped, a reassessment is also required, with creation of a new plan, perhaps with adapted goals of care. Evaluation is crucial for patient safety; there is simply no point in applying the highest quality, most contemporary treatment plan if it is not working. The evaluation stage provides time to sit back and check that the healthcare professional is doing the very best for the patient.

The nursing care plan is a written record of the entire care planning process (see 9.1 Medical Record Entries). Collating the information gathered from applying the nursing process provides a data set for a robust care plan. Once the assessment data have been collected and the goals of care made, they can be documented. Creating such a document has three main advantages: first, it supports continuity of care between staff members (see 9.9 Continuity of Care); second, it can be a valuable educational tool; and third, it can facilitate clinical governance.

8.7.7 Continuity of Care

Across the veterinary healthcare sector, there is an increase in the complexity and acuity of patients, often reflected in the need for 24-hour care. Such care inevitably leads to the requirement for transfer of information between staff members. Known colloquially by many healthcare professionals as a "handover," this can be a vulnerable point in terms of patient safety if important clinical information is missed. A detailed nursing care plan can be a valuable tool to support the handover process and in human-centered nursing it is often used as a template to format the verbal handover. Crucially, using a nursing care plan will facilitate a holistic approach to the handover. While clinical details will be shared, a care plan will also contain relevant patient-specific information such as toileting commands and nutritional preferences, details which are just as important as objective clinical information.

Continuity of care does not just apply to hospitalized patients. Across the world, human healthcare is shifting away from acute reactive nursing models to the support of chronically ill patients, often with emphasis placed on the education of patients so they are able to manage their conditions at home. It is not unreasonable to suggest that with the corresponding advances in veterinary healthcare, patients are living longer with chronic disease and requiring ongoing treatment from their owners. Veterinary nurses are ideally placed to educate and support such care and the provision of detailed nursing care plans may be an essential tool. Such care plans can be designed to include details of medication, symptoms that need monitoring, follow-up appointments and carefully curated references for clients to seek further information regarding their animals' condition. Taking the time to construct such a care plan can facilitate appropriate care for animals with chronic conditions, potentially improving their quality of life.

8.7.8 Nursing Education

Nursing care plans can also support less experienced nurses who may appreciate the written instructions for caring for their patient. This can facilitate appropriate and effective care and may enable them to seek support for planned care they do not feel adequately able to handle alone. Additionally, once care plans are finished with, if cases have been particularly unusual or have had unexpected outcomes, they can be anonymized and used as tools to support clinical discussions and analysis to support learning.

8.7.9 Clinical Governance

Care plans can also be a valuable tool for retrospective clinical audit to support clinical governance. Put simply, clinical governance is the process of checking that the care being given is to the best possible standard, usually compared to contemporary evidence-based practice and or previously agreed practice benchmarks. Postoperative nutrition is a prime example. Often a practice may agree one particular brand of food should be routinely given to patients undergoing routine elective surgery. Such decisions are often based on a combination of clinical evidence and business

models as practices enter business relationships with pet food companies. Taking steps to audit the food that animals have received after their procedures by examining the care plans can offer an insight into whether the protocol has been followed. If care plans suggest it has not been followed, then the evidence is in place to support a root cause analysis of the problem. This will identify the reason why the food is not being used and allow solutions to be put in place. Such solutions may vary from basic interventions, such as making the food more readily available, or changing the entire protocol if nurses are consistently reporting that it is not a palatable choice for their patients.

8.7.10 How to Write a Nursing Care Plan

Using the nursing process, all the relevant information that is required to nurse a patient can be gathered. The action of writing that information down creates a nursing care plan. However, time pressures and complexity of care dictate that information must be prioritized and documented in the most user-friendly fashion. Templates for nursing care plans should be created by and for individual veterinary teams, depending on their clinical priorities. A care plan document for a specialist orthopedic hospital is going to be quite different from one for an intensive care unit. When designing a care plan template, several considerations should be taken into account.

8.7.10.1 Design

Despite the clear need for care plan templates that are relevant to the type of veterinary practice, there are several essential elements that must be incorporated into any nursing care plan.

1) Patient identification (on both sides if the document is double sided).
2) A section for documenting clear concise patient goals and associated interventions.
3) Clear formatting that allows signatures and dates against entries (if document is handwritten).
4) Observations chart, so that trends and patterns may be observed over time. Also, including the observation chart streamlines the document, preventing the need for several individual documents.

While each patient is different and will require unique care plans for their needs, some elements of treatments and interventions may be duplicated for every patient. This has led to the development of standardized nursing care plan templates within human-centered healthcare. Potentially, this is something that might be applied to veterinary nursing. Consider a care plan for an elective surgical procedure – there will be a preoperative health check, potentially preoperative blood tests, preoperative medication, then postoperative care that may involve a fairly standard approach, with physiological observations taken at preset timings as the animal recovers from their anesthetic. Such templates can be designed to suit individual procedures and either handwritten or held online for digital input.

8.7.10.2 Language

Predefined language is essential on care plans to ensure that all members of the multidisciplinary team are able to clearly and quickly comprehend them. If care plans are to be used by owners for care of patients at home, clear language devoid of medical jargon is essential. Generally, it is better to steer clear of abbreviations, which may vary wildly between disciplines, languages, and cultures.

8.7.10.3 Practicalities

The use of care plans within the practice demands a few essential practical applications.

1) If documents are to be handwritten, black permanent ink should be used, with mistakes adjusted with a single line through them, so they can still be read, and corrections initialed.
2) Team members should be consulted as to where is best for the care plans to be kept, and who will be responsible for ensuring supplies. While this might seem trivial, it is an important factor in team compliance.

EXAMPLES

Nursing care plans do not need to be complicated and long-winded. One of the most useful types of care plan is used in after-hours care.

Pippa is a veterinary nurse who has just started the night shift. One of the patients she will be caring for during the night is a 10-year-old bull terrier called Bob. Bob has had two seizures in the past 24 hours and is currently recovering in the hospital, receiving medication and being monitored for any further seizure activity. Dr Barton is the veterinarian in charge of Bob's case, and she is on call overnight. As well as Bob, Pippa has several other cases each with their own individual medication regimen and care needs.

Pippa has had a comprehensive handover from the day staff and is aware that currently Bob is very unstable on his legs, does not like taking oral medication, has vomited once over the course of the day and has no patent intravenous access.

Before Dr Barton leaves the practice for the night, Pippa seeks her out to confirm a nursing care plan for Bob. There are some elements of Bob's care that Pippa and Dr Barton can plan ahead for, potentially saving time and promoting better clinical outcomes. Pippa reports that Bob has been nauseous and asks Dr Barton to prescribe antiemetic medication, in case Bob start to vomit again. In the same way, Pippa asks Dr Barton for a fitting plan, a plan of action should Bob start to seizure again. This part of the plan includes instructions about medication and details of when to call Dr Barton into the practice. During the conversation, Dr Barton remembers that the owners want to be called at any time should anything happen to Bob; this is added to the after-hours care plan.

This may seem simplistic, but it is a part of care planning that is often missed and can be the most crucial. Out-of-hours work is by nature unpredictable. Making such plans in advance, calmly and thoughtfully, will be a tremendous advantage should Bob start to seizure, just as another dog has arrived in a collapsed state. Clinical decisions have already been made and Pippa can be addressing Bob's needs with autonomy and independence while Dr Barton begins her assessment on the other emergency. Put simply, planning care in this way can result in care that is safer, more effective and delivered in a timelier manner.

TAKE-AWAYS

- Care planning is the process of establishing the needs of a patient and deciding which clinical interventions will be of benefit.
- Care planning enables an individualistic and holistic approach to patient care.
- The nursing process is a continuous cyclical activity of assessment, planning, implementation, and evaluation that facilitates structured care planning.
- A care plan is the written record of the care planning process and should include the goals of care interventions.
- Care plans can support continuity of care, learning, and development and clinical governance.

MISCELLANEOUS

Reference

1 Roper, N., Logan, W.W., and Tierney, A.J. (1996). *The Elements of Nursing*, 4e. Edinburgh, UK: Churchill Livingstone.

Recommended Reading

Ballantyne, H. (2018). *Veterinary Nursing Care Plans: Theory and Practice*. London: CRC Press.

Barrett, D., Wilson, B., and Woollands, A. (2012). *Care Planning. A Guide for Nurses*. London: Taylor and Francis.

Hall, C. and Ritchie, D. (2009). *What Is Nursing? Exploring Theory and Practice*. Exeter: Learning Matters Ltd.

Manley, K., Hills, V., and Marriot, S. Person-centred care: Principle of Nursing Practice. *Nursing Standard* 25 (31): 35–37.

Rushforth, H. (2010). *Assessment Made Incredibly Easy*. London: Wollers Kluwer Lippincott Williams and Wilkins.

Yura, H. and Walsh, M. (1967). *The Nursing Process*. Appleton-Century-Crofts: Norwalk, CT.

8.8

Care Bundles

Helen Ballantyne, PG Dip, BSc (Hons), RN, RVN

Cambridge University Hospitals NHS Foundation Trust, Cambridge, UK

 BASICS

8.8.1 Summary

Care bundles are used within human-centered healthcare to facilitate the use of strong evidence-based practice to improve clinical outcomes. They are designed to direct staff to perform a small number of crucial interventions in response to a particular condition, procedure, or set of clinical signs. As well as improving clinical outcomes, they also have the potential to improve team working, promote patient safety, facilitate clinical governance, and support staff education.

8.8.2 Terms Defined

Care Bundle: A group of evidence-based interventions related to a disease, set of clinical signs or clinical procedure that when implemented together result in better outcomes than when implemented separately.

Evidence-Based Medicine: The combination of clinical assessment with strong evidence when making clinical decisions and treatment plans.

 MAIN CONCEPTS

Care bundles are a group of evidence-based interventions related to a disease, set of clinical signs or clinical procedure that when implemented together result in better outcomes than when executed individually. They were designed in response to patient safety incidents in human-centered hospitals. A tool was required to support systematic, consistent evidence-based care to reduce the incidence of side effects of medical interventions and the variability of clinical outcomes.

Care bundles improve clinical outcomes as they provide a template of action points for staff which focus on approximately 4–6 critical tasks. They often prioritize some of the basic concepts of medicine such as asepsis or personal protective equipment, which with the increasing complexity and acuity of patient care may be forgotten. Within human-centered healthcare the use of care bundles has improved clinical outcomes and reduced the length of hospital stays and healthcare costs. Additionally, they have been credited with increasing the knowledge, skill, and confidence levels of healthcare professionals. Care bundles make information easier for the team to remember and prioritize. Memory failures can be caused through stress, situations of uncertainty and complexity and when there are multiple tasks to perform. A care bundle can direct staff to perform more effectively under difficult circumstances.

Care bundles are relatively easy to develop, implement, and audit and as such have huge potential within the veterinary profession to optimize patient outcomes and increase access to evidence-based practice as they have done in human-centered healthcare. The use of these tools can bring additional advantages, with benefits extending to the wider healthcare team. They can improve team working, contribute toward high levels of patient safety, provide a measurable record of care and support in-practice education.

One of the most well-researched clinical applications of care bundles is the treatment of the early signs of sepsis. Used widely throughout the UK National Health Service, it is called the Sepsis Six. It comprises six key interventions: three therapies and three diagnostics. They are the initiation of intravenous antibiotics and fluids, and titration of oxygen saturation levels with supplemental high-flow oxygen, monitoring of urine output and blood tests, including blood cultures (before administration of antibiotics) and lactate levels. The introduction of this care bundle was supported on a national level with education and training campaigns in hospital and universities and there was an associated increase in sepsis survival rates.

Evidence from human-centered healthcare also demonstrates the positive impact of care bundles when applied to the management of chronic disease. One example is the treatment of exacerbations of chronic obstructive pulmonary disease (COPD) in the UK, where the use of an associated care bundle has reduced the administration of intravenous corticosteroids, increased the implementation of venothromboembolism prophylaxis and increased the number of referrals to specialist respiratory services, contributing to shorter stays in hospital and better clinical outcomes.

8.8.3 Reduction of the Gap between Theory and Practice

Professional codes of conduct throughout both veterinary and human-centered medicine demand that clinicians provide care that is both adequate and appropriate. Using evidence-based practice is a key tool in supporting that objective. The practice has been defined by Sackett as "the conscientious, explicit, and judicious use of current best evidence in making decisions about the care of the individual patient" [1].

Historically, the journey of information from the laboratory bench to the consulting room or operating room in medicine, both human-centered and veterinary, has been a long and at times tortuous process. Care bundles can shorten that journey considerably.

The interventions included in a care bundle are supported by the highest level of evidence. Taking the time to construct care bundles from comprehensive literature reviews and evidence analysis means that clinical staff can implement procedures known to be the most reliable and effective for the case at hand. This not only provides the highest level of care for the patients, but supports effective resource management and profit/loss business models. Implementing proven treatment plans represents the most cost-effective approach to care, for both the owner and the veterinary practice.

8.8.4 Teamwork

There are several key characteristics of an effective healthcare team (see 8.1 Delivering Pet-Specific Care as a Team). Well-defined goals, understood by all members of staff, are crucial to collaborative work. Clear communication and open discussion are also relevant. Care bundles can support both of these elements. A preestablished care bundle dictates the goals of care for the particular intervention or treatment plan, so immediately staff members caring for the patient have a plan of action.

The use of the Sepsis Six is a prime example. Within human-centered hospitals in the UK, once a patient displays a specific set of symptoms and associated clinical parameters, the care bundle is launched. Each member of the multidisciplinary team has a role to play and is familiar with the task in hand. The nursing assistant can be gathering the relevant equipment for the administration of fluids and associated monitoring. The nurse can be measuring oxygen saturation and providing the relevant level of oxygen saturation. The phlebotomist will be taking a standard set of "sepsis blood tests" and the doctors can prescribe the relevant intravenous antibiotics. The fact that the tasks are known in advance means that they are likely to be accomplished much more efficiently. The successful treatment of sepsis, like many acute conditions, is time dependent so ensuring staff know what to do and when to do it can promote positive clinical outcomes.

The role of a care bundle in teamwork is particularly relevant in high-stress life-threatening or time-critical conditions such as anaphylaxis or sepsis. Staff members have a reference to guide their work, offsetting the potential cognitive deficit induced by high stress levels.

8.8.5 Patient Safety

The use of care bundles can contribute to an improvement in patient safety (see 7.12 Patient Safety). Within human-centered medicine there have been significant reductions in iatrogenic conditions due to the implementation of care bundles, designed specifically to prevent known side effects.

One of the original applications of the care bundle was directed toward the prevention of bloodstream infections caused by central venous catheters (CVC). The placement of CVCs is a common intervention in human-centered healthcare, with CVC lines used widely throughout intensive care units. The placement and ongoing care of a CVC requires a strict aseptic technique, but the procedure is often performed away from the formal sterile environment of operating rooms, which can potentially lead to lapses in aseptic diligence. The regularity of this procedure may also contribute to poor technique as clinicians become complacent about the invasive nature of this line when placing and caring for it.

Central venous catheter care bundles outline key steps to preserve aseptic technique. Such documents support the safe placement of CVC lines, as clinicians have clear instructions as to what they need to do to support safe and effective practice.

One of the most important principles of patient safety in healthcare is the empowerment of all staff members to speak out if they have concerns about safety (see 7.12 Patient Safety). Historically, healthcare environments have been dominated by a hierarchy with associated submissive and subservient behaviors. Staff members who perceive themselves to be lower down the hierarchy may not feel able to challenge senior members of staff about compromising patient safety (see 8.6 Nursing Leadership). The use of care bundles that have been agreed at the highest level within a hospital can offer support for people to speak out if care deviates from the bundle. If steps in the process are missing, staff have the written care bundle to support their questioning, potentially preventing an adverse event occurring as a result of not following the care bundle.

8.8.6   Measuring Patient Care

A robust care bundle can be a useful tool to measure care and support clinical governance. Whether the bundle is in paper form or online, there should be a relevant option to check off the interventions once completed, with appropriate format for explanation should an intervention not be possible. Only when all care bundle interventions have been administered together to a patient is the care bundle counted as complete. Such documents, examined in retrospect, may provide valuable information on the care a patient received which might be particularly relevant in a case with an unusual or unexpected outcome.

Such documents may also provide valuable feedback as to how easy or difficult implementing the care bundle is. Common barriers to the use of care bundles include absence or malfunction of relevant equipment, competing priorities in complex patients, and poor staff knowledge of the bundle. In an example from human-centered healthcare, an audit revealed that clinicians found it difficult to locate the sterile gloves and appropriate cleansing solution required by the CVC placement care bundle. In response to this information, CVC placement packs were designed which comprise all the relevant equipment required to fulfill the care bundle, facilitating greater adherence to the care bundle instructions.

8.8.7   Education

Both using care bundles and being part of the development process of a care bundle can be a valuable educational exercise for trainees of all disciplines. Developing a care bundle

allows the practical application of critical thinking skills as evidence must be evaluated. Being part of a team writing a care bundle can expose students to specialists which might generate formal or informal mentoring opportunities.

Using care bundles offers students a connection between theory and practice as the bundle offers a practical application of evidence-based interventions within the variable context of animal, owner, and veterinary facilities. Using care bundles while in practice can help students increase their knowledge and confidence in the clinical setting and therefore assist their transition to becoming a safe qualified practitioner.

8.8.8   Writing Care Bundles

Designing and writing a care bundle is a simple procedure that follows a standard format (see Figure 8.8.1). First, a care theme needs to be selected. A theme may be generated in a number of ways. Originally care bundles were designed in response to problem areas, so if there have been unexpected or adverse outcomes surrounding a specific intervention, disease, or set of clinical signs, designing a care bundle might help the team address the issue effectively. Alternatively, the emergence of new evidence or new technological advances may dictate changes in practice, which may be managed sensitively and effectively through the design and implementation of a care bundle.

Once the theme has been selected, every intervention that is linked to the subject should be documented. This requires conversations with all members of the multidisciplinary team to ensure that all variations of the intervention are recorded. The ultimate goal is to produce a document that all team members are happy to follow, so each needs to be given the opportunity to contribute their own way of working.

Once the list of interventions related to the procedure has been collated, evidence for each one should be examined. It is generally accepted that high-level research equates to systematic reviews and analysis of randomized controlled trials. This might be challenging, particularly

---

1. Identify a care theme
2. List all relevant tasks and practices associated with that theme.
3. Perform a literature review on each task or practice of the theme.
4. Assess evidence base for each task or practice
5. Eliminate tasks or practice that have poor evidence
6. Create a list of relevant evidence-based practices and tasks associated with the theme.

Figure 8.8.1   Six steps to writing a care bundle.

when it comes to evidence for nursing interventions. As a relatively new profession, the evidence base for the associated skills and knowledge of veterinary nursing is small.

Furthermore, nursing interventions may not often lend themselves to randomized control trials (RCTs); more often, they require a qualitative approach to ensure that the effects on the patient and their quality of life are taken into account. If high-level research is not available, lower levels should be accessed, which may include multicenter studies or opinions from well-respected bodies that are based on clinical evidence.

Evidence-based interventions cannot be applied arbitrarily, and care bundles are not to be used as an alternative to thorough assessment and clinical decision making. There are some evidence-based practices which are simply not accessible in mainstream primary veterinary practice, due to practical, financial, or logistical reasons. Within the veterinary profession, care bundles need to be designed by combining the evidence, the patient group characteristics, the clinical skill set and practice equipment availability.

Once each intervention has been assessed both against the evidence and within the context of the practice team, a decision must be made as to whether it will be included in the bundle. The number of interventions within a care bundle will vary considerably depending on the complexity of the theme, but the aim should always be to use the minimum number of action points. Too many interventions may result in their importance being diluted among a long list.

Finally, the team writing the care bundle needs to consider the practical implications of the bundle. This includes its basic format, hard copy versus online and design features such as font, color, and size. The ideal presentation is a simple and straightforward design free of too much jargon or superfluous text. Whichever format the care bundle is in, either online or in hard copy, staff members need to know where to access it and where to save the completed document.

Consider applying this entire process to infection control in operating rooms if an increase in surgical site infections has been noticed. All relevant practices associated with the infection control protocol should be listed, everything from uniform guidelines, to cleaning schedules, to use of chemical disinfectants and patient preparation. Each practice must then be checked against the relevant evidence. For example, is there evidence that staff wearing a dedicated operating room uniform can reduce the risk of infection? Is the team using disinfectants with the strongest evidence associated with them, or are they simply using the one they are familiar with?

Once the evidence has been collected, it can then be evaluated. It may have been discovered that the disinfectant being used to clean the operating room is not the product with the most evidence attached to it, but simply the cheapest product available. Therefore, a change in practice is indicated and the details of the new disinfectant are added to the care bundle.

Care bundles may differ from team to team, depending on the current priorities of the staff involved. A care bundle on peripheral cannulation for a veterinary team that has noticed an increase in their patients removing their own intravenous cannula may concentrate on the dressings used to secure the cannula. Another team may want to concentrate on the use of particular cannulas that are associated with lower levels of phlebitis, using the care bundle to remind staff to use the new equipment. A different team may want to ensure a standardized approach to hair removal after a cluster of skin irritations around cannula sites. Care bundles can be adapted as long as the interventions listed remain supported by strong scientific evidence.

8.8.9 Implementation of a Care Bundle

Implementing a care bundle can be a challenging process, as its use may require clinicians to work differently, perhaps breaking long-term habits and challenging established paradigms (see Figure 8.8.2). The process needs to be handled in a sensitive, supportive manner and should be taken into consideration at the very first stages of care bundle design. Open and effective communication at all stages of the process is essential to gather support for the new way of working.

Encouraging all relevant staff members to input and review the care bundle from its initial conception is a positive step toward smooth implementation. When people are involved from the beginning of a planned change, they are far more likely to adapt their practice and work differently. Practically, this involves taking steps to ensure all members of the multidisciplinary team are consulted. Feedback should be sought within a lenient time frame, with the opportunity for staff to offer an opinion in a variety of ways, perhaps through a direct survey, freehand review, or, if relevant, anonymously.

1. Collaborative working, with all relevant stakeholders.
2. Recruit enthusiastic and knowledgeable change makers
3. Plan education for all relevant staff members
4. Develop and publish a timeline for implementation
5. Plan audit of compliance once launched

Figure 8.8.2 Principles for implementing care bundles.

Recruiting enthusiastic and knowledgeable members of the team to support the implementation of the care bundle can be invaluable. They can disseminate information and gather support for use of the bundle. Publicizing their role means that staff members know who to approach for more information before, during, and after the implementation of the bundle.

Robust and comprehensive education is essential so all members of the team can be informed about the new care bundle, which might mean a change in working practices for some. Emphasis should be placed on the evidence for the elements of the bundle to support its use. A timeline of learning opportunities, dates of launch, audit, and review should all be published widely so team members know when and how the care bundle will be used.

The benefits to team working that the use of care bundles can bring will only be relevant if the team in question has been supported fully in their adoption of the care bundle. Robust and detailed education with theoretical concepts and simulation practice will result in a team ready and able to take full advantage of the use of the care bundle.

8.8.10 Keeping it Pet Specific

Care bundles should be used as an adjuvant to the overall plan of care, rather than instead of a plan. Implementation of a care bundle should be part of a holistic approach; it can address most of the needs of the patient, relative the condition or set of clinical signs it is experiencing, but will not take into account the potential problems that patient has or its baseline normal. As a basic example, a care bundle to support the implementation of a peripheral intravenous cannula may instruct that the skin is prepared with a specific topical antiseptic. While the evidence may instruct that the solution is the optimum product for supporting aseptic line placement, if the animal is allergic to it, its use will cause more harm than good. Care bundles encourage a standardized approach to the care of animals. However, it is important that they are used within the overall context of the patient, their owners' needs and wishes, and the practice philosophy and service availability.

EXAMPLES

Care bundles may be applied to a range of clinical scenarios; in particular, they may be highly valuable in emergency situations that may present infrequently but require complex interventions. A care bundle can summarize an evidence-based approach to the initial emergency management of a case. This might be particularly relevant should a member of the team be working independently before additional on-call support arrives. The animal will benefit from appropriate and timely interventions, which may optimize their condition and improve their prognosis. The staff member has a tool that will support them to work in a systematic and methodical manner in challenging and stressful circumstances. Examples include cesarean section, gastric dilation-volvulus, trauma, or a cat with a blocked urethra.

TAKE-AWAYS

- Care bundles are a short list of evidence-based interventions associated with a condition or set of clinical signs.
- Care bundles were originally designed to address poor clinical outcomes in human-centered medicine.
- The use of care bundles can improve clinical outcomes, support effective teamwork, promote patient safety, provide a measurable record of care and support in practice education.
- Interventions included in a care bundle should be supported by the highest level of evidence available, considered within the context of the patient, the owner, and the veterinary healthcare team.
- Design and development of a care bundle should involve all members of the team who will be using to it to support maximum engagement with its clinical application.

MISCELLANEOUS

Reference

1 Sackett, D.L., Straus, S., Richardson, W. et al. (2000). *Evidence Based Medicine: How to Practice and Teach EBM*. Edinburgh: Churchill Livingstone.

Recommended Reading

Clarkson, D. (2013). The role of 'care bundles' in healthcare. *British Journal of Healthcare Management* 19: 63–68.

Dellinger, P. (2015). The surviving sepsis campaign: where have we been and where are we going? *Cleveland Journal of Medicine* 82 (4): 237–244.

Levy, M.M., Provonost, P.J., Dellinger, R.P. et al. (2004). Sepsis change bundles: converting guidelines into meaningful change in behaviour and clinical outcome. *Critical Care Medicine* 32: 595–597.

Resar, R., Griffin, F.A., Haraden, C., Nolan, T.W. Using Care Bundles to Improve Health Care Quality. www.ihi.org/resources/pages/ihiwhitepapers/usingcarebundles.aspx

8.9

Procedure Manuals

Kurt A. Oster, MS, SPHR, SHRM-SCP

Bay State Veterinary Emergency and Specialty Services, Swansea, MA, USA

 BASICS

8.9.1 Summary

Procedure manuals and reference manuals are helpful management tools in any size or type of veterinary practice. They serve as a convenient reference tool to ensure that standards of care and standard guidelines are in place, they can be instructional in nature, and they provide a standard to hold staff accountable for counseling and coaching purposes.

Putting policies and procedures down in writing forces dialogue and promotes compromise between the members of the practice leadership. This dialogue and compromise should occur when things are calm, and people have the time to plan. All manuals should be reviewed and refreshed each year to stay current.

8.9.2 Terms Defined

Disaster Recovery Manual: Covers simple tasks such as how to function when the internet goes down or when the electricity goes out.

Doctor's Manual: Helps ensure that all doctors in a multidoctor practice are following the same basic protocols to avoid client confusion that will undermine trust in the practice.

Exam Room Assistant Manual: A resource for those veterinary assistants responsible for assisting veterinarians in appointments and other exam room procedures ranging from pedicures to emergency triage.

Laboratory Manual: A complete reference guide for technicians and doctors who may be working in the laboratory or processing samples through the laboratory.

Receptionist or Customer Service Manual: Outlines all front desk procedures in a step-by-step manner.

Safety Manual: Required for virtually all veterinary practices. It identifies hazards within the practice and delineates procedures for dealing with them.

Technician Manual: Designed to support the nurses/technicians in accomplishing their daily tasks in the back of the practice. It includes step-by-step instructions on what technical staff/nurses need to know.

 MAIN CONCEPTS

8.9.3 Developing A Manual

The first step in developing each of these manuals is to designate one individual in the practice to be the project leader. The project leader ensures that the manual will be prepared pursuant to a schedule and completed by its deadline. Every member of the manual's target group should be included in its development (in addition to the members of the practice leadership such as the practice owner, hospital administrator, or practice manager) and production. For example, if it is a reception manual, all the receptionists should contribute to it.

A brainstorming session allows everyone in the target group an opportunity to suggest topics to be included in the manual. This list of topics then becomes the Table of Contents for the manual. Each manual may cover an average of 25–50 topics.

Pet-Specific Care for the Veterinary Team, First Edition. Edited by Lowell Ackerman.
© 2021 John Wiley & Sons, Inc. Published 2021 by John Wiley & Sons, Inc.

Once the Table of Contents has been completed, the team member responsible for writing each portion of the manual should be identified. Some practices ask for volunteers to author a particular topic, whereas other practices assign topics to specific individuals. A deadline is then established for each of the authors to submit the first draft of their material. The project leader needs to review each submission for accuracy and completeness.

It is not unusual for authors to discover conflicting protocols and/or procedures within the practice, so it may be necessary for the project leader to seek clarification from the practice manager or practice owner(s). It is also quite common for authors to discover that there are multiple ways in which a specific task may be completed. An experienced manager should focus on desired outcomes rather than processes. Therefore, if all the ways identified to complete a specific task are equally as efficient and effective, then there may be a need to include them all in the manual and let individuals determine which method they like best. This is often the case in the reception manual, which includes topics that relate to completing tasks within the practice management software.

A draft copy of the manual should be prepared and distributed to each participant, as well as to the practice manager and practice owner, for final review. A comprehensive final review allows the entire practice to contribute their combined experience and insight to each of the tasks that will benefit future users (it is also an excellent refresher course for everyone involved).

The manuals may be printed, bound, and distributed to the appropriate team members, or stored on the practice network in an electronic format. Electronic copies are easier to update and less expensive to maintain. A signed receipt should be obtained for each manual distributed (or that the employee has been trained on how to access the electronic version), and the receipt should be kept in the employee's personnel file. As an alternative, some practices email electronic copies of the manuals to their team members. It is less expensive, less labor intensive and more environmentally friendly to revise and maintain electronic versions instead of hard-copy versions.

One or two printed manuals should be placed in strategic locations throughout the practice for ease of use and as part of your disaster recovery plan in case the computers are down and the team cannot access the electronic versions of the material.

EXAMPLES

The following example represents a typical entry in a procedure/reference manual. In this example, the practice is ensuring everyone understands how to charge the proper examination fee based on the number of pets the client has brought with them. This type of reference could be included in a doctor manual, a reception manual, and an exam room assistant manual, because all these team members could be required to explain these charges to a client.

XYZ Veterinary Clinic has numerous exam codes. Therefore, it is easy to understand why there has been some confusion in the past regarding the proper code to be charged for a specific type of visit. The purpose of this section is to define each type of exam code and explain its proper usage. Doctors do have discretion to increase or decrease an examination fees as they deem appropriate; however, it is important to communicate the reasoning behind any change to the appropriate receptionist. In this way, the receptionist can appear informed and be properly prepared to address client concerns (i.e., the client may question why the amount of the final invoice is different from the amount they were originally quoted).

ID	Description	Fee
107	Exam – Office Call/Exam	XX.00

This code is for our standard physical exam to be charged to our regular appointments.

ID	Description	Fee
106	Exam/Per Pet 2	XX.00
102	Exam/Per Pet 3	XX.00
112	Exam/Per Pet 4 or more	XX.50

These codes are used if multiple pets belonging to the same client are examined during the same appointment slot. Basically, you can think of them as multipet discounts. The code should be selected that represents the total number of pets in the appointment (i.e., if there are three pets, use 102, and each pet would be charged for an Exam/Per Pet 3). These discounts are not applied in a sequential order such as Exam, Exam 2 Pets, Exam 3 Pets, etc.

CAUTIONS

Avoid reference to specific staff members by name. Instead, you should refer to them by title or position. For example, instead of "Bring the sample to Sue in the lab," it should be "Bring the sample to the laboratory technician on duty."

If manuals are allowed to become dated, staff will lose confidence in them as a reference and training tool. Manuals should have a revision date and that date should always be less than one year old (establishing a reminder in your management software to update your manuals is an excellent tip). There are also numerous events that will trigger manual reviews such as the addition of new equipment and new software releases.

Maintain an off-site computer media back-up of each of the manuals which includes a cloud-based option.

TAKE-AWAYS

- The practice should make a master list of all of the types of manuals they need. The number of manuals will depend on the size, scope, and complexity of the practice.
- While each manual should have a specific project manager, the more people involved in the creation and review of the manual, the better the final product will be.
- Get visual! Pictures, clipart, screen grabs, hyperlinks, and video links all make your manual easier to read and more enjoyable which will drive staff compliance. Any manual over five topics should have a Table of Contents for easy reference.
- Manuals should be reviewed and updated as needed each year. Each update should result in a new revision date.
- Electronic manuals are easier to create, distribute, and maintain than hard-copy manuals, but at least one of each manual should be maintained in hard copy so it is available during network, internet, or power failures.

MISCELLANEOUS

Directions need to be very specific. Vagueness decreases the value of the manual and allows subjectivity to infiltrate procedures and/or protocols. Many procedures may have a short and long version in each manual. The long version is a very detailed step-by-step version designed to support someone who has never completed that specific task before, or as a tool to aid training and/or accountability. The short version is often a bulleted refresher designed to support someone who is familiar with the task but may feel a little rusty and wants to be sure they are completing the task correctly and completely.

Before revised material is put into use, it is best practice to have someone unfamiliar with the process (such as a team member from a different department) read through the material as a test. If they can complete each task without difficulty, then the manual contains all the necessary information in the proper detail. Too often, the person writing content for a manual is so familiar with the process that they skip over steps or details they take for granted that "everyone" would know.

Screen captures, photographs, and video links can improve the effectiveness and user friendliness of a manual. The ability to insert hyperlinks is another excellent reason for publishing your manuals in an electronic format rather than hard copy.

Recommended Reading

Boss, N. (2008). *How We Do Things Here: Developing and Teaching Office-Wide Protocols.* Lakewood, CO: AAHA Press.

Gawande, A. (2010). *The Checklist Manifesto.* New York: Henry Holt.

Heinke, M.L. and McCarthy, J.B. (2012). *Practice Made Perfect*, 2e. Lakewood, CO: AAHA Press.

Oster, K. (2020). Procedure manuals. In: *Five-Minute Veterinary Practice Management Consult*, 3e (ed. L. Ackerman), 146–147. Ames, IA: Wiley.

8.10

Patient and Procedure Logs

Kurt A. Oster, MS, SPHR, SHRM-SCP

Bay State Veterinary Emergency and Specialty Services, Swansea, MA, USA

 BASICS

8.10.1 Summary

Patient and procedure logs play a vital role in any practice and work best in conjunction with well-designed and well-prepared procedure manuals. Patient and procedure logs allow for the convenient storage of important data, help standardize how procedures are performed, facilitate charge capture and auditing processes, and are important if supplies such as laboratory tests kits are recalled. Practices with a well-maintained system of logs and audits may increase net revenues by as much as 10–15%.

8.10.2 Terms Defined

Audit: Methodical examination and review of practice records to assess accuracy and completeness. A large practice may have one or more staff members whose sole responsibility is to perform audits.

Hybrid Logs: These logs are a combination of patient and procedure logs.

Patient Log: Any record or list of patients that have received a specific service or product. The log generally has additional pertinent information such as excerpts from the patient's medical record and/or items helpful in the billing process (e.g., laboratory logs and new patient lists).

Procedure Log: Procedure logs help ensure that tasks have been completed and/or completed in a specific manner (e.g., a practice housekeeping checklist or a record of dates evidencing that someone has calibrated the in-house laboratory instruments).

 MAIN CONCEPTS

8.10.3 Creating a Log

Once you determine that a specific need exists, you should make a list of the data that need to be collected and the steps to be completed in order for the function to run smoothly. Quite often, logs are created in response to specific disasters that the practice leadership hopes to prevent from recurring, so the information gathering can be quick and easy. For example, most final care logs are developed after a pet that was supposed to be sent to the crematorium for a private cremation, with the ashes returned to the owner, ends up going to the pet cemetery for a group burial in an unmarked grave.

The more people involved in the creation of a log, the better the final product. It is best if multiple team members offer input and/or review drafts of the proposed log. In this way, you can ensure that a more complete and functional log is developed.

Implementation of a new log requires planning. The use of the log should be announced to the staff and they should receive training on how to complete entries and whom they should notify if they observe any discrepancies or irregularities in the log. This training also helps elevate the importance of the log with the staff, which in turn increases staff compliance and acceptance.

A specific team member should be responsible for making sure that the log is being properly completed at the required interval and that it is indeed solving the problems it was designed to solve. If the log is performing as desired, a regular schedule of audits should be implemented to maximize the log's effectiveness. If the log is

Pet-Specific Care for the Veterinary Team, First Edition. Edited by Lowell Ackerman.
© 2021 John Wiley & Sons, Inc. Published 2021 by John Wiley & Sons, Inc.

not performing as desired, it should be revised until it achieves its desired goals.

EXAMPLES

One of the simplest problems to solve in a practice through the use of logs and audits is lost revenue due to missed charges. The laboratory, for example, is a common site for lost charges, and a log that records the results of fecal exams alone can generate thousands of dollars in additional revenues for a practice each year.

The data to be collected in the log should to be determined by surveying the staff. Fecal examinations are notorious for lost charges because they are sometimes given to a receptionist, sometimes to a technician, and sometimes to the doctor. Clients may initially forget they even brought a sample with them, so you might not even get it until they are ready to leave. The staff member who sets up the sample may not be the person who reads it; therefore, it is important to have these procedures spelled out in a procedure manual, so the entire staff has the same expectation and can be held accountable for their piece of the process. Each data point collected should have a specific purpose (no one enjoys extra paperwork for no reason).

The date tells us when the test was run; the client and patient names identify the origin of the sample. Inclusion of client and patient IDs makes it easier to check in the computer that the client was charged for the examination. The initials of the staff member who set up the sample for examination help us identify that individual if there is a problem to be addressed. In many practices, the person who sets up the sample is also the person responsible for putting the proper charge on the client's invoice.

The time the sample was set up is helpful if the type of test you are running is time sensitive. For example, one popular test says the sample needs to sit for 7–15 minutes in order to be accurate. Too little time or too much time, and you could get a false-negative result.

The initials of the staff member who reads the sample and records the results are also required. In this example, results must be recorded in the log and in the patient's medical record. This is especially important for those practices that require the person who read the sample to report the results to the client. At one hospital, a staff member was reporting pollen as roundworms, so the log was essential in retesting all the samples that technician had interpreted.

The frequency of checking the log against the computer varies from practice to practice. Most practices check laboratory logs twice daily, so if a charge was missed the client can be contacted immediately and their invoice can be properly revised. Waiting days or weeks to report a billing omission to a client usually results in a lost opportunity to collect the fee as well as a less than enthusiastic client.

Sample Laboratory Log (Heartworm Test) Part 1

Client	Patient	Client ID	Date	Result	Technician
Sarah Walton	Gunner	362 598	03/31/19	Negative	Sarah S
Bill Jones	Blackie	45 826	03/31/19	Negative	Sarah S

Sample Laboratory Log (Heartworm Test) Part 2

Medical Record	Client Contacted	Assistant who called	Date	Time	Test Manufacturer	Lot Number
Yes	Yes	Jane B	03/31/19	5:21 p.m.	ABC Co	XY123
Yes	Yes	Jane B	03/31/19	5:22 p.m.	ABC Co	XY123

TAKE-AWAYS

- Logs exist to support quality assurance and compliance. They also help the practice leadership identify trends quickly.

- Logs help the practice manage product recalls in an efficient manner.
- Logs can help identify team members who need additional training, or are not fully compliant with practice policies.

- Logs support accurate charge capture and may result in increases to a practice's bottom line of 10–20% or more.
- Computer automation does not negate the need for logs and manual auditing. In many cases, the use of software increases the number of errors and omissions within a specific process.

MISCELLANEOUS

8.10.4 Cautions

Blanket policies such as "everyone is responsible for checking for missing charges" are rarely effective. When practices get busy, most staff members assume that someone else is following through because they are otherwise occupied. If everyone is responsible for completing a task, then no one is responsible for completing the task! The results can sometimes be devastating on a practice's bottom line. Thus, it is imperative that one individual ultimately owns each log and audit process to ensure compliance and accountability.

Most practices fall into a routine of only telling staff when they have made a mistake. If a log is audited and there are fewer errors than last time or no errors at all, then these results should be celebrated by the practice team. For example, one practice reinforces excellent work by giving small cash bonuses to the receptionist who has the lowest number of invoicing errors each week.

Do not fall into the trap of thinking that your computer is magically auditing all your records. Manual systems existed for decades, which gave practices ample opportunity to build in quality control procedures. Many practices abandoned these procedures when they computerized, falsely believing that all the opportunities for errors had been removed. In reality, many practice management software programs have few quality control features. Those that do are rarely set up correctly or monitored as they should be.

Those individuals charged with auditing responsibilities should record their results each and every time an audit is performed so they can look for possible trends. For example, if within a month, five technicians each miss two fecal samples, then all the technicians should probably receive some refresher training. If, however, two technicians each miss one sample and a third technician misses the remaining eight samples, then that technician should receive additional training, coaching, and/or counseling on how to properly process fecal samples.

Recommended Reading

Ackerman, L.J. (2003). *Management Basics for Veterinarians*. New York: ASJA Press.

Gawande, A. (2010). *The Checklist Manifesto*. New York: Henry Holt.

Heinke, M.L. and McCarthy, J.B. (2012). *Practice Made Perfect*, 2e. Lakewood, CO: AAHA Press.

8.11

Dental Charting

Heidi B. Lobprise, DVM, DAVDC and Jessica Johnson, DVM

Main Street Veterinary Dental Clinic, Flower Mound, TX, USA

BASICS

8.11.1 Summary

In every aspect of veterinary medicine, the accurate recording of health assessment, recognition of lesions and therapy provided generates a useful medical record. The oral cavity has its own conglomeration of indices and terminology often derived from human dentistry, with applicable variations. While often underused in some practices, becoming familiar with the terminology and their application is important for the practice team to be able to effectively communicate and record dental conditions, treatment, and instructions for our patients and clients, to provide optimal oral care.

8.11.2 Terms Defined

Calculus Index (CI): A measurement of the accumulation of calculus on the tooth surface.

Furcation Exposure (FE): Exposure of the space in between roots of a multirooted tooth that is normally covered by periodontal tissues (gingiva and bone).

Gingival Index (GI): A measurement of the extent of gingival inflammation.

Gingival Recession (GR): Loss of gingival tissue that, together with accompanying bone loss, can expose the root of the tooth and even the furcation of a multirooted tooth.

Mobility (M): An assessment of the degree of mobility of a tooth.

Modified Triadan System: A tooth numbering system used in veterinary dentistry.

Periodontal Disease Index (PD or PDI): The degree of severity of periodontal disease of a particular tooth (stage).

Periodontal Pocket (PP): The deepening of a healthy sulcus depth due to the attachment loss (AL) of periodontal tissues, measured in millimeters.

Periodontal Probe: A hand instrument used to measure the depth of a pocket or amount of root exposure (RE); marked in various millimeter increments, depending on type of probe.

Plaque Index (PI): A measurement of the accumulation of plaque on the tooth surface.

RE: Exposure of the root of a tooth that is normally covered by periodontal tissues (gingiva and bone).

Tooth Resorption (TR): Resorption of hard dental tissues – enamel, cementum, dentin.

MAIN CONCEPTS

The accurate and detailed documentation of abnormalities or pathological lesions found in the oral cavity, along with appropriate management, provides both a medical and legal record for the patient (see 9.1 Medical Record Entries).

Many dental abbreviations can be used to help capture a multitude of measurements. Full-page, two-view pictorial charts are best to allow sufficient space for writing measurements of RE and pocket depth and other lesions (see Figures 8.11.1 and 8.11.2).

These charts are species specific to capture the specific dentition of the patient. The Modified Triadan Numbering system has been developed to number and accurately identify teeth in our veterinary patients, compared to a limited tooth numbering system used for human patients (see Figure 8.11.3). A three-digit number is assigned to each

Heidi Lobprise DVM, DAVDC **Main Street Veterinary Dental Clinic** Jessica Johnson, DVM, Dental Resident

Client name:			Client #:	**Presentation:**	
Patient name:		Sex:	Patient #:		
Date:		DOB:	Pain Score VAS: pre-operative:	post-operative:	ASA:
Breed:		Wt:			

Assessment:

Radiographs: ___Full ___Partial ___None

_____
_____
_____
_____
_____
_____

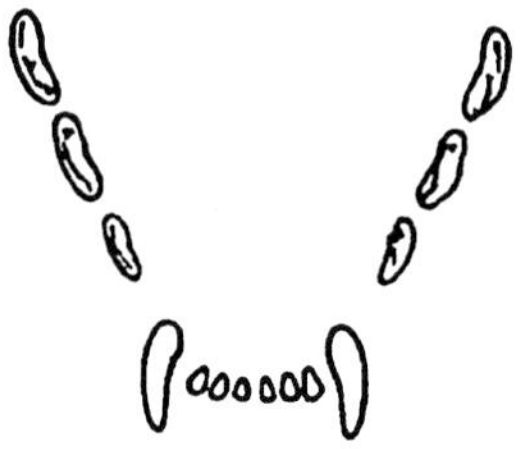

Treatment:

Clean/Polish/Fluoride ___Routine ___Extended

Periodontics	
Exodontics	
Oral Surgery	
Endodontics	
Other	
Comments:	

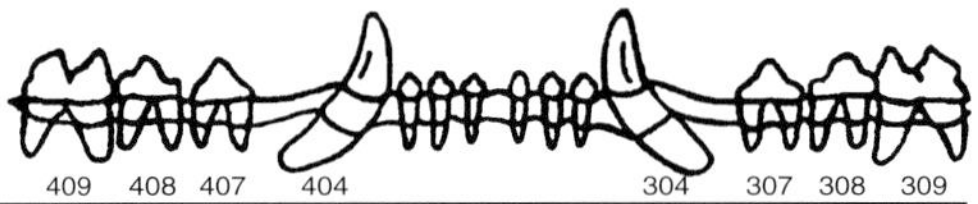

_____
_____
_____
_____
_____
_____
_____
_____
_____
_____
_____
_____
_____
_____
_____
_____
_____
_____
_____
_____
_____
_____
_____
_____
_____
_____

Peri-operative treatment:

Antibiotics:

Analgesia:

____ bupivacaine __epi ___buprenorphine mls

____ Nocita

Block	right - mls	left - mls
Infraorbital		
Caudal maxillary		
Inferior alveolar		
Mental		
local		

Diet: ____Normal ____ Soft _____

Recheck exam

Next Oral ATP
scheduled:

	GI																		
	CI																		
	PDI																		

109 108 107 106 104   204 206 207 208 209

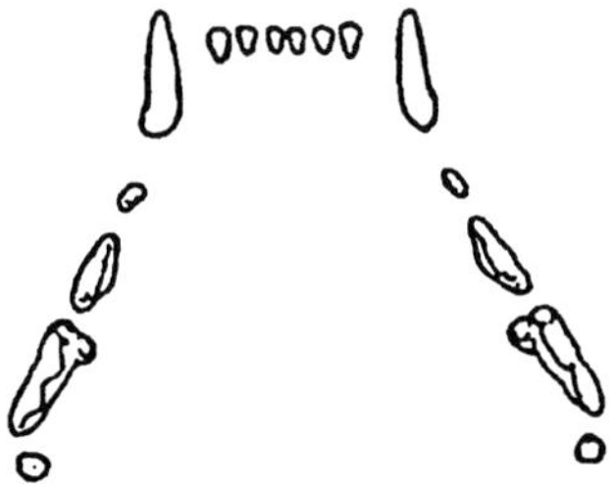

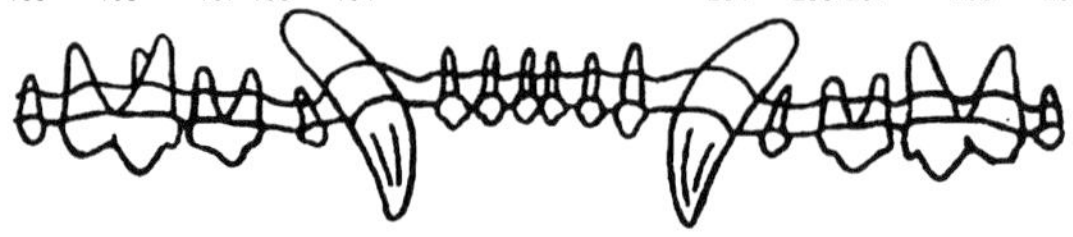

Maxilla

Right   Left

Mandible

409 408 407 404   304 307 308 309

GI											
CI											
PDI											

No sulcus or pocket probing greater than 1 mm

AVL alveoloplasty	**GE** ging enlargement	**MX** maxillary	**R/C** restoration w/ comp	**T/SN** supernumerary
AT attrition	**GR** gingival recession	**NV** non-vital	**RCT** root canal therapy	**T/U** unerupted tooth
B/E biopsy excisional	**GV** gingivoplasty	**OD** odontoplasty	**ROT** rotated	**TR** tooth resorption
B/I biopsy incisional	**M** mobile (1,2,3)	**OM** oral mass	**RP/C** root planing closed	**Type 1** inflammatory
BG bone graft	**MAL** malocclusion	**ONF** oronasal fistula	**RP/O** root planing open	**Type 2** odontoclastic
CR/A crown amput	**1** neutroclusion	**PD1** gingivitis only	**RTR** retained tooth root	**Type 3** - mixed
CTM cont to monitor	**2** mand distoclusion	**PD2** <25%attach loss	**SYM/S** symphseal sep	**VPT** vital pulp therapy
CWD crowding	**3** mand mesioclusion	**PD3** 25-50% attach loss	**T/FX** tooth fracture	**W** wedge incision
DT/P persistent decid	**MET** modified extraction	**PD4** >50% attach loss	**CCF** complicated crown fx	**X** extraction
E/D enamel defect	**Mi** missing circled	**PE** pulp exposure	**CCRF** compl crown root fx	**XS** extract section
FE furcation exposure	**MN** mandibular	**PP** periodontal pocket	**UCF** uncompl.crown fx	**XSS** extract surg

Figure 8.11.1 Feline dental chart.

Heidi Lobprise DVM, DAVDC **Main Street Veterinary Dental Clinic** Jessica Johnson, DVM Sr Resident

Client name:		Client #:	**Presentation:**	
Patient name:	Sex:	Patient #:		
Date:	DOB:	Pain Score VAS: pre-operative:	post-operative:	ASA:
Breed:	Wt:			

Assessment:

Radiographs: ___Full ___Partial ___None

_____
_____
_____
_____
_____
_____

Index	110	109	108	107	106	105	104	103	102	101	201	202	203	204	205	206	207	208	209	210
GI																				
CI																				
PDI																				

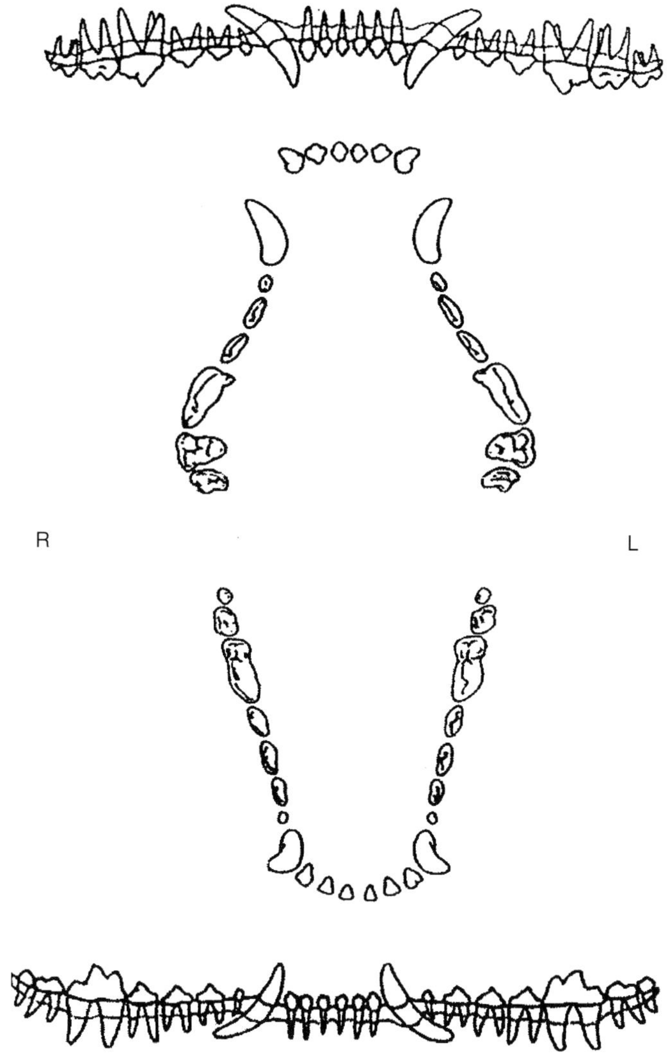

Treatment:

Clean/Polish/Fluoride ___Routine ___Extended

Periodontics _____
Exodontics _____
Oral Surgery _____
Endodontics _____
Other _____
Comments: _____

_____
_____
_____
_____
_____
_____
_____
_____
_____
_____
_____
_____
_____
_____
_____
_____
_____
_____
_____
_____
_____
_____
_____

R　　　　　　　　　　　　　　　　　　L

Peri-operative treatment:

Antibiotics: _____

Analgesia: _____

____ bupivacaine __epi ___buprenorphine

____ Nocita

GI													
CI													
PDI													
Index	411	410	409	408	407	406	405	404	403	402	401	301	302	303	304	305	306	307	308	309	310	311

Block	right	left
Infraorbital		
Caudal maxillary		
Inferior alveolar		
Mental		
local		

Diet: ____Normal ____ Soft

Recheck exam scheduled: _____

Next Oral ATP scheduled: _____

AB abrasion
AT attrition
B/E biopsy excisional
B/I biopsy incisional
BG bone graft
CR/A crown amput
CTM cont to monitor
CWD crowding
DT/P persistent decid
E/D enamel defect

FE furcation exposure
GE ging enlargement
GR gingival recession
GV gingivoplasty
M mobile (1,2,3)
MAL malocclusion
1 neutroclusion
2 mand distoclusion
3 mand mesioclusion
MET modified extraction

Mi missing circled
OD odontoplasty
OM oral mass
ONF oronasal fistula
PD1 gingivitis only
PD2 <25%attach loss
PD3 25-50% attach loss
PD4 >50% attach loss
PE pulp exposure
PRO perio prohylaxis

R/C restoration w/ comp
RCT root canal therapy
RP/C root planing closed
RP/O root planing open
RTR retained tooth root
SYM/S symphseal sep
T/FX tooth fracture
CCF complicated crown fx
CCRF compl crown root fx
UCF uncompl.crown fx

T/SN supernumerary
T/U uncrupted tooth
TR tooth resorption
Type 1 inflammatory
Type 2 odontoclastic
Type 3 - mixed
VPT vital pulp therapy
X extraction
XS extract section
XSS extract surg

Figure 8.11.2 Canine dental chart.

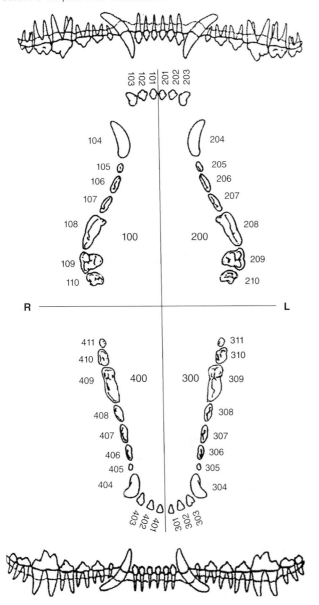

Figure 8.11.3 Modified Triadan Numbering.

tooth, with the "hundreds" place digit referring to the quadrant in the mouth.

100 – right maxilla (upper right)
200 – left maxilla (upper left)
300 – left mandible (lower left)
400 – left maxilla (lower right)

The "ones" and "tens" place digits correspond to the tooth placement within the quadrant, starting with the central incisors at the front midline and proceeding backwards around the head toward the molars.

_01, _02, _03 –	First, second, and third incisors
_04 –	Canine tooth
_05, _06, _07, _08	First, second, third, and fourth premolars
_09, _10, _11	First, second, and third molars

The large carnassial teeth (teeth for crunching) are the maxillary fourth premolars and mandibular first molars (108 and 208, 309, and 409). With up to 11 teeth per quadrant (3 incisors, 1 canine, 4 premolars and 3 M), the only perfectly full dentition is found in pigs. Dogs are missing their third upper molars (111, 211) and have 42 permanent teeth. Cats are missing their first upper premolars (105, 205) so 106 and 206 are the first "cheek teeth." They are also missing their first and second lower premolars (305, 306, 405, 406) so 307 and 407 are the first "cheek teeth." And finally, there are no second and third molars in all quadrants (110, 111, 210, 211, 310, 311, 411, 410) so 109 and 209 are the only upper molars and are very small while 309 and 409 are present, for a total of 30 teeth.

Deciduous teeth are numbered similarly except that you add 400 for each quadrant (500, 600, 700, and 800s), and there are no deciduous molars. The deciduous premolars are numbered (typically three per quadrant) from the back, e.g., 508, 507, 506, even though the last deciduous premolars have shapes similar to permanent first molar.

A SOAP style of medical record can be utilized with areas to record radiographic assessment, physical findings, assessment, and treatment provided. The most efficient way to denote these findings is "four-handed charting" with one person probing the teeth to determine periodontal pockets, GR (RE), missing teeth, etc. and calling out the measurements as a second person records the findings on the dental chart. With this coordinated effort, less anesthetic time is needed for the patient as the person examining the mouth does not have to stop to record the findings.

The extent of plaque and calculus should be recorded, either generally for the entire mouth or for individual teeth if there is a significant difference for them. The CI is commonly used. If the designation is CI 1 (C/sl), then there are slight deposits, scattered calculus covers less than one-third of the buccal (lateral) tooth surface. With moderate deposits, CI 2 (C/mod), calculus covers between one-third and two-thirds of the buccal tooth surface with minimal subgingival deposition. Heavy calculus covering greater than two-thirds of the buccal tooth surface and extending subgingivally is recorded as CI 3 (C/h). The amount of accumulated plaque is recorded by using the PI. The extent is similar to CI with slight, moderate, and heavy levels recorded as PI 1, 2, and 3. This takes a disclosing solution to accurately assess so typically it is not as clinically relevant unless copious plaque is present and should be recorded.

Any obvious swelling, mass, or abnormality in the oral cavity should be recorded, as well as any gingival overgrowth or enlargement (hyperplasia). Periodontal probing is essential, and while complete probing and recording may seem to take time when first implemented, once it becomes a part of the routine procedure, it can be done quickly. Gently insert the periodontal probe into the sulcus space at six points around the tooth and record any depths greater than normal (periodontal pockets – PP) at 2–3 mm in dogs and 0.5 mm in cats. The probe is also used to measure any RE due to GR. Adding this number to the periodontal pocket is the true extent of AL, e.g., a GR of 2 mm with a PP of 3 mm is a total of 5 mm AL. If the GR in a multirooted tooth results in exposure of the space between the roots, the extent of FE is noted (see 4.9 Periodontal Disease).

The shepherd's hook end of the probe (explorer) can be used to see if a broken tooth has an open canal or to find TR, frequently seen in cats. A defect in the enamel at the gingival margin may indicate a TR; often the TR lesion is covered by an irregular area of gingiva growing into the defect space. It is important to look for this during a conscious oral examination, as it gives you the opportunity to inform the owner that a TR may be present. Their education will continue with a discussion of what a TR is, how it will be diagnosed, and potential treatment options. This will reduce the need to discuss this at length during the anesthetic procedure.

Dental radiographs are necessary to evaluate all teeth. The explorer tip will "hang-up" in the resorptive defect if present due to the acute, rough edges. If the explorer tip just glides along the area of a tooth furcation, it may just be mild FE and not a resorptive lesion. The type of TR should be recorded. The most common type of TR in cats is the odontoclastic lesion (Type 2) – formerly known as FORL – feline odontoclastic resorptive lesion (see Figure 8.11.4). The periodontal ligament is not visible radiographically as bone has transformed or replaced root structure. A modified extraction method (crown amputation) has been shown to be sufficient for these teeth, with an attempt at full elevation after sectioning the teeth. Typically, the crown will break off, leaving a portion of resorbing root. The alveolar bone should be smoothed, and the extraction site closed after extraction. When the client understands this is a surgical procedure, they may find the phrase "crown amputation" more palatable.

Inflammatory TR (Type 1) is less common (5–10% of TR lesions in cats) than Type 2 but it is critical to differentiate them radiographically as treatment is different. The periodontal ligament is still present at those areas of the root that are not resorbing (see Figure 8.11.5). This resorption is typically due to the inflammation of periodontal disease that resorbs exposed portions of the tooth/root. These teeth have to be completely extracted with no root portion left behind. TR lesions may also be evident in dogs. It is imperative to radiograph these teeth to determine the best treatment.

Gently "palpate" the tooth to see if there is any mobility and record. If there is significant mobility, this is an indication that there is either substantial periodontal AL or a fractured root/crown. An attempt to periodontally treat mobile teeth is typically not very successful. There can be minor physiological mobility up to 0.2 mm (M0), with M1 indicating an increase in any mobility that is more than 0.2 mm but less than 0.5 mm. With a further increase in mobility of more than 0.5 mm and up to 1.0 mm, M2 is charted. M3 will refer to extensive mobility greater than 1.0 mm in any direction.

Document any chipped, worn, or fractured teeth denoting attrition (AT) and tooth fracture (T/FX). If the canal is exposed, mark it as a complicated crown fracture (CCF). A fractured tooth without canal exposure is considered non-complicated (uncomplicated (dental) crown fracture [UCF]), but the exposed dentin or initial injury can compromise the pulp, so a full evaluation (radiographs, transillumination) is still needed, along with monitoring the tooth in the future. If the tooth is discolored, does not transilluminate or has a wide canal, it may be nonvital (NV). Any tooth with a compromised pulp (open or NV) needs to be extracted or have a root canal procedure performed.

Circle any missing tooth, once radiographs are taken, to make sure it is truly missing and not just unerupted. Unerupted teeth can develop into a dentigerous cyst. If the

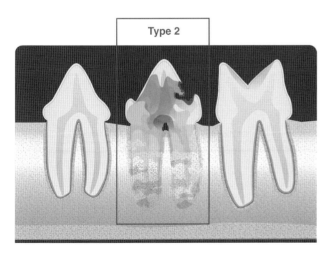

Figure 8.11.4 Type 2 TR.

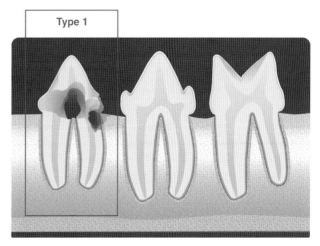

Figure 8.11.5 Type 1 TR.

roots are still present (retained), designate this by RTR. Note any crowded (CWD) or rotated (ROT) teeth as these could contribute to periodontal disease.

Overgrowth of gingival tissue can be identified by drawing in the extent of gingival enlargement (GE), and the treatment of gingivoplasty (GVP – trimming the excess gum tissue away) can also be recorded. Areas of inflammation, an oral mass (OM) or even osseous fracture can be drawn into the chart to specify location and extent. Specific treatments can also be charted, such as placing an X on the tooth to indicate it was extracted, or marking GVP for gingivoplasty of GE.

TAKE-AWAYS

- Use consistent terminology and abbreviations and markings for clear communication.
- Use full-page, two-view charting; have an abbreviation listing on the chart.
- Do four-handed charting to minimize the patient's anesthesia time.
- Combine the chart with oral photos and intraoral radiographs to provide a complete record.

- Consider converting forms to an electronic version with a "drawable" format.

MISCELLANEOUS

8.11.3 Cautions

- Ensure your writing is legible – there will be a lot to write down in a small space for complicated cases.

Recommended Reading

Lobprise, H.B. and Dodd, J.R. (2019). *Wiggs's Veterinary Dentistry, Principles and Practice*, 2e. Philadelphia: Blackwell.

Lobprise, H.B. (2007). *Five Minute Veterinary Consult: Clinical Companion – Small Animal Dentistry*, 2e. Philadelphia: Wiley-Blackwell.

Eisner, E.R., Holmstrom, S.E., and Frost, F.P. (2004). *Veterinary Dental Techniques for the Small Animal Practitioner*, 3e. Philadelphia: Saunders https://avdc.org/avdc-nomenclature/.

8.12

Preventing Animal-Related Injuries

Betsy Choder, JD, MS

VetCounsel LLC, Crown Pointe Parkway, Atlanta, GA, USA

BASICS

8.12.1 Summary

Every person who owns or works around animals is considered to have assumed the risks of being potentially injured – whether from an animal's kick, bite, scratch, or even an infectious zoonotic disease resulting from an animal's secondary sources (such as bacteria and viruses within its secretions or the bites from fleas and ticks). There are numerous ways by which domesticated and wild animals can inflict injury or harm to people, property, and other animals – regardless if the animal is acting playfully, in aggression, out of fear or simply through physical proximity. Even though a veterinarian's liability or an animal owner's liability might be at issue when injuries or damages occur to people and property, this discussion will be limited solely to ways to prevent or minimize being injured by animals at the workplace.

8.12.2 Terms Defined

Personal Protective Equipment (PPE): Any type of clothing or items used to protect an animal handler (and potentially the animal itself) from physical and health hazards. PPE includes specialized/disposable clothing, gloves, masks, protective eyewear, catchpoles, restraints, nets, prods, and other items.

Zoonotic: (Pertaining to zoonoses) a disease that can be transmitted from animals to humans; a disease that normally exists in animals but can infect humans by various routes of transmission such as contaminated needlesticks, blood-sucking insects, contact with bodily secretions, or injuries through bites/kicks/scratches.

MAIN CONCEPTS

8.12.3 Prevent Injuries by Maintaining a Safe Working Environment

In addition to being the legal duty and responsibility of the veterinary practice owner, ensuring a safe working environment for employees is essential (see 7.2 Managing the Pet-Specific Workplace). Employers are responsible for identifying workplace hazards, providing employees with proper training and protective equipment, and notifying all who enter the workplace with visible posted warning signs of potential hazards. Each workplace should also have a written safety communications manual, available to all personnel and volunteers, regarding precautions for all types of potential hazards that might be encountered, including nonanimal-related injuries.

The Occupational Safety and Health Administration (OSHA) imposes strict safety regulations on American workplaces. Although the OSHA does not address animal-related injuries directly, veterinary employers are responsible for workplace safety under the OSHA's "General Duty Clause." The broadly written clause requires an employer to "furnish to each of his employees employment and a place of employment which are free from recognized hazards that are causing or are likely to cause death or serious physical harm to employees" and, as such, veterinary employers should take proactive measures to maintain a safe working

Pet-Specific Care for the Veterinary Team, First Edition. Edited by Lowell Ackerman.
© 2021 John Wiley & Sons, Inc. Published 2021 by John Wiley & Sons, Inc.

environment. Proactive measures to minimize or prevent animal-related injuries include the following.

- *Workplace design:* Maximize available areas for placement and separation of animal cages/crates/stalls while minimizing the potential for an animal's increased stress or direct contact with other animals. It is essential to create areas for physical quarantine or separation of animals with special needs, such as those with immune-suppressed, infectious, or highly aggressive tendencies. Make clear notations in the medical record and post highly visible signs in the areas/cage/stall to warn other personnel of contagious, aggressive, fractious, or diseased animals.

- *Educate and train all personnel (including volunteers) on a continual regular basis:* Educating, training, and ensuring that all personnel adhere to safety precautions while properly approaching, handling, restraining, and treating animals is essential in a veterinary workplace. Educate all nonveterinarian personnel on animal pathogens and their transmissions. Train staff on techniques for "stress-free" methods of handling animals when able. Have policies to ensure that doors are closed and signs are clearly visible to areas where clients cannot enter, PPE is used whenever needed, and that cages/crates/stalls are securely latched to prevent animals from escaping or causing injury. Every workplace's management team should establish a culture of safety at the workplace for humans, animals, and property.

- *Use and training of PPE:* Effective training for the use of PPE is essential for every employee and volunteer in any veterinary practice. This includes training on appropriate use, putting on, taking off, and, if applicable, disposing of the protective item. (TIP: Train employees to sterilize, or dispose of PPE that has come in contact with any type of animal secretions – urine, blood, saliva, or nasal discharge – especially before handling any other animal with the same PPE.)

- *Avoid cross-contamination:* Training and adherence to prevent cross-contamination through constant disinfectant/sanitation practices is essential. All personnel should be advised to wash their hands frequently and disinfect cages/exam tables after each use, especially after coming in contact with or being exposed to an animal's saliva, blood, feces, or urine. Consider having a workplace policy that requires employees to have a second set of clothing/scrubs at the workplace or to wear PPE to avoid potential cross-contamination between animals and humans.

- *Seek medical care (compliance with state workers' compensation laws):* Depending on each jurisdiction's laws, injured employees working at veterinary facilities are oftentimes entitled, yet limited solely to receiving compensation for their injuries through the state workers' compensation system, without imposing blame or fault, as long as the injury "arises out of and in the course of employment." Employers should be aware of their state's workers' compensation requirements, including having an injured employee seek immediate medical care, regardless of how minor the injury might appear. Educate employees that even a small scratch can have serious consequences if a bacterium or virus enters the human body through the broken skin.

8.12.4 Preventing Injuries to Employees

Employees working at a veterinary facility are considered to have knowingly assumed the risks that might arise from animal-related injuries. Generally, if an animal-related injury occurs to an employee at a veterinary clinic, courts have held that employers/practice owners are not necessarily legally responsible for damages or injuries. Yet, in some situations, employers might be required to proactively advise employees who have immune-suppressed conditions or physical limitations (such as impaired use of limbs or mobility) to consult with their healthcare provider about potential hazards (such as zoonotic diseases and animal handling), to receive a physician's signed notice for "consent to work" in a veterinary facility. Depending upon the particular facts and circumstances, unless undue hardship to the employer would occur, practice owners might be required to provide reasonable accommodations for the employee to continue his or her employment.

8.12.5 Owner's/Possessor's Responsibilities

Under numerous laws, the owner (or possessor) of animals has a duty to prevent injuries or damages from occurring to other persons or property, by exercising reasonable care to keep their animal(s) under control at all times. This "control" can be achieved by ensuring the animal is restrained by a leash, a crate or a securely gated area, yet without harming the animal's safety and well-being.

8.12.6 Preventing Injuries to Client

Unlike employees, clients do not necessarily assume all risks of injuries from their own animals or other animals when visiting a veterinary facility (see 7.11 Client Safety).

In efforts to prevent any client from being injured, the following warnings and restrictions should be made.

- Take steps to ensure clients do not venture into clinical areas, or approach caged animals, in order to minimize the risks of potential injuries. Post visible warning signs on doors such as "Employees Only Beyond this Point" or "Please Keep your Pet on a Leash or in a Crate at All Times" in the lobby area or "Will Bite" on cages in the workplace.
- Advise clients about keeping their children safe. Request clients' children to remain with their parents at all times – and not to approach other clients' pets or animals' cages.
- Ask clients to allow trained employees to hold/restrain animals during examination. Unless a client's animal is known to attack or bite others when restrained by anyone other than the owner/guardian, request that the animal be handled by your trained staff (see 7.12 Patient Safety). If a client prefers to handle their own animal without relinquishing control, consider having them sign a waiver, releasing the veterinarian/clinic from liability for any potential injury by the animal that might occur to the client as a result of his/her choice.

TIP: In cases of known aggressive animal patients, request the owner's permission to (or have the owner) provide a mild sedative to the animal prior to the veterinarian's examination. Alternatively, there are "stress free" or "fear free" handling techniques that have been shown to reduce the fear and anxiety of animals without the use of medication (see 6.6 Fear Free Concepts). However, caution is still advised when handling animals, especially those that might be ill, frightened, or have fractious tendencies.

8.12.7 Educate Clients and Employees about the Potential Spread of Zoonotic Diseases

In further attempts to minimize injuries from animals, a veterinarian (or trained professional) should take the time to educate and warn nonveterinarian employees (as well as clients) about potential risks associated with zoonotic disease transmissions, especially while treating poultry, swine, reptiles, avians, equines, or companion animals (see 4.4 Preventing Infectious Diseases in the Small Animal Veterinary Hospital). People with suppressed immune systems (elderly, infants, and those with medical issues that affect their immune system) have a higher risk potential. Many types of zoonotic diseases can be fatal to humans, such as animal influenzas, anthrax, rabies, plague, and salmonella.

8.12.8 Conclusion

Animals can inflict many injuries on humans and other animals both directly (such as biting and scratching) and indirectly (such as transmitting disease-carrying bacteria or viruses). Incorporating physical barriers within the workplace with ongoing safety training protocols as well as promoting use of common-sense awareness into your daily workplace routines will help reduce the possibility of injuries and the potential for loss of productivity in your workforce, as well as preventing the potential for injuries from animals.

TAKE-AWAYS

- Prevent animal-related injuries from occurring at the workplace by maintaining a culture of safety, cleanliness, education, and training protocols for all personnel.
- Take proactive measures with clients such as posting visible warning notices (such as hazardous areas or to maintain control of their animals and their children) and educating clients on potential zoonotic diseases at home.
- Educate employees on the various pathogens that can be transmitted from animals to humans while working at a veterinary facility – and how to prevent potential exposure while handling animals.
- Use, and require the use of, PPE whenever appropriate.
- Maintain physical separation of animals, especially those with contagious, immune-suppressed or fractious qualities.

MISCELLANEOUS

8.12.9 Cautions

Design or arrange common areas to reduce the possibility of animal-to-animal (or animal-to-child/client) interactions such as using barriers/walls surrounding seating areas or having separate entrances for client intake and checkout. Reported cases have shown that animals housed together in the familiar surroundings of their home environment may attack one another when placed in strange surroundings, especially if together in same area, same cage at boarding facility or in same corral at shows. Exercise precautionary measures to minimize potential for aggressive behavior when allowing animals to socialize in unfamiliar surroundings.

Recommended Reading

Choder, B. (2020). Animal-related injuries at the workplace. In: *Five-Minute Veterinary Practice Management Consult*, 3e (ed. L. Ackerman), 772–775. Ames, IA: Wiley.

National Association of State Public Health Veterinarians/ Veterinary Infection Control Committee (2015).

Compendium of veterinary standard precautions for zoonotic disease prevention in veterinary personnel. *J. Am. Vet. Med. Assoc.* 247 (11): 1252–1277. www.nasphv.org/ Documents/VeterinaryStandardPrecautions.pdf.

8.13

Hospice and Palliative Care

Mary Craig, DVM, MBA, CHPV

Gentle Goodbye Veterinary Hospice and At-home Euthanasia, Stamford, CT, USA

BASICS

8.13.1 Summary

Animal hospice, a philosophy of care that addresses the end of life care of the pet, as well as the needs of the human caregiver, is an evolving movement that harnesses the skills and abilities of an interdisciplinary team (IDT). It includes palliative care, but also anticipates the needs of the caregivers to honor the relationship and enhance the human–animal bond, especially at the end of life.

8.13.2 Terms Defined

Activities of Daily Living (ADL**):** Daily activities that a patient normally performs (related to hygiene, exercise, play, eating and drinking, etc.) and which may require support in order to maintain quality of life (QOL).

Animal Hospice: A philosophy and/or a program of care that addresses the physical, emotional, and social needs of animals in the advanced stages of a progressive, life-limiting illness or disability as well as the mental health of the human caregivers in preparation for the death of the pet and subsequent grief.

End of Life Care: Care provided to attend to the physical, emotional, and social needs of patients in the final hours or days of their lives and, more broadly, of all patients with a terminal condition that has become advanced, progressive and incurable.

Euthanasia: The intentional termination of life through humane, AVMA-approved methods that cause as little pain, discomfort, and anxiety as possible, for the purpose of relieving an animal's suffering. The term *euthanasia* comes from the Greek words "eu" (good) and "thanatos" (death).

IDT: A transdisciplinary approach crosses disciplinary boundaries to create a holistic, collaborative, and unified team.

Palliative Care: Treatment which supports or improves the patient's QOL by relieving suffering. This term can be used when treating curable or chronic conditions, as well as during end of life care.

QOL: Quality of life refers to the total well-being of an individual animal, taking into account the physical, social, and emotional components of the animal's life.

Suffering: An unpleasant or painful experience, feeling, emotion, or sensation, which may be acute or chronic in nature. Suffering is an umbrella term that covers the range of negative subjective experiences, including (but not limited to) physical and emotional pain and distress, which may be experienced by humans and by animals.

MAIN CONCEPTS

Because pets are increasingly part of the family, it's to be expected that caregivers demand a high level of medical care for their pets. Animal hospice and palliative care, modeled after human healthcare, are a natural progression.

In all species, palliative care and hospice care are related but not the same. Palliative care can occur at all stages of life, but is especially important at end of life. It is patient-focused care to improve QOL. It might include pain control, hydration support, antinausea treatment, acupuncture, etc. Although not often named, it is a concept well understood by most veterinary care teams.

Hospice care, on the other hand, includes palliative care, but goes beyond the patient to also care for the caregiver's psychological, emotional, social, and spiritual needs, through the dying process and after the death. A fundamental guiding principle of hospice is that the patient and the family are the basic unit of care. Animal hospice often provides an option between aggressive medical intervention and immediate euthanasia. When "there's nothing else we can do," there is hospice.

8.13.3 When is Hospice the Right Choice?

Hospice isn't the right choice for all patients or all caregivers. It might be right for a patient if:

- there is a diagnosis of a terminal illness
- the decision has been made not to pursue a curative treatment
- there is a chronic illness that interferes with ADL
- curative treatment has failed
- there is a progressive illness or trauma with life-limiting health complications.

There are certain diseases and conditions that make hospice challenging. It's important, when discussing disease trajectory, to stress the unpredictable nature of disease. Diseases involving the heart, lungs, and central nervous system can take dramatic downturns and quickly become medical emergencies. If the goal of a caregiver is to avoid such an emergency, he or she might need to decide on euthanasia before the situation is critical to ensure a more controlled, peaceful passing for their pet.

Hospice also requires resources on the caregiver's part – financial, emotional, and time. For some families, there is not enough of one or more of these resource buckets to go down the hospice path. Picture the family with three small children and two working parents. It is important to discuss family dynamics and household limitations.

8.13.4 The Five Steps to a Hospice Plan

1) Asking questions and listening to the caregiver's needs, beliefs, and goals, especially as they relate to past experiences with hospice, other pets' deaths, and what they want for this pet.
2) Education about the disease process to better understand possible/probable trajectories so a caregiver can make good decisions for their pet.
3) Development of a mutually agreed personalized plan of care for the pet and caregiver.

4) Application of palliative or hospice care techniques for the rest of the pet's life with the understanding that revisions, additions, and adaptations may be needed as the disease progresses.
5) Emotional support during the care process and after death.

8.13.5 The Interdisciplinary Team (IDT)

Because the skills required to deliver hospice care extend well beyond medicine, it should and often does involve an IDT. Under the supervision of a licensed veterinarian, the IDT of providers works together to support patients and their caregivers through the dying process and after the death.

The core of the ideal IDT is the hospice veterinarian, the referring veterinarian, a veterinary technician/nurse, and a mental health professional. As needed, others may include:

- providers of physical rehabilitation
- integrated medicine practitioners
- compounding pharmacists
- massage therapists
- acupuncturists
- chaplains and spiritual counselors
- advanced pet sitters
- community volunteers.

While some of the IDT team members might be in employee relationships, most people working in animal hospice today are small businesses or volunteers that form a referral network to care for hospice families.

8.13.6 Is Hospice Instead of Euthanasia?

The hospice philosophy doesn't *preclude* euthanasia, but it does take an approach to palliative care and assessing QOL that often delays euthanasia significantly without significant suffering.

Hospice can fill a gap in care and help caregivers get to an honest place where they can let go. It's important for everyone involved to understand that there may come a point when hospice is no longer an appropriate choice if we are not effectively keeping a pet comfortable and avoiding suffering. In some cases, we're providing hospice to try to get to some finite point. It may be a college break or the end of a business trip or just getting used to a diagnosis.

The four principles of *human* hospice ethics are as follows.

1) Dying is a meaningful experience.
2) Family-centered care is more appropriate.
3) Address all aspects of suffering and protect the integrity of the patient.
4) Honor what patients find valuable and meaningful.

If we look at the death of our four-legged family members through this lens, we can more authentically honor the place they hold in our lives.

Currently, the International Association for Animal Hospice and Palliative Care (IAAHPC) offers certification programs for veterinarians and veterinary technicians, as well as a certificate program for social workers to give individuals access to advanced training in the area of hospice and palliative care.

EXAMPLES

Wally is a 13-year-old neutered male Jack Russell terrier who lived with Susan, his caregiver, a widow and a registered nurse. He was diagnosed with a renal tumor of unknown type. His nervous nature and complete unwillingness to take pills of any type lead Susan to decline surgery or further diagnostics. Susan enlisted a mobile hospice veterinarian to help them both through an unknown path forward. At the initial visit, Susan explained that she waited too long with her last dog and she didn't want Wally to die frightened at an emergency hospital. The plan they agreed on included symptomatic care as signs became apparent, emergency injectable sedation medications in case there was a crisis, and a support system for Susan that included a skilled pet sitter so she could take a long-planned family vacation, and her existing psychotherapist who was compassionate about anticipatory grief. One year later, Wally was still doing well. He had blood in his urine, but was comfortable on compounded palatable pain medication and an occasional injection of antinausea medication and still enjoyed romps on the beach and barking at the mail man.

TAKE-AWAYS

- When there is nothing else to do, there *is* something more we can do – animal hospice.
- Ideally, hospice involves an IDT to address patient needs as well as caregiver needs.
- While hospice doesn't preclude euthanasia, it often delays it until a point where patient comfort can't be maintained.
- Preparing a hospice plan requires questions and listening that delve deep into the bond shared by the human and animal.
- There is now advanced training for veterinarians, technicians, and social workers in hospice and palliative care.

MISCELLANEOUS

Recommended Reading

Gaynor, J. and Muir, W. (2008). *Handbook of Veterinary Pain Management*, 2e. St Louis, MO: Elsevier.

Pope, G. (2015). *The BrightHaven Guide to Animal Hospice*. Archangel Ink.

A.Shanan, T.Shearer, J.Pierce. *Hospice and Palliative Care for Companion Animals: Principles and Practice*: Wiley-Blackwell, Oxford, 2017

Shearer, T.S. (2011). Palliative medicine and hospice care. *Veterinary Clinics of North America: Small Animal Practice* 41 (3).

Guidelines for Recommended Practices in Animal Hospice and Palliative Care www.iaahpc.org/resources-and-support/practice-guidelines.html

8.14

Appropriate Handling of Medical Errors

Ryane E. Englar, DVM, DABVP (CANINE AND FELINE PRACTICE)

College of Veterinary Medicine, University of Arizona, Oro Valley, AZ, USA

 BASICS

8.14.1 Summary

Medical errors are infrequently discussed in veterinary practice. Few reports in the current literature describe their incidence; however, they do occur and they have the potential to cause harm, if not death, to our patients. When errors arise, they may result from cognitive limitations or system failures. As scientific knowledge advances at an accelerating rate, it may be difficult for the veterinary practitioner to maintain competency across all fields. Human error is unavoidable, and may be exacerbated by stress or decision making in emergency scenarios. Drug-based errors and communication mishaps have a substantial impact on patient care. As we, as a profession, come to terms with the reality of medical error in veterinary practice, we need to address how to manage actions on our part that endanger our patients' lives.

8.14.2 Terms Defined

Adverse Incident: A medical error that harms the patient.
Harmless Hit: A medical error that occurs, but does not harm the patient.
Near Miss: Any circumstance in which the patient would have been harmed had the medical error reached the patient.
Unsafe Condition: Any circumstance that puts a patient's safety in jeopardy.

 MAIN CONCEPTS

8.14.3   Incidence of Medical Errors in Veterinary Practice

Medical errors in human healthcare are well documented. More patients die annually from preventable medical errors than automobile accidents [1]. These statistics are less accessible in veterinary medicine because reports of error in practice are not available at the national or global level. Isolated reports suggest that medical error in the veterinary profession is more common than was once believed.

In 2004, Mellanby and Herrtage investigated the incidence of medical mistakes among recent veterinary graduates in the United Kingdom. Seventy-eight percent of survey respondents reported that they had committed at least one error or omission that negatively impacted patient care [2]. These mistakes incited feelings of guilt, stress, distress, or depression in some, but not all, respondents [2].

In the United States, a 2019 study by Wallis et al. examined reports of medical error among three veterinary practices. Between February 2015 and March 2018, 560 incident reports were identified [3]. This translated into roughly five errors every 1000 patient visits [3]. Forty-five percent of errors were relatively harmless [3]. Fifteen percent were classified as adverse incidents [3]. Adverse incidents were more likely to be reported at teaching hospitals than private practice referral or emergency hospitals [3]. Teaching hospitals were also more likely to harbor unsafe conditions [3]. Less than 2% of reported incidents caused permanent harm or death [3].

8.14.4 Causes of Medical Error in Veterinary Practice

Medical errors result from either cognitive limitations or system failures [4]. The former refers to deficiencies of the individual, whereas the latter reflects the deficiencies of the work environment.

Humans are inherently fallible. Our attention is easily diverted, and our memories are often faulty [4, 5]. This results in mistakes, even when tasks have been rehearsed.

System failures compound these deficiencies [4]. The environment must be conducive to constructive decision making. Otherwise, patient care suffers.

Efficient leadership and effective communication are also critical to patient outcomes [4, 6]. In addition, stress of production and ergonomic design impact the healthcare team's ability to perform well [4]. Failure of any one of the above sets the stage for one or more medical errors.

The most common type of medical error relates to drug dosing or administration [3]. The appropriate drug may be delivered at the wrong dose or at the wrong time, to the wrong patient, or via an inappropriate route [3].

Communication failures are second to drug-based errors [3]. Handwritten medical notes or treatment sheets may be misread. Verbal instructions may be misheard or misinterpreted.

Other types of medical error stem from [2–4, 6]:

- equipment failures
- failure to administer a prescribed treatment or perform an appropriate diagnostic test
- insufficient staffing or training
- lack of established standard operating procedures (SOP)
- misinterpretation of diagnostic tests
- misplaced or mislabeled patient biosamples
- procedural complications, such as retained surgical instruments.

8.14.5 Appropriate Handling of Medical Errors

Errors in healthcare can be reduced, but not eliminated. To reduce medical error in veterinary practice, we need to first accept and recognize that it occurs.

Recognition requires team members to self-reflect upon their actions and to exhibit transparency within a safe, constructive learning environment. Teammates must be willing to cast aside blame to focus on common ground – how to develop and implement error reduction strategies.

The old-school approach of denying medical errors is no longer applicable or relevant to today's veterinary practice.

Medical errors should be disclosed to the veterinary team and the client, and considered as teachable moments rather than badges of shame (see 7.12 Patient Safety).

Disclosure of medical errors is difficult; however, it is essential for all affected parties to move forward and heal. Disclosure of medical errors is supported by the American Veterinary Medical Association (AVMA) and Professional Liability Insurance Trust (PLIT) [7]. Given that the majority of state veterinary board complaints are due to perceived deficiencies in communication, it stands to reason that more effectively addressing veterinary medical errors should improve the veterinary–client relationship and work toward rebuilding trust [6].

Several communication models help veterinary teams to discuss medical errors with clients, including the acronym TEAM [8].

- "T" stands for truth, teamwork, and transparency.
- "E" stands for empathy.
- "A" stands for apology and accountability.
- "M" stands for management.

Our profession owes clients the truth. Clients have a right to know what happened to the patient, when, how, and why.

When medical errors are disclosed, clients are likely to question our competence or our actions. It is important that we resist the urge to become defensive. Defensiveness is instinctual; however, medical errors are not about self-preservation, they are about full disclosure.

We owe it to our clients to hear them share their experience with us. We need to see the impact of the error from their perspective.

We also owe our clients answers. We need to address concerns about how the error has impacted patient care and the anticipated consequences.

In situations that involve harmless hits or near misses, it may be tempting to minimize the medical error. However, this is inappropriate and invalidates the client's concerns about what *could* have happened.

Empathy is essential to conversations concerning medical error. So, too, is taking responsibility for the error and holding ourselves accountable [8]. Clients may be relieved to hear that attempts will be made to fix a broken system [8].

EXAMPLES

- You complete a routine castration on a 6-month-old Border collie dog, only to find that the dog presented instead for bilateral rear dewclaw removal.

- You are performing a laparotomy on a 9-month-old Great Dane dog to retrieve the abdominally located, left cryptorchid testicle. When you enter the abdominal wall via a midline incision, you inadvertently nick the urinary bladder, which was full, despite your request that it be emptied after induction of general anesthesia.
- You hospitalize a canine patient for pancreatitis, with orders that an appropriate dose of Cerenia® (maropitant citrate; 10 mg/mL) be administered subcutaneously. Your technician inadvertently administers an equivalent dose of Convenia® via the same route because the bottles are approximately the same size and are housed next to each other on the refrigerator shelf.

TAKE-AWAYS

- The veterinary profession is not immune to medical errors.
- Medical errors result from the fallibility of people and unsafe conditions.
- Drug dosing and administration, and communication-based errors are most common.
- Medical errors should be disclosed to all affected parties, with the intention of transparency, in an effort to repair client trust.
- Medical errors can be reduced if veterinary teams are willing to acknowledge and address them within a safe and constructive working environment.

MISCELLANEOUS

8.14.6 Cautions

When medical errors happen, the damage to the patient may be irreversible. It is possible that the veterinary team can rebuild trust with the client; however, repairing the relationship is not guaranteed. Clients may decide to transfer veterinary care to another provider. Clients may share their story on social media, casting you or the practice in an unfavorable light. Clients may even pursue litigation. You cannot control the client's reaction to the news of a medical error. All you can control is your response to the situation. Seek counsel from your liability insurer as needed to help you and your practice navigate uncharted waters.

References

1 Kohn, L.T., Corrigan, J., and Donaldson, M.S. (2000). *To Err Is Human: Building a Safer Health System.* Washington, DC: National Academy Press.

2 Mellanby, R.J. and Herrtage, M.E. (2004). Survey of mistakes made by recent veterinary graduates. *Vet. Rec.* 155: 761–765.

3 Wallis, J., Fletcher, D., Bentley, A. et al. (2019). Medical errors cause harm in veterinary hospitals. *Front. Vet. Sci.* 6: 12.

4 Oxtoby, C., Ferguson, E., White, K. et al. (2015). We need to talk about error: causes and types of error in veterinary practice. *Vet. Rec.* 177: 438.

5 Reason, J. (1995). Understanding adverse events: human factors. *Qual. Health Care* 4: 80–89.

6 Kinnison, T., Guile, D., and May, S.A. (2015). Errors in veterinary practice: preliminary lessons for building better veterinary teams. *Vet. Rec.* 177: 492.

7 Elkins, A.D. (2011). Veterinary medical errors: tell the truth, do it quickly. *DVM 360* www.dvm360.com/view/veterinary-medical-errors-tell-truth-do-it-quickly.

8 House, A.M. (2014). Breaking the silence: disclosing medical errors. *AAEP Proc.* 60: 270–272.

Recommended Reading

Kinnison, T., Guile, D., and May, S.A. (2015). Errors in veterinary practice: preliminary lessons for building better veterinary teams. *Vet. Rec.* 177 (19): 492.

Mellanby, R.J. and Herrtage, M.E. (2004). Survey of mistakes made by recent veterinary graduates. *Vet. Rec.* 155 (24): 761–765.

Oxtoby, C., Ferguson, E., White, K. et al. (2015). We need to talk about error: causes and types of error in veterinary practice. *Vet. Rec.* 177 (17): 438.

Wallis, J., Fletcher, D., Bentley, A., and Ludders, J. (2019). Medical errors cause harm in veterinary hospitals. *Front. Med. Sci.* 6 (12): 1–7.

8.15

Delivering Information to Clients

Brandon Hess, CVPM, CCFP

VetSupport Inc., Cincinnati, OH, USA

BASICS

8.15.1 Summary

A lot of the work that veterinary professionals do is transactional. In order to drive compliance, the value in the recommendations has to be seen. The value that is shown to clients is in the form of how it impacts them and their pet, knowledge, and/or tangible resources. All of this plays into the perceived value that the client gets from the visit. Aside from gaining compliance with clients, the other challenging communication scenario is discussing bad news. In both of these situations, empathy is a consistent need. The golden rule of communication is: speak to others the way they want to be communicated with.

8.15.2 Terms Defined

Compliance: Following through with a recommendation.
Emotional Intelligence: The capacity to perceive, assess, and positively influence one's own and other people's emotions.
Perceived Value: What someone feels they have gotten (not always financial) in return for money they have paid.

MAIN CONCEPTS

8.15.3 General Communication

Consistency in practice communication with clients is a constant battle. Not only is conveying a recommendation difficult at times, but gaining acceptance of that recommendation

is the next challenge. Communication styles differ from person to person, as does emotional intelligence, and with that comes differences in how people hear and retain information (see 8.5 How Important is Emotional Intelligence?). There are some basic aspects of communication that should be taken into consideration: verbal, nonverbal, and paraverbal.

Verbal communication is literally the words that are said. When dealing with clients, especially in stressful situations, it's important to speak clearly, using words they can understand. When too much medical terminology is used, the client can get lost in the situation and not always absorb what is being said. If there is a lack of understanding, or something is said that upsets a person, the first place you will see it is in their nonverbal reactions. Nonverbal communication encompasses things like hand position, eye contact, posture, and leg position, to name a few. If a client is confused, it will generally be seen in the head position, eye brows or with unsolicited head nodding. In uncomfortable situations, people will use responses like this when they cannot (or do not) put their thoughts into words. Lastly, paraverbal communication is the pace, tone, pitch, and inflection that are used.

Naturally, people feel more connected with someone who reminds them of themselves. For instance, a slow speaker feels overwhelmed by a fast speaker. A person who talks in a low tone of voice will feel uneasy around someone who is a very loud speaker. Something as simple as the level of communication can be important; if a client is sitting down, they will be less overwhelmed by someone sitting on the same level (or lower) than them, rather than being "talked down to."

8.15.4 Gaining Compliance

The ultimate goal is that a client takes a recommendation that is provided to them. The most impactful approach is to explain the "why" behind a recommendation before getting into the "what" or "how." In a TED Talk by Simon Sinek, he makes a profound statement: "People don't buy WHAT you do, they buy WHY you do it" [1]. This concept can be applied to veterinary medicine very easily, and clients are more receptive to hearing why they should care about the recommendation rather than what it does. The value and price are important but the client disengages more quickly once they hear the price and they may not fully appreciate the value.

A better approach that will resound clearly with a client is to talk about the "why" first. Consider creating scripts for common recommendations, following the format below.

1) *Identify the goal*: Why is the recommendation being made? What are we trying to achieve or prevent?
2) *Explain what it does*: How does the potential issue impact the client and patient?
3) *Communicate the competitive edge*: How does the product or service do what it does, and prevent the potential issue?
4) *Engage with a question*: Ensure this is an open-ended question to maximize the chance of compliance.

Scripts should not be repeated word for word; rather, they should be thought of as guidelines for consistent key communication points. An example script regarding canine influenza vaccination could look like the following.

> I noticed that Fluffy is not currently vaccinated against canine influenza (commonly called canine flu). It is our goal to protect as many of our patients against this relatively new virus as possible (GOAL). Canine influenza has very similar symptoms to kennel cough (*Bordetella*) so it can often be thought to be something it is not. It is also spread from dog to dog in the same way, which is air-borne. Luckily, the vaccine we have protects against the most common strain of canine influenza (WHAT IT DOES). The vaccination process is the same as other vaccines and it will allow Fluffy to build up immunity to the virus if he/she were exposed (COMPETITIVE EDGE). We will do the initial vaccination today and then we would need to see him/her back in ___ weeks. We have Tuesday _____ or Thursday _____ available for the booster, which one would work best for you?

8.15.5   Breaking Bad News

While sensitivity should be used when telling a client unexpected or uncomfortable information, it is also unfair to be vague. Empathy for the client must be practiced at all times [2]. It is especially important to use clear and under-

standable words. Additionally, it is helpful to check in with the client to ensure they are understanding what is being said. One way to get a client to more effectively answer a question is to ask an open-ended question (see 9.2 Asking Good Questions). Instead of "Do you have any questions?" say "What questions do you have for me?" or "What questions can I answer for you?"

8.15.6   Technology and Communication

As technology continues to advance, it will be important to adapt to client expectations. Currently, social media is dominating marketing communication, but there are still many clients who like postcard reminders. While the dominating generations within the practice's client base continue to swing toward the technology-savvy, don't forget to diversify. Use email not only as a reminder platform but also to send medical records and marketing material. Smartphone apps are also becoming more popular, and boast a much higher open rate for push notifications than emails (see 5.13 Improving Client Engagement Through Technology). Telemedicine is another growing platform to convert phone conversations to healthcare for clients who are not able/willing to come into the clinic (see 2.5 Virtual Care (Telehealth)).

EXAMPLES

Mrs Smith, a long-time client at ABC Veterinary Hospital, calls and schedules an appointment for her dog Fluffy. She has noticed Fluffy limping over the last few weeks and thinks she may have something stuck in her paw. After taking a series of radiographs, Dr Enzweiler goes into the room to discuss the results. When entering the room, Dr Enzweiler sits down on the floor with Fluffy where he can make eye contact with Mrs Smith. He informs Mrs Smith that Fluffy seems to have osteosarcoma, which is a bone cancer. He clearly communicates the treatment options, and prognosis if no treatment is provided. Even though Mrs Smith is noticeably distraught, and doesn't say much through the conversation, Dr Enzweiler asks her what questions she has about the diagnosis or treatment options. Dr Enzweiler documents the recommendations and any approved treatment in the medical record. He also makes sure to send Mrs Smith home with documents that explain the condition in case she has questions after she gets home and thinks about it.

TAKE-AWAYS

- The golden rule of effective communication is: speak to others the way they want to be spoken to. You will have to adapt to the other person's communication styles.
- Practicing empathy and using emotional intelligence will dramatically improve the way someone is perceived.
- "People don't buy what you do, they buy why you do it." Clients want to understand the "why" behind any recommendation before being told the price.
- Showing clients what is being talked about, through tangible resources, will increase understanding and compliance.

- Creating scripts, and looking at them as guidelines, will increase the consistency of messaging to clients.

MISCELLANEOUS

References

1 Sinek, S. Start with Why – How Great Leaders Inspire Action. TEDxPugetSound. www.youtube.com/watch?v=u4ZoJKF_VuA&t=440s

2 Veteos Facebook Page. Real People, Real Stories. www.facebook.com/veteos/videos/398305467598205

8.16

Dealing with Compassion Fatigue and Burnout

JoAnna Pendergrass, DVM

Medical Writer, Sandy Springs, GA, USA

BASICS

8.16.1　Summary

Compassion fatigue and burnout are common occupational stressors in veterinary practice. The same compassion and empathy for animals that attract individuals to careers in veterinary medicine can also increase the likelihood of compassion fatigue, while the work demands of clinical practice make burnout a reality for many veterinary professionals.

Compassion fatigue and burnout have an impact on more than just the individual experiencing them. These wellness issues, when not effectively managed, can also negatively impact patient care and the overall performance of a veterinary practice. Thus, both individual coping strategies and organizational solutions are needed to successfully manage and prevent compassion fatigue and burnout within the veterinary community.

8.16.2　Terms Defined

Adaptive Coping:　Positive coping strategies that provide long-term stress management.
Burnout:　The endpoint of chronic exposure to a stressful work environment.
Compassion Fatigue:　Emotional and physical depletion due to the trauma of witnessing and relieving others' suffering.
Emotion-Focused Coping:　Coping strategies that address the emotional response to a problem.

Maladaptive Coping:　Negative coping strategies that provide only short-term stress relief.
Presenteeism:　The concept that describes being present at work but being ineffective due to poor physical or mental health.
Problem-Focused Coping:　Coping strategies that address the underlying cause of a problem.

MAIN CONCEPTS

The field of veterinary medicine attracts individuals who are passionate about animal care and have high levels of compassion and empathy. Veterinarians and veterinary nurses alike often find their work rewarding and derive great satisfaction from caring for animals. However, this same compassion and empathy can increase the risk of compassion fatigue. Also, the fast-paced, high-demand environment of veterinary practice can eventually take its toll and lead to burnout.

Compassion fatigue and burnout, although similar, are not interchangeable. In broad terms, compassion fatigue results from the *type* of work being performed, while burnout is due to the work environment itself. Veterinary teams also experience compromise fatigue, which is yet another stressor (see 8.17 Dealing with Compromise Fatigue).

When left unacknowledged and unmanaged, compassion fatigue and burnout can seriously compromise an individual's physical, mental, and emotional health. In addition, compassion fatigue and burnout can negatively affect patient care and the overall performance of a veterinary practice.

8.16.3 Compassion Fatigue

The term "compassion fatigue," also known as secondary traumatic stress or vicarious traumatization, was first coined in 1992 by Carla Joinson [1], who used the term to characterize symptoms experienced by emergency room nurses. Compassion fatigue results from emotional and physical depletion from continual exposure to, and the relief of, others' suffering.

Veterinary professionals are at particularly high risk of developing compassion fatigue. Many situations in veterinary clinical practice contribute to this condition, including death, animal cruelty, and clients' financial hardships. For veterinary professionals who have grown accustomed to putting others' needs before their own, the constant demand for relieving animal suffering at the expense of personal care increases the risk of compassion fatigue.

Compassion fatigue can be experienced on individual and organizational levels. Its symptoms are listed in Table 8.16.1.

8.16.4 Burnout

Burnout results from chronic exposure to a stressful work environment. In veterinary clinical practice, workplace stresses include a lack of control over work schedule, long working hours, and client demands and expectations (see 7.2 Managing the Pet-Specific Workplace).

Burnout has long been underrecognized in veterinary medicine. However, a survey conducted at the 2012 American Veterinary Medical Association conference reported that 85% of respondents believed that burnout is an important wellness issue among veterinary professionals.

There are three dimensions to burnout: emotional exhaustion, low sense of personal achievement, and cynicism [2]. Of these, emotional exhaustion is most often associated with burnout and can increase the risk of poor physical and mental health. A low sense of personal achievement indicates that the individual no longer sees their work as meaningful. Cynicism can lead to a negative perception of, and emotional detachment from, a veterinary practice's clients. Burnout symptoms are listed in Table 8.16.1.

Table 8.16.1 Characteristics of compassion fatigue and burnout.

	Burnout	Compassion fatigue
Definition	Endpoint of chronic exposure to a stressful work environment	Emotional and physical depletion due to the trauma of witnessing and relieving others' suffering
Contributing factors	• Work overload • Inadequate pay • Co-worker conflict • Lack of control over work schedule • No acknowledgment of good work	• Moral stress • Traumatic events, including illness, euthanasia, animal cruelty, and client financial hardship
Internal feelings	• Cynicism • Emptiness • Hopelessness • Emotional and physical exhaustion • Decreased sense of personal accomplishment	• Guilt • Cynicism • Hopelessness • Powerlessness • Overburdened with others' suffering
Outward symptoms	Individual • Insomnia • Presenteeism • Substance abuse • Increased absenteeism • Emotional detachment • Troubled personal relationships • Decreased ability to process information, concentrate, and adapt Organizational • Low morale • Increased staff turnover • Reduced quality of patient care	Individual • Insomnia • Social isolation • Negative attitude • Excessive blaming • Emotional detachment • Compulsive behaviors • Poor work performance Organizational • Increased conflict • Increased absenteeism • Decreased overall performance • Negative perception of management

The workplace stressors that contribute to burnout can also increase the risk of suicide among veterinary professionals. Troublingly, veterinarians are three times as likely as the general population to commit suicide [3].

8.16.5 Solutions

Effectively managing compassion fatigue and burnout is essential to preserving the mental, emotional, and physical health of veterinary professionals. First, however, compassion fatigue and burnout must be acknowledged and not written off as simply stress or an inevitable fact of veterinary practice. Such acknowledgment is often the first step in finding and implementing healthy coping strategies.

General coping strategies can be classified in many ways, such as maladaptive/adaptive and problem-focused/emotion-focused. Maladaptive coping, such as substance abuse, is passive, unhealthy, and provides only temporary stress relief. Adaptive coping, such as self-care, is active, healthy, and offers long-term stress management. Examples of self-care include healthy eating, regular exercise, and mindfulness, which emphasizes a focus on the present and encourages self-compassion.

Problem-focused coping (e.g., devising a plan) addresses the problem's underlying cause, while emotion-focused coping (e.g., praying, journaling) addresses the emotional response to the problem. Managing compassion fatigue and burnout may require a combination of problem- and emotion-focused strategies.

General coping strategies for compassion fatigue and burnout can overlap. However, because compassion fatigue results from the type of work being performed and burnout is due to the work environment itself, specific coping strategies are also needed. For example, compassion satisfaction, which involves the practice of pausing to enjoy work successes, specifically combats compassion fatigue. Burnout management strategies include setting boundaries on work schedules, leaving work on time, finding meaning in one's work, and taking a vacation.

Resilience complements adaptive coping. It allows for a healthy emotional response to factors that increase the risk of compassion fatigue and burnout. Characteristics of resilience include self-confidence, optimism, and a firm sense of control when faced with stress or adversity. Importantly, resilience is not so much a personality trait as a skill that can be learned and improved upon.

Organizational solutions for compassion fatigue and burnout involve maintaining an even balance between job demands and job resources. Such resources include providing continuing educational and professional development, facilitating and encouraging open communication, and having debriefing sessions after particularly stressful cases.

If adaptive coping strategies are not effective, what was thought to be compassion fatigue or burnout might be depression. Clinical depression can resemble compassion fatigue or burnout but does not resolve with self-care. Depression requires the care of a medical professional.

EXAMPLES

Katherine has been a veterinarian for 10 years. Lately, she has been feeling overwhelmed with treating suffering pets and comforting grieving clients. Katherine has been isolating herself and constantly blaming her co-workers; her performance is notably suffering. A concerned colleague suggested that she may have compassion fatigue. After learning more about compassion fatigue, Katherine began regularly practicing mindfulness exercises and started a daily compassion satisfaction routine at work.

Ryan is a veterinary nurse at a busy multidoctor veterinary practice. The work seemed manageable at first, but now he feels like he has no control over his schedule. Ryan rarely gets a lunch break and, sometimes, barely a bathroom break. He frequently leaves work emotionally exhausted and is increasingly calling in sick. Ryan finally decides to take a vacation, during which he comes up with a plan to speak with the practice manager about decreasing his workload. He also commits to leaving work on time on most days and exercising regularly.

TAKE-AWAYS

- Compassion fatigue and burnout are occupational stressors within the veterinary profession that have individual and organizational impacts.
- High levels of compassion toward animals increase the risk of compassion fatigue, while the demands of clinical practice increase the likelihood of burnout.
- Compassion fatigue results from continual exposure to, and the relief of, others' suffering. Burnout results from chronic exposure to a stressful work environment.
- Mitigating compassion fatigue and burnout first requires an individual's acknowledgment of the problem, followed by the implementation of healthy coping strategies, such as self-care and compassion satisfaction.

- If coping strategies are ineffective, professional help for the treatment of clinical depression may be necessary.

MISCELLANEOUS

8.16.6 Cautions

Practicing veterinarians may have an increased likelihood of suicide due to workplace stresses and subsequent burnout.

References

1 Joinson, C. (1992). Coping with compassion fatigue. *Nursing* 22 (4): 118–120.
2 Maslach, C., Schaufeli, W.B., and Leiter, M.P. (2001). Job burnout. *Annu. Rev. Psychol.* 52: 397–422.
3 Tomasi, S.E., Fechter-Leggett, E.D., Edwards, N.T. et al. (2019). Suicide among veterinarians in the United States from 1979 through 2015. *J. Am. Vet. Med. Assoc.* 254 (1): 104–112.

Recommended Reading

Ayl, K. (2013). *When Helping Hurts: Compassion Fatigue in the Veterinary Profession*. Lakewood, CO: American Animal Hospital Association Press.
Cohen, S.P. (2007). Compassion fatigue and the veterinary health team. *Vet. Clin. North Am. Small Anim. Pract.* 37 (1): 123–134.
JAVMA News (2004). Managing and avoiding burnout: a primer for overly compassionate and overworked veterinarians. www.avma.org/javma-news/2004-08-15/managing-stress-and-avoiding-burnout
Scotney, R.L., McLaughlin, D., and Keates, H.L. (2015). A systematic review of the effects of euthanasia and occupational stress in personnel working with animals in animal shelters, veterinary clinics, and biomedical research facilities. *J. Am. Vet. Med. Assoc.* 247 (10): 1121–1130.

8.17

Dealing with Compromise Fatigue

Lowell Ackerman, DVM, DACVD, MBA, MPA, CVA, MRCVS

Global Consultant, Author, and Lecturer, MA, USA

BASICS

8.17.1 Summary

Most veterinary teams are familiar with compassion fatigue, but it is likely that compromise fatigue is every bit as common, but not as commonly discussed as an entity deserving our consideration. Pet-specific care is based on offering appropriate recommendations to clients, but at least some of those clients won't be receptive to the message and will ask us to compromise on what we believe is in the best interest of the patient. Veterinary healthcare teams are typically primed to offer first-rate medical care for their patients, but tension can arise if they are asked to compromise when clients are unprepared to accept the type of care recommended.

It can be disheartening for the entire team to regularly have to go with "Plan B," especially when a clearly superior medical option is available. It is important not to underestimate the negative impact such compromises have on the healthcare team, and the constant role that finances play in the delivery of healthcare to patients in many veterinary practices.

8.17.2 Terms Defined

Compassion Fatigue: Also known as secondary traumatic stress disorder, this is the gradual loss of compassion by people who work with individuals that are ill, suffering, or victims of trauma. This includes veterinary staff working with worried clients with sick or injured animals.

Compromise Fatigue: An extreme sense of stress associated with repeated requests to make compromises on the basis of the medical or financial management of patient care.

Hedonic Adaptation: Sometimes referred to as the hedonic treadmill, this refers to the observed tendency of individuals to return to a relatively stable level of happiness despite major positive or negative events or life changes.

Negative Stress: Also known as distress, this refers to the body's response to stress that lacks positive attributes and outcomes. Not all stress is bad, and negative stress refers to those stressors that cause anxiety or concern, are perceived as outside our coping abilities, can decrease performance, and can lead to mental and physical problems.

Plan B: An alternate strategy, often considered as a second choice to a preferred strategy.

MAIN CONCEPTS

8.17.3 Recognition

Compromise fatigue is a term first coined by Dr Lowell Ackerman in 2018 and is meant to differentiate the fatigue associated with financial compromises from the more commonly recognized compassion fatigue (see 8.16 Dealing with Compassion Fatigue and Burnout). In human medicine, the term "moral injury" is sometimes used to indicate the distress that occurs in trying to reconcile the needs of many stakeholders, including the hospital, the patient, the insurer, and the medical team.

Compromise fatigue is an insidious disorder experienced by many who work in the animal health field. Early in their careers, most animal healthcare workers focus on desirable outcomes, and the best evidence-based ways to achieve them. However, over time, as veterinarians and their teams are asked to compromise on those optimal outcomes to fit the budget of clients, a gradual shift in recommendations

Pet-Specific Care for the Veterinary Team, First Edition. Edited by Lowell Ackerman.

can occur, in which veterinary staff begin to recommend services based on their belief that pet owners won't object, rather than what is in the best interest of the animal (see 7.8 Providing Care for Those Unable or Unwilling to Pay).

Through a process sometimes referred to as hedonic adaptation, people can become accustomed to either a positive or negative stimulus, such that the emotional effects of that stimulus are attenuated over time. This can mean that we tend to continually adapt to circumstances and can shift our baseline expectations over time [1].

Compounding the problem is the fact that veterinary teams may be held responsible for less than optimal outcomes experienced, especially when they did not make or record in the medical record the appropriate recommendation, based on a belief that the client would have preferred the cheaper option.

To a certain extent, compromise fatigue should be expected, since inevitably veterinary care of companion animals must be responsive to the pet owner's ability to pay (see 2.10 Affordability of Veterinary Services). This is less of an issue in production animal medicine, in which price is always a factor, and herd health is often more relevant than patient-specific care.

Veterinarians are experiencing less job satisfaction than in the past and the top three stressors cited are time management, difficult clients, and clients' inability to pay [2]. Along with increasing job dissatisfaction, suicide rates are increasing within the profession, but the role of compromise fatigue has not really been evaluated in this regard.

8.17.4 Dealing with Compromise Fatigue

Compromise fatigue should be considered an occupational hazard in the companion animal healthcare marketplace. As such, mechanisms should be put in place to deal with this issue on a proactive basis.

The need for compromise should be anticipated in veterinary medicine, so it is worthwhile setting boundaries on where these compromises might be contemplated, and where compromise cannot be considered (see 2.2 The Role of Incremental Care). The easiest way of creating and supporting these boundaries in a hospital setting is to determine the level of care envisioned for the hospital, and then establish standards of care that reflect those beliefs (see 9.4 Standards of Care). Hospital operations manuals can formalize the process, helping to ensure that individual compromises do not adversely impact the vision for the hospital in terms of level of care delivered (see 8.9 Procedure Manuals).

Ongoing discussions and hospital team meetings should be used to clarify and refine the messaging, including what standards cannot be compromised, which might be subject to compromise with a signed waiver or "Against Medical Advice" disclaimer (with suitable notations in the medical record), and in which circumstances there might exist suitable lower-cost alternatives that can be considered with appropriate owner consent (see 10.14 Providing Cost-Effective Care for Those in Need).

It should be possible to lessen the impact of compromise fatigue when staff know the anticipated level of care expected within the practice, and clear guidelines are established regarding the suitability of compromise in certain predictable situations. Since compromise fatigue is often associated with the financial constraints of pet owners, reasonable expectations of pet care expenses should be communicated to pet owners early and often (see 5.3 What Clients Expect from the Veterinary Team, and 2.9 Anticipated Costs of Pet Care), as well as the particular healthcare risk factors for the individual pet (see 5.10 Discussing Pet-specific Care).

As part of setting reasonable expectations, veterinary teams should discuss risk management strategies with clients, such as pet health insurance (see 10.16 Pet Health Insurance), payment plans (see 10.17 – Payment and Wellness Plans), and third-party payments (see 10.18 Financing Veterinary Care).

Risk management strategies should be discussed with pet owners at the very first office visit. It is much easier to discuss potential future scenarios (such as development of a chronic disorder, visit to an emergency clinic, referral to a specialist, etc.) and how they will be paid for when there is not a crisis at hand. Clearly document in the medical record the conversation and the owner's response and have staff follow up to ensure that protection is in place.

There will always be pet owners who are indigent, so creating charitable guidelines for services and sharing resources on no-cost or low-cost alternative services are always advisable, but have appropriate conversations proactively to minimize staff compromise fatigue wherever possible (see 10.14 Providing Cost-Effective Care for Those in Need, and 2.2 The Role of Incremental Care).

 EXAMPLES

Mrs Fiona Frank presented her 11-year-old neutered male domestic shorthair, Justin, for a routine office visit at ABC Veterinary Hospital. The doctor and nurse both commented on the extent of gum disease in Justin, and recorded it in the medical record as Stage 3 periodontal disease. A recommendation was made for dental prophylaxis, with preanesthetic bloodwork, fluid therapy and dental radiography, and a verbal estimate for the services was discussed with the owner. Mrs Frank said that she would like to help Justin, but could not afford it, especially the laboratory work and fluid therapy, and asked for a less costly alternative. Dr Green wanted to help this owner, but more than that, she wanted to help Justin, who she believed would otherwise not receive the level of care he really needed. While Dr Green had some reservations, in the end she consented to compromise and perform the procedure for a fraction of the typical price, and forego the preanesthetic laboratory work as well as the fluid therapy and radiography.

Following the dental procedure, Justin recovered without event and returned home with his owner. However, about two weeks later, Mrs Frank returned Justin to the hospital and he was moribund. Bloodwork and urinalysis revealed that Justin was in kidney failure. Mrs Frank blamed Dr Green and the care that Justin had received. Dr Green reminded Mrs Frank that preanesthetic laboratory testing was declined, as was fluid therapy and radiography, but the owner was adamant that Justin was perfectly healthy before the procedure, and that she planned on making a formal complaint to the veterinary board. Dr Green admitted Justin to the hospital and provided supportive care, but Justin died two days later.

Mrs Frank did not pay her final veterinary bill and did indeed report Dr Green to the veterinary board. Their subsequent evaluation revealed that Dr Green's medical records only indicated the periodontal score and the procedures performed and that there was no evidence in the record that additional recommendations had been made, but declined. Dr Green learned the hard way that compromising standards of care as a good deed does not always have commensurate rewards in terms of customer appreciation. She was still committed to helping clients, but in the future she would ensure that everything was better documented in the medical records and that informed consent was clarified and obvious.

TAKE-AWAYS

- Compromise fatigue is associated with making compromises on the basis of the medical or financial management of patient care.

- Compromise fatigue can be insidious and can result in the best recommendations not being made with the anticipation that compromise will likely be necessary.
- Veterinary teams may be held responsible for less than optimal results following compromise, so appropriate documentation is critical.
- Compromise fatigue can be mitigated somewhat by having proactive discussions with pet owners regarding financial risk management, before problems occur.
- Do not underestimate the consequences for the hospital and staff of trying to deliver an exceptional level of care, but often having to resort to "Plan B."

MISCELLANEOUS

8.17.5 Cautions

Even having established standards of care and care pathways will not eliminate compromise fatigue entirely, since unanticipated situations will always arise. However, the goal should be to have general guidelines that provide some context as to what an acceptable compromise might be, and where compromises are not possible.

While compromise fatigue will typically improve when standards of care have been developed, some clients may still object when veterinary staff fail to accommodate their perceived financial needs. Veterinary practices need to accept that they cannot always meet the needs of every client's budget and still be true to the hospital's vision for level of care.

References

1 Stoewen, D.L. (2016). Veterinary happiness. *Can. Vet. J.* 57 (5): 539–541.
2 2015 dvm360 Job Satisfaction Survey. www.dvm360.com/view/2015-dvm360-job-satisfaction-survey

Recommended Reading

Ackerman, L: Compromise fatigue. In: Ackerman, L. (ed.) *Five-Minute Veterinary Practice Management Consult*, 3, Wiley, Ames, IA, 2020. pp. 114–115.
Kim, R.W., Patterson, G., Nahar, V.K., and Sharma, M. (2017). Toward an evidence-based approach to stress management

for veterinarians and veterinary students. *J. Am. Vet. Med. Assoc.* 251 (9): 1002–1004.

Perret, J.L., Best, C.O., Coe, J.B. et al. (2020). Prevalence of mental health outcomes among Canadian veterinarians. *J. Am. Vet. Med. Assoc.* 256 (3): 365–375.

Vande Griek, O.H., Clark, M.A., Witte, T.K. et al. (2018). Development of a taxonomy of practice-related stressors experienced by veterinarians in the United States. *J. Am. Vet. Med. Assoc.* 252 (2): 227–233.

8.18

Team Strategies for Atopic Dermatitis

Lowell Ackerman, DVM, DACVD, MBA, MPA, CVA, MRCVS

Global Consultant, Author, and Lecturer, MA, USA

 BASICS

8.18.1 Summary

Canine atopic dermatitis (CAD) is a common and often frustrating disorder to manage for both pet owners and veterinarians. While we now have many new and exciting medications to manage the associated pruritus, our approach to management hasn't changed significantly in decades: Treat the itch, try to keep the owners happy, and hope that price won't become too much of an issue in the process. If owners do push back against prices, we spend a lot of time and energy trying to manage the client's financial sensitivity as much as the patient.

To successfully manage atopic dermatitis over a pet's lifetime, it is critical that veterinary healthcare teams understand the lifelong nature of the condition, the challenges that pet owners face at home, and that they have the tools available to effectively counsel clients on this very manageable condition.

8.18.2 Terms Defined

Allergen: A substance capable of inducing an allergic reaction.

Atopic Dermatitis: The preferred term for a genetically predisposed inflammatory and pruritic skin disease with characteristic clinical presentation. Previously known by several terms, including atopy, inhalant allergies, eczema, and hay fever.

Atopic March: The natural progression and evolution of allergic manifestations that occurs over time.

 MAIN CONCEPTS

8.18.3 It's Complicated

Canine atopic dermatitis is a common condition, but not a simple one. There might be a tendency to consider allergy as a cause-and-effect relationship in which a pet breathes in some pollen and has an immediate reaction that needs to be dealt with. . . but such is not often the case. It is also critical to realize that allergy exists on a continuum, and thus benefits from early and conscientious intervention (see 9.7 Continuum of Care and Convergence Schedules).

Most atopic pets do have a genetic predisposition to develop allergies, and the clinical presentation is often characteristic (at least on a breed-specific basis), but that is typically where the simple part ends. The genetics appears to be quite complex, and there are likely many genes that impact susceptibility to allergies. Still, just like in humans, allergies do tend to run in families and there are many breeds in which allergies are commonly reported.

Another complicating factor about atopic dermatitis is that the barrier function of the skin is often compromised, allowing the facilitated penetration not only of allergens, but often of bacteria (often *Staphylococcus pseudintermedius*) and yeasts (often *Malassezia pachydermatis*) as well.

When dealing with allergic pets, it's also important to realize that while there is an inherited tendency to develop allergies, the specific types of allergies that develop (e.g., ragweed allergy, housemite allergy, etc.) are actually as much a cause of circumstance as of genetics. Allergies most commonly develop to allergens to which the individual is routinely exposed – pollens of trees, grasses and weeds, housemites, and environmental molds. In fact, a pet may start out with some pollen allergies and have problems only during certain parts of the year when those pollen counts are high, but allergies can change and perhaps half of all allergic pets end up developing year-round problems when they acquire reactions to nonseasonal allergens.

Allergies are often thought of as a nuisance, but what makes them so devastating for pet owners is that their pet is often very uncomfortable and may scratch and bite at itself until it does significant damage to the skin. Pet owners may also complain that they can't sleep at night because of the incessant scratching their pet experiences. The condition takes its toll in terms of quality of life, for both pets and their caregivers.

The simplistic view of allergies is that allergens are inhaled, cause an immediate hypersensitivity reaction and allergy antibody formation, and end up causing histamine release in the skin, which results in perceived itch, which then results in scratching. However, we know that the real picture is much more complicated. First, allergens don't need to be inhaled. In fact, in dogs, most of the allergen presentation is likely transcutaneous from allergens coming in direct contact with the skin. When dogs go outside, their fur can become a magnet for pollens and molds, and rolling on the ground only increases problems. Some allergen is also likely inhaled, and some might even be ingested. There can even be cross-reactions with food allergens. So, how allergen gets introduced into the system can be quite different in different circumstances.

Second, the old concept of immediate hypersensitivity and allergy antibody development is also somewhat antiquated. We now know that most of the initiation of allergy reactions is cell mediated and involves chemical messengers (cytokines), not allergy antibodies. Finally, much of the itch induction does not seem to be from histamine release from mast cells in the skin, but from some of those chemical messengers having effects on nerves in the skin that send a message to the brain relaying the perception of itch and causing the dog to react by scratching.

In addition to the clinical manifestations of allergy, it is important to note that dogs with atopic dermatitis may also manifest a variety of behavior problems, often directly or indirectly linked to the stress, anxiety, and irritation of the primary complaint. Thus, atopic dogs can become more hyperactive, excitable, and attention seeking. It is also important to realize that some of their behaviors, such as licking and chewing, shaking and scratching, can be stress inducing in family members as well.

8.18.4 Getting Specific

With pet-specific care, we can personalize our approach to common maladies, such as atopic dermatitis. We know that CAD is common and that there are striking breed predispositions, so our intervention can often start quite early. Those breed predispositions are influenced by gene pools, so a good place to start, if practice management software allows, is to identify the most common breeds (and crosses) in the practice for which a diagnosis of CAD has been made (see 7.9 Using Practice Management Software to Personalize Care). An alternate approach is to search medical records for patients on long-term antipruritic therapy and crudely discern breed predisposition to CAD from that information. One should not be surprised if just a dozen or so breeds are responsible for the vast majority of allergies seen in the practice.

Once the breeds most at risk in the practice have been identified, it becomes a simpler task to personalize an approach to the problem. Messaging can be further customized, since breed-specific phenotypes have been recognized. For example, boxers are more likely to have urticaria (hives) associated with their allergies, golden retrievers are more likely to develop pyotraumatic dermatitis (hot spots), dalmatians are likely to have lip involvement, and West Highland white terriers are more likely to have associated keratinization issues (seborrhea). Breed predisposition and phenotypes are important considerations, but it is also important to realize that allergies are more family based than breed based, so atopic dermatitis is seen in mixed-breed pets as well as purebreds, reflecting the likely allergy status of the parents.

Many animals are prone to allergies, but it is sufficient to start with the breeds and their crosses that have been identified to be most at risk in your particular practice. While CAD has strong genetic tendencies, it is not purely a genetic condition. There are other variables that can contribute to the clinical expression of the disorder. While most pets with CAD start to develop clinical issues between 6 months and 3 years of age, it is possible to determine animals at potential risk for allergies from birth from the breeds and their crosses that have already been identified. That doesn't mean that they will necessarily develop atopic dermatitis, but they form the basis of a population at increased risk.

Once potential risk has been identified, the management of that risk should be a top priority. Why wait until allergies start to develop over the ensuing months and years when teams can have important proactive conversations with pet owners starting with puppy and kitten visits?

A good time to start such conversations is when pets are 8 weeks of age, long before any problems are evident. At this time, the hospital team can alert the owners of at-risk breeds to be vigilant for early clinical signs, such as licking and chewing at the feet (see Figure 8.18.1), face rubbing, rashes in the armpit and groin areas, and even redness of the inner aspects of the pinnae. More specific information can be provided according to breed phenotypes for allergic manifestations. The intention is not to scare owners but to

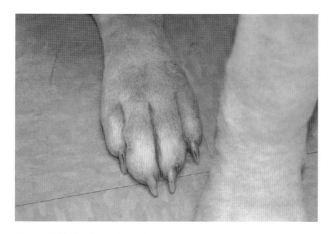

Figure 8.18.1 One of the first manifestations of atopic dermatitis is often licking and chewing at the paws.

set realistic expectations for a risk that has been identified and confirmed in the specific practice population. If such conversations were productive, it might also prompt the owner to ask what it would mean for their pet if it did develop allergies and what it might mean for them in terms of care and costs. You might think that you don't want to have those discussions during a puppy visit, but in time, you will likely realize that it was time well spent and develop resources (client handouts, website pages, trained staff, etc.) to facilitate such client education.

Pet owners can often predict the costs of such things as feeding, grooming, and boarding, but the costs of veterinary care are often much harder to predict. If we don't apprise owners of pet-related expenses that might occur in the future, we are doing them a disservice. Over the course of a lifetime, a pet could develop a chronic condition (such as atopic dermatitis, osteoarthritis, diabetes mellitus, etc.), need a referral to a specialist, or end up at an emergency clinic. While the costs of routine preventive care are relatively easy to predict, and for pet owners to afford, it doesn't take much else to happen before pet owners start to worry about the expenses associated with veterinary care. Much of this can be avoided by taking the time to have such conversations and discuss realistic expectations during puppy and kitten visits (see 2.9 Anticipated Costs of Pet Care). It can be extremely useful for hospital teams to have an appreciation of what it actually costs to manage a typical allergic pet over the course of a year, as well as over its lifetime, so owners can participate in more informed discussions.

Why have such burdensome discussions during visits when pet owners are still bonding with their new pets? It's simple. If pet owners can appreciate that every pet comes with some healthcare risks and that some of those risks can be associated with considerable expenditure, they may decide to mitigate those risks with a tool like pet health insurance (see 10.16 Pet Health Insurance), especially policies that will cover chronic care and hereditary diseases. By

having these discussions during puppy and kitten visits, when pets typically appear completely healthy, teams can help ensure that pets have few if any preexisting problems that would be excluded from insurance coverage. This is particularly important for conditions such as atopic dermatitis, where pets may start showing early evidence of allergies within a few months of those puppy visits.

If pet health insurance is in place by 8 weeks of age, general early detection testing can commence by 12 weeks of age. This might include performing genetic screening panels, which can yield DNA results for dozens of different conditions on a single sample (blood or cheek swab). Specific genetic markers for CAD may not be routinely available in most panels, but there are variant-based tests for many dermatological (ivermectin sensitivity, dermatomyositis, ichthyosis, nasal hyperkeratosis, etc.) and nondermatological (von Willebrand disease, glaucoma, degenerative myelopathy, etc.) conditions (see 3.11 Integrating Genotypic and Phenotypic Testing). At some point, there will likely be more DNA tests for risk of CAD in different breeds, and that will make an even stronger case than just breed predisposition to alert owners about potential future risks for their pets. In the meantime, there are a lot of other conditions for which early detection is possible by genetic screening, so it is worth building such an approach into standards of care, and such testing is typically done around 12 weeks of age. Such tests should not be expected to "diagnose" allergies but may help identify animals with increased risk.

By 16 weeks of age, one can start looking for phenotypic evidence (e.g., with routine use of flea combing, skin scrapings, and cytologies) as rashes develop rather than just reaching for medications, and make sure pet owners know what likely clinical presentations to be looking for at home.

8.18.5 Can We Prevent Allergic Manifestations?

At this point in time, we cannot prevent allergies from occurring, but if we intervene early, we can definitely minimize the impact of allergies on a pet's (and owner's) quality of life.

Atopic dermatitis can be attributable to the complex interactions of many different genes, and the heritability of the condition is estimated to be quite high (almost 50% in some breeds). If two allergic parents are bred, almost three-quarters of offspring may become allergic, and even one allergic parent can contribute to perhaps one-third of puppies being allergic, so clearly allergies run in families, and we can likely help prevent allergies in pups if we are willing to limit the breeding of allergic parents. This is one solution, but it is important to balance more than just one trait in selecting animals for breeding (see 3.8 Genetic Counseling).

Some circumstantial evidence supports the notion that allergies are more common now because children and pets growing up in sanitized environments may have prevented good bacteria and other environmental factors from fully conditioning the immune system, increasing the likelihood of allergies. Vaccination, and processed diets, are also sometimes blamed for their effects on a naïve immune system. These are consistent with the so-called Hygiene Hypothesis, also known as the Old Friends Hypothesis, that suggests some exposure to microbes, parasites, and toxins has positive effects on the developing immune system. Thus, there might be some benefit in cleaning but not trying to sterilize the environment in which puppies and kittens are raised, and allowing them to remain with their mother and siblings longer before weaning and sending them to a new environment.

There is some preliminary evidence that providing nutritional support in the form of diets or supplements rich in eicosapentaenoic acid (EPA) may play some role in prevention, either through its antiinflammatory properties or its effect on skin barrier function. Other nutrients such as vitamin D and zinc have been considered, but evidence-based research is needed to determine the likelihood of affecting outcomes.

For pets that have demonstrated a susceptibility to atopic dermatitis, the main strategy is to deny access of allergens to the pet. That's a challenge, but we can make a difference.

When it comes to plant pollens, flowers tend to have heavy pollens which can only travel a few meters. Because of this, allergies to most flowers are considered a rarity and most flower pollination is facilitated by insects. On the other hand, many pollinating grasses, weeds, and trees are spread in the wind, and often over many kilometers (sometimes 100 km or more), so whether those plants reside on the pet owner's property doesn't make a difference.

It may seem that the prevalence of allergies is worsening with every passing year and to a certain extent, it is – because of climate change, pollen counts are rising on a regular basis. We can't stop pollen from being spread by the wind, but since we know that most pollen enters the body directly across the skin barrier, we do have strategies that can be effective. Frequent bathing helps remove allergens from the skin and haircoat, but between baths, wiping the paws and skin with a clean damp cloth can also remove allergens before they have a chance to get absorbed. Having such a wiping protocol every time a pet reenters the house after being outside is a reasonable but somewhat labor-intensive way of keeping pollens and molds at bay.

On days with high pollen counts, it can also be helpful to keep allergic pets indoors with windows closed. The use of particulate air filters can also be helpful. Controlling populations of molds and housemites indoors can be a challenge, but since this is also an issue for people, there are plenty of great products and resources to help manage the indoor situation.

Allergic pets are also sensitive to other potential causes of pruritus such as parasites and adverse reactions to foods, so it is important to keep such pets routinely parasite free and to be aware of food sensitivities. Pets should be on year-round parasite control, and products that either have quick kill or prevent parasites from feeding are preferred.

8.18.6 Using Early Detection Effectively

It is important to realize that even though we have many diagnostic tests that we might use with atopic pets, CAD is a clinical diagnosis. As such, it is the age of onset, breed predisposition, classic clinical presentation, breed phenotype, and even response to specific medications that allow the tentative diagnosis. While we might have some genetic markers associated with risk for developing atopic dermatitis, none of these should be considered diagnostic for the condition. Genetic testing is likely to become more commonplace but for the foreseeable future, it is likely that new genetic tests may be associated with allergy risk, but won't confirm a diagnosis. Once again, atopic dermatitis is a clinical diagnosis, so it is unlikely that genetic markers will indicate anything other than risk, and should be interpreted accordingly. Similarly, while we have both intradermal and blood-based allergy tests, neither of these are diagnostic either; they just indicate the presence of allergen-specific IgE.

As was mentioned previously, atopic dermatitis typically first presents in animals with a genetic predisposition between 6 months and 3 years of age. Common clinical signs include licking and chewing at the feet, rashes in the armpits and groin areas, face rubbing, and even otitis externa. The vast majority of atopic patients have pruritus that is corticosteroid responsive. But CAD is a diagnosis of exclusion, so it is imperative that other causes of pruritus be considered, including parasites and adverse reactions to foods.

Allergy testing is available, and it can be performed by intradermal injection of allergens or can be based on blood tests, but neither of these are diagnostic tests for allergies. In fact, there is enough intralaboratory variability on blood tests that results do need to be interpreted in light of clinical history. It is also important that evidence-based guidelines be used for withdrawal times of antiinflammatory drugs prior to testing. Thus, just because an animal has reactions evident on an allergy test, this does not mean the pet is allergic, and even if it is allergic, it doesn't mean that the positive test reactions are the ultimate cause. Similarly, a proportion of typical atopic dogs may not have any positive reactions detectable on allergy tests, and this is sometimes referred to as CAD-like disease. There are many reasons for this, but the basic lesson to be learned is that allergy tests should not be used in an attempt to diagnose if a pet has allergies.

Allergy tests are typically used not to diagnose atopic dermatitis, but in animals in which atopic dermatitis has been clinically diagnosed, to discern which allergens are most likely contributing to the problem. Allergy testing is typically reserved for cases in which allergy desensitization therapy (immunotherapy, hyposensitization, allergy shots) is being contemplated, as a suggestion for which allergens should be considered for desensitization. Even then, the most important consideration is not which allergen had the highest score on testing, but rather which allergens seem to correlate best with the seasonal variability of the allergies.

Pets with atopic dermatitis tend to develop recurrent bacterial and yeast infections and so when pets develop such issues, it is important to routinely assess with cytology. It is impossible to ascertain by inspection (or smell) whether a complication is bacterial or yeast related, so using cytological confirmation is important. Once again, atopic dermatitis is a lifelong condition, so it is important to use appropriate therapies and minimize the risk of resistance developing, or not completely addressing the problem correctly.

8.18.7 Managing the Allergic Pet

Once we have done our best to identify pets in the practice which are at increased risk for CAD, invited pet owners to consider how they will afford such care if their pet is affected, and alerted owners to early clinical signs to watch for so they can notify us as soon as any problems become evident, we are actually in a very good position when it comes to disease management.

At the very earliest onset of clinical signs (or even before then, with particularly keen pet owners), teams can coach pet owners on the critical nature of preserving skin barrier function, which can affect not only allergen penetration but also susceptibility to recurrent bacterial and yeast infections. It's a perfect time for pet owners to condition their pets to accept and actually enjoy baths and other topical therapies. Very early in the course of management is also the best time to consider nutritional supplements rich in omega-3 fatty acids. These supplements often have a modest impact yet typically take many weeks for EPA to be incorporated into skin cells.

It is also very helpful if pet owners have a realistic picture of what is causing the problems and our options for addressing them. Since allergies reflect a cause-and-effect relationship between exposure to environmental allergens, those allergens crossing the skin barrier, and then allergic manifestations ensuing, there are many opportunities for client education.

When it comes to causation, it can be helpful if the pet owners can make a connection between the occurrence of substances in the environment and the cause of their pet's uncomfortable pruritic condition. In many cases, this can be aided by the clients keeping a calendar of when their pet is having problems, and being aware of what happens to be in the environment that correlates with those problems. There are now many websites and apps (e.g., http://pollen.com, http://polleninfo.com, most weather services) that track pollen counts locally and make it easy for pet owners to connect the severity of their dog's clinical signs with the quantity of specific pollen or mold in the local environment. In fact, if customer service representatives review the pollen counts each day (perhaps even displaying the counts in the reception area or on the practice's website), then clients can more easily make the connections to the environmental causes. This is important because when clients do not make the connection effectively, they may be more likely to fault the medication they are using for no longer working as well, rather than realizing that the allergic challenge might have increased, and more intervention is warranted.

When it comes to managing allergies, it is important to appreciate that there are a lot of great medications available that help manage pruritus, but for such treatment to be effective, it is critical to condition the skin to preserve barrier function, keep these pets parasite free, and use whatever tactics are necessary to minimize the contact time that allergens have with the skin surface.

Regardless of drug(s) of choice, simply treating the clinical signs of CAD is just putting a bandage on the problem. CAD is a lifelong condition. It may very well start out seasonal based on initial causative allergens, but many cases eventually become year-round. This evolution of allergic manifestations over time is sometimes referred to as the atopic "march." And, yes, since atopic dermatitis typically spans a lifetime, and allergies tend to get worse with each passing year, one not only needs a treatment strategy to manage the itchiness at the outset, but there is also a need to set realistic expectations for the pet owner, so it is possible to remain an advocate rather than an adversary and to manage the condition year after year and invoice after invoice.

Also, since allergy management is typically a lifelong pursuit, one also needs to be concerned with adverse reactions to medications, quality of life issues, and issues involved with judicious use of antimicrobials. It is very important for the veterinary healthcare team to have such discussions with owners of allergic pets so they can appreciate the role they need to play in allergy management and ensure a safe balance between effectiveness and convenience.

Allergic pets can be managed almost entirely with topical therapy but because of the frequency of intervention needed, it is inconvenient in most cases, especially on a prolonged schedule. Allergic pets can also be managed with sole medications such as corticosteroids, but given the long-term risks of such actions, it would not be recommended. Pet owners need to appreciate the goal of not only effective long-term therapy, but safe long-term therapy, and maintaining the pet's quality of life over a typical healthspan. Thus, allergies must be managed on a continuum of care, since any intervention made can affect (positively or negatively) the long-term quality of life of the patient (see 9.7 Continuum of Care and Convergence Schedules). This sets the stage for important discussions about safe long-term treatment, topical therapies over a schedule that pet owners can effectively manage, and often a combination of medications that work on different aspects of the pathophysiology of allergy. In most cases, there is no "magic bullet" and multiple strategies must be utilized to achieve optimal individualized benefit for patients.

Another point that is important to convey to owners of allergic pets is that all the therapies discussed so far are strictly symptomatic. They do not cure the condition and only serve to camouflage the problem; they are a bandage that temporarily addresses the owner's concerns and once those medications are stopped, the problem will come right back. If pet owners really want to try to make their pet less allergic over time, the only way currently of doing that is immunotherapy – introducing small amounts of the causative allergens in a controlled fashion, and making the pet more tolerant of those allergens over time. Immunotherapy (hyposensitization, desensitization) can be administered by injection or sublingually as drops, and is effective in many cases, although it typically takes many months to start taking effect, does not work in all cases, and even in cases when it is helpful, it does not necessarily allow the discontinuation of other medications although the doses needed for control may be lessened. Clients should appreciate that if they intend to invest in attempting immunotherapy, they should be committed to doing it for at least 12 months to determine efficacy.

At this point in time, we are managing the situation with a relationship-based strategy. The pet owner understands their financial commitment to the process as well as the lifelong nature of the condition and the different medical

and immunotherapeutic options for long-term management, and they are embarking on a plan to control the condition early before chronic changes complicate the process. Just think about how much easier that makes the job of the veterinary team!

Canine atopic dermatitis is common and can be frustrating, but it is also predictable and amenable to early intervention. Pet-specific care can make allergy management a much more positive experience for clients, patients, and the entire hospital team. At the same time as teams are delivering a better level of medicine and customer service, practices are also benefiting from a better healthcare model.

TAKE-AWAYS

- CAD is a diagnosis of exclusion. There are currently no diagnostic tests that will confirm a dog as being atopic.
- CAD is suspected based on factors such as age of onset, breed predisposition, classic clinical presentation, and typical responses to certain medications.
- In most cases, even though there are excellent therapies available, atopic dermatitis requires a balanced approach with numerous therapeutic modalities.
- Because atopic dermatitis is a lifelong condition, it is important that it be managed on a continuum of care since treatment choices selected at any stage can affect quality of life at later stages.
- Medications and environmental control are important but do not result in cure; immunotherapy is the only mechanism to try to make animals less allergic over time.

MISCELLANEOUS

Recommended Reading

Ackerman, L. (2018). Allergies: the personalized medicine approach. *AAHA Trends* 34 (4): 55–58.

Anturaniemi, J; Zaldivar-Lopez, S; Salvekoul, H.F.J., et al. (2020). The Effect of Atopic Dermatitis and Diet on the Skin Transcriptome in Staffordshire Bull Terriers. *Front. Vet. Sci.*, 16 October 2020. https://doi.org/10.3389/fvets.2020.552251.

Bizikova, P., Pucheu-Haston, C.M., Eisenschenk, M.C. et al. (2015). Review: role of genetics and the environment in the pathogenesis of canine atopic dermatitis. *Vet. Dermatol.* 26: 95–103.

Bizikova, P., Santoro, D., Marsella, R. et al. (2015). Review: clinical and histological manifestations of canine atopic dermatitis. *Vet. Dermatol.* 26: 79–83.

Botoni, L.S., Torres, S.M.F., Koch, S.N. et al. (2019). Comparison of demographic data, disease severity and response to treatment, between dogs with atopic dermatitis and atopic-like dermatitis: a retrospective study. *Vet. Dermatol.* 30 (1): 10–e4.

Hensel, P., Santoro, D., Favrot, C. et al. (2015). Canine atopic dermatitis: detailed guidelines for diagnosis and allergen identification. *BMC Vet. Res.* 11: 196.

Nuttal, T. (2013). The genomics revolution: will canine atopic dermatitis be predictable and preventable. *Vet. Dermatol.* 24: 10–18.

Nuttal, T.J., Marsella, R., Rosenbaum, M.R. et al. (2019). Update on pathogenesis, diagnosis, and treatment of atopic dermatitis in dogs. *J. Am. Vet. Med. Assoc.* 254 (11): 1291–1300.

Olivry, T., DeBoer, D.J., Favrot, C. et al. (2015). Treatment of canine atopic dermatitis: 2015 updated guidelines from the International Committee on Allergic Diseases of Animals (ICADA). *BMC Vet. Res.* 11: 210.

Olivry, T. and Saridomichelakis, M. (2013). Evidence-based guidelines for anti-allergic drug withdrawal times before allergen-specific intradermal and IgE serological tests in dogs. *Vet. Dermatol.* 24: 225–232.

Shou, Z., Pieper, J.B., and Kampbell, K. (2019). Intralaboratory reliability and variability for allergen-specific immunoglobulin type E serology testing. *J. Am. Anim. Hosp. Assoc.* 55: 124–129.

8.19

Team Strategies for Periodontal Disease

Heidi B. Lobprise, DVM, DAVDC and Jessica Johnson, DVM

Main Street Veterinary Dental Clinic, Flower Mound, TX, USA

BASICS

8.19.1 Summary

Periodontal disease (PD) is one of the most commonly encountered diseases in our canine and feline patients. As we learn more, we are realizing that disease present in the mouth can greatly affect the overall health of our patients. As the majority of our patients have teeth, and the minority of our clients perform home care, it is essential to increase awareness through education of our clients. If the whole veterinary team is educated on PD, how to identify it, how to treat it, and how to educate the client, the compliance of our clients will increase.

8.19.2 Terms Defined

Complete Dental Therapy: Includes dental cleaning, thorough dental examination and charting, dental radiographs, polishing and treatment (periodontal treatment, extractions), performed under general anesthesia.

Dental (Dental Prophy): Less than optimal words commonly used for the complete dental therapy experience.

Extraction: The removal of a tooth from the surrounding periodontal tissue, often through surgical means.

Home Care: Any effort a pet parent can provide to help decrease the amount of plaque and calculus forming on tooth surfaces; daily effective tooth brushing is optimal, with other methods including dental wipes and appropriate dental food, treats and chews.

Periodontal Disease (PD): Infection, inflammation, and loss of the tissues surrounding and supporting the teeth, including attached gingiva, bone, the periodontal ligament and cementum covering the root.

Tooth Resorption (TR): Resorption of dental hard tissue.

MAIN CONCEPTS

Some features of veterinary practices that promote good compliance when it comes to dentistry include educating the whole team on the benefits of a dental procedure, including front office staff, assistants and nurses/technicians, and veterinarians. That way, the whole team not only understands but believes in the benefits of oral healthcare. The whole team can also be educated on common concerns that clients have, specifically in regard to anesthesia.

The greatest tool we have to enhance the care of our patients is client communication and education. That process begins with an educated, engaged, and motivated veterinary team that understands the benefits of a mouth free of pain, disease, and infection. It is not a small endeavor to educate technicians, assistants, receptionists, and clients. The veterinarians and technicians who take the time to educate, who believe in the benefits and consistently advocate for their patients will be the ones with the most successful dental care programs. It is worth recognizing that it can be tiresome to incorporate this into almost every patient visit; however, we must remember that our clients are often unaware of the condition of their pets' mouths. It is our duty to point this out to them. There is a common misconception that "dog breath" aka "bad breath" is normal and the task to dispel that myth over and over again falls on the shoulders of the veterinary team.

Pet-Specific Care for the Veterinary Team, First Edition. Edited by Lowell Ackerman.
© 2021 John Wiley & Sons, Inc. Published 2021 by John Wiley & Sons, Inc.

The routine dental procedure is often viewed as an "elective" procedure. However, quite frequently it is an opportunity to address hidden PD. For that reason, the phrase "dental prophy" rarely applies. It is perhaps more accurate to refer to this procedure as "complete dental therapy." The clients should be well informed of what the day of surgery will look like and how they will be contacted mid-procedure to discuss the cost and treatment plan as hidden problems are found. Intraoral radiographs almost always reveal unexpected findings.

Every pet should have quality oral and dental care throughout its life stages, with an oral examination at every visit, professional care at regular intervals, and effective home care. Patients at higher risk for oral and dental diseases will likely need enhanced care, so have the pet owner consider pet health insurance (see 10.16 Pet Health Insurance), though most pets would benefit from eventual care regardless. The group at highest risk for PD are small dogs that will be less than 11 kg (25 pounds) when full grown. These dogs should have their first dental procedure by 1–2 years of age [1]. Prepare the owner for a higher incidence of dental problems as not only do they tend to have more PD, but they also tend to live longer than larger breeds, and older dogs have been shown to have a higher incidence of oral and dental disease.

Brachycephalic dogs and cats are also at higher risk of periodontal and dental disease due to crowded and rotated teeth. They also have a higher incidence of unerupted premolars that can develop into dentigerous cysts. Additional care is also needed to help manage their potentially higher anesthetic risks (see 5.12 Discussing Anesthetic Risk). As stated earlier, older dogs have a higher incidence of PD, and the frequency of oral tumors is greater in older animals. While there may be additional anesthetic risks that have to be managed, old age of itself is not a valid excuse to avoid dental treatment (see 6.17 Senior Care). For special cases with systemic issues, it is reasonable to refer geriatric patients to a dental specialist if you feel the anesthetic risk or level of dental care needed is beyond the scope of what your practice can offer. Clinics with advanced dental care experience are often more comfortable with these higher risk patients and can often decrease their anesthetic time due to the level of skill and equipment available.

Providing optimal dental care for cats can be beneficial for the patient and clinic, as they may not have regular visits as often as dogs. They will often hide problems until well advanced, so early detection of problems such as TR, which is fairly common, should be anticipated, and some may have stomatitis (severe inflammation, ulceration).

Dogs that are heavy chewers may have damaged teeth, particularly if they chew on hard objects that can be isolated in the area of the carnassial teeth. Discuss appropriate dental chews at every visit. Educate clients to avoid chews that can commonly break teeth due to hardness; if they are unable to indent a thumb nail into the product, then it is likely too hard (such as bones, antlers, and other noncompressible objects). Dogs with separation anxiety can break teeth on kennels and other items, so discuss behavioral modification and medication if needed.

Client communication and education are key in building team strategies for periodontal and dental care. The front office staff should be trained that clients who "phone-shop" for dental prices will not likely get accurate responses for dental procedures and estimates. During complete dental therapy, there can be too many variables and too many problems that will only become apparent once radiographs are taken and a full examination is done. Even a thorough initial exam will not reveal all potential problems, but by offering a complimentary oral and dental examination, you can start client education about dental care.

An important part of the communication is handling client concerns, especially about anesthesia. Anesthetic risks can be minimized with preoperative diagnostics, and any problems found can then be managed with the procedure potentially delayed until the patient is stable. In addition, individualized anesthetic and pain protocols help to minimize patient discomfort and can decrease the extent of general anesthetic drugs needed for the procedure.

Anesthetic-free dental procedure should not be recommended. Position statements from multiple organizations agree that nonanesthetic dental procedures are inappropriate for pets [2]. Adequate care cannot be provided, and the patient will likely be stressed by the procedure, whatever the claims of the provider (see 6.6 Fear Free Concepts).

Cost will be an issue with some clients (see 2.10 Affordability of Veterinary Services). Client education will include discussing how preventive care is less expensive in the long run than treating pets with significant disease, and is better for the pet's health. The client can work with the clinic's options for payment, and pet insurance can be encouraged (see 10.16 Pet Health Insurance), especially in high-risk patients (small dogs, brachycephalic dogs and cats).

For every dental patient, consider an approach to manage fear, anxiety, and stress (FAS) for both the patient and the owner. Fear Free™ methods can be employed to reduce patient FAS, particularly in previsit pharmaceuticals (see 6.6 Fear Free Concepts). Excellent communication with the owner before, during, and after the procedure can help assuage their anxiety as well (see client contact points below).

As discussed previously, the initial assessment in the examination room can only provide a partial "guestimate" on the extent of disease. While the amount of plaque, calculus, and inflammation can be assessed, dental radiographs are required to evaluate the full extent of bone and attachment loss. In the exam room, take a picture of the mouth and specific issues with the client's own cellphone; that way they can take home evidence of problems to help compliance with recommendations.

Ideally, there should be multiple client contact points on the day of the procedure. At admission, conduct a brief physical examination and discuss any diagnostic results. Review the anesthesia consent form and initial treatment plan/estimate, but make sure you can contact the owner during the procedure. Once the patient is admitted, the dental team will be contacting the owner at least three times. The first call occurs when the preoperative injection or medication is administered. Once the catheter is place, the patient is anesthetized and monitoring is started, the more complete oral examination is done. The second call is made after the full evaluation is complete, including dental radiographs and charting have identified all lesions that require treatment. Now the client can be presented with the updated treatment plan for their approval. If they do not approve specific therapy, or cannot be reached to approve these, especially extractions, they should not be performed. The third call is made when the pet is in recovery and the time for discharge can be set.

At discharge, client education continues with a review of photos and radiographs, as well as any therapy provided. This can be performed by a veterinarian or technician, depending on the clinic policy and extent of treatment. Before-and-after pictures can also be provided with the written discharge instruction. These postoperative instructions will include any medications prescribed, any recommended dietary adjustments, cautions or protection for surgical sites, and to schedule follow-up examinations. Taking the time to meet with the client to discuss the findings, treatment and postoperative care will increase the value of the procedure their pet received, as well as potentially improve compliance with recommended follow-up steps.

At the follow-up examination, typically for all patients that had any surgical procedures (extractions, etc.), the oral cavity is examined for the state of healing. In addition, the dental team can review home care options and schedule the next dental examination or procedure or set reminder.

In North America, February is traditionally considered Pet Dental Care Month. However, every month should be Pet Dental Care Month, so don't let clients wait until February if their pet really needs care. Even for those who have come annually in February, some of these patients should be seen on a more regular basis. For any dental patient, dental reminders should be set based upon the level of disease, with Stage 1 patients getting annual reminders, Stage 2 patients should be seen at nine months, and Stage 3 patients at six months. While the really diseased teeth for a Stage 4 PD patient were probably extracted, they should still be seen at 3–4 months to keep the disease from returning. This can help "adjust" the flow of patients that just come in during February.

Another way to strategize the enhancement of your dental practice is to integrate senior care and dental care throughout the year. If senior diagnostics are recent, encourage dental procedure using recent results. If dental care is needed, suggest a full diagnostic "package," especially for older pets that might be overdue for their senior care. If a dental procedure is scheduled within a reasonable time frame from diagnostic work, an incentive can be considered (discount on basic dental services).

A big challenge for many clinic strategies is scheduling procedures, as the length of time needed for any particular dental procedure can vary widely. Encourage recording the stage of PD or other dental issues found on examination. Now, the estimate of the level of disease seen in the exam room is usually based on the amount of plaque and calculus, and that is not the complete picture. Be on the watch for "red flags," oral/dental conditions that might also be present. If the gingiva or mucosa is a deep red (vermillion) above/below the tooth, that is likely an indication of a deeper infection. With broken, worn or discolored teeth, if the pulp is compromised (open canal, dark-colored tooth – dead pulp), then treatment is needed, either extraction or root canal therapy.

Transillumination can sometimes be done in the exam room to assess the vitality of a tooth. To do this, shine a bright light through (from behind) the tooth; if the light shines through the tooth and the pink of the pulp is identified, the tooth is likely vital. If the light does not shine through the tooth well and it appears dark, then the tooth is likely nonvital and needs treatment. This is similar to "candling" an egg. Also take pictures with the clinic camera or client's phone to let them take home the visual evidence that care is needed.

If Stage 3–4 or other condition is seen that needs immediate treatment, set a procedure appointment before the client leaves. This allows the dental team to get bloodwork and diagnostics started and to implement antibiotic and pain medications if needed. If a Stage 3–4 patient is not scheduled, call them back the next day to get it set. For stage 1 2 patients, the team can set up reminders to contact them in 2–4 months.

Strategies for scheduling and dental team workflow can be quite complicated. Dental procedures vary widely in the extent of disease to be managed and the amount of time needed. A patient might require just a standard dental cleaning with radiographs and polishing, and no periodontal treatment or extractions. Moderate cases may additionally involve simple extractions of loose teeth or minor periodontal treatment (closed root planning – see 4.9 Periodontal Disease). Extensive cases can involve numerous extractions or extractions of major teeth (lower canines, upper fourth premolars).

For each clinic scenario that is dependent on resources such as the staff and equipment available, determine the maximum number of uncomplicated cases that can be done in a day (e.g., no more than four procedures). Next, determine the maximum number of treatment "segments" that should be handled in a day. Divide the total time allotted for dental procedures and assign a time increment or segment that will take up that time (30–45 minutes on average). For example, if your team averages 1.5–2 segments per procedure, that would make approximately 6–8 segments if you plan on four procedures in a day. The team may then determine that they want to maximize seven segments per day.

Try to determine – prior to or at the time of scheduling – the estimated number of segments a procedure might take. For example, an uncomplicated procedure may take one segment and a moderate procedure two segments. A moderate procedure with one extended extraction may need three segments and an extensive case of severe PD with an unknown number of extractions needed (typical "small dog mouth") may take up to four segments. Once the segment slots have been filled, take no further procedures unless approved by that day's dental team. In looking at a day's schedule that already has a four-segment extensive procedure and a two-segment moderate procedure, you can only schedule one more uncomplicated case (one-segment). If all four procedures are designated as uncomplicated one-segment cases, don't fill in other slots – it is highly likely that hidden problems will be found on those "simple" cases. Also, you have determined that the maximum number of patients that can be adequately handled in a day is four. Don't compromise patient care to squeeze in one more procedure.

Managing unexpected challenges is a common problem in dental practice. Frequently, hidden lesions are found during the procedure, giving us unanticipated work beyond what the time scheduled can accommodate. Optimize team workflow to handle these "typical dental days." Often the veterinarian scheduled for dental procedures may have limited time to provide surgical treatment, with multiple patients to treat and other appointments or in-clinic treatments pending. Utilize technicians/nurses to provide the majority of dental services – prepping the patient, monitoring, cleaning, polishing, taking oral radiographs and photos.

At the beginning of each procedure, once the patient is stable, identify any "red flags" which are significant areas of disease (PD with deep pockets or loose teeth; broken or discolored teeth) that may not have been identified in the exam room, and note these on the chart. Also, quickly probe potential problem spots such as inside upper canines, around lower canines and lower first molars. Find any broken teeth with open canals (use dental explorer) or discolored teeth (transilluminate). Look for any indication of TR, especially in cats (lower third premolar is the most common site, but any tooth is possible). Communicate these finding with the attending veterinarian and once identified, these sites can be blocked with a local anesthetic and radiographed. Be flexible with the workflow of the dental procedure because if the veterinarian is only available during certain times, the cleaning and polishing can be put on hold to get the extractions done (the radiographs and blocks have already been performed). The cleaning/polishing with postextraction radiographs can be completed after the surgery.

If the unanticipated work is far beyond what can be reasonably accomplished at the time, it is appropriate to consider recommending a staged procedure. A staged procedure divides the patient's therapy into an initial phase of cleaning, assessment (probing and radiographs), polishing and any simple procedures that can be easily provided. The second phase includes any additional advanced treatment which may include surgical extractions (oral surgery) and extensive periodontal therapy. Dividing the work into two phases provides benefits for the patient. If the combined work would have required a longer single anesthetic time (over two hours), even with relatively steady physical parameters (blood pressure, body temperature), these procedures can be stressful for the patient. Getting the bulk of the infected material and debris out of the mouth will allow the remaining tissues (especially gingiva and soft tissues) to become healthier and more amenable to treatment at the second phase.

Good client communication is key to opting for a staged procedure, so providing information about this option at the beginning of any procedure is beneficial. Then communication throughout the procedure can help prepare the owner for the possibility of a staged procedure. Sometimes the patient feels so much better after the first phase that the owner neglects to return for the second phase, so be sure the owner understands the need for the additional therapy.

As discussed earlier, the two-week follow-up examination allows for visual assessment of the procedure and the healing process. This is also an excellent time to go into further detail about home care options for the pet/parent combination. The successful results of therapy are often expressed at this visit, such as "He's like a new puppy again!" or "She's eating better than she has in months!" Be sure to celebrate these successes and share with the entire clinic, to help support their efforts in encouraging owners to pursue dental care for their pets. Also share with other clients on a bulletin board, on your website, or on social media. Hearing testimonials from other pet parents can be very impactful on owners with concerns, since they had the same concerns with costs and anesthetic risks but are now enjoying the positive result. This shares the personal, emotional aspect of the benefits of good dental care beyond what we can provide on a medical level and helps to support the importance of the human–animal bond.

EXAMPLES

When Mrs Smith dropped off her dog Fluffy for a dental procedure, the information discussed at the dental consult visit was reiterated: there was moderate to heavy plaque and calculus with significant gingival inflammation, and while extractions were expected, we would not know how many until the full dental examination was completed, with radiographs. The estimate therefore was broad, with a low end covering the basic cleaning and assessment, with a few minor extractions. The high end of the estimate was still just an educated guess, but substantially more expensive.

Mrs Smith was called when the preoperative injection was given, and informed that we would be calling a second time with the updated treatment plan. Unfortunately, many of Fluffy's teeth needed to be extracted due to extensive bone loss that was not completely visible grossly but found radiographically. At the second call, the dental manager explained how severe the PD was, and that without treatment, Fluffy could even be at risk for a pathological fracture of her mandibles. It did take Mrs Smith by surprise, as she had focused on the low end of the estimate, and the total cost was more than she expected. Options for payment were discussed, as well as the possibility of staging the procedure (extracting the extremely mobile teeth and providing surgical extraction for the remainder at a later date) and she stated she needed to call her spouse for the decision to proceed.

Since the evaluation and radiographs were done fairly early in the procedure, this time was spent cleaning the teeth that would remain, providing some minor periodontal therapy and placing local blocks. Mrs Smith called back with the approval for all the work to be done that day.

At discharge, we carefully went over all the pictures and radiographs to show the extent of the disease to both pet parents, and they better understood the need for the surgery. Needless to say, at the two-week follow-up, they expressed their great appreciation, as Fluffy was now feeling and acting much better! They even scheduled the six-month dental procedure to help keep the PD under control.

TAKE-AWAYS

- If the client hears a consistent message – that oral and dental care is essential – they will believe what you believe.
- Dental procedures are often more involved than anticipated once you get in there; be prepared for staff time and owner expectations.
- Good dental care is needed for the lifetime of the pet.
- Make sure every team member has experienced the "miracle" of good dental care, whether in their own pet or participating in the care of patients.
- Be clearly aware of what aspects of PD are reversible, and which are progressive and nonreversible. Recommend intervention while problems are still reversible.

MISCELLANEOUS

8.19.3 Cautions

Many pet owners will be anxious about anesthesia and the procedure; make no guarantees for success or safety, but discuss all the measures you take to minimize risks and provide care (see 5.12 Discussing Anesthetic Risk).

Never quote a specific charge, but provide a range of charges depending on what might be realistically found after further evaluation when the pet is anesthetized.

Don't perform extractions without specific owner approval. Keeping owners informed is the best way to ensure customer satisfaction.

References

1 2019 AAHA Dental Care Guidelines for Dogs and Cats. https://www.aaha.org/globalassets/02-guidelines/dental/aaha_dental_guidelines.pdf
2 American Veterinary Dental College. Companion Animal Dental Scaling without Anesthesia. https://avdc.org/PDF/Dental_Scaling_Without_Anesthesia.pdf

Recommended Reading

Holmstrom, S.E. (2012). *Veterinary Dentistry: A Team Approach*, 2e. Philadelphia, PA: W.B. Saunders.

8.20

Team Strategies for Osteoarthritis

Mark E. Epstein, DVM, DABVP (Canine/Feline), CVPP

TotalBond Veterinary Hospitals, PC, Gastonia, NC, USA

BASICS

8.20.1 Summary

Contrary to conventional concepts, osteoarthritis (OA) is not a disease strictly of older dogs or cats. A variety of risk factors, chief among them heritable conformational problems, often begins and advances pathological joint change very early on, including in puppyhood. This creates a challenge for the veterinary team to recognize, assess, and manage OA even when (or before!) the patient is only mildly symptomatic. Fortunately, there are a number of tools to aid the clinical team in its efforts to improve both quality and length of life in dogs and cats with this condition.

8.20.2 Terms Defined

Degenerative Joint Disease (DJD): The umbrella term for damage to and degradation of hyaline cartilage and its negative consequences on joint function and comfort.

Hypersensitization: The molecular and cellular "wind-up" in peripheral tissue and dorsal horn of the spinal cord, characterized by decreased neuron firing threshold, decreased descending inhibition, recruitment of bystanding neurons and more; results in maladaptive pain.

Nociception: Pain processing with peripheral neuronal activation, transmission in the primary afferent neuron, modulation in the spinal cord, and perception in various centers throughout the brain.

Osteoarthritis (OA): A subset of DJD that occurs when the protecting cartilage on the ends of bones wears down over time.

Pain: Multidimensional unpleasant sensory and emotional experience associated with actual or potential tissue damage. Chronic pain occurs when the pain persists for three months or longer.

Pain, Maladaptive: Peripheral and central hypersensitization-induced abnormal pain, characterized by increased scope, character, and field of pain: hyperalgesia, allodynia, dysthesias.

Pain, Neuropathic: Hypersensitization and maladaptive pain that has progressed to gene expression and permanent morphological and functional changes in the peripheral and central nervous system. Pain as a disease at this point.

MAIN CONCEPTS

8.20.3 The Problem

At least 20% of all dogs are likely affected by OA, and probably many more, and most are diagnosed between 8 and 13 years old [1]; 60% of all cats and 90% of cats over the age of 10 have radiographic DJD changes [2]. Because animals are nonverbal and therefore cannot self-report their discomfort, an owner (and the veterinary team!) often under-appreciate the impact on the pet, and miss opportunities to diagnose and intervene early in life when the greatest influence can be made to modify (delay and mitigate) the disease process (see 3.12 Orthopedic Screening).

Furthermore, OA represents more than just chronic joint inflammation and pain, and includes the following additional dimensions.

- Hypersensitization
- Impact (weakness/atrophy) on the affected entire joint organ (soft tissue and even bone) due to diminished loading
- Impact on other limbs and joints due to improper (excessive) loading
- Cognitive effects – diminished learning, memory, mental agility, and even clinical depression

Fortunately, the entire veterinary team can aid in the identification of a patient affected by OA. All support staff can be trained to recognize and record risk factors, historical signs reported by the owner, and observations of patient conformation, body position, and mobility even before the veterinarian performs an orthopedic exam. This includes front desk personnel taking calls and watching pets in the reception area, technicians, and veterinary assistants escorting to the exam room and talking to owners, and animal caretakers interacting with the patients under their care.

Several clinical metrology instruments (CMI) are validated for assessment and scoring of OA in dogs, including the Canine Brief Pain Inventory (CBPI) [3] and Liverpool Osteoarthritis in Dogs (LOAD) [4]. COAST (Canine Osteoarthritis Staging Tool) [1] uniquely is a CMI that allows for identification of early (Stage 1) OA based on risk factors even in asymptomatic patients – which can drive management decisions accordingly (see Figure 8.20.1).

Risk factors for OA include:

- breed dispositions
- high body conformation score (i.e., overweight/obese)
- age (older > younger)
- activity (agility dogs vs sedentary)
- previous joint injury (e.g., cruciate) and/or surgery

- owner report of previous lameness (even if spontaneously resolved); stiffness in morning or after exercise (even if it "warms out"); for cats, diminished frequency and height of jumping.

Front desk personnel, those taking calls, emails, and other outreaches from pet owners, can immediately be alerted to a patient with prospective OA – and then set an alert for the rest of the team – by knowing at the outset only two things, breed and age, followed by cues given by the owner. It is important to bear in mind that pet owners may not recognize certain behaviors (or the lack of normal behaviors) as signs of pain, ascribing them to mere age, for example. After all, obvious signs of pain, such as limping or vocalization, may not be apparent.

Breed dispositions include heritable risk factors, such as hip and elbow dysplasia, cruciate injury, lumbosacral stenosis, luxating patellas, etc.

Owners' verbal clues may include the following.

- "Stiff, slow getting up" in the morning, after exercise
- "Have to help" get up onto the couch/bed, into the car
- "Slow on stairs" (up *or* down)
- "We started a joint supplement"
- Cats: "finally trained him not to jump up on the kitchen counter"; "he doesn't like to be held/picked up"

Once recognized, a visual notification is placed in the practice software, or if paper records or on the hospital admission/travel sheet, just a designated sticker. This can alert the rest of the team to a likely OA patient. These conversations can casually introduce the concept of prospective arthritis to the owner, when they may or may not have yet considered it a significant issue for their pet: "I wonder if she doesn't have some arthritis. We'll certainly have the doctor take a good look." If the practice has an electronic questionnaire about mobility (and/or other health) issues, it can be emailed to the owner at this point.

HIGHEST GRADE EQUATES TO COAST STAGE

	COAST Stage		
Preclinical	0	Clinically normal. No OA risk factors.
	1	Clinically normal, but OA risk factors present.
Clinical	2	Mild OA.
	3	Moderate OA.
	4	Severe OA.

Figure 8.20.1 COAST stages. *Source:* Image courtesy of Elanco.

An efficient way to ensure that the veterinary team is aware of what patients are receiving at home is to simply ask the client to put everything they are giving their pet (any and all medications, and supplements) in a bag and bring it along to the visit; the team can go through this in order to align what the client is doing with the medical records, get a hint of what the owner may have initiated unbeknownst to the hospital, and minimize the likelihood of inadvertent drug interactions. For example, some OVER-THE-COUNTER (OTC) joint supplements have aspirin in them, which may be dangerous for the pet if subsequently prescribed a veterinary nonsteroidal antiinflammatory drug (NSAID) for OA.

The orthopedic exam begins, and can be initiated visually, by any team member with observation of posture and gait. Examples include the following.

1) *Laying down*: forearms straight out? (elbow pain: elbow out to side and paw curled around)
2) *Getting up*: all four limbs simultaneously? (hip/stifle pain: up on front legs first then hoist rear quarters up; also r/o weakness, musculoskeletal, and/or neurological)
3) *Sitting*: square? (on hip: likely stifle pain but could also be hip)
4) *Standing*: hindlimbs normal angles to knee, hock? (straight-legged conformation: likely hip OA); kyphosis/bowed back, forelimbs tucked under frame, hypertrophied ("barrel chested") pectorals, atrophy? (all from chronic forward weight shift; kyphosis also from back pain)
5) *Walking*: is there a quick step? (pain in the contralateral limb); rear quarter "wiggle"? (hip dysplasia)
6) *Tail*: held high? (low: lumbosacral pain)

Once again, front desk personnel are often there at the tip of the spear, in the reception area, and as dogs are escorted to the exam room, these changes can be observed, as can another risk factor – high body condition score (BCS, i.e., overweight). And if an OA/health questionnaire has not yet been given to the owner, it can be deployed at this time for the owner to fill out while waiting for the technician.

Similar for technicians and assistants if they perform the escort, but certainly once in the exam room. Furthermore, animal caretakers can also observe such changes in patients that are staying for boarding, grooming, or other ancillary services.

About 85% of the diagnostic process for OA is in history taking. Here, technicians (and assistants, if tasked) are now at the point of the spear. If the client has not yet volunteered information, it can be prompted by the OA/health questionnaire and asking open-ended questions about the patient's activities of daily living, confirming medications or supplements the owners are giving.

If time permits and patient appropriate, the technician can deploy CBPI or LOAD to give a semi-quantitative "score" on how the OA is affecting the patient. At the very least, the technician/nurse should document historical and visual observations in the patient medical record, and alert the veterinarian accordingly.

The veterinarian will subsequently conduct the physical examination (PE), with a veterinary assistant as needed. If the patient is presenting for lameness or mobility issues, then the focus of the PE can be orthopedic and neurological in nature. However, if the patient is presenting for an annual or semi-annual wellness exam, a 2–3-minute orthopedic examination can be included in the course of the PE. As the hands move over the patient, the musculoskeletal system can be assessed for CREAPI: Crepitance, Range of Motion (ROM. decreased), Effusion, Asymmetry (one joint or limb different than contralateral), Pain, Instability.

With an accumulation of historical, orthopedic examination, and radiographic signs, minimally a COAST score can be assigned from Stage 1 (early, nonsymptomatic but with one or more risk factors), up to a maximum of Stage 4 (advanced) OA.

Communicating the degree of actual discomfort in a COAST Stage 2, or even 3 or 4, patient to their owners is not always easy, never mind explaining what is ahead for a COAST Stage 1! And in an annual or semi-annual wellness visit, there are many other things that probably require some discussion: teeth, ears, lumps, bumps, and so on. With time, attention, and resources at a premium, the veterinarian and team must convey the import of their findings and the stakes for the patient, and derive a plan in a succinct and direct but compassionate manner.

One practice tip to aid in this process is to describe OA in terms of disability, and an inevitably progressive one at that, rather than "pain," since it is the change in mobility, abilities, and activity that the owner will actually appreciate at home. In the symptomatic patient (COAST Stage 2 and greater), in fact, the appearance of the patient with regard to OA at this veterinary visit is as good as this pet is ever going to be. . .unless, that is, a management plan is undertaken, whereby clinical signs can be improved in the short run, and the disease process slowed and impact lessened over time. What we do at that visit makes a difference not just this week but for many years hence.

A second practice tip is not to overwhelm the pet owner with a long and complex discussion of OA, especially when the pet is there for something other than specifically mobility issues. A short identification and introduction is sufficient, ensure that the client is given education material, and in many cases of COAST Stage 2 and most cases of Stages 3 and 4, it can be appropriate to initiate a short course of NSAIDs. The veterinary team can say "We'll be following up in a few day to see how she is doing on the medication [and with lab test results if performed], and that's when we can have a more extensive discussion about arthritis and map out a long-term management plan at that time." A response to NSAID therapy (note that this can take up to two weeks in some dogs) will reinforce the diagnosis of OA and create the space for client acceptance of a more detailed plan. By recheck appointment, phone, email, or video chat, the veterinarian can advise on a suggested strategy. It is often during this follow-up conversation, rather than the original exam room visit, where veterinarian and pet owner collaborate and together agree on a management plan that meets the patient's needs within the client's goals and resources.

The veterinary team can then set up follow-up evaluations. This may include one or more of the following.

- Progress report from home
- Having the client regenerate CMI like CBPI or LOAD
- Return for weight check
- Return for routine lab monitoring (especially if on NSAID)
- Return for periodic consult and progress check with the veterinarian

An evidence-based approach to OA management can be derived from a number of high-quality systemic reviews and summarized in industry pain management guidelines [5, 6]. It is important to note that some of the most important modalities are nonpharmacological.

For early canine OA.

1) Puppies: decelerate growth in at-risk breeds (high-quality "large breed" dog food formulations).
2) Weight optimization: can be described as the most important of modalities (see 8.25 Team Strategies for Weight Management). Young dogs should be kept lean from the outset, and if overweight, a loss of just 6% body weight can effect improvement in dogs with OA.
3) Eicosapentaenoic acid (EPA)-rich diets in dogs, docosahexaenoic acid (DHA)-rich diet in cats.
4) Chondroprotectants (parenteral polysulfated glycosaminoglycan, PSGAG, vs nutraceuticals).
5) NSAID, including the EP-4 receptor antagonist grapiprant.

Therapeutic exercise for more advanced OA, additional modalities.

1) Adjunctive pain-modifying analgesic drugs (PMAD): for instance, amantadine, gabapentin, possibly selective serotonin reuptake inhibitors (SSRIs) (e.g., venlafaxine, duloxetine) and others. Note: tramadol has been shown to be *ineffective* in the treatment of canine OA [7].

2) Intraarticular biologics and other agents: stem cells, platelet-rich plasma (definitions and types of both products varied); new agents/products continue to be developed.
3) Anti-nerve growth factor monoclonal antibody (anti-NGF MAb) [8].
4) Physical and energy-based modalities (most evidence is cellular, molecular, and histological at this time, clinical evidence inconclusive or mixed; however, appears safe and in popular use): acupuncture, myofascial trigger point therapy, therapeutic laser, therapeutic ultrasound, pulsed electromagnetic field, extracorporeal shock wave therapy; referral for advance physical rehab including hydrotherapy.

EXAMPLES

Bernese mountain dog during puppy visits: Placed on high-quality large-breed dog food and advised to stay on adult large-breed formulation, with firm guidance on proper portions into adulthood to maintain lean body weight. Ensure good exercise program and consider nutraceutical as puppy enters adulthood. Discussion re delaying spay/neuter until after sexual maturity.

Three-year-old Labrador retriever presents for annual health visit, no complaints by owner, no conformation, gait, or PE abnormalities except for BCS of 6/9 (COAST Stage 1 due to risk factors of breed disposition and overweight). Firm guidance on weight loss plan to attain BCS 4.5–5/9 (ideally on prescription diet formulation rather than mere calorie reduction); thereafter maintain on EPA-rich diet. Place on nutraceuticals and advise regular therapeutic exercise program.

Seven-year-old Rottweiler presents for Grade 1 lameness left rear leg ("quick step" on the right rear). Patient has history of previous but spontaneously resolving lameness in same leg. Team member notices he sits on right hip (i.e., not square) with left rear leg stuck out. PE reveals BCS 7/9, medial buttress left stifle but minimal effusion and no instability (COAST Stage 2: symptomatic for chronic-active cranial cruciate injury and with history of previous injury and breed, age, and weight dispositions). NSAID for one month then reevaluation. Weight optimization to BCS 5/9 paramount. PSGAG (or alternatively nutraceutical). Minimize unrestricted activity but enhance controlled, therapeutic exercise (to include inclines/hills). EPA-rich diet. Consideration of intraarticular biologic to aid in cranial cruciate repair.

Ten-year-old 35 kg mixed-breed dog presents for semiannual visit. Owner reports she is doing really well, still goes on long walks and plays with other dog "like a puppy," although casually mentions she is stiff after resting and in the morning, and hesitant about jumping up on the couch. Team member notices she gets up on her front legs first then pulls up hindlegs, and during walk to exam room there is a "wiggle" to hind end; tail is wagging but lower rather than higher. PE reveals BCS 5/9 but mild muscle atrophy to rear legs and resists extension of both hips; objects to dorsoflexion of tail with digital pressure at lumbosacral joint. (COAST Stage 3: significantly symptomatic for hip dysplasia/OA, lumbosacral stenosis – radiographs confirm and more fully characterize – with historical, breed, and age dispositions.) NSAID for 3–6 months then reevaluation; EPA-rich diet and ensure maintains lean BCS; PSGAG (or alternatively nutraceutical). Enhance controlled, therapeutic exercise (to include inclines/hills). Consideration of one or more physical and/or energy-based modalities. Depending on response to therapies, can then consider deploying a PMAD, possible intraarticular biologics, anti-NGF MAb (if/when available).

Fourteen-year-old 20 kg mixed-breed dog with limited activity, diminished interaction with family, owner has to carry up and down stairs. Has already been placed on EPA-rich diet, chondroprotectant daily, and NSAID but owners give this intermittently rather than regularly. Team members observe obvious difficulty getting up on slick floor, stilted gait, tail low, kyphosis, and straight-legged conformation to rear legs, atrophy to rear legs and apparent hypertrophy of forequarters. PE additionally reveals BCS 6/9, limited range of motion (ROM) of carpii, elbows with thickening and discomfort upon palpation medial condylar region; myalgia/hyperesthesia along spine, resists extension of hips, crepitance in stifles and hocks. Initiate daily NSAID on sustained basis with emphasis on appropriate use and monitoring, add PMAD, place on weight optimization and gradual therapeutic exercise plan (consider referral if possible for advanced physical therapy, e.g., hydrotherapy), one or more physical and/or energy-based modalities. Strong candidate for intraarticular biologic injections and anti-NGF MAb (if/when available).

TAKE-AWAYS

- DJD and OA are present in many more dogs and cats, including young animals, than generally appreciated.
- The pathophysiology of OA in dogs is often conformational (i.e., heritable), and exacerbated by common risk factors (weight, activity, injury, age). The etiopathophysiology in cats is less well understood but still very common in cats of all ages (and in almost all cats >10 years).
- The entire veterinary team should be involved in recognizing risk factors as well as historical, conformational, mobility, and gait changes that suggest the possibility or even likelihood of OA. The clinical measurement instrument COAST allows for the identification of early (Stage 1) OA even in nonsymptomatic dogs.
- An evidence management program for at-risk or COAST Stage 1 dogs minimally includes weight optimization and can also include EFA-rich diets, chondroprotection, exercise, and short course of NSAID as needed.
- For more advanced OA, weight optimization remains paramount; EFA-rich diets, chondroprotection, therapeutic exercise, and extended courses of NSAID are also central. Other modalities such as pain-modifying analgesic drugs, physical/energy-based modalities, intraarticular biologics, and anti-NGF MAb (if/when available).

MISCELLANEOUS

8.20.4 Cautions

NSAIDs remain the most rapidly and predictably effective treatment modality for symptomatic OA (see 2.16 Pain and Pain Management). Although generally quite safe, this class does have a well-defined adverse drug effect (ADE) profile which can be exacerbated with inappropriate use. It is incumbent on the veterinary team to recognize and avoid risk factors associated with NSAID ADE (including but not limited to co-administration with corticosteroid and other NSAID), other drug interactions (including but not limited to furosemide, other nephrotoxic drugs, multiple highly protein-bound drugs), compromised patients (including but not limited to dehydration, hypovolemia/hypotension, preexisting kidney disease, gastritis/enteritis, liver dysfunction, heart disease), use of high-dose, inadequate patient monitoring, inadequate client education on ADE signs and action to take if observed [9]. Communicating to the owner safe use of NSAID (avoiding inappropriate use, recognizing ADE [vomiting most common, diarrhea, and diminished appetite], and if observed, withdrawing the NSAID then reporting to the practice) is a multilayered and shared responsibility across the veterinary team. Practice software can print out cautions, warnings, and instructions on drug labels and the invoice; technicians and veterinary assistants can share verbally and also give the NSAID client education material provided by manufacturer; similarly front desk personnel can be mindful and repeat the directive to stop the medication and call if any problems or concerns encountered. By this shared responsibility, the risk of serious NSAID ADE can be significantly minimized.

Mindfulness of veterinary team members (and pet owners) toward low-stress handling, minimizing fear, stress, and distress during hospital visits (not to mention at home) remains an all-important, but often overlooked, part of OA pain management (see Recommended Reading).

References

1 Cachon, T., Frykman, O., Innes, J.F. et al. (2018). COAST development group. Face validity of a proposed tool for staging canine osteoarthritis: canine OsteoArthritis staging tool (COAST). *Vet. J.* 235: 1–8.

2 Lascelles BD, Henry JB 3rd, Brown J, et al. Cross-sectional study of the prevalence of radiographic degenerative joint disease in domesticated cats. *Vet. Surg.* 2010;39(5):535–544.

3 Brown, D.C., Boston, R.C., Coyne, J.C., and Farrar, J.T. (2008). Ability of the canine brief pain inventory to detect response to treatment in dogs with osteoarthritis. *J. Am. Vet. Med. Assoc.* 233 (8): 1278–1283.

4 Walton, M.B., Cowderoy, E., Lascelles, D., and Innes, J.F. (2013). Evaluation of construct and criterion validity for the 'Liverpool osteoarthritis in Dogs' (LOAD) clinical metrology instrument and comparison to two other instruments. *PLoS One* 8 (3): e58125.

5 Epstein M, Rodan I, Griffenhagen G, et al. 2015 AAHA/AAFP pain management guidelines for dogs and cats. *J. Am. Anim. Hosp. Assoc.* 2015;51(2):67–84.

6 Mathews K, Kronen PW, Lascelles D, et al. Guidelines for recognition, assessment and treatment of pain: WSAVA global pain council. *J. Small Anim. Pract.* 2014;55(6): E10–68

7 Budsberg, S.C., Torres, B.T., Kleine, S.A. et al. (2018). Lack of effectiveness of tramadol hydrochloride for the treatment of pain and joint dysfunction in dogs with chronic osteoarthritis. *J. Am. Vet. Med. Assoc.* 252 (4): 427–432.

8 Webster, R.P., Anderson, G.I., and Gearing, D.P. (2014). Canine brief pain inventory scores for dogs with osteoarthritis before and after administration of a monoclonal antibody against nerve growth factor. *Am. J. Vet. Res.* 75 (6): 532–535.

9 Monteiro-Steagall, B.P., Steagall, P.V., and Lascelles, B.D. (2013). Systematic review of nonsteroidal anti-inflammatory drug-induced adverse effects in dogs. J vet intern med. *J. Vet. Intern. Med.* 27 (5): 1011–1019.

Recommended Reading

Epstein M, Rodan I, Griffenhagen G, et al. 2015 AAHA/AAFP pain management guidelines for dogs and cats. *J. Am. Anim. Hosp. Assoc.* 2015;51(2):67–84.

Mathews K, Kronen PW, Lascelles D, et al. Guidelines for recognition, assessment and treatment of pain: WSAVA global pain council. *J. Small Anim. Pract.* 2014;55(6):E10–68

Rodan I, Sundahl E, Carney H, et al. American Animal Hospital Association. AAFP and ISFM feline-friendly handling guidelines. *J. Feline Med. Surg.* 2011;13(5):364–375.

Yin, S. Low Stress Handling, Restraint and Behavior Modification of Dogs and Cats: Techniques for Developing Patients Who Love Their Visits. www.drsophiayin.com

8.21

Team Strategies for Pain Management

Tamara Grubb, DVM, PhD, DACVAA

Washington State University, Pullman, WA, USA

 BASICS

8.21.1 Summary

The most (only?) successful way to provide effective and consistent pain relief for veterinary patients is to approach pain management as a team. The team should include the front office staff/receptionists, veterinary nurses/technicians, and veterinarians. The entire team must understand, and be ready to discuss with pet owners, that animals do feel pain and that pain can negatively impact their pet's health, behavior, and welfare. Scripts/literature for client education, pain assessment systems, and analgesic protocols for acute and chronic pain must be implemented and diligently followed. Finally, for consistent pain relief and quality of life for the pet, the pet owner must be integrated into the pain management team.

 MAIN CONCEPTS

Animals cannot understand that pain can impact their health, behavior, and quality of life, they cannot request analgesic treatment and they cannot voice the efficacy, or lack thereof, of that analgesic treatment. Since the veterinary patient cannot be its own advocate, a team of people must be trained to do – and be committed to doing – all of these tasks.

The first step in building an effective pain management team is educating the team about animal pain with the goal of ensuring that every team member fervently believes that animals do feel pain and that pain can negatively impact that animal's health, behavior, and welfare (see 2.16 Pain and Pain Management). The team must also passionately believe that the veterinary practice – and all its members – are dedicated

to the relief of animal pain (see 6.14 Pain Prevention, Management, and Conditioning). The veterinary team consists of the receptionists/office staff, veterinary nurses/technicians, and veterinarians. For continued care at home, the pet owner must also be educated and integrated into the team.

The next steps in building the team include assigning specific roles for each team member, providing the training and education that the team member requires to fulfill their role and emphasizing that every team member must constantly strive to meet the practice's goal of relieving pain in every single patient.

8.21.2 Educating the Entire Veterinary Team

Education of the team can start with a review of and commitment to the American Veterinary Medical Association's (AVMA) statement on animal pain [1]. This statement can even be printed and displayed in the practice for all team members, and pet owners, to view.

American Veterinary Medical Association Statement on Pain in Animals

Animal pain is a clinically important condition that adversely affects an animal's quality of life. Drugs, techniques, or husbandry methods should be used to prevent, minimize, and relieve pain in animals experiencing or expected to experience pain. Protocols must be tailored to individual animals and should be based, in part, on the species, sex, breed, age, procedure performed, degree of tissue trauma, individual behavioral characteristics, assessment of the degree of pain, and health status of the animal.

The entire veterinary team should understand the concepts described in Figure 8.21.1 and be able to:

- communicate the fact that the sensation of pain is very similar in all mammals, which means that if a stimulus is painful to a human, it is definitely painful to an animal
- explain that, unfortunately, dogs and cats are very adept at hiding pain from humans, making it unlikely that pet owners can predictably recognize signs of pain in their pets
- explain that untreated or inadequately treated pain has a negative impact on health, behavior, and welfare of the pet
- understand, and believe, that the entire hospital team is committed to pain identification and provision of effective analgesia for all patients.

8.21.3 Role of the Receptionist/Front Office Staff

The receptionists and office staff have the unique position of often being the first person(s) to speak to the client, including potentially new clients, about pain in their pets and about the hospital team's dedication to the relief of animal pain. The office personnel need to be able to understand and to communicate the philosophies described above – that animals do feel pain, that recognition of pain in animals can be difficult and that your clinic and all its team members are dedicated to the relief of animal pain. The receptionist and office staff have the opportunity to be the first pain advocates for the pet and to convey these philosophies to pet owners in many situations, including these three common scenarios.

1) A pet owner, who is not yet a client of the practice, calls to discuss scheduling surgery for their pet and wants to know about the procedure in your practice. The office member on the call should be prepared to briefly describe the care provided to pets having surgery in the practice, with a focus on pain management. Pain management is not only the medically right thing to do for the pet, it may also set your practice apart from others in the area and this conversation can be used to emphasize both points. The entire office staff should be prepared with a script that describes the importance of pain management and the fact that, at your hospital, pain medication is provided for the pet both in the hospital and for administration at home after surgery. These scripts may also need to include an explanation of pricing if the pet owner says that the price at this clinic is higher than prices at other clinics because of the inclusion of pain-relieving therapies. A sample script is available in the examples section of this chapter.

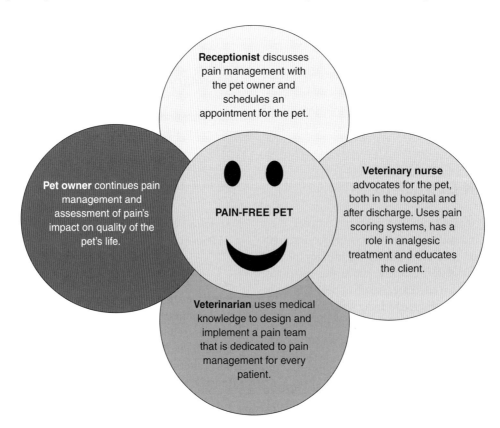

Figure 8.21.1 The team approach to pet pain management includes the receptionist, veterinary nurse, veterinarian, and pet owner.

2) A pet owner calls to inquire whether their pet should be seen by a veterinarian because of a particular disease or injury suffered by the pet. Of course, diagnoses cannot be made accurately over the phone and, in general, the office member should always schedule an appointment for the pet. However, the timing of the appointment may become more urgent if the pet owner describes something that may be painful. If this occurs, the office member should alert the client to the fact that animals feel pain and that pain can cause negative health and behavior effects. The pet should then be scheduled for the first available appointment.

3) A pet owner has questions regarding pain or the analgesic drugs as they are checking out or after they get home. When a pet is being discharged or has been discharged with pain medications, the veterinarian or veterinary nurse should discuss the medications, and the importance of giving the medications, with the pet owner. However, the pet owner may also ask questions of the front office staff, who should be able to reiterate that the pain medications are very important for the recovery of their pet from the surgery, injury, or disease. The office staff should also reiterate that the pain medications should be administered as prescribed whether or not the owner thinks that the animal is in pain. Owners should be educated that animals are very good at hiding pain, thus signs of pain often go unrecognized, but the medications were prescribed because the pet's surgery, injury, or disease is known to cause pain. Any questions that the office staff cannot answer should be referred to the veterinary nurse or veterinarian.

The office staff should also be tasked with generating, or assisting in the development of, client education material and pain management information to be posted on the hospital's website and social media pages. Accessible information can provide useful education for the client and good marketing for the hospital. As stated, pain management is not only good medicine, it can also set the practice apart from other practices and all avenues of promoting the hospital's dedication to relieving animal pain should be utilized.

8.21.4 Role of the Veterinary Nurse/Technician

As with human nurses, the veterinary nurse is generally the primary "voice," or advocate, of the patient. The nurse often spends the most time with the patient and knows the patient better than other hospital personnel. Thus, the nurse is uniquely positioned to recognize changes in behavior and well-being that might otherwise go unnoticed.

The nurse's main role is to be attentive to the patient during its entire hospital stay and to advocate for the patient if pain is potentially present. Nurses should be able to do the following with the patient.

- Assist in design and implementation of analgesic protocols for all patients, including those with chronic pain.
- Utilize pain scoring systems to assess the patient and to determine the patient's need for analgesic therapy (drugs and/or nonpharmacological therapy).
- Discuss, and be empowered to discuss, the patient's need for additional analgesic therapy with the veterinarians.
- With doctor agreement, provide basic analgesia, including bolus administration (intramuscular [IM], subcutaneous, intravenous [IV], per os or oral [PO]) of analgesic drugs, constant rate infusion initiation, and utilization of basic nonpharmacological therapy like placing ice packs on wounds or incisions. In some instances, the veterinary nurse may have advanced training or may even be a Certified Veterinary Pain Practitioner (CVPP) through the International Veterinary Academy of Pain Management (http://IVAPM.org) [2], and with doctor agreement, may be able to perform more advanced techniques like local/regional anesthetic blocks, laser therapy, basic rehabilitation exercises or massage.
- Understand the basic effects and side effects of the analgesic drugs administered to the patient and be able to discuss any concerns regarding therapy with the doctor. Concerns could include adverse effects experienced by the patient due to the drug therapy, or inadequate pain relief and the need to expand the pain therapy.

The veterinary nurse or technician, because of their medical training, should be able to take the client conversations that were initiated by the office staff to a deeper level.

Veterinary nurses should be able to discuss the following scenarios with the pet owner.

- We are absolutely, scientifically certain that animals do feel pain because they have a pain pathway or "system" that is anatomically and physiologically very similar to the pain system in humans. Thus, if a stimulus is painful to humans, it will definitely be painful to animals. This is a scientific fact, not anthropomorphism. We don't "think" animals feel pain, we "know" that animals feel pain.
- Animals hide pain from humans – and they are very good at it. This is likely because our pets evolved from wild animals that were either prey or predator. Pain could be a weakness if it limited the animal's ability to run or hide, making painful animals more likely to be preyed on. Even though we are not predators, this is a very strong instinct which has persisted in our pets. Although this may have been useful to them in

the distant past before they were domesticated, it is a detriment to them as pets. Hiding pain leads pet owners, and even veterinary professionals, to assume that animals are not feeling pain, thus they are not treated for pain.

- The owner is part of the pain team and integral to successful control of pain in the pet. Pain causes a negative impact on the patient's health, welfare, and behavior. Adequate pain management plays a very important role in health and healing after surgery, injury, or disease and pain-relieving drugs must be administered as described by the veterinarian to promote rapid return to normal health.

The veterinary nurse should also know the basic effects and side effects of the analgesic drugs discharged with the patient for treatment of either acute or chronic pain. The nurse should be able to discuss these side effects with the owner and provide guidelines of when the owner should call the veterinary hospital with concerns, if necessary.

Pain does not end when the patient is discharged from the hospital. The veterinary nurse should be available by phone or in person to discuss questions about pain and pain medication with the owner. To ensure that the owner is having no difficulty administering the analgesic drugs at home and that the pet is neither feeling pain nor having side effects from the drugs, a follow-up call should occur at a predetermined interval, for instance the day after surgery or after an appointment, for assessment of chronic pain. In most instances, the nurse can be tasked with patient follow-up and discussion of basic care. In more severe medical cases or surgeries, follow-up may need to come from the veterinarian. Regardless of who calls, as the patient's advocate, the nurse should be sure that the client receives a call. Any questions that the nurse cannot answer should be referred to the veterinarian.

8.21.5   Role of the Veterinarians

Although the veterinarians' medical knowledge is obviously important in their role on the team, the main role for the veterinarian is leadership as creator, implementer, and guide of the pain team. Without the leadership and diligent interest of the veterinarians, the team may not consistently strive to identify and treat pain in every single patient. However, an important goal is to develop a culture and a plan that the entire practice can adhere to even in the absence of the veterinarian (he/she needs a day off!). The pain team should function as a patient-centric team, not a veterinarian-centric team.

8.21.5.1   Knowledge

The veterinarians should:

- have a deeper understanding of the pain pathway so that they can design effective analgesic protocols and discuss the pathway in more depth with interested veterinary staff and/or clients
- fully comprehend the negative consequences of untreated or undertreated pain, including medical, welfare, and behavior consequences
- understand the manifestations of pain, utilization of pain scoring systems – and the limitations of the systems. If a nurse is unsure of the patient's pain level, the veterinarian should be ready to assess the patient
- have a robust knowledge of the pharmacology of analgesic drugs, including positive and negative effects, and the mechanisms of action of nonpharmacological therapy.

8.21.5.2   Leadership and Development

The veterinarians should:

- strongly believe in, advocate for, and model effective pain management as a core mission of their practice
- clearly emphasize that all personnel in the hospital are part of the pain management team and empower them to discuss all concerns regarding any pain management topic, from the clinic's philosophies to individual patient therapy
- be a good listener. Listen to the entire staff and the pet owner in order to coordinate the pain management team
- educate the entire team about animal pain, the importance of animal pain relief and their respective roles on the team. Education may require external input or attendance at meetings
- choose, implement, and guide the use of pain scoring systems and insist that every patient be scored at selected intervals. Examples of pain scoring systems are available in the resources at the end of this chapter. Coordinate training for the veterinarians and, more importantly, the veterinary nurses on appropriate use of the system
- develop, implement, and guide the use of effective acute pain management protocols, to include preemptive, multimodal, and postprocedural analgesic choices, that can be adapted to the patient's pain level. These protocols should include analgesic therapy that begins prior to surgery, continues during surgery, addresses pain in the recovery phase of anesthesia, and includes drugs to be discharged with the owner to be administered at home
- develop, implement, and guide the use of effective chronic pain management protocols and quality of life assessments

- ensure that the nurses understand the analgesic protocols and the effects and side effects of the drugs
- along with the nurse, be prepared to discuss pain and pain management with the owner for both acute and chronic pain
- along with the office staff, guide the development of client education material and website/social media messages
- continue to evaluate, reevaluate, and implement new ideas, drugs, training, etc.
- consider pain management training for themselves and the nurses through IVAPM or another pain-related group.

8.21.6 Role of the Pet Owner

The pet owner should be motivated to work with the veterinary team to ensure that the pet is not experiencing pain, either acute or chronic. Members of the veterinary team should train the pet owner on the potential signs of pain, with emphasis that animals are very good at hiding pain, and on the need for continued analgesic treatment as prescribed by the veterinarian. The owner should be encouraged to fill out quality of life "diaries" and/or to send the veterinary team videos of their pet's behavior if concerned about the pet's pain level. The owner should feel comfortable contacting the veterinary team any time that they are concerned about the pet's comfort.

EXAMPLES

A potential script for the receptionist/office staff: "Thank you for calling Ark Animal Hospital Mr Jones. At Ark, we are dedicated to the comfort of your pet and treatment here includes pain management that begins in the hospital and includes pain-relieving drugs for you to administer at home after the surgery. Thank you for your comment on our prices. If our prices are higher than other clinics it is because of the comprehensive pain management that we provide to insure your pet's comfort and well-being. We hope that you consider our care of your pet to be outstanding."

An example of a nurse conversing with a veterinarian regarding a patient that the nurse has determined to be in pain: "Dr Ree Leever, I have determined (not "I think" – I KNOW) that this patient is in pain because her heart rate is increased, she is licking incessantly at the incision and she

is hiding in the back of her cage, a behavior that is very abnormal for her." Depending on the practice and the nurse's level of training, this conversation might also include, "I recommend that we . . . (repeat the opioid dose, administer an alpha-2 agonist, start a constant rate infusion, etc. . .)."

An example of a nurse and client conversation regarding animal pain: "Yes, Mrs Smith, animals do feel pain. In fact, although it may not seem like it because animals don't want to show that they are in pain, animals feel a similar amount of pain that people feel. It is their natural instinct to hide pain, but we know that they feel pain because their pain system is very similar to the pain system of humans. We should go over the drugs that the doctor prescribed for your pet so that you understand how important they are and how you should administer them."

Leadership example: The veterinarian recognizes that either the nurses need more training on the pain scoring system or that the chosen scoring system isn't working for the team (maybe it is too cumbersome or lacks intuitive components). Rather than taking over pain scoring his/herself or allowing the team to abandon pain scoring altogether, the veterinarian holds a team meeting to explore other systems and/or better training and to choose and commit to a pain scoring system that the team can/will use.

Example of pet owner's role: A pet owner notices that their pet seems more painful today but has difficulty deciding exactly what is wrong, so they take a video of the pet's behavior and send it to the veterinary nurse or veterinarian.

TAKE-AWAYS

- The team members needed to consistently and effectively identify and treat pain in animals include the front office staff/receptionist, veterinary nurse, veterinarian, and pet owner.
- The entire team should be committed to recognizing and controlling pain in every patient.
- The fact that animals do feel pain, but often hide pain from humans, should be readily understood and communicated by every team member.
- Pain assessment and analgesic protocols should be developed for both acute and chronic pain and applied to every painful patient.
- The team must be patient-centric, not veterinarian-centric.

MISCELLANEOUS

Ideally, the efficacy of a pain scoring system to actually identify pain should be validated by research. However, many nonvalidated systems (like the Colorado State University scales) are quite useful. Lack of validation does not mean that the system does not indicate pain but only that the research proving that they indicate pain has yet to be done. Some of the validated systems are a bit cumbersome and more appropriate for research than for clinical applications. But validation does provide assurance that the scales *reliably* indicate pain.

References

1 American Veterinary Medical Association. Pain in animals. www.avma.org/KB/Policies/Pages/Pain-in-Animals.aspx
2 International Veterinary Academy of Pain Management. https://ivapm.org

Recommended Reading

Evangelista, M.C., Watanabe, R., Leung, V.S.Y. et al. (2019). Facial expressions of pain in cats: the development and validation of a feline grimace scale. *Sci. Rep.* 9 (1): 19128.

Colorado State University. Anesthesia Pain Management. http://csu-cvmbs.colostate.edu/vth/diagnostic-and-support/anesthesia-pain-management/Pages/pain-management.aspx (scroll to 'How do you know how much pain my pet is in?' to find the links)

Glasgow Pain Scales (acute and chronic, dogs and cats). www.newmetrica.com

Feline Chronic Pain (Quality of Life scale). https://painfreecats.org/the-fmpi

Canine Chronic Pain (Quality of Life scale). https://cvm.ncsu.edu/research/labs/clinical-sciences/comparative-pain-research/clinical-metrology-instruments; (scroll down to bottom and click on CSOM)

Acute pain (cats). www.animalpain.com.br/en-us/publicacoes-recomendadas.php

Grubb, T.L., Albi, M., Ensign, S. et al. (2020). *Anesthesia and Pain Management for Veterinary Nurses and Technicians.* Jackson, WY: Teton NewMedia.

Grubb, T., Sager, J., Gaynor, J.S. et al. (2020). 2020 AAHA anesthesia and monitoring guidelines for dogs and cats. *J. Am. Anim. Hosp. Assoc.* 56: 59–82.

8.22

Team Strategies for Feline Retroviral Diseases

Ryane E. Englar, DVM, DABVP (CANINE AND FELINE PRACTICE)

University of Arizona College of Veterinary Medicine, Oro Valley, AZ, USA

 BASICS

8.22.1 Summary

Two common causes of infectious diseases that impact populations of cats globally are feline leukemia virus (FeLV) and feline immunodeficiency virus (FIV). Vaccinations against FeLV and FIV are available in some but not all countries. When accessible, these immunizations limit the spread of disease between cats. However, it is essential for the veterinary team to work with clients to identify the serological status of every patient at the time of acquisition. More than one testing method may be required to be confirmatory. Repeat testing is also encouraged following exposure to cats that are either known to be infected or have unknown retroviral status. A positive retroviral status is not necessarily associated with clinical disease. Infected cats can lead high-quality, healthy lives. Open dialogue between the veterinary team and the client about effective management strategies is essential.

8.22.2 Terms Defined

Retrovirus: An infectious agent that converts its RNA into DNA after infecting a host cell. This DNA is integrated into the genetic material of the host cell, allowing the virus to replicate. When the host cell divides, each daughter cell carries copies of proviral DNA, thus spreading the infection.
Seroprevalence: The number of individuals within a population who have a positive result for a specific disease when using a blood-based diagnostic test.

 MAIN CONCEPTS

8.22.3 The Pathogenesis of Feline Leukemia Virus

Feline leukemia virus is primarily shed in nasal secretions, urine, and feces. For horizontal transmission to occur, cats must be in close proximity to one another. The oronasal route is the most typical way that cats experience horizontal transmission. However, it is possible to spread FeLV through bite wounds because the virus is also found in saliva [1]. Other activities, such as mutual grooming and the sharing of food and water bowls, increase the risk of transmission. Vertical transmission is also possible from parent to offspring.

Kittens are at greatest risk of infection. Cats develop some resistance to infection as they age [1].

8.22.4 Feline Leukemia Virus Outcomes: It's Complicated!

When a cat is exposed to FeLV, viral particles are first found in lymph tissue near the site of exposure. The presence of the p27 protein can be detected at this time through enzyme-linked immunosorbent assay (ELISA) testing.

At this early stage, the virus can integrate into the host's genome as proviral DNA. As soon as this occurs, the cat is said to be infected. Proviral DNA can be detected by polymerase chain reaction (PCR).

Monocytes and lymphocytes then carry the infection systemically. The spleen and lymph nodes are targeted during primary viremia. Infection may or may not be contained at this stage. If it is, then the cat is said to have a regressive, focal infection.

If instead the virus further replicates, then the infection spreads to the bone marrow, and the cat's leukocytes and platelets will be infected. At this point, the cat may or may not be able to halt replication of the virus. If the virus is contained, then the cat is said to have a regressive, latent infection.

If instead the virus is not contained, then a second round of viremia is triggered when FeLV-infected leukocytes and platelets enter the bloodstream. All other tissues and organs are at risk of progressive infection, and the cat will test positive on the immunofluorescent antibody (IFA) test.

Note that exposure to FeLV does not necessarily equate to active, persistent infection. The infection may also be abortive. An abortive infection is one in which FeLV is eliminated before the virus integrates into the cat's genome.

8.22.5 The Pathogenesis of Feline Immunodeficiency Virus

Saliva is the primary source of infectious material for horizontal transmission of FIV. For this reason, bite wounds remain the major risk factor for contracting this virus. Semen can also carry viral particles. However, transmission of FIV is rarely achieved via mating [2]. Vertical transmission from parent to offspring is rare among naturally infected cats, but has been experimentally produced [2].

In the acute phase of infection, the cat may develop a transient fever and swollen lymph nodes. FIV will be easily detected by PCR. After a few weeks, CD4+ (helper) and CD8+ (cytotoxic-suppressor) T lymphocytes decline, and antibodies to FIV are produced [2]. This suppresses the amount of virus circulating in the bloodstream, and cats become asymptomatic for months to years. Despite this, infected cats' immune systems become dysfunctional. They are more likely to experience chronic infections [2]. They are also five times more likely to develop neoplasia [3].

8.22.6 The Seroprevalence of FeLV and FIV

Feline leukemia virus and FIV have global presences when it comes to feline infectious disease. A 2017 study evaluated over 62,000 cats at 1396 veterinary clinics and 127 shelters throughout the United States and Canada to determine seroprevalence [4]. Seroprevalence for FeLV antigen was 3.1%; seroprevalence for anti-FIV antibody was 3.6% [4]. Adult cats, particularly intact males and those

with outdoor lifestyles, were at increased risk of contracting either disease [4].

8.22.7 The "So What?" Factor

Risk factors and seroprevalences for both FeLV and FIV are consistent with those reported previously [4]. This is concerning because guidelines were developed decades ago concerning how to prevent both retroviruses, yet FeLV and FIV remain at about the same rate in feline populations. Their persistence suggests that we need to work harder to improve serological testing and encourage clients to act on our recommendations.

8.22.8 Prevention Requires Dialogue with the Client

There is so much content to cover at new patient visits that FeLV/FIV discussions may run the risk of being cursory. However, the veterinary team needs to engage in dialogue with the client early and often concerning FeLV and FIV risk factors, testing, and vaccination protocols.

Some practitioners express concern that clients will receive information about FeLV/FIV poorly. It was not that long ago that both viruses were death sentences, and recommendations were to euthanize any cat that tested positive. This philosophy has long since expired, but some clients may recall this and be reluctant to test.

It is important that the veterinary team address concerns head on. The team may consider introducing the concept with the open-ended statement, "Tell me your experience with testing for FeLV/FIV in cats that you have owned in the past." It is also important to assess the client's knowledge: "Are you familiar with FeLV or FIV in cats?" This establishes a client-specific level of understanding, which helps the veterinary team identify gaps in knowledge.

8.22.9 Prevention Requires Discussion About Risk Factors

Any initial consultation about FeLV and FIV should explore patient- and household-specific risk factors. The following factors are associated with a strong increase in the prevalence of FeLV [2]:

- Being born to an infected queen
- Having an outdoor lifestyle
- Harboring respiratory tract or oral disease
- Sharing close contact with other cats
- Fighting with other cats

All these factors are strongly associated with a higher prevalence of FIV with one exception. Kittens born to a queen that is infected with FIV are less likely to contract the virus than those born to a queen infected with FeLV [2].

Clients need to be asked if other cats live in the household. If so, what is their lifestyle and serological status? How do these cats get along with the cat in question? It is important to explore intercat relationships to weigh each cat's risk if one member of the household is positive for disease.

8.22.10 Prevention Requires Early Detection

All cats should be tested for both viruses at the time they are acquired. Testing is not necessarily a once-in-a-lifetime event. Testing for FeLV/FIV should be repeated [2]:

- before vaccinating against either virus
- during a bout of clinical illness
- after known exposure to infected cats
- after potential exposure to infected cats.

It takes on average 30 days after exposure for an infected cat to test positive. For this reason, a patient that presents for a cat-bite abscess should be encouraged to return in 4–6 weeks for repeat testing. FeLV antigen and FIV antibodies can be identified in a matter of minutes, using a sample of whole blood, serum, or plasma. An ELISA is typically used in-house to test for p27 antigen. Alternatively, PCR can be employed to evaluate for evidence of FeLV provirus.

Tears or saliva are often inadequate to detect FeLV antigen. Tests that evaluate FeLV antigen in either body fluid typically report low sensitivity [2]. However, saliva can be used reliably through reverse transcriptase polymerase chain reaction (RT-PCR) to detect viral RNA.

8.22.11 Confirmatory Testing for FeLV and FIV

A positive point-of-care test should be confirmed using alternate methodology. A (+) FeLV result is most often confirmed via IFA, and (+) FIV result through Western blot.

Neither maternal immunity nor vaccination against FeLV creates false positives on point-of-care tests. However, cats that nursed from an infected queen do receive passive transfer of FIV antibodies. This can cause false-positive tests for FIV up to 6 months of age. It is critical that the veterinary team explain this to the client so that retesting occurs before the kitten is labeled true positive. Discordant test results are also possible.

8.22.12 Prevention Against FeLV Requires Vaccination

Vaccination plays a critical role in prevention. The American Association of Feline Practitioners (AAFP) advises that all kittens up to 1 year old be vaccinated against FeLV, as well as any at-risk adult cat [5]. Refer to the AAFP Feline Vaccination Advisory Panel Report (2013) concerning types of vaccines and vaccination protocols.

Early vaccination is advantageous because it captures cats at an age where they are most susceptible to disease (youth). Early vaccination is also protective of those whose risk factors and lifestyles may change. At the initial consultation, clients may initially share that the kitten will lead an exclusively indoor life or that it will be the only cat in a household. However, circumstances may evolve as s/he adapts to a new household. Vaccinating all kittens provides peace of mind should their lifestyles stray from what was anticipated.

There is concern among some that vaccinations may promote injection site sarcomas. The veterinary team must provide a risk–benefit analysis for each individual patient so that clients make educated choices about patient healthcare.

8.22.13 What About Vaccinating Against FIV?

Unlike FeLV, FIV vaccination is not considered to be a core immunization. In fact, FIV vaccinations are not available in Canada or the United States. Vaccine efficacy has been variable. To further complicate matters, vaccination induces antibodies that are detectable by point-of-care tests, causing a false-positive response. This could easily result in misdiagnosis. Therefore, it is critical that any vaccinated cat be labeled as such using appropriate identification. Both collars and microchips have been recommended [2].

8.22.14 Prevention Requires Environmental Management at Home

Ideally, any confirmed cat that is (+) for FeLV or FIV should be segregated in the home environment, maintained indoors, and neutered. This is not always feasible, and clients may be reluctant to separate housemates. In these situations, clients need to be encouraged to vaccinate those noninfected cats that reside in the home. When this is not possible, for instance, due to unavailability of the FIV vaccine, then sanitation is critical for limiting the spread of disease.

8.22.15 Prevention Requires Environmental Management at the Clinic

Neither FeLV nor FIV is long-lived in the environment because both viruses are very unstable outside their host [2]. Viral inactivation is easy to achieve using hospital-grade detergents and disinfectants.

Infected cats should not be allowed to contact other hospitalized cats. However, they do not require housing within isolation wards. If anything, their potentially compromised immune systems require us to shield them from those regions of the hospital that are hotbeds of infectious disease. For example, we need to limit their exposure to other cats with upper airway disease. We also need to limit their exposure to sick dogs that harbor *Bordetella bronchiseptica* and canine parvovirus because these pathogens are not limited to dogs.

Hand hygiene is essential for reducing spread of disease, as is sanitation of equipment that has come into contact with blood and/or saliva. For example, dental, anesthetic, and surgical equipment must be cleaned, then sterilized. Dosing syringes (oral or injectable) should not be shared between patients, and intravenous fluid lines and bags should not be reused. Cages should be cleaned and disinfected thoroughly, then allowed to dry before another cat is housed within that same space.

8.22.16 Prevention Requires Hospital Protocols for Blood Transfusions

The transmission of FeLV and FIV through blood has implications for transfusion medicine. No cat should be used as a blood donor without first confirming that it is negative for both viruses. It is insufficient to simply screen prospective donors for FeLV antigen and FIV antibodies. Cats that test negative on FeLV antigen tests must also undergo PCR testing because these cats may have regressive infections. Regressive infections do not show up as (+) on FeLV antigen tests; however, cats with regressive infections can still spread disease through their blood.

TAKE-AWAYS

- FeLV and FIV are common infectious diseases in cats, with worldwide distribution.

- It was once thought of as a death sentence for a cat to test positive for either virus. However, infected cats can lead quality lives.
- Maintaining an open dialogue at the initial consultation and inviting a discussion as patient risk factors and lifestyle evolve is essential.
- Early detection, environmental management, and vaccination play critical roles in reducing spread of disease, but only when the veterinary team takes the time to engage the client in discussions about each.
- Cats that test (+) for either virus have potentially compromised immunity. Preventive healthcare is key to reducing morbidity and mortality from other preventable diseases.

MISCELLANEOUS

References

1 Hartmann, K. and Levy, J.K. (2017). Feline leukemia virus infection. In: *Textbook of Veterinary Internal Medicine: Diseases of the Dog and the Cat*, 8e (eds. S.J. Ettinger, E.C. Feldman and E. Côté), 2442–2445. St Louis, MO: Elsevier.

2 Little, S., Levy, J., Hartmann, K. et al. (2020). 2020 AAFP feline retrovirus testing and management guidelines. *J. Feline Med. Surg.* 22: 5–30.

3 Hartmann, K. (2015). Role of retroviruses in feline lymphoma. *Eur. J. Comp. Anim. Pract.* 25: 4–15.

4 Burling, A.N., Levy, J.K., Scott, H.M. et al. (2017). Seroprevalences of feline leukemia virus and feline immunodeficiency virus infection in cats in the United States and Canada and risk factors for seropositivity. *J. Am. Vet. Med. Assoc.* 251: 187–194.

5 Scherk, M.A., Ford, R.B., Gaskell, R.M. et al. (2013). 2013 AAFP Feline Vaccination Advisory Panel report. *J. Feline Med. Surg.* 16: 66.

8.23

Team Strategies for Recurrent Pyoderma

Lowell Ackerman, DVM, DACVD, MBA, MPA, CVA, MRCVS

Global Consultant, Author, and Lecturer, MA, USA

BASICS

8.23.1 Summary

Recurrent pyoderma is a common and often frustrating disorder to manage for both pet owners and veterinarians. While we have many exciting medications to manage bacterial infections, our approach to management hasn't changed significantly in decades: Treat the infection with antibiotics and hope it does not recur. When it does recur, which is also common, there is a tendency to escalate the response with stronger and stronger antibiotics on the assumption that we are dealing with increasingly pathogenic organisms. There is often a quest for that "magic bullet" that will permanently address the problem.

To successfully manage recurrent pyoderma, it is critical that veterinary healthcare teams understand the microbial dynamics of such recurrent issues, the challenges and concerns that pet owners face, and the need to be rational stewards of antimicrobial therapy while effectively counseling clients on this manageable condition.

8.23.2 Terms Defined

Antimicrobial Resistance: The property of a bacterial population to survive exposure to an antimicrobial that previously would have been an effective treatment. Resistance can be conferred by mutation or gene transfer.

Atopic Dermatitis: The preferred term for a genetically predisposed inflammatory and pruritic skin disease with characteristic clinical presentation. Previously known by several terms, including atopy, inhalant allergies, eczema, and hay fever.

Folliculitis: Inflammation of the hair follicles. The term is often used to imply not only inflammation, but the involvement of bacteria.

Furunculosis: Literally the development of furuncles (boils) in the skin, but often signifying a deep folliculitis, typically with hair follicle rupture into the dermis or panniculus.

Microbiota: The population of microbes in a specific location.

Pyoderma: A skin condition associated with the production of pus. Often used synonymously with any bacterial issue involving the skin.

MAIN CONCEPTS

8.23.3 It's Not Just About Bacteria

The surface of the skin is not sterile, and it plays host to a variety of resident, transient, opportunistic, and pathogenic bacteria. It is important to understand how this occurs, since pyoderma (a term often implying bacterial infection of the skin) is commonplace, and is often a frustrating condition in veterinary practice.

Resident bacteria live and multiply on normal skin. They are located on the skin surface, and in the most superficial aspects of the hair follicles, and discourage opportunistic infections through effective competition.

Staphylococcus pseudintermedius (and to a lesser extent *S. schleiferi* and *S. aureus*) is the most important organism implicated in pyoderma of dogs, and healthy dogs are a frequent carrier of the organism. Dogs also carry the organism around the anus, genital tract, buccal mucosae, and conjunctivae. Most dogs develop their own genetically unique strains of *Staphylococcus*, present in carriage sites and in pyoderma lesions, suggesting that dogs are not routinely colonized by the staphylococci of other dogs. If this organism is present on many normal dogs and lives as a commensal organism in most cases, then the logical question should be asked as to why it is responsible for the vast majority of canine pyodermas. The answer is that since the organism is not overly pathogenic, it must be host factors that allow the organism to take hold and do its damage. Cats, in general, have different surface microbes and are not nearly as prone to recurrent pyodermas, so the remaining discussion is limited to the situation in dogs.

The term *pyoderma* is commonly used in the veterinary literature, but it is important to consider that many issues referred to as pyoderma are really associated more with overgrowth of bacteria on the skin surface rather than active infection. It is not unusual for bacterial overgrowth to evolve into infection, but it is not a foregone conclusion.

To cause pyoderma, bacteria must be able to adhere to skin cells (keratinocytes), take advantage of nutrients on the skin, compete effectively with resident organisms and overcome host defense mechanisms. Bacteria can enter from several different routes, but most penetrate through the hair follicles where there is a natural opening. There are then a number of host factors to overcome, in order for the bacteria to cause problems.

The scaly surface of the skin, the stratum corneum, itself is a lipid-rich compact barrier to the outside world. However, the openings of the hair follicles do give organisms the opportunity to push further into the follicles than normal defense mechanisms allow. Other barriers to bacterial penetration include the fur (hair coat), tight junctions between keratinocytes, the immune system, and the surface lipid barrier that influences cutaneous permeability.

Any process that disturbs the skin's barrier function will predispose to pyoderma. This includes any abrasion that removes surface barrier functions, any inflammatory process that causes epidermal disorganization, any process that affects local temperature and relative humidity on the skin, or any proliferative epidermal disease that results in keratinocyte disarray. Finally, any underlying disease that impairs immune function can predispose to pyoderma. Therefore, it is most important to investigate underlying diseases that predispose to pyoderma, rather than just responding with antibiotics.

Recurrent pyodermas refer to those situations in which a presumed bacterial skin disease responds to antibiotic therapy only to recur at some point after the antibiotic has been discontinued. While it might initially be tempting to consider that the organisms are resistant to the antibiotics used, or overly pathogenic, in the vast majority of cases the antibiotic was only temporarily suppressing the surface bacterial popu-

lation because an underlying disease had not been identified and successfully managed. Successful management of most cases of recurrent pyoderma involves not trying to eradicate surface microbes, which is an impossible task, but instead successfully managing the underlying issues.

8.23.4　Approach to Pyodermas

Pyoderma is a vague term and the clinical presentation often gives some clues as to the underlying cause(s). Pyodermas are typically characterized by their depth (superficial/surface, intermediate/superficial, deep), or by their particular characteristics.

Surface (superficial) pyodermas involve the epidermis and the outermost aspects of the hair follicles. Examples include pyotraumatic dermatitis ("hot spots"), fold pyodermas, and juvenile pustular dermatitis (often incorrectly referred to as impetigo, but much different from impetigo in children).

Intermediate (superficial) pyodermas involve deeper penetration of bacteria, and most often result in folliculitis and perifolliculitis. These most commonly occur secondary to allergies, parasites, keratinization disorders, and metabolic disorders such as hypothyroidism or hyperadrenocorticism.

Deep pyodermas involve yet deeper structures in the dermis and panniculus, including furunculosis (rupture of hair follicles with their contents discharged into the surrounding tissues), cellulitis, abscesses, and fistulating diseases (including German shepherd dog pyoderma, mycobacteriosis, etc.). These diseases reflect a more exaggerated reaction to the causes of intermediate pyodermas, a major breach in immune function, or infiltration of an organism more pathogenic than *S. pseudintermedius*.

The concept of recurrent pyoderma, once again, is that the condition responds entirely to antimicrobial therapy, only to relapse at some point after therapy has been stopped. The most common underlying causes in this regard are allergies (atopic dermatitis, adverse food reactions, parasite reactions), and mild immune compromise. Factors that shift the balance in the surface microbiota are also those that determine the likelihood of recurrence – not antimicrobial resistance. When considering the strategic approach to management, the use of antibiotic therapy is therefore not the main consideration.

8.23.5　Getting Specific

With pet-specific care, we can personalize our approach to common maladies, such as recurrent pyoderma. In some cases, we can anticipate where bacterial overgrowth is most likely to occur. For example, in pets with prominent skin folds (e.g., whole-body folds in Chinese shar-pei, facial folds in English bulldogs, etc.) there is likely to be bacterial overgrowth in the creases, and pet owners would be well advised to make cleaning those folds a regular part of health maintenance. Gentle cleansing or astringent solutions are typically all that are required to provide a lifetime of care.

The most common underlying cause for recurrent pyoderma is allergy, and atopic dermatitis accounts for a majority of cases. Fortunately (or unfortunately), atopic dermatitis tends to run in families, and there is often a striking breed predisposition, so a tendency toward bacterial overgrowth can often be predicted in these cases (see 8.18 Team Strategies for Atopic Dermatitis). It is important to realize that when allergies are the underlying cause for recurrent pyoderma, the goal must be to successfully address the underlying allergic situation – not necessarily to mount an attack against surface bacteria which are only proliferating because of the underlying inflammatory situation. If addressed early, before there is substantial barrier function disturbance, the bacterial overgrowth can usually be successfully managed entirely with topical therapies, without systemic antibiotics.

While it might seem somewhat simplistic, the use of antibiotics in many cases of recurrent pyoderma is not necessary and likely indicates a failure to be adequately proactive. Early in the course of most such pyodermas, the surface microbes are not especially pathogenic, and tend to be as responsive to topicals as they are to systemic antibiotics. Allowing damage to the skin barrier function makes control with surface cleansers more problematic, and the recurrent use of antibiotics encourages microbial resistance which not only makes the conditions harder to treat, but poses public health concerns as well (see 9.12 Judicious Use of Antimicrobials).

Once potential risk has been identified, the management of that risk should be a top priority. Owners of pets with conditions that could promote microbial overgrowth, such as allergies and skin folds, should be effectively counseled as early as possible, preferably even before the first bacterial outbreak.

A good time to start such conversations is when pets are 8 weeks of age, long before any problems are evident. At this time, the hospital team can alert the owners of at-risk pets to not only be vigilant for evidence of early clinical signs of bacterial overgrowth, but to actively embark on mitigation exercises, such as effectively cleansing inflamed areas and seeking veterinary attention before the problem requires antibiotics. The intention is not to scare owners but to set realistic expectations for a risk that has been identified and confirmed in the specific practice population. If such conversations are productive, it might also prompt the owner to ask what it would mean for their pet if they allowed the condition to progress to the point where it did require antibiotics, and why the development of microbial resistance is of concern to everyone. Most pet owners are aware of the dangers of methicillin-resistant staphylococci and can appreciate that antibiotics should be reserved for the cases that really warrant them. You might think that you don't want to have those discussions in advance, but in time, you will likely realize that it was time well spent and develop resources (client handouts, website pages, trained staff, etc.) to facilitate such client education.

8.23.6 Using Early Detection Effectively

In many cases, the early detection of recurrent pyoderma is a function of determining the contributions of underlying causes as well as perpetuating factors. Once again, it is relatively easy to appreciate that underlying causes such as allergies, parasites, skin folds, and immune compromise can lead to bacterial overgrowth on the skin surface. The use of medications that suppress the immune system (corticosteroids, etc.) can also lead to bacterial overgrowth. Once these underlying concerns have been identified, secondary bacterial overgrowth should be anticipated, and plans put in place for mitigation.

Perpetuating factors are also problematic and can lead to disease recurrence. Anything that interferes with normal skin barrier function, or changes the microbial balance on the skin surface, can lead to impairment of restoring the normal protective aspects of the skin. Areas with hair loss, with scarring (fibrosis) in the skin such as due to follicular rupture (furunculosis) or significant inflammation, or parts of the skin in which there have been hyperplastic reactions due to the pyoderma can make it progressively more difficult to resolve the situation without the chronic use of antibiotics. Veterinary teams need to be vigilant to identify problems early, before chronic changes set in that will complicate the long-term management of the condition.

Most pets today should be on year-round parasite control, which should help control at least some of the predisposing factors to bacterial overgrowth, such as fleas, demodicosis, and sarcoptic mange. In fact, some of the newer parasiticides, including the isoxazolines, may help control a variety of different parasites. Still, skin scrapings should be an important part of any work-up for a pyoderma and *Demodex* mites reside within hair follicles, and clinically can be easily confused with bacterial folliculitis;

dermatophytosis (ringworm) is another condition that can be easily confused with bacterial folliculitis.

Clinically, the process starts with macules and papules that evolve into pustules, although the pustular stage may not always be evident at the time of examination. In time, there is an outward peeling rim of scale (epidermal collarette), with central hyperpigmentation, sometimes collectively referred to as a target lesion (see Figure 8.23.1). When hair follicles rupture and discharge their contents into the underlying tissues, marked inflammation ensues, and the process is known as furunculosis.

One of the easiest and most important tests that can be used by veterinary teams is cytology. Surface lesions can be sampled (pustules, erosions, epidermal collarettes, etc.), placed on a microscope slide, and appropriately stained, and can provide a wealth of information. In early cases in which there is just bacterial overgrowth with staphylococci, coccoid bacteria will be evident, typically extracellularly. In time, more neutrophils will be found, and the bacteria may be engulfed and appear intracellularly.

Pets with atopic dermatitis and other inflammatory disorders tend to develop recurrent bacterial and yeast infections and so when pets develop such issues, it is important to routinely assess with cytology. It is impossible to ascertain by inspection whether a complication is bacteria or yeast related, so cytological confirmation is important.

When the situation is caught early enough and the bacteria can be managed with topical therapy, this may be the only testing needed to assess the bacterial contingent. However, when there is deep pyoderma, when there are complicating factors, or when systemic therapy is needed, bacterial culture and susceptibility testing is warranted.

Culture and susceptibility testing is useful when systemic therapy is being considered, but it is important to realize that because microbes are so plentiful on the skin surface, selection of causative microbes is not always assured, depending on sampling technique and laboratory factors. For example, collecting samples from an intact pustule is preferred to swabs taken of papules, crusts, or epidermal collarettes. This lessens the chance that strains of *S. pseudintermedius* will be collected that are not involved in the infection. This is important because lesions may harbor multiple *S. pseudintermedius* strains with distinct antimicrobial profiles, there is extensive strain diversity and many laboratories select a single bacterial colony to submit for susceptibility testing, and that single colony may not be representative of the bacterial strain most important clinically.

Cultures are indicated when it is believed that bacteria are clinically implicated in a problem and there has been incomplete response to empirically chosen antibiotics at an appropriate dose and over an appropriate period of time, when new lesions develop within a few weeks after complete resolution, when cytological evaluation still reveals coccoid bacteria within neutrophils, for pets that have recently received antibiotics, for deep pyodermas, and when there is a history of resistant infections for other pets (or people?) in the same household.

8.23.7 Managing the Pet with Recurrent Pyoderma

The best approach to managing the pet with recurrent pyoderma is to suspect from the outset that the problem is secondary to some underlying problem. To successfully manage the situation, it is therefore necessary to uncover the underlying problem. In rare instances, such as with sarcoptic mange, it may be possible to "cure" the underlying problem and stop the pyoderma from progressing. In most other cases, it will only be possible to "control" the underlying problem, which means the long-term control of the pyoderma hinges on the successful long-term control of the underlying problem. The most common underlying problems are atopic dermatitis, flea-bite dermatitis, adverse reactions to foods, demodicosis, hypothyroidism, hyperadrenocorticism, etc. but other underlying causes, such as compromised immune function for a variety of reasons, may be difficult to identify and correct.

The most important point for managing recurrent pyoderma, once underlying issues have been addressed and controlled, is to determine if antibiotic therapy is warranted, since antibiotics tend to be overused in many cases. The issue tends to be further complicated when veterinary teams choose the latest-generation antibiotic to try first, or use inappropriate classes of antibiotics (such as fluoroquinolones for a staphylococcal infection), or use human

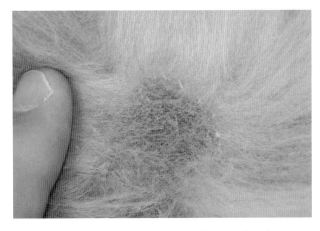

Figure 8.23.1 A common lesion of pyoderma in dogs is a peeling rim of scale with central hyperpigmentation, sometimes referred to as a target lesion.

antibiotics, most of which have not been labeled for use in animals, or selecting antibiotics for recurrent pyoderma empirically, when culture and susceptibility is indicated.

For surface (superficial) infections, treatment should involve only topical therapy, and antibiotics are rarely indicated. For superficial (intermediate) pyodermas (e.g., folliculitis), topical therapy is adequate in at least half of all cases, so systemic antibiotics may not be required at all. In these situations, topical therapy should be tried for at least two weeks; if that is not adequate, and cocci are clearly evident on cytological evaluation, a sensible antibiotic can be selected empirically and used until apparent clinical cure is evident. With first-time antibiotic therapy, sensible products include potentiated penicillins, cephalosporins, lincosamides, and potentiated sulfonamides predominantly. If these fail to control the problem, then the working diagnosis should be questioned, and further use of antibiotics should only be considered following culture and susceptibility testing. Antimicrobial peptides can provide another treatment option.

Deep pyodermas are unlikely to respond to topical therapy alone since much of the problem may be located in the deeper parts of the skin and subcutaneous fat, and antibiotic therapy should only be considered on the basis of culture and susceptibility testing. In many cases, the sample for culture may need to be collected from discharges from fistulous tracts, or macerated biopsies.

Because of the population dynamics of staphylococci, where they are capable of doubling in numbers every few hours, it is not only important to use appropriate topicals for treatment but to make sure they have adequate duration on the skin, and they are frequently repeated. Since the topicals need to make contact with the skin and hair follicles, it may be necessary to first trim the fur, to ensure adequate contact. The shampoos and rinses act to cleanse the skin surface and mechanically remove microbes, debris, and crusts that might inhibit the ingredients from directly contacting the microbes. The shampoo formulation itself may also contribute to efficacy, by enhancing residual antibacterial activity on hairs.

There are many formulations available for topically managing recurrent pyoderma, including chlorhexidine, miconazole, povidone-iodine, benzoyl peroxide, weak acids (e.g., acetic acid), bleach (sodium hypochlorite – 0.005–0.05%), ethyl lactate, and micronized silver, to name just a few options. Appropriate products should be thoroughly worked into the skin (not the fur) and allowed to remain in contact with the skin for 10–15 minutes before rinsing. In most cases, such bathing needs to be repeated 2–3 times per week to maintain effective control, with antimicrobial sprays applied in the intervals between baths.

8.23.8 The Issue of Resistance

Antimicrobial resistance is a significant issue in healthcare and must be taken seriously. It has become more common in clinical practice, likely due to repeated antibiotic use, failure to identify and control the underlying issue, and selecting inappropriate products and/or dosages for use in patients (see 9.12 Judicious Use of Antimicrobials).

While the antibiotic methicillin may not be in common use any more, the term "methicillin-resistant" still persists to indicate strains that are resistant to the beta-lactam group of antibiotics. Methicillin resistance can be transferred between microbes and confers resistance to cephalosporins, penicillins, and carbapenems, but often other antibiotics as well. Interestingly, when cultures are sent for susceptibility testing, methicillin is typically not one of the antibiotics tested for, so methicillin resistance is typically inferred from the results for oxacillin or similar antibiotic (cefoxitin, etc.).

Pyodermas caused by methicillin-resistant staphylococci are clinically indistinguishable from nonmethicillin-resistant strains, but the advice associated with each is quite different. With methicillin-resistant strains, owners should be provided with appropriate hygiene information (e.g., http://wormsandgermsblog.com) to help reduce apprehension and enhance patient care. Veterinary healthcare teams should also practice good infection control with each case of pyoderma, and this includes appropriate hand washing, cleansing, and disinfection. When methicillin-resistant cases have been confirmed, teams should use gloves and personal protective equipment and affected individuals should be sequestered from other hospital patients. Hospital staff members can be carriers of methicillin-resistant staphylococci and can cause hospital-acquired infections in hospitalized patients as well as transmitting the organisms to their own pets, and the hospital environment, so hygiene is an important concern.

Healthcare teams can help prevent the development of resistance by only prescribing antibiotics when they are absolutely needed, and according to appropriate guidelines. In many cases, topical therapies are sufficient, and the use of antibiotics can often be avoided if underlying conditions are successfully managed. Thus, in line with pet specific guidelines, antimicrobial stewardship warrants strategic initiatives with preventive approaches to make antibiotic use less necessary, early detection of potential bacterial complications when they can be resolved without antibiotics, and then evidence-based management directives with facilitated compliance to help make resistance a less likely sequel.

TAKE-AWAYS

- Recurrent pyodermas are almost always secondary to underlying causes.
- When underlying causes are not identified and corrected, pyodermas are likely to recur.
- The most common underlying causes of pyoderma are allergies and other disorders that affect the skin's barrier function.
- Most cases of recurring pyoderma can be managed without the use of systemic antibiotics.
- Veterinary healthcare teams should be vigilant in their use of systemic antibiotics, since antimicrobial stewardship is everyone's concern.

MISCELLANEOUS

Recommended Reading

Clinical and Laboratory Standards Institute. Understanding Susceptibility Test Data as a Component of Antimicrobial Stewardship in Veterinary Settings. 2019. https://clsi.org/media/3249/vet09ed1-sample.pdf

Frey, E. (2018). The role of companion animal veterinarians in one-health efforts to combat antimicrobial resistance. *J. Am. Vet. Med. Assoc.* 253 (11): 1396–1404.

Hillier, A., Lloyd, D.H., Weese, J.S. et al. (2014). Guidelines for the diagnosis and antimicrobial therapy of canine superficial bacterial folliculitis (antimicrobial guidelines working group of the international society for companion animal infectious diseases). *Vet. Dermatol.* 25: 163–175.

Larsen, R.F., Boysen, L., Jessen, L.R. et al. (2018). Diversity of Staphylococcus pseudintermedius in carriage sites and skin lesions of dogs with superficial bacterial folliculitis: potential implications for diagnostic testing and therapy. *Vet. Dermatol.* 29 (4): 291–e100.

Morris, D.O., Boston, R.C., O'Shea, K., and Rankin, S.C. (2010). The prevalence of carriage of methicillin-resistant staphylococci by veterinary dermatology practice staff and their respective pets. *Vet. Dermatol.* 21: 400–407.

Morris, D.O., Loeffler, A., Davis, M.F. et al. (2017). Recommendations for approaches to methicillin-resistant staphylococcal infections of small animals: diagnosis, therapeutic consideration and preventative measures: clinical consensus guidelines of the world association of veterinary dermatology. *Vet. Dermatol.* 28 (3): 304–e69.

Schwarz, S., Loeffler, A., and Kadlec, K. (2017). Bacterial resistance to antimicrobial agents and its impact on veterinary and human medicine. *Vet. Dermatol.* 28: 82–95.

Weese, J.S. (2012). Staphylococcal control in the veterinary hospital. *Vet. Dermatol.* 23: 292–298.

Worthing, K.A., Brown, J., Gerber, L. et al. (2018). Methicillin-resistant staphylococci amongst veterinary personnel, personnel-owned pets, patients and the hospital environment of two small animal veterinary hospitals. *Vet. Microbiol.* 223: 79–85.

8.24

Team Strategies for Otitis Externa

Lowell Ackerman, DVM, DACVD, MBA, MPA, CVA, MRCVS

Global Consultant, Author, and Lecturer, MA, USA

BASICS

8.24.1 Summary

Otitis externa is a common and often frustrating disorder to manage for both pet owners and veterinarians. While we have many exciting medications to manage bacterial and yeast infections, our past approaches to management hadn't changed significantly in decades: Treat the infection(s) with antibiotics, corticosteroids, and antifungals and hope it didn't recur. When it did recur, which was also common, there was a tendency to escalate the response with stronger and stronger products on the assumption that we were dealing with increasingly pathogenic organisms or resistance. There was often a quest for that "magic bullet" that would permanently address the problem. When medical approaches failed, surgical options remained. Thus, it is also critical to realize that otitis externa exists on a continuum, and thus benefits from early and conscientious intervention (see 9.7 Continuum of Care and Convergence Schedules).

To successfully manage otitis externa, it is critical that veterinary healthcare teams understand the anatomy, physiology, and microbial dynamics of such recurrent issues, the challenges and concerns that pet owners face, and the need to be rational stewards of antimicrobial therapy while effectively counseling clients on this difficult but manageable condition.

8.24.2 Terms Defined

Antimicrobial Resistance: The property of a bacterial population to survive exposure to an antimicrobial that previously would have been an effective treatment. Resistance can be conferred by mutation or gene transfer.

Atopic Dermatitis: The preferred term for a genetically predisposed inflammatory and pruritic skin disease with characteristic clinical presentation. Previously known by several terms, including atopy, inhalant allergies, eczema, and hay fever.

Microbiota: The population of microbes in a specific location.

Mycobiota: The population of fungal microbes in a specific location.

Otitis Externa: Inflammation of the external ear canal.

MAIN CONCEPTS

The management of ear disorders is often frustrating for both veterinarian and pet owner. Despite a plethora of ointments, drops, and flushes available, and many potent antibiotics, managing these cases can seem to be quite difficult.

Importantly, antibiotics are not the sole or even the primary answer in most instances. In the vast majority of cases, bacteria and yeasts are not the primary problem and, more specifically, the microbes cultured from the outer ear may not even represent those microbes found in the deep aspects of the canal, or the middle ear if the eardrum has been breached. Undiagnosed rupture of the eardrum is very common in chronic otitis externa. Even when the eardrum has healed over, most of the microbes responsible for keeping the problem ongoing may originate from the middle ear and, in many cases, these are not the same species isolated from samples taken from the external ear canal.

There are lots of different causes for otitis and, while it may seem surprising, true microbial causes are actually rare. While bacteria and yeasts are frequent complicating factors for ear problems, the most common underlying causes are atopic dermatitis (see 8.18 Team Strategies for Atopic Dermatitis), adverse food reactions, parasites (e.g., some ticks and mites), metabolic problems, foreign bodies, masses (tumors, polyps, etc.) and immune-mediated conditions (such as pemphigus foliaceus). Only when the correct underlying cause has been identified and managed will the ear condition be readily controlled.

While tumors of the ear canal are relatively rare and seen most commonly in older dogs and cats, inflammatory polyps may be seen in younger cats, typically 1–5 years of age. The cause is uncertain, but hereditary causes and response to prior viral upper respiratory infections is suspected. They generally cause painful otitis externa in cats, often unilaterally, but occasionally bilaterally. With otoscopy, they can typically be seen protruding through the tympanum (eardrum). They require surgical correction.

8.24.3 Understanding the Anatomy and Physiology of the Ear

To successfully treat ear canal problems, it is important to first understand some of the structures involved (see Figure 8.24.1). The external ear acts as a funnel, bringing sound toward the eardrum (tympanum). The eardrum, in turn, amplifies the sound, and relays that sound inward through tiny bones (ossicles) that transmit the sound from the eardrum to the oval window, and then to the cochlea.

The external ear includes the ear flaps (pinnae) and the horizontal and vertical canals, and the outward-facing portion of the eardrum. Inflammation of these structures is referred to as otitis externa. The middle ear consists of the inward-facing portion of the eardrum, the ossicles, and the tympanic bullae. Inflammation of these structures is referred to as otitis media. The inner ear consists of the cochlea and semicircular canals, as well as their nerve pathways. Inflammation of these structures is referred to as otitis interna.

The external ear canal is composed of two cartilage tubes, the auricular and annular cartilages, which connect the pinnae to the temporal bone. The skin lining the external ear canal is stratified squamous epithelium. There are abundant sebaceous glands in the canal epithelium, located in the superficial (papillary) dermis. There are also modified apocrine (ceruminous) glands deeper in the dermis.

The tympanic membrane (eardrum) is a sandwich with stratified squamous epithelium laterally and respiratory

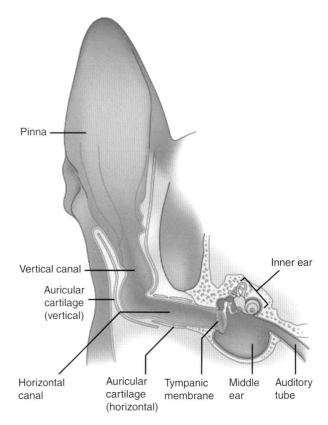

Figure 8.24.1 Basic anatomy of the canine ear. *Source:* Small Animal Dermatology, Anita Patel and Peter Forsythe, Otitis externa and otitis media in a dog, p. 325. © 2008 Elsevier.

epithelium (without goblet cells) medially. Between the two layers sits the manubrium of the malleus, in a fibrous middle layer, which then transmits vibrations along the other ossicles. The ruptured eardrum (in a noninflamed setting) requires 21–35 days to heal; in inflammatory otitis, it might require 45–60 days. There is approximately a 10 db decrease in hearing associated with eardrum rupture, but animals are not deaf simply because the eardrum gets ruptured.

The ear has normal clearance mechanisms, which involve epithelial migration, starting at the level of the eardrum and then moving outwards along the sides of the ear canals. In this way, it acts like a conveyor belt, moving material along and eventually out of the ear canal. This process can be damaged by trauma, including routine swabbing of the ear canals.

Cerumen (wax) is a collection of sebaceous and apocrine secretions and skin cells from epithelial migration. It provides lubrication, cleaning, and even some antimicrobial functions. It is important not to push wax back toward the eardrum as it can serve as an obstruction in the ear canal.

The tympanic bulla is a relatively large cavity in dogs, and sits medial to the eardrum in the middle ear cavity, like a cauldron. It is difficult to drain and provides an excellent surface for bacterial growth with associated inflammation. The bulla of the cat is separated into dorsomedial and ventrolateral compartments by a septum. Eventually, with chronic otitis, the bone of the bulla can become compromised, which is then not amenable to medical therapy.

8.24.4   It's Not Just About Microbes

The ear canal is not sterile, and it plays host to a variety of resident, transient, opportunistic, and pathogenic bacteria and fungi. It is important to understand how this occurs, since otitis externa (a term often implying infection of the external ear canal) is commonplace, and is often a frustrating condition in veterinary practice. In some cases, the primary cause has very little to do with microbes, such as when it is due to a foreign body, parasites, immune-mediated causes, or adverse drug reactions.

Resident bacteria and yeasts live and multiply in the normal ear canal. There is typically a lot of microbial diversity in the ears of healthy animals, but that diversity tends to wane in the presence of inflammation. This shift in microbial populations may be a perpetuating factor in the development of otitis externa. Thus, while many species of bacteria and fungi are found in the ears of healthy dogs, in dogs with otitis externa, it is not unusual to see competitive advantage for bacteria such as *Pseudomonas* (or *Ralstonia* which was previously included in the genus *Pseudomonas*) and yeasts such as *Malassezia pachydermatis*.

To cause otitis as a secondary event, bacteria must be able to adhere to lining cells of the ear canal, take advantage of nutrients there, compete effectively with resident organisms, and overcome host defense mechanisms.

Predisposing factors for otitis externa need to be appreciated. The ear conformation of some pets, excessive moisture in the ear canals, obstruction of the canal with masses (including tumors and polyps), and co-morbidities (including systemic diseases and otitis media) can all predispose to otitis externa. Prior treatments which have altered the microbial dynamics or the normal otic clearing mechanisms are also important predisposing factors.

Perpetuating factors are also problematic and can lead to recurrence. Anything that interferes with the normal barrier function or changes the microbial balance in the external ear canal can impair restoration of the normal protective aspects of the tissue there. When the lining of the ear canal becomes swollen, when the diameter of the canal narrows, when proliferative tissue is present, and when the eardrum is ruptured and creates an opening to the middle ear, resolving otitis externa becomes more complicated (see

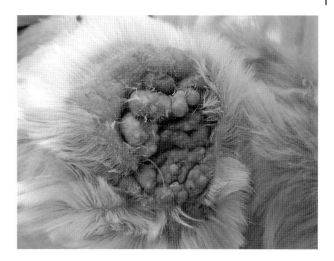

Figure 8.24.2   It is important to be proactive when managing cases of otitis externa, because chronic changes can greatly complicate management.

Figure 8.24.2). Areas with impaired epidermal migration, scarring, tissue thickening, or significant inflammation can make it progressively more difficult to resolve the situation without the chronic use of antimicrobial agents. Veterinary teams need to be vigilant to identify problems early, before chronic changes set in that will complicate the long-term management of the condition, which in some cases may necessitate surgery.

Any process that disturbs the ear canal's barrier function will predispose to otitis externa. This includes any abrasion that compromises surface barrier functions (including rough swabbing of the ear canals), any inflammatory process that causes epidermal disorganization, any process that affects local temperature and relative humidity in the ear canal, or any proliferative epidermal reaction that results in epithelial disarray. Finally, any underlying disease that impairs immune function can predispose to otitis externa, including endocrinopathies. Therefore, it is most important to investigate underlying diseases that predispose to otitis externa, rather than just responding to the clinical situation with antibiotics.

8.24.5   Getting Specific

With pet-specific care, we can personalize our approach to common maladies, such as otitis externa. In some cases, we can anticipate where microbial overgrowth is most likely to occur. For example, in pets with pendulous ears (e.g., cocker spaniel) there is likely to be microbial overgrowth in the ear canals, and pet owners would be well advised to make cleaning the ears a regular part of health maintenance. Gentle cleansing and cerumenolytic (wax-dissolving) solutions are typically all that are required to provide a life-time of care. In young dogs and cats, ear mites are not uncommon, and should be a consideration when dark discharge (often referred to as "coffee grounds") is noted clinically.

The most common underlying cause for otitis externa is allergy, and atopic dermatitis accounts for a majority of cases. Fortunately (or unfortunately), atopic dermatitis tends to run in families, and there is often a striking breed predisposition, so a tendency toward bacterial overgrowth can often be predicted in these cases (see 8.18 Team Strategies for Atopic Dermatitis). It is important to realize that when allergies are the underlying cause for otitis externa, the goal must be to successfully address the underlying allergic situation – not necessarily to mount an attack on ear canal microbes which are only proliferating because of the underlying inflammatory situation. If addressed early, before there is substantial barrier function disturbance, the microbial overgrowth can usually be successfully managed entirely with topical therapies, without systemic antibiotics.

While it might seem somewhat simplistic, the use of antimicrobials in many cases of otitis externa is not necessary and likely indicates a failure to be adequately proactive. Early in the course of most such problems, the microbes are not especially pathogenic, and tend to be as responsive to topicals as they are to systemic medications. Allowing damage to the barrier function makes control with surface cleansers more problematic, and the recurrent use of antimicrobials encourages microbial resistance which not only makes the conditions harder to treat but poses public health concerns as well (see 9.12 Judicious Use of Antimicrobials).

Once potential risk has been identified in pets, the management of that risk should be a top priority. Owners of pets with conditions that could promote microbial overgrowth, such as allergies, should be effectively counseled as early as possible, preferably even before the first episode.

A good time to start such conversations is when pets are quite young, such as at 8 weeks of age, long before any problems are evident (other than ear mites which might be evident even at this young age). At this time, the hospital team can alert the owners of at-risk pets to not only be vigilant for evidence of early clinical signs of microbial overgrowth, but to actively embark on mitigation exercises, such as effectively cleansing and soothing the ears and seeking veterinary attention before the problem requires antibiotics. The intention is not to scare owners but to set realistic expectations for a risk that can been identified in the practice population. If such conversations are productive, it might also prompt the owner to ask what it would mean for their pet if they allowed the condition to progress to the point where it did require antibiotics, and why the development of microbial resistance is of concern to everyone. Most pet owners are aware of the dangers of antibiotic resistance and can appreciate that antibiotics should be reserved for the cases that truly warrant them. You might think that you don't want to have those discussions in advance, but in time, you will likely realize that it was time well spent and develop resources (client handouts, website pages, trained staff, etc.) to facilitate such client education.

8.24.6 Using Early Detection Effectively

In many cases, the early detection of otitis externa is a function of determining the contributions of underlying causes as well as perpetuating factors. Once again, it is relatively easy to appreciate that underlying causes such as allergies, parasites, altered anatomy, and immune compromise can lead to microbial overgrowth in the external ear canal. Once these underlying concerns have been identified, secondary microbial overgrowth should be anticipated, and plans put in place for mitigation.

Most pets today should be on year-round parasite control, which should help control at least some of the predisposing factors to microbial overgrowth, such as ear mites, demodicosis, ticks, and fleas. In fact, some of the newer parasiticides may help control a variety of different parasites. Still, parasite assessment should be an important part of any workup for otitis externa and *Demodex* and *Otodectes* mites, and even some species of ticks, can reside within the external ear canal and be clinically confused with microbial involvement.

Clinically, otitis externa often starts with inflammation of the skin lining the external ear canal and that inflammation can cause tissue swelling and narrowing of the ear canal which impedes normal clearance mechanisms and creates an environment in which both bacteria and yeast can flourish.

Prior to diagnostic testing, a full clinical examination is warranted, including noting the condition of the pinnae and external ear. This often indicates whether the process is confined to the ear canal or has more systemic manifestations. Evaluation includes palpation of the external areas around the ears, which can help identify ears that are no longer pliable but might have edema, fibrosis or calcification which might help indicate the chronicity of the problem. Also, noting important history, such as seasonality of the problem, whether it is unilateral or bilateral, and whether other animals in the household are similarly affected, are important clues to diagnosis.

The first physical step in the diagnostic process is to sample exudate from both ear canals, either with swabs or aspirating with a syringe and rubber (5 Fr) tube. Samples are collected for cytological evaluation of both ears to determine the extent of involvement of bacteria, yeasts, and inflammatory cells; another set is mixed with mineral oil and evaluated for parasites. In early cases there may be just bacterial and yeast overgrowth. In time, more white blood cells will be found, and there may be evidence of large numbers of bacteria that may be engulfed and appear intracellularly; yeasts can appear in large numbers. The cytology samples from both ears are typically stained with a modified Wright stain, and sometimes with a gram stain (which can help differentiate a gram-negative *Pseudomonas* from a gram-positive *Corynebacterium*, etc.).

The next step is to visually examine all aspects of the ear canals and eardrum. When the ear canal is very inflamed and painful, it might be necessary to provide antiinflammatory therapy for 7–10 days, just to open up the ears sufficiently for full evaluation. If the ear canal needs to be flushed to allow better visualization, it is best to use saline or dilute acetic acid (1–2.5%) initially, since these are safe even if they enter the middle ear in case the eardrum is ruptured. If a wax-dissolving agent is needed, something mild like squalene can be considered. Otoscope cones can become contaminated and transfer microbes to other patients, so appropriate disinfection techniques are critical, or disposable cones can be used.

Once the ear canal and tympanum have been thoroughly evaluated, cultures may be taken from the middle ear, if indicated. It is important during this initial stage, while the pet is sedated or anesthetized, to thoroughly clean the ear canals not only so the ears can be thoroughly evaluated but also to facilitate treatment. Cleaning can not only reduce the microbial burden in the ear canal but can disrupt biofilm formation, remove debris and exudate, and facilitate the administration of otic medications. Biofilm production can be significant with *Pseudomonas aeruginosa*, may play a role in the pathogenesis of otitis externa, and, depending on the topical antibiotic used, may necessitate higher concentrations of medications.

Imaging of the middle ear is important in chronic otitis, because the tympanic bullae may become compromised. Radiographic studies (known as a bulla series) can be done but do not identify bulla damage until it is quite severe. Magnetic resonance imaging (MRI) and computed tomography (CT) are preferred for this purpose. Hand-held tympanometer measurements can also be used in conscious dogs for evaluation of the middle ear and auditory tube.

Pets with atopic dermatitis and other inflammatory disorders tend to develop recurrent bacterial and yeast overgrowth in the external ear canals and so when pets develop such issues, it is important to routinely assess with cytology. It is impossible to ascertain by inspection (or smell) whether a complication is bacteria or yeast related, so using cytological confirmation is important.

In most cases of early otitis externa due to allergies or other inflammatory disorders, antiinflammatory therapy is often more important than antimicrobial therapy. When the situation is caught early enough, the microbial component can often be managed with topical therapy, once the ear is no longer painful or inflamed. However, when there is deep involvement, when there is eardrum rupture with otitis media, when there are complicating factors, or when systemic therapy is needed, bacterial culture and susceptibility testing is warranted.

Culture and susceptibility testing is useful when systemic therapy is being considered, but it is important to realize that because microbes are so plentiful in the ear canal, selection of causative microbes is not always assured, depending on sampling technique and laboratory factors. This is important because of extensive strain diversity and the fact that many laboratories select a single bacterial colony to submit for susceptibility testing, and that single colony may not be representative of the bacterial strain most important clinically and if there is eardrum rupture, the microbes in the middle ear may not have the same profile as microbes sampled from the external ear canal. In addition, susceptibility testing is meant to predict the effects of antimicrobials administered systemically, whereas in many cases, the antibacterial dose is actually much higher for medications administered topically.

Cultures are indicated when it is believed that bacteria are clinically implicated in a problem and there has been incomplete response to empirically chosen antibiotics at an appropriate dose and over an appropriate period of time, when new problems develop within a few weeks after complete resolution, when cytological evaluation still reveals microbes and white blood cells, and for pets that have recently received systemic antibiotics for otitis externa.

Hearing loss can occur in dogs with otitis externa for a variety of reasons. The hearing loss can be conductive when the transmission or transduction of sound is compromised, such as with exudates occluding the ear canal, eardrum rupture, canal stenosis, exudates in the ear canal, etc. Hearing loss can also occur for sensorineural reasons, when inner ear alterations occur from hereditary causes, ototoxic drugs, or degenerative changes. Hearing can be assessed with brainstem auditory-evoked response (BAER) testing, but it is worthwhile employing an owner questionnaire for dogs with otitis externa to determine possible hearing changes associated with clinical, diagnostic or therapeutic interventions. Such questions might include asking about whether there are changes associated with perception of doorbells, approaching vehicles or people, pets being more difficult to rouse from sleep with noises, or even response to calls, whistles, clickers or clapping hands when not in the pet's direct line of vision.

8.24.7 Managing the Pet with Otitis Externa

The best approach to managing the pet with otitis externa is to suspect from the outset that the problem is secondary to some underlying problem. To successfully manage the situation, it is therefore necessary to uncover and successfully manage the underlying problem. In rare instances, such as with otodectic mange (ear mites), it may be possible to "cure" the underlying problem and stop the otitis externa from progressing. In cases of tumors or polyps, surgery may be curative. In most other cases, it will only be possible to "control" the underlying problem, which means the long-term control of the ear problem hinges on the successful long-term control of the underlying problem. The most common underlying problems are atopic dermatitis, adverse reactions to foods, compromised immune function, masses/tumors/polyps, and anatomical issues.

The goals of management are to:

- manage underlying problems
- keep ear canal clean
- control inflammation
- control pain
- control infection
- determine medical vs surgical candidates.

There are many medicaments that are sold for ear problems, and yet some of the simplest remedies are the most satisfying if the underlying problems have been addressed. In many cases, antiinflammatory agents are needed to reduce inflammation in the ears, decrease pain and itch, reduce glandular secretions, and reduce edema and swelling. Because the ears are initially inflamed, no topical therapies or flushes should be administered for the first week or so since this can lead to erosions and tissue maceration, and potentially can make the animal "head shy." Pain management is important during this time (see 8.21 Team Strategies for Pain Management).

The most important point for managing otitis externa, once underlying issues have been addressed and controlled, is to determine if antimicrobial therapy is warranted, since these medications tend to be overused in many cases. The issue tends to be further complicated when veterinary teams choose the latest-generation antibiotic to try first, or use inappropriate classes of antibiotics, or use human antibiotics, most of which have not been labeled for use in animals, or select antibiotics empirically, when culture and susceptibility is actually indicated.

Thorough cleaning of the ear canal is critical in the management of otitis. Not only is it important to remove debris, wax, and exudates, but purulent material deep in the ear canal often inactivates a variety of medications that can be instilled. When the ears are inflamed, sedation or anesthesia is warranted as the ears will be painful on manipulation. It is not advisable to ask owners to try to manipulate painful and inflamed ears at home, as it complicates later attempts for at-home care.

Topical medications are important in the management of otitis, but are rarely the sole therapy. Products should be selected based on cytological assessment, and whether or not the eardrum is intact. The ingredients in the topical product should match the organisms thought to be involved (e.g., *Pseudomonas*, *Staphylococcus*, *Corynebacterium*, etc.). Topical corticosteroids may be necessary as well, to help control the often very significant inflammation. Stronger topical corticosteroids may be used initially (such as fluocinolone, betamethasone), followed by more moderate products (such as triamcinolone, prednisolone, dexamethasone), and finally by weaker ones (such as hydrocortisone). It is important to appreciate that topical corticosteroids can be absorbed and have systemic effects, so their use must be strategic and monitored accordingly.

Because of the population dynamics of microbes, which are capable of doubling in numbers every few hours, it is important to use appropriate topicals for treatment, instill the appropriate volume, and have the owners massage the ears for 15–30 seconds to ensure the products get adequately distributed in the ear canal. Plucking fur from the ear canals can facilitate dispersal of medications, but can also irritate the sensitive lining, so must be considered on a case-by-case basis.

Since otitis externa tends to be a chronic issue, it is important to establish an appropriate schedule for monitoring the situation. After the initial visit, thorough cleaning and administration of medications, the pet should be evaluated 2–4 weeks later. The pet should be significantly improved, the ears less sensitive to being handled, and the owner on board with long-term control measures of any underlying problems as well as ear issues.

Ongoing monitoring should be scheduled according to the primary cause, but at each visit it is best to evaluate the ears cytologically to assess any microbial overgrowth or evidence of white blood cell infiltration. Maintenance schedules should be developed to help keep the pet comfortable, impede microbial overgrowth, and control any underlying issues. Long-term success should involve minimizing the use of antimicrobials to those absolutely needed, and also limiting systemic therapies that might have long-term side effects.

8.24.8   The Issue of Resistance

Antimicrobial resistance is a significant issue in healthcare and must be taken seriously. It has become more common in clinical practice, likely due to repeated antibiotic use, failure to identify and control underlying issues, and selecting inappropriate products and/or dosages for use in patients.

Healthcare teams can help prevent the development of resistance by only prescribing antibiotics when they are absolutely needed, and according to appropriate guidelines (see 9.12 Judicious Use of Antimicrobials). In many cases, topical therapies are sufficient, and the use of antibiotics can often be avoided if underlying conditions are successfully managed. Thus, in line with pet-specific guidelines, antimicrobial stewardship warrants strategic initiatives with preventive approaches to make antibiotic use less necessary, early detection of potential bacterial complications when they can be resolved without antibiotics, and then evidence-based management directives with facilitated compliance to help make resistance a less likely sequel.

TAKE-AWAYS

- Most cases of otitis externa are secondary to underlying causes.
- When underlying causes are not identified and corrected, otitis externa is likely to persist or recur.
- The most common underlying causes of otitis externa are allergies, parasites, anatomical issues. and other disorders that affect the ear canal's barrier function.
- Most cases of otitis externa can be managed without the use of systemic antibiotics.
- Veterinary healthcare teams should be vigilant in their use of systemic antibiotics, since antimicrobial stewardship is everyone's concern.

MISCELLANEOUS

Recommended Reading

Aufox, E.E. and May, E.R. (2019). Top 5 keys to successful management of otitis externa. *Clin. Brief*: 63–67.

Choi, N., Edginton, H.D., Griffin, C.E., and Angus, J.C. (2018). Comparison of two ear cytological collection techniques in dogs with otitis externa. *Vet. Dermatol.* 29: 413–416.

Clinical and Laboratory Standards Institute. Understanding Susceptibility Test Data as a Component of Antimicrobial Stewardship in Veterinary Settings. 2019. https://clsi.org/media/3249/vet09ed1-sample.pdf

Cole, L.K., Rajala-Schultz, P.J., and Lorch, G. (2018). Conductive hearing loss in our dogs associated with the use of ointment-based otic medications. *Vet. Dermatol.* 29: 341–344.

Frey, E. (2018). The role of companion animal veterinarians in one-health efforts to combat antimicrobial resistance. *J. Am. Vet. Med. Assoc.* 253 (11): 1396–1404.

Korbelik, J., Singh, A., Rousseau, J., and Weese, J.S. (2018). Analysis of the otic mycobiota in dogs with otitis externa compared to healthy individuals. *Vet. Dermatol.* 29 (5): 417–e138.

Mason, C.L., Paterson, S., and Cripps, P.J. (2013). Use of a hearing loss grading system and an owner-based hearing questionnaire to assess hearing loss in pet dogs with chronic otitis externa or otitis media. *Vet. Dermatol.* 24: 512–518.

Paterson, S. (2016). Topical ear treatment – options, indications and limitations of current therapy. *J. Am. Anim. Pract.* 57 (12): 668–678.

Reeder, C.J., Griffin, C.E., Polissar, N.L. et al. (2008). Comparative adrenocortical suppression in dogs with otitis externa following topical otic administration of four different glucocorticoid-containing medications. *Vet. Ther.* 9 (2): 111–121.

8.25

Team Strategies for Weight Management

Kara M. Burns, MS, MEd, LVT, VTS (Nutrition)

Lafayette, IN, USA

BASICS

8.25.1 Summary

Obesity in the pet population has reached epidemic proportions in many industrialized countries. This directly parallels the obesity epidemic in the human population. An estimated 59% of adult pets and 50% of pets over age 7 are overweight or obese [1–4].

Obesity can be defined as an increase in fat tissue mass sufficient to contribute to disease. Dogs and cats weighing 10–19% more than the optimal weight for their breed are considered overweight; those weighing 20% or more above the optimum weight are considered obese [5]. Obesity has been associated with a number of disease conditions, as well as with a reduced lifespan. Excessive caloric intake combined with decreased physical activity and genetic susceptibility are associated with most cases of obesity.

The primary treatment for obesity is reduced caloric intake and increased physical activity. This approach seems simple but with the increasing numbers of obese animals, obviously it is not simple. Obesity is one of the leading preventable causes of illness/death and with the dramatic rise in pet obesity over the past several decades, weight management and obesity prevention should be among the top health issues healthcare team members discuss with every client.

8.25.2 Terms Defined

Daily Energy Requirement (DER): The energy requirement needed for activities beyond just remaining completely at rest (e.g., activity, life-stage or physiological condition, dealing with environmental conditions). These total DERs can be approximated by multiplying the resting energy requirement (RER) by an appropriate factor given likely activity levels.

Obesity: An increase in fat tissue mass sufficient to contribute to disease.

RER: The daily energy needed to sustain essential bodily functions (e.g., respiration, circulation, digestion, metabolism) while the animal is at rest in a thermoneutral environment.

MAIN CONCEPTS

Weight management in pets, including obesity prevention and treatment, is a challenge for the veterinary healthcare team and pet owners. Clients do not always recognize that their pet is overweight or obese, nor do they know the health risks associated with being overweight or obese. Additionally, veterinary teams have a difficult time addressing the pet's obesity and the importance of weight loss because they believe the client will be personally insulted. However, it is of the utmost importance to have this discussion with the owner and truly support the pet and owner on the journey to a healthy weight. The veterinary healthcare team is the advocate for the patient, and with the myriad health risks that obesity presents, it is important to advocate for proper weight and a weight management program for the patient.

The best approach for weight management in pets is a team approach, where all team members are saying the same thing and are part of the weight management program supporting the pet owner and patient.

An effective individualized weight loss program, prescribed by the veterinarian and implemented by the entire healthcare team, provides a consistent and healthy rate of weight loss to reduce risk of disease, prevent malnutrition, and improve quality of life (see 6.15 Approaching Obesity on a Pet-Specific Basis). Weight loss is achieved through appropriate calorie restriction, diet selection, exercise, and strategies to help modify the behavior of both the pet and client. The success of any program depends on the ability of the veterinary team to partner with clients to set expectations, promote client compliance and treatment adherence, and overcome challenges presented by each pet.

8.25.3 Causes of Obesity

Obesity is caused by an imbalance of energy intake and energy expenditure. Simply stated – too many calories in, not enough calories out. Several risk factors affect energy balance. In society today, indoor pets (in North America) are typically neutered. While there are many positive health benefits associated with neutering, it is important that metabolic impacts are addressed as well (see 2.18 Population Control). Studies have demonstrated that neutering may result in decreased metabolic rate and increased food intake, and if energy intake is not adjusted, body weight (BW), body condition score, and amount of body fat will increase, resulting in an overweight or obese pet. Other recognized risk factors for obesity include breed, age, decreased physical activity, and type of food and feeding method [1, 5].

It is important for the team to recognize that specific breeds of dogs and cats are more likely to become overweight. In dogs, these include Shetland sheepdogs, golden retrievers, dachshunds, cocker spaniels, Labrador retrievers, Dalmatians, Rottweilers, and mixed breeds. In cats, mixed breeds and Manx cats are more likely to be obese compared to most purebred cats. Veterinary technicians/nurses should begin discussions on maintaining appropriate/optimal weight in pets, particularly in at-risk breeds, during the initial puppy/kitten health and wellness examinations.

8.25.4 Health Risks Associated with Obesity

There are numerous health conditions associated with obesity in pets, including osteoarthritis, diabetes mellitus (DM), cancer, skin diseases, lower urinary tract problems, hepatic lipidosis, and heart disease. It is imperative that healthcare team members discuss these risks with pet owners. Obese pets are also more difficult to manage in terms of sample collection (blood, urine) and catheter placement. Owners do not realize that obese pets may be more prone to treatment complications including difficulty intubating, respiratory distress, slower recovery time, and delayed wound healing. So, let's have that discussion.

It is widely believed that obesity affects quality of life and leads to reduced life expectancy. The dramatic impact of excess BW in dogs and cats has been demonstrated. In cats, it is estimated that 31% of DM and 34% of lameness cases could be eliminated if cats were at optimum BW. In dogs, lifespan was increased by nearly two years in those that were maintained at an optimal body condition [1, 6]. Veterinary teams need to recognize and to communicate to clients that fat tissue is not inert and that obesity is not an aesthetic condition that only affects our pet's ability to interact with us on a physical activity level. Fat tissue is metabolically active and in fact is the largest endocrine organ in the body and has an unlimited growth potential. Fat tissue is an active producer of hormones and inflammatory cytokines and the chronic low-grade inflammation secondary to obesity contributes to obesity-related diseases [6].

8.25.5 The Team Approach to Evaluating Weight and Nutrition

Obesity is a difficult disease to talk with owners about because most do not recognize (or want to admit) that their pet is overweight. All members of the healthcare team need to commit to understanding and communicating the role of weight management in pet health and disease prevention. In particular, the veterinary technician/nurse is the primary source for client education – the interface between the client, the doctor, and the rest of the hospital team – and is the key advocate for the patient.

The healthcare team should assess every patient that comes into the hospital, every time they come into the hospital, to establish nutritional needs and feeding goals. These goals will vary depending on the pet's physiology, obesity risk factors, and current health status. Designing and implementing a weight management protocol supports the team, the client, and most importantly the patient [1, 7].

The patient evaluation should include a complete history, including a detailed nutritional history, and a complete physical examination, including a complete blood count, serum chemistry, and urinalysis. Signalment data should include species, breed, age, gender, neuter status, weight, activity level, and environment. The nutritional history should determine the type of food (all food) fed, the feeding method (how much, how often), who is responsible for feeding the pet and any other sources of energy intake (no matter how small or seemingly insignificant) [1].

The veterinary assistant or credentialed veterinary nurse/technician should be leading the nutritional history. Open-ended questions, such as "Tell me what Fluffy eats in a day" should be asked along with other open-ended questions to ascertain the following information.

- Brand of food fed to the pet (try to get specific name).
- Do you feed moist or dry or both?
- Feeding method (how much, how often)?
- Does your pet receive any snacks or treats of any kind? If so, what and how often?
- Do you give your pet any supplements?
- Is your pet on any medications, including chewable medications? If so, obtain name and dosage.
- What type of chew toys does your pet play with?
- Do you feed your pet any foods or treats not specifically designated for pets (such as human foods)? If so, what and how often.
- Does your pet have ANY access to other sources of food (neighbor, trash, family member, etc.)?

Obtaining a complete nutritional history supports consistency and accuracy of patient information, provides key insights to barriers in client compliance, guides client discussion, and supports the optimal weight management program for the pet.

The veterinary assistant can weigh the pet and obtain a body condition upon the pet's arrival to the hospital. This information can then be entered into the patient's medical record by the reception team. It is helpful to use the same scale and chart the findings for the client. Body condition scoring (BCS) is important to assess a patient's fat stores and muscle mass (see 6.15 Approaching Obesity on a Pet-Specific Basis, which includes graphics for BCS in dogs and cats). A healthy and successful weight management program results in loss of fat tissue while maintaining lean body mass and consistent and accurate assessment of weight and BCS are important tools to track progress. The use of body condition charts and breed charts is helpful in discussing the importance of weight management with clients and helps them visualize what an optimal weight would look like on their pet.

The entire healthcare team should be familiar with BCS and the scoring chart used to ensure consistency in reporting and recording in the medical record.

8.25.6 Weight Management Program

As with many aspects of healthcare, designing a successful weight management program is not a "one program fits all" for our patients. The components of a successful weight management program include consistent and accurate weight measurement/patient monitoring, effective client communication, identification of compliance gaps, and utilization of tools to reinforce compliance, client and patient support and program restructure as needed.

Setting a goal for weight loss and calculating the appropriate energy intake starts with determination of the pet's ideal BW. Ideal BW is a starting goal that is adjusted for appropriate body condition as the pet loses weight. It is important to determine the number of daily calories that will result in weight loss while providing adequate protein, vitamins, and minerals to meet the pet's DER. The DER reflects the pet's activity level and is a calculation based on the pet's RER.

There are a couple of basic formulas that all technicians should memorize or have on laminated note cards in every exam room (along with a calculator). The most accurate formula to determine the RER for a cat or a dog is:

$$\text{RER kcal/day} = 70(\text{ideal body weight in kg})^{0.75}$$

or

$$\text{RER kcal/day} = (\text{kg} \times \text{kg} \times \text{kg}, \sqrt{}, \sqrt{}) \times 70$$

Once RER is determined, DER may be calculated by multiplying RER by "standard" factors related to energy needs. The calculations used to determine energy needs for obese prone pets or for pets needing to lose weight are:

Obese prone dogs	$\text{DER} = 1.4 \times \text{RER}$
Weight loss/dogs	$\text{DER} = 1.0 \times \text{RER}$
Obese prone cats	$\text{DER} = 1.0 \times \text{RER}$
Weight loss/cats	$\text{DER} = 0.8 \times \text{RER}$

Gathering the above information takes only a few minutes and is the foundation for developing a weight loss program that includes:

- target weight or weight loss goal
- maximum daily caloric intake
- specific food, amount of food, and method of feeding.

The program should also include specific protocols for monitoring the pet's weight (the reception team should schedule these before the client leaves and send reminder cards), adjusting the pet's energy intake accordingly and exercise guidelines/suggestions.

There are numerous ways for an owner to get their pet active and it is the role of the veterinary technician/nurse to discuss these with the client and determine which may work for that specific patient and client. It can and should start simply – having the owner walk their dog to the end of the driveway, for example. Also, starting to play with interactive toys with their cat for a few minutes a day would be a great way to begin to get cats more interactive and exercising. Gradually, you want to educate the owner to build up the distance and time spent exercising. If the owner is excited and takes the dog on a 5 km walk on the first day, the dog may tire easily, and the owner may find this frustrating and not want to walk with their dog again. Remember to advise owners that exercise needs to begin in moderation. By following this, a more successful outcome will result.

Effective follow-up and regular monitoring by the entire veterinary team are crucial parts of a successful weight loss program. Consider the following points.

- Train the veterinary team to provide consistent information about diet and feeding for each life stage.
- Implement multimodal client reminder systems (e.g., postcards, phone calls, emails).
- Designate specific team members for client support and follow-up encouragement.
- Recommend that clients participate in group programs (dog walking groups, agility clubs).

Once a program has begun, contact the client the next day to lend encouragement and to see if there are any initial questions. Follow up again after the first week as many get discouraged with concerns such as food refusal and begging behaviors that are best addressed early in the weight loss program. Provide clinical support from team members through frequent phone calls between weight checks. Identify and address obstacles and client concerns, satisfaction, or frustrations with the program. Follow up with the client either by telephone or an office visit every two weeks until the desired rate of weight loss is established. Monitor the patient monthly until the ideal weight has been reached and has stabilized on a long-term maintenance program. Remember to document every step in the medical record.

When following up with the patient and clients:

- ask open-ended questions to elicit client observations and concerns
- provide positive reinforcement and encouragement
- be sure to record BW and BCS in the medical record. Keep track and show the client the pet's measurements of either girth or abdominal circumference to assist in emphasizing losses
- take a picture of the patient
- create a chart to monitor and show progress.

There are several specific recommendations that support a successful weight loss program which include every member of the healthcare team:

- emphasizing feeding consistency, including feeding the pet from its designated dish only

- be sure the client is using an 8 oz measuring cup
- recommend the appropriate weight loss food and calculate the initial feeding amount
- discuss the importance of total energy intake (do not feed anything other than the recommended food at the designated amount)
- if the client wants to "treat" their pet, make appropriate recommendations and adjust the caloric intake of the base food accordingly
- encourage clients to feed their pets separately if possible
- recommend appropriate exercise for the pet
- offer your clients suggestions on ways other than food to reward or bond with their pet
- evaluate, adjust, communicate, and encourage on a consistent basis.

Every member of the veterinary team can celebrate successes. Weight prevention programs are long term. The owner will see weight loss, weight gain, and plateaus during the course of the weight prevention plan. Be sure that all team members are on the same page with the specific patient's weight protocol. Educate the owner about the highs and lows to be expected in the program. Celebrate any and all successes – whether it is 1 pound or 5 pounds. Encourage the owner when a plateau arrives, because it will! Overall, be their champion.

A successful weight management program is in the best interest of the pets. Additionally, success will greatly improve the health of the pet, reduce the potential for future health concerns, increase the level of activity of pets, and in the end will improve and strengthen the human–animal bond.

Successful weight management begins with recognition of the disease of overweight and obesity as well as the importance of weight control in our pets. It is essential that the healthcare team communicate the serious effects that even a few excess pounds can have on the health and longevity of pets' lives. Weight management should be a cornerstone of the wellness program in every clinic and the veterinary technician the champion of the program and advocate for the patient.

TAKE-AWAYS

- A nutritional assessment and recommendation should be made for every pet, every time they visit the hospital.
- Obesity in pets is a preventable epidemic.
- Every member of the healthcare team plays a role in helping patients get to a healthy/ideal BW.

- Obesity is caused by an imbalance of energy intake and energy expenditure – too many calories in, not enough calories out.
- The components of a successful weight management program include consistent and accurate weight measurement/patient monitoring, effective client communication, identification of compliance gaps, and utilization of tools to reinforce compliance, client and patient support and program restructure as needed.

MISCELLANEOUS

References

1 Burns, K.M. (2013). Why is Rocky so stocky? *NAVTA J.* (Convention Issue): 16–19.

2 Courcier, E.A., O'Higgins, R., Mellor, D.J. et al. (2010). Prevalence and risk factors for feline obesity in a first opinion practice in Glasgow, Scotland. *J. Feline Med. Surg.* 12 (10): 746–753.

3 Courcier, E.A., Thomson, R.M., Mellor, D.J. et al. (2010). An epidemiological study of environmental factors associated with canine obesity. *J. Small Anim. Pract.* 51 (7): 362–367.

4 Armstrong, P.J. and Lusby, A.L. (2011). Clinical importance of canine and feline obesity. In: *Practical Weight Management in Dogs and Cats* (ed. T.L. Towell), 3–21. Ames, IA: Wiley Blackwell.

5 Burns, K.M. and Towell, T.L. (2011). Owner education and adherence. In: *Practical Weight Management in Dogs and Cats* (ed. T.L. Towell), 173–200. Ames, IA: Wiley Blackwell.

6 Laflamme, D.P. (2006). Understanding and managing obesity in dogs and cats. *Vet. Clin. Small. Anim. Pract.* 36: 1283–1295.

7 Toll, P.W., Yamka, R.N., Schoenherr, W.D., and Hand, M.S. (2010). Obesity. In: *Small Animal Clinical Nutrition*, 5e (ed. M.S. Hand), 501–542. Topeka, KS: MMI.

Recommended Reading

American Animal Hospital Association. Weight Management Guidelines for Dogs and Cats. www.aaha.org/aaha-guidelines/weight-management-configuration/abstract

Association for Pet Obesity Prevention. www.petobesityprevention.org

Pet Nutrition Alliance. www.petnutritionalliance.org

World Small Animal Association. http://wsava.org

Body Condition Scoring, Cats. www.wsava.org/WSAVA/media/Documents/Committee%20Resources/Global%20Nutrition%20Committee/English/Cat-Body-Condition-Scoring-2017.pdf

Body Condition Scoring, Dogs. https://wsava.org/wp-content/uploads/2020/01/Body-Condition-Score-Dog.pdf

Muscle Condition Scoring, Cats. www.wsava.org/WSAVA/media/Documents/Committee%20Resources/Global%20Nutrition%20Committee/English/Muscle-Condition-Score-Chart-for-Cats.pdf

Muscle Condition Scoring, Dogs. www.wsava.org/WSAVA/media/Documents/Committee%20Resources/Global%20Nutrition%20Committee/English/Muscle-Condition-Score-Chart-for-Dogs.pdf

8.26

Team Strategies for Glaucoma

D. J. Haeussler, Jr., BS, MS, DVM, DACVO

The Animal Eye Institute, Cincinnati, OH, USA

 BASICS

8.26.1 Summary

Glaucoma is a group of ocular diseases that exhibit increased levels of intraocular pressure (IOP) that are detrimental to the maintenance of vision and health of the eye. Glaucoma is the end result due to an inadequate drainage of aqueous humor from within the eye and is one of the leading causes of not only vision loss but loss of the eye in animals. The only way to properly diagnose glaucoma in any species is to use a digital tonometer. Recognition of glaucoma in patients by the veterinary team is critical and time sensitive in order to delay loss of vision and manage comfort in the patient.

8.26.2 Terms Defined

Beta Blockers: A group of glaucoma medications utilized to reduce IOP by decreasing aqueous humor formation.

Buphthalmos: Increased size of the globe.

Carbonic Anhydrase Inhibitors: A group of glaucoma medications which inhibit the enzyme carbonic anhydrase which leads to decreased aqueous humor formation and thereby decreases IOP.

Endolaser Cyclophotocoagulation: A vision-sparing surgical procedure utilized to reduce IOP.

Enucleation: Removal of the eye, third eyelid, and conjunctival tissue.

Glaucoma: A group of ocular diseases the exhibit increased levels of IOP that are detrimental to the maintenance of vision and health of the eye.

Gonioimplant: A surgically placed device utilized to provide an alternate aqueous humor outflow pathway to reduce IOP.

Intraocular Silicone Prosthesis: Removal of the uvea, lens, and retina and placement of an intraocular silicone sphere in cases of advanced glaucoma.

Hyphema: Blood in the anterior chamber of the eye.

Hypopyon: An accumulation of inflammatory cells found in the anterior chamber of the eye.

Parasympathomimetics: A group of glaucoma medications which cause miosis, leading to a decrease in IOP by opening the iridocorneal angle.

Preiridal Fibrovascular Membrane: A network of fibrovascular membrane that forms on the anterior surface of the iris and extends into and over the iridocorneal angle.

Primary Glaucoma: Glaucoma in dogs thought to have a genetic predisposition.

Prostaglandin Analogues: A group of glaucoma medications which decrease IOP and are typically used in cases of primary glaucoma. These medications reduce IOP by increasing uveoscleral outflow.

Secondary Glaucoma: Glaucoma occurring due to any other condition except having a genetic predisposition.

Tonometer: Instrument used to measure IOP.

Transscleral Cyclophotocoagulation: A vision-sparing surgical procedure utilized to reduce IOP.

 MAIN CONCEPTS

Glaucoma is not a disease in and of itself; rather, it is a group of abnormalities that can occur within the eye in which the end result is an increase in IOP. Increased IOP can first lead to blindness and if the IOP remains elevated,

Table 8.26.1 Breeds commonly prone to primary glaucoma

American cocker spaniel	Great Dane
Basset hound	Beagle
Chow chow	Samoyed
Chinese shar-pei	Jack Russell terrier
Boston terrier	English cocker spaniel
Wire fox terrier	Cairn terrier
Norwegian elkhound	Miniature poodle
Siberian husky	

The female gender is overly represented in breeds with primary glaucoma. Age of presentation is typically 4–10 years for onset of increased IOP. If the clinician diagnoses glaucoma in one eye, it is important that both eyes have routine IOP measurements every 4–6 months to monitor for increased pressures. Patients that have primary glaucoma have an increased risk for development of glaucoma in the contralateral eye.

results in ocular pain similar to what humans feel as a migraine headache. Glaucoma can be grouped into primary and secondary glaucoma. Typically, it is thought that IOPs in the dog are considered normal if they are less than 25 mmHg; however, there is no consensus on this "cut-off" point as many ophthalmologists consider IOPs greater than 20 mmHg to be indicative of glaucoma.

Primary glaucoma is typically thought to occur in dogs with a genetic predisposition for anatomical differences which cause an inadequate outflow of aqueous, thereby leading to an increase in IOP (see Table 8.26.1).

Secondary glaucoma is typically thought to be a result of a decrease of aqueous outflow with an increase in IOP in eyes with open angles. Potential causes of secondary glaucoma include a chronically detached retina, uveitis, hyphema, hypopyon, lens luxation (both anterior and posterior), chronic progressive retinal atrophy, posterior synechia, and intraocular neoplasia. Chronically detached retinas, chronic uveitis, intraocular neoplasia, and progressive retinal atrophy result in the formation of a preiridal fibrovascular membrane. This membrane is a fibrovascular network that extends on the anterior surface of the iris and progresses into and over the iridocorneal angle which can obstruct aqueous outflow, resulting in increased IOPs.

8.26.3 Feline Patients

Secondary glaucoma is the most common type of glaucoma in cats. Most feline patients that develop glaucoma do so from chronic uveitis. It is important that the veterinary team identify uveitis, identify the underlying cause, and treat appropriately to prevent glaucoma as well as retinal detachment and loss of vision. Common causes of uveitis in

feline patients include idiopathic/immune-mediated, FeLV, FIV, FIP, fungal (cryptococcosis, blastomycosis, coccidioidomycosis), neoplasia, toxoplasmosis, and potentially bartonellosis. Primary glaucoma does occur in feline patients, but it is far more infrequent than secondary glaucoma.

Feline patients also develop a unique type of glaucoma known as aqueous misdirection syndrome. In this syndrome, aqueous is diverted into the vitreous, causing the lens to shift forward and occlude the iridocorneal angle, causing IOPs to rise. This is typically a low-grade glaucoma that causes chronic damage to the optic nerve and retina over time, leading to vision loss. Typically, IOPs are above 25 mmHg but less than 35 mmHg. The affected eye is more mydriatic than the contralateral eye and this is something that may be noticed by the client. A shallow anterior chamber is also a hallmark feature of this condition and is typically seen by the clinician, but this is not always obvious. These patients can be quite difficult to manage and removal of the lens with or without an artificial lens typically restores IOP to normal values and maintains vision. The veterinary team should advise the client that this condition needs to be addressed quickly as potentially irreversible vision loss is occurring.

Clinical signs of glaucoma can vary depending on acute versus chronic glaucoma. Acute glaucoma cases are typically cases of increased IOP diagnosed within a week after onset. Clinical signs include episcleral injection, corneal edema, dilated pupil or sluggish pupillary light response, decreased or absent menace, pain, optic disc swelling, and peripapillary edema. Chronic glaucoma are cases where increased IOP has persisted for quite some time such as for weeks, months, or longer. Clinical signs include buphthalmos, corneal edema, episcleral injection, cupping of the optic nerve, retinal vascular attenuation, and tapetal hyperreflectivity. Many times, clients will state that pets with chronic glaucoma will not eat as much or as often, will not play as much, will sleep more, and they will attribute this to the patient becoming older. The pain associated with chronic glaucoma is more of a dull pain or equivalent to a migraine but is not a sharp pain such as with a broken bone.

A few types of glaucoma can now be genetically tested for in specific breeds (see 11.3 Heritable Health Conditions – By Disease). Currently, there have been four mutations to the *ADAMTS10* gene that have been responsible for primary open angle glaucoma in the beagle as well as the Norwegian elkhound. Primary open angle glaucoma in the beagle can also be tested for to determine risk level. Two mutations associated with the *ADAMTS17* gene that cause primary open angle glaucoma in the petit basset griffon vendeen and the basset hound have also been determined. Over time, it is inevitable that more genes will be elucidated that can be tested to determine risk level for development of specific variations of glaucoma.

For the veterinary team, it is important to counsel clients as to the risk level that each of these breeds has for glaucoma (see 3.18 Breed-Related Eye Conditions). Genetic testing as well as semi-annual or annual IOP testing is important to monitor for increases in IOP as well as changes in vision. It is also important to discuss the potential for heritable traits if the client has an interest in breeding the patient.

8.26.4 Treatments

Various treatments exist for glaucoma, but the team should understand that there is never a cure for glaucoma. The goal for therapy is to preserve vision and comfort for as long as possible, but understand that eventually IOP will increase, the patient will lose vision, become blind, and a surgical therapy will likely be required to establish a pain-free way of living for the patient.

Prostaglandin analogues are utilized to reduce IOP. These medications are typically utilized in cases of primary glaucoma and the most common medications in this category are latanoprost, travoprost, and bimatoprost.

Parasympathomimetics cause a miosis in the eye which in turn decreases IOP. Pilocarpine is a parasympathomimetic but is rarely used to control glaucoma as there are more favorable medications available. Demecarium bromide is an indirect parasympathomimetic which also causes miosis and decreases IOP.

Carbonic anhydrase inhibitors reduce the enzyme carbonic anhydrase which is involved in aqueous humor formation. Reduction of aqueous humor formation reduces IOP. The most common carbonic anhydrase inhibitors include oral methazolamide, topical dorzolamide, and topical brinzolamide. Carbonic anhydrase inhibitors can be utilized in all types of glaucoma in order to decrease IOP. If oral methazolamide is utilized, side effects such as vomiting, diarrhea, and metabolic acidosis should be monitored. For this reason, oral carbonic anhydrase inhibitors have fallen out of favor compared to topical carbonic anhydrase inhibitors.

Beta blockers are an additional class of ophthalmic glaucoma medications with topical timolol maleate being the most common in veterinary medicine. This medication can be used in all types of glaucoma and is frequently used with dorzolamide. The practitioner should be cautious as this medication is systemically absorbed and can reduce the resting heart rate.

Surgical therapies for glaucoma are utilized to prevent vision loss and maintain controlled IOPs. In vision-sparing surgical procedures, many topical medications such as antiinflammatories as well as glaucoma medications continue to be used to control IOPs. Surgical therapies can be grouped into categories such as vision-sparing procedures versus comfort-restoring procedures.

8.26.5 Vision-Sparing Procedures

Transcleral cyclophotocoagulation is a procedure where laser energy is delivered from the outside of the eye across the sclera to destroy the ciliary body in order to decrease aqueous humor formation and decrease IOP.

Gonioimplants are surgical devices placed to provide an alternate pathway of aqueous humor from the inside the eye to outside the eye, thereby reducing IOP.

Endolaser is a procedure where a small endoscopic unit is placed inside the eye, the ciliary processes are visualized, and laser energy is applied to destroy the ciliary processes, thereby reducing aqueous humor formation and reducing IOP.

8.26.6 Comfort-Restoring Procedures

Prior to performing a comfort-restoring procedure, all medical options should be exhausted if the patient maintains vision. If the patient loses a menace and dazzle response, IOPs remain elevated, and the patient is uncomfortable, a comfort-restoring procedure should be considered.

Enucleation is complete removal of the eye, third eyelid, and conjunctival tissue. The eyelids are sutured closed and the patient will remain comfortable.

An intraocular silicone prosthesis is a procedure where the uvea, lens, and retina are removed and a silicone prosthesis is inserted into the patient's fibrous tunic (sclera and cornea). The patient maintains the globe, the globe moves normally, and eyelids blink normally, and IOP is eliminated, keeping the patient comfortable. This is not a prosthesis that is cleaned or removed intermittently.

Pharmacological destruction of the ciliary body involves injection of intravitreal gentamicin to destroy the retina and the ciliary body and therefore reduce or eliminate aqueous humor formation.

EXAMPLES

Example 1: A 6-year-old female spayed basset hound presents to your office with a primary concern for a blue and red right eye. The technician obtains a history and determines that the patient's right eye developed corneal edema and episcleral injection less than 24 hours ago. The patient seems to be in pain as her resting heart rate is elevated and she resists palpation on the right side of the head. The technician obtains Schirmer tear test values of 24 mm/min in the right eye and 26 mm/min in the left eye which are reported as normal. Fluorescein stain was negative in both eyes, determining that there is no concern for corneal ulceration.

The technician obtains an IOP reading using a digital tonometer after application of proparacaine and finds the IOP to be 57 mmHg. The technician notes that the patient's right eye is mydriatic, has an absent menace response, and a positive dazzle response. There is an absent direct pupillary light response to the right eye, but a positive consensual pupillary light response to the left eye. The left eye has a positive direct pupillary light response and there is a positive consensual pupillary light response to the right eye. The technician relays the findings to the attending veterinarian, who examines the patient and confirms the technician's findings. The veterinarian discusses that this is most likely primary glaucoma and administers topical latanoprost twice daily as well as oral tramadol for pain and discusses the risk for glaucoma in the left eye in the future and provides information to the client for local ophthalmologists for immediate referral to discuss further therapies which could consist of medical management, transscleral laser cyclophotocoagulation, endolaser cyclophotocoagulation, and/or gonioimplant placement. If the client declines referral, the veterinarian plans a recheck examination in two days and gives the patient a guarded prognosis.

Example 2: An 8-year-old neutered male Jack Russell terrier presents to your office with a primary concern for an acutely painful and blepharospastic left eye. The veterinary technician obtains a history and confirms that the patient's left eye is blepharospastic and the clinical sign started yesterday afternoon. Schirmer tear test values are normal at 21 mm/min in the right eye and 28 mm/min in the left eye. Fluorescein stain is performed and shown to be negative, indicating no corneal ulceration. Topical proparacaine is applied to both eyes and IOP is measured with a digital tonometer and reported to be 16 mmHg in the right eye and 45 mmHg in the left eye. Pupillary light response is positive in the right eye and positive consensual from the left to the right eye. The technician reports that the pupillary light response cannot be visualized in the left eye. The patient has mild corneal edema in the left eye and the anterior chamber appears abnormal. These results are reported and confirmed by the veterinarian.

Upon examination, the veterinarian diagnoses an anterior lens luxation of the left eye with secondary glaucoma. The veterinarian strongly recommends emergency referral to the local ophthalmologist to discuss options for an intra-capsular lens extraction to remove the lens and reduce IOPs as well as to closely examine the right eye for signs of lens instability. The veterinarian prescribes topical dorzolamide-timolol three times daily in the left eye as well as oral carprofen and oral tramadol for pain control. If the client declines referral, the veterinarian schedules a recheck in 3–5 days.

Example 3: A 2-year-old spayed female shih tzu presents to your office with a primary concern for a red left eye. The veterinary technician acquires a history and finds out the red eye occurred yesterday and the patient is squinting. Menace response and dazzle response are negative in the left eye and positive in the right eye. Pupillary light response is positive in the right and is not consensual from the left to the right. Pupillary light responses in the left eye cannot be seen due to what the technician believes is a substantial amount of blood in the left eye. Schirmer tear test is normal at 21 mm/min in the right eye and 23 mm/min in the left eye. There is no fluorescein stain uptake in either eye. IOPs are normal in the right eye at 13 mmHg and increased in the left eye at 43 mmHg. These results are relayed to the veterinarian who then confirms these findings.

The veterinarian diagnoses the patient as having a secondary glaucoma and starts the patient on topical dorzolamide-timolol three times daily to reduce the IOP and topical diclofenac three times daily to reduce inflammation. The veterinarian discusses the recommendation for referral to an ophthalmologist for further evaluation and ocular ultrasound. The veterinarian recommends a complete blood count, biochemical profile, blood pressure, potential for coagulation panel and discusses the potential to see a veterinary internist.

TAKE-AWAYS

- Glaucoma is a progressive disease in the veterinary patient. The IOPs will continue to progress beyond the point of control and the patient will eventually lose all vision and become painful.
- Identification of glaucoma by the veterinary team is important in a time-sensitive manner and can only be accurately diagnosed with a tonometer.
- It is important to determine if the glaucoma is primary or secondary and acute versus chronic as this will dictate prognosis for the client, whether further diagnostics are indicated, and appropriate treatment plans.
- If a secondary glaucoma occurs due to uveitis, hyphema, hypopyon, or neoplasia, it will be important to determine the underlying cause in order to better treat glaucoma.

- Various treatments are available to control the IOP and maintain comfort for as long as possible. Eventually, the medications will no longer be effective, and a surgical therapy will be indicated.

MISCELLANEOUS

8.26.7 Cautions

- Exercise caution when prescribing any medication with timolol as this can decrease heart rate in patients.

- Do not use latanoprost, demecarium bromide, or pilocarpine in patients with an anterior lens luxation as this will cause a miosis which will increase IOPs.
- Be aware of systemic side effects when utilizing carbonic anhydrase inhibitors such as vomiting, diarrhea, and metabolic acidosis.

Recommended Reading

Plummer, C.E. and Gelatt, K.N. (2013). *Veterinary Ophthalmology*, 5e, vol. 2, 1050–1145. Ames, IA: Wiley.

Martin, C.L. (2005). *Ophthalmic Disease in Veterinary Medicine*, 337–368. London: Manson Publishing.

8.27

Team Strategies for Diabetes Mellitus

Ryane E. Englar, DVM, DABVP (CANINE AND FELINE PRACTICE)

College of Veterinary Medicine, University of Arizona, Oro Valley, AZ, USA

BASICS

8.27.1 Summary

Diabetes mellitus (DM) is frequently diagnosed in companion animal practice. Although it is a treatable condition, medical management of DM can be complicated. Clients may be reluctant to initiate treatment if treatment options are not tailored to their lifestyle and to the patient. Clients may also become frustrated by the persistence of clinical signs in poorly regulated diabetic patients, which are at risk of developing life-threatening complications, such as diabetic ketoacidosis (DKA).

A team approach to medical management of DM is essential. Clients who feel supported in partnership with the veterinary team are more likely to initiate and continue treatment. Effective therapy requires commitment to care by both the client and the veterinary team. Successful outcomes are contingent upon both parties working together to communicate changes in the patient's status as they arise so that medically sound interventions can be made early.

8.27.2 Terms Defined

DKA: A metabolic complication of uncontrolled or poorly regulated patients with DM, in which rapid breakdown of fat leads to an accumulation of ketones in the bloodstream and urine. Body fluids become dangerously acidic, and the condition is fatal if acid–base and electrolyte imbalances cannot be corrected in a timely fashion.

DM: A medical condition that is characterized by persistent high blood glucose (BG) (sugar) levels, either due to inadequate production of insulin or inadequate sensitivity of cells to the action of insulin.

Glucosuria (Glycosuria): The condition in which blood sugar is excreted from the body in the urine. For this to occur, BG concentration has to exceed the renal tubular threshold, which is of the order of 250–300 mg/dL in cats and 200 mg/dL in dogs.

Hyperglycemia: An elevation in blood sugar that may be transitory, as occurs during times of stress, or chronic, as in cases of DM.

MAIN CONCEPTS

8.27.3 The Classic Picture of Diabetes Mellitus in Clinical Practice

Diabetes mellitus is a common endocrine condition in dogs and cats that results from dysfunctional pancreatic beta cells, reduced tissue sensitivity to insulin, or both. Because insulin is required for cellular uptake of glucose, decreased amounts of this hormone or reduced ability of the tissues to respond to it lead to persistent hyperglycemia.

Blood glucose levels continue to climb as cells are unable to make use of sugar as an energy source. In response to starvation, appetite is triggered. The affected patient initially exhibits polyphagia (PP). However, with no way to make use of ingested glucose as fuel, the body is forced to break down its own stores of fat and protein. This incites weight loss.

As soon as rising BG levels exceed the renal tubular threshold, sugar spills into the urine [1]. By the principles of osmosis, water chases the glucose into the urinary tract.

Large volumes of body fluids are excreted through the kidneys, and the patient is said to exhibit polyuria (PU). In an attempt to minimize dehydration, the patient develops compensatory polydipsia (PD), increased thirst.

8.27.4 What Does an Unmanaged Diabetic Patient Look Like?

Newly diabetic patients, prior to diagnosis, often present with histories of PU and PD, as well as weight loss in spite of PP [1].

If these clinical signs are not recognized by the client and brought to the attention of the veterinary team, then DM will progress. Protracted presentations perpetuate mobilization and breakdown of fat stores into usable fuel through lipolysis and beta-oxidation [1].

Catabolic states may lead to the development of hypercholesterolemia and hypertriglyceridemia, hepatomegaly, and hepatic lipidosis as the liver goes into overdrive to provide emergency fuel [1].

Alternative energy sources are provided by the liver in the form of three ketone bodies: acetone, acetoacetate, and beta-hydroxybutyrate (BHB) [1]. Acetone may be detectable as a distinct aroma on the breath of an unregulated diabetic. Acetoacetate and BHB are anions of relatively strong acids. As their concentrations rise, the blood becomes acidic. If unchecked, the persistence of ketonemia and ketonuria may result in an emergency state of DKA [1].

8.27.5 Risk Factors for Diabetes Mellitus

A common mistake made by the veterinary team in clinical practice is to not address DM until it happens. In truth, we need to begin the conversation about DM long before the diagnosis. This is particularly true when our patients possess one or more risk factors that we know will increase the chances of developing DM in the future.

Obesity is a well-established risk factor for the development of DM [1]. Certain breeds of companion animals also appear to be predisposed: Burmese cats of Australian or European descent, as well as Australian terriers, beagles, keeshonds, and Samoyeds [2, 3].

An appropriate time to initiate a conversation about risk factors for DM is when patients present as kittens and puppies for wellness visits. Wellness visits are an excellent opportunity for client education concerning content areas that are essential to pet health. Consider, for instance, the mastiff puppy that presents for its first visit to the veterinary clinic. We would be wise to mention breed-appropriate nutrition, specifically the need for slow and steady growth, so as to lessen the chance for development of orthopedic disease.

New puppy and kitten visits are the optimal time to emphasize the importance of maintaining an appropriate body condition score (BCS), which will reduce the patient's risk for developing DM (see 6.15 Approaching Obesity on a Pet-Specific Basis).

Likewise, if a patient belongs to an at-risk breed, then it is our responsibility to highlight breed as an additional reason why nutrition is going to be a critical aspect of that patient's lifestyle (see 11.3 Heritable Health Conditions – By Disease).

Our goal is not to frighten clients or to suggest that their new pet is defective. Each and every breed has positive and negative attributes. Our task is to highlight those attributes that we have the power to alter now with the intent of lessening risk for disease later.

Breed and BCS are not the only risk factors for the development of DM. Certain physiological states, such as pregnancy, also increase the chance that a patient will become diabetic [1]. This does not mean that we advocate against breeding, as pregnancy is a natural state.

What we do need to do is to partner with breeders to recognize that insulin resistance is more likely to occur during pregnancy. We need to emphasize the importance of maintaining bitches and queens at the appropriate BCS before they conceive and throughout pregnancy. Doing so will not eliminate the risk of DM but it will lessen the impact that insulin resistance has on the patient throughout this physiological state.

As our patients age, they may develop one or more medical conditions that induce varying degrees of insulin resistance and, as such, are risk factors for the development of DM [1, 4, 5]:

- acromegaly
- dental disease
- hyperadrenocorticism (HAC)
- hyperthyroidism (cats)
- pancreatitis
- renal insufficiency (cats).

Although our primary goal for patient health is to manage these conditions, we need to keep in mind that one or more disease processes may be linked. Patient screening for DM should be considered an essential part of medical management. Clients who are educated about the risk for DM are more likely to identify changes in patient health sooner. Being proactive helps us to diagnose and intervene early.

An open door to dialogue is an essential component of wellness that cannot be overstated. Just as the practice of human medicine has evolved to recognize predisease states, the veterinary profession is equally responsible for identifying and managing risk factors before disease develops.

Finally, the use of certain medications may incite DM. Consider, for instance, long-term corticosteroids, cyclosporine, or progestins [1]. It is our responsibility when prescribing these medications to balance the benefits against the risks and alert clients to the potential for adverse effects.

8.27.6 Client Considerations: Making the Diagnosis

As DM becomes more prevalent among human patients, the familiarity of veterinary clients with DM has grown. Many clients know someone – human or nonhuman – with DM and are more comfortable with the concept that the condition is medically manageable, even among veterinary patients.

However, not all clients are equally knowledgeable about DM. Not all clients may feel that it is within their comfort zone to initiate and maintain treatment. Many clients are looking for support and encouragement from the veterinary team. A diagnosis of DM may be uncharted territory for these clients. In other words, when a client presents a dog or cat for evaluation of PU and PD, a diagnosis of DM may seem like a life sentence if the client was expecting an easy fix.

For some clients, the prospect of managing a chronic condition may be overwhelming.

The diagnosis may be complicated by financial and/or time constraints: for instance, how does someone with a 16-hour workday fit in bi-daily injections of insulin? Or, how does someone who travels frequently out-of-state alter homecare plans to factor DM into the equation? How can we help these clients to work around their schedule to make DM management feasible? What resources are available in the immediate vicinity that we can direct them to?

8.27.7 Client Considerations: Avoid Assumptions

It is important not to make assumptions about your client when making the diagnosis of DM. Start the conversation about diagnosis by assessing the client's knowledge base. Consider asking the client:

- "What do you know about DM?"
- "What have you heard about DM in dogs (or cats)?"

Allow the client sufficient opportunity to answer your question, and set aside judgment.

Maybe what the client knows about DM is wrong. That's okay, it's not about who's right and who's wrong. It's about discovering a starting point so that you can build onto the preexisting foundation of knowledge with follow-up conversation.

Note that every client's foundation will be different. The client who has owned five diabetic cats in his lifetime is likely to know more about diagnosis and treatment than the client who has never owned a cat before, let alone a diabetic one. The client who himself is diabetic is likely to contribute far more to the conversation than someone who has never had to administer injections of any sort.

All clients are contributors; it's our responsibility to find out how they can contribute and what we can do to assist them in their efforts. Use what the client shares with you as background knowledge to amend, clarify, and/or build onto the conversation surrounding the diagnosis. The client needs to know what the impact of DM will be on the patient as well as on him/herself. Check in with the client frequently to assess for mutual understanding.

Support staff are invaluable members of the veterinary team because they can invest in time-intensive parts of the diagnostic conversation.

8.27.8 Client Considerations: Addressing Management Options

Conversations about the therapeutic approach to DM should also begin with a baseline assessment of what the client knows about the condition.

You may begin with a closed-ended question: "Do you know how we treat DM in dogs (or cats)?" Alternatively, you may open up the question to encourage the client to share details: "Tell me what you know about treatment options for DM in dogs (or cats)." This can be softened by tacking on the word *please*, or the phrase *can you please tell me*, at the beginning of this statement.

This line of questioning helps you understand how informed the client is about the condition and what an appropriate starting point is. For instance, the client who has successfully managed a diabetic dog in the past with twice-daily insulin injections does not benefit from the spiel about how insulin is administered via injectable therapy. The client already knows this and desires new information to add to his knowledge base.

For the client who is truly a novice, it is appropriate to ask for permission to discuss treatment options: "May I share with you what our typical approach is for dogs (or cats) with DM?" Remember to trim out medical jargon so that the conversation occurs at an appropriate level for the right audience.

Eliciting the client's perspective about the disease process and treatment options is a critical part of medical management.

- "How do you feel about managing Darcy's diabetes?"
- "Do the treatment options that I've outlined sound reasonable?"
- "How do you feel about changing Darcy's diet?"
- "How do you feel about administering insulin to Darcy?"
- "What is most concerning to you about Darcy's diabetes?"
- "What is your greatest concern moving forward with treatment?"
- "What more do you need from us by way of support to help you through this?"

These questions may seem soft and fluffy but they are necessary. They invite the client to share what is on his or her mind, including obstacles that may hinder compliance and adherence.

The responsibility falls upon us, the veterinary team, to acknowledge, address, and navigate concerns so that we set the client and patient up for success.

8.27.9 Getting on the Same Page Concerning Management

The typical protocol for treatment of DM involves insulin therapy and dietary management. Both arms of therapy target the patient's circulating BG concentration, with the hope of keeping this below the renal threshold for as long as possible. Reduced degrees and periods of hyperglycemia lessen glucosuria, which in turn will improve clinical signs of PU and PD.

Monitoring the diabetic patient is an essential part of medical management so that clinical signs are controlled without hypoglycemic episodes.

If the client is to be able to follow the practice's recommendations for management, then all members of the veterinary team need to be on the same page. It does not help compliance or adherence for the client to hear contradictory points of view from different team members. To achieve standardization, practices should consider adopting the most current consensus statements, such as the most recent AAHA Diabetes Management Guidelines for Dogs and Cats. This does not require all veterinarians to prescribe the same treatment for all diabetic patients. The most effective management plans are tailored to the individual rather than being cookie cutter in approach.

Based upon these guidelines, the following generalizations can be made about care for diabetic patients.

8.27.9.1 Diet

1) Dietary modification should center on the need to attain and maintain optimal body weight. Obese cats can safely achieve 0.5–2% weight loss per week, compared to 1–2% in dogs [1].
2) Simple carbohydrates should be limited to reduce postprandial (posteating) hyperglycemia.
3) High-protein diets are recommended for diabetic cats.
4) Canned diets are preferred over feeding dry diets to diabetic cats because they offer increased water content while reducing caloric density.
5) High-fiber diets are acceptable for diabetic dogs that are in need of weight maintenance or weight loss.

8.27.9.2 Blood Glucose

1) Insulin products are the mainstay of treatment. At the time of writing, two products were currently approved by the Federal Drug Administration (FDA) for use in dogs and cats: porcine insulin zinc suspension (Vetsulin®) and protamine zinc insulin (PZI). Off-label, acceptable options include glargine (Lantus®) in cats and Neutral Protamine Hagedorn (NPH; Humulin N®, Novulin N®) in dogs.
2) Non-insulin therapeutic agents, such as glipizide, may be attempted in cats whose owners decline insulin therapy. Other products, such as alpha-glucosidase inhibitors (acarbose) and incretins (glucagon-like peptide 1, GLP-1) may be used in combination with insulin to improve glycemic control.
3) The goal is *not* to normalize BG. BG will fluctuate.
4) The goal *is* to reduce the degree of hyperglycemia. Reducing hyperglycemia such that BG is lower than the renal tubular threshold, 250–300 mg/dL in cats and 200 mg/dL in dogs, will lessen glucosuria [1]. Reducing glucosuria will reduce clinical signs of PU and PD.
5) Monitoring BG is challenging and may consist of in-hospital BG curves (BGCs), at-home BGCs, hematological measurement of glycosylated proteins (fructosamine), and/or urine glucose measurements. It is critical for team members and clients to have buy-in when it comes to the recommended test of choice. At the same time, monitoring needs to be tailored to the patient and client. For instance, a client who cannot bear the sight of blood is unlikely to be successful with at-home BG monitoring. Likewise, in-hospital BGCs are of low diagnostic value in the perpetually fractious cat with stress hyperglycemia.

8.27.10   Client Education

Diabetes mellitus is a complicated metabolic condition. Client education is an essential contributing factor to case outcomes. If we do not provide the client with the tools that they need then how can we expect them to succeed?

Even team members and clients with prior experiences with DM are likely to get confused if instructions are not clear. Even when communication is clear, patients only recall about 50% of the content of a clinical encounter [6]. What can we do to assist with retention?

- We can speak slowly and insert pauses between thoughts. Rapid-fire conversations do not allow the client sufficient time to process.
- We can limit our discussions by lumping related topics into bite-sized chunks, taking care to check in with clients after the delivery of detail-rich content. Three key points is about all that we can expect clients to remember.
- We can stage discussions: share what the client needs to know now and hold off on covering the next topic until it is necessary or relevant to the client.

We also need to make specific recommendations. For example, recommendations for insulin storage and handling need to be appropriate for the prescribed insulin type.

Concerning storage, it is insufficient to tell the client that insulin cannot be exposed to heat. What does that actually mean? Clients are unlikely to ask, and if we don't share, then we risk the likelihood that storage of the insulin will be incorrect. We need to be specific with our instructions: "Do not leave inside a parked car."

Likewise, it is important to emphasize the need to refrigerate but not freeze insulin.

Concerning handling, we cannot assume that our clients read the package inserts. Instead, share the critical details. For example:

- "You need to shake Vetsulin until the suspension looks milky before you inject it."
- "You should not shake vials of PZI. You need to roll them instead."

Take this a step further and demonstrate the action to the client. Better yet, have the client demonstrate the action to you. This may seem silly but practice may save the client the cost of an insulin vial that was improperly stored or handled.

Other important client education topics for DM include:

- dose and frequency of insulin administration
- types of syringes that are compatible with the prescribed insulin

- when to administer insulin, relative to eating
- what to do about insulin administration when patients refuse to eat
- clinical signs that are suggestive of hypoglycemia
- what to do if the patient becomes hypoglycemic
- who to contact to troubleshoot after-hours emergencies.

8.27.11   What is a Realistic Goal of Treatment?

Clients of diabetic pets need to understand what the treatment aims are. This establishes reasonable expectations for care.

Remission in diabetic cats is attainable [1, 7]. Remission in cats is most likely if glycemic control is established within the first six months of diagnosis [1]. Additional factors that positively contribute to remission include a low-carbohydrate diet in combination with Lantus or detemir (Levemir®) insulin therapy [1, 7].

By contrast, the majority of diabetic dogs require exogenous insulin therapy for life. It is rare that a dog will go into remission [1]. Treatment of DM in dogs is therefore focused on controlling clinical signs rather than eliminating them.

 TAKE-AWAYS

- DM is a metabolic condition that is easily diagnosed, and can be effectively managed with a combination of insulin therapy and dietary modifications that promote a lean body weight and reduce postprandial hyperglycemia.
- Complications from DM arise when patients are poorly regulated.
- Poor regulation may result from patient incompatibility with a given product, insulin resistance, and/or lack of client compliance and adherence.
- Assessing the client's knowledge, eliciting their perspective, asking for permission to share, checking in, and educating the client are essential communication skills that facilitate clinical conversations about the diagnosis and medical management of DM.
- Team members need to work with clients to set realistic goals for monitoring and treatment. To be successful, these goals must also factor into consideration client and patient lifestyle, time and financial constraints.

MISCELLANEOUS

8.27.12 Cautions

A team approach to medical management can make the difference between the client electing to proceed with treatment for DM or electing to euthanize the patient.

Barring financial obstacles, a client who feels supported by the veterinary team is more likely to initiate and attempt treatment because they have been provided with the tools that they need to succeed.

When the veterinary team and the client are not on the same page, meaning that they are not communicating effectively, then case outcomes are likely to be compromised. Poor case outcomes, such as uncontrolled diabetic patients, represent failures not only of medical management, but also of the system itself, the team, to respond to unmet needs through problem solving.

References

1 Behrend, E., Holford, A., Lathan, P. et al. (2018). 2018 AAHA diabetes management guidelines for dogs and cats. *J. Am. Anim. Hosp. Assoc.* 54: 1–21.

2 Hess, R.S., Kass, P.H., and Ward, C.R. (2000). Breed distribution of dogs with diabetes mellitus admitted to a tertiary care facility. *J. Am. Vet. Med. Assoc.* 216: 1414–1417.

3 Rand, J.S., Bobbermien, L.M., Hendrikz, J.K. et al. (1997). Over representation of Burmese cats with diabetes mellitus. *Aust. Vet. J.* 75: 402–405.

4 Nelson, R.W. (2000). Selected topics in the management of diabetes mellitus in cats. *J. Feline Med. Surg.* 2: 101–104.

5 Davison, L.J. (2015). Diabetes mellitus and pancreatitis – cause or effect? *J. Small Anim. Pract.* 56: 50–59.

6 Hersh, L., Salzman, B., and Snyderman, D. (2015). Health literacy in primary care practice. *Am. Fam. Physician* 92: 118–124.

7 Bloom, C.A. and Rand, J. (2014). Feline diabetes mellitus: clinical use of long-acting glargine and detemir. *J. Feline Med. Surg.* 16: 205–215.

Recommended Reading

Behrend, E., Holford, A., Lathan, P. et al. (2018). 2018 AAHA diabetes management guidelines for dogs and cats. *J. Am. Anim. Hosp. Assoc.* 54: 1–21.

8.28

Team Strategies for Cancer

Samuel Stewart, DVM, DACVECC and Chand Khanna, DVM, PhD, DACVIM (Onc), DACVP (Hon)

Ethos Veterinary Health, Woburn, MA, USA

BASICS

8.28.1 Summary

Patients with cancer may have numerous co-morbidities, requiring doctors across multiple disciplines to be involved in their care. When effective, this team provides continuous care aligned with specific goals articulated by the owner. When improperly delivered, this team can be misaligned, resulting in poor continuity of care and fragmented attentiveness to the owner's needs. It can also affect the owner's compliance with the multitudes of recommendations. A solution to this issue is the implementation of a multidisciplinary team (MDT) composed of the hospital teams involved in the patient's care and a team leader. Regular meetings of the MDT allow for collective discussion of the patient's case, assuring that all members are aware of the patient's treatment plan and that all the patient's needs are being met.

8.28.2 Terms Defined

Communicative Medicine: Involvement of the owner in the discussions surrounding patient care and the development of a treatment plan to assure that the owner's needs and preferences are being met appropriately.

Co-Morbidity: Additional condition(s) co-occurring with the primary condition being evaluated and/or treated

Multidisciplinary Team: A team that consists of clinicians from multiple specialties that are involved with a given patient's care.

MAIN CONCEPTS

8.28.3 The Problem

Cancer is an aggressive and systemic disease process that may directly and indirectly affect several organ systems. Furthermore, it is a condition that most commonly occurs in older patients who may suffer from unrelated co-morbidities. As a result, these patients may present to the hospital for a multitude of reasons, such as a routine recheck appointment with their general practitioner (GP), a consultation with a surgeon to discuss the removal of a tumor, or an emergency room visit due to a complication from their chemotherapy treatment.

The above scenario results in patients with cancer requiring care from numerous clinicians and paraprofessionals in different specialties throughout the course of their diagnosis and treatment. The resulting patchwork of medical attention has the potential to result in poor continuity of care, with the owner getting differing opinions and recommendations from each staff member (see 9.9 Continuity of Care). This approach to cancer care can be stressful and confusing to both the pet and the owner. When owners feel confused about their options, they are more likely to delay or defer care, potentially leading to increased complication rates and poorer long-term outcomes for their pet. It is often the job of the patient's primary care team to help the owner navigate this often overwhelming process to assure the best outcome for the patient.

8.28.4   The Solution

A solution to the standard process of patient care is the implementation of a MDT. An MDT is a group of clinicians and paraprofessionals that include the primary care team as well as specialists across multiple disciplines that collectively coordinate their care of a cancer patient. A successful MDT approach includes regular meetings to evaluate the patient's diagnosis, treatment plan, and progress. These meetings create a unified mode of communication regarding a patient and can have a direct impact on quality of care and quality of life. In human medicine, the implementation of an MDT approach is well accepted among clinical teams, leading to improved outcomes and consistent standard of patient care.

Similarly, within the primary care team, it is important that clinicians, paraprofessionals, and customer service representatives form their own team in order to be able to take the information provided by the MDT and create appropriate consensus and messaging so that a consistent story can be communicated to clients.

Without an MDT, a single individual must summate the opinions of numerous clinicians and collate them into a singular report that has the potential to miss key recommendations and can misconstrue information to the owner. In contrast, the unified knowledge of an MDT results in more accurate opinions and recommendations being made to a patient. Additionally, the collective meeting of doctors and paraprofessionals acts as a platform for objective second opinions regarding the varied portions of a patient's care, allowing for better approaches to treatment and, ultimately, improved patient outcomes. Evidence of improved outcomes from the use of MDTs has been demonstrated in clinical trials comparing their use to the same treatments being offered outside a trial.

The implementation of an MDT has been shown to result in shorter times from diagnosis to treatment, higher rates of treatment, and improved patient adherence to clinical recommendations. As a result, long-term survival rates have been shown to increase.

8.28.5   Building an MDT

An effective MDT requires a selected individual to assume a leadership role. It will be this individual's responsibility to assure that the goals of the MDT are being met. These goals include regularly scheduled meetings, equal participation of all clinicians and paraprofessionals on the team, and maintenance of a collective team approach to patient care. The leader also has the important role of monitoring that the MDT approach is having a beneficial impact on the patient. Furthermore, this individual must act as a unifying voice when there are disagreements among team members. The GP is often a good option to be this leader, given their historical experiences with the patient and often strong relationships with the owner. The GP, in essence, acts as facilitator of a patient's care and corrects any problems that may arise.

Multidisciplinary team meetings should have a predefined structure that is meticulously followed. Figure 8.28.1 shows a basic flowchart of how MDT meetings should be conducted. Strictly following this format insures that all details of a patient's condition(s) are reviewed and assessed prior to a treatment and follow-up plan being determined. The clinician with the most knowledge about the patient should lead the review of the case during meetings. Even though there will be a designated clinician leading the conversation, it is expected that all members of the team will be actively engaged in the conversation. Following a predetermined meeting format will ensure that all clinicians involved have an in-depth understanding of the patient's treatment plan which will, therefore, reduce the potential that the owner receives differing opinions and recommendations from members of the team.

An important focus for the development of a treatment plan is communication with the owner, with special focus on allowing them to have their opinions and concerns heard by the group. The best plan for patient care requires affirmative responses from the owner on the following questions.

- Does the plan deliver a desired goal?
- Does the plan deliver acceptable risks for the owner?
- Are the costs of care feasible?

If the answer to any of these three questions is no, then a new plan should be developed and offered. This approach of involving the owner in the development of a treatment plan is referred to as communicative medicine. Veterinary medicine often focuses less on the question of "what is the matter and how to treat it," and more on "what matters and how the treatment plan will meet the owner's goals." This approach is different from the more algorithmic medicine practiced by most human clinicians.

It is important that MDT meetings occur on a previously defined regular schedule (i.e., monthly). This not only allows for better tracking of patient outcomes, but also creates the opportunity to make adjustments to the treatment plan. This regularity also makes it easier for the members to maintain their commitment to the MDT as they can allot time in their clinical schedule for the meeting(s). The advance notice of a

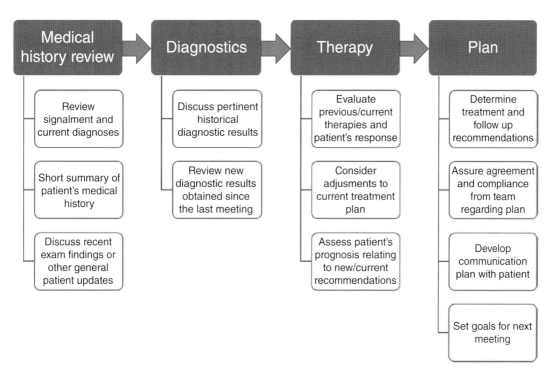

Figure 8.28.1 MDT meeting structure.

meeting provides the time needed to gather any diagnostic results or recent literature that could be important to review at the meeting. Additionally, each meeting allows the opportunity to review the decisions made at the previous meeting and evaluate their effectiveness, as well as to ensure that they were appropriately implemented.

Time constraints among clinicians is a common problem with the implementation of an MDT. To be effective, meetings should be collectively integrated into clinical schedules of every member, with an understanding of the importance of attendance. A predefined meeting agenda should be assembled and distributed to each member prior to the meeting. This will inform each member of the goals for that meeting and keeps the meeting focused and on schedule. An adequate amount of time should be allotted for each patient to be discussed during the meeting, allowing for at least 15–30 minutes of discussion per patient.

If an MDT is composed of clinicians and paraprofessionals located at different hospitals, then it is important to have a designated conference line that can be used to unify the team. Conference lines that include video capability are preferable, as this allows for easier sharing and review of documents that pertain to the discussion. These conference lines eliminate the need for clinicians to travel to other hospitals, which increases participation. Conference meetings can be scheduled on a recurring basis with preset reminders, eliminating the need for a single individual to coordinate the scheduling of each meeting. Furthermore, inviting owners to the meeting and involving them in the process will convey the value of the MDT to them.

8.28.6 Additional Benefits

In addition to the benefits to the patient, MDT meetings can also act as a valuable learning opportunity for veterinary students, interns, residents, and clinicians who are less experienced with certain disease processes. Detailed discussions of clinical patients in real-world scenarios is more engaging than traditional means of learning. MDT meetings result in a collective exchange of opinions from multiple clinicians, giving a broader view of the patient's condition than would be obtained solely from a textbook or a review given by a single clinician. Furthermore, the structure of MDT meetings does not have to be focused only on the discussion of patient care, but can also include a didactic component. This could involve a short 10–15-minute pre-prepared presentation that one of the team members can give regarding a given aspect of that patient's disease process or care.

If a patient is seen by clinicians or specialists located at different hospitals, then the opportunity to include these clinicians in the meetings will result in a closer relationship between the hospitals. This not only allows for improved patient care, but also makes it easier for patients to locate and be seen by specialists. This benefit extends beyond those patients being discussed in the MDT meetings and applies to all patients that may have circumstances where they need to be transferred between facilities.

Multidisciplinary team meetings also open the opportunity for the pursuit of research studies investigating new diagnostics and therapies. For cancer patients, this can include improved modes of monitoring for metastasis/recurrence or new formulations of chemotherapy drugs. The GP is key in the identification of eligible patients for these types of studies. MDT meetings act as a regular means to assure that the study guidelines are being appropriately followed and to closely monitor for adverse events that arise as a result of study participation. If there are clinicians from multiple hospitals involved in the meetings, then this also opens the opportunity for multicenter studies to be conducted, increasing the value of the results obtained.

8.28.7 Barriers to an MDT

Even with the known benefit of MDTs, there are still barriers to their efficacy. Poor relationships between clinicians may lead to disagreement about treatment plans or to disengagement of team members. The value of having all clinicians equally engaged in these meetings cannot be overstated, and it is imperative that a good working relationship is maintained between all members of the team. It is the team leader's duty to monitor the relationships and interactions of the members and to make sure that the team remains focused on its goals of comprehensive patient care.

There can also be barriers related to the general awareness and sharing of the MDT's existence. In order for an MDT to be successful, owners, GPs, and referral hospital staff must understand the reason for and value of a team approach to patient care. Promotion of the MDT should take these factors into consideration when offering its services to clients and the referring community. Rather than offering the MDT approach to all clients, it is recommended that specific criteria be used to select cases and clients who will be responsive to and benefit most from this type of collaborative care. Even though there are known benefits with the use of an MDT, it also needs to be understood that some clients may feel overwhelmed or frightened by a team approach to care.

Another barrier can occur in hospitals that don't possess the facilities to offer a patient all the necessary disciplines to provide their care, and that patient then needs to be referred to a different hospital that isn't a member of the MDT. Invitations should be extended to these clinicians to participate in the meetings. Having clear goals, a set schedule, and means for these clinicians to join the meetings remotely will increase the potential for them to get involved. If these outside clinicians are not interested in participating in the MDT, then their medical records associated with the patient should be obtained ahead of time to be reviewed and interpreted by the group at the next meeting. Any collective opinions and recommendations made by the MDT should then be put in a formal report and sent to the clinician so they are aware of the plans that the MDT will be discussing with the owner.

A final barrier would be the need to expediently convene an MDT for patients/clients that need to make immediate treatment decisions. This scenario would be more feasible for a patient that already has a preexisting MDT compared to a patient who hasn't had a team put together yet.

8.28.8 The Future

Even with the documented benefits of employing MDTs in patient care, there is still a lack of implementation at hospitals around the world, both human and veterinary. For many clinicians, there has been a limited amount of experience or exposure to MDTs, and they might not be fully aware of their benefit. Furthermore, the benefits of these regular meetings might not be seen clinically in the patient for a period of time, which will cause some clinicians to question the efficacy of the MDT.

A possible solution to the poor implementation of MDTs could be through the growing field of electronic medicine (e-medicine). E-medicine involves the use of electronic medical records that are contained within the cloud and can be easily accessed and shared. E-medicine allows clinicians to meet among themselves or with the owner over a digital platform regardless of the physical location of each party. Additionally, there is the growing market of at-home diagnostic and treatment modalities that link to the cloud, allowing patient data to be transmitted seamlessly to the MDT for review. Certain technologies allow for two-way communication that allows a clinical team member to adjust treatments from a distance. An example of this is the ability for some metered dose inhalers to have their delivered dose adjusted electronically from a clinician's office. App-based medicine is also becoming increasingly valuable as it is easy to use and accessible to patients and clinicians on their mobile devices.

The principles and importance of an MDT approach to patient care are essential to impart to those entering the veterinary profession. As the utilization of MDTs becomes more commonplace, the benefits of this will not only affect patients afflicted with cancer, but with any number of acute and chronic illnesses.

EXAMPLES

Copper, a 10-year-old golden retriever, presents to the emergency service at ABC Veterinary Hospital following an episode of collapse and labored breathing. He is found to have a bleeding tumor on his spleen and is referred to an emergency hospital where he is stabilized by the emergency room clinician with a blood transfusion and IV fluids. Once the patient's cardiovascular status is improved, he is transferred to a surgeon for a splenectomy. The histopathology of the spleen is consistent with an aggressive form of cancer called hemangiosarcoma. Copper is referred to an oncologist to discuss and start a chemotherapy protocol to slow the progression of his cancer. Samples of the tumor and blood samples are submitted for genomic analysis, a process known as precision/personalized medicine (PMed), which will aid in the development of a patient- and tumor-specific treatment plan (see 2.20 Cancer Precision Medicine).

While undergoing chemotherapy, Copper is evaluated by a radiologist for regularly scheduled abdominal ultrasounds to monitor for evidence of cancer progression. He is also seen regularly by his GP for routine evaluations to make sure that he is tolerating his treatment plan. In addition to his cancer diagnosis, Copper has a previous history of autoimmune disease and has been treated with multiple immunosuppressive medications over the last two years. While undergoing treatment of his cancer he continues to have regular appointments with an internal medicine specialist to monitor his autoimmune condition.

With the combination of the immunosuppressive medications and the chemotherapy, Copper's immune system becomes overly suppressed and he develops sepsis. This requires admission to the intensive care unit where he is cared for by a critical care specialist. An MDT of all of these specialists is formed to collectively develop the best treatment and follow-up plan for Copper. The MDT makes it easier to monitor his progression, assure that his owner is following the treatment recommendations that were made, and to monitor for further side effects and complications of his treatment.

TAKE-AWAYS

- Cancer patients are often afflicted with concurrent conditions that require clinicians across multiple disciplines to treat.
- An MDT composed of these clinicians allows for a group assessment of the patient's condition and a collective

process of determining recommendations to be made to the owner.

- Implementation of these teams has been shown to decrease the time from diagnosis to treatment, increase owner compliance, and improve patient outcomes.
- There can be many barriers to the formation of a successful MDT but having a group leader to identify and correct these barriers will improve success.
- The utilization of MDTs in hospitals is still low; however, there is an opportunity to better educate teams about the benefits of MDTs, thereby increasing the potential that they will employ them in pet-specific care initiatives.

MISCELLANEOUS

8.28.9   Cautions

The implementation of an MDT can prove highly valuable for the patient, owner, and clinical staff. At the same time, this approach could be unsuccessful or, worse, detrimental if there is not a commitment from all the members on the team. The decision to undertake the development of an MDT should be thoroughly discussed and planned by all who intend to be involved before its official creation. This will assure that the goals of the team will be met, and the intended benefits will be passed on to the patient.

Recommended Reading

Abdulrahman, G.O. Jr. (2001). The effect of multidisciplinary team care on cancer management. *Pan Afr. Med. J.* 9: 20.

Cancer Council SA. A multidisciplinary team approach to cancer care. www.cancersa.org.au

Haward, R.A. (2006). The Calman-Hine report: a personal retrospective on the UK's first comprehensive policy on cancer services. *Lancet Oncol.* 7 (4): 336–346.

Pillay, B., Wootten, A.C., Crowe, H. et al. (2016). The impact of multidisciplinary team meetings on patient assessment, management and outcomes in oncology settings: a systematic review of the literature. *Cancer Treat. Rev.* 42: 56–72.

Taylor, C., Munro, A.J., Glynne-Jones, R. et al. (2010). Multidisciplinary team working in cancer: what is the evidence? *BMJ* 340: c951.

Section 9

Medical Management Considerations

9.1

Medical Records

Cindy Trice, DVM

Relief Rover, Bradenton, FL, USA

 BASICS

9.1.1 Summary

Medical records are the most important documents in veterinary practice. These legal documents serve many functions including being a record of a patient's medical care and client communications, a guide for medical decisions, and a historical reference. They also transfer information between the team and can provide protection from accusations of legal or ethical violations. The format varies greatly but categories of information recorded should be consistent across practices. When writing these documents, one should keep in mind readers who will be unfamiliar with the patient. A new staff member, locum veterinarian, or referred veterinarian should be able to read medical records and clearly understand the history, physical exam findings, diagnostics, diagnoses, medications, treatments, prognosis, and client communications without having to "read between the lines" or interpret uncommon abbreviations. A common saying in veterinary medicine is that if it isn't written down in the medical record, it didn't happen!

9.1.2 Terms Defined

Definitive Diagnosis: Determination of the nature or cause of a disease.

Differential Diagnosis: Conditions with common features that are being considered as potential diagnoses. Also known as "rule-outs."

Medical Record: A chronological written account of a patient's examination and treatment that includes the patient's medical history and complaints, the veterinarian's physical findings, the results of diagnostic tests and procedures, definitive or differential diagnoses, medications and therapeutic procedures, prognoses, and follow-up plans.

Prognosis: A forecast of the probable course and outcome of a disease, especially of the chances of recovery.

Signalment: That part of the veterinary medical history dealing with the animal's age, sex, and breed.

SOAP: A common organizational technique for recording medical records. S = Subjective, O = Objective, A = Assessment, and P = Plan.

Zoonotic Disease: An animal disease that can be transmitted to humans.

9.1.3 What to Include in the Medical Record

Veterinary boards in different jurisdictions have rules and regulations regarding specific items that are required in veterinary medical records. For a complete list, contact your veterinary regulatory agency.

The most basic information that needs to be included are the pet's and client's names, signalment (age, breed, gender), and presenting complaint. Try to be as accurate as possible regarding breed. If the pet is purebred, or if you know the parentage of a mixed-breed pet, record this information. Since this is a medico-legal document, if it is a mixed-breed pet of uncertain parentage, resist the temptation to guess (e.g., collie cross) since this can confound attempts to recognize risk and predisposition to disease (see 3.19 Mixed-Breed Considerations). Instead, if parentage cannot be reliably determined, record the breed as "mixed" or other such designation.

Signalment should be followed by a thorough history. Histories should include the duration of the problem(s), list and characterization of clinical signs, medications or supplements the patient is currently taking or has recently taken (names, dosages, and frequency of administration), current diet (including any snacks, table scraps, or dietary indiscretions), amount and frequency of feedings, travel history, exposure to other pets, vaccine status, and previous medical conditions.

The physical examination should include measurable data such as body weight, temperature, heart rate, respiratory rate, and in some cases, blood pressure. Next, each organ system should be systematically examined and observations recorded, including normal results.

Following the physical exam, an assessment should be recorded in the form of a problem list along with the differential diagnoses of each problem. In addition to this, or alternatively, it may be appropriate to document a definitive diagnosis.

Based on the above information, a diagnostic and treatment plan is recorded. This should encompass all diagnostic tests, including their results and interpretation. When documenting specific treatments, include detailed descriptions of procedures, exact medications, dosages, and the time and route of administration. Make sure that all controlled substances and amounts used are recorded and match the practice logs. Nursing care plans are also an important part of complete medical records (see 8.7 Nursing Care Plans).

Follow-up and alternative treatment plans are helpful for following a medical case. Record when you expect the patient back for a recheck, or the circumstances in which they should return to the hospital or seek emergency care. Noting alternative treatment plans or further diagnostics can be helpful to jog one's memory or to help others who may pick up the case. Be sure to record all client communications in the medical record. The date, time, form of communication (in person, phone, email, text, social media, or letter) and a summary of the conversation should be noted. Note any diagnostics or treatments that were offered but declined by the client (see 8.17 Dealing with Compromise Fatigue). This can save confusion and potentially ethical or legal problems in the future. Informed consent for surgeries, dentistry, or other anesthetic or sedated procedures must be recorded (see 7.4 Getting Informed Consent). Many practices have clients sign forms and attach these to the medical record to indicate the owner's understanding of the risks. Clients should be informed of zoonotic disease risk if applicable and this should be recorded as well.

The person documenting should sign their name or initial at the end of each of their medical record entries.

9.1.4 What Not to Include in the Medical Record

It is unprofessional and ill advised to include editorial comments on clients. Notations such as "difficult client" or "never pays his bill" should never be written in an official medical record.

9.1.5 Confidentiality of Veterinary Medical Records

Be sure to understand your local jurisdiction's regulations regarding the confidentiality of medical records. In some places, the medical records can only be released to clients or other attending veterinarians unless there is written permission (see 7.6 Privacy and Confidentiality).

9.1.6 Format of Veterinary Medical Records

There are many ways to format a medical record and many practice management software systems will break the entries into specific sections to guide the user. A popular technique is the SOAP system.

The **S** stands for *subjective*. This is where we record the history and all the information that drove the client to bring their pet to the veterinarian. A thorough history will include the presenting complaint, the client's observations, current medications including supplements, diet, travel history, and previous relevant medical history.

The **O** stands for *objective*. The findings recorded in this section are objective and recorded without any assessment. Signalment, vital signs, physical exam findings, and the results of diagnostic tests. It is common practice to combine subjective and objective information in an S/O section.

The **A** stands for *assessment*. This is where you will make your assessment of the subjective and objective findings. The problem list and differential diagnoses are recorded here.

The **P** stands for *plan*. This is where all the information from the S/O/A sections is compiled and assimilated into a strategy with action items. The diagnostics and treatment plans and prognosis go here.

EXAMPLES

9.1.7 Example of SOAP Formatted Veterinary Medical Record

* Client information (name, address, phone number), the patient's name and birthday, and the date will be included in the practice management system whether digital or paper and that information will be attached to every medical record.

S/O: Rover is a 2-year-old male neutered Labrador retriever who presents for shaking his head. The shaking started about three days ago after he swam in a lake. Rover has had no coughing, sneezing, vomiting, or diarrhea. He has a normal appetite and activity level. He is current on his vaccines and has no travel history or previous medical conditions. His diet consists of three cups a day XXX brand adult maintenance kibble and four XXX brand dog biscuits daily. He gets occasional table scraps.

Physical exam: Body weight = 36 kg; T = 101.5; P = 90; R = 40. Rover is quiet, alert, responsive, and hydrated. His mucous membranes are pink and moist with a capillary refill time of <2 seconds. He has a scant amount of tartar on his teeth. His eyes are clear. He has moderate brown waxy debris in both ears and his tympanic membranes appear to be intact. He has no heart murmur or arrhythmia and his pulses are strong and synchronous. He is eupnic and his lungs are clear. His abdomen is soft and nonpainful with no evidence of masses or organomegaly. His lymph nodes are normal. His coat is healthy and clean and there are no skin lesions noted or evidence of ectoparasites. He is well muscled and ambulatory on all four limbs and has a body condition score of 5/9. No neurological abnormalities are noted.

Ear cytology results: 3+ yeast and 2+ cocci AU

A: Diagnosis: Otitis externa AU

P: Treatment plan: Flushed ears AU in clinic with XXX brand medicated ear flush.

RX: XXX brand medicated ear flush: Flush each ear daily for seven days. Allow medication to sit in ear for 5–10 minutes then wipe out any excess fluid and debris. Apply medicated drops after.

RX: XXX brand ear drops: Instill eight drops into each ear every 24 hours for seven days.

Follow-up: Recheck ears and ear cytology in 6–7 days.

Prognosis: Excellent, but recurrence possible or likely depending on exposure to underlying cause (see 8.24 Team Strategies for Otitis Externa).

Client communication: Ear cleaning and medicine application were demonstrated to the client. Discharge instructions and an information sheet on otitis externa were sent home with the client.

Cindy Trice, DVM

TAKE-AWAYS

- Be clear. Make sure that the next person to read the medical record can follow the actions and thought process of the entire case. Use a consistent format such as the SOAP or problem-oriented approach.
- Be complete. Avoid nonstandard abbreviations. Record all aspects of the case including client communications.
- Be contemporaneous. Writing medical records as close in time to the patient visit leads to more accurate and complete documentation. Ideally, records are completed the same day, so details don't get forgotten and if patients end up at another facility for further care, the records are available for review.
- Be cautious. Know your jurisdiction's legal restrictions for releasing medical records. Leave out all editorial comments on clients or other medical professionals.
- Be critical. Document your critical thought process by recording differential diagnoses and potential further recommended diagnostics or treatments. This will help jog your memory and assist others in making rational medical decisions for further care.

MISCELLANEOUS

Abbreviation

AU   Auris utraque (both ears)

Recommended Reading

Riegger M. Using S.O.A.P. is good medicine. www.dvm360.com/view/using-soap-good-medicine

Rosenberg M. Writing the right veterinary records. www.dvm360.com/view/writing-right-veterinary-records

Quizlet. Veterinary Medical Records. https://quizlet.com/106459241/veterinary-medical-records-flash-cards

Zeltzman P. Could your veterinary records get you in trouble? www.veterinarypracticenews.com/could-your-veterinary-records-get-you-in-trouble

9.2

Asking Good Questions

Amanda L. Donnelly, DVM, MBA

ALD Veterinary Consulting, LLC, Nashville, TN, USA

 BASICS

9.2.1 Summary

Asking relevant questions helps veterinary healthcare providers gain specific information about pets and the owner's relationship with their pet. By asking the right type of question at the right time, veterinary teams can enhance client engagement and tailor client education for individual pets which helps build trust. The ultimate value of asking questions lies in the ability of team members to use this communication skill to increase trust with pet owners which in turn leads to increased client loyalty and compliance.

9.2.2 Terms Defined

Client Engagement: Refers to the communication connection and relationship between a client and the veterinary business.

Client Service Representative: Employee who works at the front reception desk with primary responsibilities of answering phones and interacting with clients during the check-in and check-out process.

Closed-Ended Question: Question that can be answered with a "no" or "yes" response or a single word.

Open-Ended Questions: Questions that cannot be answered with a one-word answer.

 MAIN CONCEPTS

9.2.3 The Power of Asking Questions

To tap into the power of asking good questions, veterinarians and paraprofessional staff need to first appreciate the value of asking questions. To accomplish this objective, veterinary practice leaders should engage the entire team in a discussion, so they understand that the purpose of asking good questions is to get more pets the care they deserve and have them live long, healthy lives with their owners. This discussion is critical so team members recognize that while increasing client loyalty and compliance benefits the business, the real value is about helping pets and people.

Team training includes making sure everyone knows the difference between a closed-ended question and an open-ended question. Closed-ended questions can be answered with a "no" or "yes" response or a single word. Open-ended questions are those that cannot be answered with a one-word response.

Closed-ended questions are used extensively to gather information from clients. For example, client service representatives (CSR) may ask clients if their address has changed and veterinary assistants may ask if they need more heartworm preventive. Veterinarians frequently ask closed-ended questions such as whether the pet has vomited. All these questions can be answered with a "no" or "yes" response.

Open-ended questions invite an expanded response and as such help teams gain more information from pet owners. They're also more effective than closed-ended questions in building rapport and trust with clients. For example, the question "Tell me about Lucy's behavior the last few days" will likely lead to more information than the question "Is Lucy eating?"

Team members need to be trained to know when to ask questions and what questions are right for different client interactions. It is helpful to brainstorm as a team what questions are relevant for various client scenarios. Teams that have thought about good questions for both new and existing clients can more easily identify opportunities to ask pet owners specific questions that enhance client engagement and education.

9.2.4   Questions to Increase Client Engagement

Client engagement refers to the relationship between the veterinary practice and clients. With high levels of client engagement, pet owners feel emotionally bonded to a practice. As a result, they are more likely to visit often, accept treatment recommendations, and refer others to the business. One of the best ways to enhance client engagement is to use questions to make authentic connections with pet owners.

Aside from demonstrating an interest in another person, asking questions helps put people in the position of being better listeners. Teams sometimes lack the art of asking questions as a means to build rapport, especially with new clients. Some people have a natural ability to engage clients with questions while others may need to be more mindful about developing this habit. Here are examples of some questions that can help to build relationships.

- "How do you like living here?"
- "Why did you name your cat Peppermint?"
- "What fun plans do you have for the summer?"
- "How is your son doing in soccer?"

The following questions show you care about the client and their pet which helps build trust.

- "What kind of toys does Hannah like to play with?"
- "How did you decide to get a Jack Russell terrier?"
- "Tell me about the time you spend with Gidget?"
- "Tell me how Bucky has been doing since his last visit."

One of the challenges teams encounter is engaging with clients during busy times. It's human nature for busy employees to avoid asking questions because they think "I don't have time to listen and chat!" The trick to engaging pet owners with questions in these circumstances is to ask

closed-ended questions or questions that don't take long to answer, such as the following.

- "Did you see the soccer game last night?"
- "Have you had a long-haired dachshund before?"
- "Where did you get those lovely shoes?"
- "Are you looking forward to the end of the school semester?"

9.2.5   Questions to Enhance Client Education

Traditional models of client education have been to lecture clients on why their pet needs a particular service or product. This type of communication tends to be one-sided and paternalistic in nature. Moreover, clients may be skeptical of a standard recommendation rather than one tailored for their pet.

Newer models of veterinary–client communications promote a more collaborative approach. Studies have shown multiple positive outcomes when veterinarians use a relationship-centered care approach focused on developing a partnership with clients. One study found pet owners were more likely to adhere to treatment recommendations and had a greater level of satisfaction with this approach. Another study showed that when veterinary teams are trained to use specific communication skills such as open-ended questions, clients felt more involved in appointments and that their veterinarian was more interested in their opinion.

To provide tailored education, it's important to inquire about the client's relationship with their pet and the pet's lifestyle. For example, consider the difference between a sedentary client with an overweight poodle that eats table food and an active client with a slightly overweight retriever that routinely goes to the dog park. Both pets need to lose weight but have different environments that need to be considered when formulating a healthcare plan.

In the above instance, it would be best to ask questions such as "Tell me about Bailey's daily activities" rather than "Does he go outside?" Another good question would be to ask the client a question such as "Tell me what items seem most important to you about Jake's diet" versus asking "What do you feed Jake?"

To create dialogue and promote collaboration with pet owners, team members need to ask good questions that help to assess clients' knowledge level about their pet's medical care. Here are some examples.

- "What do you know about . . . [particular product, disease or treatment]?"
- "Tell me about your previous experience with managing allergies."
- "How did you decide to feed Bella this diet?"

Asking questions throughout the client education process helps pet owners feel heard and allows team members to provide information that is relevant and tailored to each client.

9.2.6 Questions to Discover Underlying Feelings and Motivations

Clients don't always articulate what they're thinking regarding their pet's medical care. Pet owners may experience anger, sadness, fear, guilt, or grief which can influence their decisions. Often the underlying emotions and motivations behind clients' comments or nonverbal communications aren't clear. Asking pet owners the right questions helps teams to avoid making false assumptions and often leads to greater compliance.

The following questions help uncover pet owners' feelings about care and treatment recommendations.

- "What are your thoughts about how Sadie is responding to treatment?"
- "What do you know about living with a blind cat?"
- "Tell me how you're feeling about what we've discussed so far."

9.2.7 Questions to Help Pet Owners Make Decisions

The role of the veterinary team is invaluable whether they're helping clients choose which preventive product to buy or make major decisions in life-threatening situations. It's important to *not* assume money is the reason for reluctance to accept treatment or product recommendations (see 10.15 Putting Price into Perspective). Sometimes spending money is an obstacle because clients don't understand the value of recommended care. The right questions can help clients achieve peace of mind and make decisions that are best for their family. These questions are appropriate when presenting treatment plans to clients.

- "What concerns do you have about Sophie's treatment plan?"
- "What questions do you have about the procedure?"
- "I sense you're frustrated by Tigger's response to treatment. Tell me your thoughts."
- "How can I help you make this decision?"

EXAMPLES

Mrs Smith is a new client who brings her terrier, Daisy, to ABC Animal Hospital for a preventive care exam. During check-in, the CSR asks Mrs Smith how she decided to name her dog Daisy and what plans she has for the upcoming holidays. In the exam room, a certified veterinary technician asks "Tell me about Daisy's typical day and what she enjoys doing with you" and "What concerns would you like to talk to the doctor about?" Dr Taylor engages Mrs. Smith in dialogue by asking "Tell me about Daisy's last visit to the veterinarian and how she's been doing since then" and "What is most important to you about her diet?" Dr Taylor shows Mrs Smith that Daisy has heavy tartar on her teeth and gingivitis along her back molars. Before making a recommendation for dental radiographs and a professional dental cleaning, Dr Taylor asks "Do you know what causes that dental build-up on Daisy's teeth?" and "Tell me what you know about pet oral care."

Mrs Smith likes her new veterinary team because they inquire about her relationship with Daisy, ask her thoughts, and listen to her concerns.

TAKE-AWAYS

- The value of asking questions is to help more pets get care. Good questions help build trust with pet owners which increases client loyalty and compliance.
- Open-ended questions increase client engagement which leads to pet owners feeling more emotionally bonded to a veterinary practice.
- Client education is more effective with a collaborative approach that involves pet owners in decision making.
- Open-ended questions help teams gain information and tailor healthcare recommendations for each pet and client.
- Asking questions helps pet owners feel heard and helps teams understand clients' emotions.

MISCELLANEOUS

Recommended Reading

Durrance, D. and Lagoni, L. (2010). *Connecting with Clients: Practical Communication for 10 Common Situations*, 2e. Lakewood, CO: AHAA Press.

Dysart, L., Coe, J., and Adams, C. (2011). Analysis of solicitation of client concerns in companion animal practice. *JAVMA* 238: 1609–1615.

9.3

Guidelines

Lowell Ackerman, DVM, DACVD, MBA, MPA, CVA, MRCVS

Global Consultant, Author, and Lecturer, MA, USA

 BASICS

9.3.1 Summary

Guidelines are typically created by veterinary organizations as a consensus regarding approaches or procedures. They are meant to be evidence based, but sometimes they are just general directions based on information currently available. Because guidelines are often meant to cover a variety of circumstances and geographies, they tend to be broad in their applications.

When guidelines are customized by individual practices to meet their specific circumstances, they are typically referred to as standards of care for that particular practice (see 9.4 Standards of Care), or as care pathways (see 9.6 Care Pathways).

9.3.2 Terms Defined

Guideline: Routine or sound practices, often formed by consensus within veterinary organizations.

Standard of Care: Customized directives within a practice, organization, or locality that promote and guide clinical practice. Also, in a legal sense, the level of medical care that is expected for a competent veterinary professional to deliver to a patient within a specified veterinary practice. In veterinary medicine, the term *standard of care* is often used synonymously with *protocol*.

 MAIN CONCEPTS

Guidelines are used by the veterinary profession as a "go to" resource for how to approach diagnostic testing, therapy, care pathways, and procedures. On their own, they are sometimes too generalized to be used "as is" in practice, and so are typically used as substrates on which individual practices can create standards of care.

 TAKE-AWAYS

- Guidelines are helpful resources, representing consensus statements for a variety of approaches.
- Guidelines are typically broadly written, but can be edited and customized for individual practices in the form of standards of care.
- Most guideline committees strive to make guidelines evidence based, but sometimes they just represent consensus reached as of a certain point in time.
- Guidelines are not eternal, and are meant to be updated periodically.
- Since many guidelines are meant to be applied in certain circumstances or geographies, they are not always applicable for every practice.

Guideline	Web Address
AAFP Anesthesia Guidelines	https://www.catvets.com/guidelines/practice-guidelines/anesthesia-guidelines
AAFP Antimicrobial Use	http://www.catvets.com/guidelines/practice-guidelines/antimicrobial-in-cats
AAFP Environment Needs	http://www.catvets.com/guidelines/practice-guidelines/environmental-needs-guidelines
AAFP Feline Behavior	http://www.catvets.com/guidelines/practice-guidelines/behavior-guidelines
AAFP Feline Handling	http://www.catvets.com/guidelines/practice-guidelines/handling-guidelines
AAFP Feline NSAIDs	http://www.catvets.com/guidelines/practice-guidelines/nsaids-in-cats
AAFP Feline Nursing Care	http://www.catvets.com/guidelines/practice-guidelines/nursing-care-guidelines
AAFP Feline Vaccines	http://www.catvets.com/guidelines/practice-guidelines/feline-vaccination-guidelines
AAFP Fluid Therapy	http://www.catvets.com/guidelines/practice-guidelines/fluid-therapy-guidelines
AAFP House-Soiling	http://www.catvets.com/guidelines/practice-guidelines/house-soiling
AAFP Hyperthyroidism	http://www.catvets.com/guidelines/practice-guidelines/feline-hyperthyroidism
AAFP Pain Management	http://www.catvets.com/guidelines/practice-guidelines/pain-management-guidelines
AAFP Retrovirus Testing & Management Guidelines	http://www.catvets.com/retroviruses
AAFP Retrovirus Management	http://www.catvets.com/guidelines/practice-guidelines/retrovirus-management-guidelines
AAFP Senior Care Guidelines	http://www.catvets.com/guidelines/practice-guidelines/senior-care-guidelines
AAFP Zoonoses Guidelines	http://www.catvets.com/guidelines/practice-guidelines/zoonoses-guidelines
AAFP-AAHA Feline Life Stage Guidelines	http://www.catvets.com/guidelines/practice-guidelines/life-stage-guidelines
AAHA Anesthesia and Monitoring	https://www.aaha.org/anesthesia
AAHA Anesthesia Implementation	https://www.aaha.org/professional/resources/anesthesia.aspx
AAHA Antimicrobials	https://www.aaha.org/professional/resources/antimicrobials.aspx
AAHA Behavior Implementation	https://www.aaha.org/professional/resources/behavior_management_toolkit.aspx
AAHA Behavior Management	https://www.aaha.org/professional/resources/behavior2015.aspx
AAHA Canine Life Stage Guidelines	https://www.aaha.org/caninelifestage
AAHA Canine Life Stage Implementation	https://www.aaha.org/professional/resources/canine.aspx
AAHA Canine Vaccine Guidelines	https://www.aaha.org/guidelines/canine_vaccination_guidelines.aspx
AAHA Dental Care	https://www.aaha.org/aaha-guidelines/dental-care/dental-care-home/
AAHA Dental Care Implementation	https://www.aaha.org/professional/resources/dental.aspx
AAHA Diabetes	https://www.aaha.org/guidelines/diabetes_guidelines/default.aspx
AAHA Feline Life Stage Guidelines	https://www.aaha.org/professional/resources/feline_life_stage.aspx
AAHA Fluid Therapy	https://www.aaha.org/professional/resources/fluid_therapy_guidelines_abstract.aspx
AAHA Fluid Therapy Implementation	https://www.aaha.org/professional/resources/fluid_therapy_toolkit.aspx
AAHA Infection Control, Prevention & Biosecurity Guidelines	https://www.aaha.org/aaha-guidelines/infection-control-configuration/aaha-infection-control-prevention-and-biosecurity-guidelines/
AAHA Mentoring	https://www.aaha.org/professional/resources/mentoring_guidelines.aspx
AAHA Nutritional Assessment	https://www.aaha.org/professional/resources/nutritional_assessment.aspx
AAHA Nutritional Assessment – Cats	http://www.catvets.com/guidelines/practice-guidelines
AAHA Oncology Guidelines	https://www.aaha.org/professional/resources/oncology.aspx
AAHA Oncology Guidelines Implementation	https://www.aaha.org/professional/resources/oncology_toolkit.aspx

Guideline	Web Address
AAHA Pain Management	https://www.aaha.org/professional/resources/pain_management.aspx
AAHA Pain Management Implementation	https://www.aaha.org/professional/resources/pain_management_toolkit.aspx
AAHA Preventive Care	https://www.aaha.org/professional/resources/preventive_healthcare.aspx
AAHA Referrals	https://www.aaha.org/professional/resources/referral_guidelines.aspx
AAHA Senior Care	https://www.aaha.org/professional/resources/senior_care.aspx
AAHA Weight Management	https://www.aaha.org/professional/resources/weight_management_toolkit_abstract.aspx
AAHA Weight Management Implementation	https://www.aaha.org/professional/resources/weight_management_toolkit.aspx
AAHA/AAFP Feline Vaccination Guidelines (2020)	https://www.aaha.org/aaha-guidelines/2020-aahaaafp-feline-vaccination-guidelines/feline-vaccination-home/
AAHA/AVMA Partnership for Preventive Pet Healthcare	http://www.pethealthpartnership.org/
AAHA/IAAHPC End-of-Life Guidelines	https://www.aaha.org/professional/resources/end_of_life_care_guidelines.aspx
AAHA/IAAHPC End-of-Life Implementation	https://www.aaha.org/professional/resources/end_of_life_care_toolkit.aspx
AAVMC Internship Guidelines	https://jav.ma/InternshipGuidelines
AAVMC Service Dog Guidelines	https://www.aavmc.org/assets/site_18/files/about_aavmc/service_animal_access.pdf
ABCD Anaplasma, Ehrlichia, Rickettsia Infections	http://www.abcdcatsvets.org/anaplasma-ehrlichia-rickettsia-infections/
ABCD Aspergillosis	http://www.abcdcatsvets.org/dermatophytosis-ringworm-2/
ABCD Babesiosis	http://www.abcdcatsvets.org/babesiosis/
ABCD Blastomycosis, Histoplasmosis, Coccidioidomycosis	http://www.abcdcatsvets.org/blastomycosis-histoplasmosis-coccidioidomycosis/
ABCD Blood Transfusion in Cats	http://www.abcdcatsvets.org/blood-transfusion-in-cats/
ABCD Bordetella bronchiseptica	http://www.abcdcatsvets.org/bordetella-bronchiseptica-infection-in-cats-2012-edition/
ABCD Borna Virus Infection	http://www.abcdcatsvets.org/borna-virus-infection/
ABCD Capnocytophaga canimorsus Infection	http://www.abcdcatsvets.org/capnocytophaga-canimorsus-infection/
ABCD Chlamydia felis	http://www.abcdcatsvets.org/chlamydia-chlamydophila-felis/
ABCD Cowpox	http://www.abcdcatsvets.org/cowpox-virus-infection/
ABCD Coxiellosis (Q Fever)	http://www.abcdcatsvets.org/coxiellosis-q-fever/
ABCD Cryptococcosis	http://www.abcdcatsvets.org/cryptococcosis/
ABCD Cytauxzoonosis	http://www.abcdcatsvets.org/cytauxzoonosis/
ABCD Dermatophytosis	http://www.abcdcatsvets.org/dermatophytosis-ringworm-2/
ABCD Disinfectant Choices in Feline Facilities	http://www.abcdcatsvets.org/disinfectants/
ABCD Evidence-Based Veterinary Medicine	http://www.abcdcatsvets.org/evidence-based-veterinary-medicine-2/
ABCD Feline Bartonellosis	http://www.abcdcatsvets.org/feline-bartonellosis/
ABCD Feline Calicivirus Infection	http://www.abcdcatsvets.org/feline-calicivirus-infection-2012-edition/
ABCD Feline Herpesvirus Infection	http://www.abcdcatsvets.org/feline-herpesvirus/
ABCD Feline Immunodeficiency	http://www.abcdcatsvets.org/feline-immunodeficiency/
ABCD Feline Infectious Peritonitis	http://www.abcdcatsvets.org/feline-infectious-peritonitis/
ABCD feline Influenza	http://www.abcdcatsvets.org/influenza-virus-infection-in-cats-2/

(Continued)

Guideline	Web Address
ABCD Feline Injection Site Sarcoma	http://www.abcdcatsvets.org/feline-injection-site-sarcoma-2/
ABCD Feline Leptospirosis	http://www.abcdcatsvets.org/leptospira-spp-infection/
ABCD Feline Leukemia	http://www.abcdcatsvets.org/feline-leukaemia-def/
ABCD Feline Panleukopenia	http://www.abcdcatsvets.org/abcd-guidelines-on-feline-panleukopenia-2012-edition/
ABCD Feline Rabies	http://www.abcdcatsvets.org/rabies/
ABCD Feline Viral Papillomatosis	http://www.abcdcatsvets.org/feline-viral-papillomatosis/
ABCD Francisella Tularensis	http://www.abcdcatsvets.org/francisella-tularensis-infection/
ABCD Giardiasis	http://www.abcdcatsvets.org/giardiasis/
ABCD Hemoplasmosis in Cats	http://www.abcdcatsvets.org/haemoplasmosis-in-cats/
ABCD Hepatozoonosis	http://www.abcdcatsvets.org/hepatozoonosis/
ABCD Infectious Disease in Shelter Situations	http://www.abcdcatsvets.org/infectious-diseases-in-shelter-situations-and-their-management/
ABCD Leishmaniasis	http://www.abcdcatsvets.org/leishmaniosis/
ABCD Lungworm	http://www.abcdcatsvets.org/lungworm-disease-2/
ABCD Maternally Derived Immunity	http://www.abcdcatsvets.org/maternally-derived-immunity-and-vaccination/
ABCD Matrix Vaccination Guidelines	http://www.abcdcatsvets.org/matrix-2/
ABCD Mycobacteriosis	http://www.abcdcatsvets.org/mycobacterioses/
ABCD Pasteurella multocida	http://www.abcdcatsvets.org/pasteurella-multocida-infection/
ABCD Phaeohyphomycosis and Hyalohyphomycosis	http://www.abcdcatsvets.org/rare-opportunistic-mycoses-phaeohyphomycosis-and-hyalohyphomycosis/
ABCD Pseudorabies	http://www.abcdcatsvets.org/aujeszkys-disease-pseudorabies/
ABCD- SARS-2 Coronavirus (COVID-19)	http://www.abcdcatsvets.org/sars-coronavirus-2-and-cats/
ABCD Sporotrichosis	http://www.abcdcatsvets.org/sporotrichosis/
ABCD Streptococcal Infections	http://www.abcdcatsvets.org/mycobacterioses/
ABCD Toxoplasma gondii	http://www.abcdcatsvets.org/toxoplasma-gondii-infection-2/
ABCD Tritrichomoniasis	http://www.abcdcatsvets.org/tritrichomoniasis/
ABCD Vaccination in Immunosuppressed Cats	http://www.abcdcatsvets.org/vaccination-in-immunosuppressed-cats/
ABCD Vaccines and Vaccination	http://www.abcdcatsvets.org/vaccines-and-vaccination-an-introduction/
ABCD Vaccines – Adverse Reactions	http://www.abcdcatsvets.org/Adverse-reactions-to-vaccination/
ABCD West Nile Virus	http://www.abcdcatsvets.org/west-nile-virus/
ABCD Yersinia pestis	http://www.abcdcatsvets.org/yersinia-pestis-infection/
ACVECC Advanced Life Support	http://www.acvecc-recover.org/
ACVECC Basic Life Support	http://www.acvecc-recover.org/
ACVECC Monitoring	http://www.acvecc-recover.org/
ACVECC Postresuscitation Care	http://www.acvecc-recover.org/
ACVECC Prevention & Preparedness	http://www.acvecc-recover.org/
ACVECC Resuscitation	http://acvecc-recover.org/
ACVIM Antimicrobial Use	https://onlinelibrary.wiley.com/doi/pdf/10.1111/j.1939-1676.2005.tb02739.x
ACVIM Antimicrobial Use and Antimicrobial Resistance	http://onlinelibrary.wiley.com/doi/10.1111/jvim.12562/full

Guideline	Web Address
ACVIM Blood Donor Screening for Blood-Borne Pathogens	http://onlinelibrary.wiley.com/doi/10.1111/jvim.13823/full
ACVIM Cytotoxic Chemotherapeutics	https://onlinelibrary.wiley.com/doi/full/10.1111/jvim.15077
ACVIM Ehrlichial Disease	https://onlinelibrary.wiley.com/doi/pdf/10.1111/j.1939-1676.2002.tb02374.x
ACVIM Endoscopic Biopsy	https://onlinelibrary.wiley.com/doi/abs/10.1111/j.1939-1676.2009.0443.x
ACVIM Enteropathogenic Bacteria	https://onlinelibrary.wiley.com/doi/full/10.1111/j.1939-1676.2011.00821.x
ACVIM Gastrointestinal Protectants	https://onlinelibrary.wiley.com/doi/10.1111/jvim.15337
ACVIM Helicobacter	https://onlinelibrary.wiley.com/doi/pdf/10.1111/j.1939-1676.2000.tb02243.x
ACVIM Hepatitis – Dogs	https://onlinelibrary.wiley.com/doi/10.1111/jvim.15467
ACVIM Hyperadrenocorticism	https://onlinelibrary.wiley.com/doi/abs/10.1111/jvim.12192
ACVIM Hypertension	https://onlinelibrary.wiley.com/doi/full/10.1111/jvim.15331
ACVIM Immune-Mediated Hemolytic Anemia Treatment – Dogs	https://onlinelibrary.wiley.com/doi/10.1111/jvim.15463
ACVIM Immune-Mediated Hemolytic Anemia Diagnosis – Dogs & Cats	https://onlinelibrary.wiley.com/doi/10.1111/jvim.15441
ACVIM Leptospirosis	https://onlinelibrary.wiley.com/doi/full/10.1111/j.1939-1676.2010.0654.x
ACVIM Lyme Disease	https://www.onlinelibrary.wiley.com/doi/full/10.1111/jvim.15085
ACVIM Myxomatous Mitral Valve Disease	https://onlinelibrary.wiley.com/doi/10.1111/jvim.15488
ACVIM Proteinuria	http://onllinelibrary.wiley.com/doi/10.111/j.1939-1676.2005.tb02713.x/pdf
ACVIM Seizure Management in Dogs	http://onlinelibrary.wiley.com/doi/10.1111/jvim.13841/full
ACVIM Treatment and Prevention of Uroliths in Dogs and Cats	http://onlinelibrary.wiley.com/doi/10.1111/jvim.14559/full
ACVIM Valvular Heart Disease	https://onlinelibrary.wiley.com/doi/abs/10.1111/j.1939-1676.2009.0392.x
AHS Canine Heartworm	http://heartwormsociety.org
AHS Feline Heartworm	http://heartwormsociety.org
AHS Heartworm Management	http://heartwormsociety.org
AKC CHF Testing	http://www.akcchf.org/canine-health/genetic-tests/
Association of Shelter Veterinarians – Working in Shelters	http://sheltervet.org/associations/4853/files/Standards final bookmarks_with security.pdf
AVMA – Leishmaniasis Diagnosis	http://avmajournals.avma.org/doi/abs/10.2460/javma.236.11.1184
AVMA - Compendium of Animal Rabies Prevention and Control	http://avmajournals.avma.org/doi/pdf/10.2460/javma.239.5.609
AVMA - Compendium of Measures to Prevent Disease Associated with Animals in Public Settings	https://avmajournals.avma.org/doi/abs/10.2460/javma.251.11.1268
AVMA COVID-19	https://www.avma.org/resources-tools/animal-health-and-welfare/covid-19/caring-patients-interacting-clients-covid-19
AVMA Depopulation of Animals	https://www.avma.org/resources-tools/avma-policies/avma-guidelines-depopulation-animals
AVMA Euthanasia	https://www.avma.org/resources-tools/avma-policies/avma-guidelines-euthanasia-animals
AVMA Leishmaniasis – Prevention	http://avmajournals.avma.org/doi/abs/10.2460/javma.236.11.1200
AVMA Leishmaniasis – Treatment	http://avmajournals.avma.org/doi/abs/10.2460/javma.236.11.1192
AVMA Principles of Veterinary Medical Ethics	https://www.avma.org/KB/Policies/Pages/Principles-of-Veterinary-Medical-Ethics-of-the-AVMA.aspx

(Continued)

Guideline	Web Address
AVMA Working with Animal Control and Welfare Organizations	https://www.avma.org/KB/Policies/Pages/AVMA-Guidelines-for-Veterinarians-and-Veterinary-Associations-Working-with-Animal-Control-and-Animal-Welfare-Organizations.aspx
AVMA Zoonoses	http://avmajournals.avma.org/doi/pdf/10.2460/javma.237.12.1403
Banfield State of Pet Health	www.stateofpethealth.com
CAPC (Companion Animal Parasite Council)	www.capcvet.org/recommendations/index.html
CAPC Ascarids	https://www.capcvet.org/guidelines/ascarid/
CAPC Babesiosis	https://www.capcvet.org/guidelines/babesia/
CAPC Baylisascaris	https://www.capcvet.org/guidelines/baylisascaris-procyonis/
CAPC Bedbugs	https://www.capcvet.org/guidelines/bed-bugs/
CAPC Cestodes	https://www.capcvet.org/guidelines/cestodes/
CAPC Cheyletiella	https://www.capcvet.org/guidelines/hairclasping-mite/
CAPC Coccidia	https://www.capcvet.org/guidelines/coccidia/
CAPC Cryptosporidia	https://www.capcvet.org/guidelines/cryptosporidium/
CAPC Cuterebra	https://www.capcvet.org/guidelines/cuterebriasis/
CAPC Cyclophylidea	https://www.capcvet.org/guidelines/
CAPC Cytauxzoonosis	https://www.capcvet.org/guidelines/cytauxzoonosis/
CAPC Demodicosis	https://www.capcvet.org/guidelines/demodex/
CAPC Diphyllobothrium	https://www.capcvet.org/guidelines/diphyllobothrium-spp/
CAPC Dipylidium	https://www.capcvet.org/guidelines/dipylidium-caninum/
CAPC Dracunculus insignis	https://www.capcvet.org/guidelines/dracunculus-insignis/
CAPC Echinococcus	https://www.capcvet.org/guidelines/echinococcus-spp/
CAPC Ehrlichia and Anaplasma	https://www.capcvet.org/guidelines/ehrlichia-spp-and-anaplasma-spp/
CAPC Flea Borne Rickettsiosis	https://www.capcvet.org/guidelines/flea-borne-rickettsiosis/
CAPC Fleas	https://www.capcvet.org/guidelines/fleas/
CAPC Giardia	https://www.capcvet.org/guidelines/giardia/
CAPC Heartworm (Canine)	https://www.capcvet.org/guidelines/heartworm/
CAPC Heartworm (Feline)	https://www.capcvet.org/guidelines/heartworm/
CAPC Hepatozoonosis	https://www.capcvet.org/guidelines/american-canine-hepatozoonosis/
CAPC Hookworms	https://www.capcvet.org/guidelines/hookworms/
CAPC Ixodes scapularis and Ixodes pacificus	https://www.capcvet.org/guidelines/ixodes-scapularis-and-ixodes-pacificus/
CAPC Leishmaniasis	https://www.capcvet.org/guidelines/canine-leishmaniasis/
CAPC Lice	https://www.capcvet.org/guidelines/lice/
CAPC Lungworms	https://www.capcvet.org/guidelines/lungworms/
CAPC Lyme Disease	https://www.capcvet.org/guidelines/lyme-disease/
CAPC Mesocestoides	https://www.capcvet.org/guidelines/mesocestoides/
CAPC Mosquitoes	https://www.capcvet.org/guidelines/mosquitoes
CAPC Nasal Mites	https://www.capcvet.org/guidelines/canine-nasal-mites/
CAPC Neosporosis	https://www.capcvet.org/guidelines/canine-neosporosis/
CAPC Notoedric Mange	https://www.capcvet.org/guidelines/notoedric-mite/
CAPC Otodectic Mange	https://www.capcvet.org/guidelines/otodectic-mite/
CAPC Physaloptera	https://www.capcvet.org/guidelines/physaloptera-spp/
CAPC Rocky Mountain Spotted Fever	https://www.capcvet.org/guidelines/rocky-mountain-spotted-fever/

Guideline	Web Address
CAPC Sarcoptic Mange	https://www.capcvet.org/guidelines/sarcoptic-mite/
CAPC Schistosomiasis	https://www.capcvet.org/guidelines/canine-schistosomiasis/
CAPC Spirometra	https://www.capcvet.org/guidelines/spirometra-spp/
CAPC Taenia	https://www.capcvet.org/guidelines/taenia/
CAPC Ticks	https://www.capcvet.org/guidelines/ticks/
CAPC Toxoplasmosis	https://www.capcvet.org/guidelines/toxoplasma-gondii/
CAPC Trematodes	https://www.capcvet.org/guidelines/trematodes/
CAPC Trichomoniasis	https://www.capcvet.org/guidelines/trichomoniasis/
CAPC Trichuris vulpis	https://www.capcvet.org/guidelines/trichuris-vulpis/
CAPC Trypanosomiasis	https://www.capcvet.org/guidelines/trypanosomiasis/
CAPC Urinary Tract Nematodes	https://www.capcvet.org/guidelines/urinary-tract-nematodes/
Clinician's Brief COVID-19 Owner Contact Guidelines	https://wsava.org/wp-content/uploads/2020/03/COVID-19-Owner-Contact-Guidelines-Clinicians-Brief.pdf
Clinician's Brief Decreased Tear Production in Dogs	https://www.cliniciansbrief.com/article/decreased-tear-production-dogs?utm_medium=email&utm_source=Clinician%27s+Brief+Newsletter&utm_campaign=Online+170526&ajs_uid=9120I9772801J5T
CLSI Understanding Susceptibility Test Data	https://clsi.org/standards/products/veterinary-medicine/documents/vet09/
Dermatology Allergy Testing Drug Withdrawal	https://onlinelibrary.wiley.com/doi/10.1111/vde.12016
Dermatology Canine Atopy	http://onlinelibrary.wiley.com/doi/10.1111/j.1365-3164.2010.00889.x/suppinfo
Dermatology Canine Demodicosis	http://onlinelibrary.wiley.com/doi/10.1111/j.1365-3164.2011.01026.x/pdf
Dermatology Guidelines for Diagnosis and Treatment of Superficial Folliculitis	http://onlinelibrary.wiley.com/doi/10.1111/vde.12118/full
ESCCAP Control of Ectoparasites in Dogs and Cats	http://www.esccap.org/page/GL3+Control+of+Ectoparasites+in+Dogs+and+Cats/27/#.WdVjntFryUk
ESCCAP Control of Intestinal Protozoa in Dogs and Cats	http://www.esccap.org/page/GL6+Control+of+Intestinal+Protozoa+in+Dogs+and+Cats/30/#.WdVj4NFryUk
ESCCAP Control of Vector-Borne Diseases in Dogs And Cats	http://www.esccap.org/page/GL5+Control+of+VectorBorne+Diseases+in+Dogs+and+Cats/29/#.WdVjwNFryUk
ESCCAP Superficial Mycoses in Dogs And Cats	http://www.esccap.org/page/GL2+Superficial+Mycoses+in+Dogs+and+Cats/26/#.WdVjetFryUk
ESCCAP Worm Control in Dogs and Cats	http://www.esccap.org/page/GL1+Worm+Control+in+Dogs+and+Cats/25/#.WdVjTtFryUk
FDA Judicious Use of Antimicrobials	www.fda.gov/AnimalVeterinary/SaftetyHealth/AntimicrobialResistance/JudiciousUseofAntimicrobials/default.htm
FDA Strategy on Antimicrobial Resistance	www.fda.gov/animalveterinary/guidancecomplianceenforcement/guidanceforindustry/ucm216939.htm
FDA Veterinary Feed Directive	www.fda.gov/AnimalVeterinary/ucm071807.htm
FECAVA Antimicrobial Resistance	https://www.fecava.org/policies-actions/guidelines/
ICADA Diagnosis of Canine Atopy	http://www.biomedcentral.com/1746-6148/11/196
ICADA Treatment of Canine Atopy	http://www.biomedcentral.com/1746-6148/11/210
IRIS Consensus for Diagnosis of Proteinuria	http://onlinelibrary.wiley.com/doi/10.1111/jvim.12223/full
IRIS Consensus for Immunosuppressive Therapy Absent an Established Diagnosis	http://onlinelibrary.wiley.com/doi/10.1111/jvim.12222/full
IRIS Consensus for Immunosuppressive Therapy Based on Established Pathology	http://onlinelibrary.wiley.com/doi/10.1111/jvim.12228/full

(Continued)

Guideline	Web Address
IRIS Consensus for Therapy of Glomerular Disease	http://onlinelibrary.wiley.com/doi/10.1111/jvim.12230/full
IRIS Consensus for Treatment of Serology Positive Glomerular Disease	http://onlinelibrary.wiley.com/doi/10.1111/jvim.12232/full
IRIS Grading of Acute Kidney Injury	http://www.iris-kidney.com/guidelines/grading.html
IRIS Prevalence of Immune-Complex Glomerulonephritides	http://onlinelibrary.wiley.com/doi/10.1111/jvim.12247/full
IRIS Staging of Chronic Kidney Disease	http://www.iris-kidney.com/guidelines/staging.html
IRIS Treatment Recommendations for Chronic Kidney Disease	http://www.iris-kidney.com/guidelines/recommendations.html
ISCAID Guidelines for Antimicrobial Therapy of Bacterial Folliculitis	https://www.ncbi.nlm.nih.gov/pubmed/24720433
ISCAID Guidelines for Diagnosis and Treatment Of Respiratory Disease	http://www.iscaid.org/
ISCAID Urinary Guidelines	http://www.iscaid.org/
ISFM Chronic Kidney Disease – Cats	journals.sagepub.com/doi/pdf/10.1177/1098612X16631234
ISFM Diabetes – Cats	http://www.catvets.com/guidelines/practice-guidelines
ISFM Hypertension – Cats	http://journals.sagepub.com/doi/pdf/10.1177/1098612X17693500
ISFM Population Management – Cats	http://www.catvets.com/guidelines/practice-guidelines
Leishvet Leishmania – Cats	http://www.leishvet.info/publications-and-guidelines
Leishvet Leishmania– Dogs	http://www.leishvet.info/publications-and-guidelines
VECCS CPR Guidelines	www.veccs.org
WAVD Diagnosis and Treatment of Dermatophytosis	http://onlinelibrary.wiley.com/doi/10.1111/vde.12440/full
WAVD Recommendations for Approaches to Methicillin-Resistant Staphylococci	http://onlinelibrary.wiley.com/doi/10.1111/vde.12444/full
WSAVA Animal Welfare Guidelines	https://www.wsava.org/Guidelines/Animal-Welfare-Guidelines
WSAVA Gastrointestinal	http://www.wsava.org/guidelines/gastrointestinal-guidelines
WSAVA Global Dental Guidelines	http://www.wsava.org/guidelines/global-dental-guidelines
WSAVA Global Nutrition	http://www.wsava.org/guidelines/global-nutrition-guidelines
WSAVA Global Pain	http://www.wsava.org/guidelines/global-pain-council-guidelines
WSAVA Hereditary diseases	https://www.wsava.org/Guidelines/Hereditary-Disease-Guidelines
WSAVA Liver Disease	http://www.wsava.org/guidelines/liver-disease-guidelines
WSAVA Microchip	http://www.wsava.org/guidelines/microchip-identification-guidelines
WSAVA Nutrition – Cats	http://www.catvets.com/guidelines/practice-guidelines
WSAVA Renal Standardization	http://www.wsava.org/guidelines/renal-standardization-guidelines
WSAVA Vaccination	http://www.wsava.org/guidelines/vaccination-guidelines

MISCELLANEOUS

Recommended Reading

Ackerman, L. (2020). Standards of care and care pathways. In: *Five-Minute Veterinary Practice Management Consult*, 3e, 586–593. Ames, IA: Wiley.

American Animal Hospital Association. Promoting Preventive Care Protocols: Evidence, Enactment, and Economics. www.aaha.org/globalassets/05-pet-health-resources/promoting_preventive_care_protocols.pdf

American Animal Hospital Association. Implementing Preventive Care Protocols. www.aaha.org/globalassets/05-pet-health-resources/implementing-preventive-care-protocols.pdf

Desquilbet, L. (2020). Challenges of making decisions on the basis of significant statistical associations. *J. Am. Vet. Med. Assoc.* 256 (2): 187–193.

9.4

Standards of Care

Lowell Ackerman, DVM, DACVD, MBA, MPA, CVA, MRCVS

Global Consultant, Author, and Lecturer, MA, USA

BASICS

9.4.1 Summary

In many veterinary practices, veterinarians function relatively independently and autonomously, and although some may cherish this personal freedom, it leaves client care quite variable, even within a single hospital.

Standards of care and care pathways are used to preserve best practices, so that clients receive consistent evidence-based care regardless of the level of expertise and experience of individual staff regarding both common and uncommon conditions. Standards of care and care pathways not only recognize best practices for many different preventive and treatment options, but also comprise one of the best ways of realizing appropriate hospital patient care.

9.4.2 Terms Defined

Care Bundle: A group of evidence-based interventions related to a disease, set of clinical signs or clinical procedure that when implemented together result in better outcomes than when implemented separately.

Care Pathway: Also known as clinical pathways and care maps, care pathways are evidence-based practices for specific groups of patients with a predictable clinical course in which professional intervention can be defined, optimized, and sequenced, and in which the outcomes can be measured, contributing further to evidence-based evaluation.

Evidence-Based Practice: Use of the best currently available resources (research and clinical expertise) in making decisions about patient care.

Guidelines: Routine or sound practices, often formed by consensus within veterinary organizations. A general rule intended to make the actions of its followers more predictable.

Level of Care: The intensity, appropriateness, or competence of care provided.

Spectrum of Care: The availability and accessibility of veterinary medical care regardless of the socioeconomic status of the pet owner.

Standards of Care: Customized directives within a practice, organization, or locality that promote and guide clinical practice. In a legal sense, the level of medical care that is expected for a competent veterinary professional to deliver to a patient within a specified veterinary practice. In veterinary practice, the term *standard of care* is often used synonymously with *protocol*.

MAIN CONCEPTS

9.4.3 Standards of Care (Protocols)

Most standards of care begin as guidelines, which are typically created by veterinary organizations, associations, or specialty colleges. The guidelines are general in nature to be applicable to a wide audience and geographic area (see 9.3 Guidelines). The term *standard of care* is also used in a different context, to describe the legally acceptable level of care provided by competent medical professionals (see 9.5 A Different Perspective on Standard of Care), but the discussion here is on standards as protocols, which typically evolve from guidelines.

When guidelines have been customized to meet the needs of a specific hospital or organization, it is then that they typically become referred to as standards of care. Standards of care are critical for veterinary practices and they provide the foundation for evidence-based veterinary

Pet-Specific Care for the Veterinary Team, First Edition. Edited by Lowell Ackerman.

medicine. At a time when compliance has been documented to be significantly less than estimated by most veterinarians (see 9.17 Improving Compliance and Adherence with Pet-Specific Care), standards of care are needed for the ultimate benefit of the practice as well as clients and their pets. As a subset of standards of care, care pathways can be developed for specific groups of patients with a predictable clinical course in which professional intervention can be defined, optimized, and sequenced, and in which the outcomes can be measured (see 9.6 Care Pathways).

Practice protocols and care pathways are easy to understand and comforting for clients, and they allow the hospital to use best practices, regardless of the experience levels of individual doctors and staff members. These protocols needn't be rigid, and can and should change based on circumstances and accumulated data.

Lapses in adherence to protocols can be costly for practices and potentially dangerous for clients and their pets, and may even open the hospital to liability on the basis of substandard care. Clearly, a consistent level of service is good for hospital success and good for the pet owner and pet.

It can be confusing for both clients and staff when doctors in the same practice follow different directives for routine care. If hospitals want to assure clients they are delivering a certain level of care (the intensity, appropriateness, or competence of care provided), then it is critical to also be concerned with consistency of care. Protocols allow all staff to reinforce the practice message about desirable care options and even relatively small changes in protocol adherence can make large differences in healthcare compliance . . . as well as the success of the hospital.

Although many like to believe that veterinary medicine is as much an art as a science, and nobody likes to be dictated to, standards of care allow everyone in the practice to deliver the same consistent high quality of medicine. However, it is also important to realize that not all clients can afford all standards of care, and so practices need to have some flexibility in terms of incremental care options for certain clients in need (see 2.2 The Role of Incremental Care, and 10.14 Providing Cost-Effective Care for Those in Need). This accommodation is sometimes referred to as spectrum of care.

Guidelines are commonplace in human medicine, where evidence-based standards of care are relied upon to ensure patients are receiving appropriate care within hospitals. To successfully implement standards of care into practice, it is worthwhile to first examine the potential benefit to everyone involved, including pets, their owners, and the practice itself. To be accepted by everyone as a hospital-wide standard of care, it is worthwhile building consensus, and that might involve soliciting fact-based evidence for protocols from outside experts, if necessary.

Although it is possible to create standards (protocols) for almost every medical presentation, it is best to concentrate

- Lifetime wellness schedule
- Vaccination
- Integrated parasite control
- Nutritional and weight management
- Oral healthcare and prophylaxis
- Breed-specific screening
- Prescription refills (by medication)
- Pre-anesthetic requirements
- Senior evaluation

Figure 9.4.1 Basic standards of care that are applicable for most veterinary hospitals.

on wellness protocols first, because these should be less controversial and should have the most impact on clients, pets, and practices (Figure 9.4.1). This allows doctors the personal freedom to handle most other medical presentations but agree to follow accepted standards of care for most of the routine wellness situations.

To be successful, protocols must be universal in their application to ensure compliance and positive benefit to all pets in the practice. These standards of care must not be ambiguous, or selective, or they will not be embraced by staff or clients. However, it is also important for all to realize that standards of care still need to be interpreted on a pet-specific basis, and decisions made on what is most appropriate for an individual pet. Criteria for these wellness protocols can be determined based on risk assessment, and the criteria should be easily understood by all staff members (see Figure 9.4.2).

Most pet owners have experienced accepted protocols associated with human health, so they may be even more comfortable with the concept than veterinary staff. Some of these human healthcare protocols may have to do with dental care, vaccination to enter the public school system, mammography recommendations, colonoscopy, and so on.

Different doctors within the same veterinary hospital having different standards of care for pets, without a good explanation, may create controversy among staff and clients (which doctor is right?). Therefore, the goal should be to have standards of care that can be universally adopted by all staff members, whenever medically prudent to do so. That being said, there can be different acceptable standard tiers that range from "gold standard" to a basic protocol, that all meet the ethical and professional needs of the practice but can be customized to meet the financial needs of the client (see 7.8 Providing Care for Those Unable or Unwilling to Pay).

When creating standards of care, it is important to realize that there is unlikely to be complete consensus for all given protocols. Standards of care are more about compromise for the greater good, realizing that no standard will be appropriate for all pets in all circumstances. Therefore, there needn't be endless debate on medical minutiae, and

Sample Integrated Parasite Control Protocol – Dogs

1. Fecal parasite assessment at 2 weeks, 8 weeks, 12 weeks and 26 weeks (6 months) of age, then twice yearly thereafter.
2. Deworming for roundworms and hookworms at 2, 4, 6, & 8 weeks of age with **Brand A**
3. Fecal parasite assessment at 8 weeks of age and treatment as appropriate; start core puppy parasite control with **Brand B**; if additional tick control needed, add **Brand C**
4. Fecal parasite assessment at 12 weeks of age and treatment as appropriate
5. At 6 months of age:
   * Gastrointestinal parasite screen, and treatments as appropriate
   * Continue flea +/– tick control
   * Start heartworm prevention with **Brand D** if routine parasite control does not address this parasite
6. At 12 months of age, and then semi-annually or annually:
   * Semi-annual gastrointestinal parasite screen, and treatment as appropriate
   * Semi-annual to annual heartworm testing, as indicated, and continue control
   * Regular flea/tick control; periodic screening as needed for tickborne diseases

Figure 9.4.2 Example of a standard of care for integrated parasite control.

the hospital team should instead focus on standards that are sensible and defensible, and that can be readily understood and implemented by all staff.

When a protocol is adopted, set a firm time period for when it will be reevaluated, so it becomes a dynamic process and not dogma. It is important to involve all hospital members in the discussion, because veterinarians themselves are sometimes poor judges of what clients want and what they consider to be acceptable risk. Nonveterinarians in the practice are often more likely to identify questions and concerns of the pet-owning public that might be nonmedical in nature.

As protocols are developed, it is important to keep them technologically sound, current, and consumer driven. That includes keeping protocols customized for individual patients and utilizing all available tools, including genetic screening.

Protocols are extremely important for practices, in terms of building consistency into wellness, decreasing confusion of pet owners and staff, and setting expectations regarding optimal pet care.

Care bundles are similarly important for veterinary practices (see 8.8 Care Bundles). These are evidence-based interventions associated with a condition or set of clinical signs designed to address potential poor clinical outcomes. The use of care bundles can improve clinical outcomes, support effective teamwork, promote patient safety, provide a measurable record of care, and support in-practice education.

TAKE-AWAYS

- Veterinarians like the freedom to practice their own brand of medicine, but this can be extremely confusing for clients and staff.

- Standards of care (protocols) help ensure that patients receive the same level of care regardless of the expertise or experience of individual clinicians.
- Standards of care (protocols) represent a compromise and a consensus regarding medical approaches.
- Regardless of standards, individual teams can customize approaches based on the specific needs of individual patients.
- It is important to periodically review standards so that new information can be incorporated. Standards are not meant to be dogma.

MISCELLANEOUS

9.4.4 Cautions

Standards of care, care bundles, and care pathways are intended for typical case presentations, but ultimately, care delivered must meet the specific needs of owner and patient.

Recommended Reading

Ackerman, L. *The Genetic Connection*, 2, AAHA Press, Lakewood, CO, 2011

Ackerman, L: Standards of care and care pathways. In: Ackerman, L. (ed.) *Five-Minute Veterinary Practice Management Consult*, 3, Wiley, Ames, IA, 2020, pp. 586–593.

American Animal Hospital Association-American Veterinary Medical Association Preventive Health Guidelines Task Force. Development of new canine and feline preventive healthcare guidelines designed to improve pet health. *J. Am. Vet. Med. Assoc.*, 2011; 239(5): 625–629.

American Animal Hospital Association. *Promoting Preventive Care Protocols: Evidence, Enactment, and Economics*, 2018. AAHA Press, Lakewood, CO.

American Animal Hospital Association. *Implementing Preventive Care Protocols*, 2019. AAHA Press, Lakewood, CO.

Companion Animal Parasite Council. www.capcvet.org

Partners for Healthy Pets. www.partnersforhealthypets.org

Stull, JW; Shelby, JA; Bonnett, BN; et al.: Barriers and next steps to providing a spectrum of effective health care to companion animals. *J. Am. Vet. Med. Assoc.*, 2018; 253(11): 1386–1389.

9.5

A Different Perspective on Standard of Care

Gary Block, DVM, MS, DACVIM

Ocean State Veterinary Specialists, East Greenwich, RI, USA

BASICS

9.5.1 Summary

The term "standard of care" is frequently found in both human and veterinary medical literature. Although a legal definition of standard of care (SOC) has been firmly established, there is no universally accepted medical definition of SOC. Veterinarians and the profession suffer from a lack of clear, practical, clinically relevant guidelines to help them understand and meet SOC requirements. Furthermore, a lack of consensus on what constitutes SOC will continue to hamper our profession's ability to provide optimum veterinary care and hinder the legal system (including regulatory boards) from consistently identifying, critiquing, and prosecuting cases of veterinary malpractice. There is increasing recognition that SOC should reflect a continuum of acceptable care that takes into account available evidence-based medicine (EBM), client expectations, and financial limitations that may limit available diagnostic and treatment options [1].

9.5.2 Terms Defined

Clinical Practice Guidelines (CPGs): Systematically developed statements to assist practitioner and patient decisions about appropriate medical care for specific clinical circumstances.
EBM: An approach to medical practice intended to optimize decision making by emphasizing the use of evidence from well-designed and conducted research.

Principles of Veterinary Medical Ethics (PVME): A code of ethical conduct to which American veterinarians are expected to adhere.
Tort: A wrongful act or an infringement of a right leading to civil legal liability.

MAIN CONCEPTS

In veterinary tort law, SOC has been defined as "the standard of care required of and practiced by the average reasonably prudent, competent veterinarian in the community" [2]. One court added ". . .nor does the legal standard set the threshold for liability at a particularly high level. The average or normal practitioner, not the best or most highly skilled, sets the standard" [3].

Historically, the courts have considered the veterinarian's actions in comparison to prevailing community standards or veterinarians in "similarly situated communities." This "locality rule" can create the perplexing situation where a different SOC might be required of two neighboring veterinary practices treating the same theoretical patient simply because they are located on different sides of a state border. The origin for these geographic distinctions is likely the presumed lack of access of rural and small-town practitioners to information, certain equipment, and newer medical developments. Given the increasing emphasis on (often mandatory) continuing education in veterinary medicine, online educational opportunities, and the widespread availability of internet and telemedicine consultations, this geographic SOC variability may no longer be defensible despite its persistence in many current US practice acts.

For many of these reasons, human medicine appears to be migrating from a state-mandated toward a nationally accepted SOC [4].

It is also important to contrast the legal use of the term SOC with the common use of the term to denote "gold standard" or idealized care. SOC is also used synonymously with hospital protocols, to designate the application of general guidelines in a specific setting (see 9.4 Standards of Care). These nonlegal uses of the term are frequently found in clinical veterinary journals and articles but may serve to confuse an already muddled understanding of the legal definition of SOC.

Some state practice acts specifically recommend the PVME of the AVMA as "a standard for professional conduct," a violation of which "constitutes cause for disciplinary action." Though a valuable resource for veterinarians, the PVME are too general and lack sufficient prescriptive detail to provide guidance to veterinarians with regard to the SOC in a specific clinical setting. Although EBM is becoming a more important driver of SOC, the use of EBM is still in its infancy in the veterinary profession compared to human medicine (see 2.1 Evidence-Based Veterinary Medicine and Personal Bias). National and international organizations such as the World Veterinary Association, the Royal College of Veterinary Surgeons, the American Animal Hospital Association, and AVMA-recognized specialty organizations such as the American College of Veterinary Internal Medicine all produce consensus statements, CPGs, and white papers on topics germane to their areas of expertise yet there is no requirement or even routine recommendation that these or other relevant clinical resources be considered when assessing cases of potential veterinary malpractice (see 9.3 Guidelines).

Because animals are still considered property in the eyes of the law and pet owners are entitled to decide how much to spend on their pet's care, the veterinary team are all too often faced with ill or injured pets whose owners essentially dictate what the SOC is going to be regardless of what level of care the veterinarian may endeavor to provide. Rather than trying to define some finite, minimum level of care, many are starting to recognize that the concept of "spectrum of care" may be more reasonable and clinically relevant. Rather than having the SOC be "whatever the State Board of Examiners says it is when you are sitting in front of them accused of not meeting it," spectrum of care acknowledges that the care we provide to our patients be grounded in EBM but that we must also take into account client expectations, living situation, and financial means when determining a course of care (see 10.14 Providing Cost-Effective Care For Those in Need).

In human medicine CPGs are systematically developed statements to assist practitioner and patient decision making in specific clinical situations. Unfortunately, veterinary medicine does not currently have any universally accepted CPGs for treating specific medical conditions. The existing veterinary literature only rarely includes reports of studies with outcome measures that include costs of care, quality-of-life assessments, and treatment effectiveness. Outcomes-based research is becoming increasingly important in human medicine for monitoring and improving the quality of human healthcare and veterinary medicine should make this more holistic approach to providing care a priority over the next decade [5]. Creating a centralized database of such CPGs would likely help practitioners, regulatory boards, and the legal system bring some standardization to the current inconsistently applied metrics for assessing the care veterinarians provide to their patients.

Embracing such fundamental changes to how we choose, execute, and assess the care we provide our patients will require all parties to acknowledge the shortcomings of the system as it currently exists. Any changes must continue to instill confidence in the public that veterinarians are an appropriately self-regulating profession and that a system is in place to identify and prevent malpracticing colleagues from continuing to practice.

Given the lack of clinical guidance currently available with regard to SOC and the potentially capricious nature of regulatory boards and the legal system in cases where veterinarians are accused of malpractice, veterinarians and veterinary technicians will be best served by meticulously documenting their medical records and their communications with pet owners regarding preferred therapies, client expectations, and financial limitations that impact on available treatment options.

Regardless of whether SOC, spectrum of care or CPGs become more prevalent and applicable in the future, veterinarians and veterinary technicians must continue to stay abreast of the current veterinary literature and truly commit to life-long learning including, but not limited to, partaking in regular continuing education opportunities. Failure to do so will result in the public losing faith and trust in the care we provide to their pets.

EXAMPLES

How to treat a urethral obstruction in a male cat can be an excellent example of a disease with a wide range of treatment options that are available to veterinary teams, none of which has been accepted as SOC. These disparate approaches will likely vary in success and most definitely will vary in cost but, depending on the situation, all might be reasonable choices.

- *Conservative treatment*: sedation, urinary catheter placement, subcutaneous fluids, drug therapy (prazosin, diazepam, analgesics), place and send home with open-ended tom-cat catheter.
- *No urinary catheter approach*: repeated cystocentesis PRN, sedation, analgesics, no u-cath, place cat in quiet cage until urination occurs.
- *Aggressive treatment*: complete blood count, serum chemistry profile, urinalysis with sediment, urine culture at presentation, intravenous catheter and fluids, blood gas analysis, sedation, pulse oximetry, blood pressure monitoring, epidural nerve block during indwelling u-cath placement with closed collection system, drug therapy, radiographs, or abdominal ultrasound, recheck electrolytes and renal values during hospitalization, urine culture after u-cath removal to check for nosocomial infection.

TAKE-AWAYS

- There is no universally accepted medical definition of SOC.
- A lack of consensus on what constitutes SOC will continue to hamper our profession's ability to provide optimum veterinary care.
- Spectrum of care, rather than SOC, may be a more clinically relevant concept for practicing veterinarians.
- Veterinarians and veterinary technicians must continue to stay abreast of the current veterinary literature and truly commit to life-long learning.
- Developing CPGs to help guide medical therapy should be a priority for the profession.

MISCELLANEOUS

Abbreviation

PRN   pro re nata (Latin, for "as needed")

References

1 Humane Society Veterinary Medical Association. Guiding principles to ensure access to veterinary care. www. hsvma.org/guiding_principles_to_ensure_access_ to_veterinary_care

2 Dyess v. Caraway, 190 So.2d 666 (La. 1966)

3 Turner v. Benhart, 527 SO 2d 717 (Ala 1988)

4 Willis CJ. Establishing standards of care: locality rules or national standards. AAOS Now, 2009. www.aaos.org/ news/aaosnow/feb09/ managing9.asp

5 Stull, J.W., Shelby, J.A., Bonnet, B.N. et al. (2018). Barriers and next steps to providing a spectrum of effective health care to companion animals. *J. Am. Vet. Med. Assoc.* 253: 1386–1389.

Recommended Reading

Block, G. (2018). A new look at standard of care. *J. Am. Vet. Med. Assoc.* 252: 1343–1344.

Stull, J.W., Shelby, J.A., Bonnet, B.N. et al. (2018). Barriers and next steps to providing a spectrum of effective health care to companion animals. *J. Am. Vet. Med. Assoc.* 253: 1386–1389.

9.6

Care Pathways

Lowell Ackerman, DVM, DACVD, MBA, MPA, CVA, MRCVS

Global Consultant, Author, and Lecturer, MA, USA

BASICS

9.6.1 Summary

In many veterinary practices, veterinarians function relatively independently and autonomously, and although some may cherish this personal freedom, it leaves client care quite variable, even within a single hospital.

Care pathways are used to preserve best practices regarding health management, so that clients receive consistent evidence-based care regardless of the level of expertise and experience of individual staff regarding both common and uncommon conditions.

Care pathways not only recognize best practices for many different preventive and treatment options, but also comprise one of the best ways of realizing appropriate patient care and hospital success.

9.6.2 Terms Defined

Care Bundle: A group of evidence-based interventions related to a disease, set of clinical signs or clinical procedure that when implemented together result in better outcomes than when implemented separately.

Care Pathway: Also known as clinical pathways and care maps, care pathways are evidence-based practices for specific groups of patients with a predictable clinical course in which professional intervention can be defined, optimized, and sequenced, and in which the outcomes can be measured, contributing further to evidence-based evaluation.

Evidence-Based Practice: Use of the best currently available resources (research and clinical expertise) in making decisions about patient care.

Guidelines: Routine or sound practices, often formed by consensus within veterinary organizations.

Standards of Care: Customized directives within a practice, organization, or locality that promote and guide clinical practice. In a legal sense, the level of medical care that is expected for a competent veterinary professional to deliver to a patient within a specified veterinary practice. In veterinary medicine, the term *standard of care* is often used synonymously with *protocol*.

MAIN CONCEPTS

In addition to guidelines and standards of care, "care pathways" are also important to practices, especially for chronic or lifelong conditions (see Figure 9.6.1). They help practices focus on the long-term but predictable aspects of patient care, including complications to monitor for, unexpected events, and even the point at which referral to a specialist is indicated. Also important are "care bundles," which are collections of interventions which are likely to result in better clinical outcomes. (see 8.8 Care Bundles).

Care pathways can also serve as substrates for supportive client education materials, because they can look at the medical steps and then focus on aspects of particular significance to the pet owner, such as the evolution of the condition, anticipated effect on healthspan and lifespan, whether the condition can be cured or managed, a time frame for when clinical improvement can be expected, when referral is indicated, and likely price points of extended care (veterinary visits, diagnostic testing, therapies, referral, etc.).

It's important to appreciate from a hospital perspective that care pathways don't constrain the actions of the veterinary healthcare team. They just help everyone to visualize

- Atopic dermatitis
- Glaucoma
- Diabetes mellitus
- Hypoadrenocorticism (Addison's disease)
- Hyperadrenocorticism (Cushing's syndrome)
- Osteoarthirities (degenerative joint disease)
- Congestive heart failure
- Colitis
- Keratoconjunctivitis sicca
- Seizure disorders
- Urolithiasis

Figure 9.6.1 Conditions for which hospitals might consider creating care pathways.

the likely clinical paths that a condition could take, and the decision points to be considered along those paths.

For even the most common clinical presentations, there are likely many different possible approaches. Care pathways start from a position of what is known about the condition and the most sensible ways to commence treatment. There are also bound to be decisions to be made along the path, such as when a pet does not respond as anticipated. The care pathway just serves as a roadmap of how the condition is anticipated to respond to therapy, and what to do when that doesn't happen.

For example, if a pet presents with superficial bacterial folliculitis, there are obviously many different ways to approach the situation. Should the first treatment approach be with topical therapy or antibiotic? If the hospital decides to treat empirically with antibiotic, which antibiotics are most likely to be appropriate? For what duration should the treatment continue? If the condition responds to the treatment only to recur when treatment is discontinued, what is the next step? If the condition does not respond to the empirical treatment, what is the next step?

For many of these situations, the job of the veterinary healthcare team can be much easier if there is an action plan in place, and everyone understands the next steps involved. Also, when there is an action plan in place, it is much easier for other team members, including other veterinarians who might be seeing the patient, to understand the thought processes and not inadvertently make contrary recommendations to the client.

Care pathways are not complicated to create, and they do benefit from hospital team consensus. In many cases, guidelines already exist (see 9.3 Guidelines), so it is just a matter of deciding if that information could be condensed into a short step-by-step format that could be used by the healthcare team.

Another great resource for creating care pathways are the specialists in the area to which referrals are already being sent. These specialists can often provide great insight into how common problems they see could best be handled in primary care practice, and even the ideal decision point at which to consider referral. The referral decision point is often more important than many team members realize, because ultimate success in terms of outcomes depends on referral before irreversible damage has occurred.

EXAMPLES

Sample Care Pathway – Canine Atopic Dermatitis
1) Assess and treat any microbial complications that could exacerbate pruritus.
2) Start antipruritic therapy with nonsteroidal cytokine inhibitor (Brand B), and frequent topical therapy (Brand C).
3) Schedule telephone follow-up for two weeks and clinical reevaluation for four weeks.
4) Decision tree after four weeks of therapy.
   - If doing well on therapy, continue with Brand B for another four weeks.
   - If condition not controlled, switch to corticosteroid (Brand D) for six weeks and commence both parasite control (Brand E) and elimination diet trials (Brand F).
5) Decision tree after next six weeks of therapy.
   - If still doing well on Brand B therapy, consider stopping temporarily to determine possible seasonality; restart as needed.
   - If condition well managed on corticosteroid (Brand D), but recurs when product discontinued after six weeks, either restart Brand D or consider long-term immunomodulatory alternative (Brand G).
   - If condition not well controlled, refer to specialist.
   - If condition well managed on elimination diet trial, stop diet to see if problem recurs; if so, start on diet again and consider challenge feeding.
6) If condition requires more than four months of consecutive therapy, consider allergy testing and immunotherapy and add high-EPA oil to the diet (Brand H).

Guideline:
Treatment of canine atopic dermatitis: 2015 updated guidelines from the International Committee on Allergic Diseases of Animals (ICADA). BMC Vet Res. 2015;11:210.

TAKE-AWAYS

- Care pathways allow hospital team members (and clients) to appreciate that there is a logical action plan for managing ongoing medical issues.
- Care pathways are also a good resource for practices creating client estimates for specific conditions.
- Care pathways encourage consistency of care within a hospital, and consistent messaging by hospital team members.
- Care pathways can help establish criteria for when referrals are indicated.
- Care pathways should be periodically reviewed to ensure that they encompass the most current therapeutic approaches.

MISCELLANEOUS

9.6.3 Cautions

Standards of care, care bundles, and care pathways are intended for typical case presentations, but ultimately, care delivered must meet the specific needs of owner and patient.

Abbreviation

EPA eicosapentaenoic acid

Recommended Reading

Ackerman, L. (2020). Standards of care and care pathways. In: *Five-Minute Veterinary Practice Management Consult*, 3e (ed. L. Ackerman), 586–593. Ames, IA: Wiley.

Ackerman, L. (2011). *The Genetic Connection*, 2e. Lakewood, CO: AAHAPress.

American Animal Hospital Association-American Veterinary Medical Association Preventive Health Guidelines Task Force (2011). Development of new canine and feline preventive healthcare guidelines designed to improve pet health. *J. Am. Vet. Med. Assoc.* 239 (5): 625–629. https://www.aahanet.org/Library/PreventiveHealthcare.aspx.

Companion Animal Parasite Council. www.capcvet.org

David, S.S. (2016). *Clinical Pathways in Emergency Medicine*. Cham: Springer.

Middleton, S. and Roger, A. (2000). *Integrated Care Pathways: A Practical Approach to Implementation*. London: Butterworth-Heinemann.

Partners for Healthy Pets. www.partnersforhealthypets.org

Stull, J.W., Shelby, J.A., Bonnett, B.N. et al. (2018). Barriers and next steps to providing a spectrum of effective health care to companion animals. *J. Am. Vet. Med. Assoc.* 253 (11): 1386–1389.

9.7

Continuum of Care and Convergence Schedules

Lowell Ackerman, DVM, DACVD, MBA, MPA, CVA, MRCVS

Global Consultant, Author, and Lecturer, MA, USA

BASICS

9.7.1 Summary

Pet-specific care involves the care of pets across their entire lifespan. The continuum of care explores the concept that over that lifetime of care, any intervention by the healthcare team affects everything that occurs downstream. In addition, being aware of what could happen on that continuum should prompt teams to discuss those possibilities with clients in a proactive manner.

9.7.2 Terms Defined

Big Picture: The larger context of a situation, not just what is immediately apparent.

Care Pathway: Also known as clinical pathways and care maps, care pathways are evidence-based practices for specific groups of patients with a predictable clinical course in which professional intervention can be defined, optimized, and sequenced, and in which the outcomes can be measured, contributing further to evidence-based evaluation.

Checklist: A tool intended to reduce human failure by drawing the user's attention to key tasks that must be performed in a particular order and allowing the user to mark off each task as it is performed to prevent missed steps.

Continuum of Care: The timespan over which all care is provided.

Convergence Schedule: In veterinary medicine, the coming together of different processes into the same continuum of care.

Evidence-Based Practice: Use of the best currently available resources (research and clinical expertise) in making decisions about patient care.

Guidelines: Routine or sound practices, often formed by consensus within veterinary organizations. A general rule intended to make the actions of its followers more predictable.

Standards of Care: Customized directives within a practice, organization, or locality that promote and guide clinical practice. In a legal sense, the level of medical care that is expected for a competent veterinary professional to deliver to a patient within a specified veterinary practice. In veterinary medicine, the term *standard of care* is often used synonymously with *protocol*.

MAIN CONCEPTS

9.7.3 Continuum of Care

Over the course of a pet's lifetime, every intervention by the veterinary healthcare team occurs as a discrete event along a continuum, one point in time plotted on an animal's lifespan (see Figure 9.7.1).

The concept of a continuum is useful for helping teams be aware of the consequences of actions taken. For example, if an 18-month-old golden retriever is presented for pruritus and the diagnosis is considered to be atopic dermatitis, what gets done at that visit can affect the state of the pet well into the future (see 8.18 Team Strategies for Atopic Dermatitis). If the immediate response is to treat with corticosteroids, and we acknowledge that atopic dermatitis is a lifelong condition, can we envision what the pet might be like at 10 years of age on this regimen? Potentially, it could be cushingoid, smelly, and be subject to recurrent surface infections. If we fail to start topical therapy soon

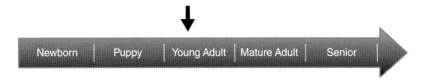

Figure 9.7.1 The care of a pet happens on a continuum. Any individual intervention (*arrow*) happens as one discrete event on that continuum, but affects everything after that event.

enough, can we predict what the impact of that compromised barrier function will be regarding susceptibility to bacterial and yeast overgrowth? For any chronic condition (atopic dermatitis, osteoarthritis, glaucoma, etc.), how pets are managed when the diagnosis is first suspected can have a major effect on how that condition is likely to progress.

The continuum concept can also help frame discussions for what could have happened prior to the diagnostic event. In our example with the 18-month-old golden retriever that we suspect has atopic dermatitis, could we have been more proactive in our approach? Could we have predicted that such an animal might be at increased risk of atopic dermatitis (golden retrievers are perceived as a breed at risk for atopic dermatitis in many parts of the world) and had conversations with owners even at puppy visits? If so, we might have counseled them on what to look for as early evidence of the condition (usually first presents at 6 months to 3 years of age, licking and chewing at the feet, rashes in the armpit and groin areas, face rubbing, etc.) and we might have even been able to convince them to start using positive reinforcement techniques so that the pet willingly accepts bathing and ear care. If the owners were told what the long-term costs might be if their pet did develop allergies, it is also possible that they would enroll in pet health insurance so they would be prepared to accept hospital team recommendations regarding long-term management (see 10.16 Pet Health Insurance).

Throughout a pet's lifetime, it will also develop issues that may or may not be predicted. However, once that information is known, it is important for the healthcare team to be aware of how it could affect future susceptibilities. For example, a pet that is found to have evidence of hip dysplasia during orthopedic screening procedures (see 3.12 Orthopedic Screening) should be considered for evidence of developing osteoarthritis later in life (see 8.20 Team Strategies for Osteoarthritis). A pet diagnosed with hyperadrenocorticism (Cushing's syndrome) should be considered at increased risk for developing diabetes mellitus as a co-morbidity (see 8.27 Team Strategies for Diabetes Mellitus). Once again, any event that occurs on a continuum of care affects things downstream, so this can help teams be aware and plan to stay ahead of those potential consequences. It pays to look past the complexity and keep in mind the "big picture." Continuum of care models help us achieve this.

9.7.4 Convergence Schedules

One of the major problems with a continuum of care concept is that there are a lot of things to do and discuss with owners, and relatively few opportunities to do so. To help make sure that everything that needs to get discussed does get discussed, it can be useful for the team to use a convergence schedule (see Figure 9.7.2). This is particularly helpful to highlight topics to be covered during puppy and kitten visits, but it can also be used with care pathways (see 9.6 Care Pathways), and personalized care plans (see 1.3 Personalized Care Plans). The schedule just makes sure that topics get covered in a timely manner, whose responsibility it is, the manner in which the contact should take place, and provides a permanent record of who was responsible for that contact and when it happened. All this information should also be reconciled with the medical record system so that there is official documentation of the contact and discussion.

TAKE-AWAYS

- Continuum of care is a great way to visualize the impact of veterinary team interactions on individual pets.
- Everything that happens during a veterinary interaction will have potential long-term implications.
- Viewing patient care on a continuum also helps envision conversations and proactive screening that should happen before issues become clinical.
- The biggest challenge of working on a continuum of care is making time to have appropriate discussions with pet owners about the actual healthcare needs of their pets.
- A convergence schedule is a form of checklist which can be developed to help staff members know what discussions should take place with pet owners, and when that contact should occur.

Patient Name   *Fluffy Smith*

What	When	How	Who	Done
Fecal Evaluation	6 weeks	Phone	CSR	2 Jun 2020
Integrated Parasite Control	8 weeks	Direct	Nurse	16 Jun 2020
Vaccination	8 weeks	Direct	Nurse	16 Jun 2020
Microchipping	8 weeks	Direct	Nurse	16 Jun 2020
Apply for Pet Health Insurance	8 weeks	Direct	Nurse	16 Jun 2020
Breed-specific issues	8 weeks	Direct	DVM	16 Jun 2020
Nutritional Counseling	12 weeks	Direct	Nurse	14 Jul 2020
Genetic Screening & Counseling	12 weeks	Direct	Nurse	14 Jul 2020
Diet & Oral Hygiene	12 weeks	Direct	Nurse	14 Jul 2020
Create Lifelong Care Plan	16 weeks	Direct	CSR	14 Jul 2020
Spay/Neuter	26 weeks	Direct	Nurse	10 Oct 2020
Heartworm testing/prevention	26 weeks	Direct	Nurse	10 Oct 2020
Behavior Counseling	26 weeks	Link	CSR	10 Oct 2020
Microchip (if not done at 8 weeks)	26 weeks	Direct	Nurse	10 Oct 2020
Health Risk Assessment	1 year	Direct	CSR	6 June 2021
Orthopedic Screening/Radiographs	2 year	Phone	CSR	1 May 2022

Figure 9.7.2   Example of a convergence schedule.

MISCELLANEOUS

9.7.5   Cautions

No matter how prepared the team is, it is not possible to predict everything that might happen in the life of a pet. It might be in boarding and acquire a respiratory infection. It may get loose from the house and sustain a traumatic injury. It might develop a cancer for which there wasn't a known predisposition. The continuum of care and convergence schedules are really meant for conditions which might be reasonably predicted.

Abbreviations

CSR   Customer service representative
DVM   Doctor of Veterinary Medicine

Recommended Reading

Ackerman, L. (ed.) (2020). *Five-Minute Veterinary Practice Management Consult*, 3e. Ames, IA: Wiley.

9.8

Ensuring Consistency of Care

I. Craig Prior, BVSc, CVJ

College Grove, TN, USA

BASICS

9.8.1 Summary

Service industries are judged on the service they provide and by the standard of their care. Client expectations of veterinary hospitals are no different. For any given veterinary service, the level of care can vary greatly from hospital to hospital and practitioner to practitioner, even within the same hospital. It is essential for the hospital's success, whether it be a single hospital or a large group, that it has a powerful mission statement, standards of care covering all the most common services or procedures performed, products dispensed, and care pathways associated with each of these. In addition to guidelines, there must be continual staff training on messaging around these guidelines. This "One Voice, One Message" approach keeps staff members uniform and the hospital recommendations consistent and helps ensure the services provided meet or exceed the hospital's mission statement.

In some hospitals, individual veterinarians may have their own way of doing things, but to ensure a promised level of care to clients, everyone needs to be on the same page, at least as far as routine standards, testing, procedures, and treatment plans go. This helps ensure that the hospital has a unified message to clients rather than individual doctors doing their own thing.

9.8.2 Terms Defined

Care Pathway: A treatment plan based upon the care guidelines explaining what is involved and showing costs involved, stored in the practice management software (PMS) system.

Core Values: Values that support the vision, shapes the culture, and reflects the values, principles, philosophy, and beliefs of the company.

Mission Statement: A formal summary of the aims and values of a company, organization, or individual.

Recommendation: A suggestion or proposal as to the best course of action, especially one put forward by an authoritative body.

Service Standards: Standards that help define the level of service that clients should expect to receive, whether in person, on the phone, or in writing, and provide a foundation for management and employee expectations and obligations.

Standards of Care: These practice-specific clinical practice guidelines are statements that include recommendations intended to optimize patient care, are informed by a systematic review of evidence and an assessment of the benefits and harms of alternative care options.

Vision: What an organization aspires to be.

MAIN CONCEPTS

Attaining a standardized, consistent level of care for clients can often be challenging (see 9.4 Standards of Care, and 9.6 Care Pathways). Hurdles to overcome are clients not always seeing the same doctor and doctors not performing procedures, services, treatments, or prescribing medications the same way. This results in deflated client expectations and experience, which in turn can be costly to both the hospital and client. For the client, if they receive different treatment plans for similar services, this can lead to confusion, extra clinic visits, and potentially increased costs. For the clinic, if the client is disappointed with the service provided or confused by the different treatment plans, then this can

---

Pet-Specific Care for the Veterinary Team, First Edition. Edited by Lowell Ackerman.
© 2021 John Wiley & Sons, Inc. Published 2021 by John Wiley & Sons, Inc.

cause a reduction in client retention, possible negative reviews via websites or social media and frustration for staff members.

In order to provide a consistent client experience, the following steps should be considered.

9.8.3 Review or Create a Mission Statement, Core Values, and Vision for the Clinic

The mission statement of the hospital is powerful. It should be considered the cornerstone for the practice – providing the image and inspiration, defining the "why" – and is the reference that guides all decision making and planning. This mission statement along with the core values will help shape the company culture, communications and consistency, and provides the basis for any action plan. It will help guide the conversation and unify staff members under a central theme (i.e., pet-specific care, treating pets as family, innovative medicine, clients first, etc.). In creating a mission statement, it should help differentiate your practice from others, it should be brief, and it should be concise – don't generalize. If creativity is not your strong point, there are companies that will help you develop a statement.

9.8.4 Establish Standards of Care and Care Pathways

Hospital teams should review available Guidelines (see 9.3 Guidelines), which should facilitate discussions of evidence-based approaches for all the most common procedures, services (including early detection), treatments, and product recommendations. The guidelines can then be customized for the individual practice, in which case they become standards of care (see 9.4 Standards of Care) and care pathways (see 9.6 Care Pathways). Establish a list of the most common procedures, services, treatments, and product recommendations, divide the list up among the team, set a framework and timeframe for completion, and then reconvene to review, discuss, and approve each one. All team members must agree to them in principle and should be following these standards as the first line when offering care to clients.

9.8.5 Messaging

Guidelines for messaging and expectations around the standards should be formulated at doctor and/or staff meetings with the understanding that all members will be held accountable for abiding by these approaches. Messaging should adhere to "One Voice, One Message," where clients hear the same clear, concise, unified message from all team members.

9.8.6 Care Pathways

Care pathways, service and product codes, and reminders should be developed and reviewed (see 9.6 Care Pathways). Creating canned treatment plans is one way to help ensure a consistent client experience across different veterinarians. Wellness plans may be developed encompassing the most important wellness guidelines of early detection and prevention for the geographic area, age, sex, species, and breed of patient. Used correctly, it takes the focus off the money and places emphasis on the medicine!

9.8.7 Service Standards

These should be developed collaboratively with the whole team, placed in writing, and become part of job descriptions for the hospital. Be concise in order to eliminate ambiguity, and standards should be measurable to a predetermined benchmark. Most importantly, they should make the hospital stand out – head and shoulders above the crowd! Consider writing standards for face-to-face client communications (greeting, departure, exam room, hospitalization of patents, discharge of patients, and conflict resolution), phone communications, written communications (including text), internal communications (between employees), and operational standards. In developing these standards, follow the examples of successful businesses (e.g., Ritz Carlton: www.ritzcarlton.com/en/about/gold-standards#Three_Steps_of_Service).

9.8.8 Training

Once completed and approved, the standards should be disseminated to the hospital team through staff meetings, staff training (can be group setting, role plays, etc.), employee handbooks, web-based training sites, and during one-on-one performance and training reviews. Building consensus among the different doctors in the practice is paramount, since if they don't embrace this evidenced-based approach, it will be exceedingly difficult for the concepts to be successfully implemented. People all learn by different methods, so it is important to add variety when communicating with employees. Staff training should be ongoing and repetitive through staff meetings, performance reviews, lunch and learns, seminars, etc., as there will be staff turnover and message "drift." Customer service representatives (CSRs), nursing staff, and kennel attendants should all understand their role in delivering these messages and recommendations to clients.

All in all, the clients should be seeing and hearing a cohesive hospital team providing superior client service and presenting clear, concise messages and recommendations to enhance the health and well-being of their pets.

EXAMPLES

A CSR brings to the attention of the practice manager (PM) that client concerns have been expressed regarding the treatment of pets. The concerns are that there are obvious different levels of care depending upon the doctor seen and, correspondingly, the costs of treatments. Clients are starting to question whether some doctors are overtreating and overcharging or, conversely, that some pets may not be receiving the care they deserve.

The PM and medical director (MD) decide to start reviewing one of the most common ailments – ear problems (otitis externa) – so access all charts with diagnostic codes for otitis externa in the last three months. Surprisingly, they find that the level of diagnostics, treatment, and charges vary greatly from doctor to doctor. Some perform no diagnostics; treatment varies from daily drops to packing medications to long-acting medication and some doctors were not even charging full exams.

The problem is presented to the medical team, and then the meeting is focused on the hospital mission statement and core values. These are very powerful and focused on best care, innovation, preserving the human–animal bond, and creating a fear-free environment. The diagnostic and treatment options being offered to clients are then discussed in relation to the mission statement, core values and vision, and the level of care the hospital is striving to offer their clients (see 8.24 Team Strategies for Otitis Externa).

All doctors agree that they need more consistency, so guidelines are reviewed for otitis externa, and a standard of care created. The Standards for Otitis Externa include a full exam, ear cytology, ± culture and sensitivity based on ear cytology results, ear cleaning if necessary, appropriate medications that are long acting if possible (and administered in-clinic) to increase compliance and adherence, and

dedication to identifying likely underlying causes. Emphasis is also placed on fear-free handling. Care pathways are created, reminders linked in the PMS, and then a general staff meeting convened. The mission statement, core values, and vision of the hospital are reviewed, and then the Standard for Otitis Externa is presented, with a thorough explanation of the "why" and "how." Team training is then instituted, and job descriptions, handbooks, websites, and marketing materials are all updated.

TAKE-AWAYS

- The mission statement of the hospital is the guiding light for ensuring consistency of care.
- Consistency of care can vary greatly between veterinary hospitals, and even among team members in the same hospital.
- Establishing standards of care can help ensure a hospital is achieving a consistent level of care across patients and practitioners.
- Cohesive team members speak with "One Voice, One Message," providing a united front to the clients.
- Ongoing and consistent team meetings including doctors keep employees focused on the hospital goals and mission statement.

MISCELLANEOUS

Recommended Reading

American Animal Hospital Association. Guidelines. www.aaha.org/pet_owner/aaha_guidelines/default.aspx

American Veterinary Medical Association. Companion animal care guidelines. http://avma.org/KB/Policies/Pages/Companion-Animal-Care-Guidelines.aspx

Companion Animal Parasite Council. http://CAPCVET.org

Heartworm Society. http://Heartwormsociety.org

European Scientific Counsel Companion Animal Parasites. http://Esccap.org

Michellig, J. (2008). *The New Gold Standard: 5 Leadership Principles for Creating a Legendary Customer Experience Courtesy of the Ritz-Carlton Hotel Company*. New York: McGraw-Hill Education.

9.9

Continuity of Care

Kurt A. Oster, MS, SPHR, SHRM-SCP

Bay State Veterinary Emergency and Specialty Services, Swansea, MA, USA

 BASICS

9.9.1 Summary

Continuity of care is a broad term that encompasses all aspects of medical record keeping and corresponding communications. Through proper documentation, all team members can track a patient's progress and respond appropriately to client concerns and issues.

Today, continuity of care has broadened to include all who have a role in patient care. There may be significant time and geographic variances, which increases the need for accurate record keeping. Care may be provided by the primary care veterinarian, the pet-owning family, the emergency hospital, numerous specialists, trainers, physical therapists, chiropractors, acupuncturists, etc.

The backbone of continuity of care and the doctor–client relationship is communication. The majority of breakdowns in patient care and customer service are rooted in incomplete, untimely, and/or incorrect communication.

9.9.2 Terms Defined

Continuity of Care: The cooperative efforts of the healthcare team and clients to ensure quality of care and beneficial outcomes over time, even when multiple healthcare professionals are involved.

SOAP: An acronym that identifies the most common data entry format used by veterinary practices. The data are generally located in the progress notes portion of a problem-oriented medical record. The letters stand for: Subjective, Objective, Assessment, and Plan.

 MAIN CONCEPTS

Continuity of care is a critical responsibility of every veterinary staff member. It is important to recognize that although the ultimate burden rests on the doctor managing the case, it is the responsibility of the entire staff to ensure that each patient receives complete and seamless veterinary healthcare. Complete, problem-oriented medical records identify the patient and document all medical information in a logical, well-organized manner. Such records define each problem while facilitating "total care of the patient." Proper medical records facilitate rapid retrieval of information and a thorough progression of care despite the involvement of multiple veterinary healthcare providers (see 9.1 Medical Records).

In many practices, the skills and talents of the support staff may be overlooked. Veterinary technicians play a significant role in helping to improve continuity of care. In many practices, the treatment technicians round simultaneously with the doctors. Technicians often have added insights on how the pet is responding (e.g., alert, lethargic, uncomfortable, or tearing out IV lines). They may also have additional input regarding how well the pet is eating, drinking, and so on. Even small tips can be helpful (for example, recommending an alternate route of administering medications). Depending upon individual skill levels and practice environments, many doctors will round with a technician if the oncoming doctor is unavailable. Many hospitals also have a technician-round journal, or nursing notes where the technicians enter helpful comments regarding each patient's care (e.g., whether or not restraint is needed and, if so, what type is the most effective).

Pet-Specific Care for the Veterinary Team, First Edition. Edited by Lowell Ackerman.
© 2021 John Wiley & Sons, Inc. Published 2021 by John Wiley & Sons, Inc.

Utilize technology as much as possible. Digital photographs can be taken and stored in most software systems. A picture is worth a thousand words, so save yourself all the writing. Photographs are an effective way to document lacerations, skin problems, masses, external parasites, dental problems, and so on. If you forget to communicate everything you wish to the doctor who is taking over the case, it is never too late to follow up with an email or voice mail message from home or on the road. Always assume that the piece of information you left out is the first question your colleague will be asked.

9.9.3 Process

To ensure continuity of care, even simple procedures such as recheck examinations require the implementation of a systematic, decision-making process. Without proper "set-up" and communication, customer service and patient care will suffer.

Before the client leaves the office, the staff, if possible, should schedule the patient's recheck examination, preferably with the same doctor. This type of immediate follow-up helps increase client compliance and improves the probability that the original doctor, rather than one of their associates, will see the patient at the recheck. When using a flexible scheduling system such as a 10-minute flex, it is important to specify the appropriate time slot for the recheck (e.g., a 10-minute or 20-minute time slot).

If, after checking your schedule, you realize that you are not scheduled or are not available when the recheck is due, check the practice schedule to determine if one of your colleagues who is on duty today will be on duty when you schedule the recheck. If so, introduce your colleague to the client and allow that doctor to have a quick look at the patient so that he or she is better informed. The client must be informed and fully understand any specific instructions that might impact the visit. For example, does the pet need to be fasted or should they not walk their pet prior to entering the hospital because a urine sample needs to be collected?

It is important to provide a detailed description of each condition your colleague will review at the recheck. The more detail you provide, the easier it makes everyone's job. For example, if you have located a mass and wish to monitor it, you should measure its exact size with calipers or a ruler. You should also mark on a diagram of the pet the exact position of the mass. Never estimate sizes, always use a calibrated measuring device. You should also document your expectations as to what the desired response or recovery should be at the time of the recheck. Have detailed

plans developed that include references to further diagnostics, treatment options, and client expectations.

Scheduling (and providing adequate time and resources) doctor rounds is an extremely important component that contributes enormously to improving the continuity of care. Regularly scheduled rounds are even more important in practices with new or less experienced doctors, in larger practices, and in 24-hour environments.

In addition to the standard morning cage-side rounds that most practices employ, larger facilities will also implement teaching rounds at the beginning or end of the day. In a 24-hour environment, rounding at the end of each shift is critical, especially because many of the cases found in a 24-hour environment typically require a higher level of care. Establishing a 24-hour schedule with intentional shift overlap is one easy way to help increase rounding compliance. Sample shifts may include 7.00 a.m. to 4.00 p.m., 3.00 p.m. to 12.00 a.m., and 11.00 p.m. to 8.00 a.m. The guaranteed overlap helps facilitate rounds.

If the practice is extremely busy and work continues into the overlap, it is generally the responsibility of the doctor coming on duty to release the doctor going off duty. Such practices ensure that the oncoming doctor is comfortable with the status of all the cases in the hospital and is able to take over their care until the next shift comes on duty.

TAKE-AWAYS

- Ensuring continuity of care is no longer the exclusive responsibility of the treating doctor. Technicians, veterinary assistants, and client service staff must all contribute to the process.
- A pet's healthcare team may extend hundreds of miles and consist of numerous individuals in addition to the general practitioner. Veterinary specialists, emergency doctors, veterinary acupuncturists, chiropractors, massage therapists, and rehabilitation technicians are just a few examples of other caregivers.
- The role of clients in their pet's treatment should not be underestimated. They administer medication, observe behavior, and approve treatment plans.
- Proper names should be recorded in any record of communication.
- Contemporary technology supports timely and accurate communication such as text messaging, emails, and digital photography, but a process must exist to ensure all this information is properly captured and entered into the pet's permanent medical record.

MISCELLANEOUS

One common test of the quality of a medical record and its ability to facilitate excellent continuity of care is the "telephone roundtable game." Many teaching hospitals require their interns to participate in this exercise each month to reinforce the importance of quality medical records as well as to demonstrate to the interns how much their record-keeping abilities will improve throughout their tenure.

The game is played by having each participant select a record of one of the cases they are managing in the hospital. The participants then sit around a table and pass their record to the doctor on their right. The facilitator then engages each doctor in a role-playing exercise by pretending to be the pet's owner and calling him or her on the telephone for a progress report. The "pet's owner" asks the doctor numerous questions, and the doctor only has the medical record and their own personal knowledge of the case (such as from rounds) from which to draw. Needless to say, the first few games are a little frightening, but after a while the medical records become more complete and the participants are much more articulate.

9.9.4 Cautions

Standardize the abbreviations that your practice uses in its medical records. Multidoctor practices employing graduates from different veterinary schools often have trouble understanding one another's abbreviations.

Always prepare clients before you turn cases over to other doctors. The more informed a client is and the more proactive communication she receives, the greater her confidence and trust level will be. If you do need to turn cases over, it is often best to identify a doctor with whom the client has had prior contact. Working from established, positive relationships is always easier than initiating new relationships, especially during stressful times (such as when a pet is hospitalized for emergency treatment).

Using vague entries such as "follow-up bloodwork" or "liver panel" instead of identifying specific tests may jeopardize the patient's life or cause the patient's owners to incur unnecessary costs (e.g., if the correct diagnostics are not done).

When documenting communication, always use the proper name of the person you spoke with. Stating "owner" or "referring veterinarian" in record entries is too vague and ambiguous to support proper continuity of care. Numerous individuals within a household may consider themselves the owner. Similarly, speaking with any doctor within the referring practice is not the same as having a conversation with a specific doctor identified by name.

Recommended Reading

Catanzaro, T. (2018). *Veterinary Medical Records for Continuity of Care and Profit*, VCI Signature Series Monograph. Davis, CA: VIN Bookstore.

Heinke, M.L. and McCarthy, J.B. (2012). *Practice Made Perfect*, 2e. Lakewood, CO: AAHA Press.

Oster, K. (2020). Continuity of care. In: *Five-Minute Veterinary Practice Management Consult*, 3e (ed. L. Ackerman), 594–595. Ames, IA: Wiley.

Robinson, G.W., Berg, J., and Skeels, M. (2003). *Path to High-Quality Care*. Lakewood, CO: AAHA Press.

Robinson, G.W., Berg, J., and Skeels, M. (2010). *Standard Abbreviations for Veterinary Medical Records*, 3e. Lakewood, CO: AAHA Press.

Uijen, A.A., Schers, H., Schellevis, F. et al. (2012). How unique is continuity of care? A review of continuity related concepts. *Family Practice* 29: 264–271.

9.10

Dispensing and Prescribing

Lowell Ackerman, DVM, DACVD, MBA, MPA, CVA, MRCVS

Global Consultant, Author, and Lecturer, MA, USA

 BASICS

9.10.1 Summary

The role of the pharmacy continues to evolve in veterinary practices, especially in the US. Dispensing still makes up a considerable proportion of revenue in many practices, but it seems to be trending downward as there is increased competition from alternate retail channels.

In most veterinary practices, dispensing is divided into prescription, over-the-counter, and diet sales. As a subcategory, parasite control products (both prescription and non-prescription) are the leaders in revenue generation, but these product sales are also most vulnerable to outside retail competition. Pharmacy management requires attention to inventory management, but also to strategic opportunities and challenges that can impact this important profit center.

9.10.2 Terms Defined

Acquisition Cost: The unit cost at which a product or service can be purchased, including any delivery fees and/or taxes.

Inventory Turnover: Also known as inventory turns, merchandize turnover, stockturn, stock turns, turns, and stock turnover, this refers to the cost of goods sold divided by the average inventory. It is a measure of the number of times inventory is sold or used within a time period.

Production: A form of commission paid to veterinarians on the basis of their revenue generation.

Shrinkage: Product reduction due to wastage, loss, or theft.

 MAIN CONCEPTS

The pharmacy has become an extremely competitive revenue center for veterinary hospitals, as the marketplace has become crowded with retailers offering similar or even identical products. There was also a time when many products sold by veterinary practices were available almost exclusively through veterinary channels, but that may just be a fond memory for many veterinarians as they are faced with a new reality in dispensing.

9.10.3 The Pharmacy as Profit Center

The main marketplace changes that have had the most impact on veterinary practices are the more mainstream sale of products through retailers, and the increased "share of voice" these retailers have with pet owners. It is now very easy for consumers to find their products of interest from various retailers, online and otherwise, and to shop for the best prices and delivery options as well.

The other aspect of dispensing that cannot be ignored if veterinarians want to dispense profitably is that inventory is not typically managed efficiently and effectively, given its critical contribution to hospital income. Thus, many practices carry too much inventory given their small retail footprint and so the typical ordering and carrying costs are often excessive given "turns" (a measure of the speed of converting inventory back to cash through sales) associated with those products. Because of this, even if such inventory generates "revenue" for the practice, it may not generate sufficient "profit" given the costs involved.

Pet-Specific Care for the Veterinary Team, First Edition. Edited by Lowell Ackerman.

9.10.4 Pricing

Most veterinary practices use a combination of mark-up, margin, and community pricing for pharmacy items (see 10.13 Approach to Pricing). Mark-up involves calculated additions to the acquisition price, margin involves calculating the profit margin on a fee after factoring in direct and indirect costs, and community pricing involves matching the price of value leaders for the same or similar products

Pet owners may not bother comparing costs on a one-time prescription (such as for treating a urinary tract infection), but for medications used chronically and those used for parasite control, comparison shopping should be anticipated.

This loss of business can be insidious, but it can also be devastating to the long-term success of the veterinary pharmacy. For instance, veterinarians may not be aware that parasite control products typically represent the majority of their prescription dispensing revenue, and may not realize the extent of the situation until they find that many clients are buying their flea and tick control products through nonveterinary channels.

In some practices, dispensing is not strictly a retail activity, and a commission (production) may be paid to veterinarians based on the products they recommend and dispense. There's nothing wrong with this in principle but since retailers don't do this, it serves as one more impediment to competitive pricing, since the veterinary price to consumers must reflect both fair pricing for the product itself, as well as the commission to be paid to the veterinarian, making the veterinary price potentially significantly higher than that of the retailer. Similarly, adding a dispensing fee is something that veterinarians have historically done, but it also inflates final product costs to the consumer when our competition does not do the same.

9.10.5 Managing Inventory Costs

The best ways for veterinarians to profitably provide dispensing is to limit the number of products stocked to those that make medical and financial sense, ensure that product recommendations are routinely made by the hospital team so that product turns are optimized, promote compliance so clients give the medications as directed and for the correct interval (including refills), and price fairly so that there are few or no obstacles to client acceptance and purchase.

From a medical standpoint, the best way of limiting inventory is to create standards of care within the hospital, and primarily stock products that satisfy those standards of care (see 9.4 Standards of Care, and 9.6 Care Pathways). Using products that ensure compliance (such as injecta-

bles) is also a great way to provide additional value to clients, who in general would prefer not to have to medicate their pets at home (see 9.14 New Treatment Modalities).

9.10.6 Partnering with an Online Pharmacy

Veterinary teams do not need to stock everything in their own pharmacies in order to provide more complete retail options to their clients. If hospitals concentrate on stocking products for which they have good turnover, profitability, and compliance, then it makes sense to let someone else shoulder the inventory costs for other products that might be used infrequently, or for which there is not adequate profit margin, or that didn't make it into the hospital's standards of care.

The only other products to stock that don't meet those criteria are emergency drugs (which are not "shopped" so do not need to be priced as commodities), and "starter" packs to commence treatment and for which longer-term therapy may eventually be outsourced (e.g., diets, parasite control products, nonsteroidal antiinflammatory drugs [NSAIDs], etc.).

Online pharmacies that work with veterinary practices allow veterinarians access to a wide range of products that can be provided for home delivery, but the inventory itself is held and managed by the online pharmacy. The online pharmacy has its base price on products for the veterinary hospital, to cover the product direct and indirect costs and a profit margin for the online pharmacy. The veterinary hospital can then establish the retail price for its clients and the difference between the base price and the retail price (less any merchant fees) is paid back to the practice as margin. In this way, practices can make at least some profit on inventory that they never have to stock. So, while there is less revenue generated, there are substantial savings on inventory costs.

Veterinarians can sometimes fool themselves into believing that they make more money selling the products from their in-house pharmacy because it is cheaper to buy the products directly from the manufacturer or distributor, but that often neglects the fact that there are very real ordering and carrying costs for inventory (often 20–45% of the direct product costs), and for many products it is actually more profitable to dispense them from an online pharmacy than to stock them in the hospital.

Online pharmacies not only allow veterinary hospitals to limit their in-house inventory expenses, but in many ways, they may actually improve profitability of dispensing in general. They virtually eliminate shrinkage (product reduction due to wastage, loss, or theft) since those products aren't available in the hospital to be diverted. Without having to contend with inventory costs, every online product sale can be profitable. The same cannot be said for in-hospital pharmacy sales.

When it comes to online pharmacies, pricing can be competitive by design. There may be less profit margin for some products than others based on retail competition, but since there are no direct or indirect inventory costs, it is possible to compete even with slim margins (see 10.13 Approach to Pricing).

Another benefit of online pharmacies is that compliance is often much improved, especially for chronic medications and parasite control products. This is a very important component of pet-specific care. Once the medication has been prescribed and the number of refills documented, it is typically the online pharmacy that follows up with clients to ensure they are getting their refills in a timely manner. Not surprisingly, this feature alone has been responsible for increased pharmacy profitability and customer satisfaction in many instances.

9.10.7 Hospital Team Considerations

Paying production (commission) on products tends to inflate the costs of those products to the consumer so is likely not sustainable in the long run as practices attempt to keep the price of products competitive for clients. Clients who purchase products outside the veterinary channel, such as buying from a retailer or an unaffiliated internet pharmacy, do little to support veterinary hospitals directly or indirectly. That represents lost opportunities for everyone concerned.

For hospitals that compensate their doctors based on production, online pharmacies can cause some trepidation as veterinarians wonder if they are going to make less money when fewer products are being dispensed directly and for which they would otherwise receive a commission. It's certainly a concern, but there are ways of structuring things to minimize that angst.

Interestingly, clients may pay the online pharmacy for products and characterize that spend as separate from the veterinary hospital, and still spend comparably at the hospital because that is their expectation. Thus, if clients are used to spending a certain amount of money during a veterinary visit, many will still spend close to that amount (perhaps opting for additional diagnostics, dental care, etc. if offered), and consider the bill from the online pharmacy as a separate expenditure.

If that doesn't happen, some hospitals have altered the percentage compensation on professional services, or even switched from revenue sharing (production) to profit sharing based on the margins that the online pharmacy pays to the hospital. Removing production altogether by paying salaries is another option worth considering, since commission sales often get harder to justify with each passing year as margins

tighten. It is worthwhile to everyone to make this a win–win situation, since it lowers costs for the hospital, which in turn allows the hospital to lower costs to clients, which itself leads to greater compliance and client satisfaction.

TAKE-AWAYS

- Veterinary hospitals need to evolve in their handling of dispensing, or they run the risk of ongoing erosion of this important revenue stream.
- Since pharmacy is still the largest revenue-generating category for most practices, veterinarians need to consider strategies to maintain a meaningful share of this dispensing revenue … or change the veterinary business model so that it is not quite so dependent on this source of income.
- Veterinary teams should focus on pharmacy items that help ensure successful outcomes and client satisfaction.
- In-house pharmacy items can be limited to those that satisfy standards of care, those that help ensure compliance, those that are profitable to keep in stock, and those considered medically necessary for practice.
- Online pharmacies can be very useful for dispensing products not routinely used, those unprofitable to keep in stock, or those where refill compliance has been problematic for the hospital.

MISCELLANEOUS

Recommended Reading

Ackerman, L. (2009). What's the future of the veterinary pharmacy? *Veterinary Forum* 26 (12): 2–17.

Ackerman, L. (2019). Ready to partner with an online pharmacy? *AAHA Trends* 35 (1): 49–53.

Ackerman, L. (2020). Pharmacy management as a profit center. In: *Five-Minute Veterinary Practice Management Consult*, 3e (ed. L. Ackerman), 622–623. Ames, IA: Wiley.

American Animal Hospital Association (2019). *Financial & Productivity Pulsepoints*, 10e. Lakewood, CO. AAHA Press.

Heinke, M.L. and JB, M.C. (2012). *Practice Made Perfect: A Complete Guide to Veterinary Management*, 2e. Lakewood, CO: AAHA Press.

Mealey, K.L. (2019). *Pharmacotherapeutics for Veterinary Dispensing*. Ames, IA: Wiley Blackwell.

Packaged Facts (2019). *Pet Medications in the U.S.*, 6e. www.packagedfacts.com/Pet-Medications-Edition-12543601.

9.11

Vaccination

Lori Massin Teller, DVM, BS (Vet Sci), DABVP (Canine/Feline Practice)

Department of Small Animal Clinical Sciences, College of Veterinary Medicine & Biomedical Sciences, Texas A&M University, College Station, TX, USA

BASICS

9.11.1 Summary

Preventing disease is much easier than treating it. Vaccination has been one of the safest, easiest, and most cost-efficient ways to prevent and control the spread of infectious diseases and has led to better health and longer lifespans. Many infectious diseases are species specific, but some can be spread between species, including to humans, making the vaccination of our pets an important component of public health. Canine distemper, parvovirus, feline herpesvirus (FHV), calicivirus, and panleukopenia still persist in much of the world and can be rampant in Asia and Africa. When one of these diseases occurs in a shelter or kennel environment, there can be widespread morbidity, and these facilities may have to temporarily close to contain the problem. It is important that the appropriate immunizations are administered at the appropriate time and in the appropriate manner to be most effective at preventing disease.

9.11.2 Terms Defined

Core Vaccines: Offer protection against highly contagious, life-threatening infections or those that pose a serious threat to human health.

DNA or Recombinant DNA Vaccine: Contains protein antigens from the virus that stimulate an immune response.

Killed or Inactivated Vaccine: Does not contain a weakened form of the live virus, but contains the antigen with an adjuvant to help stimulate the immune response.

Modified Live Virus (MLV) Vaccine: Also known as live attenuated vaccine, it contains a weakened or attenuated form of the infectious agent to stimulate an immune response.

Morbidity: Having a disease, or the clinical signs associated with a disease.

Noncore Vaccines: Offer protection against less serious infections or those that provide a regional risk.

MAIN CONCEPTS

For vaccinations to be most effective, they should be administered according to manufacturer directions and the most recent guidelines published by reputable organizations, such as the American Animal Hospital Association (AAHA) [1], the American Association of Feline Practitioners (AAFP) [2], and the World Small Animal Veterinary Association (WSAVA) [3]. Recommendations for vaccinations are divided into core and noncore immunizations. Core vaccinations should be given to all animals, regardless of their location or lifestyle, unless another medical problem precludes immunization. Veterinarians must regularly evaluate their patient's lifestyle and environment, so they can recommend and administer noncore vaccines as appropriate to best protect the animal's health.

Canine core vaccines include rabies (killed or inactivated) and MLV or recombinant distemper, parvovirus, adenovirus-2, ± parainfluenza, which can be administered in a combination vaccine. Noncore vaccines should be administered based on the dog's risk of infection and include *Leptospira*, *Bordetella bronchiseptica*, *Borrelia burgdorferi* (Lyme disease), canine influenza H3N2, canine influenza H3N8, and *Crotalus atrox* (Western diamondback rattlesnake).

Feline core vaccines include rabies (killed or inactivated) and MLV or recombinant panleukopenia, calicivirus, and herpesvirus-1. Noncore vaccines should be administered based on the cat's risk and include feline leukemia (FeLV), feline immunodeficiency virus (FIV), *Bordatella bronchiseptica*, *Chlamydophila felis*, feline infectious peritonitis, and dermatophytosis. While FeLV is not considered a core vaccine, the AAFP and WSAVA recommend that kittens receive the initial pediatric series regardless of their current or future risk. Once they have reached adulthood, they only need to be revaccinated if they are at risk of exposure. Not all of these vaccines are available in all countries.

When presented with a puppy or kitten, it is important to understand how an immature immune system processes a vaccine and to educate the client about the appropriate immunization schedule to provide the best protection. *In utero*, a minimal quantity of maternal antibodies is passed from the dam or queen to the fetuses. The newborn puppies or kittens then receive a more significant amount of maternal antibodies from the colostrum when they first begin nursing. This passive transfer of immunity does provide some initial protection, although the level of protection is dependent on the health and immune status of the mother as well as of her offspring. Over a period of several weeks, the level of maternal antibodies begins to wane, leaving the puppies or kittens unprotected from infectious pathogens. Depending on the species, the quantity of maternal antibodies transferred and absorbed, and the health of the neonate, most puppies and kittens will be left with inadequate protection starting at the age of 6 weeks and possibly up to 5 months.

Though the puppies and kittens may not have enough maternal antibodies remaining in their systems to prevent them from becoming infected, they may still have enough to interfere with their ability to respond to vaccine antigen. Maternal antibodies, even at lower levels, can neutralize the vaccine antigen or render it ineffective by impeding the immune system's ability to recognize and process the antigen. This is one of the reasons why pediatric patients are administered a series of vaccinations every 3–4 weeks until they reach 16–20 weeks of age. The final immunization in the pediatric series should be administered between 16-20 weeks in puppies and at 6 months of age in kittens.

In naïve animals that have yet to receive an immunization and that have no or low maternal antibody levels, the first vaccine administered primes the immune system. Antibodies are typically produced 10–14 days after the vaccine has been administered, though it may take up to 21 days for the maximum response. Subsequent vaccines in the series will lead to immunological memory and a stronger, quicker response to the antigen. While the first vaccination primes the system, immunity does not result until after immunological memory is in place following subsequent vaccinations.

Once a puppy or kitten has attained immunity, they will then be placed on a revaccination schedule. For core vaccines, dogs are revaccinated one year after completing the pediatric immunization series, and then every three years thereafter. Depending on the jurisdiction where the animal resides, the dog may need to be revaccinated for rabies on an annual, biennial, or triennial basis. Revaccination for noncore immunizations, such as *Leptospira*, *Borrelia*, *Bordetella*, canine influenza (both strains), and rattlesnake, typically occurs annually. Dogs that are overdue for leptospirosis, Lyme, canine influenza, and/or parenteral *Bordetella* booster and are within 18 months of a previous dose may receive a single dose booster. Dogs exceeding an 18-month interval should restart the initial two-dose series.

Dogs that are 16–20 weeks old when presented for initial vaccinations need to receive a second vaccination of canine distemper virus (CDV), canine adenovirus-2 (CAV), canine parvovirus (CPV), and, where at risk, *Leptospira*, Lyme, canine influenza virus (CIV), or rattlesnake, 3–4 weeks after the first. If a dog presents >20 weeks of age, then a single vaccination for CDV, CAV, and CPV is expected to provide immunity until the dog returns for revaccination one year later. However, *Leptospira*, CIV, Lyme, and rattlesnake vaccines need to be initially administered as a series of two immunizations, 3–4 weeks apart, regardless of the dog's age when first immunized against these diseases.

Cats that are 16+ weeks of age upon presentation for initial vaccinations should receive two doses of feline panleukopenia virus (FPV), FHV, and feline calicivirus (FCV), as well as FeLV, then be revaccinated one year later. Following that, cats should be revaccinated on a triennial basis for core vaccines except for rabies, where revaccination may be on an annual or triennial basis, depending on the vaccine used and the jurisdiction where the cat resides. For FeLV vaccines, annual or biennial revaccination is currently recommended until more is known about the vaccine's duration of immunity (DOI).

In the case of rabies immunization, jurisdictional law supersedes all else. In general, puppies and kittens should receive their first rabies immunization between 12 and 16 weeks, followed by another dose one year later. After that, almost all jurisdictions in the United States recognize a three-year revaccination interval, with a vaccine labeled for such, but it is incumbent upon the veterinarian and staff to be aware of local statutes, where municipal or state laws may dictate annual or biennial revaccination.

It is also very important that there is a minimum interval of two weeks between immunizations because there is a transient downregulation of the immune response that could potentially interfere with the effects of another vaccine given within 10–12 days of the first. It is acceptable to give the core vaccines at one appointment, then give the noncore vaccines, as long as there is a two-week interval between injections [1].

Dogs and cats should be revaccinated at the recommended intervals throughout their lives. There have been questions about the necessity of vaccinating dogs and cats in their senior years. While data are limited, it is well known that immune function can decline with advanced age in a process known as immunosenescence. Currently it is believed that while immune system function may decline, the memory cells probably maintain enough function to be protective against disease in most cases. However, this function may not be as robust as it was when the pet was younger, so at this time it is recommended that dogs and cats continue to be vaccinated based on the recommended schedules published by the AAHA, AAFP, and WSAVA.

Adverse events are uncommon, but can occur. Smaller dogs (≤10 kg) tend to be more susceptible to acute-onset adverse reactions. It is worth considering an alternative immunization schedule for these dogs to lessen side effects [4]. One alternative is to administer core vaccinations and then give the noncore vaccines two weeks later. Most adverse reactions are transient and mild; they include localized swelling, pain, pruritus, or formation of an abscess, granuloma, or seroma. Other transient reactions can include lethargy, inappetence, fever, generalized discomfort, vomiting, or diarrhea. On rare occasions, more serious adverse events may occur. These can include angioedema, urticaria, hives, collapse, dyspnea, immune-mediated hemolytic anemia or immune-mediated thrombocytopenia, cutaneous ischemic vasculopathy (more commonly associated with rabies vaccine), corneal endothelialitis (associated with CAV-1 vaccines, which are no longer available in the US), or, on extremely rare occasions, systemic anaphylaxis or death. Known or suspected adverse vaccination events should be reported to the United States Department of Agriculture Animal and Plant Health Inspection Services (USDA APHIS) Center for Veterinary Biologics, as well as to the manufacturer.

In rare cases, it is possible for a dog or cat to be vaccinated but fail to mount an appropriate immune response. The most common reason is interference from maternal antibodies. Other causes may include administering the vaccine at a lower volume or dose than recommended by the manufacturer, mishandling the vaccine before administration (i.e., not storing the vaccine properly), or the animal may be genetically predisposed to be a "nonresponder" or "low responder" [1, 2].

Another rare adverse event, occurring mostly in felines, is an injection site sarcoma (feline injection site sarcoma [FISS]) [6]. Initially it was believed that vaccines triggered the FISS, but later research has shown that any injectable drug can trigger a sarcoma. A FISS can be more difficult to remove than other soft tissue sarcomas, especially if located over the interscapular area. Generally radical resection of the mass and surrounding tissue will be needed. This is particularly difficult to accomplish over the interscapular area, and it is much more feasible to obtain surgical control if an affected leg or the tail has to be amputated vs removing tissue along the dorsum of the trunk.

For this reason, the AAFP has published guidance on the best locations to administer vaccines in cats [2]. They recommend that all immunizations be given as distally as possible on the limbs, and they further state that they should all be given subcutaneously instead of intramuscularly. Specifically, the rabies vaccine should be administered in the right hindlimb, below the stifle, the FeLV vaccine should be administered in the left hind imb, below the stifle, and the feline viral rhinotracheitis, calicivirus, and panleukopenia (FVRCP) should be administered in the right thoracic limb, below the elbow. A recent study has suggested an alternative location of administering vaccines in the cat's tail [7]. The study did not show a difference in level of response or side effects whether the vaccines were administered in the tail or in the distal limbs. It is also important to note that the use of distal limbs or tail as locations for vaccine administration is not common outside North America. The WSAVA guidelines recommend using the lateral thorax or abdomen as locations to administer vaccinations [3]. They also recommend alternating vaccine sites each time so that one year the rabies vaccine is given on the right side and the FVRCP on the left, and the next time, the rabies is given on the left and the FVRCP on the right. The WSAVA guidelines concur with those of the AAFP that immunizations be administered subcutaneously, not intramuscularly.

It is also important to note that the minimal risk of FISS is far outweighed by the benefits of protection from disease that is conferred by vaccination. While there are no specific anatomical locations recommended for the administration of canine immunizations, it is important to document route and location in the dog's medical records.

Concerns may be raised when a patient is immunocompromised because of chemotherapy for cancer or medical therapy for an autoimmune disease, or, in the case of cats, with FeLV or FIV. The benefits vs risks need to be evaluated for each patient. Where possible, a killed virus vaccine will be theoretically preferable to a modified live vaccine. In cases where immunosuppressive medications need to be administered, it would be a good idea to update any immunizations before initiating therapy to lessen risks whenever possible.

In addition to having knowledge of the patient's health status, life stage, and living environment, it's important to know what diseases are prevalent in the area where the patient lives or will be traveling to. A dog may live in the southwest US, but travel to the northeast for a summer vacation. It is important to discuss with the client the potential exposure to *Borrelia burgdorferi* and determine if vaccination is warranted.

The vaccination for FIV was a noncore vaccine for cats, but has been discontinued. In the US, FIV is seen in about 2–3% of healthy cats, and that rate obviously differs from country to country. The rate can be higher in cats that are sick or at a higher risk of infection, such as free-roaming, aggressive, male cats. The virus tends to be transmitted through bites. Casual contact is not considered an efficient way of spreading the disease, and cats that live in a stable environment where there are no acts of aggression tend not to contract the disease. Furthermore, there are different clades of FIV. In the US, clade A is found mostly along the west coast and clade B more diffusely across the country. However, the vaccine that was previously available protected against clades A and D (D has not been documented in the US). Therefore, if a veterinarian in Texas is presented with an outdoor male cat that is prone to fighting, the veterinarian will need to explain to the owner that the cat is susceptible to FIV, but the vaccine would not be likely to protect the cat from becoming infected. Other methods to keep the cat healthy will need to be discussed.

Medical record keeping and documentation are essential components to best practices surrounding immunizations (see 9.1 Medical Records). Maintaining accurate records will allow for continuity of care, help to avoid lapses in prevention of infectious disease, and allow for monitoring of potential adverse events. Documentation should include identifying information about the patient (name, breed, sex, including spay/neuter status, age, or birthdate, microchip number, rabies tag number); name and type of vaccine administered, including manufacturer and lot/serial number; date and route of administration; anatomica; site where administered; previous vaccine history; and medication the pet is receiving in case it could potentially interfere with the animal's ability to mount an immune response to the vaccine [1].

Appropriate storage and handling of vaccines is of the utmost importance to ensure maximum potency. While it may seem more efficient to reconstitute several vaccines at the start of each day, this will lead to decreased potency and less effective protection. Vaccines should not be reconstituted more than one hour before administration to maintain potency. It is also important that vaccines be stored at 2–8 °C [3]. Refrigerators in the US maintain a temperature of 4 °C. Temperatures outside this range can lead to breakdown of the vaccines and render them ineffective. Avoid using a dorm or bar-style refrigerator/freezer combination unit that has a single door and an exposed evaporator coil. These units pose a significant risk of freezing vaccines which makes them impotent.

A couple of other things to keep in mind: do not use a disinfectant to clean the patient's skin before administering an MLV because it could potentially inactivate the vaccine [3].

Intranasal and oral *Bordetella bronchiseptica* vaccines contain live gram-negative bacteria. The parenteral version is inactivated. If the intranasal or oral vaccine is inadvertently given parenterally, then cellulitis and an abscess may occur at the vaccine site. If this does happen, then the veterinarian may want to administer doxycycline for at least five days to stop bacterial replication and help prevent progression of adverse effects. Deaths have been reported from subsequent bacteremia and hepatic necrosis. It is also not recommended that oral or intranasal *Bordetella* vaccines be administered to a patient that is currently receiving antimicrobial therapy. The medication may inactivate the live virus in the vaccine and result in no or poor response to it.

EXAMPLES

Gracie is a 12-week-old, female Labrador retriever that was adopted one week ago by a family in Louisiana. The dog will mostly be a family pet, and she will accompany the owner on hunting trips. She is also scheduled to start group obedience training next week. The breeder had Gracie vaccinated against distemper, adenovirus-2, parainfluenza, parvovirus (DA2PP) when she was 9 weeks old. At presentation to the veterinary hospital, it is recommended that Gracie receive a booster against DA2PP today and then continue to receive booster vaccinations every 3–4 weeks until she is 16–20 weeks old. Today she is also old enough to receive her first rabies vaccination. Because of Gracie's expected lifestyle and her current age, she should also begin the immunization series for leptospirosis and receive her first *Bordetella* dose.

Gatsby is an outdoor, approximately 3-year-old intact male cat in Wisconsin that a client has just caught after feeding it for several weeks. The client would like to make sure the cat is healthy and add it to her household. She currently has two other adult cats that are neutered and current on rabies and FVRCP immunizations. They did receive the FeLV series as kittens, but the owner did not continue those into adulthood since the cats live only indoors.

Gatsby appeared healthy on physical exam and the veterinarian recommended testing him for FeLV and FIV. Gatsby was negative for both, and the veterinarian started the FVRCP and FeLV immunization series and administered a rabies vaccine. It was also recommended that Gatsby be kept separated from the other two cats for 14 days until it was determined that he wasn't harboring a respiratory virus, and that he be castrated. The veterinarian further recommended that since it is possible that Gatsby could have a latent FeLV infection or that the owner may choose to keep him as an indoor/outdoor cat or choose to adopt other cats in the future, she should resume vaccinating the other two cats against FeLV.

TAKE-AWAYS

- Pediatric vaccines are administered as a series to overcome the effects of maternal antibodies.
- Evaluate the patient's lifestyle at each wellness visit to determine appropriate immunizations to protect the pet's health.
- Separate the number of vaccines administered to small dogs to reduce the risk of adverse events.
- Store vaccines in a refrigerator and do not reconstitute until time to administer.
- Document route and anatomical site of vaccine administration in the medical record.

MISCELLANEOUS

References

1 Ford, R., Larson, L., McClure, K., Schultz, R., Welborn, L. 2017 AAHA Canine Vaccination Guidelines. www.aaha.org/guidelines/canine_vaccination_guidelines.aspx

2 Scherk, M., Ford, R., Gaskell, R. et al. (2013). 2013 AAFP feline vaccination advisory panel report. *Journal of Feline Medicine and Surgery* 15: 785–808.

3 Day, M., Horzinek, M., Schultz, R., Squires, R. WSAVA Guidelines for the Vaccination of Dogs and Cats. https://wsava.org/wp-content/uploads/2020/01/WSAVA-Vaccination-Guidelines-2015.pdf

4 Ford R. 2013 Canine Vaccination Guidelines: Implementing the Protocol. https://cvm.ncsu.edu/wp-content/uploads/2015/06/Ford_2013CANINEonlyVACCINEMNS.2.pdf

5 Ford R. Vaccines and Vaccinations: Update and Insights. www.oregonvma.org/files/Ford-Vaccines-Vaccination.pdf

6 Ford, R. Vital vaccination: feline injection site sarcoma. *Today's Veterinary Practice* https://todaysveterinarypractice.com/vital-vaccination-series-feline-injection-site-sarcoma.

7 Zabielska-Koczywąs, K., Wojtalewícz, A., and Lechowski, R. (2017). Current knowledge on feline injection site sarcoma treatment. *Acta Veterinaria Scandinavica* 59 (1): 47.

Recommended Reading

Day MJ, Kaekare U, Schultz R., et al. Recommendations on vaccination for Asian small animal practitioners: a report of the WSAVA Vaccination Guidelines Group. https://wsava.org/wp-content/uploads/2020/01/Recommendations-on-vaccination-for-Asian-small-animal-practitioners-report.pdf

Day, M., Horzinek, M., Schultz, R., Squires, R. 2015 Vaccination Guidelines for the Owners and Breeders of Dogs and Cats. https://wsava.org/wp-content/uploads/2020/01/WSAVA-Owner-Breeder-Guidelines-2015_1.pdf

Teller, L. (2018). Vaccination best practices. *Veterinary Team Brief*: 29–32.

Newbury S, Blinn M, Bushby P, et al. Guidelines for Standards of Care in Animals Shelters. www.sheltervet.org/assets/docs/shelter-standards-oct2011-wforward.pdf

9.12

Judicious Use of Antimicrobials

Patricia Dowling, DVM, MSc, DACVIM (LAIM), DACVCP

Veterinary Clinical Pharmacology, Western College of Veterinary Medicine, Saskatoon, Saskatchewan, Canada

BASICS

9.12.1 Summary

In recent years there have been important changes in antimicrobial therapy. There are new antimicrobials available and there is a greater database of species-specific pharmacokinetic information available for antimicrobials used in veterinary medicine, which allows for more accurate drug dosing. Concern over the continued development of bacterial resistance to antimicrobials has heightened the awareness of judicious use of antimicrobials. There is increasing veterinary oversight of antimicrobial use in animals and veterinarians are expected to document an evidence-based need for antimicrobial therapy.

9.12.2 Terms Defined

Concentration-Dependent Antimicrobials: Antimicrobials whose efficacy is associated with achieving high concentrations at the site of infection.
Minimum Inhibitory Concentration: The lowest drug concentration that inhibits bacterial growth.
Pharmacodynamics (PD**):** What the drug does to the bacteria – kill or inhibit growth.
Pharmacokinetics (PK**):** What the body does to a drug, including absorption, distribution, metabolism, and excretion.
Postantibiotic Effect (PAE**):** The period of time for whichbacterial growth remains suppressed after antimicrobial concentration has decreased below the minimum inhibitory concentration (MIC).

Time-Dependent Antimicrobials: Antimicrobials whose efficacy is associated with keeping concentrations above the bacterial MIC for some proportion of the dosage interval.

MAIN CONCEPTS

9.12.3 Considerations Before Starting Antimicrobial Therapy

9.12.3.1 Does the Diagnosis Warrant Antimicrobial Therapy?

Using antimicrobials to treat minor infections or purely viral or inflammatory diseases is irrational and expensive, can be hazardous to the patient and encourages antimicrobial resistance. Clients have come to expect antimicrobials for trivial infections or "just in case" an infection may develop. The veterinary team must resist client pressure to use or prescribe unnecessary drugs.

9.12.3.2 What Pathogens Are Likely to Be Involved?

For many infections, the likely pathogen can be successfully predicted from the history and clinical signs (e.g., urinary tract and skin infections in dogs).

9.12.3.3 What is the *In Vitro* Antimicrobial Susceptibility of the Pathogen?

The signs of some infectious diseases are so obvious that the need for microbiological identification is minimal but for those infectious diseases of unknown cause or for those attributable to pathogens with irregular antimicrobial susceptibility, there is no substitute for isolation and identification of the causative agent.

9.12.3.4 In What Part of the Body or Tissue is the Infection Located? Will the Antimicrobial Reach the Site of Infection in Effective Concentrations?

Consideration of the pathophysiology of the infection will aid in selection of effective therapy. Treatment of sequestered infections such as prostatitis or meningitis requires antimicrobials that readily cross membrane barriers. Antimicrobials characterized by low values for volume of distribution are unlikely to reach therapeutic concentrations in such sites.

9.12.3.5 Will the Antimicrobial Be Effective in the Local Environment of the Pathogen?

For some antimicrobials the local infection environment reduces their efficacy. Sulfonamides are ineffective in purulent debris, as paraamino benzoic acid (PABA) released from decaying neutrophils serves as a PABA source for bacteria and reduces the competitive effect of the sulfonamide. Aminoglycosides are ineffective in an abscess due to the acidic, anaerobic environment along with the presence of nucleic acid material from decaying cells which inactivates the aminoglycosides (see Table 9.12.1).

9.12.3.6 What Adverse Drug Reaction or Toxicities May Occur? Do the Benefits of Treatment Outweigh the Risks?

The risks of adverse reactions from antimicrobials are often underappreciated. A serious adverse reaction may complicate treatment of the original problem and even be fatal. Failure to communicate the risks of adverse drug reactions to clients is a common cause of litigation.

Table 9.12.1 Efficacy of antimicrobials in abscesses

Very effective	Moderately effective	Ineffective
Rifampin	Erythromycin (pH)	Aminoglycosides (pH, debris)
Florfenicol	Fluoroquinolones (pH)	Beta-lactams (penetration)
Tetracyclines		Sulfonamides (penetration, debris)

9.12.3.7 What Drug Formulation and Dosage Regimen will Maintain the Appropriate Antimicrobial Concentrations for the Proper Duration of Time?

Label doses only apply to label pathogens and disease states. When treating "extralabel," the dosage regimen must be adjusted for the antimicrobial susceptibility of the specific pathogen and pathophysiological changes in the patient.

9.12.4 Antimicrobial Dosage Design

Successful antimicrobial therapy relies on administering sufficient doses so that pathogens at the site of infection are killed or sufficiently suppressed that they can be eliminated by the host's immune system. An effective antimicrobial dosage regimen depends on both a measure of drug exposure (PK) and a measure of the potency of the drug against the infecting pathogen (PD).

Drug concentration at the infection site is assumed to be of major importance in determining drug efficacy. The PK parameters of an antimicrobial (absorption, distribution, metabolism, and excretion) are determined by molecular size, lipid solubility, drug pKa, local pH, specific cellular transport mechanisms, and degree of protein binding. The PK parameters used in dosage design are the area under the plasma concentration versus time curve (area under the curve [AUC]) from 0 to 24 hours, the maximum plasma concentration (Cmax), and the time the antimicrobial concentration exceeds a defined PD threshold (T). PD is the relationship between bacteria and antimicrobial and is described by the MIC, which is the lowest drug concentration that inhibits bacterial growth. In relating the PK and PD parameters to clinical efficacy, antimicrobial drug action is classified as either concentration dependent or time dependent.

Other considerations include the PAE and the drug effect on the pathogen (see Table 9.12.2). For some bacteria–drug interactions, bacterial growth remains suppressed for a period after drug concentration has decreased below the MIC and this is known as the PAE. The PAE may be the reason why dosage regimens that fail to maintain drug concentration above the MIC are still efficacious. The PAE is dependent on both the antimicrobial and the bacterial pathogen.

It is common to classify antimicrobials as bactericidal or bacteriostatic (see Table 9.12.3). For many drugs, the distinction between bactericidal and bacteriostatic is not exact, and may depend on the drug concentration attained in the target tissue and the pathogen involved.

Table 9.12.2   Postantibiotic effects

	Long PAE(>3 h)	Intermediate PAE	Short PAE (<1 h)
Gram positives	Fluoroquinolones	Aminoglycosides	
	Macrolides	Penicillins	
	Chloramphenicol	Cephalosporins	
	Tetracyclines		
Gram negatives	Fluoroquinolones		Penicillins
	Aminoglycosides		Cephalosporins
Anaerobes	Metronidazole		

Table 9.12.3   Effect of antimicrobials on bacteria

Bactericidal	Bacteriostatic
Fluoroquinolones	Chloramphenicol
Aminoglycosides	Tetracyclines
Penicillins	Macrolides
Cephalosporins	Lincosamides
Trimethoprim/sulfas	Sulfonamides

Specific situations in which a bactericidal drug may be preferred over a bacteriostatic drug include immunosuppressed patients (cancer patients), septicemia, and surgical prophylaxis.

9.12.4.1   Concentration-Dependent Antimicrobials

For antimicrobials whose efficacy is concentration dependent, high plasma concentrations relative to the MIC of the pathogen (Cmax:MIC) and the area under the plasma concentration–time curve that is above the bacterial MIC during the dosing interval (area under the inhibitory curve) ($AUC_{0-24\,h}$:MIC) are the major determinants of clinical efficacy. These drugs also have prolonged PAEs, which allows once-daily dosing with maintenance of maximum clinical efficacy. For fluoroquinolones (e.g., enrofloxacin, orbifloxacin, pradofloxacin, marbofloxacin), clinical efficacy is associated with achieving either an AUC_{0-24h}:MIC of more than 125 or a Cmax:MIC of more than 10. For aminoglycosides (e.g., gentamicin, amikacin), achieving a Cmax:MIC of more than 10 is considered optimal for efficacy. For extralabel pathogens with high MIC values, such as *Pseudomonas aeruginosa* in cases of otitis externa in dogs, achieving the optimum PK:PD ratios with oral therapy may be impossible with label or even higher than label dosages. In such cases, underdosing is ineffective and contributes to antimicrobial resistance.

9.12.4.2   Time-Dependent Antimicrobials

For antimicrobials whose efficacy is time dependent, the time during which the antimicrobial concentration exceeds the MIC of the pathogen (T>MIC) determines clinical efficacy. The penicillins, cephalosporins, most macrolides and lincosamides, tetracyclines, chloramphenicol, and potentiated sulfonamides are considered time-dependent antimicrobials. How much above the MIC and for what percentage of the dosing interval concentrations should be above the MIC still are being debated and likely are specific for individual bacteria–drug combinations. Typically, exceeding the MIC by 1–5 multiples for between 40% and 100% of the dosing interval is appropriate for time-dependent antimicrobial agents. The time that the concentration exceeds MIC should be closer to 100% for bacteriostatic antimicrobials and for patients that are immunosuppressed. Therefore these drugs typically require frequent dosing or constant-rate infusions for appropriate therapy. Exceptions are the third-generation cephalosporins cefovecin and cefpodoxime. They maintain concentrations above the target MIC for seven days (cefovecin) or 24 hours (cefpodoxime) because of a high degree of protein binding.

9.12.5   Concurrent Use of Additional Antimicrobials

Combination antimicrobial therapy is commonplace in veterinary medicine, but has rarely been demonstrated as superior to single-drug therapy in clinical trials. In addition to increased costs, there is usually also an increased risk of adverse effects from the administration of multiple antimicrobials (e.g., antimicrobial-associated diarrhea). Use of multiple antimicrobial drugs should be limited to:

- known synergism against specific organisms (e.g., beta-lactams plus aminoglycosides in the treatment of enterococcal endocarditis)

- prevention of the rapid development of bacterial resistance (e.g., trimethoprim in combination with a sulfonamide)
- extending the antimicrobial spectrum of initial therapy of life-threatening conditions (e.g., beta-lactams plus aminoglycosides to cover gram-positive, gram-negative, and anaerobic bacteria)
- treating mixed bacterial infections (e.g., cefazolin plus enrofloxacin in the treatment of pneumonia).

Known antagonistic combinations of antimicrobials should be avoided, such as penicillin with tetracycline (penicillin acts on actively dividing cell walls, while tetracyclines are bacteriostatic in action).

9.12.6 Prophylactic Antimicrobial Therapy

The relative risk of infection must warrant the use of prophylactic antimicrobials. The risks of the prophylactic drug must be less than the risk of development of disease and its consequences. In veterinary medicine, most of the risk of infection depends on the skill of the surgeon and handling practices in the hospital. Most prudent use guidelines recommend against prophylactic antimicrobial therapy for routine neutering of dogs and cats, and for routine, uncomplicated dental procedures. The organism(s) that are likely to cause the infection and their antimicrobial susceptibility should be known or accurately predicted. The antimicrobial must be administered and must distribute to the site of potential infection before the onset of infection. Therefore, choose antimicrobials that can be given intravenously and have a high volume of distribution. The duration of antimicrobial prophylaxis should be as abbreviated as possible. Most of the time, a single preoperative dose is sufficient. Prophylactic antimicrobials should be bactericidal rather than bacteriostatic. Drugs used prophylactically should not be those that would be used therapeutically.

EXAMPLES

Max is 2-year-old golden retriever who has peritonitis and septicemia after ingesting a peach pit that caused an intestinal perforation. You need broad-spectrum antimicrobial therapy to cover gram-positive, gram-negative, and anaerobic bacteria. You decide to administer gentamicin and cefazolin intravenously. Gentamicin is a concentration-dependent killer with a long PAE for gram-negative bacteria and PK/PD integration supports the dosage of 9 mg/kg every 24 hours. As cefazolin is a time-dependent killer with a short elimination half-life but long PAE for gram-positive bacteria, PK/PD integration supports the dosage of 20 mg/kg every eight hours.

TAKE-AWAYS

- Determine that antimicrobial therapy is truly indicated.
- Use culture and susceptibility testing to choose the most appropriate antimicrobial.
- Use dosage regimens based on PK/PD integration.
- Only use combinations of antimicrobials where specifically indicated for synergistic or additive effects.
- Follow prudent use guidelines for appropriate prophylactic antimicrobial therapy.

MISCELLANEOUS

Recommended Reading

Giguere, S., Prescott, J.F., Baggot, J.D. et al. (eds.) (2013). *Antimicrobial Therapy in Veterinary Medicine*, 5e. Ames, IA: Blackwell Publishing.

Toutain, P.L. and Lees, P. (2004). Integration and modeling of pharmacokinetic and pharmacodynamic data to optimize dosage regimens in veterinary medicine. *J. Vet. Pharmacol. Ther.* 27: 467–477.

9.13

Preanesthetic Considerations

Tamara Grubb, DVM, PhD, DACVAA

Washington State University, Pullman, WA, USA

BASICS

9.13.1 Summary

Preanesthetic considerations encompass much more than just drug selection for the patient. Anesthetic safety begins in the preanesthetic period. Ensuring that anesthesia will be as safe as possible includes a good physical exam (PE), history, and completion of pertinent diagnostic tests. Stabilization of the patient, either short or long term, may also be necessary. Complete preparation of all anesthetic, monitoring, and support equipment should be a major focus in the preanesthetic period. Drugs administered as preanesthetics include both sedatives and analgesic drugs, but drugs for all phases of anesthesia, including analgesia and patient support (e.g., drugs to improve blood pressure), should be calculated and readied. Adequate preparation is key to safe anesthesia and all tasks just described should be completed prior to administration of any anesthetic drugs.

MAIN CONCEPTS

Anesthesia should be thought of as four distinct and equally important phases: (i) preanesthesia; (ii) induction; (iii) maintenance; and (iv) recovery. We tend to overlook the importance of preanesthesia and recovery, yet these phases contribute as much to the overall safety and efficacy of anesthesia as induction and maintenance. The preanesthesia phase is not just about administering drugs ("premedication") but also about patient *and* equipment preparation to ensure that the patient will be as safe as possible during the entire anesthetic period. In most instances, appropriate patient preparation is more important than actual anesthetic drug selection, although drug dose is always extremely important. A checklist (see Table 9.13.1) should be used to ensure that no preparatory step is inadvertently omitted [1].

9.13.2 Preanesthetic Patient Preparation at Home

Patient preparation for anesthesia begins at home. On the day of anesthesia, the owner should be advised to withhold food ("fast") from their pet but to allow the pet access to water at all times. Fasting in most healthy patients has traditionally been done by preventing access to food, starting at just after midnight on the day of the surgery. However, this recommendation is now under scrutiny and shorter fasting times are becoming more common. It is likely that fast times of no more than six hours are adequate for most patients and this is now commonly recommended [2]. There is some evidence that a small meal (half of the normal meal volume, canned food) three hours prior to anesthesia may decrease gastric reflux [3]. However, this is not yet commonly utilized and more evidence is needed before a recommendation of feeding near the surgery time is made. Neonates that are suckling should be fasted for no more than one hour and diabetic patients are generally fasted for no more than four hours. Both groups of patients should be fed as soon as possible following return to normal swallowing in the recovery phase of anesthesia. Denying the pet water could lead to dehydration and is not recommended for any pet.

In general, all medications that the patient is currently receiving should be administered as prescribed on the day of anesthesia [2]. The exceptions are some cardiac medications

Table 9.13.1 Preanesthetic checklist [1]

Anesthesia Checklist: must be completed prior to anesthetizing any patient. Address every item. Check when complete or mark with an "x" if not required. No blanks!   ☑/X

Patient and record

Drugs administered within the last 24 hours, including those administered at home (e.g., anxiolytics, cardiac medications, etc.) discussed with the doctor and documented in chart

Fasted (document duration in record if outside recommended limits)

Physical exam (document concerns in chart)

History (document concerns in chart)

Weight (written in chart and on anesthetic record)

Laboratory work (listed in chart)

Other diagnostics (listed in chart)

Anesthetic record started with appropriate patient information and drug dosages

Pain score sheet ready for recovery

Anesthesia equipment: set up before anesthetizing patient

Oxygen tank on or oxygen line connected

Oxygen supply adequate (>200 psi in tank)

Vaporizer full

Breathing system connected (rebreathing >5 kg, 11 lb; nonrebreathing <5 kg, 11 lb)

Connect fresh gas supply line to breathing system. Check and double check this one!

CO_2 absorbent checked/changed every 6–10 hours of use or if two-thirds of crystals are blue

Machine and breathing system pressure checked to 30 cmH$_2$O

Pressure relief valve (pop-off valve) open!!!!!

Monitoring equipment: set up and check function before anesthetizing patient

Monitors turned on and all cables attached (ECG, blood pressure, ETCO$_2$, SpO$_2$)

Blood pressure cuff (correct size)

Lube or alcohol for ECG clips

Thermometer or temperature probe

Anesthesia support supplies and drugs: set up before anesthetizing patient

Mask for preoxygenation

Eye lube

IV catheter, catheter cap or line, tape, and saline (+/− heparinized) for flush

Laryngoscope

Endotracheal tubes (at least 2 sizes), cuffs leak tested, tube tie attached

Syringe to inflate/deflate tube cuff

Stylet for tubes under 5.0 mm

Lidocaine for cats (1–2 drops on each arytenoid)

Circulating warm water blanket on and covered with towel or blanket or forced air warming blanket ready

IV fluids (warmed) with appropriate drip set (15 or 60 drops/mL)

Anticipated support drugs (e.g., dopamine, atropine, etc.) calculated and ready

Warm/quiet area for recovery identified and prepared

Anesthetic and analgesic drugs

Drugs discussed with veterinarian and drug dosages calculated, including:

- Preanesthetic sedative and analgesic drugs
- Induction drug(s)
- Maintenance drug(s) (if not inhalant)
- Local anesthetic drug for local/regional block(s)
- Other analgesic drugs (e.g., constant rate infusion drugs)

Source: Grubb and Albi [1].

and insulin, whose dosages are generally decreased to decrease their impact on blood pressure or blood glucose, respectively [2]. Other drugs, such as anxiolytics and/or antiemetics, may be recommended for administration prior to leaving home. Stress/fear/anxiety can decrease anesthetic safety by increasing the dose of drugs necessary to achieve anesthesia. The higher dosages are more likely to cause adverse effects. Trazodone and/or gabapentin are commonly used as prehospital visit anxiolytics [1, 2]. Maropitant or other antiemetics should be considered for those patients likely to become nauseous or vomit during the car ride to the veterinary clinic [1, 2].

9.13.2.1 Preanesthetic Patient Preparation in the Hospital

Patient preparation in the hospital should start with a thorough PE, even in presumably healthy patients. Since animals can't self-report that they may be having health issues, it is up to the veterinary professional to identify, or rule out, those issues. An important and accurate medical adage is "More is missed by not looking than by not knowing" (Thomas McCrae MD, 1870–1935). Preparation should also include a comprehensive history, including questions about current and past health concerns, concurrent medications or supplements, and information on familial history, if available. Asking about health concerns, even for patients seen frequently at your hospital, is vital since new health concerns, or old health concerns that the owners have forgotten to mention, may be revealed. Concurrent medications, along with any adverse effects caused by the medications, need to be reviewed and the medications may need to be discontinued or changed prior to anesthesia. The owner should be asked directly whether the patient is receiving any other products or supplements. Owners often don't realize that herbal supplements, aspirin, cannabis cookies, etc. have effects that can impact anesthesia/surgery and they may not think to mention these products unless directly asked.

Familial history can be important in identifying potential heritable conditions or familial tendencies to drug reactions. This is especially important in patients whose individual response to anesthesia is unknown, as in patients undergoing their first anesthetic episode.

Diagnostic tests may be necessary to identify, rule out, or define the degree of underlying disease. Healthy patients for brief elective procedures may need only the PE and perhaps very basic lab work, for example measurement of packed cell volume (PCV) and total protein. Patients with more health concerns or extremes of age (neonate, geriatric) should have more robust testing that likely includes a full complete blood count (CBC), serum chemistry analysis, and potentially a urine analysis. Seemingly healthy geriatric pets can have a fairly high incidence of underlying disease that is discovered during preanesthetic testing, and may result in changes in the anesthetic protocol or postponement/cancelation of the anesthetic procedure [4–6].

Depending on patient need and suspected or known disease conditions, there are numerous specific diagnostic laboratory tests that may be appropriate. Examples include bile acid analysis for patients with hepatic disease, thyroid stimulating hormone (TSH) assay for patients with thyroid dysfunction, a feline leukemia test for sick cats or cats exposed to other cats with the virus, and fructosamine measurement in diabetic patients. An electrocardiogram (ECG) is recommended, especially in geriatric and compromised patients. Arrhythmias are common in these two populations and the arrhythmia may need to be treated prior to anesthesia. Advanced imaging such as thoracic/abdominal radiographs or ultrasound may also be warranted in select patients. Diagnostic tests should not be omitted. Identification of underlying disease will significantly decrease the likelihood of anesthesia-related adverse events because the anesthesia plan can be better individualized for the patient and the veterinary team can be prepared for patient-specific monitoring and support.

Patients should never be rushed to anesthesia unless they are in danger of immediate death if not anesthetized. An example of that situation is a patient who is actively hemorrhaging into its abdomen from a ruptured splenic mass. In this case, immediate abdominal surgery to control the bleeding may be the only chance the patient has for survival. Outside this type of emergency, all patients should be stabilized prior to anesthesia. Stabilization, defined as treatment of a disease or pathological condition to minimize the impact of that condition on patient safety during anesthesia, could mean treatment for several hours to several days or even weeks, depending on the condition. Examples of these scenarios are provided at the end of this topic. Risk of anesthetic death is increased as the American Society of Anesthesiologists (ASA) status (see Table 9.13.2) is increased [7]. Stabilization can decrease the ASA status, thereby decreasing the risk of anesthetic death, so the value of stabilization should never be overlooked.

Once all of the history questions and diagnostic tests are complete, and stabilization has occurred (if necessary), the anesthetic process should be explained to the pet owner. The owner should be asked if they have any concerns about anesthesia and all concerns should be thoroughly discussed (see 5.12 Discussing Anesthetic Risk).

Following a checklist (see Table 9.13.1) with all the information described in this chapter will eliminate accidental oversights in preparation that could lead to patient compromise. The checklist should be filled out in its entirety for every patient. The checklist can be laminated, filled in with information for the current patient, copied for the patient record, and then wiped clean for the next patient. But remember that the checklist is just that – a list. More detailed information on the patient's current medications, PE, and diagnostic test findings and relevant history should be documented in the patient's chart, along with any concerns for anesthesia. The checklist is used to indicate that these data have been collected and reviewed by the veterinarian. The anesthetic record should be filled out with relevant patient information, as should the pain scoring sheet to be used in recovery.

Table 9.13.2 American Society of Anesthesiologists (ASA) physical status

Status	Description
ASA 1	Normal healthy patient
ASA 2	Patients with mild systemic disease
ASA 3	Patients with moderate to severe systemic disease
ASA 4	Patients with severe systemic disease that is a constant threat to life
ASA 5	Moribund patients who are not expected to survive without the operation

Source: Grubb et al. [1, 2].

9.13.3 Preanesthetic Preparation of Equipment

The anesthetic machine should be connected to the oxygen source and the source should be checked to insure an adequate oxygen supply. The oxygen tank (small tank [E-tank] on the machine or large tank [H-tank] for hospital-wide supply) should contain at least 200 psi (pounds per square inch). The vaporizer should be filled at the beginning of the day and should be at least 50% full for every patient. The appropriate-sized breathing system (rebreathing >5 kg, 11 lb; nonrebreathing<5 kg, 11 lb) should be connected to the machine and the fresh-gas supply line (line carrying oxygen and inhalants to the breathing system) should be attached to the breathing system in the correct location. This is critical! Without this step, the patient will not be receiving oxygen and anesthetic gas. The carbon dioxide absorbent should be changed every 6–10 hours of use or when two-thirds of the granules in the canister have turned blue.

A critical step is to pressure check the machine and breathing system to a pressure of 30 cmH$_2$O (water). The machine should be checked between every patient since leaks can develop at any time. If the machine leaks, the patient will not be receiving adequate oxygen or anesthetic gases – and the anesthetic gases will not be scavenged so may be inhaled by veterinary personnel, which can create health concerns. Once the machine has been checked, the pressure relief (or "pop-off") valve must be opened! Failure to do this can result in dangerously high airway pressures within just a few minutes of connecting the endotracheal tube to the breathing system. A safer option is to have a button-type valve that requires pressing by the anesthetist to close and that opens automatically as soon as the anesthetist's finger is removed from the button.

All monitoring and support equipment (e.g., warming devices) should be set up, turned on, and checked for proper function prior to the administration of premedications. All supplies and equipment should be ready so that the team can act quickly if the patient experiences any adverse effects from the drugs, with potential need for immediate support or intervention. The middle of a crisis is not the time to determine that the anesthetic monitors are not working. Monitoring equipment should include blood pressure, ECG, end-tidal carbon dioxide (ETCO2), oxygen saturation with the pulse oximeter (SpO2), and body temperature. A mask for delivery of oxygen prior to anesthesia ("preoxygenation"), intravenous (IV) catheter supplies, and eye lube should be set out, along with endotracheal tubes with cuffs leak-checked, tube ties, and a laryngoscope. Heating pads or blankets and warmed IV fluids with the appropriate-sized drip set (15 or 60 drops/mL) should also be prepared.

Dosages for support drugs like atropine and dopamine should be calculated and drugs should be drawn up if they are to be administered, or placed nearby if use is probable but not certain. Thinking ahead, a warm, quiet area for recovery should be identified.

9.13.3.1 Preanesthetic Selection of All Anesthetic Drugs and Calculation of Dosages

Finally, drugs and drug dosages should be chosen and tailored to the patient. Drugs to be considered include anesthetic and analgesic drugs for the four phases of anesthesia (premedication, induction, maintenance, and recovery). The drugs administered in the preanesthetic phase should include sedatives and analgesic drugs. Sedatives improve anesthetic safety by allowing a decreased dosage of induction and maintenance drugs. As previously stated, most adverse drug effects are dose dependent. Preemptive analgesia (analgesia administered prior to causing pain) is important because preventing pain is more effective than treating it. Drug choices are covered in more depth in other chapters but, briefly, to choose the safest and most effective drugs for each specific patient, consider [1, 2]:

- the health of the patient (unhealthy patients generally require lower dosages of drugs and may require less potent sedatives)
- the energy/stress level of the patient (high-energy or stressed patients usually require higher dosages of drugs and may require more potent sedatives)
- the reason why patient needs anesthesia. This usually means a surgical procedure but could be imaging, bandaging, etc. The duration, invasiveness, expected amount of blood loss, and expected impact on body temperature (e.g., an abdominal procedure is likely to cause a large degree of heat loss) should all be considered. This will affect support choices more than anesthetic drug choices but could determine whether the patient can be anesthetized with injectable drugs or inhalant drugs and will impact analgesic choices
- pain level expected (more painful procedures = need for more analgesia, local blocks should always be considered, constant rate infusions or repeat boluses may be required).

 EXAMPLES

Rocky, a 7-year old male castrated Labrador retriever, was just hit by a car and obviously has a fractured femur. The owner is very scared for the dog and wants Rocky to go to surgery immediately to fix the fracture, but you explain that Rocky is not physiologically stable for anesthesia, making anesthesia much more dangerous. Rocky is in shock, is painful, has lost a lot of blood, and has cardiac arrhythmias. These all greatly increase the risk of complications or even death during anesthesia. After a night of stabilization with IV fluids and pain medication, Rocky is no longer in shock or painful, his blood loss has stabilized, and the arrhythmias are gone. Now Rocky is ready for anesthesia.

Jerry, a 12-year old male castrated domestic shorthair cat, needs a dental procedure that may be long because several teeth need to be extracted. While taking the cat's history, you discover that Jerry has been sleeping more than usual and doesn't have the energy he used to have. You listen to the heart and take thoracic radiographs and diagnose Jerry with cardiac disease. You send Jerry home on cardiac medication – along with antibiotics and analgesics for the dental disease – for 2–4 weeks of stabilization.

Missy is a 14-year-old female spayed mixed-breed dog who needs anesthesia for removal of a small mass on her left foreleg. She is friendly and very calm. Because of her age and calmness, you determine that an opioid plus a benzodiazepine will be adequate for premedication.

Spidey is a 3-year old male intact extremely nervous Australian shepherd who will be castrated today. He is so nervous in the clinic that he is hiding under a chair, panting, and trying to avoid being touched but the owner cannot bring him back another day when he is calmer. Because of this high level of stress, you decide that an opioid plus an alpha-2 agonist (dosed at the high end of the range) will be necessary for adequate premedication and recommend that the owner administer previsit anxiolytics (e.g., gabapentin or trazodone) prior to the next hospital visit.

TAKE-AWAYS

- Anesthesia should be considered as four equally important phases: preanesthesia, induction, maintenance, and recovery. The patient's needs for each phase must be addressed.
- The preanesthesia phase of anesthesia includes not only administration of sedative and analgesic drugs ("premedication") but also preparation of the patient, which may include nothing more than a PE and basic diagnostics or may require advanced diagnostics and/or stabilization.

- Preanesthesia also includes preparation of anesthesia, monitoring, and support equipment and supplies. This should be complete before the patient is anesthetized.
- Anesthetic drugs and drug dosages should be based on patient health and tailored for the individual patient. Drugs administered in the preanesthesia phase should include both sedatives and analgesics. Administration of these drugs will increase anesthetic safety.
- Checklists can ensure that important steps are not omitted, which could jeopardize patient health.

MISCELLANEOUS

References

1 Grubb, T.L., Albi, M., Ensign, S. et al. (2020). *Anesthesia & Pain Management for Veterinary Nurses and Technicians*. Jackson, WY: Teton NewMedia.

2 Grubb, T., Sager, J., Gaynor, J.S. et al. (2020). AAHA anesthesia and monitoring guidelines for dogs and cats. *J. Am. Anim. Hosp. Assoc.* 56: 59–82.

3 Savvas, I., Raptopoulos, D., and Rallis, T. (2016c). A "light meal" three hours preoperatively decreases the incidence of gastro-esophageal reflux in dogs. *J. Am. Anim. Hosp. Assoc.* 52 (6): 357–363.

4 Joubert, K.E. (2007). Pre-anaesthetic screening of geriatric dogs. *J. S. Afr. Vet. Assoc.* 78 (1): 31–35.

5 Webb, J.A., Kirby, G.M., Nykamp, S.G., and Gauthier, M.J. (2012). Ultrasonographic and laboratory screening in clinically normal mature golden retriever dogs. *Can. Vet. J.* 53 (6): 626–630.

6 Willems, A., Paepe, D., Marynissen, S. et al. (2017). Results of screening of apparently healthy senior and geriatric dogs. *J. Vet. Intern. Med.* 31 (1): 81–92.

7 Brodbelt, D.C., Blissitt, K.J., Hammond, R.A. et al. (2008). The risk of death: the confidential enquiry into perioperative small animal fatalities. *Vet. Anaesth. Analg.* 35 (5): 365–373.

Recommended Reading

Gawande, A. (2009). *The Checklist Manifesto*. New York: Metropolitan Books.

9.14

New Treatment Modalities

Lowell Ackerman, DVM, DACVD, MBA, MPA, CVA, MRCVS

Global Consultant, Author, and Lecturer, MA, USA

 BASICS

9.14.1 Summary

For most of the history of modern veterinary medicine, we have relied on "drugs" of various classes for the management of disease. Whether we are discussing antibiotics, parasite control products, or nonsteroidal antiinflammatory drugs, our focus was on these chemical agents and how they were to be dosed in our patients.

As pet-specific care expands and evolves, it will be important for veterinary teams to be comfortable with different approaches to medicine. There are a variety of these new modalities currently available, and many more to come.

9.14.2 Terms Defined

Biopharmaceutical: Also known as biologicals, these are pharmaceutical drugs derived from biological sources.
Biosimilars: Approved versions of innovator biopharmaceutical products.
Biological Response Modifier: A type of treatment that mobilizes the body's immune system to fight disease.
Exome: The protein-coding part of the genome.
Genome: All the hereditary information encoded in the DNA, including the genes and the noncoding sequences of DNA.
Legend Pharmaceuticals: Another term for prescription drugs.
Pharmacogenomics: The study of how genes affect the response to drugs.
Secretome: Proteins expressed by an organism and secreted into the extracellular space.

 MAIN CONCEPTS

9.14.3 Biopharmaceuticals

Biopharmaceuticals, also known as biologicals, are pharmaceutical drugs derived from biological sources and often behave differently from standardized synthesized pharmaceuticals. Biopharmaceuticals might include products like blood and blood products, immunotherapies, vaccines, hormones (such as insulin), allergen extracts ("allergy shots"), gene therapies, stem cell therapies, monoclonal antibodies, interleukin-based products, recombinant therapeutic proteins, fecal microbiota, and other such things.

9.14.4 Biosimilars

Compared to small-molecule pharmaceuticals, biopharmaceuticals, which consist of chemically identical active ingredients, are more complex and heterogeneous. However, just as with legend pharmaceuticals and their generic equivalents, biosimilars will become available in the veterinary marketplace, as they are in human medicine, and they must remain equivalent throughout their life cycle. Unlike generic medicines, biosimilars are unlikely to be an exact copy of the innovator product, and are assessed through a different regulatory pathway. In general, this pathway requires more testing than for small molecules, but still less than a completely new drug application.

9.14.5 Biological Response Modifiers

Biological response modifiers are substances that modify immune responses, and the most commonly applied products to date have been monoclonal antibodies. Veterinary medicine is just starting to see an increase in therapeutic antibodies being used to treat a variety of conditions (allergies, osteoarthritis, etc.) and many more are bound to be introduced. Most of these are caninized or felinized monoclonal antibodies targeting specific inflammatory mediators. In general, because the effects are so specific, these typically offer fewer side effects than traditional systemic therapies.

There are also medications that specifically target certain reactions by interfering with inflammatory mediators (such as Janus kinase inhibition), and in this way provide beneficial effects.

9.14.6 Immunotherapies

Immunotherapy refers to treatments that work by modulating the immune system, typically by either activating or suppressing responses. Allergy immunotherapy, through subcutaneous injections or sublingual drops, is one of the most common forms of immunotherapy, although the mechanism of action is still not completely understood.

Immunomodulating products tend to have fewer side effects than most drugs, although the response to therapy can be more difficult to predict. There are a variety of different forms of immunomodulators, including cytokines, interleukins, chemokines, glucans, imide drugs, and others.

9.14.7 Checkpoint Inhibitors

Checkpoint inhibitors are immunotherapies that target immune checkpoints, which are key regulators of the immune system that cancers can use to shield themselves from the body's immune responses. A variety of checkpoint inhibitors have been approved for the treatment of several human cancers, and their application in veterinary medicine is to be anticipated.

9.14.8 Stem Cell Therapies

Mesenchymal stem cell therapy involves collecting mesenchymal stem cells from patients, manipulating them, and then reintroducing them by injection into areas of disease or dysfunction. The hope is that the stem cells will undergo cell division to develop into fully differentiated cells that will result in tissue renewal.

In most cases, adult-derived mesenchymal stem cells are thought to assist in tissue regeneration and repair through a number of different mechanisms, including reducing inflammation, new blood vessel development, immune modulation, and proliferation of local stem cells at the site of injury. Transplanted stem cells may not survive long in their new locations, but it is still thought that their secretions, or secretome, may recruit stem cells to the area and enhance tissue repair. If stem cells can be manipulated so they don't initiate an immune response, it should also be possible to utilize allogeneic stem cell therapy, rather than having to harvest stem cells from individual patients.

Despite the fact that there are few studies that actually support the beneficial effects of stem cell therapy, its clinical use for conditions, especially osteoarthritis and feline stomatitis, is growing. Further investigation into potential benefits is eagerly awaited.

9.14.9 Gene Therapies

Gene therapies rely on the introduction of functional genes to treat or prevent problems. While currently experimental, they have been used in a variety of veterinary settings, including correcting inborn errors such as in certain forms of retinal dystrophy.

Gene therapy can be used to replace a defective gene that is causing or will cause issues with a normal copy of that gene, inactivate a defective gene that is acting improperly, or introduce a new gene to help fight disease or protect against disease.

9.14.10 Gene Silencers (RNA Interference)

Gene silencing is a technology in which RNA molecules inhibit gene expression or translation by neutralizing targeted messenger RNA (mRNA). This RNA interference (RNAi) can be used to treat the root cause of diseases, arresting or even reversing a condition rather than just slowing its progression. It relies on molecular messengers like RNA to switch off genes that are responsible for disease. For example, human drugs like patisiran are synthetic strands of RNA that interfere with the genes driving the rare genetic disease hereditary transthyretin-mediated amyloidosis. The high price tag on such novel therapies may preclude their use in pets for the immediate future, but gene silencers are an exciting new treatment modality.

9.14.11 Genomic Selection of Therapies

With the advent of genomic research has come the possibility of using genomic information about an individual as part of clinical diagnostic and therapeutic decision making. As pet-specific care becomes more prominent in veterinary medicine, expect that genomics, epigenomics, environmental exposure, and other inputs will play a role in more accurately guiding diagnosis and treatment.

In human medicine, genomic markers are increasingly used in cancer screening, and in guiding bespoke treatment strategies. Once the clinical utility of such genomic markers has been well documented in animals, the next step will be to incorporate them into existing standards of care.

In addition to finding individual genomic markers that are important in predicting outcomes for individuals regarding diagnostic or therapeutic screening, whole-genome sequencing will eventually allow veterinary teams to look for mutations responsible for diseases or conditions across the entire genome simultaneously.

Pharmacogenomics uses information from genome studies to determine whether or not a particular therapy might be effective. Many human drugs even have pharmacogenomics information on their labels, especially drugs used as analgesics, antivirals, cardiovascular drugs, and cancer therapeutics. The information provided in the genome, or in the exome (the protein-coding exons within genes), can help determine which drugs are likely to be effective in individuals.

9.14.12   Helminthic Therapies

In human medicine, certain nematode therapies containing hookworms (*Necator americanus*) and whipworms (*Trichuris suis*) have proven helpful for patients not only with allergies, but also with conditions such as Crohn's disease, multiple sclerosis, and asthma. It is thought that the co-evolution of helminths with hosts is associated with immune modulation of sorts, perhaps through interleukin expression. It is possible that such expression might also prove relevant in pets.

EXAMPLES

Mrs Calderon presented Jake, a 3-year-old neutered male golden retriever, to ABC Animal Hospital for problems related to his allergies. He has been treated with a Janus kinase inhibitor and Mrs Calderon was happy to avoid the use of corticosteroids, but it has been difficult to keep Jake controlled with only once-daily therapy, as specified by the doctor.

On occasion, Mrs Calderon had treated Jake twice daily with the Janus kinase inhibitor, even though she had been warned that this is not recommended and could result in certain side effects.

Dr Black understood Mrs. Calderon's frustration, and was encouraged by the response to the Janus kinas inhibitor, and suggested that they might try an immunotherapy that targets interleukin-31, similar to the Janus kinase inhibitor but this time by injection. Mrs Calderon was willing to give it a try, and liked the fact that it could be given by injection so that there was nothing she needed to administer at home.

TAKE-AWAYS

- The pharmacy is changing, and veterinary teams should anticipate new treatment modalities with which they might not be familiar.
- Just as in human medicine, there will be many different monoclonal antibody therapies introduced in veterinary medicine.
- Many new therapies will be injectable, typically administered in the hospital rather than being dispensed.
- Once these novel therapies have been proven safe and efficacious, they will likely take their place in many of our standards of care.
- Not every new therapeutic modality will be an improvement over existing therapies, so veterinary teams will need to be knowledgeable about new therapies and their potential advantages and disadvantages.

MISCELLANEOUS

Recommended Reading

Amato, N.S. Mesenchymal Stem Cell Therapy. Clinician's Brief, 2019. www.cliniciansbrief.com/article/mesenchymal-stem-cell-therapy

Cunha, A. (2017). Genomic technologies – from tools to therapies. *Genome Medicine* 9: 71.

Mealey, K.L. (2019). *Pharmacotherapeutics for Veterinary Dispensing*. Ames, IA: Wiley Blackwell.

9.15

Nutritional Counseling

Kara M. Burns, MS, MEd, LVT, VTS (Nutrition)

Lafayette, IN, USA

 BASICS

9.15.1 Summary

Proper nutrition is a critical component for maintaining the health of pets. Every patient, healthy or ill, that enters the veterinary hospital should have an evaluation of their nutritional status – this is known as the fifth vital assessment. Healthcare team members should make a nutritional recommendation based on this evaluation and effectively communicate this recommendation to clients.

Clients want information on the proper nutrition for their pets. This nutrition discussion is best had with the veterinary healthcare team. There are numerous myths and misperceptions surrounding pet nutrition which in some cases can be detrimental to the health and well-being of the pet; therefore, the healthcare team member must initiate the discussion through proper nutritional history.

9.15.2 Terms Defined

Lifestage Nutrition: Feeding animals foods designed to meet their optimum nutritional needs at a specific age or physiological state (e.g., maintenance, reproduction, growth, or senior) is known as lifestage nutrition.

Nutritional Evaluation: An in-depth evaluation of objective and subjective data related to the patient's food and nutrient intake, lifestyle, and medical history.

 MAIN CONCEPTS

Inclusion of nutrition in preventive guidelines as a vital assessment recognizes the important role nutrition plays in overall health. The positive impact of proper nutrition on health and disease is well established in all animals. Appropriate feeding throughout all life stages can help prevent diet-associated diseases, as well as assist in the management of other disease. Since good nutrition is integral to optimal pet care, it is critical to incorporate a nutritional assessment and specific nutrition recommendation into each pet visit. In order to give healthcare teams a roadmap to implementing this best client care, the American Animal Hospital Association (AAHA) released the Nutritional Assessment Guidelines for Dogs and Cats [1] in July 2010 and in April 2011 the World Small Animal Veterinary Association (WSAVA) launched the V5 Global Nutrition Guidelines [2].

Incorporating the screening evaluation described in these guidelines as the fifth vital sign in the standard physical examination requires little to no additional time or cost. Yet, incorporating nutritional assessment and recommendations into the care of companion animals helps to develop a partnership between the owner and veterinary healthcare team, with the end result being healthier pets. Further evaluation can be even more specific, including breed factors (see 3.17 Breed-Related Nutritional Issues).

The nutritional assessment considers several factors including the animal, the diet, feeding management, and environmental factors. Healthcare teams must also keep in mind that the nutritional assessment is an iterative process in which each factor affecting the animal's nutritional status is assessed and reassessed as often as required. The nutritional guidelines can be summarized into three easy to implement steps.

1) Incorporate a nutritional assessment and specific dietary recommendation in the physical exam for every pet, every time they visit.
2) For every patient, perform a screening evaluation (nutritional history/activity level, body weight and body/muscle condition score [MCS]).
3) Perform an extended evaluation for a patient with abnormal physical exam findings or nutritional risk factors such as lifestage considerations, abnormal body condition score (BSC) or MCS, poor skin or hair coat, systemic or dental disease, diet history of snacks or table food that is greater than 10% of total calories, unconventional diet, gastrointestinal upset or inadequate or inappropriate housing.

9.15.3   Nutritional Evaluation

Every animal that presents to the hospital should be assessed to establish nutritional needs and feeding goals, which depend on the pet's physiology and/or disease condition. The role of the veterinary technician/nurse is to ascertain patient history, score the patient's body condition, work with the veterinarian to determine the proper nutritional recommendation for the patient, and communicate this information to the pet owner.

The first step in evaluating a pet and determining its nutritional status is to obtain a complete history, including signalment (i.e., species, breed, age, gender, reproductive status, activity level, and environment). Next, a nutritional history should be taken to determine the quality and adequacy of the food being fed to the pet, the feeding protocol (e.g., whether the pet is fed at designated meals or has free choice, the amount of food given, the family member responsible for feeding the pet), and the type or types of food given to the pet. When evaluating a pet, the veterinary team member should ask the owner the following questions.

- What brand and type of food do you feed your pet?
- What brand and type of snacks or treats do you give your pet?
- Do you give your pet any supplements? If so, what kind?
- Is your pet receiving any chewable medications? If so, what are they?
- What type of chew toys does your pet play with?
- What human foods does your pet consume?
- Does your pet have access to other sources of food?

The owner should also be asked about the pet's access to foods, supplements, and medications and how much of each substance the pet consumes each day. Pets also may be fed by more than one family member or receive numerous treats throughout the day. All these factors play a role in proper nutrition of pets.

All members of the healthcare team should be familiar with taking a nutritional history. Through this mechanism, the team can pinpoint a breakdown in owner compliance (e.g., more than one person in the household feeding the pet, the pet getting more calories than is recommended, etc.) and begin to establish a feeding protocol to insure the pet's proper calorie consumption.

9.15.3.1   Nutritional Calculations

Veterinary healthcare teams should be comfortable with calculating the amount of food or the appropriate energy intake of the patient. The pet's daily energy requirement (DER) reflects its activity level and is a calculation based on the pet's resting energy requirement (RER).

There are a couple of basic formulas to follow when calculating amount to feed. The most accurate formula to determine the RER for a cat or a dog, regardless of the breed, is:

$$\text{RER kcal/day} = 70(\text{ideal body weight in kg})^{0.75}$$

or

$$\text{RER kcal/day} = (\text{kg} \times \text{kg} \times \text{kg}, \sqrt{}, \sqrt{}) \times 70$$

9.15.3.2   Body Condition Scoring

The health care team should document the pet's BCS and weight at every visit as part of the physical examination. Body condition scoring is a subjective assessment that is important when determining whether a dog or cat is at a healthy weight and when substantiating a diagnosis of obesity in a pet (see 6.15 Approaching Obesity on a Pet-Specific Basis). It allows healthcare team members to assess a patient's fat stores and muscle mass, helps in evaluating weight changes, and provides a value that can be used in team communication.

The two most common BCS systems are the five-point scale and the nine-point scale. Both rating scales use nine points, but the five-point scale is scored to the nearest half-point whereas the nine-point scale is scored to the whole point [2, 3]. It is important for all members of the healthcare team to use the same scoring system from the outset so as not to confuse or miscalculate the patient's weight.

Body condition is assessed beginning at the head of the pet and working toward the tail. Fat cover is evaluated over the ribs, down the topline, around the tail base, and ventrally along the abdomen. On the five-point scale, a score of 1 represents "too thin" and 5 represents "obese"; a score of 3 means "ideal." According to body composition studies in cats and dogs, a body condition of 15–25% fat is optimal; therefore, a pet with an ideal BCS has 15–25% body fat. A pet with a BCS indicating overweight has 26–35% body fat, and a pet with a BCS indicating obesity has more than 40% body fat [3].

The MCS evaluates the muscle mass of the animal. The muscle mass evaluation includes visual examination of the patient and palpation over the temporal bones, scapula, lumbar vertebrae, and pelvic bones. Assessing muscle condition is important, as muscle loss is greater in patients with acute and chronic diseases vs healthy animals deprived of food, when primarily fat is lost. Muscle loss adversely affects strength, immune function, and wound healing.

Improving owner compliance with nutritional recommendations is as simple as instituting a system for making follow-up calls. The AAHA compliance survey confirms 78% of pet owners want a reminder call but only 52% report receiving one. More than 80% of pet owners indicated that they want to discuss feeding and home care with other members of the healthcare team, not just doctors (see 8.25 Team Strategies for Weight Management). Not surprisingly, clinics that involved the healthcare team saw a 29% increase in owner compliance to nutritional recommendations.

EXAMPLES

Flounder, a 7-year-old castrated male Maine Coon cat, presents for annual wellness examination. While taking a history on the patient, the owner states that she finally taught him to not jump on the counter. The owner is quite proud of this accomplishment and announces that after six years of "shooing" him off the counter, Flounder no longer jumps up.

In-depth questioning of how Flounder acts at home has uncovered the fact that Flounder does in fact not jump up to anything. One of his favorite positions was curling up on the dining room chair in the sun but he has lately been lying in the sun on the floor of the dining room. Flounder also has not been as interactive as he used to be – playing with the owners with an interactive feather toy on a pole. He shows interest but really does not chase the feather as much as he once did. The owner attributed that to his maturity – relating it to a teenager who no longer wants to interact with their parent.

His BCS is found to be 4/5. Flounder has gained "a little" weight each year he presents to the hospital. Today he is weighing in at 22 lb (10 kg). He has gained 4 lb since a year ago.

Upon physical examination, Flounder has mats toward the caudal end of his flank and on his back end. He also has decreased range of motion in his hips and tightens when his hips are palpated. He is found to be seriously overweight. An in-depth nutritional history finds that Flounder is eating 2× his DER, as he is fed free choice, gets chicken from the kids upon returning home from school, and multiple high-calorie treats.

The veterinarian performs an orthopedic examination and a more in-depth examination of Flounder's hips confirms that he has significant decrease in range of motion. He is allowed to walk around the exam room and has a stiff gait resulting from difficulty moving in his hip area. He also is found to have decreased range of motion, crepitus, and pain in his left knee area, with some muscle atrophy.

Hemogram and chemistry are within normal limits (WNL). V/D radiographs are indicative of hip dysplasia.

The veterinarian has reviewed all the findings reported and recorded in the medical chart by the technician and has evaluated Flounder. The diagnosis by the veterinarian is hip dysplasia, obesity, osteoarthritis (OA) secondary to hip dysplasia and OA in the knees.

Nursing care and supportive therapy as determined by the veterinarian and orders written for the technician to follow through.

Flounder needs to lose weight and begin nutritional therapy aimed at decreasing pain and increasing quality of life. The veterinarian recommends a diet for OA, environmental enrichment, and a gradual weight loss treatment plan. The veterinary nurse is responsible for educating the owner regarding Flounder's obesity and the risks associated with obesity, as well as instituting the weight management program. Follow-up and open communication are crucial to the success of the weight loss program.

TAKE-AWAYS

The fifth vital assessment – every patient, healthy or ill, that enters the veterinary hospital should have an evaluation of their nutritional status.

- Healthcare team members need to make a nutritional recommendation and effectively communicate this recommendation to their clients.

- There are many myths and misperceptions surrounding pet nutrition which may be detrimental to the health and well-being of the pet.
- The veterinary healthcare team must initiate the nutrition discussion through a proper nutritional history.
- The nutritional assessment is an iterative process in which each factor affecting the animal's nutritional status is assessed and reassessed as often as needed.

MISCELLANEOUS

References

1 Baldwin, K., Bartges, J., Buffington, T. et al. (2010). AAHA nutritional assessment guidelines for dogs and cats. *Journal of the American Animal Hospital Association* 26: 285–296.

2 WSAVA Nutritional Assessment Guidelines Task Force (2011). Nutritional assessment guidelines. *Japan Society of Applied Physics* 52 (7): 385–396.

3 Burns, K.M. (2006). Managing overweight or obese pets. *Veterinary Technician*: 385–389.

Recommended Reading

Pet Nutrition Alliance http://Petnutritionalliance.org

World Small Animal Veterinary Association. Global Nutrition Guidelines. www.wsava.org/Global-Guidelines/Global-Nutrition-Guidelines

World Small Animal Veterinary Association. Nutritional Assessment Checklist. www.wsava.org/WSAVA/media/Documents/Committee%20Resources/Global%20Nutrition%20Committee/English/Nutritional-Assessment-Checklist.pdf

World Small Animal Veterinary Association. Diet History Form. www.wsava.org/WSAVA/media/Documents/Committee%20Resources/Global%20Nutrition%20Committee/English/Diet-History-Form.pdf

9.16

The Role of Nutritional Supplements in Pet-Specific Care

Kara M. Burns, MS, MEd, LVT, VTS (Nutrition)

Lafayette, IN, USA

 BASICS

9.16.1 Summary

Dietary supplements are very popular in the human population. About half of the adult population in the United States takes at least one supplement regularly [1]. Society has emphasized good health and much of the focus has been on nutritional supplementation.

The trend is not only in humans. An estimated 10–33% of dogs, cats, and horses in the US receive a daily dietary supplement. Additionally, an estimated 90% of practicing veterinarians reportedly dispense supplements in their practice [2].

The animal dietary supplement market today boasts products of all imaginable types: vitamins and minerals, herbs and botanicals, antioxidants, chondroprotective agents, and probiotics. Therefore, it is important that veterinary healthcare team members understand the regulations and safety surrounding nutritional supplements for pets.

Also known as nutraceuticals, these products are extremely popular. Veterinary teams and pet owners alike often believe that dietary supplements do not have federal regulation. On the contrary, nutraceuticals are scrutinized but it is the lack of effective monitoring and control that gives the impression of nonregulation.

What is true is that not all animal supplement products on the market comply with applicable law. The veterinary team should be aware of this as it results in many commercial products potentially containing substances that may not be safe. An additional concern is that labels may permit poorly supported if not totally unsubstantiated claims.

As many pet owners continue to use dietary supplements and nutraceuticals for their pets, it is important for the veterinary team to familiarize themselves with the gaps in regulation of dietary supplements so that they may better critically evaluate ingredients and claims prior to dispensing products to clients.

9.16.2 Terms Defined

Animal Dietary Supplement: As defined by the National Research Council (NRC), this is a substance for oral consumption by horses, dogs, or cats which can be given in or on feed or offered separately. The intent is for specific benefit to the animal by means other than provision of nutrients recognized as essential, or provision of essential nutrients for intended effect on the animal beyond normal nutritional needs, but not including legally defined drugs.

Association of American Feed Control Officials (AAFCO): Nongovernmental organization in the US that creates model animal feed laws, regulations, and ingredient definitions, which then may be adopted by individual state agencies charged with regulation of animal feed.

Dietary Supplement: A product intended to supplement the diet that bears or contains one or more of the following dietary ingredients: a vitamin, a mineral, an herb or other botanical, an amino acid, a dietary substance used to supplement the diet by increasing total daily intake.

Drug: A medication intended for use in the diagnosis, cure, mitigation, treatment, or prevention of disease or that affects the structure or function of the body.

Functional Food: Food alleged to have a health-promoting or disease-preventing property beyond the basic function of supplying nutrients.

Generally Recognized As Safe (GRAS): Substance generally recognized, among experts qualified by scientific training and experience to evaluate its safety, as having been adequately shown through scientific procedures to be safe under the conditions of its intended use.

Pet-Specific Care for the Veterinary Team, First Edition. Edited by Lowell Ackerman.
© 2021 John Wiley & Sons, Inc. Published 2021 by John Wiley & Sons, Inc.

National Animal Supplement Council (NASC**):** A trade organization comprising manufacturers of dietary supplements for companion animals and associated industries.

NRC: The working arm of the National Academies, a private body that advises the United States federal government on matters related to health and science issues.

Nutraceuticals: Dietary supplements intended for health benefits beyond prevention of essential nutrient deficiencies.

United States Food and Drug Administration (FDA**):** The federal agency responsible for regulation of foods and drugs in interstate commerce.

 MAIN CONCEPTS

It is important for the veterinary healthcare team to understand the regulatory framework surrounding dietary supplements for pets. In 1994, the Dietary Supplement Health and Education Act (DSHEA) reformed the regulations regarding the distribution of dietary supplements in the United States. This reformation resulted in an incredible growth of human and animal supplements. Prior to DSHEA, the law governing foods and drugs for human and animal use was the Federal Food, Drug, and Cosmetic Act of 1938 (FFDCA) [3]. The FFDCA stated that the distinction between a "food" and a "drug" largely depended upon the claims associated with the product.

The DSHEA altered dietary supplement regulation in numerous ways. One major change was the FFDCA amendment stated that a substance in a product that met the statutory definition of "dietary supplement" was not a food additive. This is important as the product was no longer subject to premarket clearance requirements. Essentially, the DSHEA moved the manufacturers' burden from having to prove a substance was safe prior to use to the FDA having to prove a substance was unsafe before enforcement action could be taken [3]. The result – substances with no historical use as food could now be included in products considered to be dietary supplements without regulatory recourse.

The DSHEA also altered the model for what established a drug claim. Claims to treat or prevent a disease still are not allowed under DSHEA. However, DSHEA does provide for "support" claims or claims to affect the structure or function of the body beyond its food qualities.

The FDA Center for Veterinary Medicine (CVM) in 1996 issued notice in the Federal Register stating that DSHEA was not applicable to products intended for animals. Therefore, if DSHEA did not apply to animal products, the existing provisions in FFDCA apply. Consequently, unless a supplement is considered a drug, there is no regulatory distinction between dietary supplements for animals and any other animal feed. They are simply "food." Thus, animal dietary supplements may not contain unapproved food additives. Additionally, the manufacturers cannot make claims comparative to effects on the structure or function of the body unless they pertain to accepted nutritional principles.

It is important for veterinary teams to ask pet owners if they are using some form of supplementation for their pets. Assuming the "owners will tell us" is not a good protocol to follow for a number of reasons – owners may be defensive about supplementing, may be embarrassed that they are supplementing, and may not know the interactions the supplement may have and thus not be aware of any potential harm. Human cancer patients use vitamin supplements as complementary therapy, and this use is often without the recommendation or knowledge of their physician [4–6].

The NASC has created a new term that is not in the regulatory dictionary ("dosage form animal health product") to apply to dietary supplements for animals not in the human food chain. The intent is for these products to be given status as "unapproved drugs of low regulatory priority" by CVM. This industry group has an affiliation with the FDA and strict guidelines for member companies regarding quality control and adverse event recording.

The NASC is a nonprofit industry group whose mission is "dedicated to protecting and enhancing the health of companion animals and horses throughout the US." The NASC Quality Seal program was started as part of an ongoing effort to improve and standardize the industry. "Different from the NASC logo, members must earn permission to display the Quality Seal by agreeing to adhere to NASC's quality standards, and by submitting to an independent audit to ensure compliance with our rigorous quality system requirements" (https://nasc.cc/).

9.16.3 Functional Foods and Supplements

Functional foods provide health benefits when eaten regularly. Functional foods have been shown to:

- modify gastrointestinal physiology
- promote changes in biochemical parameters
- improve brain function
- reduce or minimize the risk of developing specific pathologies.

Research in functional food consumption in pets continues as veterinary nutrition aims to better understand how dietary interventions of functional foods can be used for disease prevention and treatment [7]. There are products available that are considered functional foods and aim to mitigate potential disease conditions or aid in the management of these conditions. Healthcare teams need to decide whether a functional food is better in the specific case vs a nutraceutical.

EXAMPLES

Nutraceuticals are not considered drugs and therefore are not regulated by the FDA's guidelines. Unfortunately, nutraceuticals may be mislabeled, may contain impurities, may have variable quantities of active ingredients, or the active ingredient may not be bioavailable.

Guidelines for veterinary healthcare team members to consider regarding the recommendations for nutraceutical use by pet owners include the following [8].

- Price: less expensive supplements are likely to be lower quality.
- Lot number and expiry date.
- Monograph within the US Pharmacopeia: allows for documenting accuracy of ingredient labeling.
- Safety and efficacy claims: if there is a claim of medical benefit on the label, a New Animal Drug Application (NADA) number should be with the product. This is a legal mandate.
- Ingredient list: all ingredients should be listed in order by weight.
- Proper instructions for use.
- Scientific evidence supporting manufacturer's claims: this is a bonus as some manufacturers have begun providing data for their specific products through independent scientific studies.
- Testimonials vs valid research.
- Ignore the "satisfied user" testimonials
- If no scientific research is available to supporting the claims, do not use.
- Membership of NASC (www.nasc.cc). Member companies are likely to have better quality products.

TAKE-AWAYS

- Dietary supplements are very popular in the human and animal populations.

- Not all animal supplement products on the market comply with applicable law.
- Regulations do not ensure efficacy.
- Functional food consumption in pets continues as veterinary nutrition aims to better understand how dietary interventions can be used for disease prevention and treatment.
- It is important for veterinary healthcare team members to follow guidelines when discussing dietary supplements with pet owners and when discussing a specific supplement with the product manufacturer.

MISCELLANEOUS

9.16.4 Cautions

Safety and efficacy evaluation can be difficult. Healthcare team members are encouraged to ask manufacturers their formulations. Questions to be asked prior to the veterinarian prescribing a nutraceutical include the following [8].

1) What studies have been done to prove the product does what it claims?
2) Does the product contain what it claims? Is the product bioavailable?"
3) Were the studies *in vivo* or *in vitro*?
4) Were the studies completed in the target species?
5) Did the study use the same dose as is contained in the final product?
6) Were the studies well controlled?
7) Were the studies published in a peer-reviewed journal?
8) What other medications is my patient receiving, and how might the nutraceutical in question interact with them?
9) Has a margin of safety been established?

References

1 Supplements: A Scorecard. www.health.harvard.edu/staying-healthy/supplements-a-scorecard
2 Freeman, L.M., Abood, S.K., Fascetti, A.J. et al. (2006). Disease prevalence among dogs and cats in the United States and Australia and proportions of dogs and cats that receive therapeutic diets or dietary supplements. *Journal of the American Veterinary Medical Association* 229 (4): 531–534.
3 Dzanis, D.A. (2012). Nutraceuticals and dietary supplements. In: *Applied Veterinary Clinical Nutrition* (eds. A.J. Fascetti and S.J. Delaney), 57–68. Ames, IA: Wiley Blackwell.

4 Burns, K.M. (2010). Therapeutic foods and nutraceuticals in cancer therapy. *Veterinary Technician*: E1–E7. https://pdfs.semanticscholar.org/91a3/9d11efa978ed3a1290d50dfabebb4b0a3169.pdf.

5 Metz, J.M., Jones, H., Devine, P. et al. (2000). Cancer patients use unconventional medical therapies far more frequently than standard history and physical examination suggest. *Cancer Journal* 7: 149–154.

6 Bernstein, B.J. and Grasso, T. (2001). Prevalence of complementary and alternative medicine use in cancer patients. *Oncology* 15: 1267–1272.

7 Di Cerbo, A., Morales-Medina, J.C., Palmieri, B. et al. (2017). Functional foods in pet nutrition: focus on dogs and cats. *Research in Veterinary Science* 112: 161–166.

8 Wynn, S., Bartges, J.W., Hamper, B., et al. When diets aren't enough – supplements and nutraceuticals. Proceedings of CVC Meeting, San Diego, 2009.

9.17

Improving Compliance and Adherence with Pet-Specific Care

I. Craig Prior, BVSc, CVJ

College Grove, TN, USA

BASICS

9.17.1 Summary

Compliance and adherence are measures of how well the veterinary team is communicating with clients or caring for their patients. It is based upon the care guidelines set up by the veterinary practice for the health of patients and good of clients, as well as the financial guidelines set by the practice manager and clinic owner for the continued health of the practice. The best source of new business for the veterinary practice is not bringing in new clients but more completely serving the existing client and patient base. Veterinary teams need to ask pointed questions and tactfully direct conversations with pet owners in order to better understand each situation, recommend treatments and services based on this, and prescribe medications that will set the client up for success at home. After a visit, it is critical that a hospital has multiple touch points with the client to follow up on the visit and set reminders regarding return visits and on-time administration of medications provided.

9.17.2 Terms Defined

Adherence: The extent to which patients take medications prescribed, involving the pet owner in filling and refilling the prescription; administering the correct dose, timing and use; and completing the prescribed course. Adherence is a term applied specifically to medications; it does not refer, for example, to recommendations for wellness checks, diagnostic screenings, and so on.

Compliance: The extent to which pets receive a treatment, screening, or procedure in accordance with accepted veterinary healthcare practices. Compliance involves both veterinary staff performing and/or recommending treatments, screenings, and procedures and pet owner follow-through.

MAIN CONCEPTS

There are many factors that affect compliance and adherence to a prescribed medication or a medical or surgical procedure [1]. Some of the more common factors that affect adherence include the client's perceived image of the human–animal bond, ability of the client to administer the medication, cost of the treatments, and/or lack of firm recommendations from the clinic staff. The lack of a firm recommendation often diminishes the value or the need for the service or product being discussed with the client. Clients often feel "guilt" giving medications to their pets or agreeing to have procedures or surgeries performed on their pets. This feeling can cause a client to believe they are negatively affecting the relationship between them and their pet and can lead to them either not having the procedure performed or not giving the prescribed medication correctly. Clients oftentimes will not openly express this concern with veterinary staff, which is why it is important to ask strategic questions to elicit any hesitations or preferences the client may have regarding a veterinarian's recommendations or treatment plan.

Additionally, it is important to take the client's lifestyle into consideration as it may affect their ability to administer medication to a pet, timing of medication administration (BID, TID, QID), type of medication (pill, capsule, topical, liquid, etc.), and duration of administration. Cost should always be evaluated with a client, but it should be properly communicated in a way that shows the value and reason behind the price point (see 10.15 Putting Price into Perspective). Simply providing a list of tests/services/medications and the price does not effectively communicate the reason behind what is being recommended and may not lead to the proper "buy-in" from the client.

Lastly, consider the client experience – are team members dressed professionally, are they presenting the recommendation in a professional manner, is the hospital clean, modern, quiet, and supportive of the image you're trying to portray? All in all, the majority of these challenges are easily overcome with improved client communication and engagement before they enter the clinic, during their visit, and follow-up thereafter.

Client engagement should start before the client even sets foot in the hospital. Walk through the hospital looking at it from the client perspective and review the flow of a visit. Although a full hospital remodel is not always a viable option, there are many things that can be done to improve client perceptions – a fresh coat of paint, new flooring, moving financial discussions away from the check-in counter to exam rooms, designating an exam room as a consultation room/end of life room, separate dog and cat waiting areas, dedicated cat exam rooms, moving client payment to exam rooms instead of the front desk, monitor the sound levels – look at ways to reduce noise. Review the clinic website – is it easy to navigate? Does it give the client clear expectations regarding their visit, the flow of their visit, financial responsibilities, your clinic care guidelines? Is the client able to request or schedule an appointment online/by app/text? If the client calls in to book an appointment, does the CSR (client service representative) set clear expectations, walk the client through the visit, financial responsibilities, what to bring (stool sample, all medications), etc.? Does your clinic offer telehealth or telemedicine? Having these options provides a value-added service for your clients, further bonding them to your clinic and adding a touchpoint to reinforce client expectations when they visit the clinic. Once the client reaches the clinic, time management becomes very important. Hopefully appointments are running on time but if they are not, communicate openly and honestly with the owner, offering solutions (drop-offs, rescheduling), and be time-aware during the appointment.

In the appointment the veterinary team needs to educate the owner on what is occurring as well as ask open-ended questions that may gain them new understanding into the client/patient's situation (see 9.2 Asking Good Questions). Once it is determined that a treatment plan is needed, create one based on the clinic's care guidelines (or use a canned treatment plan), but do not automatically default to the medication/procedure/surgery that is the cheapest. Draw up the treatment plan, explain it to the client, and finish by asking "Is this the level of care you want for (pet's name) today?" (It is important to note that this is not being called an "estimate," as the word "estimate" can automatically bring about a negative connotation of expense in the client's mind. "Treatment plan" focuses on medicine and care.)

After asking an open-ended question, pause and wait for the client to answer as oftentimes they need a minute to process what was offered to them. Asking open-ended questions helps determine the ability, wants, and needs of the client. A few examples of open-ended questions are: "What are your concerns today?" "How may I further help you make a decision?" "Tell me what's important to you regarding . . .?" "What do you know about . . .?" "Tell me your experience with managing . . ." "How do you think (pet's name) is responding to . . .?" Once the pockets of resistance are identified (i.e., lack of understanding or merely noncompliant), then solutions may be implemented or strategies developed to overcome them. Working together toward these solutions and strategies – veterinarian with the medical recommendations and education and client with their level of comfort and ability to implement them – improves adherence to and compliance with the desired treatment plan.

Other solutions that improve compliance and adherence include client education resources (web-based, videos, printed handouts, brochures, or longer in-person discussions), financing options for more expensive procedures, pet health insurance, wellness plans, smart device apps for medication reminders, longer-acting or injectable medications and/or different administration options (included simple treat-based administration), in-hospital vs home care options, house call options or even referral. Reducing the number of times a day a client has to medicate their pet will increase adherence – in different studies, it was found that up to 25% of clients may not give sufficient doses for optimal treatment, less than 33% dosed at the correct interval [2], and less than 25% were able to comply with once-daily dosing completely [3].

Clients should always be asked to bring all medications (including parasiticides and supplements whether prescribed by the hospital or obtained elsewhere) that the pet is on to biannual visits. This not only helps to update the medical record, allowing the veterinary team to know what else the client is using that is not purchased through the clinic, but also allows the staff to understand the administration habits of the owner (adherence) and be sure there are no contraindications between medications (e.g., aspirin and NSAIDs – client may be giving aspirin without the veterinarian's knowledge).

Medical/surgical discharge should be done in an exam room, without the patient present (as this is a large distraction to the client), and again using open-ended questions to determine the client's level of understanding. At this time client payment should be dealt with and the next medical/surgical progress exams or telemedicine consult should be scheduled. After all this is complete, the patient should be brought to the owner.

However, the clinic's job is not yet over; following up with the client/patient is crucial. The veterinary support team should call/text/email or provide a telemedicine consult to the client two days and one week post discharge or following commencement of new medications. The team members should again use open-ended questions to determine client adherence, with the patient record updated and any issues relayed to the attending veterinarian. Reminder apps are now available for the veterinary field. Introduce clients to them, help them set the app up and enter medications, especially parasiticides and other long-term medications. Hospitals should have an online store with auto-ship capabilities – this is ideal for those clients with poor adherence.

Improving compliance and adherence in the veterinary practice is multifaceted, and involves such areas as standards of care, staff training, client education, leveraging practice management software capabilities, and data analysis.

9.17.3 Standards of Care

The veterinary team involved in improving compliance and adherence must first develop a list of treatments, procedures, screening, and products that they feel are essential for improving or maintaining the health of their patients (see 9.4 Standards of Care). These may include but are not limited to:

- allergy testing and treatment (see 8.18 Team Strategies for Atopic Dermatitis)
- behavior counseling (see 6.8 Managing Routine Procedures to Minimize Problems)
- core vaccinations (see 9.11 Vaccination)
- dental prophylaxis (see 8.19 Team Strategies for Periodontal Disease))
- ear evaluation and treatment (see 8.24 Team Strategies for Otitis Externa)
- FeLV and FIV control (see 8.22 Team Strategies for Feline Retroviral Diseases)
- parasite prevention and treatment (see 4.5 Prevention and Control of Parasites)
- early detection programs (see 4.7 Embracing Early Detection)
- microchipping

- nutrition counseling (see 9.15 Nutritional Counseling)
- senior wellness screening (see 6.17 Senior Care)
- reproductive control (see 2.18 Population Control)
- infectious disease control (see 4.3 Prevention and Control of Infectious Diseases).

These treatments, procedures, etc. must all be realistic, attainable, and based on best medicine principles.

9.17.4 Staff Training

Clients should receive specific, firm recommendations from the hospital team instead of a list of choices. Recommendations are based upon concepts of best medicine, and are limited, concise, and consistent. When provided with too many choices, clients can become overwhelmed, and may turn to the internet for further clarification.

The hospital team must adhere to the "One Voice, One Message" principle – all team members, no matter what their position in the practice, must be on the same page, educated on the key points, key messages, and key client "take-aways." Formulating and regularly reviewing a set of key customer questions often helps staff members lead clients to key recommendations of services or products. For example:

"What's your tolerance to fleas and ticks (and mosquitoes)?" The client's answer is typically: "None." The staff member's reply should be: "Then we recommend (product X)." Additionally, asking the client what they currently use on their pet and when they last gave or applied it helps to determine the level of client adherence and allows the staff to then make better recommendations.

9.17.5 Client Education and Engagement Strategies

A multifaceted client engagement strategy is critical as a hospital will have different client populations to reach and each of those populations will respond to different platforms. These may include social media posts (Facebook, Twitter, Instagram, Snapchat), posters, handouts, mailings, emails, text messages, reminders (postcard, email, and text), YouTube videos, in-house seminars, etc. The more creative and personalized a clinic can be to their client base, the better, but it is important to write in terms that clients will understand, excluding overly technical medical jargon. Educational materials are available from many different sources, e.g., http://capcvet.org, http://petsandparasites.org, http://petdiseasealerts.org, etc. as well as from industry, and can often be tailored to your practice.

9.17.6   Data Mining

Select services, treatments, surgeries, and product sales, measured either as quantity or percentage of revenue, should be examined at a minimum every six months (compliance). Most practice management software systems are able to run these reports if set up properly (see 7.9 Using Practice Management Software to Personalize Care). There are also third-party companies that will provide these reports, and some pharmaceutical companies will even cover the expense, and provide the reports. Once the hospital reports are received, compare them to available industry benchmarks for reference and comparison. Opportunities should be apparent, and strategic planning can then be devised and implemented.

EXAMPLES

A 4-year-old mixed-breed spayed female dog was brought in for a skin condition, characterized by follicular papules, pustules, and epidermal collarettes. After the exam, diagnostics were performed (after presenting a treatment plan to the client and receiving approval) – skin scraping, skin cytology, and dermatophyte culture. The tentative diagnosis was a probable bacterial folliculitis, the condition was discussed, and a recommendation for a culture and sensitivity was given to the client but then declined by them.

The client was sent home with an antibacterial shampoo – the pet to be bathed every other day, and antibiotics to be given every eight hours daily for two weeks, with a recommendation for a medical progress exam at that time. The client did not schedule or call for a medical progress exam, but did return a month later, complaining that the condition was no better. Upon further discussions, it was ascertained that she did not bathe the dog, and still had over a week's worth of antibiotics left as she was unable to administer them to the dog.

Compliance and adherence could have been improved if after the diagnosis and before medications were dispensed, open-ended questions regarding adherence were posed to the owner: "How easy is (pet's name) to bathe?" "Terrible!! I've never been able to bathe her!!" "The medication I would like to prescribe for her requires it to be given three times daily orally – what are your thoughts around that?" "Well, I've always had trouble giving her any type of medi-

cine, but we're going out of town for a week, and the pet sitter is only coming by the house twice a day."

At this point, the veterinarian can offer two solutions – for the owner, when in town, to bring the pet by the clinic (or a groomer) twice weekly for medicated baths (potentially selling a package of baths at a discount), and to offer a long-acting injectable antibiotic. The client accepts both, and before she leaves, bathing appointments and a medical progress exam are scheduled, and call reminders are set up for the hospital staff to follow up with her in one week to ensure that she has no further questions or concerns and the client is also texted the day before the medical progress exam to remind her of the appointment next day.

9.17.6.1   Intestinal Parasite Screening

As a general guideline, the typical number of intestinal parasite screenings (IPSs) in a clinic should represent about 50% of all exam visits (wellness and sick pet). The statistic can be calculated from practice management software by determining the total number of clinical visits, and the total number of IPSs in the same period. In the author's practice, the first time IPS compliance was run, the result was 33%. This discrepancy was discussed at a meeting involving the practice owner (myself), the practice manager, doctors, lead receptionist, and lead technician. Care guidelines were updated to perform an IPS at the first visit of all new patients, at every semi-annual exam, at least twice during puppy and kitten wellness visits, 2–4 weeks after intestinal parasite treatment (as appropriate), and with every visit involving pets with vomiting and/or diarrhea (as medically appropriate). The practice management reminder system was updated to provide reminders for all these situations and staff members were trained – receptionists reminded every client to bring a stool sample whenever they came in for a visit and technicians incorporated the need for IPS into their conversations with owners and collected samples during the visit if not provided by the owner. Compliance rose to 48%.

After three years, compliance dropped again, this time to 38%. Three factors contributed to this, the first two being staff turnover and message drift, reinforcing the need for ongoing regular staff training. The last reason was that there had been a software update that had created a glitch with the reminder system, so not all reminders were being sent. If it was not for compliance testing, the software glitch would not have been discovered and corrected. Six months later, compliance had returned to its former acceptable level.

TAKE-AWAYS

Simplifying protocols where possible (e.g., frequency of administration, lifestyle adaptation) leads to less staff confusion and less client confusion and improves compliance and adhesion.

- Client education, improving client communication, and modifying client beliefs are essential and ongoing elements that should be fundamental parts of every client interaction.
- Remain neutral (unbiased) – speaking on a level the client can understand or providing written information on a fifth grade level.
- Compliance is an essential element of measuring the health and profitability of the practice, the level of patient care, identifying if team members are adhering to the "One Voice, One Message" concept, and helps reinforce desired client behavior.
- Evaluating adherence and compliance on a regular basis determines the level of success and reveals untapped opportunity.

MISCELLANEOUS

9.17.7 Cautions

Most practice management software will run compliance percentage using a denominator such as "last exam." It's important to understand how this number changes with the numerator as the product or service being measured – the denominator will change with time, even days, hence altering the percentage. Therefore, it is important that compliance testing should be run on the same dates each year to obtain accurate percentages.

References

1 American Animal Hospital Association. Compliance Study Executive Summary 2009. www.aaha.org/public_documents/. . .complianceexecutivesummary.pdf

2 Maddison, J.E. (2008). Medication compliance in small animal practice. *Insights Vet. Med.* 6 (3): 1–5.

3 Amberg-Alraun, A., Thiele, S., and Kietzmann, M. Study of the pet-owners compliance in a small animal clinic. *Kleintierpraxis* 49 (6): 359–366.

Recommended Reading

American Animal Hospital Association. Compliance Study Executive Summary 2009 www.aaha.org/public_documents/. . ./complianceexecutivesummary.pdf

Section 10

Practice Management Considerations

10.1

Strategies for Success with Pet-Specific Care

Jason C. Nicholas, BVETMED (Hons)

Independent Consultant, Author and Speaker, Co-founder, Preventive Vet, Portland, OR, USA

BASICS

10.1.1 Summary

A pet-specific care (PSC) approach is better for patients, clients, and the practice. PSC helps teams deliver better care and health for patients, as well as better engagement and value for clients. This can translate to better job satisfaction for the team and increased revenues for the practice.

10.1.2 Terms Defined

Care Plans: Long-term outline of the examinations, diagnostics, procedures, monitoring, and other care that a pet may need and most benefit from throughout its life.
Health Risk Assessment (HRA): A comprehensive system for helping to determine a specific patient's risks for developing particular diseases and conditions, or suffering from toxicities and other emergencies.
Wearables: Smart collars and other technological accessories that we can put on pets to measure, monitor, and track their vitals, activity levels, and other diagnostically important variables.

MAIN CONCEPTS

10.1.2.1 Client Education is Crucial

With PSC, teams need to be proactive in educating clients and helping them see how it benefits them and their pets. It's important for clients to understand that a personalized approach to their pet's care, though perhaps a bit more time-consuming and costlier up front, is far better for their pet's long-term health, comfort, and safety *and* will save them time, money, and heartbreak in the long run (see 1.2 Providing a Lifetime of Care). Good and early communication of these benefits will help to increase client "buy-in."

10.1.2.1.1 Strategies and Tools to Educate Clients on PSC

- Write a client education piece explaining PSC, including "how" and "why" your practice uses it to help your clients and their pets (see 5.10 Discussing Pet-Specific Care). *Tip:* Submit an adapted version of your blog post to your local newspaper for publication. This can make for great (and free) marketing for your practice!
- Create a short video where you and your team talk about why you believe in and practice PSC. Include success stories of cases that benefited from the PSC approach. Put the video prominently on your practice website, share it on your practice's social media pages, and add it to the rotation of the videos that play on your waviting and exam room TV monitors. *Tip:* If you can get the clients whose pets are featured in the stories to speak about the case on camera too, all the better!
- Ensure that everybody on your practice team – *everybody* – is well versed in PSC and why it's your practice's approach to pet care. You never know when or with whom the conversation will come up. It's helpful if everyone also has a success story or two that they can share with clients when asked. Everybody can tell their favorite, or there can be a few that are discussed at team meetings that everybody shares.

10.1.2.2 Make it Easier for your Clients to Say "Yes"

Ensuring that your clients are educated on and aware of the benefits of your PSC approach is the first step to getting client buy-in. The next step is making it as easy as possible for them to see the benefits and value for them, and to say "yes" to the PSC approach and your recommendations.

10.1.2.2.1 Strategies to Help Clients Say "Yes"

Create personalized care plans for your patients and review them with your clients (see 1.3 Personalized Care Plans). Care plans are a long-term outline of the examinations, diagnostics, procedures, monitoring, and other care that you are anticipating a pet will need and most benefit from throughout their life. Each pet's plan is informed by their signalment, risk assessment, physical examination, diagnostic, historic, and other data (see below). A patient's care plan is adapted over time, as needed, based on their most current data, lifestage developments, health conditions, and other influencing factors. Care plans help clients see the big picture and understand the rationale for your recommendations. They also help clients plan and budget for their pet's anticipated care.

- Offer and utilize payment plans (see 10.17 Payment and Wellness Plans). Not only do payment plans help clients spread the costs of their pet's care, they make it more likely that a client will come in for their recommended exams and agree to more of your diagnostic, therapeutic, and other recommendations. Work with your payment plan provider to customize offerings as much as possible.
- Utilize and promote pet health insurance to your clients at the earliest stage of their relationship with your practice (see 10.16 Pet Health Insurance). Pet health insurance can help clients better comply with a PSC approach, as well as making it easier for them to authorize the level of care necessary in the event of an illness or emergency.

10.1.2.3 Gather as Much Data as Possible (and as Early as Possible)

Pet-specific care depends on data. You gather data all the time in your practice – physical exam findings, diagnostic test results, etc. – but there's so much more data to be had! And these additional data can hold a treasure trove of insight that can help you and your clients plan for and provide the best level of care for their pets (see 7.10 Analytics and Informatics, and 10.8 Using Practice Data as a Credibility-Boosting Tool).

10.1.2.3.1 Strategies and Tools to Gather More and Better Data

- Get patient histories and updates prior to appointments. The best histories are thorough, detailed, and time-consuming. Appointments are often too short and already jam-packed with all that needs to be evaluated and covered, making a truly comprehensive history difficult to obtain in the exam room. (Not to mention that you've then got to type/write it all into the medical record!) Save yourself time and get the best history possible by having clients fill in a thorough history or update form *prior* to their appointment. They complete the form in the comfort of their own home, where they can actually go and look at the name of the food and treats they're giving their pets, the medication and supplement names and dosages, and all the other important, yet "often-forgotten-in-the-exam-room" details (see 2.7 Risk Assessment). They can text, email, or upload their completed form to you prior to coming in, saving you time and making it easier for you to provide the best advice and plan at the time of the appointment. *Tip:* Try incentivizing your clients by offering them a small reward if they've submitted their completed history and update forms prior to the visit. Having this information in advance won't just make your time in the exam room more efficient (which is a money saver for the practice), it'll also make it more likely that you'll pick up on risk factors or problems that otherwise would have been missed and might lead to additional testing or treatment recommendations (i.e., revenue generators).
- Early life genomic (DNA) testing can help you make the best healthcare recommendations for your patients (see 3.6 Genetic Testing). It can also help your clients get a better idea of what problems or concerns they might expect with their pet in the future. Genetic testing in veterinary patients isn't perfect, but when done through a reputable company and when the results are interpreted with the help of a client's veterinarian, such testing can be an important part of determining and planning a pet's lifetime care plan (see 1.2 Providing a Lifetime of Care).
- Promote "wearables." You may use an activity tracker or smart watch to help monitor your own activity and health, but don't forget that more and more of these devices for pets are hitting the market on a regular basis. While the logistics of using a wearable on a pet may not be as straightforward as they are on people, they're still a practical and useful tool for gathering and trending important health data on your patients (see 2.5 Virtual Care (Telehealth)). This could include activity level and heart rate changes in an arthritic pet you've started on a new pain management and/or weight control program,

monitoring activity level in an epileptic patient throughout the day to detect possible unobserved seizure activity, trends in heart and respiratory rates in a patient with diagnosed cardiac disease, or in any number of other scenarios.

EXAMPLES

Jackson was a 3-year-old Labrador retriever. During the history taking at his annual wellness exam, his veterinarian learned that the owner's husband had just been started on the "keto diet" by his own doctor due to concerns about weight and prediabetes. Astutely, Jackson's veterinarian cautioned the owner about the dangers that xylitol, commonly used as a sweetener for people on "keto" and other low-carb diets, poses to dogs. Thankfully they did, because when Jackson counter-surfed the batch of keto-friendly peanut butter cookies later that month, his owners had already known to replace the xylitol called for in the recipe with erythritol. As a result, Jackson just had to deal with a little bit of digestive upset following this dietary indiscretion, rather than the severe hypoglycemia and acute hepatic necrosis he possibly would have suffered from had xylitol been his people's low-carb sweetener of choice.

Felix's owners didn't initially notice anything wrong with their 9-year-old Doberman pinscher, but a trend of increasing heart and respiratory rates and decreased daily activity levels recorded by his smart collar prompted a visit to their veterinarian. Felix's veterinarian suspected a splenic mass during physical examination, which was confirmed on ultrasound. The risk of acute rupture and bleed was discussed and it was decided to do a splenectomy. Felix had been screened (negative) for von Willebrand's disease as a puppy and had had a few uncomplicated surgeries throughout the years, so presurgical lab work was submitted and surgery was scheduled for the following day. Felix recovered well from his surgery and the histopathology report showed his splenic mass to be benign.

TAKE-AWAYS

- Educating clients about and promoting your practice's PSC approach helps get client "buy-in" and engagement, which is crucial to the successful use of PSC in practice.
- Using and promoting payment plans and pet health insurance makes it easier for clients to say "yes" to your PSC approach.
- Data are key! The more (good) patient data you have, the more accurate and helpful your risk assessments and pet care plans can be.
- Utilize technology both to promote your practice's use of PSC and to gather more and better patient data, and to do it earlier and more often.
- A PSC approach firmly solidifies you and your practice as an integral part of a pet's lifetime care team and clearly shows your clients that you, not their local pet supply store or "Dr Google," are their most trusted advisor when it comes to their pet's health and well-being.

MISCELLANEOUS

Recommended Reading

Canine Inherited Disorders Database. University of Prince Edward Island. http://cidd.discoveryspace.ca

Gough, A., Thomas, A., and O'Neill, D. (2018). *Breed Predispositions to Disease in Cats and Dogs*, 3e. Ames, IA: Wiley.

Knesl, O., Lavan, R., Horter, D., and Holzhauer, J. Pet Wellness Report: Canine Health Risk Assessment – A Review of 7,827 Cases. www.aaha.org/globalassets/02-guidelines/canine-life-stage-2019/pwr_canine_health_risk_assessment_technical_bulletin.pdf

New data supports value of veterinary health risk assessments. http://veterinarybusiness.dvm360.com/new-data-supports-value-veterinary-health-risk-assessments

10.2

The Importance of Practice Differentiation

Lowell Ackerman, DVM, DACVD, MBA, MPA, CVA, MRCVS

Global Consultant, Author, and Lecturer, MA, USA

 BASICS

10.2.1 Summary

Practice differentiation is the process of distinguishing your hospital, products, and services from others, to make them more appealing to your target market. As competition in an area increases, differentiation becomes more important to ensure an adequate share of new clients, as well as creating brand loyalty.

To be effective, differentiation must be valued by clients. A differentiation attempt that is not perceived is not effective. Without adequate differentiation, products and services often become perceived as commodities.

When clients cannot perceive a difference between practices, they can be tempted to differentiate based on price (i.e., who offers the services at the lowest price). Differentiation on its own does not make clients unaware when a price premium is presented. It just makes them less sensitive to competing offers because of the value they attribute to the differentiated offering.

Pet-specific care provides a unique opportunity to differentiate a practice based on customized and personalized care, which provides a service approach that is difficult to replicate from other sources.

10.2.2 Terms Defined

Differentiation: The process of distinguishing your hospital, products, and services from others, to make them more attractive to your target market.

Omnichannel Consumer: Consumers looking for a consistent marketing message, both online and offline.

Target Market: A particular type of client that the practice wants to attract.

 MAIN CONCEPTS

10.2.3 The Veterinary Marketplace

For pet owners, the veterinary marketplace tends to be fairly homogenous, and this contributes to the commoditization of veterinary services – the perception that services offered at one hospital are likely comparable to those offered at most other hospitals. Most veterinary practices in a given community offer similar services, and dispense similar products, often for very similar fees, and this can foster a belief among pet owners that there is not much difference between veterinary practices.

When this is the case, and pet owners don't see much of a difference between veterinary practices, they might decide to choose goods and services based solely on price. After all, if one practice is very much like another, why pay a premium at one location when you can likely get comparable service at a lower price point elsewhere? Consumers may not choose the very cheapest competitor, believing that the lowest price may be associated with some inferior aspect, even if they can't discern this, but consumer psychology suggests that in the face of no clear differentiation, they will likely choose one of the mid-priced alternatives, avoiding the highest and lowest priced options, unless they are appropriately differentiated.

There are relatively few examples of clear-cut differentiation in veterinary practice. Clients expect to pay more when they are referred to a specialist, or when they need to take their pet to an emergency clinic, but otherwise there is little to differentiate one primary care practice from another, and this complicates the process of trying to charge appropriately without clients (or staff) complaining (see 10.15 Putting Price into Perspective).

In times past, veterinarians used to be the keepers of veterinary medical information, and so clients were compelled to come to veterinarians for information that they couldn't obtain elsewhere. This is no longer the case. There is an extensive assortment of noncurated pet health information online, most of it available for free, so veterinarians cannot rely on access to information to be their sole differentiator in the marketplace.

For clients, there is more information available on the internet than ever before, and yet it has become almost impossible for them to know what is actually the most relevant. This provides a unique opportunity for veterinary teams to curate the appropriate information, and differentiate their practices in the process by providing pet-specific care, something that pet owners would have difficulty replicating from other nonveterinary providers, and for which veterinary teams are uniquely qualified.

10.2.4 The Retail World

In most sectors of the retail world, differentiation allows customers to perceive a clear relationship between value and price, and to select accordingly. Most consumers know that whether they are considering a restaurant for dining, buying a car, television or timepiece, or deciding whether to wear haute couture or bargain-basement fashion, price exists along a spectrum – they can go cheap, expensive, or anywhere in between and likely find an option with which they can be satisfied.

When we compare this to the veterinary marketplace, it is clear that this spectrum of price and quality is much compressed with veterinary options. If the qualifications of one graduate veterinarian in primary care practice are very much like the qualifications of most graduate veterinarians, and if they are all using similar-quality equipment, medications, vaccinations, and approaches, it can be difficult for pet owners to discern why they should pay more at one practice, if they don't see a discernible difference.

It is this relative uniformity of veterinarians and veterinary practices that leads to commoditization of veterinary services, and a hesitancy to spend more when differentiation is not evident. After all, in the retail world, when clients perceive something to be clearly a commodity, they tend to naturally gravitate to getting the best deal they can, which might even involve making the purchase online rather than buying from a "bricks-and-mortar" establishment.

It is important not to lose sight of the fact that pet owners actively differentiate pet services, even if they don't or can't discern differentiation in veterinary services. Many actively select certain pet foods, accessories, over-the-counter products, and a variety of ancillary pet services (grooming, boarding, etc.) on the basis of perceived value and price.

10.2.5 Pareto Principle

The Pareto Principle is a crude rule of thumb that suggests that the majority of effects (about 80%) are actually due to a small number of events (about 20%). It is therefore sometimes referred to as the 80/20 rule.

This principle suggests some wide-ranging considerations when it comes to veterinary practice, such as that 80% of a practice's revenue likely comes from about 20% of its clients, or that 80% of a hospital's retail revenue likely comes from about 20% of its products.

If the Pareto Principle is true, even approximately, then a small segment of your client base is actually responsible for a large share of your revenue stream. This segment is often your core or "A" clients, and often the target market for differentiation. Core clients are those aligned with your mission (e.g., those seeking pet-specific care), not necessarily their spending patterns in any given year (see 10.4 Client and Patient Segmentation).

It is important to realize that the Pareto Principle is simply a rule of thumb, and almost no hospitals will have exactly an 80/20 spilt between effects and events. It really just suggests that while your differentiated services may only appeal to a small niche of clients (e.g., new pet owners, pet parents, etc.), that small group of clients can nonetheless provide outsize returns for your practice. Veterinary teams sometimes get bogged down with what the majority of clients want, when it is actually an aligned subset of clients that may be driving most of the success in a practice.

10.2.6 Making Differentiation Work

For differentiation to work, it is necessary to define a target market of desirable "core" customers and develop messaging that will resonate with them (see 10.6 Target Marketing and Targeted Client Outreach). Most veterinary hospitals utilize a "one-size-fits-all" approach, which will only appeal to generic pet owners, not your target audience.

With differentiation, there is no need to ignore the remainder of the practice population and so it is also important to create conversion pathways to transition willing typical clients to being "core" clients. In this way, develop ways to convert "D" clients to "C" clients, "C" clients to "B" clients, and "B" clients to "A" clients.

Today's consumers are fickle, so don't take customer loyalty for granted. Businesses need to prove and reprove their value to clients with every interaction. Copycat competition is to be expected. Businesses must continually evolve and innovate to stay ahead of the competition.

Alignment of staff is critical to the process (see 8.4 Alignment – The Key to Implementing Pet-Specific Care). Differentiation needs to be specific enough that staff understand the distinctions and are able to communicate them effectively with clients.

Clients today are omnichannel consumers, so it is important that they receive consistent messages across all your marketing efforts, including your website, in-hospital materials, conversations with staff, standards of care, etc.

Businesses must be able to measure and illustrate the value delivered to clients. It is not enough that the hospital thinks the differences should be valued. Clients are only prepared to pay a premium when they clearly value the differentiation offered.

When differentiation is introduced to a practice, it is important to realize that it will not appeal to everyone. The goal is to cultivate clients whose interests align with the practice, not to convince all clients that they should immediately embrace the new offering.

EXAMPLES

Veterinary hospitals can differentiate themselves across a spectrum of attributes. Here are just a few.

- Pet-specific care
- Expertise/specialization
- Hours of operation
- Financing options
- Customer service
- Accessibility
- Reputation
- VIP/loyalty programs
- Niche services
- Value/quality/price
- Trendiness
- User interface/user experience

TAKE-AWAYS

- Consumers are prepared to spend more on some goods and services than on others, if they can make appropriate value distinctions.

- Differentiation is critical for practice success, but the differentiation may appeal to only a relatively small percentage of existing customers.
- The Pareto Principle suggests that a change that is applied across a small subset of clients may generate major benefits for a practice.
- Differentiation is in the eye of the beholder; clients must perceive and appreciate the value of the offering.
- Practices that provide pet-specific care offer differentiated services that would be difficult for pet owners to replicate elsewhere.

MISCELLANEOUS

10.2.7 Cautions

A hospital's differentiation strategy should change and evolve along with its clients and competitors. It is best to have a strategic plan to stay ahead of the curve.

Recommended Reading

Ackerman, L. (2020). Practice differentiation. In: *Five-Minute Veterinary Practice Management Consult*, 3e (ed. L. Ackerman), 416–417. Ames, IA: Wiley.

Greyser, S.A. and Urde, M. (2019, January-February). What doe your corporate brand stand for? *Harvard Business Review*: 81–89.

Liozu, S.M. (2016). *Dollarizing Differentiation Value: A Practical Guide for the Quantification and the Capture of Customer Value*. Value Innoruption Advisors Publishing https://valueinnoruption.com/.

Lodish, L.M. and Morgan, H.L. (2015). *Marketing that Works: How Entrepreneurial Marketing Can Add Sustainable Value to any Sized Company*, 2e. Upper Saddle River, NJ: Pearson FT Press.

Saunders, G.L. (2011). *Developing New Products and Services: Learning, Differentiation and Innovation*. New York: Business Expert Press.

Williams, R.L. Jr. and Williams, H.A. (2017). *Vintage Marketing Differentiation: The Origins of Marketing and Branding Strategies*. London: Palgrave Macmillan.

10.3

Pet-Specific Outreach

Linda Wasche, MBA, MA

LW Marketworks, Inc., Sylvan Lake, MI, USA

BASICS

10.3.1 Summary

Marketing has always been about meeting customer needs and wants. The obvious reality is that not every consumer's needs and wants are the same. A basic tenet of successful marketing is to create and make available products and services that appeal to various consumer segments based on knowledge of the customer's preferences, lifestyle, problems, frustrations, and other influences. Products and services that try to be "everything to everyone" often end up appealing to no one.

This goal of the marketing process was expressed very well by business consultant and visionary Peter Drucker who said, "The aim of marketing is to know the customer so well, the product or service fits them and sells itself" [1]. This notion certainly applies to pets that come in all shapes and sizes with a variety of health and wellness concerns.

10.3.2 Terms Defined

Marketing Process: The steps involved in developing, producing, and delivering products and/or services to a targeted group.
Market Segments: Parts or pieces of an overall market for a product or service that share common traits, needs, and circumstances.
Outreach: A means of connecting with and communicating with a target; part of the promotion phase of marketing.

Pet-Specific: Pertaining to, and relevant to, the needs and concerns of different pet types based on variables such as breed, size, color, lifestyle, geographic region, health risks, and so on.

MAIN CONCEPTS

In reaching out to any audience, the more that is known about that audience, the greater the chance the sender or source has of creating a message that is meaningful and relevant. In other words, the message means something to the recipient. This basic principle of effective communication applies to every form of marketing outreach.

Outreach uses a message – or content – to connect with a target. In the words of Jamie Turner, founder and chief content officer of the 60-Second Marketer, "The only way to win at content marketing is for the reader to say, 'This was written specifically for me'" [2].

While pets are not the direct recipients of marketing content or messages, they are recipients of veterinary services. When asked about who the target market is for marketing efforts, veterinarians will often say, "Well, pets, of course." Wrong answer. The practice that tries to reach all pets in the same way is missing out on opportunities to be meaningful and relevant to one of the largest and most consistently-growing markets on the planet. Pet product manufacturers already understand the benefits of pet-specific marketing. Look carefully the next time you are at a pet supplies store. You will see pet foods, treats, and other products that are directed to pets by:

- age
- lifestyle

- size/weight
- breed
- health condition.

In promoting these products, you will also see website content, TV and print commercials, special programs and other outreach tools directed to the variety of market segments based on these variables (see 10.4 Client and Patient Segmentation). What is more appealing – a generic one-size-fits-all dog food or a food that is geared to your need for a grain-free, all-natural, hypoallergenic food for small dogs with skin allergies?

This same principle of pet-specific targeting can be applied to veterinary practice outreach. Practices might believe that they are practicing pet-specific outreach simply by seeing different types of pets. While a practice might provide services by happenstance to a variety of pets, this is not pet-specific outreach. Outreach is a proactive means of reaching out and connecting with a target. For a practice, common forms of outreach include – or should include – a variety of channels.

- Website
- Special events
- Targeted campaigns
- Social media content
- Email content
- Lobby library/printed content
- On-hold message
- Local publicity
- Community involvement
- Clinics/screenings

By making these forms of outreach pet specific, a practice strongly increases their relevance to the target.

The entire market of "pets" can be segmented based on a number of variables. A few obvious ones are based on life stages. Some practices may offer special exams or "packages" that cater to such pets. That's great, but practices can do much better by taking the notion of pet-specific outreach a step further.

Identifying reachable pet segments should be based on a common need of the pet. Practices should be asking, "What does the segment experience in terms of health concerns and need for veterinary services?" This information can come from veterinary content found in publications and online resources that address common health concerns based on various pet variables, such as breed (see 10.7 Breed-Specific Marketing). Ideally, though, the practice should be able to consult its own practice management software for the answers (see 7.9 Using Practice Management Software to Personalize Care). Practices that segment their patients based on shared traits and related

health concerns are better prepared to meet the needs of those market segments.

Pet-specific segmentation might be based on such traits as:

- breed
- size
- age
- lifestyle
- geography
- color
- genotype
- phenotype.

Determine how such traits can affect the pet's health needs. View the table below for examples, but keep in mind that there are many more ways to segment a practice's pet patients.

Variable	Segment	Health risk
Size	Certain large breeds	Osteosarcoma
Size	Overweight cats	Diabetes mellitus
Color	Orange tabby cats	Resorptive disease
Breed	Maine Coon cat	Cardiomyopathy
Geography	Mississippi River valley	Blastomycosis
Lifestyle	Dogs that hike in the desert	Desert toads
Genotype	DNA test positive for vWD variant	Blood clotting issues
Phenotype	Early evidence of hip dysplasia	Osteoarthritis

Any of the above represent potential targeted segments for a veterinary practice. Of course, there are many more based on the variables listed above. Each practice should come up with its own targeted segments based on these factors.

- *Practice growth opportunity*: does the segment offer growth potential for the practice?
- *Underserved segments*: which segments are being underserved – or poorly served – by other practices?
- *Overlooked segments*: which services have been ignored by other practices?
- *Competitive advantage*: which segments offer the practice the ability to pursue competitive edge in the marketplace?

In answering the above, practices should consider the following.

- *Veterinary outlook*: what is being reported in professional journals and at conferences? What health issues are on the upswing, thus creating more demand? Cancer? Heart disease? Diabetes? Certain infectious diseases? Which types of pets are most likely to be affected?

- *Patient attraction*: what trends and patterns do you see in your client database? Are you seeing more thyroid disease in certain types of cats? Are more pets getting arthritis? At the same time, are there certain pet segments that your practice would like to see more of? Is your practice viewed as the place to take senior pets which require a lot of care? If not, where are these pets going and why not to your practice?
- *Anecdotal information*: gather staff input on opportunities for pet-specific outreach. Are more pet parents asking for a particular type of service? Are you turning away pets due to a lack of expertise? Are pet parents going to other practices for certain services and treatments?
- *Community needs*: based on factors such as geographic location, local activities and seasonal/weather changes, what are pets in your community susceptible to? What local conditions affect health and welfare?

Be sure to take into account your staff's expertise. If you do not have a veterinarian or veterinary technician with special expertise in geriatric pets, then do not target this segment until the team has been properly trained and developed such expertise. Or, if you have a staff member with a special interest for which he or she is willing to pursue additional training, consider targeting this area.

Once a practice has defined its targets, it should consider the form of outreach to effectively connect with the target. More than one form of outreach is advised. In all cases, keep in mind that once is not enough. It will take repetition and consistency to cut through the increasing clutter facing today's consumers.

Refer back to the earlier list of possible outreach channels. In determining which forms of outreach to choose, practices should first determine the following.

- *Goals*: how will the practice measure success?
- *Resources*: what is practical given the practice's resources and facilities?
- *Measurements*: how will response to pet-specific initiatives be tracked and measured?
- *Continuity*: how will the practice maintain contact with pet parents who respond to the initiative? (A single point of contact is a waste of time! How will you keep the momentum going?)

Pet-specific outreach results in content and messaging that are more likely to resonate with pet parents than a "one-size-fits-all" approach (see 5.2 Meeting Client Needs). Not only is this approach more meaningful and relevant to the segment, it also does a lot for a practice's credibility and ability to differentiate itself from the competition. There is a huge difference between saying "Oh yes, we see them all – we do everything you need for pets" and "If you have a senior pet, we would love to enroll them in our arthritis early detection program to help spot the signs early when there are more options for management."

EXAMPLES

There are many examples of client-specific outreach. A few of them are listed below.

- Target the growing number of pets that are living longer and getting arthritis. Consider conducting a gait analysis clinic to determine if a pet may be exhibiting signs. Orthopedic screening is an excellent way to detect pets at risk, before they are actually having any gait issues. Develop and offer alternative forms of pain reduction and treatment including exercise classes, dietary changes, weight reduction, rehabilitation, and vitamins/supplements. Targeted messages should provide pet parents with reminders, tips, and notices of special events.
- Target certain breeds of cats and dogs that are more susceptible to heart disease (see 11.3 Heritable Health Conditions – By Disease). Develop a heart health initiative to promote healthy eating, exercise, and annual echocardiograms for at-risk breeds. There are many such initiatives that can be undertaken, including for pets at risk of other conditions, such as glaucoma (see 10.5 Early Detection Campaigns).
- Target pets that share recreational experiences with their pet parents. More pets are camping, running, hiking, and exploring. Such pets are susceptible to injuries, predators, and exposure to a variety of infectious agents. Provide seasonal content directed to various outdoor activities in the form of targeted email newsletters, special workshops, and preventive care videos.

TAKE-AWAYS

- Pet-specific outreach is more meaningful and relevant to pet parents than a generic one-size-fits-all approach.
- Pet-specific outreach should be based on a number of variables including pet health concerns, breed, genetic susceptibility, geographic location, the local community, and other factors that affect a pet's likelihood of and risk for disease.

- Veterinary literature contains lots of information on disease rates of occurrence and trends and patterns taking place in the general pet population.
- There is no single magic form of outreach; instead practices should rely on a combination of "touch points" via a variety of channels.
- Outreach efforts should coincide with practice goals for patient attraction.

 MISCELLANEOUS

Abbreviation

vWD   von Willebrand disease

References

1 Brenner, M. Marketing is Business: The Wisdom of Peter Drucker. www.pharma-iq.com/drucker/strategic-marketing-the-customer/articles/marketing-is-business-the-wisdom-of-peter-drucker

2 Elias, B. 47 Content Marketing Quotes that Will Make You a Better Marketer. www.activecampaign.com/blog/content-marketing-quotes

10.4

Client and Patient Segmentation

Linda Wasche, MBA, MA

LW Marketworks, Inc., Sylvan Lake, MI, USA

BASICS

10.4.1 Summary

Practices that try to be everything to everybody are on risky ground. Successful businesses profile customers and segment the market so they can tailor products and services to meet the needs and preferences of each segment. For veterinary practices, knowing who their clients and prospects are is essential to practice positioning and to planning and pricing the right mix of services. The result is a practice that's in sync with its clients and the marketplace and is positioned to deliver meaningful value better than the competition. On the other hand, practices that attempt to "cast a wide net" and appeal to everyone offer little that's compelling to anyone. It's difficult to form a meaningful connection with a client or prospect with a "one size fits all" approach.

10.4.2 Terms Defined

Client or Market Niche: A subset of a client or market segment that possesses like characteristics. An example of a client or market niche is pet owners who go camping with their dogs.

Client Profiling: Understanding a practice's existing client (and patient) base by grouping together pet owners based on a variety of like traits and attributes. These resulting client "segments" are then assumed to have similar needs and wants based on these attributes.

Client Segmentation: Using client profile data to categorize existing clients (and patients) into groups with similar characteristics.

Market Segment: A reachable part of a group or market that is identified as a result of market segmentation. A market segment can be identified from a variety of traits and characteristics that can include geographic location; demographic characteristics (objective, measurable traits like gender, income, age and education); psychographic characteristics (a segment's lifestyle, values and attitudes); and behaviors that pertain to the usage of a particular service or product.

Market Segmentation: The process of splitting or segmenting the pet owner market into identifiable parts or segments that share similar traits. Market segmentation makes it easier for any business to identify and reach out to its most likely and/or lucrative targets.

MAIN CONCEPTS

There are numerous advantages for practices that profile their client base and segment their market. They can:

- better understand client needs and wants
- more easily define and deliver value
- focus client retention and growth efforts on predetermined targets
- determine what types of clients the practice currently attracts and cannot attract
- identify targets for outreach and business development efforts

- more easily define marketing goals and track/measure results
- identify opportunities among particular pet owner segments and niches (see 7.9 Using Practice Management Softward to Personalize Care)
- save money by avoiding misguided marketing and marketing missteps.

Profiling a practice's client base and segmenting the local pet owner market are essential to client retention, client attraction, and practice growth. The clients a practice attracts, and seeks to attract, must be in alignment with the practice's business goals.

Profiling might have some negative connotations in criminal justice, but it helps a practice position and define itself in the marketplace. If it doesn't know its targets, a practice will have a difficult time developing a market identity that will resonate with anyone.

It's also important for a practice to be able to plan and structure its service mix (services should ideally be "client focused," meaning they should be defined taking into account the needs of particular pet owner segments). Otherwise, practices end up offering a list of veterinary services that mean something to the practice but little or nothing to the pet owner (see 10.2 The Importance of Practice Differentiation).

A practice needs to be able to deliver relevant services. Different pet owner segments seek out different standards or tiers of care. If service delivery is out of alignment with a segment, they will go elsewhere.

Pricing of services is also dictated somewhat by targeting. Without knowing who it's targeting, a practice has no clue how to set prices. Prices are a big factor in influencing how pet owners perceive the value of a practice's services and set their expectations (see 10.15 Putting Price into Perspective).

Segmentation is helpful in defining and delivering value. What represents value varies from segment to segment. If pet owners do not feel they are receiving value, they will go elsewhere.

Finally, segmentation facilitates communication with clients and prospects. Pet owners interpret generic service reminders as sales messages from the practice. On the other hand, segmentation enables a practice to reach out with information that's meaningful and valuable: "Sign up for our new glaucoma screening program for early detection of this devastating eye disease that is common in your pet's breed."

What types of clients and patients is a practice seeing now? Practice management software makes it easy to enter customized variables, run reports, and obtain a variety of client data (see 7.9 Using Practice Management Software to Personalize Care). Practices should first determine what

they want to know. This will differ for each practice and should be based on the practice's goals, observations, financial performance in various sectors, hunches, market opportunities, and other factors.

Most practices track some type of client frequency data. They may know how many dogs they see, number of cats, number of muliti-pet households, number of single households, and so on. Beyond this, it's valuable for practices to break these segments down further. For example, for dogs, how many puppies, geriatric, or performance pets is the practice seeing?

Practices can easily cross-tabulate data to further profile their client and patient base. Figure 10.4.1 shows how a practice that wants to better understand the relationship that clients have with their pets can compare differences based on species. In this simple example, practices can better understand how clients view a pet's role in the family, which can translate to how important the pet is to the family, how much the family may be willing to spend on veterinary care, interest in various types of messaging about pet care, and so forth.

Using the same example, practices can further profile clients by further segmenting data (see Figure 10.4.2). Pets viewed as family members can be further segmented by the variable "pet activities" to identify what the pet does as part of the family. In this example, the practice is identifying pets that participate in family vacations and those that are involved in some form of sport or recreation. Understanding the role that pets play in client families enables practices to tailor services as well as messaging directed to these groups. In addition, based on the response a practice gets, it may want to reach out to these segments as part of its client attraction efforts. Additionally, such variables can be

		Pet owner relationship with pet	
		Family member	Pets are pets
Species	Dog		
	Cat		

Figure 10.4.1 Use client and patient segmentation to discern the role of pets in the family, by species. Using the "2 × 2" matrix as a guide, practices can cross-tabulate client data. This approach can be used with multiple sets of variables.

Figure 10.4.2 Client and patient segmentation based on pet activities, by species.

Population	Trends
Pet owners	• Living longer • More mobile • More single households • Pets are children • Stressed/less leisure time
Pets	• Living longer • Getting fatter • More kidney/heart disease • Considered family member • More performance pets • Popularity of big dogs

Figure 10.4.3 Sample pet owner trends.

tracked to help the practice identify service growth areas, areas in decline, greatest revenue to the practice, and so on.

Profiling enables practices to tailor and distribute communications to particular segments of their client/patient base (e.g., cat owners, puppy owners, etc.). Practices that use patient profile data to track illness and health conditions can also use this information to report on trends and emerging health concerns. Being able to say "Our data shows an X percent increase in feline heart disease" is a powerful message for a practice to send, especially to clients who are on the fence about wellness exams. It also helps the practice position itself as an authority, build credibility, and create news for local media (see 10.8 Using Practice Data as a Credibility-Boosting Tool).

Segmenting the pet owner market is similar to profiling and segmenting a practice's client base. However, the practice is focusing its attention externally and looking for opportunity in the marketplace. Practices have to ask themselves which segments represent the greatest opportunity to attract new clients and grow the client base. However, it's never enough to say, "Well we don't have a lot of small dogs at the practice so let's try to get more small dogs." Instead, a practice must first get a good handle on where opportunity exists by becoming familiar with pet owner trends and related needs and preferences. Understanding trends helps practices recognize changes in everything from human–pet relationships to health concerns and issues affecting various species and breeds (see Figure 10.4.3). For example, the fact that pets are living

longer has opened up tremendous opportunity for practices given that longevity (as in humans) leads to age-associated health concerns such as arthritis and kidney disease. The fact that there is a growing number of single households in the US represents a segment in which pets take on the role of companion or child.

Such rigor also helps facilitate the search for pet owner segments not being served, or being underserved, by the competition. A practice that understands how a particular group of pet owners views local veterinary services has an advantage over its competition in servicing this segment.

Similarly, segmentation is also useful when looking for "gaps" in service delivery, such as services that are not being delivered or being poorly delivered. In some cases, there may be a lack of a particular type of veterinary service that pet owners seek. For example, a practice might determine that owners of pet rabbits have nowhere to go for dental care as no practice in the area has yet claimed the role of rabbit dental expert. The underlying issue is that rabbits are more frequently becoming house pets just like cats and dogs. As a result, they are getting better care and living longer. Older rabbits are prone to tooth spurs and abscesses that can be serious, requiring removal and oftentimes surgery. The practice could carve out a lucrative niche by recognizing an unmet need and attract clients from throughout the region.

Understanding the marketplace paves the way for practices to identity and target market segments (see 10.6 Target Marketing and Targeted Client Outreach).

Trends, along with local market intelligence, help practices determine whether or not to pursue a particular segment. There are numerous ways in which pet owners (and any market) can be segmented.

Geographic location and where pet owners originate from and how far they are willing to go are considerations that all practices take into account. For small animal practices, this is calculated as drive time, for which the typical standard is 10–15 minutes to get to an urban or suburban practice. However, if a practice is perceived to offer a meaningful difference or advantage that no one else offers, this drive time can be considerably longer. An example is the niche practice, specialty practice, or emergency clinic. For specialty practices, the typical acceptable drive time is 45 minutes; however, again, drive time becomes less important when clients perceive a difference. It's not unusual for certain specialty practices to draw clients from considerable distances.

Geographic location also pertains to type of setting such as urban, suburban, or rural. Where a pet owner resides plays a big role in pet and owner lifestyle and related veterinary needs.

Another method of segmentation is to separate clients and patients by demographic traits. For humans, there are numerous demographic traits that marketers consider. Veterinary practices might take into account traits like gender, age range, type of household, and number of pets, all of which will have different needs as a result. With regard to pets, practices might target services/programs to such pet demographic traits as species, breed, size of pet, known predisposition to disease, and health problem/condition.

There are also psychographic or lifestyle traits that include personal beliefs, values, and outlook, as well as likes and dislikes when it comes to activities and pastimes. These traits will also very likely influence a person's choice of pet and acceptable veterinary practice. Oftentimes values and likes/dislikes are related. For example, a person who is passionate about the environment will probably spend more time in nature/natural settings. A person who is passionate about the environment and spends time in nature and has a dog probably has a large dog like a golden retriever or other hearty breed, and probably takes that dog hiking and camping. A person who is sedentary may read a lot and is more likely to have a lap dog.

Practices should also take into account client usage, which pertains to frequency of visits and purchases of such things as pet food. A broader definition of usage can extend to a segment's participation in the pet community. Active participants are more likely to share information through Facebook likes, social media sharing, blogging/reblogging, and so on (see 7.5 Connecting with Clients Through Social Media). Highly engaged pet owners are a desirable target because they are more likely to become advocates for the practice.

There is one more type of segment that may not appear on traditional lists of ways to segment a market. Consider the influence that others can have on customers or, in this case, clients. Influencers, or thought leaders, include anyone in a position to have an impact on someone else's deci-

sions and choices. For pet owners, there are many. Pet supplies retailers, pet groomers, pet boarding and day-care facilities, shelters, and rescue groups can all be considered trusted sources by people who have pets. Their opinions can be valuable when it comes to choosing other pet-related services. Segmenting and targeting influencers is a smart choice for any practice.

Using segmentation variables, a practice can identify a variety of pet owner segments. These segments should match the local marketplace and where the practice spots opportunity. By further defining characteristics among these variables, a practice can pinpoint market segments that have identifiable needs as a result of these characteristics.

Such information provides a focus for practices to develop:

- services to reach out to the needs of the segment
- a possible point of difference to distinguish a practice from others
- information that is much more meaningful and valuable because it focuses on the needs of the segment
- multiple ways to engage clients in related discussions; something to talk to them about.

Once a market segment is targeted, just like with any marketing effort, tracking/measuring results is critical. Segmentation makes measurement much easier because a practice knows who is responding to its efforts. The practice that does not segment its market, and tries to reach everyone, will have little idea among whom its efforts are resonating.

Segmentation allows a practice to determine:

- how the segment responds to services and programs directed its way
- what client feedback says about whether or not the segment feels its needs and expectations are being met
- if the segment was accurately defined or if it should be narrowed or broadened
- the impact that the segment is having on the practice's bottom line.

Additionally, practices that measure client satisfaction will be able to compare client satisfaction among various segments. For example, a practice may be getting a good response from dog owners, but may not score as highly among clients with cats.

TAKE-AWAYS

- Practices that understand their clients and know who they are – based on standard methods of customer segmentation – are able to develop services and outreach to appeal to these segments.

- Practice management software makes it easy to identify and track a variety of market segments, their representation and contribution to practice goals.
- The clients and pets being targeted should be based on not only who a practice already sees, but on practice growth opportunities in the local market.
- Methods of segmenting clients and pets include geographic location, demographic traits, lifestyle, and the role that they play in the local pet community.
- Segmentation makes it much easier for a practice to track and measure its performance and ability to attract market segments with a high level of need for veterinary services.

CAUTIONS

Practices should not assume that just because they have the desire to reach out to a certain market segment that an opportunity is there. The practice has to first identify the need and then tailor its services or develop new services to meet the need – not the other way around. Or, a practice may notice a competitor pursuing a particular market segment and follow suit. What is successful for one practice may not work for another. That's why understanding pet owner trends, the local marketplace, and your competition is so important. Look for opportunity first, and then define the segment, as opposed to targeting the segment and hoping that the opportunity is there.

MISCELLANEOUS

Recommended Reading

Best, R.J. (2009). *Market-Based Management: Strategies for Growing Customer Value and Profitability*, 5e. Upper Saddle River, NJ: Pearson Prentice Hall.

Sheth-Voss, P., Carreras, Ismael E. How informative is your segmentation? https://protobi.files.wordpress.com/2012/01/information-and-segmentation.pdf

Wasche, L. (2020). Client and patient segmentation. In: *Five Minute Veterinary Practice Management Consult*, 3e (ed. L. Ackerman), 402–405. Wiley, Ames, IA.

10.5

Early Detection Campaigns

Linda Wasche, MBA, MA

LW Marketworks, Inc., Sylvan Lake, MI, USA

BASICS

10.5.1 Summary

For many veterinary practices, the regular office examination is the best opportunity for early disease detection. But it is also important to realize that for some pets, the interval between these examinations may be too long for early detection and optimal intervention. And, of course, this assumes that the pet parent makes it into the practice consistently for such recommended evaluations.

Veterinary visits actually seem to be trending downward, so simply telling clients they should come in for recommended evaluations may not always be successful. Pet owners may believe that it is actually in the veterinarian's best interest – not theirs – to bring in the pet for all such recommended visits. Or, they might neglect such examinations with excuses such as "my pet's not sick" or "even I don't see the doctor that often."

Pet parents are not necessarily seeing the value in preventive care visits and "because s/he needs her/his shots" is not necessarily a compelling enough reason to make the appointment in some cases. Instead, veterinary practices have to look for meaning and relevancy in a compelling reason that goes beyond the regularly recommended examination.

10.5.2 Terms Defined

Campaign: An organized effort that involves a connected series of initiatives designed to bring about a particular result.

Early Detection: Evaluating patients for early evidence of issues, ideally before they become problematic.

Engage: What a target does when a campaign or like effort is in their best interest. In other words, it is meaningful and relevant to them and they understand and recognize the benefit.

Target: The particular market segment that is the focus or intended recipient of campaign efforts and messages.

MAIN CONCEPTS

Human medicine has made great strides at reaching out to patients with early detection campaigns. Such campaigns focus on major illnesses and health concerns that can be prevented or treated with early intervention. Hospitals, governments, and nonprofit health associations have been successful at reminding humans to:

- get a mammogram at appropriate intervals. Deaths from breast cancer have been decreasing in the past few decades, as a result of treatment advances, earlier detection through screening, and increased awareness. When mammograms should be started, and the interval at which they should be conducted, can be customized based on individual risk factors
- get regular dental care and address problems early, before they result in chronic irreversible damage
- get a colonoscopy at appropriate intervals. Deaths from colon cancer have also been decreasing over the past few decades, as a result of increased awareness, early detection screening, and the removal of polyps while still precancerous. When colonoscopies should first be started,

and the interval at which they should be conducted, can be customized based on individual risk factors.

There are many more such examples. The results make it obvious that getting patients to play a role in their own health is effective, not only at reducing the occurrence of diseases, but at engaging and involving patients.

So, why not similar campaigns directed at veterinary patients and pet parents? For whatever reason, veterinary medicine has lagged behind when it comes to proactive patient outreach and has instead, in many cases, rested on its laurels with periodic examinations, vaccinations, and parasite control.

Advising pet parents to come in periodically for examinations is not enough. Instead, practices need to elevate the seriousness of proactive screening while boosting awareness of the advanced capabilities of veterinary medicine (see 4.7 Embracing Early Detection). The reality is that pets often face the same diseases and health concerns as humans. It's also true that veterinary medicine has access to many of the equivalent diagnostics and treatments as human medicine. However, it is still not unusual for pet owners to say things like "I didn't know a cat could get diabetes" or "I didn't know a dog could get heart disease."

An early detection campaign is intended to raise the alert to pet parents in a manner that focuses on the disease or health condition along with the pet's welfare. In this way, it is not seen as self-serving to the veterinary practice ("Be sure to book your pet's wellness exam"), and is seen as reaching out to achieve a pet health goal. So, instead of telling pet parents that "if they love their pet" they will bring Fluffy or Fido to the practice for an examination, an early detection campaign engages them by making detection and management of the disease front and center.

A campaign is an organized effort that includes a series of connected initiatives created to bring about a particular result. An early detection campaign:

- focuses on a desired goal or outcome (with milestones to celebrate success)
- elevates awareness about a disease or health condition
- provides a means of confronting or managing the disease or health condition
- reaches out to a target or targets who are most likely to be affected
- is a process that integrates multiple messages through multiple channels.

An early detection campaign doesn't simply tell pet parents "be sure to get your cat tested for diabetes." Instead it works to engage pet parents by appealing to their self-interest and the interest of their pet by offering:

- information (what they probably didn't know before, including applicable risk factors)
- convenience (ability to easily act on what is being offered)
- belongingness (they are not alone)
- peace of mind (their veterinary team has it covered)
- involvement (they are able to do something)
- ability to act (opposite of helplessness).

An early detection campaign reaches out to a target through multiple channels with multiple tools (see 10.6 Target Marketing and Targeted Client Outreach). Instead of simply reaching out to "pets," such a campaign targets pets that are most susceptible to the particular problem. For example, heart disease affects certain breeds of dogs more than others, including Cavalier King Charles Spaniels, which are prone to degenerative valvular disease. Certain breeds, such as Doberman Pinschers, are prone to dilated cardiomyopathy. In cats, diabetes occurs more often in older neutered males, and especially those that are overweight and fed a diet high in carbohydrates. In addition, certain cat breeds, such as the Burmese, might also be more prone to diabetes mellitus.

Each disease or health issue will have its more susceptible targets (see 1.2 Providing a Lifetime of Care). In reaching out to such targets, an early detection campaign does not rely on a single tactic, but rather reaches out through multiple touch points. Single tactics may produce short-lived results, but may not be effective in the long run. An early detection campaign, on the other hand, seeks to change how and what pet owners believe when it comes to caring for their pets, and a timetable under which such care should be delivered (see 1.3 Personalized Care Plans).

An added benefit of such a campaign is that it helps to position the practice as an expert – and champion – in tackling disease or a health concern that is the focus of the campaign. The practice that is taking a stand to boost early detection and intervention for canine cancers is seen as knowing something about canine cancer, and wanting to minimize its impact on pets. The practice that reaches out to the local community in an effort to help owners recognize and treat osteoarthritis in their pets is more likely to be seen as having expertise in treating this highly debilitating condition. In this way, the campaign elevates perceptions of the practice as not just another generalist practice but as having substantive condition-centric expertise.

EXAMPLES

There are numerous early detection campaigns that can be developed based on pet disease and health conditions. Here are a few examples.

Campaign goal: Reduce occurrence of feline diabetes mellitus while boosting early detection and management.

Possible campaign elements:

- Campaign objectives: more cats receiving early treatment, fewer euthanasias due to diabetes.
- Warnings signs on website, in handouts, or on lobby poster.
- Diabetes screenings for senior and high-risk cats (perhaps in conjunction with National Diabetes Month?).
- Series of informative emails (or incorporate into practice newsletter if one is being produced).
- Preventing diabetes workshops with a focus on feline nutrition.
- Local media publicity focused on the feline diabetes problem.
- Recognition for cats/cat parents that are successfully managing diabetes at home.
- Chart of which cat breeds are more susceptible, and what risk factors are most likely to predispose to diabetes
- Collaboration with local pet-related businesses/organizations (groomers, rescues, and pet supplies retailers) to help with early detection.

Campaign goal: Increase early diagnosis and treatment of canine arthritis.

Possible campaign elements:

- Campaign objectives: fewer pets living with pain; more pets receiving appropriate care and treatment.
- Early detection of conditions that can predispose to arthritis, such as hip dysplasia.
- Gait analysis clinic for dogs.
- Special exercise/mobility classes for dogs with arthritis.
- Warning signs/what to spot at home as website content, on lobby posters, emails.
- Special laser and massage therapy "spas."
- Recognition for pets who are still active despite living with arthritis.
- Local media publicity on pets getting arthritis "just like humans" and what to do about it.
- Collaboration with local pet-related businesses/organizations (groomers, pet supplies retailers, rescues).

- Make early detection campaign pet-centric by targeting those pets most likely to be affected by certain disease and illnesses. Be proactive to identify such problems before they become clinical.
- Campaigns operate in the pet's interest by focusing on disease reduction and early detection as opposed to the veterinarian's perceived self-interest.
- Use a campaign approach that relies on more than one tactic and instead, incorporates multiple touch points through a variety of initiatives and channels.
- Gauge the impact of the campaign so that the practice can report on milestones and successes.

MISCELLANEOUS

Recommended Reading

Cat Diabetes & Health. www.petcathealth.info/cats-likely-suffer-diabetes.

Early detection important for treating pet's heart disease. https://vetmed.illinois.edu/pet_column/early-detection-important-treating-pets-heart-disease

American Cancer Society. Key Statistics for Colorectal Cancer. www.cancer.org/cancer/colon-rectal-cancer/about/key-statistics.html,

Olcott, M. The real reason veterinary visits are declining and four easy things you can do about it. http://content.vitusvet.com/blog/the-real-reason-veterinary-visits-are-declining-and-what-you-can-do-about-it

Reinberg, S. Melanoma rates rising for boomers, falling among young. https://consumer.healthday.com/cancer-information-5/skin-cancer-news-108/melanoma-rates-rising-for-boomers-falling-among-young-730792.html

US Breast Cancer Statistics. www.breastcancer.org/symptoms/understand_bc/statistics

TAKE-AWAYS

- Human health has successfully reduced occurrences of serious disease and illness through targeted early detection campaigns; however, veterinary medicine lags behind in embracing this concept.

10.6

Target Marketing and Targeted Client Outreach

Linda Wasche, MBA, MA

LW Marketworks, Inc., Sylvan Lake, MI, USA

BASICS

10.6.1 Summary

Practices that assess the market, choose their targets, and focus their marketing efforts have greater success than practices trying to be everything to everyone. Target marketing enables practices to address clients and prospects that are the best match for their services; focus marketing efforts to avoid wasting time and resources; develop a positioning strategy that is meaningful and postures the practice to attract and retain the right clientele; develop a service mix that is in alignment with the needs of a practice's targets; and more easily track and measure results.

10.6.2 Terms Defined

Commodity: Services and goods that are easily interchanged due to lack of perceived differences among targets. When services or goods become viewed as a commodity, consumers shop on price alone because they view everything else as equal.

Marketing: The process of developing and delivering services and/or products matched to the needs of consumers with the ability, desire, and means to acquire them. Marketing includes service/product development, pricing, distribution, and promotion.

Positioning Strategy: Defining a practice and creating a market identity that is in alignment with the needs and desires of the practice's targets. A practice's positioning is conveyed through every way in which it interacts with pet owners, including the practice's facility, visual devices and symbols, people, services, and service

delivery. All these elements work together to create an understanding of what pet owners can expect when they walk in the door.

Service Mix: The selection of services a practice offers that should be in alignment with, and reflective of, the needs of its targets. When services are structured around the needs of a target, it's easier for the target to understand the benefit or advantage they will gain from using the service.

Target Marketing: Identifying select target markets and directing marketing efforts to these targets. It is the opposite of mass marketing in which all customers and prospects are treated the same.

MAIN CONCEPTS

Marketing professionals have known for years that mass market appeals only work for homogenous products or services with broad market appeal. These are typically low-cost and low-risk (less customer remorse if they are dissatisfied) products and services that are easily interchangeable and considered commodities. Still, even widely marketed goods and services are often promoted through targeted campaigns.

Once a practice has defined its targets (see 10.4 Client and Patient Segmentation), it's ready to tailor its marketing efforts to reach out to these targets. Practices must start with a good grasp of each target's needs, wants, and preferences. These are related to what defines and distinguishes the target in the first place; for example, cat owners will have different needs from dog owners, and so on. Note that what a target is looking for often changes over time, as the target group's needs evolve, new needs arise, or new choices become available in the marketplace.

Once the target's needs are understood, target marketing is done by creating ways to deliver value to the target using targeted services, targeted programs, and targeted information.

Most practices offer the same types of veterinary services. When services are not targeted, most clients have a difficult time relating to or understanding the need for services such as surgery, chemotherapy, dental care, radiography, ultrasound, and so on. In fact, in most cases, clients hope that their pet will never need any of these!

Practices must look for ways to create and orient services to make them meaningful and relevant to a target. In other words, they must specifically target their services.

For owners interested in pet-specific care, existing services can be bundled to create tailored packages appealing to different targeted segments. Although these "bundles" may contain the same services a practice offers now on an à la carte basis, they are repackaged to create meaning and obvious value for the segment. Examples include:

- senior pet exams for older pets
- healthy living packages for overweight pets
- pre-travel exams for pets who vacation with their owners
- glaucoma screening for breeds at risk
- cat and dog exams based on breed-specific health concerns.

The same principles can be used to create or add new services that reach out to client targets.

- Sports medicine for active/performance pets.
- Hospice care for terminally ill pets (see 8.13 Hospice and Palliative Care).
- Osteoarthritis early detection and care (see 8.20 Team Strategies for Osteoarthritis).

Consider specialized education or study for a veterinarian or staff member who may be interested in reaching out to a particular client target (for example, a trained pet hospice nurse on staff that has affiliated with a local clinical psychologist for client grief counseling).

Another way to deliver value to clients is through targeted programs. Engaging today's pet owners must occur on their terms (see 5.4 The Changing Nature of Pet Owners). Given that pet owners can easily access information from multiple sources, they are more likely to act based on what they've learned from other sources instead of what their veterinarian has told them to do. Developing targeted programs adds value and helps to build client relationships through information/education, participation in the practice (through events, workshops, etc.), access to other pet owners, and so on. Client programs should have meaning and relevancy to a particular client segment and

are a great way to engage clients without being seen as pushing or selling services.

Create programs based on the traits and needs of particular pets, such as:

- pets with chronic conditions
- geriatric pets
- pets with breed-specific health problems
- pets with behavior issues.

Create programs based on client situations, such as:

- multiple pet homes
- families with new puppies or kittens
- rescue group foster care homes
- homes with young children.

Use programs as a platform for delivering value to clients and prospects through:

- workshops, seminars, and events
- blogs, including guest blogs by clients
- support groups
- special education/instruction
- patient specials and special offers
- related social media posts.

Finally, practices that target outgoing information are more likely to have an impact. Due to information overload, consumers have become adept at disregarding messages that they consider a waste of time and at capturing those that mean something to them. Practices that target their marketing are more likely to get through the filters. Instead of sending out "one size fits all" reminders, practices should engage clients with information that's relevant to their pets or households by varying newsletter content to reach out to different pet owner targets; creating specialized bulletins or newsletters tailored to particular segments (e.g., cats, big dogs, purebreds, senior pets, performance pets, etc.); developing information pieces and/or website content tailored to different pet health concerns and issues; creating useful videos that reach out to specific pet owner issues and concerns; or reaching out to different client segments via Facebook, Twitter, and other social media.

Another benefit of target marketing is that practices will find it easier to track and measure results. Practices can gauge which targets are most responsive to various initiatives and which, for whatever reason, are not.

Target marketing also enables clients to capture meaningful client feedback. By targeting particular client groups for surveys, focus groups, interviews, and other client feedback measurement tools, practices will gain a better understanding of which groups' needs are being met and which are not. This is superior to simply putting clients into one big group and lumping responses together.

EXAMPLES

One feline-only practice has reached out to families whose cat has a terminal illness or is near the end of life. The practice's end-of-life and hospice care program targets clients whose cats are considered family members and who are looking for options to euthanasia but have concerns about their pet comfort. The end-of-life care program, which offers palliative care and helps clients monitor their pet's quality of life, fits hand in hand with another of the practice's targets: clients with pets with serious illnesses and chronic conditions who value support with end of life considerations.

 TAKE-AWAYS

- Practices that offer the same services as everyone else are at risk of their services being viewed as a commodity – easily interchangeable with those of other practices.
- Targeting veterinary services makes them meaningful and relevant to the client by tailoring them to pets' needs.
- Targeted programs go beyond veterinary services to add value and engage clients through useful information/education and participation in events, workshops, clinics, and other means of outreach.
- Client information that is targeted, versus "one size fits all," is more likely to get the attention of pet families.
- Targeting also makes it easier for practices to track and measure the results of marketing efforts.

 MISCELLANEOUS

10.6.3 Cautions

Practices must make sure that they're prepared to service a particular segment before reaching out to it. This means putting in place the right expertise and experience, procedures and protocols, internal communication, and client information. It's easy to lose client trust when a service area or program lacks clarity or credibility. Making whatever you do real before introducing it to clients is a must.

To effectively perform target marketing, it is important to appropriately "flag" patient features in the practice management software so that pets with similar needs can be easily located for marketing campaigns (see 7.9 Using Practice Management Software to Personalize Care). For example, although features such as species, breed, age, and gender are easily segmented within practice management software, others are not routinely designated for later recall. Some of these important segments might include periodontal score, body condition score, pain score, diagnosis, and therapy. Once this type of information is routinely entered and flagged within the software, it is possible to recall all patients with a specific feature to be sent targeted marketing materials.

Recommended Reading

Best, R.J. (2009). *Market-Based Management: Strategies for Growing Customer Value and Profitability*, 5e. Upper Saddle River, NJ: Pearson Prentice Hall.

Wasche, L. (2020). Target marketing and targeted client outreach. In: *Five Minute Veterinary Practice Management Consult*, 3e (ed. L. Ackerman), 406–407. Ames, IA: Wiley.

10.7

Breed-Specific Marketing

Peter Weinstein, DVM, MBA

PAW Consulting, Irvine, CA, USA

BASICS

10.7.1 Summary

Marketing refers to the activities used by a hospital to get a pet owner to act on a need for their pet. In most cases, marketing activities are general and impersonal. Breed-specific marketing is personalized to the pet owner and their pet, including both purebred and mixed-breed pets. By personalizing the marketing efforts, the client realizes that the practice has customized their experience, thus strengthening the bond between the practice and the pet owner.

Retention marketing, acquisition marketing, and referral marketing are all components of the marketing mix, but they usually lack anything to create a stronger bond. Breed-specific marketing is focused on educating the pet owner about the diseases, conditions, and problems that a particular breed or mix of breeds displays more frequently as a result of a congenital, hereditary, or other predilection. By sharing knowledge with a pet owner, they can start to act earlier to diagnose or treat and it minimizes the surprises that everyone dislikes.

10.7.2 Terms Defined

Acquisition Marketing: Marketing to pet owners that are not your clients to get them to choose your practice for their veterinary care.

Breed-Specific Marketing: Educating clients about the pertinent risks relevant to their specific pet in order to encourage proactive engagement. Breed-specific marketing

also refers to programs created to educate and inform clients about their pet's risks based upon that breed's associated risk factors.

Marketing: Getting people who have a specific need to know, like and trust you, your products, and your services.

Referral Marketing: Marketing to your clients and other local businesses to get them to refer their friends, family, and co-workers to your practice for veterinary and other care that your practice provides.

Retention Marketing: Marketing specifically to your existing clientele to get them utilize your services.

MAIN CONCEPTS

10.7.3 Foundation

If marketing is getting people who have a need to know, like and trust you, there are certain things you can do to get clients to know you; this is the basis of acquisition marketing. This involves doing everything to get a pet owner to choose your practice over all others and to become a client of your practice (see 10.6 Target Marketing and Targeted Client Outreach). Once they have experienced your practice, it is imperative to retain them as clients as long as they have their current pet and then the next pet or pets. There are many components to retention marketing that practices use to keep their clients satisfied and coming back for more. One of the more relevant components of retention marketing is education marketing. In education marketing, you use all your marketing tools to teach your clients how to be responsible pet owners.

10.7.4 What is Breed-Specific Marketing?

In the current environment, where all information is readily available on the internet, it is more imperative than ever for the veterinary practice to be the primary source for accurate and relevant information for pet owners on the care of their pets. Whether the pet is a dog, cat, or other species, there are tendencies that veterinarians see in conditions that pets develop. Skin, ear, and eye problems in cocker spaniels are an example of medical disorders that are overrepresented in this breed And in mixed breeds in which the cocker spaniel is a genetic component. Developmental joint problems are more likely in Labrador retrievers and any mix breed with Labradors.

To be the primary source for pet owner education, veterinarians must take a proactive approach to client education on wellness care, preveative care, and breed-specific care. And it should start early in the pet's life. Create a system to share the various problems that a breed might develop at the various puppy visits and continue to have this conversation at subsequent annual visits. However, you must go beyond this.

Create an ongoing breed-specific education marketing program that reaches out to pet owners with customized marketing pieces on a regular basis. An email that provides details on a single high-risk condition for that breed can be sent out quarterly or more often if desired. Letters with information can also be created and mailed regularly. Even text messages can be a part of the education program.

Of course, the aim is not to scare pet owners but rather to teach and let them know that your practice can help them with early diagnosis and treatment. Additionally, too much knowledge in any one message is daunting and could be detrimental to your efforts. Keep it simple, focused, directed, and customized, such as: "Did you know that Goldie and other golden retrievers have a very high risk for developing hip dysplasia? Hip dysplasia is. . .."

There are hundreds of different breeds of dogs and cats not including the other species you see in practice. Start with the top 20 registered breeds in your area or, better yet, use your practice management software to see which breeds are most represented as patients in your practice. With this information in hand, you need to do some research on breed predilections (see 11.4 Heritable Health Conditions – By Breed). There are a number of books and websites that are great resources to help you create your own breed-specific education pieces. Do not just refer people to somebody else's website. This is your chance to strengthen your bond with your clients with personalized and customized information.

You can host your own breed-specific education pieces on your website and refer people to your website to supplement the conversations, handouts, emails, letters, and texts you use. This is also great team-based healthcare delivery as your client service team, technicians, and assistant team can all be a part of the education process.

10.7.5 Why Breed-Specific Marketing?

In a competitive marketplace, there are many ways to differentiate your practice (see 10.2 The Importance of Practice Differentiation). Price, location, service, value, and relationships are among things clients look for. Most practices offer the same or similar product mix and service mix to the pet owner, so you have to use every skill you have to get your new clients and retain them for the duration. In general, educated clients are more likely to say "yes" to their pet's needs since they can make decisions from a position of knowledge and not emotion. By providing information to a client about what their pets need and why they need it, you can differentiate yourself from competitive practices that only focus on providing services. The process of education often starts with basic puppy or kitten care and usually ends there except for annual wellness visits or sick pets. That needs to change.

If you are looking for a means to make your practice stand out and focus on the needs of pets individually, breed-specific marketing puts you ahead of the competition who aren't having these discussions. Every piece of knowledge you share creates a great level of trust for the client with the practice. This is another example of transparency in communication while concurrently helping with early diagnosis and treatment. So, the answer to the question "why do breed-specific marketing?" is to add value, educate, build trust, and differentiate from other practices.

10.7.6 How to Do Breed-Specific Marketing

Breed-specific healthcare starts with helping pet owners to select their pet (see 3.10 Advising Clients on Selecting an Appropriate Pet). This is a discussion about clinical issues that are prevalent as well as behavioral issues that are possible and probable without appropriate training. Do your clients come to you for advice when choosing their next pet? If not, why not? Do you let them know that you and your team are there to help them make a right choice based upon lifestyle and pet health? Step one in breed-specific marketing is being there to help choose pets that are best for the client.

10.7.6.1 What, Who, When, How to Perform Breed-Specific Marketing

Before you get started, you'll need the following.

1) A digital camera – clients love pictures of their pets. Take one at least every year and add it to the record.
2) Create breed-specific handouts and information about the what and why of each breed and their specific conditions.
3) Timeline for each visit and what to address at each visit from the list of conditions relevant to the breed.
4) Timeline for educational sends using social media, text, email, snail mail, etc., to be sent between visits.
5) A breed-specific spreadsheet that includes #3 and 4 above (see Figures 10.7.1 and 10.7.2).

10.7.6.2 Action Items

1) Search your database for your most frequent breeds and work on the content to support them as they are the breeds that you will see in the future as well. Start adding the next tier of top breeds after you have completed your most frequent list.

Puppy to one year
Discussions and education pieces on:
    Hip dysplasia (radiographs)
    Elbow dysplasia (radiographs)
    Progressive retinal atrophy (genetic testing, ERG)
    Subaortic stenosis (stethoscope, radiographs, ultrasound)
    Von Willebrand disease (genetic testing and vWF)

One year to six years
Discussions and education pieces on:
    Conditions noted for *Puppy to one year* plus:
    Atopic dermatitis
    Ear infections
    Epilepsy
    Hypothyroidism
    Cancer – lymphosarcoma, osteosarcoma, mastocytoma, hemangiosarcoma
    Bloat and/or GDV
    Cataracts (based on genetic testing results)

Over seven years
Discussions and education pieces on:
    Conditions noted for ages *Puppy to seven years* plus:
    Senior screening
    Cognitive impairment
    Senior care

Figure 10.7.1 Example of a checklist for breed-specific life stage marketing.

2) Start the conversation about breed-specific marketing with each new puppy or kitten.
3) Take a picture on each visit.
4) Follow up with each puppy and kitten on a regular basis with new information and knowledge using all the tools that you have, including text, postcard, email, letter, phone call, conversation, virtual care, etc.
5) For patients that have not been included in your breed-specific program as puppies/kittens, based upon their age, start to integrate the program into the

	ACTION	<6 months	6 months to 18 months	18 months to 7 years	>7 years
Hip dysplasia	Radiographs	Conversation	Email		
Elbow dysplasia	Radiographs	Conversation	Email		
Progressive retinal atrophy	Eye Exam, Genetic screening	Conversation Email		Conversation Email Letter	Conversation Email
Bloat/GDV	Gastropexy	Conversation Email	Conversation	Email	Text
Cancer	Exam Labwork Radiographs			Conversation Email Text	Conversation Email
Hypothyroidism	Thyroid profile		Conversation Email	Conversation Email Text	Conversation Email Text

Figure 10.7.2 Example of a breed-specific marketing plan

regular visits (better yet, add a breed-specific visit to the schedule).

6) For patients that have not been included previously, start them on a series of educational pieces based upon their age and breed and communicate with them using all the tools that you have, including text, postcard, email, letter, phone call, conversation, virtual care, etc.

7) Marketing pieces should be educational, informational, easy to read, not too long, graphically appealing, customized to include the pet's name, and include a call to action.
   - Did you know that golden retrievers like Goldie have a much higher risk of developing certain cancers? We can work with you and Goldie to identify cancer risk early which improves survival and ….
   - Goldie, as a middle-aged golden retriever, has a higher than average risk of developing hypothyroidism – a condition where the thyroid gland produces too little of its thyroid hormone. These conditions may manifest themselves… and we can easily test Goldie for this condition and get her started on treatment if needed.

8) Marketing should be done at least quarterly to keep your practice top of mind to the client.

9) You can include a motivation to action which could be free food, nail trim, discount, etc.

10) Measure your success by tracking the marketing that you do and its related costs and the number of additional tests, radiographs, exams, etc. that you perform.

10.7.6.3 External Marketing

Social media is a great tool to promote your focus on breed-specific education and care. While many social media posts show cute puppy and kitten pictures or new clients and patients, here is an opportunity to educate your clients and potential clients about their pets and their healthcare needs (see 7.5 Connecting with Clients Through Social Media).

With so many breeds of dogs and cats and so many medical and behavioral conditions prevalent, you should dedicate one post per week on all your social media platforms to a "Breed-Specific Did You Know That. . ..?" If you have had a success story where a condition was diagnosed early, allowing for earlier intervention, highlight that story. If you have situations where earlier intervention via earlier diagnosis could have been beneficial, highlight that as well. Take advantage of the graphical and interactive nature of social media to tell stories and seek stories on breed-specific conditions to help clients and potential clients know and understand their pet's health better.

10.7.7 Final Thoughts

Every day that you are not communicating with your clients is a day that they can be cajoled to look for another veterinarian to save money or find a stronger relationship than they currently have. By reaching out on a routine basis and providing knowledge and expertise, you are keeping them away from Dr Google while concurrently showing how much you care about the health of their pet. The worst thing that a client can say to you is, "I didn't know that! Nobody told me about this being a problem." A fully transparent educational marketing program will help clients prepare for inevitabilities if they occur or be wary of things that might be on the horizon. And most importantly, this puts you top of mind on a regular basis when you reach out.

Breed-specific healthcare replaces the depersonalized and commoditization of veterinary care with a form of personalized and customized care. Consider it as a way to provide "designer medicine" for your clients who are looking for added value from their veterinary experience.

10.7.8 Future Thoughts

The increasing accuracy of genetic testing for breed identification will allow pet owners to have a better understanding of the breed composition of their mixed-breed pet and will give veterinarians greater understanding about what conditions might be of greater risk to a pet given the likely genetic make-up. There is also an increasing amount of research on conditions they might be carrying genetically (see 3.4 Predicting and Eliminating Disease Traits). This testing provides another tool for veterinarians to discuss the risks and benefits of inherited conditions.

Drug sensitivity testing is another developing option with breed-specific aspects. Sensitivities to ivermectin, milbemycin, and loperamide are just a few of the potential drug reactions that can be tested for by looking for a mutation in the MDR1 gene. In the future, we should be able to use genomics to identify drugs most likely to be beneficial (or not) in individual patients with specific genetic markers.

 TAKE-AWAYS

- Create a breed-specific marketing system for your practice that includes client education resources and a schedule for ongoing education using both direct marketing and social media marketing.

- Starting with puppy and kitten visits, share breed predilections with pet owners, focusing at this age on developmental abnormalities.
- Create annual breed-specific foci recognizing that certain breed predilections do not become evident until a pet gets older, e.g., hypothyroidism, glaucoma, keratoconjunctivitis sicca, etc.
- Mixed-breeds, whether dogs or cats, should be a part of the breed-specific marketing if you know the breeds that make up the gene pool. Just because a pet is a mixed-breed doesn't mean that they are immune to breed-specific conditions; in fact, they are at risk of getting any or all of the different breeds' problems, depending on how they are inherited.
- Monitor the number of additional diagnostic screening tests performed in response to your education programs to measure how your marketing is working. Adjust as needed.

MISCELLANEOUS

10.7.9 Cautions

Don't ignore mixed breeds (see 3.19 Mixed-Breed Considerations). This is such a large component of your patient list that you need to focus on them as being at risk for a multitude of issues and they aren't necessarily safe because they are a mutt (or moggie).

Don't overmarket. Send small bite-size information snippets written at an easy to understand level. Pictures or videos are a great adjunct.

Abbreviations

ERG   Electroretinogram
GDV   Gastric dilation/volvulus
vWF   von Willebrand factor

Recommended Reading

Ackerman, L. (2011). *The Genetic Connection*. Lakewood, CO: AAHA Press.

Benchmarks 2020. A Study of Well-Managed Practices. WTA Veterinary Consultants, 2019, http://wellmp.com

10.8

Using Practice Data as a Credibility-Boosting Tool

Linda Wasche, MBA, MA

LW Marketworks, Inc., Sylvan Lake, MI, USA

 BASICS

10.8.1 Summary

Veterinary practice management software enables practices to track multiple pet variables. The resulting data not only make it easy to develop and disperse targeted messaging and programs, but are a valuable tool for boosting practice credibility as well as level of patient care.

A typical veterinary practice's software is capable of tracking and tabulating:

- prevalence of diseases/health conditions
- types of patients most commonly affected (by species, breed, lifestyle, and so on)
- treatments and outcomes.

Such data are often underutilized by veterinary practices, which is unfortunate. They can be used to:

- identify high-risk/most vulnerable patients
- show patterns and trends in disease occurrence
- track outcomes
- develop more insightful diagnoses and treatments.

The resulting information can be used to boost the trust and confidence that pet parents have in the practice as well as increase quality of care.

10.8.2 Terms Defined

Credibility: The quality of being trusted and believed; being convincing or believable.

Data: Information collected for reference or analysis. Practice management software allows practices to establish data collection variables and to analyze data using these variables.

Variable: An element, feature, or factor. For our purposes, variables include patient traits and characteristics, health conditions, treatment options, outcomes, and other factors that can be measured and analyzed.

 MAIN CONCEPTS

In human medicine, data are used to predict epidemics, analyze patient characteristics, cure disease, identify the most effective treatments, profile patients for preventive care initiatives, identify predictive events in disease outbreaks, avoid preventable deaths, and much more. Data are used to understand as much as possible about a patient to pick up early warning signs of serious illness when treatment is far simpler (and less expensive) than if it had not been spotted until later [1].

Human healthcare providers also use data in human interventions and preventive care initiatives. Instead of simply reminding human patients to "get their wellness exam," physicians can target 40-year-old females with a family history of (or genetic markers for) breast cancer to let them know, with a great deal of certainty, how likely they are to experience the same disease, at what age, and what they can do about it. Or similarly, human medicine can target 30-year-old males with a family history of colon cancer and suggest recommended diagnostics based on the projected likelihood of the patient getting the disease.

Pet-Specific Care for the Veterinary Team, First Edition. Edited by Lowell Ackerman.
© 2021 John Wiley & Sons, Inc. Published 2021 by John Wiley & Sons, Inc.

Physicians use data not only to tailor care but to build a more compelling and meaningful reason for patients to pay attention to and act on their advice. Instead of encouraging patients to "come and see the doctor" – seen as self-serving to the physician – patients are appealed to in an effort to act in their own best interest. In human medicine, data are the basis for numerous patient outreach initiatives and campaigns that do exactly that. It's more effective to convey that "The five-year survival rate for colorectal cancer found at the local stage is 90%" [2] than it is to simply say, "Come on in for your colonoscopy."

In veterinary medicine, electronic recording systems were originally used for record keeping and billing. However, a wealth of data can be captured for research as well as for developing evidence-based approaches to clinical practice and the subsequent improvement of animal health [3]. The veterinary practice that uses data to connect with pet parents tells a much more compelling story (see 7.9 Using Practice Management Software to Personalize Care). It also boosts its credibility as a veterinary services provider by using the practice's own data to share its expertise.

Useable data are being captured by practice management software each time a practice sees a pet and records the pet's signalment, diagnosis, and/or treatment. It's up to the practice to analyze the data and put it to use. Practices can easily track diagnoses and cross-tabulate them by any number of variables including species, breed, age, and size of pet. Table 10.8.1 outlines an example of a simple frequency analysis that could be compiled to track the occurrence of diabetes, in this case, in felines. Data can be easily cross-tabulated in the software to obtain data across multiple variables – breed and age, for example. Such data can also be used to track occurrence rate fluctuations during the course of months or years, as well as seasonal variances.

Table 10.8.1 provides an illustration of how a practice can track the occurrence of diabetes mellitus in felines. Of course, this can be done using any health condition and any

variables that the practice finds meaningful to the particular disease or health condition. In any case, it enables the practice to stand on firm ground when discussing the occurrence of a disease and what pet parents can do about it. So, instead of saying "Sure, we treat feline diabetes. We do it all," a practice can say, for example, "In the past four years, we have seen the rate of diabetes mellitus increase 120 percent in cats that are 7 years or older. Our data show that breeds such as Burmese and Russian Blue make up more than half of the patients we are treating for this disease. Remember that when caught early, feline diabetes is highly manageable."

The practice that shares such data – with clients and the local community:

- adds substance and believability to its message
- demonstrates its experience/expertise in diagnosing and treating a particular disease
- appears as proactive versus reactive in diagnosing and managing a disease
- comes across as more authoritative and credible
- can target messages and programs to high-risk/most vulnerable patient groups.

Practices might wonder how to go about sharing such data. There are numerous channels for using data to provide meaningful and relevant content to pet parents.

Use data in *social media*. Most practices post messages to social media such as Facebook and Twitter. These are very simple media in which including data will strengthen and add substance to posts (see 7.5 Connecting with Clients Through Social Media). For example, instead of posting "February is National Dental Health Month. Don't forget your pet's dental exam," think about how data might make this plea stronger. Consider: "Of the 2200 cats we saw last year, 1900 suffered from periodontal disease. Of these, more than half were under the age of 3."

Use data as part of *website content*. The purpose of your website is to provide a means of getting acquainted with

Table 10.8.1 Example: occurrence of feline diabetes

Diabetes	Species Qu.		Breed[a] Qu.		Age Qu.		Size Qu.	
	Feline	?	Burmese	?	<3	?	<2.5 kg	?
			Russian blue	?	3–7	?	2.5–5 kg	?
			Norwegian forest cat	?	8–12	?	5–7 kg	?
			Abyssinian	?	13–20	?	>7 kg	?
			Other	?	>20	?		
	Canine		(Fill in)					
	Exotic		(Fill in)					

[a] The breeds listed in this example are all considered to experience higher rates of diabetes mellitus than other feline breeds [4].

your practice before a new client walks in the door. It is also a resource for existing clients to turn to with questions and concerns. Many practice websites contain sections on various diseases and health conditions as well as breed-specific content, age-related health concerns and so on. Consider incorporating data into all of these areas.

Use data in *pet parent communication*. Many practices publish electronic newsletters or send periodic emails – in the form of alerts or reminders – to pet parents. Some provide printed fact sheets and information pieces. Again, instead of just telling pet parents what to do, make messages more credible with data. A practice in the American Midwest might send out an alert about the dangers of blue-green algae on freshwater lakes and ponds. Consider how much more powerful this message would be by stating how many dogs the practice treated but could not save last spring/summer due to this terrible, but often underreported health hazard.

Use data to create local *publicity*. Publicity is coverage in news outlets: TV, radio, newspapers, magazines, and online news sources. It's different from advertising in that it is not paid for, but instead is earned because of the newsworthiness of the information.

News media love to use data which is considered factual and credible. There are any number of opportunities for a veterinary practice to place news on such topics as:

- increases in occurrence of a particular disease
- decrease in disease given certain pet owner practices
- winning the battle against a certain disease, etc.

Finally, use data as the basis for local *outreach campaigns*. There is tremendous potential for a practice that uses data to create a campaign focused on a data-driven goal (see 10.6 Target Marketing and Targeted Client Outreach). Such a goal might be to reduce occurrences of feline diabetes mellitus, increase early detection – and survival rate – for dogs with osteosarcoma, detect early evidence of hip dysplasia in breeds at risk, or reduce occurrence of feline kidney disease. In such a campaign, the practice leads the charge to make a difference for pets in the community. Campaigns include a multichannel effort that, in the course of striving for the goal, serves to raise awareness, engage clients and rally pet parents around a common cause (see 10.5 Early Detection Campaigns.)

EXAMPLES

There are numerous examples of using pet diagnostic and treatment data to benefit a practice. Tracking the occurrence of multiple diseases and health conditions

can help pet parents recognize the significance of early detection (see 4.7 Embracing Early Detection). Examples include increases and decreases in prevalence of heart disease, cancers, diabetes, thyroid disease, arthritis, kidney disease, pancreatitis, Lyme disease, leptospirosis, liver disease, and so on.

TAKE-AWAYS

- Put to use data that your practice is already capturing.
- Use data to make a more compelling reason for pet parents to follow standards for preventive care and early detection.
- Incorporate data into messaging to add credibility and build practice trust.
- Pattern efforts on numerous successful human health initiatives.
- Target messaging and programs to high-risk patient segments.

MISCELLANEOUS

References

1 Marr, B. How Big Data is Changing Healthcare. www.forbes.com/sites/bernardmarr/2015/04/21/how-big-data-is-changing-healthcare/

2 American Cancer Society. Key Statistics for Colorectal Cancer. www.cancer.org/cancer/colon-rectal-cancer/about/key-statistics.html

3 Jones-Diette, J., Brennan, M.L., Cobb, M. et al. (2016). A method for extracting electronic patient record data from practice management software systems used in veterinary practice. *BMC Vet Res.* 12: 239. www.ncbi.nlm.nih.gov/pmc/articles/PMC5073902.

4 Öhlund, M., Fall, T., Ström Holst, B. et al. (2015). Incidence of diabetes mellitus in insured Swedish cats in relation to age, breed and sex. *Journal of Veterinary Internal Medicine* 29: 1342–1347. www.ncbi.nlm.nih.gov/pmc/articles/PMC4858030.

Recommended Reading

Raghupathi, W. and Raghupathi, V. (2014). Big data analytics in healthcare: promise and potential. *Health Inf Sci Syst.* 2: 3. www.ncbi.nlm.nih.gov/pmc/articles/PMC4341817.

10.9

Laboratory Considerations

Kara M. Burns, MS, MEd, LVT, VTS (Nutrition)

Lafayette, IN, USA

BASICS

10.9.1 Summary

Many veterinary hospitals today provide in-house laboratory testing. However, the extent of in-house laboratory testing in a veterinary hospital varies dependent upon the philosophy of the hospital owner and veterinary team. Additionally, as new and advanced equipment and tests become available, the amount of in-house laboratory testing may change. Some veterinary hospitals will run everything in-house that they possibly can. Other hospitals find they use their laboratory primarily for emergency/critical care purposes. Essentially, all clinics find it necessary to utilize a blend of their in-house laboratory and a reference laboratory to meet the needs of their clients.

The question that some practices struggle with is "Do I send it out or run it in-house?" Other hospitals struggle with the fact that each doctor randomly decides where to perform testing – there is no set protocol. Deciding on what the appropriate mix should be depends on several factors. Once these factors are understood and researched, it becomes easier to make an appropriate decision on the combination. The choice is an individual one, partially based upon practice philosophy, culture, practice set-up and size, and the results of researching the issue.

10.9.2 Terms Defined

In-House Laboratory Services: All laboratory testing that can be readily completed at the hospital by the hospital team: chemistry profiles, complete blood cell counts, urinalysis, intestinal parasite testing, cytology, in-house testing kits, and so on.

Integrated Diagnostic Systems: Diagnostic tests that are linked to practice software; often entering the diagnostic code will both order the test (in-house or outside) and input the charge for the test. Results typically are downloaded into the medical record and manual entry is not required.

Outsourcing (Laboratory Testing): Laboratory testing that is sent out to be completed by an outside company, typically a reference laboratory.

Real Time (Laboratory Testing): Laboratory testing performed at the hospital (in-house), by the hospital team, for immediate results.

Workflow Dynamics: How the flow of work is organized to occur at the business place/hospital. This may or may not be the most efficient; the status quo is often evaluated to come up with a process that might lead to better efficiencies or better customer service.

MAIN CONCEPTS

The following issues, pros, and cons, should be considered when deciding the correct mix of laboratory services for a specific practice.

10.9.3 Cost

A fundamental question that arises when comparing in-house to reference laboratory services is the cost comparison.

- From a cost accounting standpoint alone, when all aspects are added in, it typically costs more to run testing in-house versus sending to the reference laboratory.
- When you consider such factors as reagent cost, labor, and wasted reagents, it is typically more costly to perform testing in-house.
- A clinic's ability to negotiate pricing for in-house reagents and outside laboratory services will likely impact the cost differential, but it would not be unusual for there to be upwards of a 25% difference. The difference typically is significant and should be considered.

10.9.4 Accuracy

Many clinics rely on in-house testing for critical care/sick pet visits because they need quick answers – but are these results as accurate as they would be if they were sent to the reference laboratory? How do they compare? Can you expect an in-house laboratory station to get as good results as those performed by a reference laboratory? Can the quality control of an in-house laboratory compare with that of a reference laboratory? In addition, when it comes to intestinal parasite testing or performing a urinalysis, can your technical crew compare with the expertise of reference laboratory technicians who spend most of their time preparing and reading samples?

- There is not much argument that blood chemistry results run in-house or at the outside laboratory yield comparable results. In-house, however, may have limitations on the scope of available tests and panels.
- Hemogram results from the reference laboratories likely yield more reliable results on a consistent basis.
- Regarding results for fecal and urine samples, preparation, handling, and experience of the reader have a big impact on the final result.
- The reference laboratory provides a degree of quality control on these samples; in-house this is more likely to be variable and also would be expected to vary depending on how reliably the equipment is calibrated.
- Overall, the biggest areas of discrepancy/reader error are hematology and tests that require use of the microscope.

10.9.5 Efficiency

Besides cost and accuracy, clinics must carefully consider the issue of efficiency and any potential impact this will have on customer service. There are several ways to look at efficiency – staff time, doctor time, and potential client wait time. Does it make sense for a practice to take up time processing/reading blood, fecal, and urine samples in real time while a client is waiting? Does that answer change if the patient is sick vs healthy?

10.9.6 The Argument for Outsourcing

Many clinics see the value (time-wise) of sending out routine wellness tests: blood, urine, and stool. If the patient does not have a pressing medical concern, it makes sense to send testing that is not time sensitive to a reference laboratory.

- The results from these tests are not vital and not time sensitive, so outsourcing them to the reference laboratory saves valuable time – for the veterinary team and the client – as they do not have to wait around for results. Instead, they can leave and be informed later of the laboratory results. Consider, for example, the wellness fecal. To properly prepare and accurately read this sample is time consuming; instead, the team member could be focusing on client care, education, and allowing the client to leave the practice in a timely manner. Another issue that may occur is the sample is performed in-house but not real time. Consider that during busy days, fecal samples may accumulate waiting for technician availability, only to be read much later or when time allows. When this occurs, accuracy may be adversely affected.
- Clinics that prefer outsourcing believe it is efficient, and a good use of team and client time.

10.9.7 The Argument for In-House Testing

Based on the previous discussion and the touting of efficiency, why is there a growing body of practices that prefer real-time testing and immediate results? Although many clinics outsource routine laboratory work, there is a small but growing percentage of clinics that prefer processing results immediately with clients present. These practices see major advantages to this

- They find it efficient to run almost all laboratory work in house because they can give the client results right away, explain the results, and educate clients as needed.
- They feel there is much value in this approach, as the client can readily discuss results and better understand the purpose of the tests performed.
- When results are available right away, the doctor does not need to reconnect with the owner to discuss them

and does not need to leave messages the client may not understand.

- For preanesthetic laboratory testing, the pet can be admitted and the laboratory work performed prior to anesthesia. This is convenient for the client and provides up-to-date results for the clinician.
- When practices have invested heavily in in-house laboratory equipment, they can only achieve cost efficiency by running as many samples as possible through that equipment.

Advances in technology are making the real-time approach more feasible and realistic for many clinics. The new analyzers often use minimal amounts of blood, require minimal preparation, have faster turnaround time (5–10 minutes), and have the potential to run multiple samples at one time.

- Practices that fully embrace this approach may have all samples collected from pets before the doctor sees the pet, and results are ready before the pet leaves.
- Clinics that focus on workflow dynamics prefer the efficiency of this system; if a problem is detected, medication or treatment can be provided at the time, rather than inconveniencing the client to return and potentially letting a problem linger.
- It is also often much easier for the team or doctor to educate clients when they are there and can see the actual results.
- Another benefit and time saver is that if laboratory testing and reports occur on a real-time basis, then there are no inefficiencies associated with reviewing accumulated patient laboratory work, remembering the specifics of each case, and then telephoning the clients to discuss the results.

10.9.8 Best Mix for the Hospital

Many factors influence the proper mix of in-house and outside laboratory services for a practice. For many clinics, sending out all laboratory tests except critical care cases makes sense; it keeps the client flow running smoothly, allowing the team to focus on the client rather than running tests. In addition, it's cost effective for the clinic and client, allows for expanded testing, and is very accurate. Laboratory results are typically downloaded directly into the client's medical record, if the system is fully integrated.

In contrast, clinics that prefer running testing in-house likely charge a little more for what they consider a premium service. They feel that having results at the time of the clinic visit provides excellent service to clients and

allows for prompt treatment of problems and saves the clinic time by not relegating additional work (file review, client call-back) to the next day. In addition, most in-house blood analyzers now integrate/download results right into practice management software, another time saver versus manually entering results.

The mix a practice ultimately chooses is influenced partially by practice philosophy that is based on the aforementioned factors – *cost*, *accuracy*, and areas of *efficiency* – which they feel will work best for their clinic. Practices can change the mix from time to time as well; a clinic that upgrades equipment may be excited to switch to real-time results.

The size of a clinic often influences what works best. A multidoctor practice that is trying to improve workflow dynamics may find it easier to have results done in-house so that the next day, if different doctors are at the hospital, they do not need to interpret results on cases they did not see. Practice culture may also dictate the mix: "That's the way we've done it for years," may be the attitude.

Clients want it all – fast and accurate results that are cost efficient. To meet these expectations, the veterinary team can provide the following:

- a diagnostic base of wellness services
- protocols for early disease detection
- standards of care with chronic disease management
- real-time results during consultations.

Patient care can be promoted with an in-house lab and consequently provide fast relief to the patient [1].

As the expectation of rapid results intensifies, it is important for the veterinary team to recognize that the best time to establish informed consent (see 7.4 Getting Informed Consent) and discuss a treatment plan is while the client is still in the practice. The immediate review of diagnostic results helps reinforce the perception of value and strengthen the trust in the veterinary team needed to create an effective therapeutic plan.

Additionally, a practice's operations can be improved considerably through the reduction of team member time spent on phone consultations to deliver next-day results from reference labs.

Most clinics tend to be hybrids. Many send noncritical blood samples to the reference laboratory, but they may run fecal and urine samples in the clinic. Others send the majority of this work to the reference laboratory, but they may run preanesthetic bloodwork in-house on the morning of the procedure. Other hospitals may hire a consultant to analyze their workflow to help determine the best approach for their clinic. There really is not a right or wrong mix; a lot of the decision making may be based on the actual veterinary team and practice philosophy.

TAKE-AWAYS

- A point to consider when comparing in-house to reference laboratory services is the cost comparison of performing a test in-house vs sending that same test to the outside laboratory.
- Clinics need to consider the need for in-house testing for critical care/sick pet visits (quick answers) vs the accuracy of the results.
- Clinics need to consider the issue of efficiency and the potential impact this may have on customer service.
- Veterinary healthcare teams must discuss in-house testing vs outsourcing and develop a protocol that meets the practice's standard of care and the client's expectations.
- Clients want it all. Therefore, most hospitals develop a hybrid protocol.

MISCELLANEOUS

Reference

1 Riolo, C.A. Benefits of in-house labs. www.veterinarypracticenews.com/benefits-of-in-house-labs/

Recommended Reading

Antech Insights (2011). *July Focus: In-House vs. Reference Lab Testing, Part I*. Chapel Hill, NC: Antech Diagnostics.

Antech Insights (2011). *July Focus: In-House vs. Reference Lab Testing, Part II*. Chapel Hill, NC: Antech Diagnostics.

Metzger, F. 10 reasons to test in house. www.dvm360.com/view/10-reasons-test-house

SafePath Laboratories, LLC. Cost of In-house Testing for Veterinary Diseases vs Cost of Send Out Laboratory Testing. https://safepath.com/cost-of-in-house-testing-for-veterinary-diseases-vs-cost-of-send-out-laboratory-testing

10.10

Making Referrals Work

Suzanne Russo, DVM, MS

College of Veterinary Medicine, Midwestern University, Glendale, AZ, USA

BASICS

10.10.1 Summary

Veterinary medicine has become increasingly specialized and will continue to be so into the foreseeable future. As a result, we have many resources to help us deliver optimal healthcare for our patients and the families that care for them. With so many opportunities to partner with specialty healthcare, it is critical for general practitioners and specialists to develop processes and procedures within their practices that support the most advantageous relationships between their clients and their referral partners of choice.

Many of the specialties that are available in human medicine are now available for our veterinary patients, from private specialty practice as well as academic institutions. Specialty practices rely on general practitioner referrals for much of their caseload and revenues. The benefits of these relationships are vital to the quality of healthcare that our veterinary patients receive – failure to refer appropriately ultimately harms patients.

10.10.2 Terms Defined

Board Certification: The recognition of a veterinarian's expertise in a particular specialty or subspecialty of veterinary medicine, as determined by a certifying body within the profession. Board certification typically follows an approved residency program in the specialty as well as passing certifying examinations in the specialty.

Primary Care Veterinarian: A veterinarian who is the primary contact for a pet owner and manages the medical needs of the pet. Also known as a first-opinion veterinarian or general practitioner.

Referral: The transfer of patient care from one clinician or hospital to another, upon request.

Specialist: A clinician highly skilled in a specific medical discipline.

MAIN CONCEPTS

General practitioners (GPs) are most often the first step in the healthcare continuum and provide routine diagnosis and treatment of illnesses and injuries in addition to preventive care – ideally pet-specific care.

When patients require or would benefit from additional diagnostics and/or specific types of treatment, there is a duty to refer them to others who have advanced knowledge and/or capabilities. Examples of needs that could benefit from referral include the following.

- Advanced imaging techniques such as magnetic resonance imaging (MRI) or computed tomography (CT).
- Physical rehabilitation services for orthopedic problems.
- Complex medical cases (e.g., endocrine diseases, cancer, heart disease, etc.) that would benefit from a consult with a recognized expert.
- Chronic conditions that would benefit from a complete work-up and long-term management plan.
- Complex/advanced surgical cases.
- Medical or surgical cases that require hospitalization and 24-hour monitoring and care with advanced equipment such as ventilators, blood gas analyzers, dialysis.
- Other conditions that would benefit from specialized skills and equipment.

10.10.3 The Process

It is important for GPs to develop strong relationships with the specialists in their geographic area that they trust to provide the best care possible to their patients in addition to excellent customer service for their clients. GPs should consider the specialists they have selected to work with as an extension of their own practice in terms of patient care and client service.

The best way to build these relationships is via ongoing direct and indirect communication, such as at continuing education meetings, online forums, and hospital visits. It is also important to maintain these relationships through frequent outreach for feedback on what is working well and what needs to be improved from the perspective of both the GP and the specialist.

The decision regarding what cases and when to refer should be based on what is in the best interest of the patient. The recommendation from the primary care veterinarian should be made on the basis of the pet-specific needs of the patient and client. The referring GP should then prepare the client for the actual referral process and the estimated costs associated with the initial examination by the specialist; the final decision on whether or not to seek specialty care should rest solely with the client after discussions with the primary care practice. It is not the job of the referring veterinarian (rDVM) to decide what makes economic sense for the client and they should avoid using judgmental language, such as saying that specialists can be "very expensive." That being said, it is important to provide the client with information of what to expect in terms of specialist services and costs and to appreciate that such services may not be within everyone's budget (see 2.10 Affordability of Veterinary Services).

Ideally, there should be referral coordinator(s) on staff at the specialty practice specifically for:

- scheduling consultations and describing what is involved and the associated costs
- making sure all the proper referral forms and medical records are available in advance
- explaining to the client and referring hospital the protocols associated with any need to repeat laboratory testing or imaging that might have initially been done at the primary care hospital
- ensuring client and referring GP communication is timely and complete
- scheduling hospital visits to the referring GPs periodically to make sure any challenges are identified and addressed in a timely manner.

All specialists should be willing to discuss cases, at least in a general sense, by telephone, remotely, and in person whenever possible and practical. Each case provides a teaching opportunity for both – the GP will learn more about how to manage complex cases and will be encouraged to refer more often and at the appropriate time, and the specialist will gain additional cases from other doctors within the practice (improved clinic penetration) and other practices in the area (improved market share), as well as better understand the needs of GPs in the area for continuing education topics.

All specialists should be involved in development and execution of the business and marketing plans for their specialty services. It is not just the referral coordinator's job. There are, however, many challenges to fostering these ongoing relationships.

- Specialty hospitals can be large and can hamper communication and allow inconsistencies between services (hospital within a hospital). Make sure all departments have a unified, consistent business and marketing plan for their referral relationships.
- Get to know all the doctors at referring and potentially referring hospitals – visits, surveys, continuing education events, etc. A big consideration in the referral process is that individual doctors at a primary care hospital may refer to individual specialists at different specialty hospitals. This can make for difficult and inconsistent referral relationships, and requires an extra layer of referral management.
- The specialty hospital should endeavor to give the referring veterinarian an experience they cannot get elsewhere, such as continuing education for GPs and technicians, lunchtime rounds, prompt consultations, etc.
- Invite primary care veterinarians to "rounds" at the specialty hospital, the process of reviewing case details with the next hospital shift ("This is Sparky Jones . . . Sparky is a patient of Dr Smith at Compassionate Veterinary Hospital and Dr Smith sent Sparky to us for. . .."). It is important to review with an attorney what information needs to be confidential to protect client privacy, and what can be legitimately disclosed (see 7.6 Privacy and Confidentiality).
- On an ongoing basis, specialists should retrieve the data from their top referring general practices based on caseload, identify the individual doctors and what services they are using. This helps determine clinic penetration (the percentage of possible doctors in the primary care practice that are referring), the market share (the percentage of referring hospitals in the total market area of possible referring clinics), as well as the breadth of the referrals within referring hospitals (are they only referring to the dermatology service, but not surgery, etc.?). This provides substrate for discussions of how the referral relationship can be enhanced and improved.

- The goal is for all GPs in a given primary care practice to be referring cases to all available specialties in a specialty service, and for those primary care practices to be exceptionally well serviced by the specialty practice.

Building strong specialty referral relationships is in everyone's best interest – the patient, the client, and the veterinary team.

TAKE-AWAYS

- Appropriate and efficient referral strategies and procedures are essential to practicing the highest quality of medicine and ensuring the best patient outcomes.
- Every referring general practitioner should feel like their specialty referral hospital partner is an extension of their practice.
- The best referral partnerships require strong personal relationships and provide the highest level of patient care in addition to supporting mutual growth for both practices.
- All doctors in both practices must be engaged and supportive of the activities necessary to build strong referral relationships to ensure the process is functioning at the highest level.
- Feedback is critical to the referral process. Most bad experiences with a referral are due to communication inadequacies rather than poor medicine. Make sure all parties have the information they need to make appropriate informed decisions, and act promptly on any negative feedback.

MISCELLANEOUS

10.10.4 Cautions

While many referrals happen smoothly and in the way they should, it is important to remember that self-referral is also an option for clients and can add a layer of complexity to the referral process.

Clients may hear about specialty medicine from a variety of sources and decide to self-refer, or contact specialists directly for appointments. In some cases, they can complicate matters even more by requesting that primary care veterinarians not be notified of the visit, or not be provided with a referral report. Most of the time, it is because they don't want their regular veterinarian to know that they don't have complete confidence in how the case has been managed to date, but no matter what the reason, it creates a dilemma that needs to be managed by the specialty hospital, respecting the rights of the pet owner but also wanting to be supportive of the primary care hospital.

Referrals happen best when they are part of a well-conceived care pathway (see 9.6 Care Pathways), and the clients understand potential outcomes that would warrant referral, and how that referral will be handled. When clients understand that referral is not a sign of failure but rather a routine part of medical care (and potentially available whenever a client would like a second opinion), such awkward situations can be kept to a minimum.

Recommended Reading

2013 AAHA Referral and Consultation Guidelines. www.aaha.org/aaha-guidelines/referral-configuration/referral/

Burrows, C.F. (2008). Meeting the expectations of referring veterinarians. *Journal of Veterinary Medical Education* 35 (1): 20–25.

Choder, B. (2020). Legal duty to refer. In: *Five-Minute Veterinary Practice Management Consult* (ed. L. Ackerman), 832–833. Ames, IA: Wiley.

10.11

Financial Benefits of Pet-Specific Care

Michael R. Dicks, PhD

AE Consulting, Arvada, CO, USA
Erupt, LLC, Kodak, TN, USA

BASICS

10.11.1 Summary

The gap between the care pets need and what they receive has grown through three decades. Accessibility, affordability, and perceived value are three factors important in this growing gap. Pet-specific care guidelines that consider the knowledge and skills of the veterinary team, the current scientific evidence regarding the safety and efficacy of available treatments, recommendations or "best practice" guidelines, practice-specific goals, and the culture, available resources, and goals, values, and resources of the client will help close the gap and improve practice performance.

10.11.2 Terms Defined

Accessibility: The ease of reaching and approaching.
Care Guidelines (Care Recommendations): The set of processes and practices that meet the needs of both the pet and the pet owner.
Willingness to Pay: Maximum amount of money a consumer thinks a product or service is worth.

MAIN CONCEPTS

The gap between the care that pets need and that provided has been growing over the last three decades. Many

factors have been identified as contributors to this problem including slow and variable growth in household incomes, rising prices of veterinary products and services at rates greater than inflation, increasing pet ownership in areas with limited access to veterinary hospitals, and increasing tests and treatments over that deemed medically required.

The care that pets need is defined by veterinary practices based on the knowledge, training, and experience of the veterinary team within the practice. These care recommendations reflect what is believed to provide the best healthcare for pets. However, pet owners may have limited knowledge of the risks associated with not adhering to recommendations as well as their ability or willingness to pay for these practices.

The risks associated with not adhering to care recommendations fall into two camps: the risk to the health and well-being of the animal, and the risk to the financial well-being of the owner. The ability to pay is simply a function of the cost of services versus the household's income and the relative importance of other budget expenditures (see 2.10 Affordability of Veterinary Services). Willingness to pay, on the other hand, is more complicated, with factors such as the degree of human–animal bond, cultural values, and knowledge of pet healthcare outcomes that are weighed against the price of services that impact the care decisions (see 7.8 Providing Care for Those Unable or Unwilling to Pay).

10.11.3 Fewer Pets Receiving Care

Data published by the American Veterinary Medical Association (AVMA) and the US Bureau of Labor Statistics (BLS) show that over the last 15 years, veterinary

Pet-Specific Care for the Veterinary Team, First Edition. Edited by Lowell Ackerman.
© 2021 John Wiley & Sons, Inc. Published 2021 by John Wiley & Sons, Inc.

medical prices have increased 91%, while the US rate of inflation has increased 35% (see Figure 10.11.1) [1]. During this period, mean wages of Americans have increased only 1.8%. Likewise, as shown in Figure 10.11.1, as veterinary prices outpaced other consumer costs, the percentage of pets not visiting the veterinarian has increased.

While an increasing number of pets are not visiting the veterinarian, the gap between the preventive and medical (curative and palliative) care recommended and the care provided has also been increasing. While not widely measured, there have been attempts to define this increasing gap for both. For preventive care, an IDEXX study in 2016 (see Figure 10.11.2) indicated that the value of care required over an average 12-year lifespan for a canine was $17700

and that in review of the records of roughly 10 000 practices, the average canine received only $3600 of that preventive care over that same 12-year lifespan [2]. The American Animal Hospital Association preventive care guidelines and average prices were used and included wellness exam, vaccines, parasiticides, dental exams, and nutrition.

In a similar study of 600 practices by Henry Schein, the gap between pet healthcare needs and that provided in preventive care was more than the total revenue for the practice [3]. In numerous analyses of the share of the wellness market acquired by veterinary practices, AVMA's economics division found that on average, veterinary practices only capture 20–25% of the potential preventive care market for their business area.

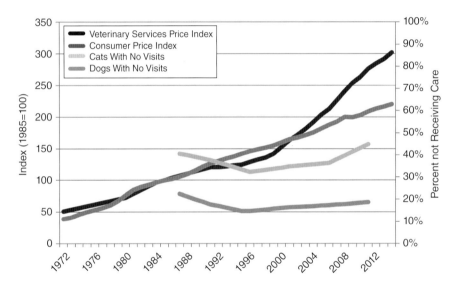

Figure 10.11.1 Relative price of veterinary service and pet visits. *Source:* Adapted from Dicks et al. [1].

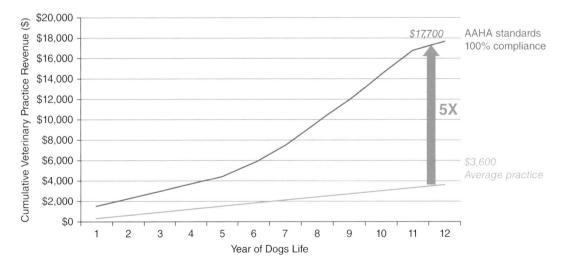

Figure 10.11.2 Lifetime revenue from typical 12-year-old dog.

In examining a specific preventive parasiticide, Animalytix found that dog owners were providing roughly 25% of the recommended heartworm medication [4]. Across major US metropolitan areas, the average months of heartworm coverage ranged from less than one month to roughly four months while the recommended preventive dosage is for 12 months of coverage.

The gap between the recommended palliative and curative care for pets and the care provided is well known to veterinarians but not well documented. However, a three-year study by Mississippi State University regarding pet health insurance found evidence that household incomes, human–animal bond (see 2.14 Benefits of the Human–Animal Bond), and pet health insurance (see 10.16 Pet Health Insurance) affected the amount of care selected and the cost of care that would move the care decision from treatment to euthanasia (see Figure 10.11.3) [5].

10.11.4 Growing Gap Implications

These studies indicate that pets are not receiving the healthcare that veterinarians believe they should receive.

The combination of the increasing number of pets unseen by veterinarians with the gap between recommended and provided care is a problem for the animal, animal owner, veterinarian, and veterinary practice.

If preventive care recommendations are tied to prevention of specific adverse health outcomes, then the health of the animals not meeting these recommendations is compromised. Where medical care recommendations are not followed, pet and pet owner well-being is compromised. The compromised health of the animal increases the cost of pet ownership, may reduce pet life expectancy and the bond between the pet and the pet owner. For the veterinary practice, the failure of clients to follow care recommendations not only represents the missed financial opportunity associated with the care gap, but also suggests a failure to adequately establish the veterinarian–client relationship such that the primary source of animal health information is no longer (if it ever was) the veterinary team. This less than optimum veterinarian–client relationship adversely affects veterinarian well-being by increasing both burnout and secondary traumatic stress and has adverse implications for the financial sustainability of the practice.

Not well documented is the relative importance of the various factors that may influence the client's pet healthcare decisions. Clients may not understand the risk to the animal or their own financial risk of not following the care recommendations, they may not agree with the recommendations because of their relationship to the animal or their primary source of information is not the veterinary team, or they simply can't afford to pay for the recommended level of prevention.

The demographics of animal owners and veterinarians are rapidly changing, and new business models that enable veterinary practices to provide preventive, curative, and palliative care that is accessible and affordable and meets the needs of the local community must be constantly examined (see 5.4 The Changing Nature of Pet Owners).

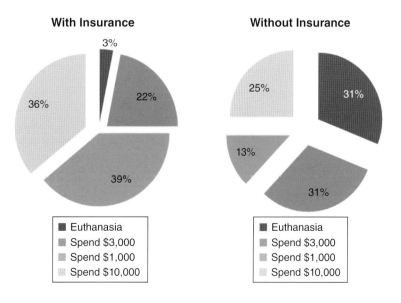

Figure 10.11.3 Pet health expenditures with and without pet health insurance. *Source:* Based on Williams et al. [5].

With Insurance

3%
22%
36%
39%

- Euthanasia
- Spend $3,000
- Spend $1,000
- Spend $10,000

Without Insurance

25%
31%
13%
31%

- Euthanasia
- Spend $3,000
- Spend $1,000
- Spend $10,000

EXAMPLES

10.11.5 Financial Impacts of Pet Specific Care

Because preventive care is often a larger share of total revenue than medical care and has been more broadly studied, an example of a "wellness bundle" is used to give the practicing veterinarian a template for examining the financial impacts of the gap between their pet-specific care recommendations and the care their client's pet receives (see Figure 10.11.4). The "routine capture" refers to those preventive products and services that are common to a wellness visit and include the wellness exam, vaccines, fecal exam, and blood tests for infectious agents. The actual case provided below indicates a total cost of $177.30 for this bundle, which is close to the national average transaction cost of $168. By including the shopped products, parasiticides and pet food, the annual cost is boosted to $1055.03. Finally, by including the average annual cost of every third-year dental exam, total costs are increased to $1227.40, giving a 12-year lifetime expenditure of $14 732.

While the difference in total cost between the entire bundle of services and the routine capture is $1050, the difference in the gross profit is $556, representing a loss of more than $1 million for the average veterinarian seeing 1800 patients per year.

A larger question is the willingness of pet owners, at various levels of household income and human–animal bond, to spend roughly $100 per month on their pet and how many more households would purchase the entire wellness bundle at a lower total cost (see 10.17 Payment and Wellness Plans). Without changing the total profit of the practice, the entire bundle could be provided for less than $750 annually or $60 per month. This may improve the care pets currently being seen receive and increase the number of pets visiting the veterinary hospital.

TAKE-AWAYS

- The care that is recommended for pets by the veterinary team exceeds the care that they receive, and this gap is growing.
- The gap consists of two components – pets that are visiting the veterinary hospital and not purchasing from the hospital the recommended products and services, and pets that are not visiting the hospital.
- Household incomes, level of human–animal bond, veterinary product and service prices and the value that pet

Annual Budget	Vet	Cost	Profit	%Profit
Annual Well Pet Pysical	$54.00		$54.00	100%
Heartworm test	$43.00	$15.00	$28.00	65%
DA2PPV, 3yr	$8.00	$3.00	$5.00	63%
Bordatella	$8.00	$6.00	$2.00	25%
Rabbies, 3yr	$9.33	$6.00	$3.33	36%
Fecal	$20.00	$5.00	$15.00	75%
Blood Test	$35.00	$16.00	$19.00	54%
Flea and Trick (Simparica)	$247.13	$75.79	$171.34	69%
Heartworm (Pro Heart 6)	$314.71	$112.00	$202.71	64%
Proplan	$315.86	$228.00	$87.86	28%
Dental	$172.67	$77.70	$94.97	55%
Total	**$1,227.70**	**$544.49**	**$683.21**	**56%**
12 Year total	**$14,732**	**$6,534**	**$8,199**	**56%**
Routine Capture	$177.33	$51.00	$126.33	71%
Heartworm/Flea and Tick/Nutrition	$1,055.03	$466.79	$588.24	56%
Plus Dental	$1,227.70	$544.49	$683.21	56%

Figure 10.11.4 Typical preventive dog care bundle budget.

owners place on the risk of not following the recommendations are all important factors in care decisions.

- The combined impact of these factors on care decisions represents a very large financial opportunity for veterinary practices.
- Research is needed to determine the importance of each of these factors in the care decision to aid veterinarians in capturing those opportunities.

MISCELLANEOUS

References

1 Dicks, M.R., Bain, B., and Knippenberg, R. 2017 AVMA Report on the Market for Veterinary Services. AVMA, October 18, 2017.

2 IDEXX. Personal communications from presentation at the 2016 Annual Meeting of the American Animal Hospital Association, August 5–8, San Antonio, Texas.

3 Burdett, D. Increasing Client Compliance. Presentation at the 2016 Annual Meeting of the American Veterinary Medical Association, Practice Management Core CE program, August 5–8, San Antonio, Texas.

4 Ragland, C. (2019). Veterinary Meeting Expo (VMX). State of the Industry Presentation, January 19–23, Orlando, Florida.

5 Williams, A., Coble, K.H., Williams, B. et al. Consumer Preferences for Pet Health Insurance. Paper presented at Southern Agricultural Economics Association (SAEA) Annual Meeting, San Antonio, Texas, February 8, 2016.

10.12

Dashboards and Key Performance Indicators

Mark J. McGaunn, CPA/PFS, CFP®

McGaunn & Schwadron, CPA's, LLC, Medfield, MA, USA

BASICS

10.12.1 Summary

The perfect key performance indicator (KPI) is designed to provide a window into both the financial and nonfinancial operating parameters of a veterinary practice. In practice, the high level a financial statistic or nonoperating parameter is, the more interpretation that is required to determine its usefulness. A KPI should not be so vague as to provide no real direction for practice owners to take and not so specific that actions based upon its result are so limited that it provides no meaningful impact. KPIs can be designed to provide a window into operational performance, patient care success and failures, and even marketing campaign wins and losses. The most successful KPI measurement programs always compare to a preset benchmark that has been custom designed by practice owners and management to truly evaluate real-life results versus aspirational goals. KPI programs are best designed to reach all levels of care and all levels of staffing.

10.12.2 Terms Defined

Business Intelligence (BI): BI is the accumulation, analysis, reporting, budgeting, and presentation of business financial and operational data. The goal of utilizing BI for a veterinary hospital is to increase the visibility of hospital operations and financial status to better lead and manage the hospital.

Executive Dashboard: An executive dashboard is a reporting tool that provides visual displays of an organization's financial and operational KPIs, metrics, and data. The objective of developing an executive dashboard is to provide healthcare executives instant summarized visibility into business performance across all business lines.

KPI: A KPI is a type of performance measurement that helps determine how an organization or department is performing. A good KPI should be well defined, quantifiable, thoroughly communicated, and crucial to achieving strategic goals.

MAIN CONCEPTS

Veterinary practice owners and management must be aware of the dynamics in their ever-changing healthcare delivery model. Each is subject to its own constantly changing environment – diminishing patient visit volumes, competitive equipment and supply costs, and qualified staffing shortages.

An executive dashboard is a summation, typically on one page, of several important KPIs, those designated by practice owners or management to be the defining metrics of success or failure. Veterinary practice executives first need to ask what goal their organization is trying to accomplish. Practice managers may believe that the only goals that their organization is trying to measure are purely financial. It has been the experience in human healthcare organizations that vast efforts have been designed to measure the delivery, adequacy, and safety results of the actual medicine employed. Whole teams of trained healthcare technicians in teaching hospitals work as part of the risk management enterprise effort to measure and improve the delivery of medical care and reduce untoward results.

Dr. Atul Gawande, a best-selling author and physician practicing in Boston, designed studies in intensive care

Pet-Specific Care for the Veterinary Team, First Edition. Edited by Lowell Ackerman.
© 2021 John Wiley & Sons, Inc. Published 2021 by John Wiley & Sons, Inc.

units to reduce the number of both intubated patients' infection rates and hospital-wide infection rates related to the simple act of hand washing. These KPIs were indeed very specific and could fit on one page so that all staff and management could understand the magnitude and impact of improving these specific KPIs. Simple protocols resulted that both patients and staff were aware and continually reminded of the simple protocols that resulted. Hospitals around the globe employed Dr. Gawande's methods of KPI measurement specificity and obtained successful results.

The advantage that large institutions enjoy in healthcare stems from the fact that they can deploy significant resources to the task of creating BI. Whole teams of data analysts can be tasked with collecting, aggregating, and analyzing raw data from various departments (see 7.10 Analytics and Informatics). Those data could be in the form of emails, spreadsheets, text messages, and extracted raw data from practice management software. Data could also be in the form of questionnaires sent to staff, practitioners, administrators, patients, and vendors.

Once those data are tabulated in a meaningful format, the reports are sent to the data stewards, those individuals whose job it is to ensure the process is completed in a timely manner. They also review the analysis and confirm the accuracy of the data in comparison to established benchmarks. There are also companies whose sole job is to make the executive reporting or dashboard tools to be easily interpreted and pleasing graphically. Most veterinary practice managers do not have access to this type of resource so they must rely on either self-developed spreadsheets or outside third-party software programs to accumulate their data.

Once determined and agreed upon by both veterinary practice owners and staff (as buy-in is needed across all levels of management and practitioner), all must agree on how long is appropriate to measure the KPI. Is it for a specific window in time such as weeks, months, quarterly, annually or repeated periodic times during the year? Agreement must also be reached on how to interpret the data, because if the data are accumulated and not able to be interpreted, possibly against a budgeted or targeted amount, then the process is set for failure. So, the right staff level should be assigned to be the champion of the data interpretation process.

Measuring and interpreting KPIs can be a very time-consuming process. The data accumulation process is one limiting factor why many entities do not realize KPI platforms or executive dashboards. Even very small healthcare entities have data residing in different locations – practice management software, financial software, marketing software, etc. If the data from a veterinary practice management system is difficult to extract once, let alone at various

periods or continually across the course of the calendar year, the operating insight that management and practice owners were expecting to receive may be difficult to obtain. Integrated software data visualization programs, such as VetSuccess Daily Dashboard, iVet360, and Analytix Insight360, provide automated tools to extract and analyze financial and operation data in a clearly laid out format with comparisons to prior period data.

EXAMPLES

10.12.3 Financial KPIs

10.12.3.1 Days Cash on Hand

The days cash on hand metric is equivalent to the number of days that a veterinary practice could continue to pay its operating expenses, including payroll and vendors, given the amount of cash available. The formula is ([Cash and Equivalents] $\times$ 365 days)/(Total Operating Expenses-Annual Depreciation). Most nonhealthcare entities strive for 90–180 days, but most veterinary practices operate on much more stringent cash positions.

10.12.3.2 Current Ratio

A more relevant metric for cash adequacy is the current ratio, which measures the ability to pay current liabilities (vendor payable, lease payments, and loan payments) with cash, receivables, and inventory. The current ratio should be at least 1:1.

10.12.3.3 Profit Centers

Key performance indicators that track individual profit centers such as retail, pet food, pharmacy, vaccinations, dentistry, and surgery, from both a revenue side and cost side, are valuable to track so that a gross profit could be estimated for each profit center. The format of the AAHA/VMG chart of accounts (www.aaha.org/professional/resources/chart_of_accounts.aspx) is a good tool on both the revenue delineation and cost of sales breakout formats to categorize data for this type of analysis. Staffing and direct costs can then be allocated for more genuine profit analysis. As in all cost accounting measurement projects, there is some arbitrary allocation of overhead and indirect costs that may make seemingly profitable centers show a loss. So this is a valuable exercise to undertake.

10.12.3.4 Production Per Veterinarian

Production per doctor is a gross metric or KPI that in and of itself may show trends or suggest other patterns by doctor and the hospital that can be relevant. It should be noted that production also includes price increases that have transpired across the measurement period and net realizable increases must take that into account as this KPI may suggest that production on a real basis is flat or declining.

10.12.3.5 Average Transaction Charge (ATC) or Revenue Per Patient Visit

A most overutilized statistic, it is still relevant in a global context, though a deeper dive is needed to determine if medical protocols are being adhered to, discounts or missed invoice charges (unintentional or intentional) are occurring, etc.

10.12.3.6 Number of Transactions

This metric can be measured by hospital and on an individual veterinarian basis. Various studies have shown a significant number of hospitals experiencing year-over-year declines in the number of transactions. This may be indicative of a decline in the number of new patients, or a trend in new patients making fewer wellness visits and mechanisms that are poorly designed to increase those numbers.

10.12.3.7 New Patients

New patients are the lifeblood of any growing veterinary practice. New patient activity data can be indicative of marketing effort success, patient recall efforts, patient engagement efforts, and current pet owner referral program success. As in any KPI metric development, absolute numbers could indicate a deficiency in efforts but relative comparisons to prior years and prior providers could indicate positive trends regardless. The goal is for continued success in reaching new patients and retaining those new patients to be fully active participants in their pet's healthcare.

10.12.3.8 Building Capacity Ratio

This metric attempts to determine if the patient volume has outgrown the physical building space. There is a wide variety of discussion in the veterinary practice management community of when a veterinary practice has reached its capacity. Some practice management consultants view less than $350 dollars of revenue per square foot per year as an adequate volume to continue practice in the same space, with $400–500 per square foot of revenue per year as a moderate indicator that there may be a need for more physical space. Over $600 per square foot could be a strong indicator of the need additional hospital space. While space may not be easy to obtain in the short run, additional capacity can be generated by extending hours in the short term assuming staffing is easily obtainable to do so.

10.12.3.9 Equipment Utilization and Payback Time

From an accounting context, high-dollar assets such as endoscopy units, digital and dental X-ray units, ultrasound, surgical and therapeutic lasers, and other significant expenditures are overpriced if they are not being fully utilized as they were intended before purchase. Tracking the utilization and revenue generation of each high-dollar asset post purchase is necessary to ensure that those dollars were wisely expended. Most equipment vendors have calculators that show the profit experienced from "average" use post installation, but very few veterinary hospitals perform posttransaction utilization studies to analyze performance. Many therapy lasers rest unused in quiet hospital rooms, like dentists who purchase $150,000 CEREC machines to manufacture in-house crowns, then realize they prefer their favorite laboratory technician to make the crown over their own artistry. Low utilization rates of these assets also detract from top-line revenue and bottom-line profitability. High utilization rates potentially indicate cases where additional dollars should be spent in order to prevent increased wait times for necessary veterinary procedures.

10.12.4 Medical/Clinical KPIs

10.12.4.1 Medical Errors

Most physician-based healthcare systems look at hospital incidence which could be patients acquiring infections, transfusion reactions, bed sores, or postoperative failures such as dyspnea and hemorrhage or hematomas. They also analyze postoperative and postprocedural death rates, which are indicative of how the hospital is performing regarding the quality of care and sites that potentially require immediate corrective courses of action. In our experience, we have not witnessed veterinary dashboard programs that generate any KPI related to medical errors or incidents. Checklists or protocols can be instituted in veterinary hospitals to have a positive effect on these potential untoward events.

10.12.4.2 Wellness Compliance

Various automated tools in some practice management software programs and third-party software can analyze the relative compliance of a hospital's patient base, and even target a particular veterinarian's patient base as a subset for varying side-by-side performance data. Compliance factors should be utilized to determine overall compliance with senior care, core vaccinations, nutrition, heartworm and other parasitic compliance, etc. (see 9.17 Improving Compliance and Adherence with Pet-Specific Care)

10.12.4.3 Medication/Infusion Errors

With the volume of medications, varying administrative paths and dosages, a busy veterinary hospital is a prime candidate for a medication error. Reporting protocols and tracking protocols are necessary to be a window into this potential source of harm for patients in hospital and those prescribed medications for home administration. The result may be the institution of better education for pet owners checking medication orders that have been filled from a quality control standpoint or more focused veterinarian to technician communication in the treatment environment.

10.12.4.4 Active Patients Percentage

This KPI looks at the number of patients residing in practice management software that have been seen in the past 12 months. Some programs count active patients as being seen in the past 18 months, which dentistry uses as a metric, but in the life of a canine or feline patient, that is equivalent to not being to the doctor in 10.5 years. It is also indicative of lapsing awareness of the practice that needs to be reactivated through text, email, or by a telephone call from the practice reception team.

10.12.4.5 Canine/Feline Comparison

Some KPIs developed by veterinary practices track the numbers of canine and feline patients. In the Fear Free Certification movement, the possibility of increasing the number of feline and canine patients that were not comfortable visiting a veterinary hospital before is a reality (see 6.6 Fear Free Concepts). So, these metrics should be tracked, especially since there is a movement to have feline-only exam rooms and entire wings of hospitals to encourage feline owners to visit more frequently.

10.12.4.6 Patient Versus Staff Ratio

While most hospitals consider the support staff to veterinarian ratio as the defining metric for staffing efficiency, it assumes that a high ratio equates to inefficiency; that is, that technicians and assistants are not being effectively utilized for revenue generation (billable patient services). However, most industries measure provider numbers to recipient numbers (cruise ship guests per crew member, students to classroom teacher, not teachers to custodial staff). Thus, the number of providers and total staff should be matched to patients to see if there is adequate coverage during the hours of care provision.

10.12.4.7 Patients Who Leave Without Being Seen

Particularly relevant in an emergency hospital environment, but equally relevant to a small animal or urgent care facility, this KPI tabulates the number of pet owners who were unwilling to wait the requisite amount of time subsequent to the triage process to be seen by a veterinarian. With this KPI one could determine that more staffing of technicians or veterinarians or treatment rooms is necessary, or that there was inefficiency built into the system of treatment scheduling. Whether it's not adequately assigning enough time to previous appointments in the schedule or staffing is not adequate, this indicator produces those at the far reach of the bell curve.

10.12.4.8 No-Shows

Even with the advent of social media, reminder programs, and practice management software that has complete patient access data such as cellphone, home phone, and email address, there are still patients who are no shows for scheduled appointments for their pets. With the mantra of finding the right pet owners as clients for your practice, continued no-shows should be met with the progressive form of discipline ultimately ending in expulsion from your practice client roster. There are more than enough patients out there who do desire your top-notch provision of healthcare. However, you still need to measure the occurrence of no-show appointments and delve into the reason for them, whether they were staff related, pet related, unforeseen circumstance, or no valid reason.

10.12.4.9 Unfilled Schedule Slots

Though the incidence of unfilled time blocks in your schedule should be minimal, there are instances where you were unable to fill open time slots for a variety of reasons. Tracking needs to be done and each instance of attempts to fill and ultimate failure or success noted. There is cloud software available now that automates a modern wait list feature to send messages to patients via their contact preference regarding last minute appointment cancelations and openings. This is a valuable tool to minimize any unfilled space in your schedule at the last minute which also increases both your revenue and profitability for each appointment filled.

10.12.4.10 Average Patient Rooms in Use at One Time

The goal of this metric is to look at occupancy rates, like hotel room occupancy analysis, and see how well hospital square footage designated as examination rooms is being utilized. If there are consistently underutilized exam rooms in the hospital, a more detailed examination could be made to determine if more patients could be seen using either current staffing or slightly enhanced staffing to maximize all available space. This KPI data should be analyzed over a short period of time immediate to the designation of this KPI needing to be used or it could trend over certain periods of time to see consistency of utilization.

10.12.4.11 Patient Wait Time

Patient wait time is analyzed by many healthcare environments, including veterinary hospitals. Patient wait time is a direct influencer of patient satisfaction scoring mechanisms. The goal of every veterinary hospital is to minimize the wait time between each discrete transportation event from arrival until departure from the hospital. Both the average wait time between checking in and seeing a veterinarian and the average wait time from entering the hospital until checking in and seeing a staff member in an exam room should be recorded. However, averages in this instance do not do this metric justice; the outliers, both positive and negative, should be recorded as well because in this instance, like water purity, 99.9% water purity means that 0.01% of the time the water was impure. If you were a patient with a significant wait time, the average may still be excellent, and that patient's experience may not be reflective of the other patients' wait time experience.

10.12.4.12 Pet Owner Satisfaction

Whether it's defined by pet owner surveys post appointment or surveys sent to a wide variety of patients in the active patient base, the pet owner satisfaction metric may accurately describe the overall satisfaction of pet owners at the hospital. However, similar to the average 1–3% direct mail success rate, pet owner satisfaction surveys may only accurately project the opinions of highly motivated pet owners or those on the other extreme who may have experienced negative encounters. As in all surveys, all data need to be analyzed and verified, while each experience needs to be evaluated and responded to individually.

TAKE-AWAYS

- Veterinary healthcare executives need to focus more on what is needed for the future success based on KPI derivation than those results that happened in the past. So more predictive indicators need to be developed rather than reactive KPIs.
- Appealing presentation of visual data is almost as important as the data itself. Colors, shapes, and patterns should be employed in dashboard development.
- Targets or benchmark goals need to be meaningful, attainable, and understood by staff.
- More time should be spent on developing action plans in response to data summaries than in aggregating and sourcing KPI data.
- After an effective BI program has been instituted at a typical human hospital, adverse events are reduced 7%, patient satisfaction increases 15%, and staff productivity increases with a drop in corresponding overtime of 11% (http://Infosys.com).

MISCELLANEOUS

10.12.5 Cautions

Manually aggregating medical and financial performance data could lead to significant inaccuracies. According to one study, 88% of all Excel spreadsheets in the study contained formula errors [1]. It is therefore necessary for somebody in the BI effort to check and review data after tabulation to ensure accuracy. So, data validation is a key role for someone in the organization. This process is more complicated with desktop or server practice management programs, but with the upgrade of many practice management software systems to cloud-based versions complete with APIs for seamless integration, this data-gathering process may get easier as time goes on.

Clear communication related to goals and resulting feedback needs to be outlined during the KPI development process. Results should not be used in a punitive fashion but should result in positive change in both financial and clinical areas with the goal of patient care enhancement.

Many doctors will not enter targets or goals to achieve. The best BI platforms display trended actuals versus targets – including target variances – and visually appealing, color-coded graduated assessments of developed metrics to progress targets.

Reference

1 Marketwatch. 88% of spreadsheets have errors. www.marketwatch.com/story/88-of-spreadsheets-have-errors-2013-04-17

Recommended Reading

McKinsey and Company. Ahead of the curve: The future of performance management. | www.mckinsey.com/business-functions/organization/our-insights/ahead-of-the-curve-the-future-of-performance-management

10.13

Approach to Pricing

Lowell Ackerman, DVM, DACVD, MBA, MPA, CVA, MRCVS

Global Consultant, Author, and Lecturer, MA, USA

BASICS

10.13.1 Summary

There are many different methods by which veterinary services can be priced. Mark-up pricing is commonly used in veterinary practices and involves taking the acquisition cost of the product and multiplying it by a mark-up percentage (or a mark-up factor) to arrive at a retail price for customers. Margin (cost-plus) pricing is a basic pricing method in which all the costs of providing a product or service are calculated, including direct and indirect costs of overhead, labor, and materials, and then a profit margin is added once all costs have been recovered to arrive at the retail price.

Because of marketplace competition, veterinarians frequently price goods and services on the basis of benchmarking to other sellers of similar goods and services (sometimes referred to as community pricing). This is convenient, but is fraught with a number of hazards [1, 2]. Other businesses may be undercharging for the service, so you could be losing money by matching prices. Other businesses may be overcharging for the service, so there may be opportunities that would result in a competitive advantage. In many cases, practices "bundle" their prices (examination, anesthesia, surgery, medications), so it may be difficult to discern the true cost of providing services.

With pet-specific care, clients tend to be more engaged with the veterinary practice in the care of their pets. It is important for those clients to appreciate that they are receiving exceptional value with this approach, and so pricing must be carefully considered.

10.13.2 Terms Defined

Acquisition Cost: The wholesale price at which a good or service can be acquired for resale.

Community Pricing: Establishing a price for a good or service based on the prices charged by others.

Loss Leader: Products or services sold at a loss to attract customers to potentially purchase other products or services.

Margin Pricing: Also known as cost-plus pricing, this involves taking all the direct and indirect costs in providing a good or service and adding a set amount or percentage that corresponds to a gross profit margin to arrive at a retail price.

Markup Pricing: Pricing based on taking the acquisition cost and increasing it by percentage or factor to arrive at a retail price.

Materials: Costs associated with providing products used for a service, including both direct and indirect costs.

Overhead: Costs of operating a business, even if no clients avail themselves of any services.

Profit Margin: The (gross) profit margin is the difference between the total cost to the practice of delivering a product or service, and the final price to the client. It is typically expressed as a percentage.

MAIN CONCEPTS

The true cost of providing veterinary goods and services is often shocking given that most veterinary practices undercharge for their professional services (but may overcharge for retail items and laboratory tests to compensate). This is a chronic problem and translates not only to the relatively low profit margins for many veterinary hospitals, but also to what the practices can then afford to pay employed veterinarians, paraprofessional staff, receptionists, and practice managers (see 7.2 Managing the Pet-Specific Workplace).

Clients may not know what the price of veterinary products or services should be, but they often have some knowledge of signpost items, things they have purchased in the past that might be considered an approximation. Clients might use the prices of signpost items to form an overall impression of prices quoted, thereby giving at least an impression to guide the purchase of items when they have less actual price knowledge [3]. In some instances, the disconnect between what clients know about the prices of signpost items (such as their own medicated shampoos, or flea control products they see at a pet store) can lead them to believe that veterinary products or services are overpriced, so attention must be given to value-based prices, especially those considered shoppable. Consider also that small charges applied to many invoices (e.g., a token charge to cover medical waste) can have a profound impact on revenue generation and profit without materially affecting total cost for clients.

Pricing in the retail marketplace tends to be more dynamic that just establishing a single price for services. In many cases, offering tiered solutions (good, better, best) allows clients to select the level of service they prefer, and often results in higher revenue generation for veterinary practices [4]. It's also important to realize that when adjusting fees, certain goods and services (especially those considered shoppable) are more price sensitive than others; tweaking nonsensitive prices can achieve the same goals as general price increases without alarming clients or staff.

Today's consumers are not passive price takers, so it is important to price goods and services in a manner that is considered fair, and that focuses on relationships over transactions [5]. If at all possible, prices should be set in ways that encourage customer behavior that benefits both the practice and the pet owner (see 10.15 Putting Price into Perspective). Businesses that are transparent about how they make their money tend to foster engagement and build trust with clients, which in turn leads to better client satisfaction and retention.

With continued use, value-based approaches to pricing will help veterinary teams charge appropriately or stop performing services for which they cannot be adequately compensated to cover costs and make a fair return on investment.

10.13.3 Mark-Up

Although mark-up is currently the most common pricing model used in veterinary practice, it has several disadvantages. Applying a fixed mark-up percentage to the acquisition cost has uneven effects depending on the acquisition cost. So, inexpensive medications that are "marked up" remain inexpensive and provide very little profit potential for the practice, whereas the same mark-up applied to more expensive goods and services tends to inflate the retail price to the customer, without providing commensurate value.

In today's competitive retail environment, practices may attempt to use mark-ups for commodities (products) that are significantly higher than those used by retailers for the same or similar items, potentially making veterinary prices seem artificially higher than competitors.

Mark-ups tend to amplify the costs of products or services that tend to be more expensive or used to treat larger animals, while minimizing the prices of less expensive goods or services for those used to treat smaller animals, unrelated to value delivery. Mark-ups applied to acquisition costs tend to work best on moderately priced goods and services in which there is minimal variability in price, or when different mark-ups are used in a tiered fashion, based on acquisition price.

Paying employed veterinarians (associates) a commission (production) on such items to be marked up forces the final retail price to be even higher to the consumer without providing additional value than was gained from the office visit. Using mark-up makes it easy to calculate a retail price, but additional calculations would be necessary to determine indirect costs and profit margin.

10.13.4 Margin

Margin (cost-plus) pricing is used to price a good or service based on full cost recovery plus a gross profit "margin" that could be a percentage or a fixed amount. Margin pricing accounts for all the direct and indirect costs associated with providing a good or service and then adds a gross profit margin.

Margin pricing does not penalize an animal that needs a more expensive product or service and does not artificially discount less expensive goods or services or those intended to treat smaller animals. Margin pricing intends to achieve full cost recovery for delivering a good or service, and then add a fair gross profit margin based on the value delivered. The main disadvantage to margin pricing in a typical veterinary setting is that the pricing is competitive so doesn't readily accommodate paying production (commission) "off the top." It is designed for full cost recovery and a predictable profit margin.

10.13.5 Value Pricing

Most clients today are value shoppers, so it is important that we do not place any obstacles in the way of providing the care needed for their pets. This is extremely important regarding pet-specific care, since we are asking them to be more involved and engaged with the care of their pets. If we want our clients to be informed, that also includes being informed and educated about the costs of healthcare, including prevention, early detection, and disease management with facilitated compliance.

Consumers spend money on fancy coffees, indulgences for their pets, premium diets, online shopping extravaganzas, and prioritized delivery, so spending money is not an issue if they see the value in their purchases. For many pet owners, it is difficult to appreciate the value in veterinary offerings, so we must be able to demonstrate that value.

When veterinarians sell products or services for which there is a "shoppable" alternative, the pricing should really reflect comparable pricing with perhaps a slight premium for convenience or a legitimate explanation for why the product/service price is not comparable with what they might find elsewhere. It is better to disclose such information up front, since most clients won't begrudge paying slightly more to buy from a veterinary clinic than a retailer. In fact, some may willingly pay a premium just so they don't have to go to a retailer to get the product.

In addition to pricing based on acquisition costs, there are two other charges that are common in the industry but make it difficult to compete with retail alternatives.

Paying employed veterinarians (associates) a commission (production) on the sale of products and diagnostic tests is commonplace but makes it extremely difficult to be comparable in price to other entities that do not pay such commissions (essentially everyone else). Similarly, a dispensing fee on medications is not charged by the majority of other retailers, so makes it difficult for veterinary practices to be price-competitive in an apples-to-apples comparison. In the end, veterinary practices will need to make some tough decisions regarding these types of discrepancies. There was a time when these strategies made sense for struggling veterinary practices, but the marketplace has changed, and business models may also need to change to be sustainable.

There are many strategies that can be used to be competitive, since we really want our retail business to help drive professional services, rather than using professional services as a loss leader to drive retail sales. Veterinary practices should rely on their expert professional services for profit and use ancillary services (e.g., pharmacy, laboratory) for customer service, convenience, and retail profit, and to support additional professional services that can be provided at professional service rates.

TAKE-AWAYS

- Today's pet owners are value shoppers, so pricing should reflect the value that they receive from their interactions with veterinary practices.
- Not all clients will search for less expensive alternatives that might be available, but the practice staff should be confident that if there are any major discrepancies, there are valid reasons for them.
- Professional services provided should be more profitable than ancillary services; if not, there is something wrong with the veterinary business model.
- Disclose pricing early in the process. Nobody likes surprises when it comes to costs.
- Some clients will always want the cheapest alternative, but most clients will spend the money needed to keep their pet healthy and happy. Make the case and let owners decide what they value most.

MISCELLANEOUS

References

1 Ackerman, L. (2009). What's the future of the veterinary pharmacy? *Veterinary Forum* 26 (12): 2–17.

2 Ackerman, L.J. (2002). *Business Basics for Veterinarians*. New York: ASJA Press.

3 Anderson, E. and Simester, D. (2003). Mind your pricing cues. *Harvard Business Review* 81 (9): 96–103.

4 Mohammed, R. (2018). The good-better-best approach to pricing. *Harvard Business Review* 96: 106–115.

5 Bertini, M. and Gourville, J.T. (2012). Pricing to create shared value. *Harvard Business Review* 90: 96–104.

Recommended Reading

Ackerman, L.J. (2003). *Management Basics for Veterinarians*. New York: ASJA Press.

Ackerman, L.J. (2020). Pricing strategies. In: *Five-Minute Veterinary Practice Management Consult*, 3e (ed. L. Ackerman), 474–477. Ames, IA: Wiley.

Mohammed, R. (2018). The good-better-best approach to pricing. *Harvard Business Review* 96: 106–115.

10.14

Providing Cost-Effective Care for Those in Need

Gary Block, DVM, MS, DACVIM

Ocean State Veterinary Specialists, East Greenwich, RI, USA

 BASICS

10.14.1 Summary

Many pets reside in homes where family members live at or below the poverty line and many more live with people often described as "the working poor." Decreasing animal pain and suffering and improving animal welfare are core pillars of our veterinary oath. Failure to make veterinary care financially accessible to as many people as possible is an abdication of that oath. In addition, clients' inability to afford care for their pets is routinely cited as one of the greatest sources of stress and job dissatisfaction for veterinarians. Without a paradigm shift in how we provide veterinary care, pet ownership and its attendant veterinary care could soon become a luxury that only the affluent can afford.

10.14.2 Terms Defined

Human–Animal Bond: A mutually beneficial and dynamic relationship between people and animals that is influenced by behaviors that are essential to the health and well-being of both.

Spectrum of Care: A continuum of care that takes into account available evidence-based medicine, client expectations, and financial limitations that may limit diagnostic and treatment options.

 MAIN CONCEPTS

10.14.3 The Problem

A flourishing human–animal bond, greater societal recognition of the value animals bring to our lives, and continued advances in the technology veterinary medicine can bring to our beloved pets would seem to be the perfect recipe for improving animal welfare. Unfortunately, these same factors that have allowed veterinarians to do some remarkable things (cancer chemotherapy, magnetic resonance imaging [MRI], and cardiac pacemakers to name a few) have also resulted in a progressively larger percentage of the pet-owning public being effectively "priced out" of receiving quality veterinary care (see 2.10 Affordability of Veterinary Services).

The 2017–2018 edition of the AVMA (*American Veterinary Medical Association*) *Pet Ownership and Demographics Sourcebook* found that only 47.2% of cat owners brought their animals in for routine or preventive care at least once a year [1]. The 2018 publication of *Access to Veterinary Care: Barriers, Current Practices, and Public Policy* found that dogs and cats living in lower-income households and with younger pet owners are most at risk for not receiving recommended care. The overwhelming barrier for all groups of pet owners and all types of care is financial, with 80% unable to obtain preventive care due to financial constraints, 74% for sick care, and 56% for emergency care [2].

Pet-Specific Care for the Veterinary Team, First Edition. Edited by Lowell Ackerman.
© 2021 John Wiley & Sons, Inc. Published 2021 by John Wiley & Sons, Inc.

Society, and the veterinary team in particular, needs to do a better job of educating the public as to the responsibilities and costs associated with pet ownership. Most people considering adding a dog or cat to their home are not aware of the approximate cost for a lifetime of care, feeding, and veterinary expenses for the average dog and cat (see 2.9 Anticipated Costs of Pet Care). Faced with this knowledge, some people may reasonably reconsider their decision to add a pet to their household. A 2017 report found only 31% of veterinarians discussed the anticipated costs of veterinary care with pet owners *prior* to their pet getting sick or injured [3].

10.14.4 The Solution

Veterinary education has historically taught students "gold standard" medicine. This was not surprising given that the majority of clinicians in academia were board-certified specialists and that many were not routinely seeing referrals of clients with severe financial limitations. Universities have started addressing this gap in student education by providing "community practice" rotations, more externships, and by acknowledging that the profession needs to do more to improve access to veterinary care (see 9.5 A Different Perspective on Standard of Care).

In the last decade, many veterinarians have created successful business models that specifically cater to low-income clients (see 6.5 Opportunities and Challenges of Providing Services for Low-Income Families). Some of these practices utilize sliding scale fee structures and some use financial means testing to ensure that only the neediest clients can take advantage of reduced cost care. Many veterinary medical associations have successfully started financial assistance programs and some hospitals now administer their own financial assistance funds for needy clients. Pet owners and hospitals should be aware and avail themselves of the many state and national financial assistance funds that are available to pet owners in need.

Another way in which we can provide care to more patients is by promoting the concept of "spectrum of care" rather than the outmoded and often nebulous concept of "standard of care." The former acknowledges that the care we provide to our patients has to ideally be grounded in evidence-based medicine but that we must take into account circumstances such as client expectations, living situation, and financial means when determining a course of care (see 2.2 The Role of Incremental Care). A continuum of treatment options may thus be medically and legally acceptable in a particular clinical situation. Other examples for helping clients afford care is to ensure your

hospital has a variety of payment and financing options available. Pet health insurance is becoming more prevalent and may allow clients to afford what previously might have been prohibitively expensive care (see 10.16 Pet Health Insurance).

Veterinarians should adhere to the mantra of "you miss more things by not looking than by not knowing." What this means is that many health issues in our patients can be identified sooner and less expensively by getting a detailed and comprehensive medical history and performing a thorough physical exam. Examples of commonly forgotten and often elucidating exam components include the rectal exam, fundic exam, and palpation of the thyroid glands in older cats. One of the best ways to save clients money is to stay current and up to date on the veterinary literature. Many diseases and conditions can be diagnosed and managed more easily and less expensively than they might have been in the past. Another important concept for the veterinary team to embrace is that tests should not be performed if it will not change the way you treat your patient.

Other simple ways to provide more cost-effective care include the following.

- Sending out laboratory work for stable patients. This is usually less expensive than processing samples in-house.
- Veterinary generic drugs are bio-equivalent medications that can be a less expensive option for some clients.
- Many effective, over-the-counter medicines such as antacids, antihistamines, and antidiarrheals are available at local drugstores without a prescription.
- "Big Box" store pharmacies can sometimes provide prescriptions of common drugs at prices that simply cannot be matched by a veterinary practice.
- Reputable, online veterinary pharmacies can be a good source for expensive long-term medications for clients as their bulk purchasing power allows them to offer these medications less expensively.
- Avoid "injectophilia" (the pressure to give injections simply because they are rapid acting). Even though an injection will enter the bloodstream a little faster, a stable patient can wait for the oral medicine to take effect if price is a serious issue.
- Familiarize yourself with alternative drugs that have similar efficacy or spectrum of activity but are less expensive.
- Ask your drug company representatives for free samples, discount coupons, and rebates. Pass these savings on to your neediest clients.
- While referring to a specialty hospital or university can save the life of a critically ill or injured pet, if it's a choice

between you and a textbook vs euthanasia/certain death, you have nothing to lose by trying. Don't be afraid to do something out of your comfort zone if finances preclude referral, as long as clients appreciate the compromise being made.

- Sometimes doing nothing is the best way to save your clients money. For example, a stable cat with an upper respiratory infection, which doesn't have a fever and is still eating, requires nothing but keeping his eyes and nose clean, and the owner to call you if he gets worse.

Clients not being able to afford recommended care for their pets is consistently noted as a major source of burnout and compassion fatigue (see 8.16 Dealing with Compassion Fatigue and Burnout). On the other hand, repeatedly being asked for lower-cost care options can also be a source of stress for veterinary healthcare teams (see 8.17 Dealing with Compromise Fatigue). Establishing acceptable but less expensive ways to provide quality care can benefit pet owners, pets, and the entire veterinary team.

EXAMPLES

Parvovirus infection in puppies is associated with high morbidity and, in untreated dogs, high mortality as well. Historically, infected dogs were routinely admitted for aggressive in-hospital care and in many cases, unless hospitalization was financially feasible, euthanasia was recommended. Recent studies have shown that outpatient therapy with subcutaneous fluids, antiemetics, antibiotics, potassium supplementation, and nutritional support is associated with survival rates of over 75% [4].

In referral practices, cystoscopy is often used to visualize and obtain a biopsy sample for dogs with bladder or urethral tumors. While extremely effective in obtaining a definitive diagnosis, anesthesia and cystoscopy are not inexpensive. Newer molecular technology options, using a DNA-based assay, can diagnose a common cause of tumors in dogs – transitional cell carcinoma – by identifying a mutation in malignant cells shed in the urine. Sample collection is simple and the test is highly sensitive and specific. Used appropriately and in a timely fashion, this test may result in earlier diagnosis and at considerably lower cost [5].

Addison's disease (hypoadrenocorticism) is associated with an excellent long-term prognosis. Unfortunately, monthly desoxycorticosterone pivalate injections can be expensive and with lifetime therapy required, some animals are euthanized simply due to the client's financial limitations. Newer studies have demonstrated that the routinely recommended every-25-day injection schedule can actually be gradually modified by lowering the dose and increasing the duration between injections. This can lower costs associated with treatment up to 50% over the lifetime of the pet [6].

TAKE-AWAYS

- Veterinary medicine is becoming prohibitively expensive for a progressively larger percentage of the pet-owning public.
- Veterinary education must do a better job creating graduates who can provide a spectrum of care options to their clients.
- Better history taking, physical exams, and diagnostic testing can streamline the diagnostic process and ultimately save clients money.
- Don't do tests if it won't change the way you treat your patient.
- Finding medically appropriate but less expensive ways to treat our patients will decrease stress and improve the mental health of the entire veterinary team.

MISCELLANEOUS

References

1 AVMA Pet Ownership and Demographics Sourcebook: 2017–2018. www.avma.org/PracticeManagement/Documents/AVMA-Pet-Demographics-Executive-Summary.pdf

2 Access to Veterinary Care: Barriers, Current Practices, Public Policy. http://avcc.utk.edu/avcc-report.pdf

3 Kipperman, B.S., Kass, P.H., and Rishniw, M. (2017). Factors that influence small animal veterinarians' opinions and actions regarding cost of care and effects of economic limitations on patient care and outcome and professional career satisfaction and burnout. *Journal of the American Veterinary Medical Association* 250: 785–794.

4 Venn, E.C., Preisner, K., Boscan, P.L. et al. (2017). Evaluation of an outpatient protocol in the treatment of canine parvoviral enteritis. *Journal of Veterinary Emergency and Critical Care* 27 (1): 52–65.

5 Sentinel Biomedical. www.sentinelbiomedical.com/braf-vets

6 Jaffey, J.A., Nurre, P., Cannon, A.B. et al. (2017). Desoxycorticosterone pivalate duration of action and individualized dosing intervals in dogs with primary Hypoadrenocorticism. *Journal of Veterinary Internal Medicine* 31 (6): 1649–1657.

Recommended Reading

Moses, L., Malowny, M.J., and Boyd, J.W. (2018). Ethical conflict and moral distress in veterinary practice: a survey of north American veterinarians. *Journal of Veterinary Internal Medicine* 32 (6): 2115–2122.

10.15

Putting Price into Perspective

Lowell Ackerman, DVM, DACVD, MBA, MPA, CVA, MRCVS

Global Consultant, Author, and Lecturer, MA, USA

 BASICS

10.15.1 Summary

Veterinary practices, and the staff who work in them, depend on the revenues generated from services to provide salaries, money for practice reinvestment, and a return on investment. Accordingly, getting paid for services rendered is every bit as important as the level of customer service and the quality of medical care provided.

Veterinary costs are a relative bargain for the pet-owning public when compared to similar costs in the human healthcare arena. However, most veterinary practices would counter that clients (and staff) resist attempts to increase fees, and that it is a continual challenge to attempt to practice high-quality medicine while keeping prices artificially low. This is only true, however, if veterinary medicine is a commodity in the minds of clients, and those services are interchangeable at any number of clinics. This also happens because clients often benchmark services against procedures that are already highly subsidized. For example, a client might have difficulty understanding why a laparotomy costs so much more than an ovariohysterectomy, when presumably the ovariohysterectomy likely requires as much or more effort. This is the fault of veterinary pricing policies, and messaging used with clients, not the whim of the pet-owning public (see 10.13 Approach to Pricing).

Similarly, something that veterinary teams might consider a commodity transaction – the purchase of a dog or cat – is viewed quite differently by many pet owners. Although veterinary teams might scoff at the "quality" of animals found in a pet store, clients willingly spend hundreds and sometimes thousands of dollars acquiring a pet, and often on impulse. These new owners typically buy the pet as a full cash transaction, with little tendency to price shop to see if they can get a better deal elsewhere.

10.15.2 Terms Defined

Commodity: Product that is interchangeable with another product of the same type. The price is a function of supply and demand.

Prophy: Colloquial term for a dental prophylaxis procedure.

 MAIN CONCEPTS

10.15.3 Allowing Clients to Make Informed Choices

A major problem associated with any sales transaction is prejudicially making assumptions about what the client can afford and what services they would choose if given appropriate information. The fact is that when clients pay for a consultation, they are entitled to that consultation, which should include the appropriate options and the costs involved. Armed with all the appropriate information, the client is then prepared to make an informed decision of how they would like to proceed.

There are certainly clients who will select a path that is less expensive than the optimal route, but it is critical that the client make that decision and not the veterinary team. Similarly, if the client would have selected the optimal route but the veterinary team did not recommend it because a personal judgment was made that the client couldn't afford the service, then a terrible injustice was done to the client and to the pet.

10.15.4 Payment at Time of Service

For many years, veterinarians offered care with easy payment terms, and so there are still clients who expect financing options (although they do not expect such options from other businesses). The easiest way to correct the situation is to make the terms of service obvious from the start and to feel comfortable speaking with clients about financial matters. This is often a point of concern, because many veterinary team members do not feel comfortable talking about money with clients and therefore are prone to making bad decisions in this regard. Two of the most common mistakes include offering credit (often without charge) or discounting the service that was likely already offered at a bargain price (see 2.11 Discounting in Veterinary Practice). If the services were priced fairly (see 10.13 Approach to Pricing), then only the hospital loses in this scenario.

Veterinary practices should endeavor to increase transparency in setting expectations for visits, so clients can logically anticipate what their veterinary bill is likely to be for routine visits so they can plan accordingly (see 1.2 Providing a Lifetime of Care, and 2.9 Anticipated Costs of Care). When clients cannot reasonably predict what veterinary charges are likely to be, it makes it difficult to plan ahead for paying for them.

10.15.5 Delivering Value

In most circumstances, consumers make purchase decisions on the basis of value, not price. The value may be perceived rather than actual, but clients select on the basis of value, nonetheless. Thus, it is critical that veterinary hospitals deliver value, and not try to sell goods and services as commodities. Commodities are only bought and sold on the basis of supply and demand. People willingly pay for goods and services that they value. For commodities, it is fine to shop around for the best price, because there is little difference in quality. The value added by a veterinary practice is the entire reason for the veterinary visit, and the premise on which veterinary services are offered – the continued health of animals.

Not all clients want the same things, and some clients are prepared to pay for additional features, and some for less, so most retailers benefit from tiered solutions (good, better, best). Veterinarians would be well served to consider similar strategies. There is no doubt that some clients are financially challenged, and need to make decisions on the basis of a spectrum of care, but they still want value, even on

basic care options (see 10.14 Providing Cost-Effective Care for Those in Need).

10.15.6 Including Pet Owners in the Healthcare Team

Most consumers are unwilling to pay for services that they do not understand. Therefore, one of the most valuable tools to making owners aware of optimal medical care and its costs is to incorporate those pet owners into their pet's healthcare team. If they understand the process and are part of the solution, they will also bear responsibility for those costs.

10.15.7 Milestones for Payment

Nobody likes surprises, so clients should be kept abreast of any possible changes in a patient's status, especially if they will affect the amount on the final bill, and clients should be able to anticipate payment points that correspond to milestones in the treatment-to-discharge pathway. This can be facilitated by:

- creating estimates for all patients that will be admitted for any procedure. Standard estimates can actually be created for commonly performed procedures, but should have realistic ranges so that the final bill should not be more than 10% above the estimated price
- establishing payment in full at time of discharge for all outpatient and day procedures. Clients should be aware of this prior to dropping off their animals. Establishing in advance how the bill will be paid can save time at discharge and also will confirm with the owner that payment will be expected at that time
- establishing payment points for animals that will be hospitalized for longer than one day. It is important to create a reasonable estimate, and also to request payments that correspond to points between admission and discharge. For example, for an expensive hospitalization, one might ask for one-half of the estimated final bill in advance, another quarter after a given number of days (when a better estimate of prognosis might be possible), and the final quarter upon discharge. During daily communication with the owner, a more up-to-date accounting can be provided, and the owner asked for additional funds (if warranted) in concert with the agreed-upon proposal. It is also important for clients to sign appropriate waivers that there might be unforeseen complications that may

affect the anticipated outcome and the estimates of cost. Taking the time to get properly informed consent in advance is extremely helpful if things do go wrong, and if costs escalate for unanticipated reasons (see 7.4 Getting Informed Consent).

10.15.8 Accommodate Clients' Financial Needs

In some instances, clients would authorize the work that needs to be done, but simply cannot afford to have everything done and paid for at one time (see 2.10 Affordability of Veterinary Services, and 10.14 Providing Cost-Effective Care for Those in Need). There are several ways to manage this situation.

- Plan to have the same amount of work done, but space out the procedures (if medically feasible) to allow the client to budget (see 2.2 The Role of Incremental Care). For example, if a pet needs a dental "prophy" and practice protocols require the animal to have a preanesthetic blood panel, consider collecting the blood sample first, and then schedule the dental procedure for a future date that would better meet the budgeting needs of the client.
- If a significant portion of the bill is for pharmaceuticals, consider performing the medical procedures and authorizing a prescription for the medications that can be filled elsewhere (including an affiliated online veterinary pharmacy). In some cases, this may lessen the hospital invoice to the client significantly, and allow them to proceed with the medical care recommended (see 9.10 Dispensing and Prescribing).
- Establish prepayment plans that spread the charges out over time rather than requiring a lump sum at time of service. For nonemergency situations, especially wellness programs, this is an excellent way to allow clients to budget and for practices to collect fully on the services provided (see 10.17 Payment and Wellness Plans).

Although nobody anticipates the need for expensive healthcare intervention, they appreciate that it is a possibility, so they should manage this risk accordingly. This topic is covered in greater detail in 10.16 Pet Health Insurance, but if more pet owners had appropriate insurance, and if veterinary teams routinely recommended it, veterinary teams would have fewer complaints about getting paid for services rendered. As long

as clients believe that pet healthcare will continue to be inexpensive and readily affordable, there is no real need for insurance. It is worthwhile for veterinary teams to discuss the reasonable costs of pet healthcare over an animal's lifetime (see 2.9 Anticipated Costs of Pet Care), including possible visits to specialists and emergency clinics. Clients could then choose to mitigate those risks, and likely many more would choose to properly insure their pets.

EXAMPLES

Donna Smith has complained to Dr Jones that she spends about $x yearly on her dog, Spike, but that there must be a less expensive way to care for him. Many times, she buys a year's worth of supplies, such as heartworm prevention, and sometimes she even forgets to give the medication and then needs another blood test.

Dr Jones asked if it would be helpful if they provided a package service that included two clinical examinations a year, any needed vaccines and/or titers, a heartworm test and a fecal evaluation, and the care be charged $y monthly instead of lump sums during semi-annual office visits. Donna agreed that it would. To help with the heartworm prevention issue, Dr Jones even administered an injectable preventive so that Donna would not need to remember when to administer the medication at home.

TAKE-AWAYS

- Most consumers are value shoppers, so price is a consideration but not necessarily the main predictor of their actions.
- Veterinary teams should endeavor to provide guidance to pet owners as to the likely costs associated with pet ownership (including potential development of common chronic conditions, emergencies, need for referrals) so they can plan accordingly.
- Veterinary teams must be comfortable talking with pet owners about hospital policies regarding payment, so everyone is clear on expectations.
- Risk management strategies like pet health insurance are best implemented when pets are young (preferably 8 weeks of age) when there are no problems evident that would be excluded from coverage.

- Nobody likes to be surprised with costs they weren't expecting. Help pet owners plan in advance for pet health, and there will be fewer awkward conversations to be had with owners who were unprepared.

MISCELLANEOUS

10.15.9 Cautions

If clients do not see the value in services provided, they will be resistant to paying for those services. Similarly, if clients do not see the inherent value in their pet, they will be unable to see the value in veterinary services recommended. The best driver of clients valuing their pets is the human–animal bond (see 2.14 Benefits of the Human–Animal Bond), so this bond should be promoted and validated by practices at every opportunity (see 2.15 Promoting the Human–Animal Bond).

Recommended Reading

Ackerman, L.J. (2002). *Business Basics for Veterinarians*. New York: ASJA Press.

Ackerman, L.J. (2003). *Management Basics for Veterinarians*. New York: ASJA Press.

Ackerman, L.J. (2020). Getting paid for services rendered. In: *Five-Minute Veterinary Practice Management Consult*, 3e (ed. L. Ackerman), 542–543. Ames, IA: Wiley.

Carlson, D., Haeder, S., Jenkins-Smith, H. et al. (2020). Monetizing bowser: a contingent valuation of the statistical value of dog life. *J. Benefit-Cost Anal.* 11: 131–149.

Mohammed, R. (2018). The good-better-best approach to pricing. *Harv. Bus. Rev.* 96: 106–115.

Stull, J.W., Shelby, J.A., Bonnett, B.N. et al. Barriers and next steps to providing a spectrum of effective health care to companion animals. *J. Am. Vet. Med. Assoc.* 253 (11): 1386–1389.

10.16

Pet Health Insurance

Lowell Ackerman, DVM, DACVD, MBA, MPA, CVA, MRCVS

Global Consultant, Author, and Lecturer, MA, USA

BASICS

10.16.1 Summary

Pet health insurance (PHI) is an important method by which pet owners can manage the financial risks of pet healthcare. In fact, it is the most useful risk management strategy in countries and marketplaces where it is available. PHI is not only important when clients need to have access to funds for covering care at the primary care veterinarian, but also becomes progressively more important as clients require services from specialists and emergency clinics, centers that tend to be significantly more costly than primary care practices. Pet-specific care typically signifies that pets will receive more care than they are currently, so PHI is a tool that allows clients to be able to afford this enhanced level of care.

Properly utilized, PHI provides pet owners with peace of mind that they have planned ahead for the eventualities that we often don't want to think about, but that nonetheless are an unavoidable part of pet ownership.

10.16.2 Terms Defined

Benefit Schedule: Summary of covered services, benefit limitations, and applicable co-payments provided in an insurance policy.

Co-Pay: Specified amount of covered services that is the insurance policyholder's responsibility.

Deductible: Amount an individual must pay for health services before the individual's insurance company starts to pay.

Discount Plans: Not insurance. Instead, this is a service by which pet owners pay a fee to receive discounted services from participating veterinarians.

Exclusion: A condition that is not covered under an insurance policy.

Indemnity Insurance: System of health insurance in which the insurance carrier reimburses the insured individual for medical expenses after care has been provided.

Insurance Coverage: Insurance coverage, or cover, is the amount of risk or liability that is protected in an insurance contract.

Managed Care: Healthcare system under which healthcare professionals are organized into a group or "network" to manage the cost, quality, and access to healthcare.

Third-Party Payment: Monetary reimbursement for medical services from someone other than the client/patient.

MAIN CONCEPTS

10.16.3 Why Should We Make Clients Aware of Pet Health Insurance?

Most pet owners typically do not have separate savings to use when their pets require unanticipated veterinary services, so it is natural that they will want to find ways to manage those unanticipated costs as effectively as possible.

In human medicine, it is widely appreciated that it is necessary to manage the risks associated with high healthcare bills by having insurance, either as indemnity insurance, managed care, or socialized medicine.

It might seem counterintuitive, but people don't buy insurance to save money – they purchase insurance for the peace of mind that comes with knowing that if the unexpected happens, they will have the resources available to do what needs to be done.

Even in markets in which PHI has been available for many years, many pet owners may still be unaware of the service and, in some instances, only hear about it after a problem occurs, which then becomes a preexisting condition and potentially invalidates future coverage for that problem.

10.16.4 What is Pet Health Insurance?

It is important to realize that indemnity insurance is not the same as human healthcare insurance, managed care or discount plans. The major PHI companies are indemnity insurers (property and casualty insurance), in which clients pay for veterinary services and then submit claims to the insurance company for reimbursement. With indemnity insurance, pet owners can visit the veterinarian or the specialty or emergency clinics of their choice, and the veterinarian and veterinary hospital are only required to provide the service, not process any paperwork (other than signing a claims form and providing clients with the information they need to submit with the claim). In some cases, the claims can be initiated by the veterinary practices themselves, and some even provide near-instantaneous reimbursement to enrolled hospitals.

Discount plans are not insurance at all. They are buying groups that sell discounted services to pet owners and then rely on a network of veterinarians to provide discounts in exchange for being promoted within the network. It is currently unclear if there is any real benefit for participating veterinarians, because the discount may exceed the profit margin on services offered. The premise is that discounted services attract new clients (the premise of all discounts), but that does not necessarily translate to profit for participating veterinary practices (see 2.11 Discounting in Veterinary Practice).

Managed care plans have not been promoted in the veterinary marketplace, and given their lack of popularity with doctors and patients on the human side, will likely not be warmly welcomed in veterinary medicine.

Veterinarians do not need to promote specific insurance companies, but it is certainly worthwhile for them to notify clients that PHI exists as a viable option and help them research the products available in their area so they can have intelligent discussions with clients about risk management (see Figure 10.16.1). Owner compliance tends to be higher when veterinarians can provide information about the pros and cons of specific policies, reflecting features that would be of most concern to pet owners. In addition, owners are 50% more likely to enroll in PHI if their veterinarian actively recommends it [1].

Compare Insurance Plans				
Coverage	Sample	Plan A	Plan B	Plan C
Accidents & illness	✔			
Emergency & specialty visits	✔			
Genetic and "predisposed" conditions	✔			
Ongoing care for chronic conditions	✔			
Clinical visits & diagnostic tests (not including wellness care)	✔			
Pre-clinical screening	✔			
Telehealth (Virtual Care)	✔			
Prescription medications	✔			
Surgeries & hospitalization	✔			
Rehabilitative, Acupuncture, & Chiropractic Care				
Vaccinations, parasite control, and routine wellness exams	Optional add-on			
Annual Limit	Unlimited			
Exclusions	None			
Deductible	Annual			
Co-pay	10%			
Price				

Figure 10.16.1 Resources that can be used to compare insurance plan features.

Clients (and veterinarians) should be aware of the terms of insurance policies, such as whether heritable conditions are covered, whether the insurance is offered on a benefit schedule or based on a veterinary invoice, whether the care of chronic conditions and heritable issues is covered, whether there is an annual limit, whether the pet is covered for its entire life, and whether there are exclusions in the policy.

All insurance policies define what is covered in the policy, and also what is excluded from coverage. The most common exclusion is for preexisting conditions, problems that have been identified in the pet prior to the insurance policy taking effect. For example, if a pet has osteoarthritis prior to being covered by insurance, it should be anticipated that the ongoing care of osteoarthritis will be excluded from policy coverage. This is one of the reasons why it is so important that pets have insurance coverage early in life, when nothing is considered preexisting and the pet appears completely healthy.

Some PHI policies extend the concept of exclusion to conditions known or believed to have a heritable component. So, if a certain breed is known to be "predisposed" to certain ailments, coverage of those conditions may be excluded in some policies. The best way to safeguard against this is to recommend policies that clearly state that genetic problems are covered by the policy (as long as they are not preexisting). It should be expected that such policies will be slightly more expensive, but they are often well worth it, since it can be disappointing to pet owners to have insurance, only to learn that conditions that pose considerable risk might not be covered. This is particularly relevant concerning pet-specific care. Similarly, some policies can appear cheaper if they don't offer chronic care coverage. So, for example, if a pet develops diabetes mellitus during the policy term, it will be covered, but when the term renews, the medical condition could be considered "preexisting" and excluded from further coverage. Everyone wants to save money on insurance but such short-term savings are rarely worth it. If at all possible, recommend policies that will provide ongoing care for chronic conditions, as well as coverage for hereditary conditions.

10.16.5 What Gets Reimbursed?

Deductibles are set dollar amounts that are "deducted" from the insurance reimbursement. Some policies have deductibles that apply per incident, while others might have an annual deductible, so that once that amount is reached, further deductibles won't apply for the remainder of the term. Deductibles are meant to keep premiums affordable, by ensuring that pet owners have some stake in the process.

Co-pays reflect the relative proportion of the covered amount to be paid for by the insurance company and the pet owner. For example, while there are a variety of possible co-pays, depending on what pet owners would like the premium to be, a typical co-pay may be that the insurance company will reimburse 90% of the covered amount, after the deductible, while the pet owner will be responsible for 10%. If owners are prepared for higher co-pays, they will likely see slightly lower premiums, but they will be paying for a higher percentage of their pet's care.

Some insurance policies provide renewable lifelong care, albeit possibly with per-year or per-incident limits. However, as indicated earlier, some policies with nonlifetime provisions may cover a condition during the course of a policy year but upon renewal in the subsequent year, the condition might be excluded as "preexisting" and no longer covered. It is important to appreciate this distinction because lifelong care is one of the most important reasons to consider PHI in the first place.

Originally, PHI was intended more for catastrophic coverage, and later for lifelong care, but some policies today also provide regular-care options, such as vaccination, parasite control, and even dental cleaning. In other instances, this type of wellness coverage can be an "add-on" to more traditional policies.

It is worthwhile for veterinary teams to understand treatment terms and any diagnostic codes for the insurance policies that they recommend. This makes it easier for the insurance company to match what was done at the veterinary hospital with conditions for which there is coverage, which in turn facilitates the process of the client being reimbursed. Policy information is provided on the websites of most insurance companies, or can be requested by contacting the insurance company directly. Only some indemnity insurance companies still use benefit schedules; some set annual limits, regardless of illness or condition.

10.16.6 Integrating Insurance Into Practice Standards

Pet health insurance is an important component of allowing clients to manage their pet healthcare costs. It also allows clients to have veterinary care provided at the time it is needed without worrying about financing those costs by other means.

Pet health insurance also tends to be highly effective at increasing compliance with veterinary recommendations and allowing increased expenditures on veterinary medical services by pet owners [2].

Pet health insurance is also a valuable "perk" for veterinary hospital employees. It allows them to get veterinary care, including visits to specialists and emergency centers, without having to request discounts or informal consultations. This is one of the best ways to ensure that staff are ambassadors for excellent pet healthcare. Otherwise, many employees of veterinary practices may not be able to afford the care they are supposed to recommend to clients (see 7.2 Managing the Pet-Specific Workplace). PHI is a much-requested benefit from a variety of companies and clinics. In many cases, the employees pay for the plans themselves, but receive a group discount by buying the insurance through their employers.

Discussions about PHI should take place as early as possible (typically when pets are about 8 weeks of age), before any conditions occur that might be considered preexisting. Waiting until an incident has already occurred can be costly for clients. Similarly, the discussion should take place before the client encounters a situation that might involve a hefty healthcare bill. Most owners are unaware that they might eventually need levels of care that could be beyond their means (see 2.9 Anticipated Costs of Pet Care).

Clients could save money specifically for the purpose of paying these bills when they arise, but most don't. While it might be possible to replicate coverage by making contributions to a pet-specific savings account each month, it is important to realize that almost nobody takes this kind of disciplined approach to saving for a pet's healthcare needs. In addition, it would take years to save enough funds to cover potential veterinary expenses, especially given that it is not possible to predict when those funds will actually be needed.

Sooner or later, most pets are going to develop medical problems that require ongoing medical care and monitoring (e.g., osteoarthritis), need a referral to a specialist, or have a mishap that requires a visit to an emergency clinic. For most people, having a PHI policy is the best way to deal with those likelihoods. PHI plays the role of taking the cost of pet healthcare out of available discretionary funds, and turns it into a budgeted affordable expense. Without such insurance, it can be very expensive to provide the type of care that most pet owners would prefer.

The true value of PHI, as it currently exists, is that it is truly a third-party payment. Clients visit their veterinary hospitals, veterinarians provide services, clients pay their bills and then submit them to the insurance company, and the insurance company reimburses the pet owner. This allows veterinarians to practice high-quality medicine and help clients afford high-quality healthcare, without veterinarians being directly involved in the financing of that care.

As part of the arms-length relationship between insurance companies and veterinarians, it is important for the hospital to be a client advocate, but to avoid direct intervention in the insurance process unless it is just to clarify the diagnosis made or the treatment provided.

Part of the advantage of third-party payment is the independence that this affords veterinary teams. As an advocate for the client and patient, the veterinary team should encourage clients to plan for unanticipated pet health expenses. The practice can facilitate this process by having clients compare available policies and select the one that best meets their needs. If the client later has a dispute with the insurance company over a claim, the veterinary team should remain impartial and not be viewed as an agent of the insurance company, which clearly they are not.

It is helpful to both the client and the practice if hospital teams have basic knowledge of what different recommended insurance policies offer, so they can help clients select a plan appropriate for them (see Figure 10.16.1). Insurance policies can be confusing to understand but assisting clients in making valid comparisons enables them to select a suitable product for their specific circumstances, as well as basing decisions on value rather than just price. Sometimes offering tiered solutions (good, better, best) can get clients past the initial decision of whether or not to get PHI, and instead focus on which policy best meets their needs. Clients need to understand the trade-offs in going for a policy that might be cheaper but does not really meet their needs. In the end, clients need to be satisfied with the coverage they receive for the amount of money they are prepared to pay.

EXAMPLES

Strudel, a 4-year-old miniature schnauzer, had been continuously insured since puppyhood without any insurance claims. In fact, Strudel's owners had considered discontinuing the insurance because it hadn't been used, but continued it on the advice of their veterinarian. A few months later, Strudel was admitted to ABC Veterinary Hospital with acute abdominal pain that was later confirmed to be pancreatitis. Strudel was hospitalized for three days, maintained on intravenous therapy, and then finally released. The hospital bill was considerable, more than the total insurance premiums paid to date. Strudel's owner, Mrs Park, put the charge on her credit card and promptly submitted the bill to her PHI company. Within a few weeks, she received her reimbursement, in which the vast majority of the bill was covered, after the deductible and co-pay.

TAKE-AWAYS

- Pet health insurance is an important risk management strategy, especially for unanticipated healthcare expenses.
- Pet health insurance is not a money-saving mechanism. It is designed to cover the risk of healthcare expenses that are not anticipated.
- Pet health insurance gives clients peace of mind that they will have the resources to do what is needed when healthcare issues arise.
- Two of the most important features that should be included in a PHI policy are coverage for chronic conditions and for hereditary disorders.
- To be most effective, PHI policies should be started when animals are young (typically around 8 weeks of age), when they are unlikely to have any problems that would be considered preexisting.

MISCELLANEOUS

True indemnity insurance is a highly regulated industry, and each state has its own licensing procedure. Many insurance look-alikes abound in the pet marketplace, but are not bound by the same regulations as the insurance companies. These can be confusing for pet owners and veterinarians alike, but most are discount plans without the same regulatory safeguards in place.

Insurance can be a confusing topic for owners, and it is worth making suggestions as to the types of companies available (not all insurance plans are necessarily available in all locations) that offer indemnity insurance. One of the ways of keeping premiums comparatively low is that PHI is not typically sold by agents, and there has been relatively little direct marketing to the public previously.

Other forms of pet insurance do exist, but are not related to healthcare coverage and so are not discussed further here. For example, liability insurance is available to cover damage done to property and people by pets (see 4.12 Homeowner Insurance Considerations), there are insurance products that would cover the theft of a pet, and even forms of life insurance that would pay out if an animal dies.

10.16.7 Cautions

In the context of pet-specific care, it is important that hospital teams understand any limitations policies might have about preclinical screening. It should be expected that

some policies will be more generous than others when it comes to evaluating pets that might have certain risk factors but no actual clinical signs of disease. For example, a pet may have risk factors for the development of glaucoma (such as genetic testing results or breed predisposition) and ideally the policy should cover additional diagnostics for monitoring the pet, even though there is not yet a clinical diagnosis of glaucoma.

Because indemnity insurance is true third-party coverage, it is important that veterinary teams and veterinary hospitals not make any representations regarding the insurance company, such as assuring clients that the care being provided will be covered. If there are any questions about coverage, the clients should contact the insurance company directly.

It is critical that veterinarians maintain their ethical standing with third-party payer companies and with clients. Clients sometimes ask veterinarians to provide fraudulent documentation that would allow them to recoup expenses from insurance companies. Veterinarians should never comply with such requests, but should offer to make available legitimate records that are a truthful rendering of the situation.

References

1 North American Pet Health Insurance Association (NAPHIA). State of the Industry Report. www.naphia.org

2 Flietner, M.B. (2017). Study: insurance brings pets in the door. *Trends Magazine* (January): 53–55.

Recommended Reading

Ackerman, L.: Why pet health insurance is important for the profession. www.ecronicon.com/eco19/pdf/ECVE-02-ECO-04.pdf

Ackerman, L. (2020). Pet health insurance. In: *Five-Minute Veterinary Practice Management Consult*, 3e (ed. L. Ackerman), 544–547. Ames, IA: Wiley.

Ackerman, L.J. (2018). Response to "do we need pet insurance.". *AAHA Trends* 34: 9–10.

American Veterinary Medical Association (AVMA). AVMA Guidelines on Pet Health Insurance for Pet Owners. www.avma.org/resources-tools/avma-policies/pet-health-insurance

North American Pet Health Insurance Association. Pet Insurance Buying Guide. https://naphia.org/find-pet-insurance/insurance-buying-guide

10.17

Payment and Wellness Plans

Lowell Ackerman, DVM, DACVD, MBA, MPA, CVA, MRCVS

Global Consultant, Author, and Lecturer, MA, USA

BASICS

10.17.1 Summary

Payment plans, sometimes referred to as wellness plans or concierge plans, are tools used to make veterinary visits more affordable by spreading charges on a regular recurring basis rather than submitting larger client invoices at time of service.

10.17.2 Terms Defined

Concierge Medicine: A doctor–client–patient relationship in which medical care is provided for an agreed-upon fee and array of services.

Driver: An aspect of a business that leads to change in other aspects of a business, usually in a positive fashion.

Insurance: A form of risk management in which reimbursement for specified veterinary expenses is guaranteed in exchange for premium payments.

Payment Plan: A bundled medical plan in which specified veterinary services are provided and paid for in installments or pre-paid, rather than at time of service. Sometimes referred to as wellness plans or concierge plans.

Wellness: The pursuit of good health.

MAIN CONCEPTS

10.17.3 Premise

It is generally appreciated that pet owners want predictability of veterinary care expenditures and would appreciate opportunities to pay for those services over time rather than all at once [1]. Many clients who use payment plans appreciate the ability to budget for anticipated veterinary care and spread the annual costs over periodic (often monthly) payments.

Veterinary practices often entertain payment plans to encourage clients to commit to a recommended array of services, improving compliance and smoothing out cash flow more evenly over the course of a year rather than changing with seasonal trends. With pet-specific care, it is not unusual that clients spend more money, especially on prevention and early detection, and such payment plans allow pet owners to more easily budget available funds over time.

Payment plans can include any services to which the practice and the client are in agreement. They are entirely customizable. Typically, payment plans cover services over a 12-month period, but that, too, is customizable.

The most common payment plans are for "wellness" visits, and might include the number of visits during the plan period (from one to unlimited), vaccinations, parasite testing, certain diagnostics (e.g., heartworm testing, DNA screening, titers, etc.), identification (e.g., microchipping), and other services.

Payment plans are not limited to preventive care, and can also be used in care pathways (see 9.6 Care Pathways), for which expenses can be readily predicted, and even for accounts receivable, to provide an option for clients who carry a balance but hope to continue to utilize veterinary services.

The number of clinic visits provided in a payment plan can be quite variable, even unlimited. Virtual care (telehealth) may also be incorporated into these plans (see 2.5 Virtual Care (Telehealth)). The rationale for providing more clinic visits than is customary is to remove any barrier to the client coming in for attention, with the realization that it is the clinic visit that is the "driver" for additional medical services.

Research has demonstrated that the extent to which customers use the products they have already paid for helps determine whether they will repeat the purchase the next year [2]. Consumers feel compelled to use products and services that they have paid for, to avoid feeling that they've wasted their money. This approach benefits both pet owners, who want their pets to be cared for, and veterinary clinics that want to provide that care. This consumption also affects switching costs, since it would be difficult for clients to "un-bundle" their services if they were considering changing clinics.

Veterinary proponents of payment plans assert that clients seek veterinary attention more often and earlier when they have a payment plan, and that this makes clients less price conscious, removing one important barrier to more comprehensive and regular veterinary care. When this happens, client traffic in the clinic typically increases, more incidental problems are caught and treated earlier, and pet owners have more opportunities for purchasing their medications, diets, and supplies at the hospital, typically as ancillary spend to the payment plan, and sometimes included in a plan.

10.17.4 Implementation

Currently, perhaps 20% or so of small animal veterinary practices offer some form of payment plans to their clients [3]. Many more have contemplated such plans but were uncertain how to best implement them.

The working concept for most plans involves a commitment of the pet owner to make installment payments toward an agreed-upon bundle of services to be provided by the veterinary hospital. Other clients might be prepared to pay for the entire plan period up front in order to be assured a bundle of services at a fixed price, or associated with a slight prepayment discount.

The veterinary practice must decide on the number of plans that will be offered, which might be determined by life stage (see 1.2 Providing a Lifetime of Care), plan status (e.g., silver, gold, platinum, etc.), species, care pathway, and any number of other determinants.

For each plan, the practice needs to determine the total price for the bundle over the plan period (typically, one year). Once the fair retail price has been determined, the practice has the option of whether to offer a discount on that amount, as an incentive for owners to commit to the full array of services. In many premium plans, the service list typically includes more than most clients would otherwise request during the plan period, so discounts are offset somewhat by a higher starting fee. For example, the Companion Animal Parasite Council (CAPC; www. capcvet.org) recommends fecal evaluation 2–4 times during the first year of life, and then once to twice yearly in

adults. Whereas many clients might have fecals evaluated perhaps once a year, the premium plans can actually cover the full CAPC recommendation, bundled into a manageable payment plan.

Practices also have the option to charge an upfront administrative fee to enact the plan, either as a fixed amount or as a percentage of the plan total. This "enrollment fee" reflects the pet owner's commitment to the process, perhaps even implying a sense of membership or community, and provides the hospital with some initial revenue to defray the costs associated with services provided before full payment is received.

The payment plan itself is not just a way for clients to defer their veterinary expenses. It is meant to be a contract that guarantees revenues for the hospital as well as providing affordable payment options for pet owners. Once a practice has elected to initiate payment plans, it needs to create a marketing plan, train staff, set performance targets, and carefully measure return on investment (ROI).

10.17.5 Administration

In addition to creating and pricing plans, the hospital must decide how they intend to collect recurring payments and how they are going to reconcile payments with services provided in the practice management software (PMS). For example, if a payment plan includes two office visits, vaccinations, and fecal and heartworm testing, the practice needs to be aware that when the client presents for a third office visit during the course of the plan period, this is outside the plan and must be billed separately.

Practices can decide to administer the plans themselves, with payment collected on a recurring basis, but they must maintain security standards (e.g., Payment Card Industry [PCI]) as required by law to protect the financial integrity of their clients (see 7.13 Keeping Client Information Secure).

Practices can also make arrangements with their credit card merchant accounts for processing recurring payments, and with banks to debit clients' accounts for the appropriate amounts during the plan period. There are also commercial alternatives that will handle payment processing for a fee. Depending upon the company selected, payment plans can be created for payments made with credit cards or automatic bank drafts (ACH). Some of these companies even provide instant credit analysis as part of their service.

A final approach is to consider utilizing a full-service company that processes payments, tracks plan utilization, provides sample plans, and may even integrate with some PMS.

EXAMPLES

Mrs Franklin brought in her Maine Coon cat, Franny, to ABC Veterinary Hospital and while she was waiting for her appointment, she read a brochure for the hospital's Concierge Plans, a form of annual payment plan. They even had some breed-specific plans, and the receptionist explained that for Franny, they could construct an initial plan that would include up to four office visits per year, telehealth consults, fecal evaluation, year-long parasite control, all vaccinations, microchipping, baseline laboratory values (blood and urine), viral profile, heartworm testing, and a genetic screening panel that included hypertrophic cardiomyopathy, polycystic kidney disease, and spinal muscular atrophy. The receptionist provided an estimate of the retail value of those services and offered two options for payment: a 10% discount on the total for prepayment of the entire amount, or a monthly payment plan could be created and implemented for either credit card or bank draft processing, for a separate upfront enrollment fee. In subsequent years, different plans would be created based on Franny's particular needs.

TAKE-AWAYS

- Payment plans can be a convenient way for pet owners to spread the cost of care over an extended time period.
- The coverage within payment plans needs to be carefully articulated so owners are not confused about what is covered and what is not.
- Payment plans are not limited to use just during wellness visits in the first year of life. They can be used whenever total fees can be clearly predicted.
- It is important for clients to realize that payment plans are not insurance and cannot be used for anything outside the scope of the agreement.
- Payment plans can be convenient for clients and hospitals as long as the terms of the agreement are clear to everyone.

MISCELLANEOUS

10.17.6 Cautions

All veterinary hospitals in the United States, of any size, that process, store, or transmit credit card information must be PCI compliant for keeping clients' payment card data secure. This is particularly relevant for payment plans if the practice intends to store client payment card data for entry on a recurring basis.

Another major issue that requires clarification with many clients is that payment plans should not be confused with pet health insurance (see 10.16 Pet Health Insurance). Clients need to realize that payment plans cover only the specified procedures that constitute the plan itself. They do not cover unanticipated medical issues that are not specifically detailed in the plan. They also don't include visits to other veterinary practices, including emergency facilities and specialists. Payment plans should be associated with contracts that clearly detail the responsibilities, benefits, and limitations of such programs.

Most payment plans cannot guarantee that there won't be any payment defaults, so practices need to also have a process in place to deal with situations in which some services have been rendered but payments have been interrupted or discontinued. Some corporate services will assist with nonsufficient funds (NSF) transactions, expired credit cards, and other such issues.

There also need to be processes in place when clients move, a pet dies, or in some other circumstance, when payments will end before the plan period and it is necessary to reconcile payments made with services already provided.

Employee (associate) veterinarians that are paid on production (commission) must be confident that the practice has a system in place to assure their fair compensation when clients come in for services not associated with invoices. The most common approach is to credit them on the basis of the discounted price at time of service, but as long as there is mutual agreement, many different compensation models could work.

Some practices significantly discount the total payment plan amount as an enticement for clients to commit to the full complement of recommended services. They might also discount ancillary services as part of the loyalty program. Because veterinary profit margins might be lower than the discounts offered, it is important to track these programs to ensure that they are, in fact, profitable for the practice. If the benefits of payment plans are clearly explained to clients, discounting need not be a significant part of such programs. Discounts are typically not necessary if the plan itself provides adequate value.

It is not unusual that clients do not fully utilize all services in a payment plan. Although in some ways this might seem attractive as money is collected without providing services, it is important to remember that one of the reasons for offering payment plans is to actually deliver a high level of veterinary care, so clients should be encouraged and reminded to fully utilize the services provided in their plans.

Practices must consider strategies for ongoing renewal of plans, so they are not perceived as being limited to puppy/kitten visits. There is no reason why payment plans cannot be used in adults, or with standardized approaches to care.

Payment plans are not suitable for all clients. In many communities, there are still pet-owning families that have neither credit cards nor bank accounts, making them unsuitable participants in payment plans.

Payment plans are not a guarantee of profitability for a practice. If the practice has problems with customer service, communications skills, staff alignment, or administrative oversight, payment plans can contribute more problems than they will solve.

Abbreviation

ACH   Automated Clearing House

References

1 Volk, J.O., Felsted, K.E., Thomas, J.G. et al. (2011). Executive summary of the Bayer veterinary care usage study. *Journal of the American Veterinary Medical Association* 238: 1275–1282.

2 Gourville, J. and Soman, D. (2002). Pricing and the psychology of consumption. *Harvard Business Review* (September): 91–96.

3 Tumblin, D. Benchmarks 2019 – A Study of Well Managed Practices®. www.wmpb.vet

Recommended Reading

Ackerman, L. (2020). Payment (wellness) plans. In: *Five-Minute Veterinary Practice Management Consult*, 3e (ed. L. Ackerman), 548–549. Ames, IA: Wiley.

Boone, D. and Hauser, W. The Veterinarian's Guide to Healthy Pet Plans: How to Design, Implement and Measure Your Way to Preventive Care Plan Success. www.lulu.com/en/us/shop/wendy-hauser-dvm-and-debbie-boone-bs-ccs-cvpm/the-veterinarians-guide-to-healthy-pet-plans-how-to-design-implement-and-measure-your-way-to-preventive-care-plan-success/ebook/product-1e8m46w8.html

Partners for Healthy Pets. Monthly payment preventive healthcare plans. www.partnersforhealthypets.org/preventive_pet_healthcare.aspx

Salzsieder, K. What wellness plans can be for your veterinary practice. www.dvm360.com/view/what-wellness-plans-can-be-your-veterinary-practice

Tumblin, D. (2012). 8 mistakes to avoid in your wellness plans. *Veterinary Economics* 53 (10): 18–22.

10.18

Financing Veterinary Care

Lowell Ackerman, DVM, DACVD, MBA, MPA, CVA, MRCVS

Global Consultant, Author, and Lecturer, MA, USA

BASICS

10.18.1 Summary

Pet owners have a lot of options when it comes to paying veterinary invoices; most pay with credit cards, checks, or cash. There are also many clients who cannot afford to pay for their veterinary services this way, and so other mechanisms have become available to help clients in this regard. While similar to other forms of credit, veterinary-specific third-party financing allows clients to pay for services with a variety of other options.

10.18.2 Terms Defined

Accounts Receivable: Monies due to a company for goods sold or services rendered for which payment has not yet been received.

Economic Euthanasia: A situation in which euthanasia is selected principally on the basis of a pet owner's unwillingness or inability to pay for needed veterinary care.

MAIN CONCEPTS

10.18.3 Risk Management

It is important to help clients appreciate the potential healthcare costs for a pet over its entire lifespan (see 2.9 Anticipated Costs of Pet Care). When that is done properly, pet owners can then assess their potential options for being able to pay for those veterinary services.

The most common risk management strategies are pet health insurance (see 10.16 Pet Health Insurance) and payment and wellness plans (see 10.17 Payment and Wellness Plans).

Pet health insurance is a great mechanism for helping to pay for unanticipated expenses, such as the treatment of diseases, emergencies, and even referrals to specialists. Some pet health insurance policies will also cover more routine "wellness" care, either as part of the policy or on an add-on basis. The pet health insurance itself is pet specific and while coverage is based on the particular policy selected, it can be used at virtually any veterinary facility, not just with the primary care hospital at which the pet is being seen for routine care.

Payment plans, on the other hand, are typically arranged by a specific veterinary facility for a specific pet, and for a specific array of services. The coverage is typically for anticipated care, and allows pet owners to spread the costs of this anticipated care over periodic payments (usually monthly). Most payment plans established by veterinary hospitals are only applicable for services performed at that specific hospital (or affiliated hospitals).

For clients who don't necessarily have the financial wherewithal to pay for their veterinary care all at once with cash, check, or credit card, and whose veterinary bills might not be covered by pet health insurance or payment plans, other options have become available.

10.18.4 Options Available

Many pet owners do not plan ahead for healthcare issues, and also may find that they don't have access to sufficient funds to provide the care they would like for their pets (see 2.10 Affordability of Veterinary Services).

When pet owners are confronted with veterinary expenses they can't afford, they may turn to the veterinary hospital for solutions. In most cases, it is not an ideal situation for veterinarians to accept delayed payments, and in many clinics the number of clients that would avail themselves of such services would create accounts receivable issues (see 7.8 Providing Care for Those Unable or Unwilling to Pay).

Pet health insurance requires that pet owners have policies in place before care is needed, or such coverage is likely to be dismissed for "preexisting" conditions. Payment plans are simply a tool for pet owners to spread anticipated expenses over an established time interval. This leaves at least some clients with a need for a program that is flexible enough to be used with either anticipated or unanticipated pet care expenses, and be able to spread those costs predictably over an interval of time.

Veterinarians are not in the financing business and probably shouldn't be extending credit to clients, but there are several financial institutions that are ready to provide such veterinary-specific funding to our most credit-worthy clients.

Unfortunately, without such options, veterinarians would likely find themselves in even more predicaments where they have to make life-or-death decisions, not because there are no medical options but because clients cannot afford to pay for them, at least not up front or all at once (see 6.5 Opportunities and Challenges of Providing Services for Low-Income Families). Sometimes this results in the death of the pet as a financial alternative. This is sometimes referred to as "economic euthanasia" and serves the interest of neither the veterinary hospital nor the client.

10.18.4.1 Third-Party Financing

The goal of third-party financing is laudable – helping pet owners to be able to afford the care their pets need, and allowing veterinarians to focus on the delivery of excellent healthcare with minimal involvement in financing. There are a variety of third-party financing options, but most involve either credit cards, loans, or payment plans.

10.18.4.1.1 Veterinary-Specific Credit Cards
Private-label credit cards are available through several different financial institutions (such as CareCredit, Wells Fargo and Citibank in the US) and pet owners may be aware of them because they are also used for financing different human healthcare needs (such as dentistry, chiropractic, and vision care).

Veterinary-specific credit cards can be used at different locations, but only for veterinary expenses, and only at providers that are part of the company's network. These credit cards typically provide a revolving line of credit that can be used to pay for veterinary services within the company's network of enrolled providers.

Veterinary hospitals accepting such credit cards typically pay an administrative fee to be part of the network, as well as merchant fees on the credit card purchases. Each company has its own financing options, but most provide no-interest (for the pet owner) loans if the debt is paid in full within the established payback period, and fixed monthly payments at established interest rates for longer periods.

In most instances, credit approval is quick for credit-worthy clients and can be accomplished online, by app, or by telephone in real time. Once the application has been approved, the cardholder can use the card for purchases at veterinary clinics up to the approved limit. The approval rate for such cards may be higher than for typical credit cards, but credit-worthiness of the client is the major determinant.

When a client has been approved and uses such a card, the veterinary hospital typically receives its payment within a few days, less the administrative fees. With most of these programs, the financial relationship is between the financing company and the cardholder, so veterinarians get paid even if the client defaults.

The benefit to veterinary hospitals is that it allows credit-worthy clients who might not have the ability to pay for all needed services at once to pay for them over time through an independent financing option.

10.18.4.1.2 Loans and Payment Plans
Other options for third-party financing include loans and payment plans. There are now several companies established to provide loans and payment plans for pet owners, including Medical Financing (http://medicalfinancing.com), First Look (http://firstlookapproval.com), ClearGage (http://cleargage.com), LoanHero (http://loanhero.com), PetLoans (http://petloans.com), Prosper (http://prosper.com), Scratch (http://scratchpay.com), Varidi (http://varidi.com), VetBilling (http://VetBilling.com) and Veterinary CreditPlans (http://extendcredit.com/veterinary). There is often considerable flux within the industry, with companies entering and exiting the marketplace, and names changing with corporate mergers and acquisitions.

Payment terms vary significantly depending on the credit-worthiness of the pet owner. Some require automatic withdrawal for client's bank accounts, and most of the processing and administrative fees are paid by the borrower. Sometimes hospitals are required to pay a fee with each transaction but in most instances, there are no start-up or subscription fees. Payment to the practice typically occurs as soon as the service is rendered.

10.18.4.2 Other Veterinary Assistance Programs

There is now a plethora of financing options available to clients that are only bounded by a pet owner's imagination.

There are a variety of crowdfunding platforms where pet owners can appeal to others for for-profit funding, the largest of which to date is GoFundMe (http://gofundme.com). However, there are many others including PlumFund (http://Plumfund.com), Waggle (http://waggle.org), and YouCaring (http://youcaring.com). Expect this marketplace to continue evolving, and it is necessary to verify the integrity of such lending platforms.

Assistance for pet owners is also available through a variety of programs including the Pet Fund (http://petfund.com), Humane Society of the United States (http://humansociety.org), American Society for the Prevention of Cruelty to Animals (http://aspca.org), and Feline Veterinary Emergency Assistance (http://fveap.org). Programs are also available that function solely on a local level (e.g., http://face4pets.org), so it is worthwhile doing an extensive search to uncover resources that may be applicable.

There are also a variety of charitable organizations that provide financial assistance on a breed-specific basis. Examples include LabMed (http://labmed.org) for Labrador retrievers, and WestieMed (http://westiemed.org) for West Highland white terriers.

In some instances, it might even be possible for veterinary hospitals to create a not-for-profit foundation to benefit clients who are unable to afford needed care.

TAKE-AWAYS

- Third-party financing can be very useful for pet care not covered by pet health insurance or clinic payment plans.
- The most common financing options include credit cards, loans, and payment plans.
- Third-party financing is most appropriate for clients who are deemed credit-worthy.
- Most veterinary practices are not in a position to extend credit to the number of clients who are unprepared or unable to pay for veterinary services.
- Third-party financing is just one strategy for helping clients deal with the costs of veterinary care and discussions regarding costs should ideally happen before such care is needed.

MISCELLANEOUS

10.18.5 Cautions

While there are many financing options available for pet owners, it is unlikely that solutions exist for every potential situation.

There is a difference between clients who don't have the means to afford needed care for their pets, and those who have the means but choose not to prioritize the needs of their pet over other expenditures. However, both cases can prove difficult for veterinary hospitals, since there is still a pet in need of care. In many cases, hospitals need to provide tiered services that will be able to address pet needs, even if not in an optimal fashion (see 2.2 The Role of Incremental Care, and 10.14 Providing Cost-Effective Care for Those in Need). This is sometimes discussed in terms of a spectrum of care

If a veterinary financing company deems your client not to be credit-worthy, believe them, and fight the temptation to be the lender of last resort. This is not a sustainable approach to providing such care.

The best way to address the situation proactively is to address financing needs early with clients, even at puppy and kitten visits, and encourage the owner to plan ahead, if at all possible. It's also better if the practice has a plan in place for how to best accommodate clients with spending limitations (see 6.5 Opportunities and Challenges of Providing Services for Low-Income Families).

Open book management can be enlightening for the hospital team to help with the realization that individual veterinary hospitals are not in the position of being able to routinely finance veterinary care for clients (see 7.2 Managing the Pet-Specific Workplace).

There is no doubt that having discussions about finances is not easy, especially when it involves the life of someone's beloved pet (see 5.11 Discussing Finances for Pet-Specific Care).

Realize the stress that comes from having to provide alternatives to an established standard of care (see 8.17 Dealing with Compromise Fatigue).

Avoid the temptation to extend credit to clients unless you are prepared to research how such a process can be done legally, while protecting the financial security of clients. If considering doing so, develop a credit application and have it reviewed by an attorney, and learn what recourse you might have if the client defaults on the debt.

Recommended Reading

Ackerman, L. (2020). Third-party financing. In: *Five-Minute Veterinary Practice Management Consult*, 3e (ed. L. Ackerman), 550–551. Ames, IA: Wiley.

Boss, N. (1999). *Educating Your Clients From A to Z: What to Say and How to Say It*. Lakewood, CO: AAHA Press.

Heinke, M.L. and McCarthy, J.B. (2012). *Practice Makes Perfect: A Guide to Veterinary Practice Management*, 2e. Lakewood, CO: AAHA Press.

Wilson, J.F. (1988). *Law and Ethics of the Veterinary Profession*. Yardley, PA: Priority Press.

Section 11

Appendices

11.1

Finding More Information on Pet-Specific Care Topics

Lowell Ackerman, DVM, DACVD, MBA, MPA, CVA, MRCVS

Global Consultant, Author, and Lecturer, MA, USA

Additional Book Resources

Ackerman, L. *The Genetic Connection*, 2. AAHAPress, Lakewood, CO, 2011

Ackerman, L. *Five-Minute Veterinary Practice Management Consult*, 3, Wiley Publishing, Ames, IA, 2020

Ackerman, L. *Proactive Pet Parenting: Anticipating pet health problems before they happen.* Problem Free Publishing, 2020.

Ackerman, L. *Problem Free Pets: The ultimate guide to pet parenting.* Problem Free Publishing (Dermvet), 2020.

Bell, J; Cavanagh, K; Tilley, L; Smith, F. *Veterinary Medical Guide to Dog and Cat Breeds.* Teton NewMedia, Jackson, WY, 2012.

Berndt, ER; Goldman, DP. *Economic Dimensions of Personalized and Precision Medicine.* University of Chicago Press, Chicago, IL, 2019.

Boss, N: *How We Do Things Here: Developing and Teaching Office-Wide Protocols.* AAHAPress, Lakewood, CO, 2008.

Boss, N. *Educating Your Clients From A to Z*, 2. AAHA Press, Lakewood, CO, 2011

Carini, C; Fidock, M; van Gool, A: *Handbook of Biomarkers and Precision Medicine.* Chapman and Hall/CRC, Boca Raton, FL, 2019.

Clark, R. *Medical, Genetic and Behavioral Aspects of Purebred Cats.* Forum Publications, Alresford, UK, 1992

Clark, R; Stainer, JR. *Medical and Genetic Aspects of Purebred Dogs*, 2. Forum Publications, Alresford, UK, 1994

Clinician's Brief. Algorithms to Guide Your Diagnosis and Treatment. www.cliniciansbrief.com/algorithms

Cote, E. *Differential Diagnosis of the Dog and Cat. An Excerpt from Clinical Veterinary Advisor*, 3, Elsevier, St Louis, MO, 2015

Cullis, P. *The Personalized Medicine Revolution: How Diagnosing and Treating Disease Are About to Change Forever.* Greystone Books, Vancouver, Canada, 2015

Englar, RE: *Common Clinical Presentations in Dogs and Cats.* Wiley Blackwell, Ames, IA, 2019.

Englar, R.E. *A Guide to Oral Communication in Veterinary Medicine.* 5M Publishing, 2020.

Gerber, M. E. and Weinstein, P. *The E-Myth Veterinarian: Why Most Veterinary Practices Don't Work and What to Do About It.* Michael E. Gerber Companies, Carlsbad, CA, 2015.

Gladwell, M. *The Tipping Point: How Little Things Can Make a Big Difference.* Back Bay Books, New York, 2002

Gough, A; Murphy, K: *Differential Diagnoses in Small Animal Medicine*, 2, Wiley Blackwell, Ames, IA, 2015

Gough, A; Thomas, A; O'Neill, D. *Breed Predispositions to Disease in Dogs and Cats*, 3. Wiley Blackwell, Ames, IA, 2018.

Hays, P. *Advancing Healthcare Through Personalized Medicine.* CRC Press, Boca Raton, FL, 2017.

McKenzie, BA. *Placebos for Pets? The Truth About Alternative Medicine in Animals.* Newmachar, UK: Ockham Publishing; 2019.

Nicholas, FW. *Introduction to Veterinary Genetics*, 3, Wiley Blackwell, Ames, IA, 2010.

Ostrander, EA; Giger, U; K Lindblad-Toh (eds). *The Dog and its Genome.* Cold Spring Harbor Laboratory Press, Cold Spring Harbor, NY, 2006.

Padgett, GA. *Control of Canine Genetic Diseases.* Howell Book House, Nashville, TN, 1998.

Parker, K: *A Practical Guide to Managing Employee Performance in Veterinary Practices.* AAHAPress, Lakewood, CO, 2017.

Pothier, KC. *Personalizing Precision Medicine. A Global Voyage From Vision to Reality.* Wiley, Ames, IA, 2017.

Prainsack, B: *Personalized Medicine: Empowered Patients in the 21st Century?* NYU Press, New York, 2017

Prendergast, H. *Front Office Management for the Veterinary Team*, 3. Elsevier, St Louis, MO, 2019

Silverman, J., Kurtz, S., Draper, J. *Skills for Communicating with Patients*, 2. Radcliffe Publishing, Oxford, UK, 2005

Snyder, M: *Genomics and Personalized Medicine: What Everyone Needs to Know*. Oxford University Press, Oxford, UK, 2016

Thompson, MS: *Small Animal Medical Differential Diagnosis*, 2, Elsevier, St Louis, MO, 2014.

Topol, E: *Deep Medicine: How Artificial Intelligence Can Make Healthcare Human Again*. Basic Books, New York, 2019

Vella, CM; Shelton, LM; McGonagle, JJ; Stanglen, TW. *Robinson's Genetics for Cat Breeders & Veterinarians*, 4. Butterworth-Heinemann, London, 1999

Willis, MB. *Practical Genetics for Dog Breeders*. Howell Book House, Nashville, TN, 1992.

Website Resources

Organization	Website
American Animal Hospital Association (AAHA)	www.aahanet.org
American Association of Feline Practitioners (AAFP)	www.catvets.com
American Kennel Club Canine Health Foundation	www.akcchf.org
American Veterinary Medical Association (AVMA)	www.avma.org
American Association of Animal Poison Control	www.aapcc.org
ASPCA Animal Poison Control Center	www.aspca.org/apcc
Best BETs for Vets	http://bestbetsforvets.org
British Veterinary Association Health Schemes	www.bva.co.uk/chs
Canine Health Information Center (CHIC)	www.ofa.org/about/chic-program
Canine Inherited Disorders Database	https://cidd.discoveryspace.ca/
CATalyst Council	www.catalystcouncil.org
Cat Friendly Clinic	https://catfriendlyclinic.org
Cat Friendly Practice	https://catvets.com/cfp/cfp
Cat Healthy	www.cathealthy.ca
Centers for Disease Control	www.cdc.gov
Companion Animal Parasite Council	www.capcvet.org
Dog Breed Health	www.dogbreedhealth.com
DVM 360	www.dvm360.com
Fear Free Pets	www.fearfreepets.com
Food and Drug Administration (FDA)	www.fda.gov
FDA Center for Veterinary Medicine	www.fda.gov/drugs
FEMA Disaster Assistance	www.fema.gov
Genetics Home Reference (NIH)	https://ghr.nlm.nih.gov
Indoor Pet Initiative	https://indoorpet.osu.edu
International Cat Care	https://icatcare.org
International Collaboration on Dog Health & Welfare	https://dogwellnet.com
Medline Plus	www.medlineplus.gov
National Pesticide Information Center	www.npic.orst.edu
North American Pet Health Insurance Association	www.naphia.org
One Health Certificate Course (WSAVA)	Jav.ma/onehealth
Online Mendelian Inheritance in Animals	http://omia.org
Orthopedic Foundation for Animals	www.ofa.org
Partners for Healthy Pets	www.partnersforhealthypets.org
PennGen Genetic Testing Directory	http://bit.ly/2YWXBsc
Personalized Medicine Coalition	www.personalizedmedicinecoalition.org
Pet-Specific Care	www.petspecificcare.com

Organization	Website
Problem Free Pets	www.problemfreepets.com
Pet Health Partnership	www.pethealthpartnership.org
Universities Federation for Animal Welfare	www.ufaw.org.uk
USDA APHIS Emergency Operations	www.aphis.usda.gov/emergencyresponse
USDA Center for Veterinary Biologics	http://Bit.ly/VetBiologics
VeNom Coding	http://venomcoding.org
Veterinary Support Personnel Network	www.vspn.org
Veterinary Information Network (VIN)	www.vin.com
Veterinary Virtual Care Association	www.vvca.org
Winn Feline Foundation	www.winnfelinefoundation.org
World Small Animal Veterinary Association	www.wsava.org

Pet Information and Images

Organization	Website
American Cat Fancier's Association	www.acfacat.com
American Kennel Club (AKC)	www.akc.org
AKC clubs	https://webapps.akc.org/club-search#/
AKC Rescue	www.akc.org/dog-breeds/rescue-network/contacts
American Rare Breed Association	www.arba.org
Australian National Kennel Council	http://ankc.org.au
Canadian Cat Association	www.cca-afc.com
Canadian Kennel Club	www.ckc.ca
Cat Fancier's Association	www.cfa.org
Cat Time	www.cattime.com
Continental Kennel Club	https://ckcusa.com
Dog Time	www.dogtime.com
Fédération Cynologique Internationale	www.fci.be
Fédération Internationale Féline	www.fifeweb.org
French Kennel Club	www.scc.asso.fr
	www.chiens-online.com
German Kennel Club	www.vdh.de/ueber-den-vdh/wir-ueber-uns
Kennel Union of South Africa	www.kusa.co.za
Swedish Kennel Club	www.skk.se/en
The International Cat Association	www.tica.org
The Kennel Club	www.thekennelclub.org.uk/
United Kennel Club	www.ukcdogs.com

11.2

Abbreviations

Lowell Ackerman, DVM, DACVD, MBA, MPA, CVA, MRCVS

Global Consultant, Author, and Lecturer, MA, USA

AAFCO	Association of American Feed Control Officials	aPTT	Activated Partial Thromboplastin Time
AAFP	American Association of Feline Practitioners	ARVC	Arrhythmogenic Right Ventricular Cardiomyopathy
AAHA	American Animal Hospital Association	ASA	American Society of Anesthesiologists
AAVMC	Association of American Veterinary Medical Colleges	ASPCA	American Society for the Prevention of Cruelty to Animals
AAVSB	American Association of Veterinary State Boards	AST	Aspartate Aminotransferase
		ATC	Average Transaction Charge
ABCD	Advisory Board on Cat Diseases	ATP	Adenosine Triphosphate
ACCT	American Car-Chasing Terrier	AU	Auris Utraque (Both Ears)
ACH	Automated Clearing House	AUC	Area Under The Curve
ACL	Anterior Cruciate Ligament	AV	Atrioventricular
ACTH	Adrenocorticotrophic Hormone	AVMA	American Veterinary Medical Association
ACVAA	American College of Veterinary Anesthesia And Analgesia	BCS	Body Condition Score
		BF	Body Fat
ACVD	American College of Veterinary Dermatology	BG	Blood Glucose
		BGC	Blood Glucose Curve
ACVECC	American College of Veterinary Emergency and Critical Care	BHB	Beta-Hydroxybutyrate
		BLS	(United States) Bureau of Labor Statistics
ACVIM	American College of Veterinary Internal Medicine	BMR	Basal Metabolism Rate
		BP	Blood Pressure
ADE	Adverse Drug Event	BPH	Benign Prostatic Hypertrophy
ADL	Activities of Daily Living	BUN	Blood Urea Nitrogen (Urea)
ADR	Adverse Drug Reaction	BW	Body Weight
AHS	American Heartworm Society	C/T	Click And Treat
AKC	American Kennel Club	CAD	Canine Atopic Dermatitis
AKC CHF	American Kennel Club Canine Health Foundation	CAPC	Companion Animal Parasite Council
		CAV	Canine Adenovirus-2
AKI	Acute Kidney Injury	CBA	Cost–Benefit Analysis
AL	Attachment Loss	CBC	Complete Blood Count
ALD	Angular Limb Deformities	CBD	Cannabidiol
ALP	Alkaline Phosphatase	CBPI	Canine Brief Pain Inventory
ALT	Alanine Aminotransferase	CCC	Classical Counterconditioning
API	Application Programming Interface	CCF	Complicated Crown Fracture (Exposed Canal)

CCLR	Cranial Cruciate Ligament Rupture		DOI	Duration of Immunity
CCU	Critical Care Unit		DRA	Differential Reinforcement of an
CD	Compulsive Disorder			Alternative Behavior
CDS	Cognitive Decline Syndrome		DRI	Differential Reinforcement of an
CDV	Canine Distemper Virus			Incompatible Behavior
CE	Continuing Education		DS	Desensitization
CHF	Congestive Heart Failure		DSH	Domestic Shorthair
CI	Calculus Index		DSHEA	Dietary Supplement Health and Education
CIV	Canine Influenza Virus (Any Strain)			Act
CKD	Chronic Kidney Disease		DVM	Doctor of Veterinary Medicine
CLSI	Clinical and Laboratory Standards Institute		EAP	Emergency Action Plan
CMI	Clinical Metrology Instruments		EBM	Evidence-Based Medicine
CNS	Central Nervous System		EBV	Estimated Breeding Value
CO	Cardiac Output		EBVM	Evidence-Based Veterinary Medicine
COAST	Canine Osteoarthritis Staging Tool		ECG	Electrocardiogram
COGS	Cost of Goods Sold		ECI	Emotional Competency Inventory
COPS	Cost of Professional Services		ECPA	Electronics Communications Privacy Act
COX	Cyclooxygenase		ECVAA	European College of Veterinary
CPD	Continuing Professional Development			Anaesthesia and Analgesia
CPE	Continuing Professional Education		ED	Elbow Dysplasia
CPG	Clinical Practice Guidelines		EFT	Electronic Funds Transfer
CPV	Canine Parvovirus		EHR	Electronic Health Record
CQI	Continuous Quality Improvement		EI	Emotional Intelligence
CREAPI	Crepitance, Range of Motion, Effusion,		EIA	Emotional Intelligence Appraisal
	Asymmetry, Pain, Instability		EIC	Exercise-Induced Collapse
CRI	Constant Rate Infusion		ELDU	Extralabel Drug Use
CRM	Customer (Client) Relationship		EMR	Electronic Medical Record
	Management		EOL	End of Life
CSF	Cerebrospinal Fluid		EPA	Eicosapentaenoic Acid
CSOM	Client-Specific Outcome Measure		EPA	Environmental Protection Agency
CSR	Customer (Client) Service Representative		EPI	Exocrine Pancreatic Insufficiency
CT	Computed Tomography		EQ	Emotional Intelligence
CTA	Call to Action		EQ	Emotional Quotient
CTR	Click-Through Rate		ER	Emergency Room
CVC	Central Venous Catheter		ERG	Electroretinogram
CVM	Center For Veterinary Medicine (at the		ESCCAP	European Scientific Counsel Companion
	FDA)			Animal Parasites
DA2PP	Distemper, Adenovirus Type 2,		ESCI	Emotional and Social Competency Inventory
	Parainfluenza, Parvovirus		$ETCO_2$	End-Tidal Carbon Dioxide
DCM	Dilated Cardiomyopathy		ETS	Environmental Tobacco Smoke
DER	Daily Energy Requirement		FAQ	Frequently Asked Questions
DHA	Docosahexaenoic Acid		FAS	Fear, Anxiety, Stress
DICOM	Digital Imaging and Communications in		FB	Foreign Body
	Medicine		FCV	Feline Calicivirus
DISHAA	Disorientation, Interactions, Sleep–Wake		FDA	(United States) Food And Drug
	Cycles, Housetraining, Anxiety, Activity			Administration
DIVAS	Dynamic Interactive Visual Analogue Scale		FE	Furcation Exposure
DIY	Do It Yourself		FECAVA	Federation of European Companion
DJD	Degenerative Joint Disease			Animal Veterinary Associations
DKA	Diabetic Ketoacidosis		FeLV	Feline Leukemia Virus
DM	Diabetes Mellitus		FEMA	Federal Emergency Management
DNA	Deoxyribonucleic Acid			Administration

FFDCA	Federal Food, Drug, and Cosmetic Act		ICP	Infection Control Program
FHV	Feline Herpesvirus		ICS	Incident Command System
FIC	Feline Interstitial Cystitis		ICU	Intensive Care Unit
FISS	Feline Injection Site Sarcoma		ID	Identification
FIV	Feline Immunodeficiency Virus		IDP	Individual Development Plan
FNA	Fine Needle Aspirate		IGTV	Instagram TV
FORL	Feline Odontoclastic Resorptive Lesion		IM	Intramuscular
FPV	Feline Panleukopenia Virus		IOP	Intraocular Pressure
FSH	Follicle-Stimulating Hormone		IOT	Internet of Things
FT	Full Time		IPS	Intestinal Parasite Screen
fT4	Free Thyroxine Level		IQ	Intelligence Quotient
FTE	Full-Time Equivalent		IRIS	International Renal Interest Society
FVRCP	Feline Viral Rhinotracheitis, Calicivirus, and Panleukopenia		ISCAID	International Society for Companion Animal Infectious Diseases
GDV	Gastric Dilation/Volvulus		ISFM	International Society of Feline Medicine
GE	Gingival Enlargement		IT	Information Technology
GGT	Gamma-Glutamyl Transferase		IUD	Intrauterine Device
GI	Gastrointestinal		IV	Intravenous
GI	Gingivitis Index		IVDD	Intervertebral Disk Disease
GN	Glomerulonephropathy		JAVMA	Journal of the American Veterinary Medical Association
GnRH	Gonadotropin-Releasing Hormone			
GP	General Practitioner		JIT	Just in Time (Inventory)
GPO	Group Purchasing Organization		KCS	Keratoconjunctivitis Sicca
GR	Gingival Recession		KPI	Key Performance Indicator
GRAS	Generally Recognized As Safe		LBM	Lean Body Mass
GVP	Gingivoplasty		LH	Luteinizing Hormone
GWAS	Genome-Wide Association Studies		LOAD	Liverpool Osteoarthritis in Dogs
H_2O	Water		LP	Luxating Patella
HAB	Human–Animal Bond		LRT	Lower Respiratory Tract
HAI	Hospital-Acquired Infection		LTV	Lifetime Value
Hb	Hemoglobin		M	Mobility, Tooth (M0–3)
HCM	Hypertrophic Cardiomyopathy		MA	Megestrol Acetate
Hct	Hematocrit		Mab	Monoclonal Antibody
HD	Hip Dysplasia		MAP	Mean Arterial Pressure
HHS	US Department of Health and Human Services		MBTI	Myers-Briggs Type Indicator
			MCS	Muscle Condition Score
HIPAA	Health Insurance Portability and Accountability Act 1996 (HIPAA)		MCT	Mast Cell Tumor
			MD	Medical Director
HIV	Human Immunodeficiency Virus		MD	Medical Doctor
HK	High Potassium		MDR	Multidrug Resistance
HMP	Human Microbiome Project		MDT	Multidisciplinary Team
HPC	Hospice and Palliative Care		MIC	Minimum Inhibitory Concentration
HRA	Health Risk Assessment		MLV	Modified Live Virus
IA	Intraarticular		mmHg	Millimeters of Mercury (Pressure)
IAAHPC	International Association for Animal Hospice and Palliative Care		MPA	Medroxyprogesterone Acetate
			MRI	Magnetic Resonance Imaging
IASP	International Association for the Study of Pain		mRNA	Messenger Ribonucleic Acid
			MSCEIT	Mayer-Salovey-Caruso Emotional Intelligence Test
IBD	Inflammatory Bowel Disease			
ICADA	International Committee on Allergic Diseases of Animals		MSDS	Material Safety Data Sheet
			MVD	Mitral Valve Disease
ICC	International Cat Care		Na/K	Sodium/Potassium

NADA	New Animal Drug Application		POS	Point of Service
NASC	National Animal Supplement Council		PP	Periodontal Pocket
NGF	Nerve Growth Factor		PP	Polyphagia
NIH	National Institutes of Health		PPE	Personal Protective Equipment
NMDA	N-Methyl-D-Aspartate		PR	Public Relations
NPH	Neutral Protamine Hagedorn		PRA	Progressive Retinal Atrophy
NPS	Net Promoter Score		PRA	Prostaglandin Receptor Antagonist
NRC	National Research Council		PRN	*Pro Re Nata* (Latin for "As Needed")
NSAID	Nonsteroidal Antiinflammatory Drug		ProBNP	Pro B-Type Natriuretic Peptide
NSF	Nonsufficient Funds		PSA	Prostate-Specific Antigen
NT-proBNP	N-Terminal Pro B-Type Natriuretic Peptide		PSC	Pet-Specific Care
OA	Osteoarthritis		PSGAG	Polysulfated Glycosaminoglycan
OCC	Operant Counterconditioning		psi	Pounds Per Square Inch
OCD	Obsessive Compulsive Disorder		PU	Polyuria
OFA	Orthopedic Foundation For Animals		PU/PD	Polyuria/Polydypsia
OM	Oral Mass		PVME	Principles of Veterinary Medical Ethics
ONF	Oronasal Fistula		PVP	Previsit Pharmaceuticals
ORF	Open Reading Frame		PVQ	Previsit Questionnaire
OSA	Osteosarcoma		PZI	Protamine Zinc Insulin
OSHA	Occupational Safety and Health Administration		QA	Quality Assurance
			QC	Quality Control
OTC	Over The Counter (Medications That Do Not Require a Prescription)		QoL	Quality of Life
			RBC	Red Blood Cell
OVE	Ovariectomy		RCT	Randomized Controlled Trial
OVH	Ovariohysterectomy		rDVM	Referring Veterinarian
PA	Performance Appraisal		RE	(Dental) Root Exposure
PACS	Picture Archiving and Communications System		RER	Resting Energy Requirement
			RI	Reference Interval
PAE	Postantibiotic Effect		RMR	Resting Metabolic Rate
PCI	Payment Card Industry (Data Security Standard)		RMW	Regulated Medical Waste
			RNA	Ribonucleic Acid
PCR	Polymerase Chain Reaction		RNAi	Ribonucleic Acid Interference
PD	Periodontal Disease		ROI	Return on Investment
PD	Pharmacodynamics		ROM	Range of Motion
PD	Polydipsia		RP/C	Root Planing, Closed
PDI	Periodontal Disease Index (1–4)		RP/O	Root Planing, Open
PDL	Periodontal Ligament		RV	Rabies Virus
PE	Physical Examination		RVN	Registered Veterinary Nurse
PHI	Pet Health Insurance		SA	Sinoatrial
PI	Plaque Index		SBP	Systolic Blood Pressure
PII	Personally Identifiable Information		SCC	Squamous Cell Carcinoma
PIMS	Pet Information Management System		SD	Standard Deviation
PIMS	Practice Information Management Software		SDMA	Symmetric Dimethylarginine
			SDS	Safety Data Sheet
PK	Pharmacokinetics		SEM	Search Engine Marketing
PKD	Polycystic Kidney Disease		SEO	Search Engine Optimization
PLIT	Professional Liability Insurance Trust		SMART	Specific, Measured, Achievable, Realistic, and Timed
PM	Practice Manager			
PMAD	Pain-Modifying Analgesic Drug		SMS	Short Message Service
PMed	Precision/Personalized Medicine		SNOMED	Systematized Nomenclature of Medicine
PMS	Practice Management System/Software		SNP	Single Nucleotide Polymorphism
PO	Per Os (Oral)		SOAP	Subjective/Objective/Assessment/Plan

SOC	Standard of Care	UPC	Urine Protein/Creatinine
SOP	Standard Operating Procedures	URT	Upper Respiratory Tract
SpO$_2$	Oxygen Saturation as Measured by Pulse Oximeter	USDA	United States Department of Agriculture
		USP	Unique Selling Point
SSRI	Selective Serotonin Reuptake Inhibitor	UTI	Urinary Tract Infection
STS	Secondary Traumatic Stress	UX	User Experience
STT	Schirmer Tear Test	VBM	Veterinary Behavioral Medicine
SUEIT	Swinburne University Emotional Intelligence Test	VCPR	Veterinarian–Client–Patient Relationship
		VHT	Veterinary Healthcare Team
SWOT	Strengths, Weaknesses, Opportunities, Threats	VNI	Veterinary Nurse Initiative
		VOHC	Veterinary Oral Health Council
T4	Thyroxine	VPC	Ventricular Premature Contraction
TA	Trade Area	VTE	Veterinary Time Equivalent
TCC	Transitional Cell Carcinoma	VTM	Veterinary Team Member
TEIQue	Trait Emotional Intelligence Questionnaire	VTS	Veterinary Technician Specialist
T/FX	Fractured Tooth	VUCA	Volatile, Uncertain, Complex, and Ambiguous
TLI	Trypsin-Like Immunoreactivity		
TOD	Target Organ Damage	vWD	Von Willebrand Disease
TP	Total Protein	vWF	Von Willebrand Factor
TPMT	Thiopurine Methyltransferase	WAVD	World Association for Veterinary Dermatology
TPR	Temperature, Pulse, and Respiration		
TPR	Total Peripheral Resistance	WBC	White Blood Cell (Total Leukocyte Count)
TQM	Total Quality Management	WGS	Whole-Genome Sequencing
TR	Tooth Resorption	WHO	World Health Organization
tT4	Total Thyroxine Level	WNL	Within Normal Limits
UA	Urinalysis	WOM	Word of Mouth
UCF	Uncomplicated (Dental) Crown Fracture	WSAVA	World Small Animal Veterinary Association
UI	User Interface	X	(Tooth) Extract

11.3

Heritable Health Conditions – By Disease

Lowell Ackerman, DVM, DACVD, MBA, MPA, CVA, MRCVS

Global Consultant, Author, and Lecturer, MA, USA

The following are just some of the conditions recognized in purebred dogs and cats that are thought to have a heritable component. The goal here is not to list all potential disorders, nor all the breeds that might be affected by them, but to provide a very brief synopsis of what the conditions are, and some of the breeds that have been recognized with the disorders. The breeds listed are just a sampling, and more breed-specific listings can be found elsewhere (see 11.4 Heritable Health Conditions – By Breed). Also, affected breeds are listed in alphabetical order, not in order of prevalence, since risk can differ on a geographic basis.

It is important to realize that many of the conditions listed represent groups of disorders and even conditions with the same name may be associated with different genetic variants and modes of inheritance.

Even with these cautions, it is worthwhile to have access to this type of information, since genotyping has allowed many "new" disorders to be better characterized, so even a brief introduction can be a welcome start to the process.

Acanthosis Nigricans

Description: A poorly understood condition in dogs in which the skin becomes blackened, specifically in the axillary and groin areas. It may represent a breed tendency to hyperpigmentation in inflamed skin rather than a distinct entity.

Breeds: Dachshund

Accessory Pathway Arrhythmias

Description: Abnormal cardiac muscle fibers that can cause the heart to contract, independent of the atrioventricular node. This can lead to arrhythmias such as Wolff–Parkinson–White syndrome. A mode of inheritance has not been determined, but breed predisposition has been recognized.

Breeds: Labrador retriever

Achromatopsia

Description: Also known as cone degeneration and hemeralopia, this is a cause of day blindness in dogs. This is an inherited trait characterized by degeneration of the cones in the retina. The condition does not progress to complete blindness because the rods remain unaffected. In most breeds the inheritance is believed to be autosomal recessive. Several genetic mutations have been characterized, and DNA testing is available for some of those breed-specific variants.

Breeds: Alaskan malamute, (miniature) American shepherd, Australian cattle dog, Australian shepherd, dachshund, German shepherd dog, German short-haired pointer, Great Dane, Labrador retriever, (miniature) poodle, (standard) poodle, Siberian husky

Acne

Description: A dermatologic condition in which there is a deep inflammatory reaction around the hair follicles on the chin and adjacent areas. It is not necessarily heritable, but breed predisposition has been recognized.

Breeds: Boxer, Doberman pinscher, English bulldog, Great Dane, pug, Rottweiler; Domestic shorthair, Persian

Acquired Aurotrichia

Description: Also known as gilding syndrome, this is a condition in which the color of the coat changes from normal to gold, especially along the topline. Most dogs are 2–3 years of age when the condition is first detected.

Breeds: 🐕 **Miniature schnauzer**

Acral Lick Dermatitis

Description: Also known as lick granuloma, this is a disorder in which dogs continue to lick at their limbs, abrading the skin and creating ulcers and raw, weeping areas. Once thought to be caused by boredom, more contemporary views suggest a disorder of sensory nerves or a compulsive disorder.

Breeds: 🐕 **Doberman pinscher, German shepherd dog, golden retriever, Great Dane, Irish setter, Labrador retriever**

Acral Mutilation Syndrome

Description: A bizarre sensory neuropathy, part of the hereditary sensory autonomic neuropathies (HSANs), in which animals lose pain sensation in their toes and chew at their feet and do extensive damage and even mutilation. It results from an autosomal recessive mutation of the GDNF gene, and DNA testing is available for some variants. A similar condition has been reported in Czechoslovakian shorthaired pointers.

Breeds: 🐕 **(English) cocker spaniel, English pointer, English springer spaniel, French spaniel, German shorthaired pointer**

Acute Respiratory Distress Syndrome

Description: An autosomal recessive disorder of the ANLN gene that then eventuates in fibrotic and metaplastic changes in the lungs. The condition can be exacerbated by other environmental factors such as infection. DNA testing is available.

Breeds: 🐕 **Dalmatian**

Adrenal Sex Hormone Imbalance

Description: Sometimes called alopecia X, it has been reported as a familial dermatosis in several breeds.

Abnormal adrenal steroidogenesis may result in adrenocortical hyperprogestinism and hyperandrogenism.

Breeds: 🐕 **Chow chow, keeshond, Pomeranian, poodle, Samoyed**

Aggression (Periodic)

Description: A breed-specific condition in which aggression appears periodically, with or without seizures. It is believed to be inherited as a co-dominant trait, and is highly associated with certain genetic markers.

Breeds: 🐕 **Belgian Malinois**

Aggression (Rage Syndrome)

Description: A form of dominance aggression that seems to be familial and is extremely dangerous. These cases have been likened to episodic dyscontrol, a form of epilepsy.

Breeds: 🐕 **English springer spaniel**

Alanine Aminotransferase (ALT) Activity

Description: ALT is an enzyme used to assess liver function. Some dogs tend to have lower levels of the enzyme, yet typically within normal range. This seems to be characterized by a mutation in the GPT gene, and affected dogs might have low ALT levels even in the face of active liver disease. Genetic testing is available, but breed validation and clinical significance have not yet been conclusively demonstrated.

Alaskan Husky Encephalopathy

Description: A rare neurodegenerative encephalopathy, associated with a mutation in the SLC19A3 gene and transmitted as an autosomal recessive trait. DNA testing is available.

Breeds: 🐕 **Alaskan husky**

Albinism, Oculocutaneous

Description: An inherited disorder of melanin biosynthesis, caused by breed-specific autosomal recessive mutations primarily affecting the SLC45A2 and OCA2 genes. Most of the hypopigmentation is limited to the skin and irises; most affected dogs are not deaf. DNA testing is available for some breed-specific variants.

Breeds: 🐕 **Doberman pinscher; German spitz, Great Dane, Leonberger, Lhasa apso,, Pekingese, Pomeranian; Rottweiler;** 🐈 **Siamese**

Albinism, Waardenburg Syndrome

Description: True albinism is rare in dogs and is inherited as an autosomal recessive trait. These conditions may be associated with neurological or ocular problems. Waardenburg syndrome is associated with deafness, white coat, and blue or heterochromia iridis. Albinos have melanocytes, but lack the tyrosinase necessary to synthesize melanin. In cats, the condition is associated with the white (W) color gene, but not necessarily with breed predispositions.

Breeds (Waardenburg): 🐕 **Bull terrier, collie, Dalmatian, Great Dane, Sealyham terrier**

Alexander Disease

Description: A rare hereditary neurodegenerative disorder resulting in astrocyte dysfunction and neurological compromise. In the Labrador retriever it results from an autosomal dominant mutation in the GFAP gene, and DNA testing is available.

Breeds: 🐕 **Bernese mountain dog, Chihuahua, Labrador retriever, miniature poodle, Scottish terrier**

Amaurotic Idiocy

Description: Also known as lipoidystrophy, this is an inborn error of metabolism in which defective enzymes lead to accumulation of abnormal amounts of glycosphingolipoids in the brain. It is presumed to be inherited as an x-linked recessive trait.

Breeds: 🐕 **German shorthaired pointer**

Amelogenesis Imperfecta

Description: Also known as familial enamel hypoplasia, this is an autosomal recessive congenital enamel hypoplasia, evident in both deciduous and permanent teeth and associated with brown mottling of the enamel. The condition is autosomal recessive, associated with several

different breed-specific variants (ENAM, ACP4, SLC24A4) and genetic testing is available for some of those variants.

Breeds: 🐕 **Akita, Italian greyhound, Parson Russell terrier, Samoyed**

Amyloidosis

Description: A group of diseases characterized by the accumulation of an abnormal protein (amyloid AA) in tissues or by the distribution of the deposits. Localized syndromes usually affect one organ, whereas systemic syndromes affect more than one organ and include reactive, immunoglobulin-associated, and heredofamilial syndromes. A genetic basis is suspected in some cases.

Breeds: 🐕 **Afghan, beagle, black and tan coonhound, Brittany spaniel, Chinese shar-pei, collie, English foxhound, Treeing Walker coonhound, Walker American foxhound;** 🐈 **Abyssinian, Balinese, Oriental shorthair, Siamese, Somali**

Anasarca

Description: Anasarca refers to a generalized edematous condition seen in newborn pups. It is most commonly reported in the English bulldog, where affected animals are referred to as walrus pups.

Breeds: 🐕 **Affenpinscher, American Eskimo dog, Belgian Tervuren, Boston terrier, Clumber spaniel, English bulldog**

Anesthetic Metabolism

Description: Not a true anesthetic sensitivity, but some dogs have a genetic mutation associated with the production of CYP2B11 which is an enzyme responsible for breaking down several thiobarbiturates as well as propofol. This can cause sustained plasma concentrations of these agents and delayed recovery compared to animals without the mutation.

Breeds: 🐕 **Borzoi, English bulldog, golden retriever, greyhound, Labrador retriever, Scottish deerhound, whippet**

Arachnoid Cyst

Description: A rare spinal cyst that causes spinal cord compression in the area of its presence, and predictable neurological deficits depending on that location. The cause is not known, but breed predisposition has been recognized.

Breeds: 🐾 **French bulldog, pug, shih tzu**

Aseptic Meningitis

Description: Also known as necrotizing vasculitis and meningitis, this refers to noninfectious inflammatory conditions characterized by mononuclear periarterial inflammation and vascular thrombosis of vessel walls of the meninges. There may be cross-over with the condition referred to as meningitis and arteritis as both are relatively poorly characterized. Mode of inheritance has not been determined.

Breeds: 🐾 **Bernese mountain dog, boxer, Nova Scotia duck tolling retriever**

Arterial Thromboembolism

Description: A disorder is which clots lodge in the major vessels, particularly the aorta. This is more common in cats than dogs. The cause has not been conclusively demonstrated, but breed predispositions are evident.

Breeds: 🐾 **Abyssinian, American shorthair, Birman, British shorthair, Chartreux, Cornish Rex, Devon Rex, Egyptian Mau, Maine Coon, Norwegian forest cat, Persian, Ragdoll, Siberian forest cat, Sphynx**

Asthma (Feline)

Description: A chronic progressive respiratory disease associated with labored breathing and bronchoconstriction. The cause is presumed to be at least partly due to allergies, and while breed predisposition has been recognized, no mode of inheritance has been determined.

Breeds: 🐾 **Himalayan, Siamese**

Atherosclerosis

Description: A vascular disease in which fatty deposits accumulate in the arteries, causing them to narrow and occlude blood supply. Often associated with hypercholesterolemia and hypothyroidism. Mode of inheritance has not yet been determined.

Breeds: 🐾 **Doberman pinscher, miniature schnauzer, Shetland sheepdog**

Atlantoaxial Instability

Description: A congenital disorder in which the top two cervical vertebrae are not properly aligned and connected, causing instability of the joint in this region of the neck. The result is abnormal bending of this portion of the neck, which can cause pressure or compression of the spinal cord.

Breeds: 🐾 **Bichon frisé, Chihuahua, Japanese chin, Pekingese, Pomeranian, shih tzu, toy poodle, Yorkshire terrier**

Atopic Dermatitis

Description: The canine version of hay fever, atopic dermatitis is an extremely common condition. It is believed to be a heritable predisposition to develop allergic reactions to ordinary environmental substances such as pollens, molds, and house dust. Atopic dermatitis is considered to have a strong genetic component, and heritability has been estimated to be 0.47. As in people, the mode of inheritance is not clear. However, if the parents are allergic, the offspring are highly likely to be allergic as well.

Breeds: 🐾 **Bichon frisé, Boston terrier, boxer, Cairn terrier, Chinese shar-pei, chow chow, (American) cocker spaniel, Dalmatian, English setter, German shepherd dog, golden retriever, Irish setter, Labrador retriever, Lhasa apso, miniature poodle, miniature schnauzer, pug, Scottish terrier, shih tzu, Skye terrier, (English) springer spaniel, West Highland white terrier, wire fox terrier;** 🐱 **Abyssinian**

Atresia Ani

Description: A congenital disorder in which the anus is not patent at birth. It is rare, and a genetic basis has not been determined, but breed predisposition has been recognized.

Breeds: 🐾 **Boston terrier, Finnish spitz, Maltese, miniature poodle**

Atrial Fibrillation

Description: An arrhythmia involving the atria. In many cases it is secondary to underlying heart disease, but can also present as a primary event in some animals. A genetic basis has not been determined, but breed predisposition has been recognized.

Breeds: 🐕 **Doberman pinscher, Great Dane, Irish wolfhound, English mastiff, Newfoundland, old English sheepdog, Rottweiler**

Atrial Rupture

Description: A rare form of heart disease in which the left atrium ruptures, resulting in hemopericardium. A genetic basis has not been determined, but breed predisposition has been recognized.

Breeds: 🐕 **Shetland sheepdog**

Atrial Septal Defect

Description: Atrial septal defect is a congenital cardiac anomaly resulting in communication through the interatrial septum. Currently, a genetic basis for the disorder has not been documented. Clinical signs may be absent with small defects or may include exercise intolerance, dyspnea, and syncope. The prognosis often worsens when atrial septal defect is associated with other congenital anomalies.

Breeds: 🐕 **Airedale terrier, Belgian Tervuren, boxer, Doberman pinscher, old English sheepdog, miniature poodle;** 🐈 **Domestic shorthair**

Atrioventricular Block

Description: An arrhythmia associated with disruption of the normal conduction of the electrical impulses within the heart. A genetic basis has not been determined, but breed predisposition has been recognized.

Breeds: 🐕 **Afghan hound, chow chow, German wirehaired pointer, Polish Owczarek Nizinny, West Highland white terrier**

Atrophic Membranous Glomerulopathy

Description: A poorly characterized congenital renal disease. Atrophic membranous glomerulopathy in Rottweilers seems to be distinct from other glomerulopathies, and renal failure occurs between 6 and 12 months of age.

Breeds: 🐕 **Rottweiler**

Audiogenic Reflex Seizures

Description: This refers to seizures that are triggered by environmental factors, most commonly high-pitched sounds. A genetic basis has not been determined, but breed predisposition has been recognized.

Breeds: 🐈 **Birman**

Autoimmune Lymphoproliferative Syndrome

Description: A rapidly progressive, nonneoplastic but lethal lymphoproliferative disease causing lymphadenomegaly, splenomegaly, and lymphocytic apoptosis. There is some similarity to Canale–Smith syndrome in humans. The condition is autosomal recessive, reflecting a mutation of the FASLG gene, and DNA testing is available.

Breeds: 🐈 **British longhair, British shorthair**

Autoinflammatory Disorders

Description: A family of conditions that result from the dysregulation of mediators upregulating the innate immune system. One subtype is the periodic familiar fever seen in Chinese shar-pei, and likely the recurrent inflammatory pulmonary disease of collies, but the conditions occur along a spectrum. A genetic basis has not been determined, but breed predisposition has been recognized. DNA testing is available for shar-pei autoinflammatory disease. It is considered autosomal dominant with incomplete penetrance, and the mutation is associated with the MTBP gene.

Breeds: 🐕 **Chinese shar-pei**

Axonal Dystrophy

Description: Also known as nervous system degeneration, this is a rare disease and a type of leukodystrophy, or disease of the white matter of the central nervous system. This disease causes axonal degeneration with spheroid formation throughout the spinal cord. It is inherited in an autosomal recessive manner and clinical signs generally become apparent at a young age, from 4 to 16 weeks old.

Breeds: 🐕 **Ibizan hound**

Bald Thigh Syndrome

Description: An alopecia of unknown origin, but limited to a single dog breed. The condition affects the lateral and caudal thighs and is associated with a noninflammatory hair loss. Changes evident on histopathology resemble those of endocrinopathies, but no causative endocrine imbalance has yet been identified.

Breeds: 🐕 **Greyhound**

Bernard–Soulier Syndrome

Description: An autosomal recessive bleeding disorder that affects the platelet receptor for von Willebrand factor on the GP9 gene. DNA testing is available.

Breeds: 🐕 **American cocker spaniel, English cocker spaniel**

Black Hair Follicular Dysplasia

Description: Black hair follicular dysplasia is a tardive (not apparent at birth) hereditary alopecia in dogs that have at least some black fur. The condition is inherited as an autosomal recessive trait in most breeds. DNA testing is available for some variants of the condition.

Breeds: 🐕 **American cocker spaniel, basset hound, beagle, bearded collie, border collie, Cavalier King Charles spaniel, dachshund, Gordon setter, Jack Russell terrier, large Münsterländer, papillon, pointer, saluki, schipperke, as well as mixed breeds**

Blaschko's Lines Disorders

Description: The lines of Blaschko are a pattern of lines on the skin that represent the developmental growth pattern during epidermal cell migration. They are typically invisible unless there are associated skin conditions that highlight their location. A condition in Rottweilers appears to be x-lined recessive and bears resemblance to congenital hemidysplasia with ichthyosiform nevus and limb defects (CHILD) seen in people. A similar x-linked condition seen in Labrador retrievers and associated with variants in the NSDHL gene causes a proliferative lymphocytic infundibular mural folliculitis and dermatitis with prominent follicular apoptosis and parakeratotic casts.

Breeds: 🐕 **Labrador retriever, Rottweiler**

Border Collie Collapse

Description: A form of exercise-induced collapse, Border collie collapse is usually seen in dogs after several minutes of strenuous activity. Affected dogs tend to develop a stiff stilted gait and may collapse. This is a different genetic mutation than the similar condition seen in Labrador retrievers (exercise-induced collapse).

Breeds: 🐕 **Border collie**

Borzoi Retinopathy

Description: A nonprogressive ophthalmic condition generally seen in young dogs, from around 6 months of age onwards. This condition does not cause blindness, and probably does not affect vision at all in many dogs.

Breeds: 🐕 **Borzoi (Russian wolfhound)**

Bouvier Des Flandres Myopathy

Description: A rare degenerative myopathy, with many features shared with the familial form of dysphagia and megaesophagus seen in the breed. Clinical signs in affected young adults include regurgitation, exercise intolerance, generalized muscle atrophy, and a peculiar gait; megaesophagus is common.

Breeds: 🐕 **Bouvier des Flandres**

Brachycephalic Airway Obstructive Syndrome (BOAS)

Description: Also known as brachycephalic syndrome, this consists of anatomical abnormalities that may include stenotic nares, tortuous turbinates, caudally displaced maxillae and elongated soft palate, everted laryngeal saccules, and hypoplastic trachea. All brachycephalic breeds likely have at least some degree of increased upper airway resistance.

Breeds: 🐕 **Boston terrier, boxer, Cavalier King Charles spaniel, Chinese shar-pei, English bulldog, French bulldog, Lhasa apso, Norwich terrier, Pekingese, pug, shih tzu, Staffordshire bull terrier;** 🐈 **Exotic, Persian**

Brachygnathism

Description: Brachygnathia, also known as overshot jaw and mandibular distoclusion, is a malocclusive condition in which the mandible is significantly shorter than the maxillae. It is seen in a great number of breeds.

Breeds: 🐕 **Afghan hound, akita, American cocker spaniel, Australian shepherd, basset hound, beagle, bearded collie, bichon frisé, bloodhound, bouvier des Flandres, Brittany spaniel, Cavalier King Charles spaniel, Chesapeake Bay retriever, Chihuahua, Chinse shar-pei, collie, dachshund, Dalmatian, Dandie Dinmont terrier, Doberman pinscher, English cocker spaniel, English foxhound, English setter, fox terrier (smooth and wire), German shepherd dog, German shorthaired pointer, German wirehaired pointer, giant schnauzer, Great Dane, Great Pyrenees, greyhound, Ibizan hound, Irish setter, Italian greyhound, Jack Russell terrier, Maltese, miniature schnauzer, Norfolk terrier, Norwegian elkhound, Norwich terrier, old English sheepdog, otter hound, Pembroke Welsh corgi, poodle (standard), pug, Rottweiler, saluki, Scottish terrier, Sealyham terrier, Shetland sheepdog, silky terrier, soft-coated wheaten terrier, Tibetan spaniel, Tibetan terrier, whippet**

Bronchiectasis

Description: This refers to the irreversible sequel of dilated bronchi, typically following prolonged bronchitis. A genetic basis has not been determined, but breed predisposition has been recognized.

Breeds: 🐕 **American cocker spaniel, English springer spaniel, miniature poodle, Siberian husky, West Highland white terrier**

Calvarial Hyperostotic Syndrome

Description: A progressive nonneoplastic proliferative bone disease affecting the skull of young dogs. The condition is often self-limiting. A mode of inheritance is not known but a breed predisposition is recognized

Breeds: 🐕 **Bullmastiff**

Cardiomyopathy (Arrhythmogenic Right Ventricular)

Description: An inherited cardiomyopathy often associated with right ventricular infiltration and ventricular arrhythmias. There is some similarity to arrhythmogenic cardiomyopathy in humans. DNA testing is available to help

identify pets at increased risk for the condition. A similar condition has been reported in the English bulldog.

Breeds: 🐕 **Boxer, English bulldog**

Cardiomyopathy, Dilated

Description: Dilated cardiomyopathy (DCM) is a defect of the heart muscle in which the heart muscle becomes thin and stretched, much like a balloon. In this condition, the heart is not an effective pump, and eventually affected dogs succumb to heart failure. Doberman pinschers are affected more than all other breeds combined, and most dogs with DCM are male. The condition is believed to be familial in many breeds. In some breeds, a nutritional mechanism has also been implicated. There are a variety of genetic variants that have been characterized on a breed-specific basis and genetic testing is available to help predict risk for several of them.

Breeds: 🐕 **Airedale, American bulldog, American cocker spaniel, Australian shepherd, basset hound, borzoi, boxer, bullmastiff, Dalmatian, Doberman pinscher, dogue de Bordeaux, English cocker spaniel, giant Schnauzer, golden retriever, Great Dane, Irish wolfhound, Leonberger, Neapolitan mastiff, New Zealand huntaway, Newfoundland, St Bernard, Scottish deerhound, standard poodle, standard schnauzer;** 🐈 **Abyssinian, Balinese, Burmese, Siamese**

Cardiomyopathy, Hypertrophic

Description: Canine hypertrophic cardiomyopathy is quite rare in dogs, but a hereditary form has been reported. It is a disease affecting the heart muscle that eventuates in left ventricular cardiac muscle thickness.

Breeds: 🐕 **English pointer**

Cardiomyopathy, Hypertrophic – Feline

Description: A tendency to cardiac disease that is inherited as a result of breed-specific mutations in the cardiac myosin-binding protein C gene (MYBPC3). Familial forms have also been recognized, and as variants of other genes (such as MYH7). The MYBPC3 mutations are autosomal dominant with variable expressivity and DNA testing is available for breed-specific variants.

Breeds: 🐈 **American shorthair, British shorthair, Chartreux, Cornish Rex, Devon Rex, Egyptian Mau, Maine Coon, Norwegian forest cat, Persian, Ragdoll, Siberian forest cat, Sphynx**

Catalase Deficiency

Description: Also known as hypocatalesemia and acatalasia, these are rare autosomal recessive disorders of red blood cells, in which catalase (which breaks down oxidative free radicals) is reduced or absent. The condition is largely asymptomatic, but can be associated with oral ulceration and necrosis. The condition in the beagle is autosomal recessive, the genetic mutation has been characterized, and DNA testing is available.

Breeds: 🐕 **Beagle, American foxhound**

Cataracts

Description: Cataracts are opacities of the lens of the eye. Although cataracts have many causes, many cataracts are inherited. Cataracts can be further subdivided by stage, mode of inheritance, and age of onset. Breeds may be susceptible to more than one form of cataract. DNA testing is available for some forms of cataracts, especially those associated with the HSF4 gene.

Breeds: 🐕 **Australian shepherd, Boston terrier, (wire) fox terrier, French bulldog, Staffordshire bull terrier and many others;** 🐈 **Bengal, Himalayan**

Centronuclear Myopathy

Description: A congenital neurological disorder associated with mutations of the PTPLA gene. It is inherited as an autosomal recessive trait and DNA testing is available. A similar condition in the Great Dane is associated with an autosomal recessive mutation of the BIN1 gene and DNA testing is available.

Breeds: 🐕 **German hunting terrier (jagdterrier), Great Dane, Labrador retriever**

Cerebellar Abiotrophy

Description: Also known as cerebellar degeneration, cerebellar abiotrophy results from selective cell death of Purkinje cells, granule cells, or both and is an inherited trait in many breeds. In the beagle and vizsla, genetic mutations (SPTBN2) have been characterized for neonatal cortical cerebellar abiotrophy, the trait is autosomal recessive, and DNA testing is available.

Breeds: 🐕 **Airedale terrier, American Staffordshire terrier, Australian kelpie, beagle, Bern running dog, Bernese mountain dog, Border collie, Brittany spaniel, bullmastiff, bull terrier, Carlin pinscher, English springer spaniel, Finnish hound, German shepherd dog, Gordon setter, Irish setter, Kerry blue terrier, Labrador retriever, miniature poodle, old English sheepdog, rough collie, Scottish terrier, vizsla;** 🐈 **Domestic shorthair, Siamese**

Cerebellar Ataxia

Description: A family of heritable neurological conditions in which clinical signs are attributed to cerebellar pathology. There are potentially many causes, and those that are genetic are likely due to a variety of breed-specific mutations with varying modes of inheritance. In addition, several forms of cerebellar ataxia are actually manifestations of other broader conditions, such as canine multiple system degeneration or neuronal ceroid lipofuscinosis, so are covered in more detail in those sections.

Cerebellar Ataxia (Autophagy)

Description: An inherited breed-specific form of cerebellar ataxia. Causative mutations in the RAB24 and ATG4D genes have been implicated as autosomal recessive conditions in breed-specific entities. DNA testing is available for specific variants.

Breeds: 🐕 **Gordon setter, Lagotto Romagnola, old English sheepdog**

Cerebellar Ataxia (Familial)

Description: Familial cerebellar ataxia with hydrocephalus has been reported in bullmastiffs and is believed to be inherited as an autosomal recessive trait.

Breeds: 🐕 **Bullmastiff**

Cerebellar Ataxia (Hound)

Description: A form of cerebellar degeneration most commonly seen in hounds. One variant seen in the Finnish hound and Norrbottenspets is caused by a mutation of the

SEL1L gene. It is autosomal recessive, and DNA testing is available. It is likely that other forms of hound ataxia are also associated with breed-specific variants.

Breeds: 🐕 **Beagle, Finnish hound, (American) fox-hound, (English) foxhound, harrier, Norrbottenspets**

Cerebellar Ataxia (Italian Spinone)

Description: An autosomal recessive form of cerebellar ataxia has been documented in the Italian spinone (spinone Italiano). Affected dogs appear normal at birth and in the young puppy stage, but become progressively more uncoordinated with age, and most are euthanized before 1 year of age.

Breeds: 🐕 **Italian spinone**

Cerebellar Ataxia (Jack Russell Terrier)

Description: Another autosomal recessive form of cerebellar ataxia. Affected pups are evident by 2–4 weeks of age with progressive incoordination, head bobbing, wide-based stance, and stumbling. The condition is progressive, but pups can be kept alive with excellent supportive care. This condition is different from the poorly characterized late-onset ataxia and spinocerebellar ataxia also seen in these breeds.

Breeds: 🐕 **Jack Russell terrier, Parson Russell terrier**

Cerebellar Ataxia (Neonatal)

Description: Sometimes referred to as Bandera's syndrome, pups are normal at birth and nurse well, but eventually they display tremors and head bobbing. They continue to grow and develop, and although they may make some improvement in their clinical signs, they remain physically challenged. The condition is inherited as an autosomal recessive trait, the variant has been characterized in the *GRM1 gene, and DNA testing is available.*

Breeds: 🐕 **Coton de Tulear**

Cerebellar Ataxia (Spongy Degeneration)

Description: Breed-specific variants of cerebellar ataxia associated with autosomal recessive mutations in the ATP1B2 and KCNJ10 genes. Affected pups tend to demonstrate neurological abnormalities early in life with rapid progression.

Breeds: 🐕 **Belgian Malinois, Belgian shepherd, Dutch shepherd**

Cerebellar Ataxia (X-Linked)

Description: Cerebellar ataxia has been documented as an x-linked recessive trait (XCA) in English pointer dogs. Clinical signs begin at about 12 weeks of age and progress from an awkward gait with disorientation and nystagmus to marked ataxia by 16 months of age.

Breeds: 🐕 **English pointer**

Cerebellar Cortical Degeneration

Description: A degenerative juvenile form of cerebellar abiotrophy. The condition in the vizsla results from mutations of the SNX14 gene and is inherited as an autosomal recessive trait. In the beagle, a similar condition due to mutations of the SPTBN2 gene causes cerebellar dysfunction to a limited extent. DNA testing is available for both variants. Hereditary neuronal abiotrophy has also been documented in the Swedish Lapphund dog.

Breeds: 🐕 **Beagle, Swedish Lapphund, vizsla**

Cerebellar Degeneration (Feline)

Description: A relatively rare autosomal recessive trait that has been described in cats, associated with extensive destruction of Purkinje cells. Cerebellar dysfunction becomes evident by 7–8 weeks of age, with ataxia, and becomes progressively worse, but not fatal, although most kittens are eventually euthanized. See also cerebellar abiotrophy.

Breeds: 🐈 **Domestic shorthair, Persian, Siamese**

Cerebellar Hypoplasia

Description: A definite pattern of inheritance has not been established. Dogs with cerebellar hypoplasia have an early onset of hypermetria, ataxia, and intention tremor. Cerebellar hypoplasia also occurs in cats, but most commonly associated with feline panleukopenia infection.

Breeds: 🐕 **Airedale, chow chow, Irish Setter, wire fox terrier**

Cerebellar Hypoplasia (Dandy–Walker Malformation)

Description: A familial nonprogressive ataxia due to inferior cerebellar ataxia. The mutation in the VLDLR gene has been characterized in Eurasiers as autosomal recessive, and DNA testing is available.

Breeds: 🐕 **Eurasier**

Cerebellar Hypoplasia (Vermian Hypoplasia)

Description: A subtype of cerebellar hypoplasia, similar clinically to Dandy–Walker syndrome in humans. Clinical signs, noted at about 2 weeks of age, include ataxia, dysmetria, intention tremors, and, in some dogs, vestibular signs.

Breeds: 🐕 **Australian shepherd, Boston terrier, bull terrier**

Cerebral Dysfunction

Description: A poorly characterized neurological disorder in which the genetic mutation causes a structural change of transporter systems for neurotransmitters, which in turn impairs a variety of central nervous system functions. The condition is transmitted as an autosomal recessive trait, the genetic variant has been characterized, and DNA testing is available.

Breeds: 🐕 **Stabyhoun**

Cervical Vertebral Instability

Description: Also known as cervical vertebral malformation and articulation, cervical spondylomyelopathy, and wobbler syndrome, it is caused by an instability in the intervertebral disks in the neck area. The mode of inheritance is unknown for all breeds but has been suggested to be autosomal recessive in the Great Dane, Doberman pinscher, and borzoi, and familial in basset hounds and bullmastiffs.

Breeds: 🐕 **Basset hound, beagle, boxer, borzoi, bullmastiff, chow chow, Doberman pinscher, fox terrier, German shepherd dog, golden retriever, Great Dane, Great Pyrenees, Irish setter, Irish wolfhound, Labrador retriever, old English sheepdog, Rhodesian ridgeback, Rottweiler**

Chediak–Higashi Syndrome

Description: An autosomal recessive trait in cats with a dilute smoke-blue color, and the irises tend to be yellow-green. The main characteristic is the presence of abnormally large azurophilic granules in a variety of cell types, especially leukocytes. A similar condition in which prominent granulation of normal size is apparent in the leukocytes of Birman cats is transmitted as an autosomal recessive trait but is considered completely asymptomatic.

Breeds: 🐈 **Persian, Birman**

Chiari Malformation

Description: A caudal occipital malformation that creates a narrowing of the space around where the cervical spinal cord meets the brain. It predisposes the affected pet to other problems, such as syringomyelia. A genetic basis has not been determined, but breed predisposition has been recognized.

Breeds: 🐕 **Brussels griffon, Cavalier King Charles spaniel, Chihuahua, English toy spaniel**

Chinese Shar-Pei Immunodeficiency

Description: A poorly described entity characterized by defects in both cell-mediated and humoral immune responses. Affected animals develop an intermittent fever and a variety of systemic disorders, including ulcerative colitis, pyoderma, and demodicosis.

Breeds: 🐕 **Chinese shar-pei**

Cholesterol Ester Storage Disease

Description: Also known as Wolman disease, this is a rare lysosomal storage disease (LSD) associated with a deficiency of lysosomal acid lipase. The result is an accumulation of triglyceride and cholesterol esters within macrophages of the liver and spleen, with death occurring before 1 year of age.

Breeds: 🐕 **Fox terrier**

Chondrodysplasia (Dominant)

Description: An inherited form of dwarfism associated with an FGF4-retrograde insertion in canine chromosome 18. It is a dominant trait that influences the short-leg stature associated with many canine breeds.

Breeds: 🐕 **Basset hound, dachshund, Pembroke Welsh corgi, Scottish terrier, West Highland white terrier, and others**

Chondrodysplasia (Recessive)

Description: A disorder of bone and cartilage with different forms, modes of inheritance, clinical signs, and causative genetic mutations. Mutations in the genes responsible for proteins that impact the growth plates can have varying effects on conformation and risks for other issues. In the Karelian bear dog and Norwegian elkhound, it is associated with an autosomal recessive mutation of the ITGA gene (ITGA10), and DNA testing is available.

Breeds: 🐕 **Chinook, Karelian bear dog, Norwegian elkhound; other forms seen in Alaskan malamute, miniature poodle, Samoyed, Labrador retriever, Scottish deerhound, English pointer, Great Pyrenees, Irish setter**

Chondrodysplasia (Feline)

Description: Also known as achondroplasia, this feline form of chondrodysplasia is quite unlike the clinical condition in dogs, as the head is not affected as part of the process. It appears to be transmitted as an autosomal dominant trait, and it is presumed that it is likely homozygous lethal, with kittens dying *in utero* if they carry two copies of the gene variant. The feline condition does not seem to be associated with an increased risk of developing intervertebral disk disease.

Breeds: 🐈 **Munchkin**

Chondrodystrophy

Description: A form of dwarfism also associated with undershot jaw and dental abnormalities, caused by an FGF4-retrograde insertion in canine chromosome 12 (different from that causing chondrodysplasia), and also associated with increased risk of intervertebral disk disease. For breeds in which both chondrodysplasia and chondrodystrophy are evident (such as basset hounds, dachshunds, Welsh corgis, and Scottish terriers), DNA testing and counseling can be used to reduce the prevalence of inherited intervertebral disk disease while still preserving the short-legged attributes of the breed.

Breeds: 🐕 **Australian cobber dog (Labradoodle), basset hound, beagle, bichon frisé, Cardigan Welsh corgi, Cavalier King Charles spaniel, Chesapeake Bay retriever, Chihuahua, Chinese crested, (American) cocker spaniel, coton de Tulear, dachshund, Dandie Dinmont terrier, English springer spaniel, French bulldog, Havanese, Jack Russell terrier, Nova Scotia duck tolling retriever, Pekingese, Pembroke Welsh corgi, miniature and toy poodle, Portuguese water dog, Scottish terrier, shih tzu**

Choroidal Hypoplasia (Collie Eye Anomaly)

Description: More commonly referred to as collie eye anomaly, this refers to the incomplete development of the eye, and is inherited as an autosomal recessive mutation of the NHEJ1 gene, but a cluster of genes may influence the severity and susceptibility. Because the condition is present at birth, pups can be checked as early as 5–6 weeks of age, although 6–10 weeks is preferred. DNA testing is available.

Breeds: 🐕 **Australian shepherd, bearded collie, Border collie, Boykin spaniel, Chinook, collie, English shepherd, Hokkaido, Lancashire heeler, Nova Scotia duck tolling retriever, Great Pyrenees, Pyrenean shepherd, ryukyu inu, Shetland sheepdog, silken windhound, (longhaired) whippet**

Chronic Inflammatory Hepatic Disease

Description: Also known as chronic active hepatitis, this is a catch-all phrase for myriad liver diseases that result in inflammatory hepatitis, bile duct proliferation, fibrosis, and cirrhosis. A familial association has been inferred in some breeds for this progressive hepatopathy marked by chronic inflammation, fibrosis, and copper accumulation.

Breeds: 🐕 **Bedlington terrier, cairn terrier, Cavalier King Charlies spaniel, (American) cocker spaniel, Dalmatian, Doberman pinscher, English springer spaniel, German shorthaired pointer, Great Dane, Jack Russell terrier, Labrador retriever, Samoyed, Scottish terrier, Skye terrier, West Highland white terrier**

Chronic Obstructive Pulmonary Disease (COPD)

Description: Also known as chronic bronchitis, this is a feline lower airway disease in which the airways become inflamed, not attributable to any underlying problems. There is little evidence to suggest a heritable basis, other than breed predispositions have been recognized.

Breeds: 🐈 **Balinese, Domestic shorthair, Siamese**

Ciliary Dyskinesia

Description: Also known as immotile cilia syndrome and Kartagener's syndrome, primary ciliary dyskinesia is a condition in which the hair-like cilia in the respiratory passages, in the middle ear, and on the sperm cannot perform their needed functions. The cause is abnormal function of ciliary microtubules resulting from the absence of one or both of the inner and outer dyneim arms. The genetic mutation has been characterized for several breeds (NME5, *CCDC39,* etc.) as autosomal recessive traits, and DNA testing is available for those variants (Alaskan malamute, old English sheepdog, etc.).

Breeds: 🐕 **Alaskan malamute, bichon frisé, Border collie, Chinese shar-pei, chow chow, dachshund, Dalmatian, Doberman pinscher, English pointer, English springer spaniel, golden retriever, Newfoundland, Norwegian elkhound, old English sheepdog, Rottweiler, Staffordshire bull terrier**

Cleft Palate/Cleft Lip

Description: Congenital defects of the hard and soft palates may be inherited traits with incomplete penetrance in a variety of breeds. An autosomal recessive mode of inheritance has been documented for cleft palate in the Nova Scotia duck tolling retriever, associated with mutations of the DLX6 gene. Cleft palate and cleft lip can result from either hereditary or environmental causes, and there are likely breed-specific mutations responsible for the condition.

Breeds: 🐕 **Beagle, berger blanc Suisse (white Swiss sheepdog), boxer, Boston terrier, Brittany spaniel, cairn terrier, (American) cocker spaniel, dachshund, English bulldog, English toy spaniel, French bulldog, German shepherd dog, Labrador retriever, Nova Scotia duck tolling retriever, Pekingese, pointer, St Bernard, (miniature) schnauzer, shih tzu**

Cobalamin Malabsorption

Description: Selective malabsorption of vitamin B12 has been reported as an inherited trait in several breeds of dog, with different genetic variants implicated, most affecting the AMN or CBN genes. Most are inherited as autosomal recessive traits. The diagnosis may be suspected in a young breed at risk with proteinuria and a nonregenerative anemia with poikilocytosis and anisocytosis. There is some similarity to Imerslund–Grasbeck syndrome in people. Several mutations have been characterized, and DNA testing is available for specific variants.

Breeds: 🐕 **Australian shepherd, beagle, Border collie, Chinese shar-pei, German shepherd dog, giant schnauzer, Komondor, Staffordshire bull terrier**

Colitis

Description: Colitis refers to inflammatory disorders of the large intestine. Of the numerous variants reported, only histiocytic ulcerative colitis seems to have a strongly familial basis.

Breeds: 🐕 **Boxer, French bulldog**

Collagenolytic Granuloma

Description: Also known as canine eosinophilic granuloma, is believed to be an immune-mediated disorder with some resemblance to Wells' syndrome in people. Possible triggers include insect bites, environmental, or food allergies and even some infectious agents. It is believed to be a familial trait and an inherited susceptibility to collagen injury.

Breeds: 🐕 **Cavalier King Charles spaniel, Siberian husky**

Color Dilution Alopecia

Description: This condition describes the patchy, poor hair coat that can develop in animals bred for unusual hair color, especially those described as "blue" and "fawn." The condition is believed to be associated with the interplay of different factors with the double-recessive allele on the D coat color locus. The affliction, however, cannot be determined only by the dd homozygous recessive allele, because not all color-diluted dogs develop associated hair coat problems. DNA testing is available for the D (dilution) locus.

Breeds: 🐕 **American Staffordshire terrier, Australian shepherd, Barbet, beagle, Bernese mountain dog, Boston terrier, Chihuahua (blue), chow chow (blue), curly-coated retriever, dachshund (blue), Doberman**

pinschers (blue, red), Great Dane (blue), German pinscher, Irish setter (fawn), Irish water spaniel, Italian greyhound (blue), large Münsterländer, miniature pinscher (blue), miniature schnauzer, Newfoundland, Portuguese water dog, Rhodesian ridgeback, saluki, schipperke (blue), Shetland sheepdog (blue), silky terrier, sloughi, standard poodle (blue), Thai ridgeback, whippet (blue), Yorkshire terrier (gray-blue)

Complement (C3) Deficiency

Description: C3 deficiency is a rare autosomal recessive disorder in which affected animals are prone to recurrent bacterial infections and to renal amyloidosis or type 1 membranoproliferative glomerulonephritis.

Breeds: Brittany spaniel

Congenital Blindness

Description: A rare autosomal recessive disorder associated with multiple ophthalmic anomalies such as microphthalmia, retinal dysplasia, and anterior segment dysgenesis.

Breeds: Doberman pinscher

Copper Hepatopathy

Description: An inherited condition in which dogs are prone to developing liver disease in association with inherited metabolic defects that cause copper to accumulate in the liver and leads to toxicity. In the Bedlington terrier, it is an autosomal recessive condition associated with the COMMD1 (MURR1) gene, although other genes may act as modifiers. In Labrador retrievers and perhaps Doberman pinschers, the ATP7B variant appears to be significant; ATP7A may act as a modifier. Genetic testing is available for specific breed-related variants.

Breeds: Beagle, Bedlington terrier, Dalmatian, Doberman pinscher, Labrador retriever, Skye terrier, West Highland white terrier

Cor Triatriatum

Description: Cor triatriatum is a congenital anomaly associated with a persistent membrane that divides the atrium into two chambers. The condition affecting the right chamber, cor triatriatum dexter, has been reported in dogs.

The membrane impedes venous flow and typically results in ascites.

Breeds: Chow chow

Corneal Dystrophy

Description: A constellation of corneal conditions that are bilateral, noninflammatory, and inherited; they involve the corneal epithelium, stroma, or endothelium. The opacities can be due to lipids, calcium, or dystrophic changes. All have their own breed predispositions, and perhaps modes of inheritance as well. Posterior polymorphous dystrophy in the American cocker spaniel typically does not lead to corneal edema, while endothelial dystrophy observed in the Boston terrier, Chihuahua, and other breeds is often associated with progressive corneal edema.

Breeds: Airedale, Boston terrier, Chihuahua, American cocker spaniel, dachshund, Doberman pinscher, St Bernard, Shetland sheepdog, Yorkshire terrier

Corneal Dystrophy (Macular)

Description: A form of corneal dystrophy due to accumulations of glycosaminoglycans in the cornea. The cause is a mutation in the canine carbohydrate sulfotransferase-6 (CHST6) gene, and the condition is transmitted as an autosomal recessive trait. DNA testing is available.

Breeds: Labrador retriever

Corneal Sequestrum

Description: An ophthalmic condition mostly seen in cats, in which there develops a pigmented lesion in the central cornea. A genetic basis has not been determined, but breed predisposition has been recognized.

Breeds: Birman, Burmese, Colorpoint shorthair, Himalayan, Persian, Siamese

Corticosteroid Polymorphisms

Description: Response to corticosteroid therapy has been correlated with the presence of certain polymorphisms of the glucocorticoid receptor gene (NR3C1). Depending on the polymorphism present, patients may show either increased sensitivity to glucocorticoid-induced adverse effects or resistance to their therapeutic effects.

Cranial Deformity

Description: A potentially lethal problem seen with Ojos azules cats homozygous for the dominant blue eye color. To avoid the lethal consequences of homozygotes, the breed is perpetuated by mating those with blue eyes with nonblue-eyed cats.

Breeds: Ojos azules

Craniofacial Deformity (Burmese Head Defect)

Description: A congenital craniofacial deformity that is transmitted as an autosomal recessive trait in the Burmese, associated with a mutation in the ALX1 gene. Breed-specific DNA testing is available.

Breeds: American shorthair, Bombay, Burmese

Craniomandibular Osteopathy

Description: A bizarre proliferative bone disease that typically affects the lower jawbone (mandible), the tympanic bullae, and occasionally other bones of the head. It is believed to be transmitted as an autosomal dominant trait with incomplete penetrance, at least in terriers, for which there is a DNA test. The condition, at least in some breeds, is due to a mutation in the SLC37A2 gene. The mode of inheritance in most other breeds is not known with any certainty.

Breeds: Australian shepherd, Border terrier, Boston terrier, cairn terrier, Great Pyrenees, Lancashire heeler, Scottish terrier, West Highland white terrier; other forms reported in the following breeds: boxer, bullmastiff, bull terrier, Catahoula leopard dog, Doberman pinscher, English bulldog, fox terrier, German wirehaired pointer, golden retriever, Great Dane, Great Pyrenees, Irish setter, Kerry blue terrier, Labrador retriever, Shetland sheepdog, Skye terrier, Staffordshire terrier, and Weimaraner

Cruciate Ligament Disease

Description: A common orthopedic problem in dogs that could be due to acute trauma or ligament degeneration. While a mode of inheritance is not known for certain, there is a definite breed predisposition for the condition.

Breeds: Bullmastiff, kuvasz, mastiff, Newfoundland, Rottweiler, Staffordshire terrier

Cryptorchidism

Description: Cryptorchidism refers to testicles that have not descended into the scrotum. It is believed to be at least partially hereditary, and it is commonly seen in many breeds as well as mixed-breed animals. In all likelihood, cryptorchidism will likely be found to be a sex-limited autosomal trait and will likely involve more than one gene.

Breeds: Border collie, boxer, cairn terrier, Chihuahua, English bulldog, German shepherd dog, greyhound, Lakeland terrier, Maltese, miniature dachshund, miniature schnauzer, old English sheepdog, Pekingese, Pomeranian, Shetland sheepdog, Siberian husky, silky terrier, toy and miniature poodle, whippet, Yorkshire terrier; Persian

Cutaneous and Renal Glomerular Vasculopathy

Description: A poorly understood ulcerating disease often referred to as "Alabama rot" and "Greenetrack disease." A breed predisposition is likely, although it has been reported in many breeds. The ultimate cause remains elusive, but infectious and immune-mediated causes are being considered, in addition to genetics.

Breeds: Greyhound

Cutaneous Asthenia

Description: Also known as Ehlers–Danlos syndrome and dermatosparaxis, this condition refers to a group of related biochemical disorders that affect the strength of collagen, the fibrous connective tissue of the body. Mutations in any of a number of genes (ADAMTS2, TNXB, COL5A1, etc.) can give rise to one of the variants of cutaneous asthenia in dogs and cats. In general, mutations in collagen structural genes result in dominant forms of the disorder, whereas gene mutations for enzymes that process procollagen are typically recessive.

Breeds: Australian kelpie, beagle, boxer, dachshund, English setter, English springer spaniel, Garafian shepherd dog, German shepherd dog, greyhound, Irish setter, keeshond, Manchester terrier, St

Bernard, schnauzer (miniature), soft-coated wheaten terrier, Pembroke Welsh corgi, cross-breeds; 🐈 Burmese, domestic shorthair

Cyclic Hematopoiesis

Description: Originally known as gray collie syndrome, this involves a regulatory defect of hematopoietic stem cells in the bone marrow. The condition occurs principally in silver-gray collie pups but has occasionally been reported in other breeds. In the collie, the condition is autosomal recessive and due to a mutation in the AP3B1 gene; DNA testing is available.

Breeds: 🐕 **Collie (gray), (American) cocker spaniel, Border collie, Pomeranian**

Cystic Renal Dysplasia and Hepatic Fibrosis

Description: A rare ciliopathy that results in fatal cystic renal dysplasia and hepatic fibrosis. The cause is believed to be a mutation in the INPP5E gene, which is likely transmitted as an autosomal recessive trait. DNA testing is available.

Breeds: 🐕 **Norwich terrier**

Cystinuria

Description: A group of genetic disorders associated with mutations of the SLC7A9 and SLC3A1 genes with breed-specific presentations and modes of inheritance. For example, the condition in miniature pinschers and Australian cattle dogs is autosomal dominant, while that in the Newfoundland is autosomal recessive. In the cat, variants of SLC7A9 and SLC3A1 have also been characterized. DNA testing is available for several breed-specific variants in dogs, and cats.

Breeds: 🐕 **American bulldog, American Staffordshire terrier, Australian cattle dog, Australian shepherd, basenji, basset hound, bichon frisé, boxer, bullmastiff, Chihuahua, dachshund, English bulldog, fox terrier (smooth, wire), French bulldog, Irish terrier, Kromfohrlander, Labrador retriever, Landseer, mastiff (English), miniature pinscher, Newfoundland, Scottish deerhound, Scottish terrier, silky terrier, Staffordshire bull terrier, Tibetan spaniel, Welsh corgi (Cardigan, Pembroke);** 🐈 **Domestic longhair, Maine Coon, Siamese, Sphynx, domestic shorthair**

Dalmatian Bronzing Syndrome

Description: Potentially an inherited defect of uric acid metabolism, similar to gout in people. Although the mode of inheritance has not been determined with certainty, the condition is limited to the Dalmatian and associated with excessive uric acid excretion (see hyperuricosuria); a bacterial folliculitis is likely also involved. DNA testing is available to detect hyperuricosuria in certain breeds.

Breeds: 🐕 **Dalmatian**

Darier Disease

Description: Also known as familial benign pemphigus and Hailey–Hailey disease, this is a rare skin condition that starts in young pups, usually at only a few months of age. It is presumed to be autosomal dominant with incomplete penetrance.

Breeds: 🐕 **Doberman pinscher, English setter**

Deafness (Canine)

Description: Inherited deafness is a sensorineural deafness resulting from degeneration of inner ear structures and neurons of the spiral ganglion, with clinical signs apparent from a few weeks to a few months of age. Predominantly white, merle, and piebald coat coloring predisposes dogs to inherited deafness. Genetic testing is available to determine merle and piebald genotypes. A mutation has been characterized for deafness in the Doberman pinscher (MYO7A) and DNA testing is available. There is also a linkage-based test for adult-onset deafness in Border collies.

Breeds: 🐕 **Dalmatian, American foxhound, Australian shepherd, Border collie, collie, (dappled) dachshund, Dunker, (harlequin) Great Dane, old English sheepdog, Shetland sheepdog, beagle, bulldog, bull terrier, Doberman pinscher, English setter, Great Pyrenees, greyhound, Samoyed, Sealyham terrier**

Deafness (Feline)

Description: Hereditary deafness is most commonly reported in white cats with blue eyes, associated with the autosomal dominant white pigment (W) gene and not with albinism. Whether the cat is heterozygous or homozygous for the W gene, the blue eyes and deafness have incomplete penetrance and are likely influenced by additional genes.

Breeds: 🐱 **Cornish Rex, Devon Rex, Exotic, Highland fold, Manx, Oriental shorthair, Persian, Scottish fold, Turkish angora**

Degenerative Myelopathy

Description: A group of inherited disorders of the SOD1, SOD1BA, and SOD2 genes (as well as the modifier gene SP110) that increase the breed-specific risks for a progressive debilitating spinal disease. The mode of inheritance is autosomal recessive in most cases, and DNA testing is available, but interpretation must be done on a breed-specific basis.

Breeds: 🐕 **Bernese mountain dog, boxer, Chesapeake Bay retriever, Dutch Kooiker dog, German shepherd dog, Pembroke Welsh corgi, Rhodesian ridgeback, and others**

Delayed Postoperative Bleeding

Description: Delayed postoperative bleeding is a mild bleeding disorder in which spontaneous hemorrhage is not seen, but clotting seems to be impaired following surgery or trauma. The cause has not been determined but seems to be one of enhanced fibrinolysis. It is not rare in predisposed breeds.

Breeds: 🐕 **Greyhound, Scottish deerhound**

Demodicosis

Description: Also known as demodectic mange or red mange, this is an inflammatory disease of the hair follicles that appears to be attributable in part to the presence of *Demodex* mites and in part to an inherited or acquired immune defect. The mode of inheritance is unknown, but breed predilections exist for the juvenile form of the disease.

Breeds: 🐕 **Afghan hound, beagle, Boston terrier, boxer, bull terrier, Chihuahua, Chinese shar-pei, collie, dachshund, Dalmatian, Doberman pinscher, English bulldog, English pointer, German shepherd dog, Great Dane, Lhasa apso, old English sheepdog, pit bull terrier, pug, Rottweiler, Staffordshire terrier. Adult-onset demodicosis may be seen more commonly in the English bulldog, miniature poodle, shih tzu, and West Highland white terrier**

Dermatomyositis

Description: Dermatomyositis is an inflammatory disease of the skin, muscle, fat, and sometimes blood vessels. The cause is multifactorial and at least three different genes are involved in susceptibility to the disease; genetic testing is available for some of the breeds affected and can determine a relative risk level for developing the disease. In breeds other than the collie and Shetland sheepdog, the condition is sometimes referred to as dermatomyositis-like disease.

Breeds: 🐕 **Australian cattle dog, basset hound, Beauceron shepherd, Belgian Tervuren, chow chow, collie, Garafian shepherd dog, German shepherd dog, Jack Russell terrier, kuvasz, Lakeland terrier, Portuguese water dog, Pembroke Welsh corgi, Rottweiler, Shetland sheepdog**

Dermoid

Description: Congenital collections of cutaneous tissue (skin, hair follicles, sebaceous glands, fat) found on the conjunctiva or cornea. A mode of inheritance has not been confirmed, but breed predilection is recognized.

Breeds: 🐕 **Affenpinscher, dachshund, Dalmatian, Doberman pinscher, German shepherd dog, golden retriever, St Bernard;** 🐱 **Burmese**

Dermoid Sinus

Description: Dermoid sinus refers to an abnormal tunnel that forms between the skin surface and the spinal column. The mode of inheritance is unknown for all breeds; the mutation has been determined in the Rhodesian ridgeback and Thai ridgeback, and DNA testing is available.

Breeds: 🐕 **Boxer, chow chow, Kerry blue terrier, Rhodesian ridgeback, Siberian husky, Thai ridgeback, Yorkshire terrier, shih tzu**

Diabetes Mellitus

Description: Insulin-dependent diabetes mellitus (IDDM) seems to involve a genetic predisposition to developing an autoimmune process, resulting in destruction of beta cells in the pancreatic islets of Langerhans. In some breeds, it has even been characterized as an autosomal recessive trait (dmdm), causing islet cell hypoplasia. An association has been identified to three haplotypes of the dog leukocyte antigen that might confer increased susceptibility, but specific genetic mutations have not yet been characterized.

Breeds: 🐕 **Alaskan malamute, Australian terrier, beagle, cairn terrier, chow chow, dachshund, Doberman pinscher, English springer spaniel, Finnish spitz, golden retriever, keeshond, Labrador retriever, miniature pinscher, miniature and toy poodles, miniature schnauzer, old English sheepdog, poodle, pug, Samoyed, schipperke, Swedish elkhound, Swedish lapphund, Tibetan terrier, West Highland white terrier;** 🐈 **Abyssinian, Burmese, Norwegian forest cat, Russian blue, Tonkinese**

Diffuse Idiopathic Skeletal Hyperostosis

Description: Diffuse (or disseminated) idiopathic skeletal hyperostosis is a poorly characterized disorder in the dog that resembles the condition of the same name in humans and is sometimes referred to as Forrestier's disease. The condition can be difficult to differentiate from spondylosis deformans and typically involves ossification of soft tissues, such as ligaments, joints, tendons, and muscles. Breed predispositions exist.

Breeds: 🐕 **Boxer, Great Dane, Leonberger**

Dihydropyrimidinase Deficiency

Description: A very rare feline inborn metabolic syndrome characterized by dihydropyrimidinuria. The condition is caused by a mutation in the DPYS gene. DNA testing is available.

Breeds: 🐈 **Domestic shorthair**

Diskospondylitis

Description: Inflammatory reaction of intervertebral disks, often associated with osteomyelitis. It often occurs as a secondary event but not in all cases. A genetic basis has not been determined, but breed predisposition has been recognized.

Breeds: 🐕 **Doberman pinscher, English bulldog, German shepherd dog, Great Dane, Labrador retriever, Weimaraner**

Distichiasis

Description: Distichiasis refers to eyelashes that may project toward the surface of the eye from abnormal locations, such as the openings of specialized (Meibomian) glands in the eyelids. The condition is suspected to be a genetic disorder, and there are strong breed predispositions, but the mode of inheritance is unknown.

Breeds: 🐕 **American cocker spaniel, American Staffordshire terrier, beagle, boxer, Chesapeake Bay retriever, curly-coated retriever, English bulldog, English cocker spaniel, flat-coated retriever, French bulldog, golden retriever, Lhasa apso, Pekingese, pug, St Bernard, Shetland sheepdog, shih tzu, Sussex spaniel, Tibetan terrier, toy and miniature poodles**

Dry Eye Curly Coat Syndrome

Description: An autosomal recessive genetic disorder associated with congenital dry skin, and later development of keratoconjunctivitis sicca (KCS), footpad hyperkeratosis, and abnormal claw development. The genetic variant has been characterized (FAM83H) and DNA testing is available.

Breeds: 🐕 **Cavalier King Charles spaniel**

Dungd

Description: A fatal neonatal disorder seen in Gordon setters is thought to be the result of an inborn error in metabolism. Breeders have referred to this condition as DUNGd (Darned Unnamed New Genetic disease). The condition is progressive, and by 5–6 weeks of age they are unable to stand; death is inevitable.

Breeds: 🐕 **Gordon setter**

Dysmyelinogenesis

Description: Dysmyelinogenesis refers to abnormal myelination, and hypomyelinogenesis implies a lack of myelin in the nervous system. There are a variety of breed-specific manifestations that differ in clinical presentation and mode of inheritance, including both x-linked and autosomal varieties.

Breeds: 🐕 **Bernese mountain dog, chow chow, Dalmatian, lurcher, Samoyed, English springer spaniel, Welsh springer spaniel, Weimaraner;** 🐈 **Egyptian Mau**

Dystocia

Description: Difficulty in the birthing process. It is mainly seen in small pets and those with conformation issues (e.g., brachycephalic features).

Breeds: 🐾 **Boston terrier, boxer, English bulldog, Cavalier King Charles spaniel, Chihuahua, Clumber spaniel, dachshund, Danish/Swedish farmdog, Great Dane, greyhound, Irish wolfhound, Maltese, Pekingese, Rhodesian ridgeback, schipperke, miniature schnauzer, Scottish terrier, shih tzu, Staffordshire bull terrier, Yorkshire terrier**

Eccentrocytosis

Description: A defect noticed in erythrocytes, most commonly associated with onion or garlic toxicities and a few other conditions with oxidative damage such as ketoacidotic diabetes, T-cell lymphoma, and vitamin K antagonist intoxication. Some breed susceptibilities have been recognized.

Breeds: 🐾 **Boxer, English setter, whippet**

Eclampsia

Description: Also referred to as puerperal tetany, the cause is postwhelping hypocalcemia; it is most common several weeks after parturition when milk demand tends to be highest. Breed predisposition has been recognized, but it can happen in any animal.

Breeds: 🐾 **Chihuahua, miniature pinscher, miniature poodle, Pomeranian, shih tzu**

Ectodermal Defect

Description: Ectodermal defect is a hereditary congenital alopecia observed from birth. Hair follicles are totally absent, and associated adnexa in the alopecic skin and abnormal dentition are commonly reported.

Breeds: 🐾 **Beagle, Belgian Groenendael, cocker spaniel, Lhasa apso, miniature poodle, whippet**

Ectodermal Dysplasia-Skin Fragility Syndrome

Description: An inherited skin condition associated with nonimmune-mediated acantholysis due to mutations in the gene encoding protein plakophilin-1 (PKP1). It is inherited as an autosomal recessive trait and ulcerative manifestations are most evident in areas of friction or trauma. Genetic testing is available for specific variants.

Breeds: 🐾 **Chesapeake Bay retriever, German shepherd dog**

Ectodermal Dysplasia (X-Linked)

Description: A rare dermatological condition transmitted as an XCA and presenting as symmetrical areas of hairlessness with decreased lacrimation and missing or misshapen teeth. A substitution mutation in the ectodysplasin A (EDA) gene has been identified in dogs and DNA testing is available.

Breeds: 🐾 **Berger blanc Suisse (white Swiss sheepdog), German Shepherd dog, Shiloh shepherd**

Ectopic Ureters

Description: Ectopic ureters are characterized by the termination of one or both ureters at a site other than the craniolateral aspect of the trigone of the bladder. Breed predispositions have been recognized, but not a mode of inheritance to date.

Breeds: 🐾 **Border terrier, briard, English bulldog, fox terrier (smooth, wire), golden retriever, Brussels griffon, Entelbucher mountain dog, Labrador retriever, miniature and toy poodle, Newfoundland, Siberian husky, Skye terrier, soft-coated wheaten terrier, West Highland white terrier**

Ectropion

Description: Ectropion refers to eyelids that are turned out and often appear to be drooping. It is a breed characteristic in many breeds and accepted as "normal," but also presents as a common ophthalmic problem in other breeds. Because the lids do not conform to the eyeball, affected dogs may be prone to conjunctivitis.

Breeds: 🐾 **Basset hound, black and tan coonhound, bloodhound, boxer, bull terrier, bullmastiff, Chinese shar-pei, chow chow, English setter, English springer spaniel, flat-coated retriever, Gordon setter, Irish setter, Labrador retriever, Leonberger, Newfoundland, St Bernard, Sussex spaniel**

Elbow Dysplasia

Description: Elbow dysplasia refers not to one disease but rather to an entire complex of disorders that affect the elbow joint. Several different processes might be involved, including ununited anconeal process (UAP), fragmented medial coronoid process (FCP), osteochondrosis of the medial humeral condyle, incomplete ossification of humeral condyle, and others. The different forms of elbow dysplasia appear to be inherited independently. In addition, dogs with elbow dysplasia are at increased risk for hip dysplasia, and vice versa, with the risk increasing with the grade of dysplasia observed at each site.

Breeds: 🐾 **Affenpinscher, Afghan hound, Airedale terrier, Alaskan malamute, American Eskimo dog, Australian shepherd, basenji, basset hound, beagle, bearded collie, Belgian Malinois, Bernese mountain dog, Border collie, Boykin spaniel, Catahoula leopard dog, Glen of Imaal terrier, Great Pyrenees, kuvasz, Parson Russell terrier, puli, Samoyed, spinoni Italiano, Stabyhoun, Tibetan spaniel, vizsla, Weimaraner**

Elbow Dysplasia (FCP)

Description: The most common form of elbow dysplasia, in which part of the elbow joint breaks away from its bony anchor. Although the genetics of the condition are not well characterized, breed predispositions are evident.

Breeds: 🐾 **Basset hound, Bernese mountain dog, bouvier des Flandres, bullmastiff, chow chow, German shepherd dog, golden retriever, Gordon setter, Irish wolfhound, Labrador retriever, mastiff, Newfoundland, Rottweiler, St Bernard**

Elbow Dysplasia (Incomplete Ossification of Humeral Condyle)

Description: A form of elbow dysplasia in which ossification fails to occur completely, causing the bone to become weak, and affected dogs may suffer from spontaneous fractures after even minor trauma.

Breeds: 🐾 **American cocker spaniel, Boykin spaniel, Brittany spaniel, Cavalier King Charles spaniel, Clumber spaniel**

Elbow Dysplasia (Osteochondrosis of the Medial Humeral Condyle)

Description: Strong evidence has supported the contention that osteochondritis dissecans (OCD) of the elbow is an inherited disease, likely controlled by many genes. The medial aspect of the lower humerus (condyle) retains thicker cartilage longer than the lateral aspect, and, therefore, this site is more prone to osteochondrosis.

Breeds: 🐾 **Chow chow, German shepherd dog, golden retriever, Great Dane, Labrador retriever, Newfoundland, Rottweiler**

Elbow Dysplasia (UAP)

Description: UAP occurs when the bone growth center in the anconeal process of the elbow fails to unite with the ulna of the foreleg. Changes result from loss of the stabilizing effect of the anconeal process and from inflammation within the joint. Males are affected about twice as frequently as females, but the genetics of the condition are still uncertain.

Breeds: 🐾 **Basset hound, Bernese mountain dog, bloodhound, bullmastiff, Chinese shar-pei, chow chow, English setter, German shepherd dog, golden retriever, Great Dane, Great Pyrenees, Irish wolfhound, Labrador retriever, mastiff, Newfoundland, pointer, Pomeranian, Rottweiler, St Bernard, Weimaraner**

Elliptocytosis

Description: A condition of misshapen erythrocytes that are oval to elliptical in shape, and lack a central concavity. In hereditary elliptocytosis, the finding is usually incidental in animals being evaluated for other reasons. The condition likely results from a beta-spectrin mutation altering the molecular structure of the erythrocyte membrane. It at least some cases, it appears to be autosomal dominant and associated with a variant of the SPTB gene. DNA testing is available for some variants.

Breeds: 🐾 **Chow chow, golden retriever, Labrador retriever, silky terrier, mixed-breed dogs**

Endocardial Fibroelastosis

Description: Cardiac disease associated with marked thickening of the endocardium. A genetic basis has not been determined, but breed predisposition has been recognized.

Breeds: 🐾 **American pit bull terrier, boxer, English bulldog, Great Dane, Labrador retriever, springer spaniel;** 🐈 **Burmese, Siamese**

Entropion

Description: Entropion occurs when the eyelids turn in toward the eye, often resulting in abrasive damage to the cornea. A heritable or conformational form is considered to be a polygenic trait with various subtypes. The exact mode of inheritance has not been determined.

Breeds: 🐕 **Airedale terrier, American cocker spaniel, bullmastiff, Chinese shar-pei, chow chow, mastiff, vizsla, English bulldog, English cocker spaniel, French bulldog, Great Dane, Newfoundland, Pekingese, Rhodesian ridgeback, St Bernard, spinoni Italiano, Tibetan spaniel, wirehaired pointing griffon;** 🐈 **Persian**

Epidermal Dysplasia

Description: Epidermal dysplasia refers to a serious form of keratinization disorder (seborrhea) that reflects a defect in development of skin cells (keratinocytes). Although the mode of inheritance in unknown, the disorder is believed to be a genetically determined and complicated by secondary microbial infections.

Breeds: 🐕 **West Highland white terrier**

Epidermolysis Bullosa (EB)

Description: EB refers to a group of mechanobullous diseases of unknown etiology and involves structural defects at various levels of the basement membrane zone. Congenital and acquired forms have been recognized. The three major categories, based on the location of blistering within the basement membrane zone, are epidermolysis bullosa simplex (epidermolytic EB); junctional epidermolysis bullosa (JEB); and dystrophic epidermolysis bullosa (DEB). The mutation has been characterized for recessive DEB (COL7A1) and for epidermolytic EB in the Eurasier breed (PLEC); DNA testing is available for some breeds. See also epidermolysis bullosa acquisita which is an immune-mediated disease.

Breeds: 🐕 **Akita, Beauceron shepherd, Great Dane, Eurasier, Central Asian shepherd dog, German longhaired pointer, German shorthaired pointer, German wirehaired pointer, golden retriever**

Epidermolysis Bullosa Acquisita

Description: An immune-mediated disease in which autoantibodies target a specific basement membrane zone antigen in anchoring fibrils. The result is a vesicular, bullous, and ulcerative dermatitis.

Breeds: 🐕 **Great Dane**

Epidermolysis Bullosa (Dystrophic)

Description: A group of rare inherited blistering skin diseases associated with genetic mutations of the COL7A1 gene. Manifestations are typically evident shortly after birth. The condition is transmitted as an autosomal recessive trait, the variant has been characterized in the Central Asian shepherd, and DNA testing is available.

Breeds: 🐕 **Akita, Beauceron, Central Asian shepherd, golden retriever**

Epidermolysis Bullosa (Epidermolytic EB)

Description: Epidermolytic EB in the form of epidermolysis bullosa acquisita has been described, with evidence of circulating autoantibodies targeting collagen VII epitopes. A variant of the PLEC gene has been characterized in the Eurasier, and DNA testing is available.

Breeds: 🐕 **Eurasier, Great Dane**

Epidermolysis Bullosa (JEB)

Description: JEB and a milder form (mitis JEB) has been identified. A subtype of JEB – epidermolysis bullosa junctionalis progressiva (nonlethal localized JEB) – has been described in German shorthaired pointers as an autosomal recessive trait. It primarily affects the footpads and pinnae; DNA testing is available.

Breeds: 🐕 **German shorthaired pointer, German longhaired pointer, German wirehaired pointer, poodle, mixed breed;** 🐈 **Domestic shorthair**

Epilepsy

Description: Epileptic seizures have many classifications, and it appears that there is a genetic basis for the disorder in some breeds. While it is presumed that many cases are autosomal recessive with incomplete penetrance and likely influenced by modifier genes, this information is not confirmed for most breeds. However, the heritability is presumed to be high in susceptible breeds.

Breeds: 🐕 **Beagle, Belgian sheepdog, Belgian Tervuren, Bernese mountain dog, boerboel, Border collie, Border terrier, Brussels griffon, Chinook, dachshund, (miniature wire-haired) dachshund, English**

springer spaniel, German shepherd dog, golden retriever, Irish wolfhound, Italian greyhound, Jack Russell terrier, keeshond, Labrador retriever, papillon, Parson Russell terrier, schipperke, standard poodle, vizsla, Welsh terrier, wirehaired pointing griffon

Epilepsy (Juvenile)

Description: A focal remitting seizure disorder that typically abates by 4 months of age. The condition is caused by a mutation in the Lgi2 gene, and is autosomal recessive in nature. DNA testing is available.

Breeds: 🐕 **Lagotto Romagnolo**

Epilepsy (Lafora Body)

Description: Also known as glycoproteinosis and alpha-glucosidase deficiency, this is a rare neurodegenerative disease known to be autosomal recessive in several breeds. The genetic defect results in the accumulation of Lafora bodies in cells in the brain, skin, liver, and skeletal and cardiac muscles that then result in monoclonic and tonic–clonic seizures and progressive neurological dysfunction. The condition is caused by mutations in the EPM2B (NHLRC1) gene, and DNA testing is available for some breeds.

Breeds: 🐕 **Basset hound, beagle, Chihuahua, (miniature wirehaired) dachshund, English pointer, French bulldog, miniature poodle, standard poodle, (Cardigan) Welsh corgi, (Pembroke) Welsh corgi**

Epilepsy (Myoclonic)

Description: An inherited neurological disorder caused by mutation to the DIRAS1 gene. It is inherited as an autosomal recessive trait and causes myoclonic seizures and photosensitivity. The mutation has been characterized (DIRAS1) and DNA testing is available.

Breeds: 🐕 **Rhodesian ridgeback**

Epilepsy (Phenobarbital Resistant)

Description: A form of epilepsy involving polymorphisms in the ABCB1 gene, which often acts in an autosomal dominant manner. A single nucleotide substitution seems to confer phenobarbital resistance in this breed. DNA testing is available.

Breeds: 🐕 **Border collie, koolie**

Epilepsy (Psychomotor)

Description: An unusual breed-specific focal seizure in which the prominent ictal manifestation appears to be fear. It is presumed to be inherited as an autosomal recessive trait.

Breeds: 🐕 **Boerboel**

Epileptoid Cramping Syndrome

Description: Also known as Spike's disease, this is a disorder of movement in which affected dogs suffer variable periods of abnormal muscle activity involving muscles of the body, limbs, head, and neck and also the intestines. The severity and duration of episodes vary greatly between individuals. In some dogs, it may be associated with dietary gluten.

Breeds: 🐕 **Border terrier**

Episodic Falling Syndrome

Description: An inherited neuromuscular condition associated with mutations of the BCAN gene which influence synapse stability and nerve conduction velocity. It has an autosomal recessive mode of inheritance and episodes are typically triggered by exercise, stress, and excitement. DNA testing is available.

Breeds: 🐕 **Cavalier King Charles spaniel**

Eversion of Cartilage of Nictitating Membrane

Description: An ophthalmic condition associated with scrolling of the third eyelid, which can predispose to conjunctivitis. A genetic basis has not been determined, but breed predisposition has been recognized.

Breeds: 🐕 **German shorthaired pointer, Great Dane, Irish wolfhound, Leonberger, Newfoundland, Weimaraner**

Exercise-Induced Collapse

Description: An autosomal recessive neuromuscular disorder associated with mutations of the dynamin 1 (DNM1) gene. Affected animals develop episodic limb weakness, ataxia, and collapse induced by intense exercise. DNA testing is available for some variants.

Breeds: 🐕 **Bouvier des Flandres, Boykin spaniel, Catahoula leopard dog, Chesapeake Bay retriever, Clumber spaniel, (American) cocker spaniel, (English) cocker spaniel, curly-coated retriever, flat-coated retriever, German wirehaired pointer, Hungarian wirehaired pointer, Labrador retriever, old English sheepdog, vizsla, (Cardigan) Welsh corgi, (Pembroke) Welsh corgi**

Exercise-Induced Metabolic Myopathy

Description: An inherited disorder of muscle metabolism associated with a genetic mutation of the ACADVLD gene. It is inherited as an autosomal recessive trait and results in generalized weakness, muscle pain and episodes on collapse from exercise. DNA testing is available.

Breeds: 🐕 **German hunting terrier (jagdterrier)**

Exocrine Pancreatic Insufficiency (EPI)

Description: This is believed to be the final sequela to protracted immune-mediated atrophic lymphocytic pancreatitis. A genetic predisposition seems likely, but a mode of inheritance has not been determined with certainty in most breeds.

Breeds: 🐕 **Afghan hound, Airedale terrier, akita, Bedlington terrier, German shepherd dog, greyhound, collie, beagle, English setter, chow chow, Cavalier King Charles spaniel, Czechoslovakian wolfdog, greyhound, Newfoundland, Weimaraner, West Highland white terrier**

Facial Dermatitis

Description: Idiopathic feline facial dermatitis is a poorly characterized disorder associated with facial crusting and exudation. A genetic basis has not been determined, but breed predisposition has been recognized.

Breeds: 🐈 **Himalayan, Persian**

Factor I Deficiency (Fibrinogen Deficiency)

Description: Factor I, or fibrinogen, is the substrate for thrombin and the precursor of fibrin. Afibrinogenemia,

dysfibrinogenemia, and hypofibrinogenemia are subtypes, but since most case reports have not provided sufficient information to distinguish between dysfibrinogenemia and hypofibrinogenemia, it might be best to categorize the clinical severity as mild to severe rather than to worry about distinctions of terminology. Bleeding diathesis can be severe and require infusions of plasma or cryoprecipitate. Both autosomal recessive and autosomal dominant forms have been described in other species.

Breeds: 🐕 **Bernese mountain dog, borzoi, boxer, collie, German shorthaired pointer, St Bernard, vizsla**

Factor II Deficiency (Prothrombin Deficiency)

Description: Factor II, or prothrombin, is synthesized in the liver and is converted to thrombin by the action of the prothrombinase complex. Prothrombin deficiency is extremely rare in dogs. The condition is suspected when the activated partial thromboplastin time (aPTT) and prothrombin time (PT) are prolonged and the thrombin time (TT) is normal. The diagnosis is confirmed by analysis of factor II activity.

Breeds: 🐕 **Boxer, (American) cocker spaniel, (English) cocker spaniel, otterhound**

Factor VII Deficiency

Description: Factor VII deficiency is a relatively rare mild bleeding disorder with an autosomal recessive mode of inheritance. Animals rarely suffer from spontaneous hemorrhage but, rather, display easy bruising or postsurgical oozing. DNA testing is now available for breed-specific variants.

Breeds: 🐕 **Airedale terrier, Alaskan klee kai, Alaskan malamute, beagle, American foxhound, Bernese mountain dog, boxer, English bulldog, Finnish hound, German wirehaired pointer, giant schnauzer, Irish water spaniel, Japanese spitz, miniature schnauzer, papillon, Scottish deerhound, Sealyham terrier, Welsh springer spaniel**

Factor VIII Deficiency (Hemophilia A)

Description: Factor VIII deficiency is one of the most common inherited coagulopathies of dogs and cats, reported in almost all breeds. It is transmitted as an XCA and mutations are breed specific. The degree of factor VIII deficiency determines the extent of bleeding. Although hemophilia A has been reported in almost all breeds, DNA testing is variant specific.

Breeds: 🐕 **Akita, Alaskan malamute, Australian shepherd, beagle, berger blanc Suisse (white Swiss sheepdog), boxer, Boykin spaniel, Brittany spaniel, Chihuahua, American cocker spaniel, collie, dachshund, English bulldog, English setter, French bulldog, German shepherd dog, German shorthaired pointer, golden retriever, greyhound, Havanese, Irish setter, Labrador retriever, Lhasa apso, Manchester terrier, old English sheepdog, miniature poodle, Samoyed, miniature schnauzer, Shetland sheepdog, Shiloh shepherd, Siberian husky, vizsla, Weimaraner, Sloughi;** 🐈 **Havana Brown**

Factor IX Deficiency (Hemophilia B)

Description: Hemophilia B, also known as Christmas disease, affects many breeds of pets, and different gene mutations have been documented. The condition in different breeds likely results from different mutations in the factor IX gene. The disorder is transmitted as an XCA, regardless of the actual gene mutation present. DNA testing is available on a breed-specific basis.

Breeds: 🐕 **Airedale terrier, Alaskan malamute, American cocker spaniel, bichon frisé, black and tan coonhound, bull terrier, cairn terrier, Doberman pinscher, French bulldog, German shepherd dog, German wirehaired pointer, golden retriever, hovawart, Jack Russell terrier, Labrador retriever, Lhasa apso, old English sheepdog, Rhodesian ridgeback, St Bernard, Scottish terrier, Shetland sheepdog;** 🐈 **British shorthair, domestic shorthair, Siamese**

Factor X Deficiency

Description: Also known as Stuart–Power trait, this is a rare coagulopathy transmitted as an autosomal dominant trait, with incomplete penetrance. Individuals homozygous for the gene are usually stillborn or die within the first weeks of life with massive hemorrhage.

Breeds: 🐕 **American cocker spaniel, Jack Russell terrier**

Factor XI Deficiency

Description: Also known as plasma thromboplastin antecedent deficiency, or Rosenthal syndrome, this condition is

rare in dogs. The mode of inheritance in this species has not been confirmed, but is presumed to be autosomal recessive, although the mutations are breed specific. DNA testing is available for some variants.

Breeds: 🐕 **Great Pyrenees, Kerry blue terrier, English springer spaniel, Weimaraner**

Factor XII (Hageman Factor) Deficiency

Description: Also known as Hageman factor, this is transmitted as an autosomal recessive trait in dogs and cats. Fortunately, most animals with factor XII deficiency do not experience abnormal bleeding, so the deficiency is detected during evaluation for other problems.

Breeds: 🐕 **Chinese shar-pei, German shorthaired pointer, miniature poodle, standard poodle;** 🐈 **American shorthair, American longhair, Siamese**

Familial Nephropathy

Description: A varied group of congenital renal diseases that tend to have breed-specific clinical presentations and modes of inheritance. They tend to result in proteinuria, but clinical manifestations are condition specific. Familial nephropathy in American and English cocker spaniels is an inherited disease of glomerular basement membrane zone (type IV) collagen that results in progressive and irreversible renal failure. It is inherited as an autosomal recessive trait, the genetic variant has been identified, and DNA testing is available. In the English springer spaniel, it is also an autosomal recessive trait, the genetic variant has been characterized to the *COL4A4 gene, and DNA testing is available*. The conditions in the Nova Scotia duck tolling retriever and Samoyed are inherited as x-linked traits.

Breeds: 🐕 **Beagle, boxer, bullmastiff, bull terrier, chow chow, (American) cocker spaniel, Dalmatian, Doberman pinscher, dogue de Bordeaux, English cocker spaniel, English springer spaniel, Irish terrier, miniature schnauzer, Newfoundland, Norwegian elkhound, Nova Scotia duck tolling retriever, Pembroke Welsh corgi, Rottweiler, Samoyed, shih tzu, soft-coated wheaten terrier, Welsh springer spaniel**

Familial Shar-Pei Fever

Description: Also known as autoinflammatory disease, this is a chronic inflammatory disease associated with mutations in the MTBP gene. The mode of inheritance is believed to be autosomal dominant with incomplete penetrance. There is some similarity to familial Mediterranean fever in humans.

Breeds: 🐕 **Chinese shar-pei**

Familial Vasculopathy

Description: Familial vasculopathy is a rare and poorly understood condition that often starts in pups 6–8 weeks of age. The disorder is thought to be one of immune responsiveness but has not been fully characterized. It is presumed to have an autosomal recessive mode of inheritance in the German shepherd dog.

Breeds: 🐕 **Beagle, Dalmatian, German shepherd dog**

Fanconi Syndrome

Description: A family of inherited kidney diseases associated with genetic mutations of the PAN1 gene that result in proximal renal tubular dysfunction. This results in the urinary loss of essential metabolites such as glucose, amino acids, and phosphates. It is inherited as an autosomal recessive trait with variable expressivity. DNA testing is available for some variants.

Breeds: 🐕 **Basenji; idiopathic forms seen in Afghan hound, Border terrier, Doberman pinscher, Irish wolfhound, Labrador retriever, Norwegian elkhound, (miniature) schnauzer, Shetland sheepdog, Yorkshire terrier**

Feline Gastrointestinal Eosinophilic Sclerosing Fibroplasia

Description: An inflammatory gastrointestinal disease of cats characterized by eosinophilic masses in the stomach, intestines, and regional lymph nodes. The cause is not known, but there is a breed predisposition recognized.

Breeds: 🐈 **Ragdoll**

Feline Hyperesthesia Syndrome

Description: Also known as rolling skin disease, this is a poorly characterized skin disorder in which cats respond (periodically) in an exaggerated manner when touched. It

is not known whether this represents a behavioral disorder, a seizure disorder, or some peripheral neuropathy. A breed predisposition has been recognized.

Breeds: 🐈 **Burmese, Himalayan, Siamese**

Feline Lower Urinary Tract Disease (FLUTD)

Description: Also known as feline urological syndrome, this is a relatively common problem of adult cats associated with stranguria and dysuria. There are a variety of underlying causes. There is little evidence to suggest the problem is heritable, but breed predisposition has been recognized.

Breeds: 🐈 **Abyssinian, Persian, Siamese**

Feline Orofacial Pain Syndrome

Description: A bizarre and poorly understood condition in cats in which there is pawing at and rubbing at the face. The term is typically used for situations in which an underlying disorder (such as dental issues) has not been identified. A genetic basis has not been determined, but breed predisposition has been recognized

Breeds: 🐈 **Burmese**

Femoral Artery Occlusion

Description: Thrombosis of the femoral arteries is considered a primary form of vascular disease rather than just an extension of thromboembolism. Fortunately, the condition rarely results in any clinical signs because dogs have extensive collateral circulation in their hind limbs via lateral circumflex femoral and distal caudal femoral arteries.

Breeds: 🐕 **Cavalier King Charles spaniel**

Fibrocartilaginous Embolic Myelopathy

Description: A debilitating spinal disease in which emboli of fibrocartilaginous material obstructs the spinal canal and causes acute compression of the spinal cord, typically of the lower back. A breed predisposition has been recognized

Breeds: 🐈 **St Bernard, (miniature) schnauzer**

Fibrodysplasia Ossificans

Description: Also known as myositis ossificans, this is a rare progressive musculoskeletal disorder associated with heterotopic bone deposition. At least one genetic variant of the ACVR1 gene has been characterized. The condition bears similarities to fibrodysplasia ossificans progressiva in humans.

Breeds: Domestic shorthair

Flank Sucking

Description: Flank sucking is a poorly understood condition in which a dog sucks on a patch of skin on its flank. A hereditary component is suspected but not yet proven.

Breeds: Doberman pinscher

Fold Dermatitis

Description: The pyoderma that results in folds of skin that are continually traumatized by friction and do not have adequate ventilation. There are many different varieties, often breed specific.

Breeds: Bloodhound, Boston terrier, boxer, Chinese shar-pei, (American) cocker spaniel, English bulldog, English springer spaniel, French bulldog, Neapolitan mastiff, Pekingese, pug

Follicular Dysplasia

Description: Follicular dysplasia refers to a collection of breed-specific clinical entities associated with abnormal hair loss or defective follicle formation. This classification represents several unrelated conditions that share certain clinical features. Most of these disorders are poorly characterized, and the most striking feature is the breed predisposition. Examples include very breed-specific conditions, such as mucinous lymphoplasmacytic alopecia in the Norwegian lundehund and follicular lipidosis in the Rottweiler and dachshund. In boxers, the follicular dysplasia is sometimes associated with an interface dermatitis. Most variants are likely breed specific.

Breeds: Airedale, Alaskan malamute, American water spaniel, boxer, Chesapeake Bay retriever, Chihuahua, curly-coated retriever, dachshund, Doberman pinscher, English springer spaniel, greyhound, Irish water spaniel, Norwegian lundehund, Portuguese water dog, Rottweiler, Siberian husky, Weimaraner

Footpad Hyperkeratosis

Description: An inherited autosomal recessive trait most often associated with a mutation of the FAM83G gene that causes the accumulation of keratinized tissue on all footpads in young dogs. There are many causes of footpad hyperkeratosis, but this genetic variant has similarities to epidermolytic palmoplantar keratoderma in humans. A similar autosomal recessive condition involves the KRT16 gene in the dogue de Bordeaux. DNA testing is available for certain variants in specific breeds.

Breeds: Dogue de Bordeaux, Irish terrier, Kerry blue terrier, Kromfohrländer, German hunting terrier (jagdterrier)

Fucosidosis

Description: A devastating and fatal disease associated with an inherited deficiency of the enzyme alpha-L-fucosidase. The condition is transmitted as an autosomal recessive trait, and genetic testing is available.

Breeds: English springer spaniel

Galactosialidosis

Description: Galactosialidosis is an extremely rare form of sphingolipidosis characterized by a combined deficiency of alpha-galactosidase and beta-neuramidase enzyme activity caused by a peptide mutation.

Breeds: Schipperke

Gallbladder Mucocele

Description: A hepatobiliary disorder associated with mutations of the ABCB4 gene which then results in biliary mucus accumulation and bile duct obstruction. The mutation in Shetland sheepdogs is autosomal dominant with incomplete penetrance. DNA testing is available for some breed-specific variants. Most other cases likely result from progressive biliary sludging.

Breeds: 🐕 Border terrier, cairn terrier, Chihuahua, (American) cocker spaniel, (English) cocker spaniel, miniature poodle, miniature schnauzer, Pomeranian, Shetland sheepdog; cats

Gastric Carcinoma

Description: Gastric carcinoma is a malignant stomach cancer with a noted breed predisposition. it is an aggressive cancer and most cases have metastasis by the time a diagnosis is confirmed.

Breeds: 🐕 American Staffordshire terrier, Belgian Tervuren, Belgian Groenendael, bouvier des Flandres, chow chow, collie, Leonberger, Norwegian elkhound, Norwegian lundehund, Nova Scotia duck tolling retriever, Staffordshire bull terrier, standard poodle

Gastric Dilation And Volvulus (Bloat)

Description: Also known as bloat, this occurs when air gets swallowed (when susceptible dogs exercise, gulp their food or water, or are stressed), the stomach becomes distended with air, and then the stomach can twist on itself (volvulus or torsion) to be medically catastrophic. A mode of inheritance has not been determined, although breeds with a deeper and narrower thorax have an increased risk.

Breeds: 🐕 Boston terrier, (American) cocker spaniel, German shepherd dog, Great Dane, greyhound, Irish setter; many other breeds

German Shepherd Dog Pyoderma

Description: An aggressive, deep pyoderma that has a heritable component and an autosomal recessive inheritance has been suggested. An immunological imbalance is presumed to be associated with defective T-helper cells. The condition resembles a deep infection but with poor response to most antibiotic regimens or recurrence once a course of therapy has been discontinued.

Breeds: 🐕 German shepherd dog, and crosses

Glanzmann Thrombasthenia

Description: A family of inherited bleeding diseases associated with mutations of the ITGA2B gene and inherited in an autosomal recessive manner. The severity of bleeding episodes is quite variable. DNA testing is available on a breed-specific basis.

Breeds: 🐕 Great Pyrenees, otterhound

Glaucoma

Description: Glaucoma is caused by an increase in fluid pressure in the eye. Anything that interferes with drainage of fluid inside the eye can result in glaucoma, and not all cases have a genetic basis. Nevertheless, primary glaucoma does occur in several breeds, and inherited glaucoma is of three distinct types: (i) narrow angle, (ii) open angle, and (iii) goniodysgenesis. The primary open angle variants have been best characterized and DNA testing is available for some variants.

Breeds: 🐕 Afghan, akita, Alaskan malamute, American cocker spaniel, basset hound, beagle, Bedlington terrier, bouvier des Flandres, chow chow, dachshund, Dalmatian, Dandie Dinmont terrier, English cocker spaniel, English springer spaniel, Entlebucher mountain dog, Great Dane, keeshond, Maltese, miniature pinscher, miniature poodle, Newfoundland, Norwegian elkhound, saluki, Samoyed, schnauzer (miniature and giant), Sealyham terrier, shiba inu, shih tzu, Siberian husky, standard poodle, toy poodle, Welsh springer spaniel, Welsh terrier, West Highland white terrier, wire fox terrier; 🐈 Burmese, Siamese

Glaucoma (Congenital)

Description: A early-onset form of feline glaucoma in which intraocular pressure may be elevated, even by 8 weeks of age. In most breeds, it is characterized by mutations of the LTBP2 gene, and DNA testing is available for breed-specific variants.

Breeds: 🐈 Burmese, Persian, Siamese

Glaucoma (Goniodysgenesis)

Description: A form of glaucoma caused by a mutation in the olfactomedin-like 3 (OLFML3) gene. The condition is transmitted as an autosomal recessive trait, and DNA testing is available.

Breeds: 🐕 Border collie

Glaucoma, Primary Open-Angle Glaucoma (POAG)

Description: POAGs are often associated with breed-specific mutations of specific genes, such as ADAMTS10 and ADAMTS17. Most are transmitted as autosomal recessive traits and some risks can be identified by DNA testing. Some forms of POAG can be associated with other conditions, such as primary lens luxation (for example, in the Chinese shar-pei).

Breeds: Basset hound, basset fauve de Bretagne, beagle, Norwegian elkhound, pettit basset griffon Vendeen, Chinese shar-pei

Globoid Cell Leukodystrophy

Description: Globoid cell leukodystrophy, also known as galactocerebrosidosis or Krabbe disease, is a family of LSDs associated with mutations in the galactocerebrosidase (GALC) gene. The course is progressive and invariably fatal. It is inherited in an autosomal recessive manner. Genetic variants have been characterized and DNA testing is available.

Breeds: Australian kelpie, basset hound, beagle, bluetick hound, cairn terrier, Dalmatian, Irish setter, Irish red and white setter, miniature poodle, Pomeranian, West Highland white terrier; Domestic shorthair cat

Glomerulonephritis (Immune-Mediated)

Description: Immune-mediated glomerulonephritis can result from many causes, but hereditary forms have been recognized in some breeds. It is likely that the mutations are breed specific, as are the modes of inheritance.

Breeds: Bernese mountain dog, greyhound, soft-coated wheaten terrier

Glomerulosclerosis

Description: A poorly characterized congenital renal disease in which there is scarring of the glomeruli, which results in proteinuria. There are both genetic and nongenetic causes.

Breeds: Newfoundland

Glucocerebrosidosis

Description: A rare LSD caused by a deficiency of the glucocerebrosidase enzyme which results in neurological disease. The condition is characterized by Wallerian degeneration of cerebral, cerebellar, and spinal cord white matter. It is suspected to have an autosomal recessive mode of inheritance.

Breeds: Australian silky terrier, Australian terrier

Gluten-Sensitive Enteropathy

Description: Also known as wheat-sensitive enteropathy, this is a hereditary defect in small intestinal mucosal function associated with a sensitivity to or intolerance of gluten. It appears to be familial.

Breeds: Irish setter

Glycogen Storage Disease Type IA

Description: Also known as von Gierke disease, this is an inherited metabolic disorder resulting from a deficiency in the enzyme glucose 6-phosphatase-alpha (G6Pase) and inherited as an autosomal recessive trait. The result is hypoglycemia and the accumulation of glycogen and fat in the liver and kidneys. The mutation has been characterized in the *G6PC* gene, and DNA testing is available.

Breeds: Maltese

Glycogen Storage Disease Type II

Description: Also known as Pompe disease, this is a rare autosomal recessive condition caused by an acid alpha-glucosidase deficiency. The enzyme deficiency results in an accumulation of glycogen in tissues. The mutation has been characterized in the GAA gene, is transmitted as an autosomal recessive trait, and DNA testing is available.

Breeds: Finnish lapphund, Lapponian herder, Swedish lapphund

Glycogen Storage Disease Type III

Description: Also known as Cori's disease, this LSD is inherited as an autosomal recessive trait. Genetic testing is available.

Breeds: Akita, German shepherd dog

Glycogen Storage Disease Type IIIA

Description: A glycogen storage disease inherited as an autosomal recessive trait. It is caused by a mutation of the glycogen debranching enzyme gene (AGL). It is a progressive and debilitating disorder associated with glycogen accumulation in the liver and in muscles. The mutation has been characterized in the AGL gene, and breed-specific DNA testing is available.

Breeds: Curly-coated retriever, (miniature) dachshund

Glycogen Storage Disease Type IV

Description: Also known as glycogenosis type IV, this is a glycogen storage disease of cats, caused by a mutation of the GBE1 gene. It is inherited as an autosomal recessive trait. Affected animals develop progressive neuromuscular degeneration. DNA testing is available.

Breeds: Norwegian forest cat

GM-1 Gangliosidosis (Canine)

Description: Also known as Norman–Landing disease, this LSD caused by a mutation of the GBE1 gene is inherited as an autosomal recessive trait and refers to an enzyme deficit (beta-galactosidase) that allows toxic substances (GM-1 ganglioside) to build up in nerve cells. It is a progressive and fatal neurodegenerative disorder. DNA testing is available for some variants.

Breeds: **Alaskan husky, beagle, Portuguese water dog, shiba inu, Siberian husky, (English) springer spaniel**

GM-1 Gangliosidosis (Feline)

Description: GM-1 gangliosidosis belongs to the sphingolipidosis subgroup of the LSDs. This disorder is inherited as an autosomal recessive trait. The genetic mutation for some variants of feline GM-1 gangliosidosis (GLB1) have been characterized and DNA testing is available for some of those variants.

Breeds: **Balinese, Burmese, domestic shorthair, korat, Oriental, Peterbald, Siamese, Thai**

GM-2 Gangliosidosis (Canine)

Description: GM-2 gangliosidosis is inherited as an autosomal recessive trait and refers to mutations of the HEXB gene that allow toxic substances to build up in nerve cells. There are also subgroups recognized, each with its own breed-specific mutations. DNA testing is available for some variants.

Breeds: **German shorthaired pointer, golden retriever, Japanese chin, (miniature) poodle, (toy) poodle, shiba inu**

GM-2 Gangliosidosis (Feline)

Description: GM-2 gangliosidosis is inherited as an autosomal recessive trait and refers to an enzyme or activator deficit (hexosaminidases) that allows toxic substances to build up in nerve cells. A distinct GM-2a variant has also been recognized. Breed-specific variants have been characterized (GLB1), and DNA testing is available for some of those variants.

Breeds: **American shorthair, Burmese, Japanese domestic cat, korat**

Gracilis Or Semitendinosus Myopathy

Description: Myopathy of the gracilis or semitendinosUs muscles is a rare and poorly understood entity. Affected dogs are typically adults, and they develop a characteristic hindlimb lameness with shortened stride and leg rotation.

Breeds: **Belgian sheepdog (Groenendael), German shepherd dog**

Greyhound Alopecia

Description: A bilaterally symmetrical regional alopecia that involves the outer aspects of the thighs (bald thigh syndrome), and occasionally the ventrum; otherwise asymptomatic.

Breeds: **Greyhound**

Growth Hormone-Responsive Dermatoses

Description: A rare endocrine disorder purportedly related to growth hormone deficiency in adult dogs. It bears much similarity to the conditions known as alopecia X and adrenal sex hormone dermatosis, and these terms probably all describe the same poorly characterized entity.

Breeds: **American water spaniel, chow chow, keeshond, miniature and toy poodles, Pomeranian, Samoyed**

Hairlessness (Congenital Hypotrichosis)

Description: Hairlessness from birth can occur in different breeds, associated with breed-specific genetic mutations.

Breeds purposely bred to be hairless typically represent the heterozygous state (Hrhr) of an autosomal semidominant trait which is believed to be lethal in the homozygous form. However, in the American hairless terrier (rat terrier), the hairlessness is transmitted as an autosomal recessive trait, with affected animals being homozygous (haha). In the Mexican hairless, hairlessness is inherited by an autosomal dominant trait (Hm), and litters may include both hairless and coated individuals. In breeds not intended to be hairless, hypotrichosis is a congenital, and probably hereditary, problem. Variants in the SGK3 and FOXI3 genes have been implicated in some hairless breeds. DNA testing is available for some breed-specific variants.

Breeds: 🐕 **Abyssinian sand terrier (African hairless dog), American hairless terrier, Mexican hairless (Xoloitzcuintli), Peruvian Inca Orchid, Chinese crested dog, and Turkish naked dog; occasionally seen in basset hound, beagle, Belgian shepherd, bichon frisé, cocker spaniel, French bulldog, Labrador retriever, Lhasa apso, rat terrier, Rottweiler, Scottish deerhound, toy poodle, whippet, Yorkshire terrier;** 🐈 **Sphynx**

HEART BLOCK

Description: Cardiac disease associated with failure in electrical conductivity within the heart. Classified as first-degree, second-degree, and third-degree heart block depending on the location and extent of the problem. A genetic basis has not been determined, but breed predisposition has been recognized.

Breeds: 🐕 **Catahoula leopard dog, chow chow**

Hemivertebra

Description: Hemivertebra results when the vertebra does not develop properly, typically because of persistence of the notochord or lack of ossification. It is most frequently seen in the screw-tailed breeds where it can be subclassified into subtypes, which often have their own breed predispositions. In the German shepherd dog and German shorthaired pointer, hemivertebra occurs as an autosomal recessive disorder.

Breeds: 🐕 **American Eskimo dog, basset hound, Boston terrier, cairn terrier, Doberman pinscher, English bulldog, French bulldog, German shepherd dog, German shorthaired pointer, Pekingese, pug, Rottweiler, Scottish terrier, Yorkshire terrier**

Hemophagocytic Syndrome

Description: Also known as hemophagocytic lymphohistiocytosis, this condition is a hyperinflammatory disorder that can be a primary inherited immune incompetency or occur secondary to underlying infections or cancer. A genetic basis has not been determined, but breed predisposition has been recognized

Breeds: 🐕 **Tibetan terrier**

Hemorrhagic Gastroenteritis

Description: Acute episodes of vomiting and diarrhea associated with gastrointestinal blood loss. A genetic basis has not been determined, but breed predisposition has been recognized.

Breeds: 🐕 **Maltese, miniature pinscher**

Hepatocerebellar Degeneration

Description: A poorly characterized disorder seen in puppies that affects both the cerebellum and the liver. Affected animals are usually evident by 6 weeks of age with signs consistent with cerebellar ataxia; most do not live past 6 months of age. It appears to be transmitted as an autosomal recessive trait.

Breeds: 🐕 **Bernese mountain dog**

Hereditary Myopathy (Feline)

Description: A heritable form of myopathy in the Devon Rex cat associated with muscle weakness. It is transmitted as an autosomal recessive trait, and the variant has been identified in the COLQ gene. DNA testing is available for some breed-specific variants.

Breeds: 🐈 **Devon Rex, Sphynx**

Hereditary Nephritis (Dominant)

Description: An autosomal dominant form of the disease, similar to Alport syndrome, has been recognized as a breed-specific variant of hereditary nephritis, likely associated with a mutation of the pkd1 locus. The variant in the Dalmatian is similar to but distinct from that of the bull terrier.

Breeds: 🐕 **Bull terrier, (miniature) bull terrier, Dalmatian**

Hereditary Nephritis (X-Linked)

Description: Also known as Alport syndrome, this is an inherited kidney disease that progresses toward kidney failure and is associated with mutations in the COL4A5 gene. The condition in the Samoyed is transmitted as a x-linked recessive trait and genetic testing is available.

Breeds: 🐕 **Samoyed**

Hernia (Hiatal)

Description: Problems that result when gastrointestinal organs breach the diaphragm and occupy the chest cavity. A genetic basis has not been determined, but breed predisposition has been recognized.

Breeds: Chinese shar-pei, English bulldog

Hernia (Inguinal)

Description: Inguinal hernias may arise as a result of congenital inguinal ring anomalies or trauma. They are most common in males, but any mode of inheritance has not been determined.

Breeds: 🐕 **Basenji, basset hound, cairn terrier, Pekingese, West Highland white terrier**

Hernia (Perineal)

Description: A musculoskeletal problem in which the muscles of the pelvic floor weaken, and allow an opening for abdominal contents to poke through in the area of the perineum. A genetic basis has not been determined, but breed predisposition has been recognized.

Breeds: 🐕 **Afghan hound, Australian kelpie, Boston terrier, bouvier des Flandres, boxer, Chinese shar-pei, collie, old English sheepdog, Pekingese, (Cardigan) Welsh corgi, (Pembroke) Welsh corgi, Yorkshire terrier**

Hernia (Peritoneopericardial)

Description: Peritoneopericardial diaphragmatic hernia involves abdominal contents that are herniated into the pericardial sac because of direct communication between the peritoneal and the pericardial cavities. It is the most common congenital defect involving the pericardium of dogs and cats. It is not known if the condition is heritable, but breed predisposition has been recognized.

Breeds: 🐕 **Weimaraner;** 🐈 **Himalayan, Maine Coon, Persian**

Hernia (Umbilical)

Description: Congenital umbilical hernias are the most common abdominal hernias in dogs and the result of congenital inguinal ring anomalies or trauma. They are believed to be inherited in many cases and are more common in males, but the mode of inheritance remains unknown.

Breeds: 🐕 **Airedale terrier, basenji, basset hound, cairn terrier, Pekingese, pointer, Weimaraner, West Highland white terrier**

Heterochromia Iridis

Description: Sometimes referred to as odd-eyed, the situation in both dogs and cats where each eye has a different color. In most instances it is associated with white coloring, merling, harlequin, or piebaldism. In most instances the different eye colors are not associated with health issues, but the animal may be at higher risk of partial or total deafness.

Breeds: 🐕 Australian cattle *dog*, Australian shepherd, Border collie, Catahoula leopard dog, Chihuahua, dachshund, Dalmatian, Great Dane (harlequin), Shetland sheepdog, shih tzu, Siberian husky; 🐈 British shorthair, Cornish Rex, Devon Rex, Japanese bobtail, Munchkin, Persian, Scottish fold, Siamese, Sphynx, Turkish angora, Turkish van

Hip Dysplasia

Description: Hip dysplasia is an abnormal development of the hip (coxofemoral) joint and is actually a tardive genetically transmitted tendency to develop laxity of the hip joints. The mode of inheritance is polygenic, likely influenced by several different genes. Nongenetic factors play an important role in expression as well. Genetic markers have been identified that can help determine risk on a breed-specific basis.

Breeds: 🐕 **Airedale terrier, Alaskan malamute, bearded collie, Bernese mountain dog, bloodhound, Border collie, bouvier des Flandres, Brittany spaniel, bullmastiff, Chesapeake Bay retriever, chow chow, English bulldog, German shepherd dog, German**

wirehaired pointer, golden retriever, Gordon setter, Great Dane, Great Pyrenees, keeshond, kuvasz, Labrador retriever, mastiff, Neapolitan mastiff, Newfoundland, Norwegian elkhound, old English sheepdog, pointer, Portuguese water dog, Rottweiler, St Bernard, Samoyed, (giant) schnauzer, Treeing Walker coonhound; American bobtail, American shorthair, American wirehair, Devon Rex, Himalayan, Maine Coon, Persian

Histiocytosis

Description: Cutaneous histiocytosis, hystiocytic sarcoma, and systemic histiocytosis (also known as disseminated histiocytic sarcoma) are related histiocytic disorders of antigen-presenting cells. Histiocytic sarcoma seems to result from a combination of genetic and environmental elements, and genetic markers are associated with risk of developing this cancer in specific breeds.

Breeds: Bernese mountain dog, Doberman pinscher, flat-coated retriever, golden retriever, keeshond, Labrador retriever, Rottweiler, (miniature) schnauzer

Hydrocephalus

Description: Hydrocephalus is a condition in which the brain swells from the accumulation of cerebrospinal fluid (CSF). The cause can be either congenital or secondary to some obstructive process in the outflow of CSF. Although the mode of inheritance for hydrocephalus has been determined in cats, only a familial trend in brachycephalic and small dogs has been documented. Largely unrelated to hydrocephalus, cerebral ventriculomegaly has been reported in English bulldogs, often as an incidental finding. Mode of inheritance has not been determined. In young bullmastiffs, hydrocephalus has been described in association with cerebellar ataxia.

Breeds: Boston terrier, cairn terrier, Chihuahua, English bulldog, Lhasa apso, Maltese, Manchester terrier, miniature poodle, papillon (phalene), Pekingese, Pomeranian, pug, shih tzu, toy poodle, Yorkshire terrier; Balinese

Hyperadrenocorticism (Cushing's Syndrome)

Description: Hyperadrenocorticism, also known as Cushing's syndrome, results when the body produces too much cortisol, its own form of cortisone. Most cases result from a tumor (not usually malignant) in the pituitary gland (pituitary-dependent hyperadrenocorticism) while a small percentage of cases arise from tumors (half are malignant) on the adrenal glands (adrenal-dependent hyperadrenocorticism), located near the kidneys.

Breeds: Australian shepherd, Australian terrier, beagle, Bedlington terrier, boxer, Boston terrier, cairn terrier, (American) cocker spaniel, dachshund, Dandie Dinmont terrier, German shepherd dog, Jack Russell terrier, miniature poodle, miniature schnauzer, standard schnauzer, silky terrier, West Highland white terrier, Yorkshire terrier

Hyperhomocysteinemia

Description: This can occur as a primary or secondary event. Elevated homocysteine levels can be seen in some breeds, but can also be an inflammatory marker for heart and kidney disease, as well as hypothyroidism. A genetic basis has not been determined, but breed predisposition has been recognized.

Breeds: Greyhound

Hyperlipidemia (Hypercholesterolemia)

Description: An inherited tendency to high cholesterol levels. Most are secondary to underlying problems such as nephrotic syndrome, hypothyroidism, and cholestasis, but familial forms have been recognized

Breeds: Collie, Doberman pinscher, Great Pyrenees, Rottweiler, Shetland sheepdog

Hyperlipidemia (Hypertriglyceridemia)

Description: An inherited tendency to high triglyceride levels, typically with prevalence and severity increasing with age. May predispose to pancreatitis, corneal dystrophies, seizures, neuropathies, and even cerebral atherosclerosis.

Breeds: Beagle, Briard, (miniature) schnauzer; Burmese

Hyperoxaluria (Canine)

Description: A group of disorders in which genetic mutations result in the liver producing excessive oxalates, which can result in kidney damage. Primary hyperoxaluria type I is the most common form seen in dogs. The mutation has been characterized (AGXT) as an autosomal recessive disorder in the coton de Tulear and DNA testing is available. A similar condition has been reported in the Tibetan spaniel.

Breeds: 🐕 **Coton de Tulear, Tibetan spaniel**

Hyperoxaluria (Feline)

Description: Also known as oxalosis II, this is an autosomal recessive kidney disease associated with deficiencies of the enzymes D-glycerate dehydrogenase and glyoxylate reductase caused by a mutation in the glyoxylate reductase (GRHPR) gene. Affected cats develop kidney failure associated with oxalate crystal deposition by 5–9 months of age. Genetic variants have been characterized, and DNA testing is available.

Breeds: 🐈 **Domestic shorthair**

Hyperparathyroidism

Description: An endocrine condition associated with breed-specific mutations and modes of inheritance. It leads to stunted growth, polyuria, polydipsia, and muscle weakness. Congenital hyperparathyroidism in the keeshond is inherited as an autosomal dominant trait with incomplete penetrance, and DNA testing is available on a breed-specific basis.

Breeds: 🐕 **Dachshund, German shepherd dog, golden retriever, keeshond;** 🐈 **Siamese**

Hyperphosphatemia

Description: Benign familial hyperphosphatemia bears significant resemblance to benign persistent familial hyperphosphatemia in humans. The mode of inheritance is not known precisely but is autosomal and likely recessive. It can result in spurious elevations of serum alkaline phosphatase, unrelated to any form of liver disease.

Breeds: 🐕 **Scottish terrier, Siberian husky**

Hypertension

Description: High blood pressure, or hypertension, has been reported in dogs and cats. Guidelines now exist for the identification, evaluation, and management of systemic hypertension in both species.

Breeds: 🐕 **Greyhound, Labrador retriever, Siberian husky**

Hypertrophic Gastritis

Description: A rare form of gastritis characterized by pronounced rugal folds and glandular hyperplasia. Other than in the Dutch partridge dog in which it appears to be heritable, it is only seen randomly in other breeds.

Breeds: 🐕 **Drentse patrijshond (Dutch partridge dog)**

Hypertrophic Osteodystrophy

Description: Also known as Moeller–Barlow disease and metaphyseal osteopathy, this is a developmental condition affecting primarily young, rapidly growing large-breed dogs. The condition is thought to be familial, but a mode of inheritance has not been determined.

Breeds: 🐕 **Akbash dog, Bernese mountain dog, borzoi, boxer, Doberman pinscher, German shepherd dog, golden retriever, Great Dane, Irish setter, kuvasz, Labrador retriever, Rottweiler, Weimaraner**

Hyperuricosuria

Description: An inherited tendency to excrete large amounts of uric acid into the urine. It is transmitted as an autosomal recessive trait, the condition is caused by a mutation in the SCL2A9 gene, and DNA testing is available.

Breeds: 🐕 **Alaskan husky, American bulldog, American bully, American pitbull terrier, American Staffordshire terrier, Australian cattle dog, Australian shepherd, beagle, black Russian terrier, boerboel, bulldog, Catahoula leopard dog, collie, Dalmatian, Danish-Swedish farmdog, French bulldog, German hunting terrier, German shepherd, giant schnauzer, Jack Russell/Parsons terrier, Kromfohrländer, Labrador retriever, Lagotto Romagnolo, Large Münsterländer, South African boerboel, spaniel de Pont-Audemer, Spanish water dog, Swedish vallhund, vizsla, Weimaraner; many others**

Hyperuricosuria (2,8-Dihydroxyadenine)

Description: A form of hyperuricosuria associated with a mutation in the APRT gene. The mode of inheritance is presumed to be autosomal recessive, and only homozygotes develop 2,8-dihydroxyadenine uroliths. DNA testing is available.

Breeds: 🐕 **Native American Indian dog**

Hypoadrenocorticism (Addison's Disease)

Description: A endocrine disorder for which inherited juvenile forms have been recognized. Familial hypoadrenocorticism has been described, and inherited as autosomal recessive traits in at least some breeds. DNA testing is breed specific.

Breeds: 🐕 **Airedale terrier, American Eskimo dog, basset hound, beagle, bearded collie, Bernese mountain dog, cairn terrier, American cocker spaniel, Great Dane, Great Pyrenees, Leonberger, Nova Scotia duck tolling retriever, Pomeranian, Portuguese water dog, poodle (miniature, standard), Rottweiler, St Bernard, soft-coated wheaten terrier, English springer spaniel, Wachtelhund, West Highland white terrier**

Hypokalemic Periodic Polymyopathy

Description: Also known as Burmese hypokalemia, this is an unusual cause of muscle weakness that is autosomal recessive and associated with mutations of the WNK4 gene. DNA testing is available for breed-specific variants.

Breeds: 🐈 **Australian mist, Bombay, Burmese, Tonkinese, Burmilla, Cornish Rex, Devon Rex, Singapura, Sphynx, Tiffanie**

Hypomagnesemia

Description: There are a variety of underlying causes for magnesium depletion, but low magnesium levels may also be seen in association with certain breed predispositions. It is believed that brachycephalic breeds, such as the English bulldog, may be predisposed to arterial hypertension and obstructive sleep apnea, which can be associated with chronic magnesium (Mg) depletion. Occasionally other breeds area also affected.

Breeds: 🐕 **Collie, English bulldog**

Hypomyelination

Description: Also known as shaking puppy syndrome, this is a group of neurological disorders that result in delayed myelination that eventuates in tremors. These are breed-specific hereditary disorders that may differ in genetic mutations, clinical characteristics and modes of inheritance (x-linked in springer spaniels, autosomal recessive in

Weimaraners, etc.). DNA testing is available for some breed-specific variants. Also, see the entry for Alexander disease for more information on the hypomyelination variant seen in Bernese mountain dogs.

Breeds: 🐕 **Bernese mountain dog, English springer spaniel, Weimaraner**

Hypoparathyroidism

Description: A hormonal imbalance most often associated with a lymphocytic infiltration of the parathyroid levels, resulting in hypocalcemia and elevated blood phosphorus levels. A genetic basis has not been determined, but breed predisposition has been recognized.

Breeds: 🐕 **St Bernard, (toy) poodle, (miniature) schnauzer, Scottish terrier**

Hypophosphatasia

Description: A skeletal disease associated with an autosomal recessive defect in the alkaline phosphatase gene, ALPL. The condition is characterized by reduced serum alkaline phosphatase activity and defective mineralization of bone and teeth. DNA testing is available.

Breeds: 🐕 **Karelian bear dog**

Hypospadias

Description: An abnormal opening of the urethra. A mode of inheritance is not known, but there is a breed predisposition.

Breeds: 🐕 **Boston terrier, German shepherd dog**

Hypothyroidism

Description: Hypothyroidism is a complex syndrome associated with a progressive deficiency of thyroid hormone. It is the most common of the endocrine disorders seen in dogs, with clear familial tendencies, but a mode of inheritance has not been determined in most breeds.

Breeds: 🐕 **Afghan hound, Airedale terrier, Alaskan malamute, beagle, boxer, borzoi, Chinese shar-pei, chow chow, (American) cocker spaniel, dachshund, Doberman pinscher, English bulldog, golden retriever, Great Dane, Irish setter, Irish wolfhound, miniature schnauzer, Newfoundland, Pomeranian, poodle, Shetland sheepdog and many others**

Hypothyroidism, Congenital

Description: A group of disorders in which breed-specific genetic mutations in the thyroid peroxidase (TPO) gene result in the failure to produce typical thyroid hormones. The result is an enlarged thyroid gland (goiter) and clinical signs collectively known as cretinism. It most breeds, the thyroid disorder is inherited as autosomal recessive traits. Several breed-specific genetic variants have been characterized, many on the TPO gene, and DNA testing is available for those variants.

Breeds: 🐕 American foxhound, fox terrier (toy), French bulldog, rat terrier, Spanish water dog, Tenterfield terrier; 🐈 Domestic shorthair

Hypotrichosis (Canine)

Description: Hairlessness refers to congenital alopecia and is covered as a separate topic, but hypotrichosis denotes not necessarily an absence of fur, but less fur than would typically be anticipated. In breeds not intended to be hairless, hypotrichosis is a congenital, and probably hereditary, problem. Variants in the SGK3 allele have been implicated in some breeds.

Breeds: 🐕 Basset hound, beagle, Belgian shepherd, bichon frisé, (American) cocker spaniel, French bulldog, Irish water spaniel, Labrador retriever, Lhasa apso, poodle (toy, miniature), Rottweiler, Scottish deerhound, whippet, Yorkshire terrier

Hypotrichosis (Feline)

Description: A condition of feline hairlessness that is autosomal recessive in nature and associated with a mutation of the FOXN1 gene in the Birman. The result is not only hairlessness, but affected cats also have a shortened lifespan. DNA testing is available. Other forms of hypotrichosis in other breeds have also been recognized.

Breeds: 🐈 Birman, Devon Rex

Ichthyosis

Description: A condition in which the surface of the skin becomes covered with thick, tenacious scale. There are several genetic mechanisms and several different variants of both epidermolytic and nonepidermolytic ichthyoses. DNA testing is available for several distinct breed-specific variants, such as in the American bulldog (NIPAL4), Jack Russell terrier (TGM1), golden retriever (PNPLA1), Norfolk terrier (KRT10), Great Dane (SLC27A4), German shepherd dog (ASPRV1), etc. The condition "milk crust" may refer to a transient form of golden retriever ichthyosis.

Breeds: 🐕 American bulldog, American pit bull terrier, American Staffordshire terrier, Cavalier King Charles spaniel, Doberman pinscher, German shepherd dog, golden retriever, Great Dane, Irish setter, Irish terrier, Jack Russell terrier, Labrador retriever, Norfolk terrier, Parson Russell terrier, Rhodesian ridgeback, Rottweiler, soft-coated wheaten terrier, standard poodle, West Highland white terrier, Yorkshire terrie,

Idiopathic Multifocal Osteopathy

Description: A poorly documented condition characterized by multifocal absence of bone in the skull, cervical spine, and proximal extremities. Some of the characteristics are shared with human osteolysis syndromes, particularly Winchester syndrome and vanishing bone disease.

Breeds: 🐕 Scottish terrier

Immune-Mediated Hemolytic Anemia

Description: A loss of red blood cells due to immune-mediated destruction, either as a primary or secondary event. A genetic basis has not been determined, but breed predisposition has been recognized.

Breeds: 🐕 Airedale terrier, bichon frisé, cairn terrier, American cocker spaniel, collie, Finnish spitz, Labrador retriever, Maltese, miniature pinscher, miniature schnauzer, old English sheepdog, Parson Russell terrier, saluki, Shetland sheepdog, (English) springer spaniel, vizsla

Immune-Mediated Inflammatory Myopathy

Description: An apparent polymyopathy associated with autoantibodies and cytokines targeting skeletal muscle. Similar conditions have been reported periodically, but in certain breeds are thought to be familial.

Breeds: 🐕 Pembroke Welsh corgi, vizsla

Immune-Mediated Polyarthritis

Description: This represents a diverse collection of disorders that could be breed specific, idiopathic, or considered as reactive immune-mediated nonerosive polyarthritis. Similar presentations can represent a manifestation of systemic lupus erythematosus, or be secondary to underlying events. The end result is immune complex deposition in joint tissue.

Breeds: 🐕 **Akita, American Eskimo dog, beagle, Bernese mountain dog, boxer, German shepherd dog, German shorthaired pointer, Labrador retriever, Weimaraner**

Immune-Mediated Rheumatic Disease

Description: A group of diseases characterized by antibodies targeting body functions. The most common manifestation is polyarthritis. A genetic basis has not been determined, but breed predisposition has been recognized.

Breeds: 🐕 **Nova Scotia duck tolling retriever**

Immune-Mediated Thrombocytopenia

Description: An autoimmune disease in which platelets are targeted, resulting in impaired clotting and susceptibility to prolonged bleeding times. A genetic basis has not been determined, but breed predisposition has been recognized.

Breeds: 🐕 **Airedale terrier, (American) cocker spaniel, old English sheepdog**

Immunodeficiency Syndrome

Description: This term has been used for poorly characterized disorders of the immune system, for which more specific causative terminology has been lacking. They likely represent different entities with breed-specific features. In Chinese shar-pei, this includes deficiencies of multiple immunoglobulin classes and cell-mediated responses. In Rottweilers, there is increased susceptibility to parvovirus infection, and perhaps to other infections as well. The condition in Weimaraners seems to be associated with immunoglobulin deficiencies and susceptibility to infection and possibly adverse reactions to vaccines.

Breeds: 🐕 **Chinese shar-pei, Rottweiler, Weimaraner**

Immunoglobulin A (IGA) Deficiency

Description: Selective IgA deficiency is the most common specific immunoglobulin deficiency in dogs. Clinically, IgA deficiency can manifest as surface infections, including recurrent respiratory infections, urinary tract infections, and skin infections.

Breeds: 🐕 **Akita, beagle, Chinese shar-pei, German shepherd dog, American cocker spaniel, chow chow, dachshund, Dalmatian, golden retriever, hovawart, Irish setter, miniature schnauzer, Norwegian elkhound, Nova Scotia duck tolling retriever, Rottweiler, West Highland white terrier**

Immunoproliferative Enteropathy

Description: A poorly understood familial disorder characterized by chronic intermittent bouts of diarrhea, anorexia, and weight loss. It is really a syndrome, associated with an immune-mediated intestinal condition (lymphoplasmacytic enteritis), protein loss through the intestines (protein-losing enteropathy), abnormal digestion of nutrients (maldigestion), poor absorption (malabsorption), and increased concentrations of immunoglobulin A (IgA) in the bloodstream.

Breeds: 🐕 **Basenji**

Improper Coat (Furnishings)

Description: A breed-specific term used in the Portuguese water dog to reflect an undesirable variation in the coat affecting texture and appearance, including a lack of furnishings (moustache, eyebrows). It is transmitted as an autosomal recessive trait, the mutation to the RSPO2 gene has been characterized, and DNA testing is available. While improper coat is a term applied to the Portuguese water dog, it is important to realize that alterations to furnishings can be associated with mutations to the RSPO2 gene in many different breeds.

Breeds: 🐕 **Portuguese water dog**

Inflammatory Bowel Disease

Description: A chronic inflammatory reaction in the gastrointestinal tract that results in diarrhea, weight loss, and sometimes, abdominal pain and discomfort. Genetics may play some role, but other factors (e.g., adverse food reactions) likely are of more importance.

Breeds: 🐕 Border collie, boxer, Clumber spaniel, Dutch shepherd, greyhound, Norwegian elkhound, Peruvian Inca Orchid, Portuguese water dog, Rottweiler, sloughi, Weimaraner, West Highland white terrier, Yorkshire terrier; 🐈 Siamese

Inflammatory Myopathy

Description: A rare condition of young dogs characterized by muscle tremors, pelvic limb stiffness, progressive weakness, and severe muscle atrophy. In the Dutch shepherd, it appears to be caused by a mutation within a disease-associated mitochondrial transporter gene and is transmitted as an autosomal recessive trait. DNA testing is available for some variants.

Breeds: 🐕 Boxer, Dutch shepherd, Newfoundland

Inflammatory Pulmonary Disease

Description: Also known as recurrent inflammatory pulmonary disease, this is an inherited lung disease associated with recurrent pneumonia. The genetic mutation (AKNA) has been characterized, and DNA testing is available.

Breeds: 🐕 Collie

Inherited Myopathy

Description: Also known as central core myopathy, this is a rare degenerative muscle disorder that tends to manifest itself before 1 year of age. The genetic variant has been characterized to the BIN1 gene, and the condition is transmitted as an autosomal recessive trait. Breed-specific DNA testing is available.

Breeds: 🐕 Great Dane

Intersex, Chromosomal

Description: Chromosomal intersex, resulting from abnormalities in chromosomal sexual differentiation, is rare in dogs and cats and is thought not to have a genetic basis. Examples include Klinefelter syndrome (XXY), Turner syndrome (XO), X trisomy (XXX), chimeras, and mosaics.

Breeds: 🐕 Doberman pinscher

Intersex, Gonadal

Description: Gonadal intersex results from sexual differentiation abnormalities in the gonads, including XX sex reversal, limited to dogs with XX chromosome constitution. Sexual reversal refers to animals in which chromosomal sex and gonadal sex differ. Those with an XX chromosome complement (hereditary XX sex reversal) can have the external appearance of a female and ovotestes internally. True hermaphrodites possess characteristics of both sexes. The old term pseudohermaphroditism was used for situations when the animals was born with primary sex characteristics of one sex but developed the secondary sex characteristics different from what would be expected on the basis of the gonadal tissue (ovary or testis).

Breeds: 🐕 Basset hound, beagle, (American) cocker spaniel, (English) cocker spaniel, German short-haired pointer, Jack Russell terrier, Kerry blue terrier, Norwegian elkhound, Parson Russell terrier, Pekingese, (miniature) poodle, pug, soft-coated wheaten terrier, Weimaraner

Intervertebral Disk Disease

Description: A debilitating condition of the intervertebral disks, especially more prevalent in chondrodystrophic breeds. The most common breed affected is the dachshund. An FGF4 mutation is associated with this condition and with chondrodystrophy, and can be used to help determine risk in a breed-specific manner.

Breeds: 🐕 Basset hound, beagle, bichon frisé, Cavalier King Charles spaniel, Chesapeake Bay retriever, Chihuahua, Chinese crested, (American) cocker spaniel, coton de Tulear, dachshund, Dandie Dinmont terrier, English springer spaniel, French bulldog, Havanese, Jack Russell terrier, Lhasa apso, Nova Scotia duck tolling retriever, Pekingese, Pomeranian, poodle, Portuguese water dog, shih tzu, Welsh corgi and many others; 🐈 British shorthair, Persian

Intestinal Villus Atrophy

Description: This refers to loss of villus absorptive ability in the small intestine. In most cases, this is due to other disease processes, such as parvovirus infection, gluten sensitivity, or as a secondary event to infiltration to inflammatory or neoplastic cells. In some instances, there may be a breed predisposition as a primary cause.

Breeds: 🐕 Bouvier des Flandres

Iris Cysts

Description: Also known as uveal cysts, these structures are usually asymptomatic although secondary changes can potentially impact vision and intraocular fluid drainage and rarely can progress to pigmentary uveitis. Iris cysts are common in dogs, but some breeds are believed to be predisposed. The condition in cats is almost always benign, and occurs later in life.

Breeds: 🐕 **American bulldog, Boston terrier, golden retriever, Irish red and white setter, Irish wolfhound, Newfoundland;** 🐈 **Burmese**

Iris Hypoplasia and Coloboma

Description: A developmental disorder in which the iris fails to develop properly. A genetic basis has not been determined, but breed predisposition has been recognized. Iris colobomas are congenital holes that develop because of iris thinness. On their own they do not affect vision, but can predispose to other problems.

Breeds: 🐕 **Pug, Sussex spaniel**

Iris Sphincter Dysplasia

Description: A congenital anomaly in which there is abnormal development of the muscles responsible for pupillary contraction, resulting in pupillary dilation. The mode of inheritance is not yet known.

Breeds: 🐕 **Dalmatian**

Irish Wolfhound Respiratory Disorder

Description: A familial respiratory disorder most often associated with rhinitis and bronchopneumonia. This disorder is poorly characterized, and believed to be heritable, but a mode of inheritance has not been determined.

Breeds: 🐕 **Irish wolfhound**

Iron-Deficiency Anemia

Description: A rare form of familial iron-deficiency anemia that tends to be resistant to iron supplementation, purportedly due to overproduction of hepcidin which impairs iron absorption. The condition is presumed to be transmitted as an autosomal recessive trait, caused by a mutation in the TMPRSS6 gene. DNA testing is available.

Breeds: 🐕 **American cocker spaniel, English cocker spaniel**

Juvenile Cellulitis

Description: Juvenile cellulitis, also known as juvenile pyoderma and puppy strangles, is a disease of young dogs (usually younger than 6 months) that likely has an immunological pathogenesis. Clinically, the condition involves swelling and inflammation of the face and submandibular lymph nodes.

Breeds: 🐕 **Australian terrier, dachshund, English pointer, golden retriever, Gordon setter, (yellow) Labrador retriever, Lhasa apso**

Juvenile Encephalopathy

Description: Also known as juvenile brain disease, this serious neurological disorder has an early onset at 6–12 weeks of age. Early manifestations include seizures, but then progress to irreversible brain damage. The genetic variant has been characterized, the condition is transmitted as an autosomal recessive trait, and DNA testing is available.

Breeds: 🐕 **Jack Russell terrier, Parson Russell terrier**

Keratoconjunctivitis Sicca

Description: KCS, or dry eye, is a common condition in dogs. It results from reduction in the amount of watery tears produced by the lacrimal glands. Although KCS is believed to have a familial component, a mode of inheritance has only been determined for a few variants.

Breeds: 🐕 **Bloodhound, Boston terrier, bull terrier, Cavalier King Charles spaniel, Chihuahua, Chinese pug, chinese shar-pei, chow chow, Clumber spaniel, (American) cocker spaniel, (English) cocker spaniel, English bulldog, English setter, Gordon setter, Kerry blue terrier, Lhasa apso, miniature dachshund, miniature poodle, miniature schnauzer, Pekingese, pug, Sealyham terrier, shih tzu, Welsh terrier, West Highland white terrier, Yorkshire terrier and many others**

Klippel–Trenaunay Syndrome

Description: A rare congenital disorder involving discolored patches on the skin, excess bone and soft tissue growth, and venous malformation. Mode of inheritance is not known

Breeds: 🐕 **Border collie**

Laryngeal Paralysis

Description: Hereditary laryngeal paralysis is characterized by failure of vocal folds and arytenoid cartilage to abduct properly during inspiration. The disorder has been described as hereditary, but presentation and mode of inheritance tend to be breed specific. Laryngeal paralysis can also be a feature of other inherited disorders, including laryngeal paralysis associated with polyneuropathy. Different genetic variants have been determined in specific breeds, and DNA testing is available for some of those variants.

Breeds: 🐕 **Black Russian terrier, bouvier des Flandres, bull terrier, (miniature) bull terrier, Dalmatian, English bulldog, Great Pyrenees, Leonberger, Rottweiler, Siberian husky**

Laryngeal Paralysis and Polyneuropathy

Description: Inherited neurological disorders caused by mutations to the RAB3GAP1 gene, and inherited as an autosomal recessive trait. It bears some resemblance to Charcot–Marie–Tooth disease in people. DNA testing is available for some breed-specific variants

Breeds: 🐕 **Alaskan husky, black Russian terrier, bouvier des Flandres, Dalmatian, Great Pyrenees, Irish setter, Labrador retriever, Leonberger, Rhodesian ridgeback, Rottweiler**

Late-Onset Ataxia

Description: Sometimes referred to as spinocerebellar ataxia, this is a condition that affects pets between 6 and 12 months of age. It starts with incoordination and balance issues, and progresses to more generalized disability. The condition is transmitted as an autosomal recessive trait, the variant has been characterized in the CAPN1 gene, and DNA testing is available.

Breeds: 🐕 **Jack Russell terrier, Parson Russell terrier**

Legg–Calvé–Perthes Disease

Description: Also known as aseptic necrosis of the femoral head, this is a disorder of the hip joint seen in young, small-breed dogs., Typically, the disease is seen in dogs between 4 and 12 months of age, and in most cases, only one leg is affected. A genetic trend has been suspected, involving an autosomal recessive trait with incomplete penetrance.

Breeds: 🐕 **Affenpinscher, Australian shepherd, bichon frisé, Border terrier, cairn terrier, Chihuahua, dachshund, Lhasa apso, Lakeland terrier, Manchester terrier, miniature pinscher, miniature poodle, pug, silky terrier, toy poodle, West Highland white terrier, Yorkshire terrier and many others**

Leishmania Susceptibility

Description: An inherited susceptibility to visceral leishmaniasis caused by *Leishmania* infection. The condition is associated with specific single nucleotide polymorphisms in the SLC11A1 gene. Ibizan hounds appear to be more resistant to infection than other breeds.

Breeds: 🐕 **Beagle, boxer, (American) foxhound, German shepherd dog, Rottweiler**

Lens Luxation

Description: Lens luxation refers to abnormal displacement of the lens and is believed to be a heritable trait in most breeds, even though it may not be detected until adulthood. In many, it is a reflection of an autosomal recessive mutation in the ADAMTS17 gene, and genetic testing is available to help determine risk for this variant in certain breeds.

Breeds: 🐕 **American Eskimo dog, American hairless terrier, Australian cattle dog, Australian stumpy tail cattle dog, Border collie, Brittany spaniel, bull terrier, Chinese crested, Chinese shar-pei, fox terrier (smooth and wire), German hunting terrier, Italian volpino, Parson (Jack) Russell terrier, Lakeland terrier, Lancashire heeler, miniature bull terrier, Norwich terrier, petit basset griffon Vendeen, rat terrier (American hairless terrier), Sealyham terrier, Tibetan terrier, Welsh terrier, Yorkshire terrier abd many others;** 🐈 **Siamese**

Lentigo

Description: Also known as pigmented epidermal nevus, lentigo is a relatively rare condition in which black spots appear on the skin. The mode of inheritance is not known with certainty but is suspected to be autosomal dominant with incomplete penetrance. There is some resemblance to epidermodysplasia verruciformis in humans and the condition may be associated with papillomavirus infection.

Breeds: 🐕 **Pug, (miniature) schnauzer**

Leproid Granuloma

Description: Also known as canine leprosy, this is a granulomatous disease associated with mycobacteria. There is a noted breed predisposition, but it is thought this might be due to short coats and potential spread of organisms by biting insects, rather than genetically transmitted susceptibility.

Breeds: 🐕 **Boxer, Doberman pinscher, fox terrier (smooth, wire), Staffordshire bull terrier**

LEPTOSPIROSIS SUSCEPTIBILITY

Description: Leptospirosis is a common infectious disease, and there are many predisposing factors. It is not known with any certainty whether this is a breed predilection to infection, but certain breeds have been so designated.

Breeds: 🐕 **Bernese mountain dog, German shepherd dog**

LETHAL ACRODERMATITIS

Description: A fatal skin disorder, often associated with immune compromise and inherited as an autosomal recessive trait. A likely genetic mutation has been characterized in the MKLN1 gene, and DNA testing is available.

Breeds: 🐕 **Bull terrier, miniature bull terrier**

LETHAL ASTROCYTOSIS

Description: An early-onset lethal neurological disease characterized by astrocyte swelling in the white matter. It is presumed to be inherited as an autosomal recessive trait in Gordon setters.

Breeds: 🐕 **Gordon setter**

Leukocyte Adhesion Deficiency, Type I

Description: Also known as granulocytopathy syndrome, Hagemoser–Takahashi syndrome, and beta-2 integrin adhesion molecule deficiency, these are rare autosomal recessive disorders that result from an inherited lack of certain leukocyte integrins that are critical for leukocytes adhering to, and migrating through, endothelial cells. The result is profound immunodeficiency. Some mutations have been characterized and genetic testing is available for those variants.

Breeds: 🐕 **Irish red and white setter, Irish setter;** 🐈 **Domestic longhair**

Leukocyte Adhesion Deficiency, Type III

Description: A combined defect of leukocytes and platelets with some similarity to Scott syndrome in humans. It is believed to be transmitted as an autosomal recessive trait. The condition is the result of a mutation in the gene encoding for Kindlin-3, which is a signal transduction protein vitally important for mediating integrin activation in leukocytes and platelets. Affected dogs are at risk for spontaneous hemorrhage or excessive bleeding following injury. The gene defects have been characterized in some breeds (FERMT3), and genetic testing is available.

Breeds: 🐕 **Berger blanc Suisse (white Swiss sheepdog), German shepherd dog, Greater Swiss mountain dog, Shiloh shepherd**

Leukodystrophies

Description: Leukodystrophies are so named because they primarily affect the white matter in the nervous system. The leukodystrophies differ so dramatically between breeds that each should be considered as unique breed-specific entities associated with different mutations and modes of inheritance. These include entities like breed-specific leukodystrophies, leukoencephalomyelopathy, spongiform leukoencephalomyelopathy, spongiform encephalopathy, oligodendroglial dysplasia, hereditary ataxia, hound ataxia, nervous system degeneration, central axonopathy, hereditary myelopathy, spongiform leukodystrophy, and fibrinoid leukodystrophy. DNA testing is available for several breed-specific variants.

Breeds: 🐕 **Afghan hound, Australian cattle dog, beagle, Bernese mountain dog, bullmastiff, Dalmatian, (American) foxhound, (smooth) fox terrier, harrier hound, Ibizan hound, Jack Russell terrier, Labrador retriever, Leonberger, (miniature) poodle, Rottweiler, Samoyed, Scottish terrier, Shetland sheepdog, (Australian) silky terrier**

Leukoencephalomyelopathy

Description: A family of metabolic neurological disorders associated with myelin degeneration and inability to control body movement. There are likely many different genetic variants, but a mutation in NAPEPLD is responsible for the autosomal recessive condition in Rottweilers and Great Danes, and a mutation has also been determined for the condition in schnauzers. The autosomal recessive variant causing the condition in Leonbergers is a different mutation of the same gene, and DNA testing is available.

Breeds: 🐕 **Afghan hound, Dalmatian, fox terrier, Great Dane, Jack Russell terrier, Leonberger, (miniature) poodle, Rottweiler, schnauzer (standard, miniature), West Highland white terrier**

Lichenoid-Psoriasiform Dermatitis

Description: A relatively benign condition in which wart-like bumps appear on the skin, usually on the inner ear flaps, or the abdomen, or both. The mode of inheritance is unknown, but the condition is seen almost entirely in the English springer spaniel.

Breeds: 🐕 **English Springer spaniel**

Ligneous Membranitis

Description: This is a rare chronic inflammatory disease of the mucous membranes associated with plasminogen deficiency. Clinically, puppies develop severe proliferative conjunctivitis, gingivitis and tracheitis, and many are euthanized. It appears to be inherited as an autosomal recessive trait. In the Maltese, it appears to be caused by a mutation of the PLG gene.

Breeds: 🐕 **Maltese, Scottish terrier**

Lipoprotein Lipase Deficiency

Description: Lipoprotein lipase deficiency results in hyperchylomicronemia in cats and is inherited as an autosomal recessive trait in domestic cats. Affected kittens have delayed growth rates and subnormal body fat mass. It is likely that different mutations exist because not all cats with hyperchylomicronemia test positive for the characterized mutation.

Breeds: 🐈 **Domestic shorthair**

Lissencephaly

Description: Lissencephaly is a congenital condition of the brain in which the normal convoluted appearance is absent, and the brain surface is smooth. It is believed to be genetically transmitted in at least some breeds and is a developmental disorder of neuronal migration and proliferation.

Breeds: 🐕 **Beagle, (wire) fox terrier, Lhasa apso, Irish setter**

Lumbosacral Disease

Description: A narrowing of the vertebral canal in the lumbosacral area with associated compression of nerve roots. A genetic basis has not been determined, but breed predisposition has been recognized.

Breeds: 🐕 **Kuvasz**

Lumbosacral Stenosis

Description: A spinal condition of both dogs and cats in which there is narrowing of the vertebral canal or vertebral foramen, causing lower back pain. The condition is typically secondary to other processes, but breed predispositions have been recognized in dogs.

Breeds: 🐕 **Belgian Malinois, greyhound**

Lumbosacral Transitional Vertebrae

Description: A congenital anomaly between the last lumbar and first sacral vertebrae, which can predispose to cauda equina syndrome. A genetic basis has not been determined, but breed predisposition has been recognized.

Breeds: 🐕 **Berger blanc Suisse (white Swiss sheepdog), German shepherd dog, Greater Swiss mountain dog, Labrador retriever, Rhodesian ridgeback;** 🐈 **Japanese bobtail**

Lundehund Syndrome

Description: An inherited gastroenteropathy resulting in malabsorption, protein-losing enteropathy, intestinal lymphangiectasia, and inflammatory bowel disease. It is inherited as an autosomal recessive trait, based on a mutation of the LEPREL1 gene. DNA testing is available. There is marked clinical variability in the expression of this trait.

Breeds: 🐾 **Norwegian lundehund**

Lung Lobe Torsion

Description: Lung lobe torsion is a rare condition seen in both dogs and cats in which a lung lobe rotates around the bronchus and vascular supply, creating a potentially life-threatening event. A genetic basis has not been determined, but breed predisposition has been recognized.

Breeds: 🐾 **Afghan hound, pug**

Lupoid Onychopathy

Description: Lupoid onychopathy, also known as (symmetrical) lupoid onychodystrophy, is a claw disorder characterized by onychomadesis and onychodystrophy (onychorrhexis, onychomalacia, onycholysis) of multiple digits (often all 18 claws).

Breeds: 🐾 **Bearded collie, boxer, Doberman pinscher, English setter, German shepherd dog, Gordon setter, greyhound, Irish setter, giant schnauzer, Rottweiler, Weimaraner**

Lupus Erythematosus (Discoid)

Description: Also known as cutaneous lupus erythematous and lupus-like disease of the nasal planum, this is a form of lupus erythematosus which is limited to manifestations in the skin, and systemic involvement is absent. More specifically, discoid lupus tends to be limited to the area around the nose, and is often associated with depigmentation. Clinically it may appear similar to mucocutaneous pyoderma. See also vesicular cutaneous lupus erythematosus and exfoliative cutaneous lupus erythematosus, which are covered separately.

Breeds: 🐾 **Alaskan malamute, Brittany spaniel, collie, German shepherd dog (especially white dogs), German shorthaired pointer, Rottweiler, Shetland sheepdog, Siberian husky**

Lupus Erythematosus (Exfoliative Cutaneous)

Description: Also known as lupoid dermatosis, exfoliative cutaneous lupus erythematosus presents with exfoliative lymphocytic interface dermatitis. It is believed to be

inherited as an autosomal recessive trait, and the mutation has been characterized. DNA testing is available.

Breeds: 🐾 **German shorthaired pointer**

Lupus Erythematosus (Mucocutaneous)

Description: A form of lupus erythematosus with juxtamucosal erosive lesions and a characteristic interface dermatitis. In addition to their dermatological clinical presentation, affected animals might also have dyschezia and dysuria associated with the location of the erosions.

Breeds: 🐾 **German shepherd dog**

Lupus Erythematosus (Systemic)

Description: An inflammatory disease in which the immune system attacks an animal's own tissues. It can have many different presentations depending on the systems attacked.

Breeds: 🐾 **Collie, Finnish spitz, German shepherd dog, Nova Scotia duck tolling retriever, poodle, Shetland sheepdog, Spitz**

Lupus Erythematosus (Vesicular Cutaneous)

Description: Vesicular cutaneous lupus erythematosus is a rare disease typically of adult dogs, and the primary lesions are transient vesicles or bullae that easily rupture to leave an erosive-ulcerative dermatitis, most often distributed in the groin, axillae, ventral abdomen, and mucocutaneous junctions. The condition resembles subacute cutaneous lupus erythematosus (SCLE) in humans. Earlier cases were likely reported as ulcerative dermatosis, and perhaps even as bullous pemphigoid.

Breeds: 🐾 **Border collie, collie, Shetland sheepdog and their crosses**

Lymphangiectasia

Description: A condition characterized by dilation of the lacteals in the small intestinal villi, which eventuates in compromise of the absorptive ability of the intestines. The result is often protein-losing enteropathy, lymphopenia, and hypocholesterolemia. While most cases of lymphangiectasia are idiopathic, some breed-specific forms have been recognized.

Breeds: 🐾 **Basenji, Chinese shar-pei, Norwegian lundehund, Rottweiler, soft-coated wheaten terrier, Yorkshire terrier**

Lymphedema

Description: Primary lymphedema has been reported in several breeds and is presumed to be caused by developmental defects in the lymphatic system and lymph nodes. A mode of inheritance has not yet been determined.

Breeds: 🐾 **Belgian Tervuren, borzoi, English bulldog, German shepherd dog, German shorthaired pointer, Great Dane, Labrador retriever, old English sheepdog, (miniature) poodle, Rottweiler**

Lymphoproliferative Diseases

Description: Lymphoproliferative diseases are a group of disorders associated with lymphocytosis. The most common causes are leukemia and lymphoma. There are often breed predilections recognized, but mode of inheritance is unclear.

Breeds: 🐾 **Airedale terrier, Australian shepherd, Cavalier King Charles spaniel, Chinese shar-pei, Irish wolfhound, shih tzu, Siberian husky, Yorkshire terrier**

Lysosomal Storage Disease (Lagotta Romagnolo)

Description: LSD Lagotto Romagnolo type is associated with a mutation of the ATG4D gene. The result is a neurodegenerative disease especially of the cerebellum. It is inherited as an autosomal recessive trait and DNA testing is available.

Breeds: 🐾 **Lagotto Romagnolo**

Macroblepharon

Description: Also known as eryblepharon and diamond eye, this condition is characterized by an abnormally wide opening of the eyelids, which reduces protection of the eye and can predispose to corneal ulceration. A genetic basis has not been determined, but breed predisposition has been recognized.

Breeds: 🐾 **Belgian Tervuren, Belgian shepherd, dachshund (long haired), Doberman pinscher, German shepherd dog, miniature dachshund (Smooth haired, wire haired, long haired), old English sheepdog, Rottweiler, Vizsla**

Macrocytosis

Description: Familial macrocytosis and dyshematopoiesis is a rare condition in which red blood cell macrocytosis is also associated with hypersegmented neutrophils.

Breeds: 🐾 **Miniature poodle**

Macrothrombocytopenia

Description: An asymptomatic thrombocytopenia associated typically, but not always, with large to giant platelets. Two mutations have been identified in the beta-1-tubulin gene, one of which is recessive, while the other one is dominant. DNA testing is available for breed-specific variants.

Breeds: 🐾 **Bichon frisé, boxer, cairn terrier, Cavalier King Charles spaniel, Chihuahua, (American) cocker spaniel, English toy spaniel, Havanese, Jack Russell terrier, Labrador retriever, Maltese, Norfolk terrier, (standard) poodle, shih tzu**

Malassezia Dermatitis

Description: A yeast dermatitis that occurs secondarily to an underlying problem such as allergy or a keratinization disorder. It is not known if the breed predisposition seen reflects the microbe or the underlying condition

Breeds: 🐾 **Basset hound, Chinese shar-pei, (American) cocker spaniel, English setter, (miniature) poodle, shih tzu, (Australian) silky terrier, West Highland white terrier;** 🐱 **Devon Rex**

Malignant Hyperthermia

Description: A metabolic disorder of skeletal muscle characterized by hypercatabolism and muscle contracture. An episode can be triggered by various factors. The condition is autosomal dominant and reflects a mutation to the RYR1 gene. DNA testing is available for some breed-specific variants.

Breeds: 🐕 **Border collie, American cocker spaniel, collie, Doberman pinscher, English pointer, greyhound, Labrador retriever**, St Bernard

Malocclusion

Description: Malocclusion refers to any abnormality in how the upper and lower teeth meet. Malocclusion often results from achondroplasia, a defect in cartilage growth and development. Specific forms of malocclusion and their inheritance and acceptability must be interpreted on a breed-specific basis.

Breeds: 🐕 **Afghan hound, Australian shepherd, basset hound, Belgian Tervuren, borzoi, Boston terrier, boxer, bull terrier, bullmastiff, cairn terrier, Chesapeake Bay retriever, collie, dachshund, English bulldog, English toy spaniel, French bulldog, German shepherd dog, Kangal shepherd dog, miniature poodle, Pekingese, Scottish terrier, Shetland sheepdog, shiba inu, (miniature) schnauzer, (standard) schnauzer, shih tzu, soft-coated wheaten terrier, and many more**

Mannosidosis (Alpha)

Description: A LSD caused by a deficiency of an enzyme that would typically break down complex sugars in the lysosome. It is a progressive disorder that is invariably fatal and is transmitted in cats as an autosomal recessive trait. The mutation of the MAN2B1 gene has been characterized in Persians, and DNA testing is available.

Breeds: 🐈 **American shorthair, Persian**

Mannosidosis (Beta)

Description: A LSD caused by a deficiency of an enzyme that would typically break down complex sugars in the lysosome. It is a progressive neurological disorder that appears to be transmitted in dogs as an autosomal recessive trait. The mutation of the MANBA gene has been characterized.

Breeds: 🐕 **German shepherd dog**

Masticatory Myositis

Description: Masticatory myositis, also known as eosinophilic myositis and atrophic myositis, is an immune-mediated disease in which antibodies are directed against type II M fibers in masticatory muscles.

Breeds: 🐕 **Cavalier King Charles spaniel, Doberman pinscher, Dutch shepherd, German shepherd dog, golden retriever, Labrador retriever**

May–Hegglin Anomaly

Description: An autosomal dominant form of thrombocytopenia associated with mutations on the MYH9 gene. The condition is largely subclinical but may cause prolonged bleeding time and bruising. DNA testing is available.

Breeds: 🐕 **Pug**

Megaesophagus

Description: Esophageal motility disorders consist of congenital megaesophagus, esophageal hypomotility, and esophageal dysfunction. Congenital megaesophagus seems to be inherited in a breed-specific manner and mode of inheritance, especially in the wire fox terrier (autosomal recessive) and miniature schnauzer (autosomal dominant with incomplete penetrance).

Breeds: 🐕 **Bouvier des Flandres, Chinese shar-pei, (smooth) fox terrier, (wire) fox terrier, German shepherd dog, golden retriever, Great Dane, greyhound, Irish setter, Labrador retriever, Newfoundland, (miniature) schnauzer, Shiloh shepherd;** 🐈 **Siamese**

Membranoproliferative Glomerulonephritis

Description: A poorly characterized congenital renal disease where deposits of antibodies infiltrate the glomerular basement membrane zone. It is poorly characterized in dogs, but breed predispositions have been recognized.

Breeds: 🐕 **Beagle, Doberman pinscher, (miniature) schnauzer**

Meningitis-Arteritis

Description: Most cases of meningitis and meningoencephalomyelitis occur as a result of infection. Some breed-specific forms, however, seem to have a heritable basis.

Steroid-responsive meningitis-arteritis is an immune-mediated inflammatory disease affecting the leptomeninges and associated arteries. The condition is characterized by profound neck pain, fever, and stilted gait; sometimes there can be associated polyarthritis.

Breeds: 🐕 **Beagle, Bernese mountain dog, Border collie, boxer, Jack Russell terrier, Nova Scotia duck tolling retriever, petit basset griffon Vendeen, Weimaraner, (Pembroke) Welsh corgi**

Meningitis (Aseptic)

Description: Bernese mountain dog aseptic meningitis is a severe necrotizing vasculitis that is not uncommon in the Bernese mountain dog population, although a mode of inheritance has not been determined. The age of onset is 3–12 months, with sudden onset of fever, cervical rigidity, spinal pain, and stilted gait.

Breeds: 🐕 **Bernese mountain dog**

Meningoencephalitis

Description: Meningoencephalitis refers to inflammation of the brain and meninges and has a variety of causes. The nonsuppurative condition in greyhounds seems to be familial and is progressive and often fatal. A suppurative pyogranulomatous meningoencephalitis has been described in the German shorthaired pointer. Similar but distinct conditions have been seen in the pug, Maltese, and Yorkshire terrier (see meningoencephalitis, necrotizing).

Breeds: 🐕 **German shorthaired pointer, greyhound**

Meningoencephalitis (Necrotizing)

Description: Also known as pug encephalitis, this is a hereditary neurological disease associated with mutations in at least three dog leukocyte antigen gene markers (DRB1, DQA1, DQB1). The mode of inheritance is considered autosomal recessive with incomplete penetrance in the pug, and DNA marker tests are available to help predict risk of disease.

Breeds: 🐕 **Chihuahua, French bulldog, Maltese, papillon (phalene), Pekingese, Pomeranian, pug, shih tzu, Yorkshire terrier**

Menkes Syndrome

Description: A rare X-linked condition in which copper accumulates in the liver and is deficient in most other tissues of the body. It is caused by an ATP7A gene defect. The result is kinky hair, degenerative neurological disease, and failure to thrive.

Breeds: 🐕 **Labrador retriever, Australian cobber dog (Labradoodle)**

Merling

Description: Merling is a color pattern, and the merle gene (M) is dominant, so dogs heterozygous for the trait (Mm) retain the pattern. Animals that are genotypic homozygotes (MM) may be white in coloration and have an increased incidence of deafness, blindness, and sterility.

Breeds: 🐕 **American bully, American pit bull terrier, American Staffordshire terrier, Australian shepherd, Beauceron, Bergamasco sheepdog, Border collie, Catahoula leopard dog, Chihuahua, (American) cocker spaniel, collie, dachshund, dunker, koolie, (Hungarian) mudi, old English sheepdog, Pomeranian, Pyrenean shepherd, Shetland sheepdog, (Cardigan) Welsh corgi**

Metatarsal Fistulae Syndrome

Description: A focal deep nodular to diffuse pyogranulomatous dermatitis with fistulous tracts. The condition sometimes goes into spontaneous remission, but otherwise responds best to immunomodulatory therapy such as cyclosporine, tacrolimus, or corticosteroids.

Breeds: German shepherd dog, greyhound, Weimaraner

Methemoglobin Reductase Deficiency

Description: Methemoglobin reductase deficiency results in methemoglobinemia, which can cause brown mucous membranes, weakness, and, potentially, hypoxia. Fortunately, most dogs with methemoglobin reductase deficiency are asymptomatic. A genetic connection is presumed, but a mode of inheritance not yet determined.

Breeds: American Eskimo dog, borzoi, Chihuahua, English setter, Pomeranian, (miniature) poodle, (Pembroke) Welsh corgi, and some mixed-breed dogs

Microcytosis

Description: Microcytosis can be associated with portosystemic shunts (PSS) or with deficiencies of iron, pyridoxine, or copper, and a presumed inherited microcytosis also has also been reported. The animals are clinically normal and have a low mean corpuscular volume (MCV), without concurrent anemia.

Breeds: Akita, shiba inu

Microphthalmia

Description: Microphthalmia denotes the condition of a congenitally small eye. In the soft-coated wheaten terrier, the mutation to the *RBP4 gene* and mode of inheritance (autosomal recessive with variable expressivity) have been determined, and DNA testing is available. In most other breeds, the inheritance is thought to be autosomal recessive. Microphthalmia can also occur in association with other genetic issues.

Breeds: Akita, Australian shepherd, beagle, Bedlington terrier, black Russian terrier, Border collie, borzoi, Cavalier King Charles spaniel, (American) cocker spaniel, collie (rough and smooth), dachshund, Dalmatian, Doberman pinscher, English toy spaniel, English mastiff, English springer spaniel, Great Dane, Irish terrier, Labrador retriever, Lakeland terrier, old English sheepdog, poodle (miniature, standard, toy), Portuguese water dog, St Bernard, (miniature) schnauzer, Shetland sheepdog, Rottweiler, Samoyed, Siberian husky, soft-coated wheaten terrier, Tibetan spaniel

Mitochondrial Myopathy

Description: Mitochondrial myopathy is a rare metabolic disorder first reported in young Clumber and Sussex spaniels, although similar conditions have been described in other breeds. Although the cause is still a matter of some debate, inheritance is believed to play at least some role, and the condition is thought to be associated with abnormal mitochondrial function. If inheritance is indeed cytoplasmic, affected males should not transmit the disorder to their offspring, but females can.

Breeds: Clumber spaniel, German shepherd dog, Jack Russell terrier, old English sheepdog, Parson Russell terrier, Sussex spaniel

Mitral Valvular Disease (Endocardiosis)

Description: Chronic mitral valvular disease is the most common acquired cardiac abnormality in dogs. The process is degenerative, most typically involving the atrioventricular valves and resulting in mitral regurgitation, rupture of the chordae tendineae, and, potentially, left-sided heart failure. There is thought to be a genetic tendency to experience degeneration of the collagen in the heart valves.

Breeds: Afghan hound, beagle, Boston terrier, bull terrier, Cavalier King Charles spaniel, Chihuahua, (American) cocker spaniel, dachshund, fox terrier, German shepherd dog, Great Dane, Japanese chin, Maltese, Pekingese, (miniature) poodle, (toy) poodle, (miniature) schnauzer, Yorkshire terrier and many others

Mitral Valve Dysplasia

Description: A congenital malformation of the mitral valve complex, which is more common in cats than dogs. A genetic basis has not been determined, but breed predisposition has been recognized.

Breeds: Boxer, bull terrier, German shepherd dog, golden retriever, Great Dane; Sphynx

Mucinosis

Description: A condition in which the supporting network under the skin is replaced in areas by mucin, which is a secretion with the texture of mucus. The mode of inheritance is unknown, but all Chinese shar-pei have more subcutaneous mucin than other breeds. In this breed, the mucinosis is due to hyaluronic acid deposition and is often associated with high levels of hyaluronic acid in serum.

Breeds: Chinese shar-pei, Doberman pinscher, Labrador retriever, Shetland sheepdog

Mucocutaneous Pyoderma

Description: A distinct form of inflammatory disease primarily affecting the lip margins, and sometimes other mucocutaneous junctions and nasal planum. There is a lymphocytic infiltration that suggests some immunological component, but the condition often responds to systemic and topical antibiotics. It may occur sporadically in different breeds, but there is a breed predisposition for the German shepherd dog.

Breeds: German shepherd dog

Mucolipidosis II

Description: This is a LSD caused by deficient activity of the enzyme N-acetylglucosamine-1-phosphotransferase, which leads to a failure to internalize enzymes into lysosomes. The trait is autosomal recessive and the causative point mutation (GNPTA) has been characterized. DNA testing is available.

Breeds: American shorthair, domestic shorthair

Mucopolysaccharidosis I

Description: Also known as Hurler' syndrome and Scheie syndrome, this is a rare connective tissue disease caused by a deficiency of lysosomal alpha-L-iduronidase due to mutations of the MPSI gene. It is autosomal recessive and DNA testing is available.

Breeds: Plott hound; American shorthair

Mucopolysaccharidosis II

Description: Also known as Hunter syndrome, this is a rare disease associated with a deficiency of iduronate sulfatase. Transmission is believed to be x-linked.

Breeds: Labrador retriever

Mucopolysaccharidosis IIIA

Description: A family of inherited LSDs in which mutations of the SGSH gene bear some resemblance to human Sanfilippo syndrome. The traits are autosomal recessive in nature and the cerebellar neuronal degeneration is progressive. Unlike most other LSDs, clinical signs may not be evident until adulthood. Genetic variants have been characterized and DNA testing is available.

Breeds: Dachshund, New Zealand huntaway

Mucopolysaccharidosis IIIB

Description: Mucopolysaccharidosis IIIB reflects an enzyme deficiency leading to intracellular accumulations of heparan sulfate and is transmitted as an autosomal recessive trait. The condition is caused by mutations to the NAGLU gene, and DNA testing is available.

Breeds: Schipperke

Mucopolysaccharidosis VI

Description: Also known as Maroteaux–Lamy disease, this is a rare disease of connective tissue that is inherited in a breed-specific manner as a mutation of the arylsulfatase B gene. Most of the conditions are caused by mutations of the ARSB gene, and DNA testing is available for breed-specific variants.

Breeds: Great Dane, miniature pinscher, poodle (miniature, moyen, standard, toy), (miniature) schnauzer, (Pembroke) Welsh corgi; American shorthair, Balinese, Birman, domestic shorthair, Javanese, Oriental shorthair, Peterbald, Ragdoll, Siamese, Thai, Tonkinese

Mucopolysaccharidosis VII

Description: A family of inherited LSDs in which mutations of the GUSB gene result in dwarfism, skeletal dysmorphism, and organomegaly. The traits are autosomal recessive in nature and bear resemblance to Sly syndrome in humans. Several genetic variants have been characterized and DNA testing is available for breed-specific variants in both dogs and cats.

Breeds: Berger blanc Suisse (white Swiss sheepdog), Belgian Malinois, Belgian sheepdog, Brazilian terrier, German shepherd dog, Shiloh shepherd; Domestic shorthair

Multidrug Resistance 1

Description: The multidrug resistance 1 (MDR1) gene codes for a protein (P-glycoprotein) responsible for keeping certain drugs out of the brain. The most common manifestation of this mutation is a neurological adverse reaction to certain medications. This is an autosomal recessive condition associated with a mutation of the ABCB1 gene, and genetic testing is available.

Breeds: 🐕 **Australian cattle dog, Australian shepherd, Australian stumpy-tail cattle dog, berger blanc Suisse (white Swiss sheepdog), Border Collie, Chinook, collie, English shepherd, German shepherd dog, golden retriever, Labrador retriever, McNab shepherd (McNab Border collie), old English sheepdog, Shetland sheepdog, silken windhound, whippet**

Multifocal Retinopathy

Description: Canine multifocal retinopathy (CMR) is a group of breed-specific autosomal recessive disorders, bearing some resemblance to the human dominantly inherited condition, Best vitelliform macular degeneration. The condition is typically detected around 4 months of age and is associated with multifocal, almost circular patches of elevated retina; in most cases, it is not believed to have a profound effect on vision. There are also some breed-specific as well as idiopathic forms that have been recognized. For those in which the variant has been identified, DNA testing is likely available. Borzoi retinopathy seems to represent a unique idiopathic chorioretinopathy unique to the breed, and possibly unrelated to the other forms of multifocal retinopathy (CMR1, CMR2, CMR3). It may be better classified as retinal degeneration.

Breeds: 🐕 **Borzoi**

Multifocal Retinopathy (CMR1)

Description: An autosomal recessive form of the disorder, associated with a mutation of the BEST1 gene. Changes in the fundus are typically evident before 4 months of age. DNA testing is available for several variants.

Breeds: 🐕 **American bulldog, American bully, Australian shepherd, boerboel, Brazilian terrier, English bulldog, bullmastiff, cane corso dog, dogue de Bordeaux, French bulldog, Great Pyrenees, Havanese, Perro de Presa Canario**

Multifocal Retinopathy (CMR2)

Description: An autosomal recessive form of multifocal retinopathy associated with a unique mutation of the BEST1 gene, which is a gene necessary for retinal pigment epithelium (RPE) function.

Breeds: 🐕 **Coton de Tulear**

Multifocal Retinopathy (CMR3)

Description: An autosomal recessive form of multifocal retinopathy, associated with a unique form of the BEST1 gene. It is a breed-specific mutation but with clinical presentation very similar to the other forms of the disease.

Breeds: 🐕 **Finnish lapphund, Lapponian herder, Swedish lapphund**

Multiple Skeletal Defect Syndrome

Description: Also known as skeletal lethal, this is/was a severe and often lethal (to males) musculoskeletal condition transmitted as an x-linked recessive trait. All male offspring had skeletal abnormalities and cleft palate; female heterozygotes had crooked legs and syndactyly, but typically not the cleft palate. It is believed that this was a very limited trait and may no longer be a breed health concern.

Breeds: 🐕 **Australian shepherd**

Muscular Dystrophy (Autosomal)

Description: A cause of muscular dystrophy that is transmitted as an autosomal recessive trait and caused by a mutation of the COL6A1 gene. Genetic testing is available.

Breeds: 🐕 **Landseer**

Muscular Dystrophy (Feline)

Description: A uniquely feline x-linked hypertrophic muscular dystrophy with some resemblance to Duchenne/Becker muscular dystrophy, but with lack of fat infiltration and the presence of prominent hypertrophy of both muscle fibers and muscle groups. The genetic mutation has been characterized.

Breeds: 🐈 **American shorthair, Devon Rex**

Muscular Dystrophy (LIMB GIRDLE)

Description: This represents a heterogeneous group of inherited autosomal myopathies that primarily affect voluntary muscles of the shoulders and hips. The genetic mutation of sarcoglycan has been characterized in the Boston terrier, and on the COLQ gene in Sphynx and Devon Rex cats, and DNA testing is available for breed-specific variants.

Breeds: 🐕 **Boston terrier, Chihuahua, (American) cocker spaniel;** 🐈 **Devon Rex, Sphynx**

Muscular Dystrophy (X-Linked)

Description: Similar to Duchenne muscular dystrophy, this reflects an x-linked dystrophin deficiency muscle weakness and atrophy. The underlying defect is a variety of breed-specific mutations of the dystrophin genes. Genetic testing is available for specific variants.

Breeds: 🐕 **Alaskan malamute, Brittany spaniel, Cavalier King Charles spaniel, German shorthaired pointer, golden retriever, Groenendaeler (Belgian shepherd), Irish terrier, Japanese spitz, Labrador retriever, Norfolk terrier, old English sheepdog, Rottweiler, Samoyed, (miniature) schnauzer, Weimaraner, (Pembroke) Welsh corgi**

Musculotendinopathy

Description: A tendency toward athletic injuries, especially involving the origin of the gastrocnemius muscle. There is a breed predisposition, but this appears to be more of an athletic predisposition than a breed predisposition.

Breeds: 🐕 **Border collie, Labrador retriever**

Musladin–Leuke Syndrome

Description: Musladin–Leuke syndrome, also known as Chinese beagle syndrome, is a multisystemic genetic disease that can involve bone, muscle, skin, and heart. It is inherited as an autosomal recessive trait, but the clinical presentation has much variability and even carriers may develop some subtle signs of the disorder. The genetic variant has been characterized in the ADAMTSL2 gene, and DNA testing is available.

Breeds: 🐕 **Beagle**

Myasthenia Gravis (MG) (Acquired)

Description: MG is a disease affecting the interaction of nerves and muscles. Both congenital and acquired forms

occur in the dog. Acquired immune-mediated MG has definite breed predilections but likely a more complex mode of inheritance than the congenital form.

Breeds: 🐕 **Akita, German shepherd dog, golden retriever, Labrador retriever, Newfoundland**

Myasthenia Gravis (Congenital)

Description: MG, also known as myasthenic syndrome, is a disease affecting the interaction of nerves and muscles. Both congenital and acquired forms occur in the dog. Congenital MG results from an autosomal recessive defect in the nicotinic acetylcholine receptors, which causes a transmission error at the junction of nerve and muscle. Most are the result of breed-specific mutations in the COLQ gene.

Breeds: 🐕 **English springer spaniel, (smooth-haired miniature) dachshund, (smooth) fox terrier, Jack Russell terrier, Labrador retriever, old Danish pointing dog (Gammel Dansk hønsehund), Parson Russell terrier, Samoyed**

Myasthenic Syndrome (Feline)

Description: Also known as hereditary myopathy, this refers to a group of disorders that affect the transmission of nerve signals at the neuromuscular junction. These disorders are breed specific and are likely caused by a variety of genetic mutations. The general result is muscle weakness. Megaesophagus is also common. Some mutations have been characterized (COLQ) and DNA testing is available for breed-specific variants.

Breeds: 🐈 **Abyssinian, Devon Rex, Siamese, Somali, Sphynx**

Mycobacterium Avium Susceptibility

Description: Mycobacterial susceptibility has been reported in association with an interleukin or RAMP protein deficiency. Although most dogs are relatively resistant to avian mycobacteria, affected dogs are prone to developing systemic disease, including diarrhea, weight loss, lymphadenomegaly, and nasal discharge. A variant of the CARD9 gene has been identified that is associated with increased susceptibility in the miniature schnauzer.

Breeds: 🐕 **Bassett hound, (miniature) schnauzer;** 🐈 **Abyssinian, Siamese**

Myelodysplasia

Description: Also known as myelodysplastic syndrome, this condition is characterized by ineffective hematopoiesis. The result is often a nonregenerative anemia and often pancytopenia.

Breeds: 🐕 **Alaskan malamute, Chihuahua, Dalmatian, English bulldog, Labrador retriever, Rottweiler, Samoyed, Siberian husky, Weimaraner**

Myoclonus

Description: Familial myoclonus is a rare condition of muscular hypertonicity in which animals, when stimulated, fall to their side and exhibit extensor rigidity and opisthotonos.

Breeds: 🐕 **Labrador retriever**

Myopia

Description: Also known as near-sightedness or short-sightedness, myopia has been documented in dogs. There is little evidence on which to base a mode of inheritance, but breed predisposition has been recognized.

Breeds: 🐕 **Collie, English springer spaniel, German shepherd dog, (toy) poodle, Rottweiler, (miniature) schnauzer**

Myositis Ossificans

Description: A rare muscle disorder characterized by bone formation within muscles, often in areas of trauma. The cause is not known with any certainty, but the condition in people is believed to have a hereditary component.

Breeds: 🐕 **Doberman pinscher, Rottweiler;** 🐈 **Maine Coon**

Myostatin (MSTN) Deficiency

Description: MSTN deficiency, also known as double muscling or "bully," refers to a mutation in the MSTN gene and results in heavy muscling. The mutation has been characterized and DNA testing is available.

Breeds: 🐕 **Whippet**

Myotonia Congenita

Description: A disorder of skeletal muscle characterized by delayed relaxation of the muscle fiber. In many of the conditions in dogs and in cats, the mutations are autosomal recessive variants of the CLCN1 gene and DNA testing is available for breed-specific variants in both dogs and cats.

Breeds: 🐕 **Australian cattle dog, Australian shepherd, Australian stumpy-tailed cattle dog, chow chow, (American) cocker spaniel, Great Dane, Labrador retriever, Rhodesian ridgeback, Samoyed, (miniature) schnauzer, Staffordshire bull terrier, West Highland white terrier;** 🐈 **Domestic shorthair**

Myotubular Myopathy

Description: A rare cause of rapidly progressive weakness and muscle atrophy in young animals. As an X-linked trait, it primarily affects male pups. The mutation in the MTM1 gene has been characterized and DNA testing is available for breed-specific variants. Similar conditions have been reported in the affenpinscher.

Breeds: 🐕 **Affenpinscher, Labrador retriever, Rottweiler**

Narcolepsy and Cataplexy

Description: Narcolepsy and cataplexy are two sleep disorders recognized in dogs. Narcolepsy is an autosomal recessive trait in most dogs with breed-specific variants of the HCRTR2 gene. Genetic testing is available for certain breed-specific variants.

Breeds: 🐕 **Afghan hound, Airedale terrier, Alaskan malamute, American Eskimo dog, beagle, Chihuahua, dachshund, Doberman pinscher, Irish setter, Labrador retriever, (miniature) poodle, Rottweiler, St Bernard, (giant) schnauzer, English springer spaniel, (Pembroke) Welsh corgi**

Nasal Arteritis

Description: An inflammatory reaction of the arterioles in the nasal philtrum that can lead to ulceration and hemorrhage. A genetic basis has not been determined, but breed predisposition has been recognized

Breeds: 🐕 **Basset hound, Newfoundland, St Bernard, (giant) schnauzer**

Nasal Parakeratosis

Description: Hereditary nasal parakeratosis is a crusting skin disease that affects the nasal planum and is the result of genetic mutations of the SUV39H2 gene. It is inherited as an autosomal recessive trait. Many conditions can cause the nose to be crusty, but this genetic variant is often clinically evident by 1 year of age. DNA testing is available for some breed-specific variants.

Breeds: 🐕 **Greyhound, Labrador retriever**

Nasodigital Hyperkeratosis

Description: An idiopathic keratinization disorder affecting the nasal planum and footpads. A genetic basis has not been determined, but breed predisposition has been recognized.

Breeds: 🐕 **Boxer, Boston terrier, (American) cocker spaniel, English bulldog**

Nasopharyngeal Dysgenesis

Description: A congenital nasopharyngeal stenosis associated with abnormally thickened palatopharyngeal muscles that results in dyspnea, often requiring surgical correction. A mode of inheritance has not yet been determined.

Breeds: 🐕 **Dachshund**

Necrotizing Encephalopathy

Description: A rare neurodegenerative disorder with some resemblance to subacute necrotizing encephalopathy (Leigh syndrome) in humans. The condition is considered to be familial and is presumed to be autosomal recessive in nature. The polioencephalomyelopathy seen in the Australian cattle dog is likely a distinct entity. Subacute necrotizing encephalopathy is a fatal breed-specific neurodegenerative disorder in the Yorkshire terrier. The genetic mutation has been characterized, and DNA testing is available.

Breeds: 🐕 **Alaskan malamute, American Staffordshire terrier, Australian cattle dog, Yorkshire terrier**

Necrotizing Myelopathy

Description: A progressive inherited spinal disease. There are likely different genetic variants of the condition, but the variant in the Dutch Kooiker dog is believed to be autosomal recessive in nature.

Breeds: 🐕 **Afghan hound, Dutch Kooiker dog, Great Dane**

Nemaline Myopathy

Description: An inherited congenital polymyositis that causes muscle weakness, tremors, and exercise intolerance in young animals, associated in the American bulldog with an autosomal recessive mutation in the NEB gene. DNA testing is available for breed-specific variants.

Breeds: 🐕 **American bulldog, Border collie, schipperke**

Neonatal Encephalopathy with Seizures

Description: Neonatal encephalopathy with seizures is a fatal developmental brain disease. It is transmitted as an autosomal recessive trait, and most affected puppies die shortly after birth. DNA testing is available.

Breeds: 🐕 **Poodle (miniature, moyen, standard, toy)**

Neonatal Isoerythrolysis

Description: An immune-mediated blood disorder associated with an incompatibility between the antibodies present in a mother's milk, and the blood type of the offspring. More common in cats than dogs, kittens born with blood type A develop immune-mediated reactions when they consume colostrum from mothers with type B blood.

Breeds: 🐈 **Birman, British shorthair, Cornish Rex, Devon Rex, Exotic, Highland fold, Japanese bobtail, Norwegian forest cat, Persian, Scottish fold, Somali, Turkish angora, Turkish van**

Neuroaxonal Dystrophies

Description: Neuroaxonal dystrophies are inherited errors of metabolism resulting in swellings (or spheroids) along a region of the axon. They may be primarily inherited or may occur secondarily to other disease processes. The inherited forms are mainly autosomal recessive in nature. The mutation in the papillon has been characterized (PLA2G6) and in the giant schnauzer (mitofusin 2), Rottweiler (*CLCN1*) and Spanish water dog *(TECPR2),* and DNA testing is available. Most mutations are anticipated to be breed specific.

Breeds: 🐕 **Border collie, boxer, bullmastiff, Chihuahua, collie, German shepherd dog, Jack Russell terrier, Labrador retriever, papillon (phalene), Parson Russell terrier, Rottweiler, (giant) schnauzer, Spanish water dog**

Neuronal Ceroid Lipofuscinosis

Description: Also known as Batten disease and amaurotic idiocy, these conditions are members of the lipidosis subgroup of the LSDs. There are several different forms evident in dogs and cats (NCL 1, 2, 4a, 5, 6, 7, 8, 10, 12, A) with different clinical presentations, different breed predispositions, and breed-specific genetic testing. Severe neuronal loss in the cerebral cortex and the cerebellum is a hallmark in most breeds. Most seem to be inherited as autosomal recessive traits. Many genetic variants have been characterized and have DNA tests available. Other forms have yet to be further characterized.

Breeds: 🐕 **Alpine dachsbracke, American bulldog, American cocker spaniel, American pit bull terrier, (miniature) American shepherd, American Staffordshire terrier, Australian cattle dog, Australian blue heeler, Australian shepherd, Border collie, bull terrier, Chihuahua, Chinese crested, dachshund, Dalmatian, English cocker spaniel, English setter, golden retriever, Gordon setter, Irish setter, Irish red and white setter, Japanese retriever, koolie, Labrador retriever, miniature bull terrier, Polish lowland sheepdog, (miniature poodle), saluki, (miniature) schnauzer, Tibetan spaniel, Tibetan terrier, Welsh corgi, Yugoslavian shepherd dog;** 🐈 **American shorthair, Siamese**

Neuronal Degeneration

Description: Also known as multisystem neuronal degeneration, canine multiple system degeneration, and progressive neuronal abiotrophy, this is a progressive degenerative disease that can involve the brain, spinal cord, and peripheral nerves. It has some resemblance to familial juvenile-onset Parkinson's disease in people. This likely represents different conditions in different breeds, but it is recognized as autosomal recessive in the Great Pyrenees, and genetic testing is available. In the Chinese crested, the condition is

due to a mutation in the *SERAC1 gene and transmitted as an autosomal recessive trait.*

Breeds: 🐕 **Chinese crested, (American) cocker spaniel, Great Pyrenees, Jack Russell terrier, Kerry blue terrier**

Neutrophil Bactericidal Anomaly

Description: A rare condition considered an autosomal recessive trait. Normal bacterial phagocytosis by neutrophils is present, but bactericidal activity is partially reduced. The principal presentation includes recurrent respiratory infections.

Breeds: 🐕 **Doberman pinscher**

Neutrophil Granulation Defect

Description: This trait involves the presence of atypical granules in the cytoplasm of neutrophils, but neutrophil function is not adversely affected. It is presumed to be inherited as an autosomal recessive trait.

Breeds: 🐈 **Birman**

Niemann–Pick Diseases

Description: Also known as sphingomyelinosis, the Niemann–Pick diseases are characterized by accumulation of sphingomyelin and cholesterol in tissues. Niemann–Pick disease type A (NPA) exhibits a sphingomyelinase deficiency. Niemann–Pick type C (NPC) in the boxer is characterized by a cholesterol transport defect. The autosomal recessive conditions present with ataxia, head shaking, hypermetria, dysequilibrium, and hepatomegaly. At least two variants (NPC1 and NPC2) have been characterized in cats.

Breeds: 🐕 **Boxer, miniature poodle;** 🐈 **Balinese, domestic shorthair, Siamese**

Nodular Dermatofibrosis and Renal Cystadenocarcinoma

Description: A cutaneous marker for an internal malignancy that is believed to be transmitted as an autosomal dominant trait in the German shepherd dog. The homozygous mutation is thought to be a lethal trait, so most affected dogs are heterozygotes. The condition is associated with a mutation in the BHD (Birt–Hogg–Dubé) folliculin gene and DNA testing is available.

Breeds: 🐕 **Berger blanc Suisse (white Swiss sheepdog), boxer, German shepherd dog, golden retriever, Shiloh shepherd, mixed-breed dogs**

Noise Sensitivity

Description: All pets can be sensitive to noises, such as fireworks and gunshots, but some breeds tend to have higher sensitivity than others. A mode of inheritance has not been proposed, but breed predisposition has been recognized.

Breeds: 🐕 **Lagotto Romagnolo, Norwegian buhund, soft-coated wheaten terrier**

Nonspherocytic Hemolytic Anemia

Description: This rare condition is associated with a shortened life span of red blood cells, and is presumed to have an autosomal recessive mode of inheritance. The severity of the condition in different breeds is clinically quite different, and may represent different genetic mutations and modes of inheritance.

Breeds: 🐕 **Beagle, (miniature) poodle**

Obesity (Pro-Opiomelanocortin [POMC])

Description: While obesity or adiposity is common in the pet population, genetic causes have also been identified. Mutations in the POMC gene disrupt beta-MSH (melanocyte-stimulating hormone) and beta-endorphin and consequently cause an increase in body weight, adiposity, and food motivation. The trait is believed to be transmitted in an autosomal recessive manner. The adiposity gene (POMC) has been characterized and DNA testing is available.

Breeds: 🐕 **(American) cocker spaniel, flat-coated retriever, Labrador retriever**

Ocular Melanosis

Description: An eye condition characterized by the accumulation of melanocytes and pigment in the iris, choroid, and sclera. Typically occurring in older dogs, it is considered heritable in the cairn terrier and is recognized periodically in other breeds.

Breeds: 🐕 **Boxer, cairn terrier, Labrador retriever**

Oculoskeletal Dysplasia

Description: An inherited form of retinal dysplasia associated with dwarfism and other clinical manifestations. It is considered an autosomal recessive trait caused by mutations on the COL9A3 gene in the Labrador retriever and COL9A2 in the Samoyed, and DNA testing is available. Skeletal dysplasia 2 has also been reported in the Labrador retriever in association with the *COL11A2 gene, and* DNA testing is available. Oculoskeletal dysplasia 3 has also been recognized, the gene variant characterized, and DNA testing available for the Northern Inuit and Tamaskan dog breeds.

Breeds: 🐕 **Labrador retriever, Samoyed**

Oligodontia (Missing Teeth)

Description: Anodontia is the complete absence of teeth, and oligodontia refers to several missing teeth, but not all. Oligodontia is common in many breeds and mode of inheritance has been determined for some.

Breeds: 🐕 **Affenpinscher, Afghan hound, Airedale terrier, bearded collie, Bedlington terrier, Belgian Tervuren, Border terrier, borzoi, Brittany spaniel, Chinese crested, Clumber spaniel, Dandie Dinmont terrier, Doberman pinscher, smooth fox terrier, wire fox terrier, German shepherd dog, Great Dane, Havanese, Jack Russell terrier, keeshond, Kerry blue terrier, komondor, Labrador retriever, Lhasa apso, Maltese, Manchester terrier, Norwegian elkhound, Norwich terrier, Pomeranian, miniature poodle, standard poodle, Rottweiler, Shetland sheepdog, shih tzu, Skye terrier, Swedish vallhund, Tibetan terrier, West Highland white terrier, xoloitzcuintli**

Optic Nerve Colobomas

Description: These refer to pits on the optic disk, which can also be associated with choroidal hypoplasia or other ocular anomalies. They appear to be familial but a mode of inheritance has not been confirmed.

Breeds: 🐕 **Australian shepherd, basenji, Brussels griffon, (American) cocker spaniel, curly-coated**

retriever, dachshund, **Glen of Imaal terrier**, **Labrador retriever**, **Norfolk terrier**, **Shetland sheepdog**

Optic Nerve Hypoplasia and Micropapilla

Description: Optic nerve hypoplasia is a congenital underdevelopment of the optic nerve, causing blindness; micropapilla is a small optic disk not associated with blindness. Optic nerve hypoplasia seems to be inherited, but a mode of transmission has not been determined in most breeds.

Breeds: Afghan, **Alaskan malamute**, **Australian shepherd**, **beagle**, **Belgian shepherd**, **Belgian Tervuren**, **borzoi**, **bullmastiff**, **(American) cocker spaniel**, **(English) cocker spaniel**, **collie**, **dachshund**, **flat-coated retriever**, **German shepherd dog**, **golden retriever**, **Gordon setter**, **Great Pyrenees**, **greyhound**, **Irish setter**, **Irish wolfhound**, **keeshond**, **Labrador retriever**, **miniature pinscher**, **miniature poodle**, **miniature schnauzer**, **Norfolk terrier**, **Nova Scotia duck tolling retriever**, **old English sheepdog**, **poodle (standard, toy)**, **pug**, **puli**, **St Bernard**, **Shetland sheepdog**, **shih tzu**, **soft-coated wheaten terrier**, **Tibetan spaniel**, **whippet**

Organic Aciduria

Description: A group of inherited metabolic disorders with abnormal amino acid metabolism and the accumulation of acids that are not typically present. See methylmalonic aciduria and L-2 hydroxyglutaric aciduria for breed-specific information. In addition, suspected primary organic aciduria has been reported in standard poodles, acyl-CoA dehydrogenase deficiency in Cavalier King Charles spaniels, and a condition in Shetland sheepdogs similar to Kearns–Sayre syndrome in people. Individual cats have also been diagnosed with organic aciduria

Breeds: **Cavalier King Charles spaniel**, **poodle (standard)**, **Shetland sheepdog**

Organic Aciduria (L-2 Hydroxyglutaric Aciduria)

Description: A specific form of organic aciduria characterized by elevated levels of L-2-hydroxyglutaric acid in urine, plasma, and CSF. The condition is transmitted as an autosomal recessive trait in the Staffordshire bull terrier and

Yorkshire terrier, due to different mutations in the L2HGDH gene, and DNA testing is available for breed-specific variants.

Breeds: **Staffordshire bull terrier**, **West Highland white terrier**, **Yorkshire terrier**

Organic Aciduria (Methylmalonic Aciduria)

Description: An organic aciduria in which methylmalonic and/or malonic acid accumulate in the urine. As an inborn error of metabolism, it can be associated with neurodegenerative disease. It can also be seen secondary to disorders in cobalamin metabolism.

Breeds: **Border collie**, **Labrador retriever**, **Maltese**

Osteochondritis Dissecans

Description: A disorder of growth cartilage that occurs in specific locations and is prevalent in specific breeds. The term osteochondrosis or osteochondritis itself is a matter of controversy because the initial process does not involve bone. Focal failure of endochondral ossification leads to retention of cartilage rather than conversion to bone. The etiology is complex, with trauma, genetics, growth rates, nutrition, and ischemia all having a role. Genetic factors clearly do have a role, and breed predispositions have been recognized for specific forms of the disorder.

Osteochondritis Dissecans (Elbow)

Description: OCD of the elbow has strong evidence for being an inherited disease, likely controlled by many genes. It is only one of the conditions (osteochondrosis of the medial humeral condyle) that can result in elbow dysplasia (see elbow dysplasia).

Breeds: **Bearded collie**, **chow chow**, **German shepherd dog**, **golden retriever**, **Great Dane**, **Labrador retriever**, **Newfoundland**, **Rottweiler**

Osteochondritis Dissecans (Hock)

This is a rare form of osteochondrosis. Most dogs are 6–12 months of age when they are first affected, developing progressive hindleg lameness. Both legs are affected in approximately 40% of cases. More than 70% of all cases have occurred in the Rottweiler and Labrador retriever. Most cases of tarsal OCD involve the medial trochlear ridge, except in the Rottweiler, in which the lateral trochlea is most commonly affected. Unlike most other forms of OCD, males do not seem to be overrepresented in this entity.

Breeds: 🐾 **Australian cattle dog, bull terrier, bullmastiff, golden retriever, Irish setter, Labrador retriever**, Rottweiler

Osteochondritis Dissecans (Shoulder)

Description: OCD of the humeral head is a common cause of foreleg lameness and arguably the most prevalent form of osteochondrosis in the dog. Trauma in the shoulder joint is believed to damage the articular cartilage and form a cartilage flap in the caudal-central region of the humeral head. Males are affected approximately twice as frequently as females.

Breeds: 🐾 **Afghan hound, Bernese mountain dog**, boxer, **Chihuahua, Dalmatian, Doberman pinscher, English setter, German shepherd dog, German shorthaired pointer, golden retriever, Great Dane, Great Pyrenees**, greyhound, **Irish setter, Irish wolfhound, kuvasz, Labrador retriever, mastiff**, large **Münsterländer, Newfoundland**, old English sheepdog, **pointer, (miniature) poodle, (standard) poodle, Rhodesian ridgeback, Rottweiler, St Bernard, Samoyed, Siberian husky, vizsla**, whippet

Osteochondritis Dissecans (Stifle)

Description: The most common presentation is hindleg lameness that becomes worse after exercise. Most affected dogs develop problems by 5–7 months of age. Of the cases reported, approximately three-quarters are males. Osteochondrosis of the physis between the apophysis and the cranioproximal tibial diaphysis has been suggested as a cause of avulsion of the tibial tuberosity in Doberman pinschers, greyhounds, and Rottweilers.

Breeds: 🐾 **Akita, Border collie, boxer, bullmastiff, bull terrier, chow chow, collie, Doberman pinscher, German shepherd dog, German wirehaired pointer, golden retriever, Great Dane, greyhound, Irish wolfhound, Labrador retriever, mastiff, Newfoundland, (standard) poodle, Rottweiler, Samoyed, (giant) schnauzer, Staffordshire bull terrier**

Osteochondrodysplasia (Canine)

Description: The term osteochondrodysplasia refers to a developmental abnormality of cartilage and bone resulting from delayed endochondral ossification (formation of bone from cartilage). Although most dogs are not crippled by the disorder, affected animals have a higher incidence of arthritis and joint pain. In most variants, the condition is transmitted as an autosomal recessive trait. In poodles, the condition results from mutations in the SLC13A1 gene.

Breeds: 🐾 **Akita, Alaskan malamute, American water spaniel, Australian shepherd, German shepherd dog, Great Pyrenees, Havanese, Irish setter, Labrador retriever, Norwegian elkhound, perro de presa Canario, (miniature) poodle, (toy) poodle, Samoyed, Scottish deerhound, Shetland sheepdog**

Osteochondrodysplasia (Feline)

Description: Scottish fold cats have a dominantly inherited osteochondrodysplasia involving malformation in the distal forelimbs, distal hindlimbs and tail, and progressive joint destruction. This appears to be associated with the TRPV4 gene. DNA testing is available.

Breeds: Highland fold, Scottish fold

Osteochondromatosis

Description: A skeletal condition characterized by abnormal development of endochondral bones. In some cases, it is capable of transitioning into malignant forms. Osteochondromatosis is more common in the cat (where there does not seem to be a breed predisposition but an association with feline leukemia virus or transmissible feline sarcoma) than the dog, but in dogs the variant has been determined in the EXT2 gene.

Breeds: 🐾 **American Staffordshire terrier**

Osteogenesis Imperfecta

Description: Osteogenesis imperfecta is a collection of rare heritable conditions associated with bone brittleness. Affected dogs have structural abnormalities in type I collagen. Different breed-specific variants are associated with mutations of different genes (COL1A2, SERPINH1, etc.) and with different modes of inheritance. DNA testing is available for some variants.

Breeds: 🐕 Beagle, Bedlington terrier, chow chow, dachshund, German shepherd dog, golden retriever, Norwegian elkhound, (miniature) poodle

Otitis Externa

Description: An inflammatory disorder of the external ear canal, potentially involving many different underlying factors such as predisposition to other underlying conditions (e.g., allergies), anatomical variations, fur in the ear canal, etc. Otitis externa is common in many dog and cat breeds, and even in many mixed-breed animals.

Breeds: 🐕 Brittany spaniel, Chinese shar-pei, (American) cocker spaniel, German shepherd dog, Labrador retriever, (miniature) poodle, Shetland sheepdog, Siberian husky

PAIN SYNDROME

Description: Beagle pain syndrome, also known as polyarteritis, affects beagles from 5 to 10 months of age and results in fever, depression, reluctance to move, and intense cervical hyperesthesia. In all likelihood, it is a manifestation of juvenile polyarteritis syndrome. A mode of inheritance has not been determined, but there is a striking breed predisposition.

Breeds: 🐕 Beagle

Pancreatitis

Description: Acute pancreatitis is commonly encountered in dogs, and there is a clear breed predisposition in dogs, if not evidence for outright inheritance. Variants of the SPINK1 gene may be associated with the development of pancreatitis, at least in miniature schnauzers.

Breeds: 🐕 Airedale terrier, Alaskan malamute, Australian terrier, boxer, cairn terrier, Cavalier King Charles spaniel, American cocker spaniel, collie, dachshund, smooth fox terrier, Lhasa apso, (miniature) poodle, (standard, miniature) schnauzer, schipperke, Yorkshire terrier; 🐈 Pixie-bob, Siamese

Panniculitis

Description: An uncommon inflammatory disease of the subcutaneous fat of dogs caused by a variety of underlying disorders. Genetics does not appear to play a primary role, but some breeds may be predisposed. Breed-specific variants include pedal panniculitis of German shepherd dogs, and vaccine-induced focal panniculitis in poodles.

Breeds: 🐕 Australian shepherd, Brittany spaniel, Chihuahua, collie, dachshund, Dalmatian, German shepherd dog, Pomeranian, (miniature) poodle

Pannus

Description: Also known as chronic superficial keratitis, this is a condition in which pigment and blood vessels grow across the cornea, appearing like a dark film. Genetics is believed to play some role, but environmental factors are also important. There is some association with a specific haplotype (HLA-DRB1) in the German Shepherd dog.

Breeds: 🐕 Airedale terrier, Australian kelpie, Australian shepherd, Belgian Malinois, Belgian sheepdog, Belgian Tervuren, bloodhound, Border collie, Chinese shar-pei, chow chow, dachshund, Dalmatian, Dutch shepherd, English bulldog, German shepherd dog, golden retriever, greyhound, Irish red and white setter, löwchen, miniature pinscher, Pekingese, (English) pointer, pug, Shetland sheepdog, shih tzu, Siberian husky, Tibetan spaniel

Panosteitis

Description: An inflammatory condition that affects the leg bones. The condition affects males more frequently than females and is often recurrent or periodic in nature.

Breeds: 🐕 Basset hound, Bernese mountain dog, Chinese shar-pei, Dalmatian, Doberman pinscher, English springer spaniel, German shepherd dog, giant schnauzer, Great Dane, Great Pyrenees, Irish wolfhound, Labrador retriever, (English) mastiff, Rottweiler, St Bernard and many more

Paroxysmal Dyskinesias

Description: Paroxysmal dyskinesias are episodes of abnormal involuntary hyperkinetic movements or muscle tone. Most canine variants are believed to be breed specific and autosomal recessive in nature, and actual gene mutations (e.g., PIGN) have been determined for some breeds, so DNA testing is available for some of these variants.

Breeds: 🐕 Bichon frisé, Border terrier, Cavalier King Charles spaniel, Chinook, Doberman pinscher, English bulldog, Jack Russell terrier, Labrador retriever, markiesje, Norwich terrier, soft-coated wheaten terrier, Scottish terrier

Parvovirus Susceptibility

Description: It is appreciated that certain breeds seem to be more prone to parvovirus infection, perhaps associated with some form of immune dysfunction. A mode of inheritance has not been determined.

Breeds: 🐕 Doberman pinscher, German shepherd dog, Rottweiler

Patellar Luxation

Description: Patellar luxation refers to the condition in which the kneecap slips out of its usual resting place and lodges on the medial or lateral aspect of the knee. Medial patellar luxation is evident in young dogs and is considered a heritable trait. Lateral patellar luxation, also referred to as genu valgum, also demonstrates breed predisposition.

Breeds: 🐕 Affenpinscher, Boston terrier, cairn terrier, Chihuahua, (American) cocker spaniel, Great Dane, Irish wolfhound, papillon, Pekingese, Pomeranian, (miniature) poodle, (toy) poodle, Rottweiler, St Bernard, (Australian) silky terrier, Yorkshire terrier, and many others; 🐈 Abyssinian, Cheetoh, Cornish Rex, Devon Rex, Maine Coon, Siamese, Tonkinese

Patent Ductus Arteriosus (PDA)

Description: The most common congenital heart defect in dogs, inherited as a polygenic threshold trait with a high rate of heritability in some breeds. This defect occurs when the normal fetal connection between the nonfunctional lungs and the aorta fails to close after birth, resulting in blood being shunted into the pulmonary artery and over-perfusing the lungs. Females often outnumber males.

Breeds: 🐕 Bichon frisé, Chihuahua, Border collie, (American) cocker spaniel, collie, English springer spaniel, German shepherd dog, keeshond, Kerry blue terrier, Maltese, Pomeranian, (miniature) poodle, (toy) poodle, rottweiler, Shetland sheepdog, and Yorkshire terrier and many others; 🐈 Persian

Pectinate Ligament Dysplasia

Description: A developmental disorder of the pectinate ligament and iridocorneal filtration angle, which can predispose to closed-angle glaucoma. A genetic basis has not been determined, but breed predisposition has been recognized.

Breeds: 🐕 Leonberger, (English) springer spaniel, (Welsh) springer spaniel

Pectus Excavatum

Description: Also known as funnel chest, this is a congenital developmental anomaly in which there is deviation of the sternum. Most cases are congenital but not necessarily heritable, although the condition was reported to affect Welsh terrier littermates.

Breeds: 🐕 Welsh terrier; 🐈 Munchkin

Pelger–Huet (PH) Anomaly

Description: A hereditary defect of white blood cells. The mode of inheritance is not known for certain, but it is presumed to be autosomal dominant with incomplete penetrance, at least in the Australian shepherd. Dogs that receive a PH gene from both parents usually die before they are born, and survivors are considered immune cripples.

Breeds: 🐕 Australian cattle dog, Australian shepherd, black and tan coonhound, basenji, Border collie, Boston terrier, (American) cocker spaniel, foxhound, German shepherd dog, redbone coonhound, Samoyed, mixed-breed dogs

Pemphigoid (Bullous)

Description: Pemphigoid refers to a complex of blistering conditions characterized by autoantibody deposition at the junction between the epidermis and dermis, with blister formation immediately deep to the epidermis. Canine bullous pemphigoid is a more generalized form of the disease, and cicatricial pemphigoid tends to be more localized.

Breeds: 🐕 Collie, dachshund, Doberman pinscher, Shetland sheepdog

Pemphigoid (Mucous Membrane)

Description: Also known as cicatricial pemphigoid, this is an erosive-ulcerative immune-mediated disease association with circulating autoantibodies to basement membrane zone antigens. The most common areas of involvement are the oral cavity, nose, periocular areas, and genitalia.

Breeds: German shepherd dog

Pemphigus

Description: A complex of blistering disorders characterized by autoantibody deposition within the epidermis. Variants include pemphigus vulgaris, pemphigus foliaceus (PF), pemphigus erythematosus (PE), and pemphigus vegetans, of which only PF and PE have recognized breed predispositions.

Pemphigus Erythematosus

Description: A localized form of pemphigus often resulting in a vesiculopustular to erosive-ulcerative crusting nasal dermatosis.

Breeds: Collie, German shepherd dog, Shetland sheepdog

Pemphigus Foliaceus

Description: A more generalized form of pemphigus often resulting in a vesiculopustular to erosive-ulcerative dermatosis which can occur anywhere on the body. This is the most common form of pemphigus diagnosed in dogs and cats.

Breeds: Akita, bearded collie, Chinese shar-pei, chow chow, collie, dachshund, Doberman pinscher, English springer spaniel, Finnish spitz, German shepherd dog, Newfoundland, schipperke, Shetland sheepdog; Domestic shorthair, domestic longhair, Himalayan, Maine Coon, Persian, Siamese

Perianal Fistulae

Description: A condition in which draining tracts form around the anus. Most likely it is an inflammatory or immune-mediated condition of the glands surrounding the anus or the tracts that drain them. The condition affects males twice as often as females, and there are strong breed predispositions. Genetic markers have been identified and can be used to help assess risk in susceptible dogs.

Breeds: German shepherd dog, Irish setter, Leonberger, Shiloh shepherd

Peripheral Neuropathies

Description: Peripheral neuropathies are a collection of neurological disorders affecting the peripheral nervous system, but not necessarily exclusively. Individual conditions are often quite distinct, and typically breed specific.

Breeds: Alaskan malamute, Border collie, bouvier des Flandres, Dalmatian, German shepherd dog, Great Dane, Italian spinone, Leonberger, Rottweiler

Peripheral Neuropathy (Alaskan Malamute Polyneuropathy)

Description: Hereditary polyneuropathy is believed to be an autosomal recessive trait and is seen in Alaskan malamutes. It results in paraparesis between 6 and 18 months of age, with gradual progression to the front limbs. The condition is due to a mutation of the NDRG1 gene, and DNA testing is available.

Breeds: Alaskan malamute

Peripheral Neuropathy (Dancing Doberman Disease)

Description: A progressive neuromuscular disease of unknown etiology, but genetics likely plays some role because the condition is seen only in the Doberman pinscher. A mode of inheritance, however, has not been determined. Most dogs have exaggerated hindlimb reflexes, and some have conscious proprioceptive deficits and muscle atrophy.

Breeds: Doberman pinscher

Peripheral Neuropathy (Distal Sensorimotor)

Description: A gradually progressive polyneuropathy characterized by paraparesis that proceeds to tetraparesis and muscle atrophy. There are some similarities to hereditary motor and sensory neuropathy (HMSN) type II in humans and the condition also resembles Rottweiler polyneuropathy. In the Great Dane, the chronic, progressive, symmetrical distal polyneuropathy is associated with axonal degeneration and segmental demyelination.

Breeds: 🐕 **Bouvier des Flandres, Chesapeake Bay retriever, Great Dane**

Peripheral Neuropathy (Giant Axonal Neuropathy)

Description: Giant axonal neuropathy is considered to be an autosomal recessive trait in German shepherd dogs. It is not strictly a peripheral neuropathy; the CNS can be involved as well. Affected dogs develop paraparesis at just over a year of age, with progression to the front legs, proprioceptive deficits, hypotonia, and muscle atrophy.

Breeds: 🐕 **German shepherd dog**

Peripheral Neuropathy (Golden Retriever)

Description: A different axonopathy and neuronopathy has also been reported in animals that lack proprioceptive ataxia or proprioceptive positioning deficits seen in other peripheral neuropathies in the breed. The condition is characterized by lower motor neuron paresis.

Breeds: 🐕 **Golden retriever**

Peripheral Neuropathy (Greyhound Polyneuropathy)

Description: A polyneuropathy seen in greyhounds that results in muscle weakness, exercise intolerance, and an unusual bunny-hopping gait. The disorder is caused by a mutation in the NDRG1 gene and is transmitted as an autosomal recessive trait. DNA testing is available.

Breeds: 🐕 **Greyhound**

Peripheral Neuropathy (Hypertrophic Neuropathy)

Description: Also known as demyelinative neuropathy, hypertrophic neuropathy is likely an autosomal recessive disorder of recurrent demyelination and remyelination.

Affected dogs develop pelvic limb ataxia by 2 months of age, quickly progressing to tetraplegia. Although individuals seem to improve over 1–2 months, weakness often remains.

Breeds: 🐕 **Tibetan mastiff**

Peripheral Neuropathy (Hypomyelinating Neuropathy)

Description: Hypomyelinating neuropathy is suspected to be a heritable neuropathy characterized by reduced myelination in peripheral nerves. Affected dogs have hindlimb ataxia by 2 months of age, but progression is minimal.

Breeds: 🐕 **Golden retriever**

Peripheral Neuropathy (Leonberger Polyneuropathy)

Description: A family of polyneuropathies affecting the Leonberger, and caused by distinct mutations of the ARHGEF10 and GJA9 genes. LPN1 is autosomal recessive, while LPN2 is autosomal dominant with incomplete penetrance. There are some similarities to Charcot–Marie–Tooth disease in humans. DNA testing is available for some breed-specific variants.

Breeds: 🐕 **Leonberger, St Bernard**

Peripheral Neuropathy (Progressive Axonopathy)

Description: Progressive axonopathy in the boxer is believed to be an autosomal recessive disorder, with axonal swellings in spinal nerve roots and lateral and ventral funiculi of the spinal cord. Affected dogs develop pelvic limb ataxia as pups, and this ataxia progresses to the front limbs by 1 year of age. Similar conditions have been documented in other breeds.

Breeds: 🐕 **Border terrier, boxer, golden retriever, Great Pyrenees**

Peripheral Neuropathy (Rottweiler Polyneuropathy)

Description: A distal sensorimotor polyneuropathy is believed to be an autosomal recessive trait seen in Rottweilers. The condition results in distal axonal degeneration in both motor and sensory fibers, with secondary demyelination. Paraparesis is seen in adult dogs, eventually progressing to tetraparesis. There are some similarities to HMSN type II in humans.

Breeds: 🐕 **Rottweiler**

Peripheral Neuropathy (Sensory Ataxic Neuropathy)

Description: Sensory ataxic neuropathy is an inherited neurological disorder caused by a mutation in mitochondrial DNA. As such, it is passed from mother to offspring. The disorder is due to a deletion in the mitochondrial tRN-Tyr gene, which leads to mitochondrial dysfunction and progressive loss of neurons. DNA testing is available.

Breeds: 🐕 **Golden retriever**

Peripheral Neuropathy (Sensory Neuropathy)

Description: Sensory neuropathy is thought to be an autosomal recessive loss of axons in primary sensory nerves. Affected animals develop ataxia by 2 months of age, with diminished pain perception. Although the condition is nonprogressive, urinary and fecal incontinence, and genital self-mutilation can be extremely problematic. Sensory neuropathy in the Border collie is transmitted as an autosomal recessive trait, the mutation has been characterized, and DNA testing is available.

Breeds: 🐕 **Border collie, (longhaired) dachshund**

Peripheral Neuropathy (Warburg Micro Syndrome I)

Description: An inherited form of breed-specific polyneuropathy associated with ocular abnormalities and neuronal vacuolation. They are associated with mutations in the RAB3GAP1 gene, and inherited as autosomal recessive traits. Breed-specific DNA testing is available.

Breeds: 🐕 **Alaskan husky, black Russian terrier, boxer, Rottweiler**

Persistent Atrial Standstill

Description: A lack of atrial activity resulting from a failure of atrial depolarization. It some cases, it is suspected to be due to Emery–Dreifuss muscular dystrophy, and

underlying cardiac pathology, such as myocarditis, may be present. Breed predisposition has been recognized.

Breeds: 🐕 **Border terrier, (English) springer spaniel**

Persistent Mullerian Duct Syndrome

Description: A form of pseudohermaphroditism, inherited as an autosomal recessive trait, in which there is a mutation of the gene responsible for the normal regression of female Mullerian structures in males. Normal-appearing males have oviducts, a uterus, and a cranial vagina in addition to male sex organs. Affected animals may produce normal amounts of Mullerian inhibiting substance (MIS) but the MIS receptor is absent or defective. The disorder has been characterized to the MISRII gene, is transmitted as an autosomal recessive trait, and DNA testing is available.

Breeds: 🐕 **Bassett hound, (miniature) schnauzer**

Persistent Primary Vitreous and Persistent Hyaloid Artery

Description: These refer to vascular remnants of the hyaloid artery or primary vitreous that persist. The heritability is not known in most affected breeds, but there are recognized breed predispositions for both conditions.

Breeds: 🐕 **Bloodhound, bouvier des Flandres, Doberman pinscher, English toy spaniel, Irish setter, Labrador retriever, (standard) schnauzer, Siberian husky, soft-coated wheaten terrier, Staffordshire bull terrier, and many more**

Persistent Pupillary Membranes (PPM)

Description: PPM are remnants of fetal eye tissue that, before birth, cover the pupil and provide a blood supply for the developing lens. While the mode of inheritance is still undefined in most breeds, breed predispositions are recognized.

Breeds: 🐕 **Australian cattle dog, Australian shepherd, basenji, bichon frisé, collie, chow chow, Doberman pinscher, English cocker spaniel, mastiff, miniature bull terrier, miniature longhaired dachshund, Nova Scotia duck tolling retriever, old English sheepdog, (standard) poodle, Scottish terrier,**

Staffordshire bull terrier, (Cardigan) Welsh corgi, (Pembroke) Welsh corgi, West Highland white terrier and many more

Persistent Right Aortic Arch

Description: A vascular ring anomaly in which the aorta is formed by the right fourth aortic arch instead of the left fourth aortic arch. In this anomaly, the esophagus and trachea are encircled by a vascular ring consisting of the aorta on the right, the pulmonary trunk and base of the heart ventrally, and the ligamentum arteriosum on the left. Mode of inheritance is unknown, but breed predispositions have been recognized.

Breeds: Australian shepherd, Boston terrier, (American) cocker spaniel, German shepherd dog, Great Dane, greyhound, Irish setter

Pes Varus

Description: An angular limb deformity involving the distal tibia turning inward, typically around 5–6 months of age. A genetic basis has not been determined, but breed predisposition has been recognized.

Breeds: Dachshund

Phosphofructokinase (PFK) Deficiency

Description: Also known as Tauri disease and glycogen storage disease VII, this is a genetic disease that interferes with the metabolism of glucose in the body. It results in exercise intolerance, anemia, fever, and muscle disease. It is inherited as an autosomal recessive trait, breed-specific mutations of the *PFKM gene* have been characterized, and genetic testing is available for some variants.

Breeds: Boykin spaniel, (American) cocker spaniel, (English) cocker spaniel, (English) springer spaniel, Wachtelhund (German spaniel), whippet

Piebaldism

Description: A form of partial albinism characterized by discrete patches of white skin (leukoderma). It arises from mutations in the c-kit gene. Genetic testing can identify piebald trait in several breeds.

Breeds: Boxer, bull terrier, collie, Great Dane, Italian greyhound, Shetland sheepdog

Pigmentary Uveitis

Description: An inflammatory eye disease characterized by deposits of pigment in the iris and anterior lens capsule. A genetic basis has not been determined, but breed predisposition has been recognized.

Breeds: Golden retriever

Pituitary Dwarfism (Hypopituitarism)

Description: Pituitary dwarfism is inherited as a simple autosomal recessive trait, caused by a mutation in the LHX3 gene. The earliest indication tends to be a failure to grow and retention of a puppy coat compared with littermates. The clinical signs are variable depending upon the extent of pituitary impairment. DNA testing is available for some breed-specific variants.

Breeds: Chow chow, Czechoslovakian wolf dog, Finnish spitz, German shepherd dog, Karelian bear dog, miniature pinscher, Saarloos wolf dog, toy pinscher, Weimaraner

Platelet D-Storage Pool Disease

Description: This is an inherited platelet disorder, suspected to be autosomal recessive in nature. Affected dogs have moderate to severe bleeding episodes after minor trauma, venipuncture, and surgery.

Breeds: (American) cocker spaniel

Pneumocystosis

Description: A poorly understood respiratory infection associated with *Pneumocystis carinii* pneumonia. Stunting of growth does not seem to be a feature of this disorder. The mode of inheritance has not yet been determined, but males are more often affected.

Breeds: Cavalier King Charles spaniel, dachshund

Polycystic Kidney Disease (PKD) (Canine)

Description: A collection of cystic renal diseases often with breed-specific variants and modes of inheritance. The condition has been reported in many breeds, and a strong familial tendency has been reported in several. The condition can progress to renal failure if the cysts enlarge and compress the renal parenchyma. In some breeds, the condition is also associated with dilatation of the intra- and extrahepatic bile ducts. The genetic variants have been characterized in some of these breed-specific entities, and DNA testing is available for those variants. The condition is considered to be autosomal dominant with incomplete penetrance in the bull terrier.

Breeds: 🐕 **Beagle, bull terrier, cairn terrier, West Highland white terrier**

Polycystic Kidney Disease (Feline)

Description: PKD is a relatively common cause of kidney failure in cats, and the heritable form typically causes cysts that can be documented by 12 months of age, although renal failure does not occur until later in life. Hepatic cysts and cardiac lesions are sometimes also present. The heritable condition is transmitted as an autosomal dominant trait with incomplete penetrance, the mutation has been characterized, and breed-specific DNA testing is available. This is most commonly seen in Persian cats, but many breeds have been periodically affected.

Breeds: 🐈 **American shorthair, British longhair, British shorthair, Birman, Burmilla, Chartreux, Colorpoint shorthair, Exotic shorthair, Himalayan, Maine Coon, Persian, Ragdoll, Russian blue, Scottish fold, Selkirk Rex, Siamese, Snoeshoe, Sphynx, Turkish angora, Turkish van**

Polycystic Liver Disease

Description: A poorly characterized group of disorders in which cysts are recognized within the liver parenchyma. Some are congenital, some may occur in adults, and others are associated with PKD. A genetic basis has not been determined, but breed predisposition has been recognized.

Breeds: 🐕 **Beagle, bull terrier, cairn terrier, West Highland white terrier;** 🐈 **Persian**

Polydactyly

Description: Polydactyly refers to the presence of extra toes, and true polydactyly is a congenital abnormality inherited as an autosomal dominant trait of the Pd gene, with

incomplete penetrance. Some cats are bred specifically for this trait. The prevalence is much less in dogs, where it is typically associated with mutations of the *LMBR1 gene*.

Breeds: 🐕 **Australian shepherd, Great Pyrenees, Norwegian lundehund, St Bernard;** 🐈 **Maine Coon; many others**

Polydontia

Description: Polydontia can be attributable to supernumerary or extra teeth, or to retained deciduous teeth, and the condition is prevalent in some breeds. However, the actual mode of inheritance has not been characterized in most instances.

Breeds: 🐕 **Affenpinscher, Border terrier, boxer, Brussels griffon, bull terrier, bullmastiff, Chihuahua, (English) cocker spaniel, collie, Doberman pinscher, English bulldog, golden retriever, greyhound, komondor, Labrador retriever, Maltese, Irish setter, Italian greyhound, Manchester terrier, papillon, Rottweiler, West Highland white terrier, Yorkshire terrier**

Polyendocrinopathy

Description: An immune-mediated genetic disease in which multiple endocrine organs are targeted for autoimmune attack. The condition is rare but bears some resemblance to Schmidt's syndrome in people.

Breeds: 🐕 **Italian greyhound**

Polymicrogyria

Description: A developmental disorder in which dogs are born with many smaller gyri on the surface of the brain. It appears to be a familial trait, but a mode of inheritance has not yet been determined.

Breeds: 🐕 **Standard poodle**

Polymyositis

Description: A systemic inflammatory muscle disease of adult dogs. Polymyositis can also appear as a component of other immune-mediated diseases such as systemic lupus erythematosus

Breeds: 🐕 **Boxer, Newfoundland, vizsla, (Pembroke) Welsh corgi**

Polyneuropathy

Description: A collection of peripheral nerve disorders, often with breed-specific features. See also peripheral neuropathy. *Polyneuropathy in the Alaskan malamute is an autosomal recessive trait and the genetic mutation to the NDRG1 gene has been characterized and DNA testing is available.* There is some similarity between the manifestations of polyneuropathy seen in young Bengal cats and chronic inflammatory demyelinating polyneuropathy in people. There is also a central-peripheral distal axonopathy seen in Birman cats, and an axonal neuropathy reported in young Snoeshoe cats. DNA testing is available for some variants on a breed-specific basis.

Breeds: 🐕 **Alaskan husky, Alaskan malamute, black Russian terrier, bouvier des Flandres, greyhound, Rottweiler, St Benard, Italian spinone, Leonberger;** 🐈 **Bengal, Birman, Snoeshoe**

Polyneuropathy, Leonberger 1 (LPN1)

Description: *A juvenile polyneuropathy, sometimes referred to as Leonberger polyneuropathy 1 (LPN1) in the Leonberger and St Bernard is autosomal recessive, characterized by a mutation to the ARHGEF10 gene, and DNA testing is available. The condition is usually first evident between 2 and 3 years of age, with severe progression.*

Breeds: 🐕 **Leonberger, St Bernard**

Polyneuropathy, Leonberger 2 (LPN2)

Description: *Leonberger polyneuropathy 2 is autosomal dominant, the mutation on the GJA9 gene has been characterized, and DNA testing is available. This polyneuropathy is usually first evident at around 6 years of age.*

Breeds: 🐕 **Leonberger**

Polyneuropathy (Neuronal Vacuolation – Spinocerebellar Degeneration)

Description: An autosomal recessive neurological condition associated with a variant in the RAB3GAP1 gene. DNA testing is available.

Breeds: 🐕 **Black Russian terrier, Rottweiler**

Polyradiculoneuropathy

Description: Also known as coonhound paralysis, this is a group of inflammatory diseases of the nerve roots and peripheral nerves. Often associated with acute reactions to racoon saliva or other antigens.

Breeds: 🐕 **Black and tan coonhound, bluetick coonhound, redbone coonhound, West Highland white terrier**

Porphyria

Description: Porphyria refers to a variety of disorders in which pigment is deposited in skin and teeth, and anemia may be present. There are several forms recognized in cats, including different forms associated with the HMBS and UROS genes. At least some variants of inherited porphyria appear to be autosomal recessive in nature, and DNA testing is available for some breed-specific variants.

Breeds: 🐈 **American shorthair, Siamese**

Portal Vein Hypoplasia

Description: Also known as hepatic microvascular dysplasia, this refers to a vascular developmental anomaly of the portal vein in dogs and cats. It's nonprogressive but can occur alone or in association with PSS. A genetic basis has not been determined, but breed predisposition has been recognized.

Breeds:, 🐕 **Cairn terrier, (American) cocker spaniel, dachshund, Lhasa apso, Maltese, (miniature) poodle, (toy) poodle, shih tzu, Spanish water dog, West Highland white terrier, Yorkshire terrier**

Portosystemic Shunts

Description: Congenital PSS are vascular anomalies that divert portal venous blood directly to the systemic venous circulation, bypassing the liver. Different types of shunts likely have different breed-specific presentations and modes of inheritance.

Breeds: 🐕 **Australian cattle dog, bichon frisé, Border collie, cairn terrier, (American) cocker spaniel, dachshund, Dandie Dinmont terrier, Havanese, Irish wolfhound, Jack Russell terrier, Lhasa apso, Maltese, Pekingese, poodle, pug, (miniature) schnauzer, shih tzu, (Australian) silky terrier, Yorkshire terrier and many more;** 🐈 **Himalayan, Persian**

Postoperative Hemorrhage

Description: A hereditary platelet disorder associated with mutations in the P2RY12 gene that result in platelet dysfunction and postoperative bleeding. It is inherited as an autosomal recessive trait. DNA testing is available is available for the Greater Swiss mountain dog. A similar condition is seen in greyhounds, but the genetic cause in that breed has not yet been determined.

Breeds: Greater Swiss mountain dog, greyhound

Prekallikrein Deficiency

Description: Also known as Fletcher trait, this is a rare inherited clotting disorder associated with mutations of the KLKB1 gene. The condition may be mild or even subclinical, not being evident until there is injury or surgery, in which delated clotting is noted. It is inherited as an autosomal recessive trait in shih tzus, and DNA testing is available.

Breeds: Poodle, shih tzu

Primary Secretory Otitis Media (PSOM)

Description: Sometimes referred to as "glue ear," this is a poorly defined disorder of the middle ear that is typically associated with pain localized to the head and neck, ataxia, facial paralysis, nystagmus, head tilt, hearing loss, facial pruritus, and potentially even seizures. A breed predisposition has been recognized.

Breeds: Cavalier King Charles spaniel

Prognathism

Description: Also known as undershot jaw and mandibular mesioclusion, this occurs when the mandible is significantly longer than the maxilla. In some animals it constitutes a normal breed characteristic. Prognathism is commonly seen in many breeds of dogs, but the mode of inheritance has not been determined.

Breeds: Afghan hound, akita, American Eskimo dog, American Staffordshire terrier, Australian shepherd, beagle, Belgian sheepdog, Boston terrier, (American) cocker spaniel, English bulldog, French bulldog, Cavalier King Charles spaniel, Lhasa apso, Pekingese, pug, shih tzu and many others; Burmese, Persian

Progressive Retinal Atrophy (PRA)

Description: PRA refers to several inherited disorders affecting the retina and resulting in blindness. PRA is thought to be inherited in most breeds, with each breed demonstrating a specific age of onset and pattern of inheritance. The condition is potentially even more frustrating because certain breeds may be prone to more than one form of PRA.

Progressive Retinal Atrophy (Type A)

Description: A breed-specific variant of PRA that is actually less common in the breed than type B. The genetic mutation has been characterized, and DNA testing is available. The condition is transmitted as an autosomal recessive trait.

Breeds: Miniature schnauzer

Progressive Retinal Atrophy (TYPE B)

Description: A breed-specific variant of PRA that is presumed to be inherited as an autosomal recessive trait with incomplete penetrance. The mutation has been identified, and appears to be a more common cause of PRA in the breed than type A. The mutation has been characterized and DNA testing is available.

Breeds: Miniature schnauzer

Progressive Retinal Atrophy (Bardet–Biedl Syndrome)

Description: An inherited retinopathy associated with genetic mutations to the BBS4 gene. It is inherited as an autosomal recessive trait. DNA testing is available.

Breeds: Puli

Progressive Retinal Atrophy (Central)

Description: Also known as retinal pigment epithelial dystrophy (RPED), this is a poorly characterized disorder of retinal pigmented epithelium resulting in progressive retinal degeneration and photoreceptor degeneration. There appears to be different breed-specific modes of inheritance and clinical presentations.

Breeds: 🐕 **Black and tan coonhound, Border collie, boxer, Briard, Chesapeake Bay retriever, (American) cocker spaniel, (English) cocker spaniel, collie, English pointer, English setter, (wire) fox terrier, German shepherd dog, golden retriever, Irish setter, keeshond, Labrador retriever, Polish owczarek nizinny, redbone coonhound, Shetland sheepdog, (English) springer spaniel, (Cardigan) Welsh corgi**

Progressive Retinal Atrophy (PRA-CNGA1)

Description: A breed-specific form of adult-onset PRA degenerative eye disease caused by mutations of the CNGA1 gene and transmitted as autosomal recessive traits. The earliest manifestation is often night blindness. DNA testing is available.

Breeds: 🐕 **Shetland sheepdog**

Progressive Retinal Atrophy (Cord 1)

Description: A form of PRA controlled by mutations of the RPGRIP1 gene, generally transmitted as autosomal recessive traits with incomplete penetrance. In this cone-rod dystrophy, the cones are affected first before the rods, which is the opposite order from most other forms of PRA. This is analogous to the cone-rod dysplasia 4 (crd4) variant, although breeds listed as predisposed may differ in the veterinary literature.

Breeds: 🐕 **Beagle, Boykin spaniel, Chihuahua, curly-coated retriever, dachshund (miniature longhaired, miniature smooth, miniature wirehaired, standard longhaired, standard smooth, standard wirehaired), field spaniel, French bulldog, Labrador retriever, Labradoodle, (English) springer spaniel**

Progressive Retinal Atrophy (Cord 2)

Description: A form of PRA controlled by mutations of the NPHP4 gene, generally transmitted as an autosomal recessive trait. In this cone-rod dystrophy, the cones are affected first before the rods, which is the opposite order from most other forms of PRA.

Breeds: 🐕 **Wire-haired dachshund**

Progressive Retinal Atrophy (Cone-Rod Dysplasia)

Description: A group of PRA disorders associated with degeneration of both cone and rod cells. There are several different variants (crd1, crd2, crd3, crd4, crd-SWD), mostly involving breed-specific mutations of the NPHP4, PDE6B, ADAM9, and IQCB1 genes. The variant crd4 is analogous to the cord1 disorder and crd1 has been reclassified as rcd1b. All seem to be transmitted as autosomal recessive traits, and DNA testing is available for many on a breed-specific basis.

Breeds: 🐕 **American pit bull terrier, American bully, American Staffordshire terrier, Australian cobber dog (Labradoodle), beagle, Boykin spaniel, Chihuahua, dachshund, field spaniel, French bulldog, Glen of Imaal terrier, Labrador retriever, papillon, phalene, Portuguese podengo pequeno, (English) springer spaniel, Staffordshire bull terrier**

Progressive Retinal Atrophy (Dominant)

Description: A form of PRA controlled by mutations in the RHO (rhodopsin) gene, and the only form transmitted as an autosomal dominant trait. Affected animals may have demonstrable night blindness early in life, but do not typically lose all of their sight until around 2 years of age. The genetic variant has been characterized, and DNA testing is available.

Breeds: 🐕 **Bullmastiff, (English) mastiff**

Progressive Retinal Atrophy (Early Retinal Degeneration)

Description: An early-onset autosomal recessive hereditary form of PRA associated with mutation in the STK38L gene and characterized by abnormal photoreceptor development and rapid retinal degeneration. DNA testing is available. The condition bears some resemblance to human Leber congenital amaurosis.

Breeds: 🐕 **Norwegian elkhound**

Progressive Retinal Atrophy (EARLY-ONSET)

Description: A breed-specific early onset variant of PRA that is inherited as an autosomal recessive trait. Currently a mutation has been determined and DNA test available, but it is presumed that other forms of early onset disease may exist in the breed

Breeds: 🐕 **Portuguese water dog**

Progressive Retinal Atrophy (PRA-GR)

Description: A family of late-onset forms of PRA specific to the golden retriever and caused by at least two different mutations to the SLC4A3 gene (PRA-GR1 and PRA-GR2). They are transmitted as autosomal recessive traits and DNA testing is available for both variants.

Breeds: 🐕 **Golden retriever**

Progressive Retinal Atrophy (IG-PRA1)

Description: A breed-specific late-onset form of PRA that has clinical similarities to other forms of the condition, specifically progressive rod-cone degeneration and cone-rod degeneration-3. It is transmitted as an autosomal recessive trait. DNA testing is available.

Breeds: 🐕 **Italian greyhound**

Progressive Retinal Atrophy (NECAP1)

Description: A breed-specific variant of PRA that leads to retinal degeneration and blindness. The mutation has been characterized and DNA testing is available.

Breeds: 🐕 **Giant schnauzer**

Progressive Retinal Atrophy (PAP1)

Description: A breed-specific form of late-onset PRA degenerative eye disease caused by mutations of the CNGB1 gene and transmitted as autosomal recessive traits. The earliest manifestation is often night blindness. DNA testing is available.

Breeds: 🐕 **Papillon, phalene**

Progressive Retinal Atrophy (PRA3)

Description: A breed-specific form of PRA degenerative eye disease caused by mutations of the FAM161A gene and

transmitted as autosomal recessive traits. The earliest manifestation is often night blindness.

Breeds: 🐕 **Tibetan terrier, Tibetan spaniel**

Progressive Retinal Atrophy (PRA4)

Description: A breed-specific form of PRA, transmitted as an autosomal recessive trait.

Breeds: 🐕 **Lhasa apso**

Progressive Retinal Atrophy (PRA-B)

Description: An early-onset form of PRA in cats that is characterized by photoreceptor destruction early in life. It is transmitted as an autosomal recessive trait, the genetic variant has been characterized, and DNA testing is available.

Breeds: 🐈 **Bengal**

Progressive Retinal Atrophy (PRA-BAS)

Description: A late-onset form of PRA specific to the basenji and caused by a mutation to the SAG gene. It is transmitted as an autosomal recessive trait and DNA testing is available.

Breeds: 🐕 **Basenji**

Progressive Retinal Atrophy (PRA-DS)

Description: Also known as gPRA, this is a breed-specific form of generalized PRA degenerative eye disease caused by mutations of the CCDC66 gene and transmitted as autosomal recessive traits. The earliest manifestation is often night blindness. DNA testing is available.

Breeds: 🐕 **Schapendoes**

Progressive Retinal Atrophy (PRA-PD)

Description: An early-onset form of feline PRA associated with early photoreceptor loss. This so-called Persian-derived (pd) form of early-onset PRA is associated with mutations to the AIPL1 gene, with some similarities to Leber's congenital amaurosis. It is seen most commonly in the Persian, but other breeds may also be affected. The condition is transmitted as an autosomal recessive trait, the genetic variant has been characterized, and DNA testing is available.

Breeds: 🐱 **Birman, British longhair, British shorthair, Chartreux, Colorpoint shorthair, Cornish Rex, Exotic, Himalayan, Javanese, Munchkin, Ocicat, Oriental shorthair, Persian, Peterbald, Ragdoll, Russian blue, Siamese, Scottish fold, Selkirk Rex, Singapura, Somali, Thai, Turkish angora**

Progressive Retinal Atrophy (PRCD)

Description: Progressive rod-cone degeneration is one of the most common forms of PRA and is similar to retinitis pigmentosa in humans. In prcd, the rods are the first to lose their function and then the cones, so that night blindness precedes total blindness. It is inherited as an autosomal recessive trait. Breeds susceptible to prcd have the same gene mutation, even though the severity, age of onset, and characteristics may differ between breeds.

Breeds: 🐕 **American Eskimo dog, Australian cattle dog, Australian shepherd, Australian stumpy tail cattle dog, barbet, black Russian terrier, Bolognese, bolonka zwetna, Chesapeake Bay retriever, Chinese crested dog, (American) cocker spaniel, (English) cocker spaniel, Entlebucher cattle dog, field spaniel, Finnish lapphund, golden retriever, Karelian bear dog, kuvasz, Labrador retriever, Lapponian herder, Manchester terrier, markiesje, mi-ki, Norwegian elkhound, Nova Scotia duck tolling retriever, Pomeranian, Tibetan terrier, poodle, Portuguese water dog, (giant) schnauzer, schipperke, (Australian) silky terrier, Yorkshire terrier**

Progressive Retinal Atrophy (RDAC)

Description: This refers to breed-specific inherited disorders affecting the photoreceptors in the eye. An inherited late-onset blindness (rdAc) involves a mutation of the CEP290 gene and is autosomal recessive. Genetic testing is available for breed-specific variants

Breeds: 🐱 **Abyssinian, American curl, American wirehair, Balinese, Bengal, Cornish Rex, Colorpoint shorthair, Javanese, Munchkin, Ocicat, Oriental shorthair, Peterbald, Siamese, Singapura, Somali, Tonkinese**

Progressive Retinal Atrophy (RDY)

Description: This refers to breed-specific feline disorders affecting the photoreceptors in the eye. An early-onset autosomal dominant photoreceptor degeneration (Rdy) involves a mutation of the CRX gene. Genetic testing is available for breed-specific variants

Breeds: 🐱 **Abyssinian, Ocicat, Somali**

Progressive Retinal Atrophy (Rod-Cone Dysplasia)

Description: Rod-cone dysplasia is a family of PRA eye disorders in which there is degeneration first of the rods, and then later the cones. The different forms are due to breed-specific autosomal recessive mutations in different genes, such as rcd1 (PDEB), rcd1a (PDE6B), rcd1b (PDE6B), rcd2 (RD3), rcd3 (PDE6A), and rcd4 (C2orf71), each variant with different breed predispositions. DNA testing is available for several variants.

Breeds: 🐕 **Australian cattle dog, Chinese crested dog, collie, English setter, Gordon setter, Irish setter, Irish red and white setter, Japanese spitz, (small) Münsterländer, (large) Münsterländer, old Danish pointer, (standard) poodle, Polish lowland sheepdog, Pomeranian, sloughi, (Cardigan) Welsh corgi, (Pembroke) Welsh corgi, Tibetan terrier**

Progressive Retinal Atrophy (Rod Dysplasia)

Description: An early-onset form of PRA that is transmitted as an autosomal recessive trait. Electroretinographic changes to the cones are typically evident by 6 weeks of age, and the ophthalmoscopic diagnosis can be made by 1–2 years of age.

Breeds: 🐕 **Norwegian elkhound**

Progressive Retinal Atrophy (Vallhund)

Description: A breed-specific variant of PRA that is presumed to be inherited as an autosomal recessive trait. The mutation is believed to involve the MERTK gene, and genetic testing indicates increased risk of PRA in the relevant breed.

Breeds: 🐕 **Swedish vallhund**

Progressive Retinal Atrophy (X-Linked)

Description: A group of PRA disorders that are inherited as x-linked traits. There are different varieties (such as PRA-XL1, PRA-XL2, and PRA-XL3) based on breed-specific mutations, often of the RPGR gene. DNA testing is available on a breed-specific basis.

Breeds: 🐕 **Border collie, Samoyed, (miniature) schnauzer, Siberian husky, Weimaraner**

Prolapsed Gland of the Nictitans

Description: Also known as "cherry eye" or "haw," this refers to an enlarged gland at the base of the nictitating membrane that is displaced from its normal position. Although the breed predisposition seems clear-cut, a heritable nature has not been proven.

Breeds: 🐕 **Basset hound, beagle, bloodhound, Boston terrier, boxer, bull terrier, Chinese shar-pei, (American) cocker spaniel, English bulldog, Lhasa apso, Neapolitan mastiff, Newfoundland, (miniature) poodle, St Bernard, shih tzu and many more;** 🐈 **Burmese**

Proliferative Episcleritis

Description: Also known as nodular fasciitis, nodular episcleritis, nodular granulomatous episclerokeratitis, and fibrous histiocytoma, this is likely an immune-mediated familial inflammatory disease in which fleshy masses are seen on the cornea, sclera, nictitating membrane, lips, and conjunctivae.

Breeds: 🐕 **Border collie, (American) cocker spaniel, collie, golden retriever, (miniature) poodle, Shetland sheepdog**

Proptosis

Description: Proptosis occurs when the eye protrudes from the orbit. In many cases, it is due to trauma, but several breeds, especially those which are brachycephalic, have a tendency toward proptosis due to the shallow orbits in these breeds.

Breeds: 🐕 **Lhasa apso, Pekingese, pug, shih tzu**

Protein-Losing Enteropathy

Description: This term refers to a collection of small intestinal diseases that result in the loss of plasma and proteins into the gastrointestinal tract. Some may be primary conditions, such as congenital intestinal lymphangiectasia, while others are likely secondary to underlying problems, such as immunoproliferative enteropathy.

Breeds: 🐕 **Basenji, Maltese, Norwegian lundehund, soft-coated wheaten terrier, Yorkshire terrier**

Protein-Losing Nephropathy

Description: Breed-specific variants of glomerulonephritis, often with different modes of inheritance. In the soft-coated wheaten terrier, there are at least two different mutations (NPHS1, KIRREL2) associated with disease susceptibility and DNA testing is available.

Breeds: 🐕 **Airedale terrier, Bernese mountain dog, golden retriever, Labrador retriever, soft-coated wheaten terrier**

Pseudohyperkalemia

Description: A false elevation of potassium caused by some peculiar blood cell properties in breeds that have higher cellular levels of potassium than other breeds. It is mainly of concern in that it can lead to spurious laboratory results and can also make animals more prone to onion toxicity.

Breeds: 🐕 **Akita, Chinese shar-pei, shiba inu, tosa inu**

Pulmonary Artery Dissection

Description: A rare but catastrophic condition in which the pulmonary artery ruptures and blood is discharged into the mediastinum, typically causing sudden death. It may occur as an individual disorder, or as a complication of PDA or surgery to correct pulmonic stenosis. A genetic basis has not been determined, but breed predisposition has been recognized.

Breeds: 🐕 **Weimaraner**

Pulmonary Fibrosis

Description: Sometimes called Westie lung disease, this refers to a poorly characterized condition in which the underlying problem is thought to be exposure to pollutants or allergens; genetics likely plays at least some role.

Breeds: 🐕 **American Staffordshire terrier, bichon frisé, bull terrier, cairn terrier, Jack Russell terrier, Scottish terrier, shih tzu, Staffordshire bull terrier, West Highland white terrier, Yorkshire terrier**

Pulmonic Stenosis

Description: Pulmonic stenosis refers to a stricture or incomplete opening through the pulmonic valve in the heart. In most cases, the underlying defect is pulmonic valve dysplasia. Many dogs with pulmonic stenosis are asymptomatic but do have a heart murmur. As they get older or if the condition is severe, they show evidence of exercise intolerance, fainting (syncope), coughing (rarely), or fluid accumulation in the body. A mode of inheritance is not known. In the English bulldog, pulmonic stenosis is associated with, and probably caused by, a coronary artery anomaly.

Breeds: 🐕 **Beagle, boxer, Boykin spaniel, Chihuahua, (American) cocker spaniel, English bulldog, fox terrier, keeshond, (English) mastiff, miniature schnauzer, Samoyed, West Highland white terrier and many more**

Pyloric Stenosis

Description: A narrowing of the pyloric canal, such as by congenital antral hypertrophy, resulting in partial or complete obstruction to the outflow of ingesta from the stomach to the small intestines.

Breeds: 🐕 **Boston terrier, boxer, Maltese**

Pyruvate Dehydrogenase Phosphatase 1 Deficiency

Description: An autosomal recessive disorder associated with exercise intolerance, postexercise collapse, and occasionally neurological signs. It is caused by a point mutation of the PDP1 gene and DNA testing is available.

Breeds: 🐕 **Clumber spaniel, Sussex spaniel**

Pyruvate Kinase Deficiency (Canine)

Description: An inherited trait associated with the shortened lifespan of red blood cells. In most breeds, it is inherited as an autosomal recessive trait, associated with mutations of the PKLR gene, and DNA testing is available on a breed-specific basis.

Breeds: 🐕 **American Eskimo dog, basenji, beagle, cairn terrier, Labrador retriever, pug, West Highland white terrier**

Pyruvate Kinase Deficiency (Feline)

Description: An inherited trait associated with the shortened lifespan of red blood cells. In most breeds, it is inherited as an autosomal recessive trait, associated with the PKLR gene, and DNA testing is available on a breed-specific basis.

Breeds: 🐈 **Abyssinian, American shorthair, American longhair, Bengal, domestic longhair, Egyptian Mau, La Perm, Maine Coon, Norwegian forest cat, Ocicat, Savannah, Siberian forest cat, Singapura, Somali**

Raine Syndrome

Description: A form of dental hypomineralization associated with severe tooth wear and pulpitis. It is inherited as an autosomal recessive trait in Border collies, the mutation has been characterized, and DNA testing is available.

Breeds: 🐕 **Border collie**

Recurrent (Seasonal) Flank Alopecia

Description: A skin condition involving bilaterally symmetrical truncal hair loss that waxes and wanes on a seasonal basis. There is often a striking breed predisposition, although the genetic nature has not yet been confirmed.

Breeds: 🐕 **Airedale terrier, bearded collie, boxer, English bulldog, (miniature) schnauzer and others**

Renal Agenesis

Description: A rare condition in dogs in which there seems to be a familial failure of the kidneys to develop properly. The mode of inheritance is not known. Bilateral agenesis is fatal, but unilateral agenesis may remain inapparent as long as the animal maintains adequate renal function.

Breeds: 🐕 **Beagle, Doberman pinscher, Shetland sheepdog**

Renal Dysplasia

Description: A developmental disorder in which the kidneys fail to develop properly and eventually experience impaired function. There are both heritable and nonheritable causes. In some breeds, the condition is thought to be autosomal dominant with incomplete penetrance and in others autosomal recessive. In yet other breeds, it is just recognized as a familial trait.

Breeds: 🐕 **Akita, Alaskan malamute, Bedlington terrier, Bernese mountain dog, chow chow, (American) cocker spaniel, (English) cocker spaniel, collie, Doberman pinscher, Dutch Kookier dog, German shepherd dog, golden retriever, Gordon setter, harrier, Havanese, Kangal shepherd dog, keeshond, Lhasa apso, Norwegian elkhound, (miniature) poodle, (standard) poodle, Portuguese water dog, miniature schnauzer, Samoyed, Shetland sheepdog, shih tzu, soft-coated wheaten terrier, Tibetan terrier, Weimaraner, West Highland white terrier**

Renal Dysplasia and Hepatic Fibrosis

Description: Also known as diffuse cystic renal dysplasia and hepatic fibrosis, this is a debilitating and often fatal breed-specific condition, transmitted as an autosomal recessive trait. The genetic mutation has been characterized in the INPP5E gene, and DNA testing is available.

Breeds: 🐕 **Norwich terrier**

Renal Glucosuria

Description: A defect in proximal renal tubular reabsorption of glucose that results in glucosuria without hyperglycemia. The condition is asymptomatic but may pose concerns for those trying to determine the cause of the glucosuria since there is clinical similarities to Fanconi syndrome. It appears to be transmitted as an autosomal recessive trait.

Breeds: 🐕 **Basenji, Norwegian elkhound, Scottish terrier, mixed-breed dogs**

Renal Telangiectasia

Description: A vascular anomaly characterized by multiple dilated renal blood vessels. Affected dogs present with episodes of hematuria during adulthood.

Breeds: 🐕 **Pembroke Welsh corgi**

Retinal Dysplasia

Description: An abnormal development of the retina that is evident at birth. The condition can exist on its own or be associated with other genetic issues (such as skeletal achondrodysplasia). Most forms of retinal dysplasia are congenital, due to breed-specific genetic mechanisms, and best documented at 12–16 weeks of age, when the retina is mature. Retinal dysplasia can also be part of oculoskeletal dysplasia, which is believed to be inherited as an autosomal dominant trait with incomplete penetrance. DNA testing is available to help predict risk for this disorder.

Breeds: 🐕 **Affenpinscher, Afghan hound, Airedale terrier, Akbash dog, akita, Alaskan malamute, American pit bull terrier, American Staffordshire terrier, American water spaniel, German shepherd dog, Labrador retriever, Samoyed, (English) springer spaniel, Bedlington terrier, Sealyham terrier and many others;** 🐈 **Balinese**

Rhinitis/Bronchopneumonia

Description: A poorly characterized respiratory disorder of adult Irish wolfhounds, starting with rhinitis and proceeding to recurrent bouts of pneumonia. It is believed that the underlying disorder may closely resemble ciliary dyskinesia, and ciliary dysfunction has been documented. A similar condition appears to occur in the Scottish deerhound.

Breeds: 🐕 **Irish wolfhound, Scottish deerhound**

Rickets

Description: Hereditary vitamin D-resistant rickets is the result of an autosomal recessive mutation of the VDR gene in which there is not a deficiency in vitamin D, but rather an end-organ resistance to the active hormone. The result is hypocalcemia, secondary hyperparathyroidism, and hypomineralization of bone. DNA testing is available for breed-specific variants.

Breeds: 🐕 **Pomeranian;** 🐈 **Domestic shorthair, Siamese**

Ridgelessness

Description: The ridge in Rhodesian ridgebacks is a dominant trait. Since homozygosity for the ridge gene predisposes dogs to dermoid sinus, there are many heterozygotes which carry less risk. In a small proportion of heterozygotes, ridge formation will be suppressed, creating a small chance of a heterozygote without ridges. When two heterozygotes are bred, a proportion of the litter will be ridgeless. Since such animals are homozygous for ridgelessness, when bred together they will not produce ridged offspring. DNA testing is available for ridgelessness.

Breeds: 🐕 **Rhodesian ridgeback**

Sacrocaudal Dysgenesis

Description: A malformation of the sacrocaudal vertebrae and spinal cord segments that is believed to be inherited in at least some breeds. Clinical signs are apparent by 4–6 weeks of age.

Breeds: 🐕 **Boston terrier, English bulldog, pug,;** 🐈 **Manx**

Schnauzer Comedo Syndrome

Description: Also known as "schnauzer crud," this syndrome is a keratinization disorder that affects hair follicles, primarily along the topline. The mode of inheritance is not known with certainty but there is a striking breed predisposition.

Breeds: 🐕 **Miniature schnauzer**

Scott Syndrome

Description: An autosomal recessive canine platelet procoagulant deficiency that can be a cause of recurrent hemorrhage because the platelet defect results in impaired thrombin formation. The condition is transmitted as an autosomal recessive trait and DNA testing is available for this form of hemorrhagic diathesis.

Breeds: 🐕 **German shepherd dog**

Scottie Cramp

Description: A paroxysmal hyperkinetic disorder believed to be transmitted as an autosomal recessive trait. The disease involves a functional defect in the neural pathways that control muscle contraction. While the condition is most prevalent in the Scottish terrier, similar conditions have been reported in other breeds, including the Norwich terrier, Cesky terrier, Dalmatian, and Labrador retriever.

Breeds: 🐕 **Scottish terrier**

Sebaceous Adenitis

Description: A collection of inflammatory skin diseases that have in common a destruction of hair follicle elements, especially the sebaceous glands. It likely represents several different breed-specific conditions that share some common clinical or pathological findings. The mode of inheritance likely also varies on a breed-specific basis.

Breeds: 🐕 **Airedale, akita, American Eskimo dog, basset hound, Bernese mountain dog, chow chow, (American) cocker spaniel, collie, dachshund, Dalmatian, Doberman pinscher, German shepherd dog, golden retriever, Havanese, hovawart, Irish setter, Labrador retriever, Lhasa apso, Maltese, miniature pinscher, old English sheepdog, Pomeranian, (miniature) poodle, (standard) poodle, (toy) poodle, St Bernard, Samoyed, Scottish terrier, shih tzu, (English) springer spaniel, (Welsh) springer spaniel, vizsla, Weimaraner**

Seborrhea

Description: True primary seborrhea is an inherited defect of the skin and how it orients itself. Thus, the defect is inherent in the skin itself and is not an internal disorder. The mode of inheritance is not known with certainty.

Breeds: 🐕 **Afghan hound, Airedale terrier, basset hound, cairn terrier, (American) cocker spaniel, Chinese shar-pei, dachshund, Doberman pinscher, German shepherd dog, golden retriever, Irish setter, Labrador retriever, (standard) poodle, Rottweiler, (English) springer spaniel, West Highland white terrier**

Sensory Neuropathy

Description: An inherited sensory neurological disease that is progressive and debilitating. In the Border collie, the variant has been characterized as an autosomal recessive variant of the FAM134B gene, and DNA testing is available. It is likely that many of the sensory neuropathies will be associated with breed-specific mutations and modes of inheritance.

Breeds: 🐕 **Border collie, Brittany spaniel, (long-haired) dachshund, (wire) fox terrier, German short-haired pointer, Jack Russell terrier, (English) pointer, Siberian husky, (Pembroke) Welsh corgi, whippet**

Severe Combined Immunodeficiency (Autosomal Recessive)

Description: A heterogeneous group of immune disorders in which there is failure of both the humoral and cell-mediated immune systems, associated with genetic mutations with an autosomal recessive mode of inheritance. The genetic variants tend to be quite breed specific such as in the Frisian water dog (RAG1) and Jack Russell terrier (PRKDC). DNA testing is available.

Breeds: Frisian water dog (wetterhoun), Jack Russell terrier, Parson Russell terrier

Severe Combined Immunodeficiency (X-Linked)

Description: A heterogeneous group of immune disorders in which there is failure of both the humoral and cell-mediated immune systems, associated with genetic mutations with an x-linked mode of inheritance. The genetic variants tend to be quite breed specific and reflect mutations to the IL2RG gene. DNA testing is available.

Breeds: Bassett hound, (Cardigan) Welsh corgi, (Pembroke) Welsh corgi

Shaker Syndrome

Description: Also known as generalized tremor syndrome, little white shaker syndrome, corticosteroid-responsive tremor syndrome, and generalized sporadic acquired idiopathic tremors, this is a poorly understood condition of young dogs that involves intention tremors of the head and limbs, hypermetria, and ataxia. Despite the breed predisposition, a genetic cause has not been determined, and at least half of affected dogs are not white.

Breeds: Beagle, bichon frisé, dachshund, Finnish spitz, Maltese, miniature pinscher, (miniature) poodle, Samoyed, shih tzu, West Highland white terrier, Yorkshire terrier

Short Tail

Description: Also known as brachyury and bobtail, this is an autosomal dominant trait in several breeds of dog, controlled by a T-box transcription factor involved in development of the embryo. The mutation has been identified and genetic testing is available.

Breeds: Australian cattle dog, Australian shepherd, Australian stumpy-tail cattle dog, Austrian pinscher, boxer, braque du Bourbonnais, Brazilian terrier, Brittany spaniel, Catahoula leopard dog, Croatian sheepdog, Danish/Swedish farm dog, Great Pyrenees, Jack Russell terrier, Kangal shepherd dog, Karelian bear dog, mudi, Polish owczarek nizinny, Pyrenean shepherd, schipperke, Spanish water dog, Swedish vallhund, (Pembroke) Welsh corgi

Sialocele

Description: Also known as a salivary mucocele, these are cystic structures that become apparent as swelling under the neck. The mode of inheritance is not known, but there are breed predispositions recognized.

Breeds: Dachshund, German shepherd dog, (miniature) poodle, (Australian) silky terrier

Sick Sinus Syndrome

Description: Sick sinus syndrome is a clinical syndrome associated with irregular discharge of the sinoatrial node, causing severe bradycardia. It is characterized by periods of sinus arrest, which may be clinically apparent or may result in dizziness or syncope. Animals recover soon after the attack. Sudden death is a rare sequel.

Breeds: Miniature schnauzer, West Highland white terrier

Signal Transduction Disorders

Description: Also known as hereditary thrombopathy (or thrombopathia), this describes breed-specific diseases in which platelets fail to aggregate properly. Mutations have been characterized, and genetic testing is available for breed-specific variants.

Breeds: American Eskimo dog, basset hound, Finnish spitz, Landseer

Sinus Tachycardia

Description: Sinus tachycardia can be secondary to a variety of underlying factors (stress, pain, exercise, etc.), or it can be a variation of normal in specific animals. Some animals tend to have elevated heart rates for unknown reasons, and there is at least some breed predisposition for this.

Breeds: 🐕 **Yorkshire terrier**

Skeletal Dysplasia

Description: Skeletal dysplasia 2 is a form of disproportionate dwarfism associated with an autosomal recessive (with incomplete penetrance) mutation in the COL11A2 gene. It should be clinically differentiated from retinal dysplasia/oculoskeletal dysplasia (RD/OSD), which is caused by a different genetic mutation. DNA testing is available for skeletal dysplasia 2 in the Labrador retriever. Similar conditions have also been recognized in the Newfoundland, Chesapeake Bay retriever and Nova Scotia duck tolling retriever.

Breeds: 🐕 **Labrador retriever**

Small Intestinal Bacterial Overgrowth (SIBO)

Description: Also known as antibiotic-responsive diarrhea (ARD), this is poorly understood and characterized, but is often considered to be an important cause of chronic diarrhea in specific breeds.

Breeds: 🐕 **Beagle, German shepherd dog, Norwegian lundehund**

Spherocytosis

Description: Hereditary spherocytosis associated with spectrin deficiency has been associated with hemolytic anemia and osmotic fragility of erythrocytes. It is considered an autosomal dominant trait that has been reported in Dutch golden retrievers.

Breeds: 🐕 **Golden retriever**

Spiculosis

Description: A hair follicle defect in which hairs are brittle and thickened and form nodules known as spicules. Although the mode of inheritance is unknown, the condition has been breed limited.

Breeds: 🐕 **Kerry blue terrier**

Spina Bifida

Description: Part of the spinal dysraphism group of neurological disorders, this is a developmental failure in part of the vertebra. The condition is thought to be heritable, but a mode of inheritance is currently not known.

Breeds: 🐕 **Beagle, Boston terrier, boxer, English bulldog, Chihuahua, Dalmatian, French bulldog, pug, Samoyed;** 🐈 **Manx**

Spinal Dysraphism

Description: Also known as myelodysplasia, this is a form of neural tube defect that causes neurological disease in pups. It is likely that the condition is the result of many different breed-specific mutations, and in the Weimaraner there is an autosomal recessive mutation of the NKX2–8 gene; DNA testing is available on a variant-specific basis.

Breeds: 🐕 **Alaskan malamute, Dalmatian, German shepherd dog, golden retriever, Rottweiler, Weimaraner, West Highland white terrier**

Spinal Muscular Atrophy (Canine)

Description: A collection of breed-specific inherited neuromuscular diseases in which motor neurons are affected preferentially but not necessarily exclusively. They probably represent a spectrum disorder, from focal degeneration to multisystemic disease for a variety of different breed-specific mutations and modes of inheritance. In the Brittany spaniel, it appears to be inherited as an autosomal dominant trait with incomplete penetrance.

Breeds: 🐕 **Bloodhound, Brittany spaniel, cairn terrier, (American) cocker spaniel, Doberman pinscher, German shepherd dog, griffon briquet Vendeen, (English) pointer, Rottweiler, saluki, Swedish lapphund**

Spinal Muscular Atrophy (Feline)

Description: An inherited neuromuscular disease caused by the death of the spinal cord neurons that activate skeletal muscles of the trunk and limbs. It is autosomal recessive and caused by a mutation of the LIX1-LNPEP gene; DNA testing is available.

Breeds: 🐈 **Maine Coon**

Spinocerebellar Ataxia

Description: A progressive neurological disease associated with mutations of the KCNJ10 gene and with tremors and deteriorating neurological function. It is inherited as an autosomal recessive trait. DNA testing is available for breed-specific variants.

Breeds: 🐕 **Alpine, dachsbracke, (smooth-haired) fox terrier, (toy) fox terrier, Jack Russell terrier, Parson Russell terrier, Tenterfield terrier**

Spinocerebellar Ataxia (Myokymia And Neuromyotonia)

Description: Associated with different mutations of the *KCNJ10 gene, m*yokymia refers to muscle twitching, and neuromyotonia involves additional neurological manifestations such as muscle stiffness and cramping. This early-onset form of spinocerebellar ataxia may have multiple gene mutations involved with the clinical presentation on a breed-specific basis. It is presumed to be autosomal recessive in nature. See also late-onset ataxia.

Breeds: 🐕 **Basenji, Chihuahua, fox terrier, fox terrier (miniature, smooth, wire), Jack Russell terrier, Parson Russell terrier, Tenterfield terrier**

Splenic Torsion

Description: A condition caused when the spleen twists on its blood supply, either as an independent event or associated with gastric dilation/volvulus. A genetic basis has not been determined, but breed predisposition has been recognized.

Breeds: 🐕 **English bulldog, German shepherd dog, Great Dane**

Spondylocostal Dysostosis

Description: Also known as comma defect, this is a skeletal growth disorder associated with truncal shortening, hemivertebrae, and rib anomalies. It is inherited as an autosomal recessive trait due to a mutation in the HES7 gene. Genetic testing is available.

Breeds: 🐕 **Miniature schnauzer**

Spondylo-Epiphyseal Dysplasia Tarda

Description: Spondylo-epiphyseal dysplasia tarda is a rare congenital anomaly that is believed to be x-linked recessive, resulting in abnormally short legs and body length, and painful ambulation.

Breeds: 🐕 **Danish farm hound, Swedish farm hound**

Spondylosis Deformans

Description: A common degenerative spinal condition characterized by osteophyte production that results in bone spurs or ridges that bridge the intervertebral disk space. It is possible that genetics may play a role, at least in some cases.

Breeds: 🐕 **Boxer, flat-coated retriever, German shepherd dog**

Spontaneous Chronic Corneal Epithelial Defects

Description: Also known as indolent ulcers and ulcerative keratitis, these are chronic superficial ulcers that most often appear in middle-aged animals and may be associated with an abnormality in the adhesive mechanism of the corneal epithelium to the stroma. A mode of inheritance is not known, but a breed predisposition has been recognized.

Breeds: 🐕 **Boxer, golden retriever, keeshond**

Spontaneous Pneumothorax

Description: The situation where air accumulates in the pleural spaces, and it is not associated with traumatic injury. It can occur secondary to underlying lung disease, but in certain situations, it can be associated with breed predisposition.

Breeds: 🐕 **Siberian husky**

Stargardt Disease

Description: An inherited eye disease leading to vision loss and blindness and resulting from a mutation in the ABCA4 gene. It is transmitted as an autosomal recessive trait. DNA testing is available.

Breeds: 🐕 **Labrador retriever**

Startle Disease (Hyperekplexia)

Description: A hereditary neurological disorder associated with mutations in a variety of genes, especially SLC6A5. The SLC6A5 variant is inherited as an autosomal recessive trait, and results in prominent startling in response to touch or sound. DNA testing is available for some variants.

Breeds: 🐕 **Irish wolfhound, greyhound**

Stationary Night Blindness

Description: Also known as hereditary retinal dystrophy, RPED, and Leber congenital amaurosis, this is a nonprogressive night blindness due to early rod degeneration that is apparent by 5–6 weeks of age. The condition is autosomal recessive in most breeds studied, and DNA testing is available for some breed-specific variants. See similar conditions under progressive retinal atrophy.

Breeds: 🐕 **Beagle, Briard, (standard) poodle, Shetland sheepdog**

Sterile Pyogranuloma

Description: An idiopathic granulomatous reaction in the skin, unassociated with microbial infections. There is a recognized breed predisposition, but no known mode of inheritance.

Breeds: 🐕 **Collie, English bulldog, Great Dane**

Stiff Skin Syndrome

Description: Perhaps related to scleroderma, this is a condition characterized by dermal fibrosis resulting in induration of the skin with or without other manifestations (joint, internal organs, vascular). It bears some resemblance to Musladin–Leuke syndrome in beagles.

Breeds: 🐕 **West Highland white terrier**

Stomatocytosis

Description: An inherited defect in red blood cells in which there is reduced or absent membrane protein (stomatin), which in turn promotes hemolytic anemia. The genetic defect may be associated with other abnormalities as well, such as chondrodysplastic dwarfish in the Alaskan malamute and hypertrophic gastritis (Ménétrier syndrome) in the Drentse patrijshond. The condition in standard schnauzers is usually asymptomatic. The mode of inheritance in the Drentse patrijshond is believed to be autosomal recessive. Genetic variants are likely breed specific.

Breeds: 🐕 **Alaskan malamute, Drentse partrijshond, Pomeranian, (miniature) schnauzer, (standard) schnauzer**

Strabismus

Description: Abnormal positioning of the eyeball. One manifestation is the appearance of the animal being cross-eyed (convergent) such as in the Siamese, or pointing outward (divergent) such as in the Boston terrier. Mode of inheritance in pets has not been determined, but breed predisposition has been recognized.

Breeds: 🐕 **Boston terrier;** 🐈 **Balinese, Himalayan, Persian, Siamese**

Subaortic Stenosis

Description: A congenital heart disease involving a narrowing or stricture just below the aortic valve. The stricture is usually an abnormal fibrous ring of tissue that results in a reduction in blood flow from the heart, which causes the cardiac muscle to overwork and thereby increases the heart's oxygen needs. Breed predisposition is recognized.

Breeds: 🐕 **Bouvier des Flandres, boxer, bull terrier, English bulldog, German shepherd dog, German shorthaired pointer, golden retriever, Great Dane, Newfoundland, Rottweiler, Samoyed and many more**

Sudden Acquired Retinal Degeneration Syndrome (SARDS)

Description: A sudden cause of blindness in dogs with associated pupillary dilation. The cause is unknown with certainty (neuroendocrine? autoimmune?), but there does appear to be a breed predisposition.

Breeds: 🐕 **Brittany spaniel, dachshund, pug, (miniature) schnauzer, (English) springer spaniel**

Superficial Necrolytic Dermatitis

Description: Also referred to as hepatocutaneous syndrome, necrolytic migratory erythema (NME), and diabetic dermatopathy, this is a potentially fatal condition that manifests in the skin but is associated with an underlying hepatic disorder, and occasionally as a result of a glucagon-secreting pancreatic tumor (glucagonoma). Breed predisposition is recognized.

Breeds: 🐕 **Border collie, (American) cocker spaniel, Lhasa apso, (miniature) schnauzer, Scottish terrier, Shetland sheepdog, West Highland white terrier**

Syringomyelia

Description: A condition in which fluid-containing cavities develop in the spinal cord, caused by various primary problems such as abnormalities in the caudal fossa (Chiari malformations), which can be familial. They are likely influenced by genes of more than one locus.

Breeds: 🐕 **Brussels griffon, Cavalier King Charles spaniel, Chihuahua, English toy spaniel, Maltese, papillon, phalene, pug, Yorkshire terrier**

Tail Chasing

Description: Tail chasing is not an unusual pursuit in dogs, but compulsive tail-chasing behavior has been variously described as a subepileptic episodic behavior, a neuro-pathological disorder, a psychosis, an opioid-mediated compulsive disorder, and a displacement behavior. An intense spinning and whirling disorder has been described in terriers.

Breeds: 🐕 **American Staffordshire terrier, bull terrier, (miniature) bull terrier, Jack Russell terrier, Kangal shepherd dog, shiba inu**

Taillessness (Feline)

Description: Taillessness is inherited as a dominant trait in the Manx (M), but it is a lethal trait in that heterozygotes are tailless, but homozygotes usually die before birth. Thus, no pure breeding strains of Manx exist, and when two Manx cats are bred, litter size is typically lower, reflecting mortality of those homozygous for taillessness. Spina bifida can be a complication of taillessness, although the prevalence of this possible sequela has not been determined.

Breeds: 🐈 **American bobtail, Cymric, Japanese bobtail, Manx**

Tapetal Degeneration

Description: A recessively inherited condition in which degeneration of the tapetum does not affect vision in any way and, therefore, is not associated with blindness.

Breeds: 🐕 **Beagle**

Temporomandibular Joint Dysplasia

Description: A malformation of the temporomandibular joint that results in increased range of motion of the dysplastic mandible. It can just be an incidental finding, or result in joint instability, subluxation, and locking of the jaw. A genetic basis has not been determined, but breed predisposition has been recognized.

Breeds: 🐕 **Basset hound, Cavalier King Charles spaniel, (American) cocker spaniel, Gordon setter, Irish setter**

Tetralogy of Fallot

Description: Tetralogy of Fallot has four components: ventricular septal defect, overriding of the interventricular septum by the aorta, pulmonic stenosis, and right ventricular hypertrophy. This affliction is uncommon but breed predisposition has been recognized. The condition is rare enough, though, that relative risks cannot be reliably assigned for these breeds. A hereditary component has been established in the keeshond as a severe manifestation of conotruncal hypoplasia.

Breeds: 🐕 **Border terrier, English bulldog, (wire) fox terrier, golden retriever, keeshond, Labrador retriever, (toy) poodle, Siberian husky**

Thrombasthenic Thrombopathia

Description: Canine thrombasthenic thrombopathia is an autosomally inherited platelet function defect seen in breed-specific presentations. The gene defects are distinct in the affected breeds, and DNA testing is available.

Breeds: 🐕 **Great Pyrenees, otterhound**

Thrombopathia

Description: An inherited bleed disorder associated with breed-specific platelet abnormalities. Most are inherited as autosomal recessive traits, with breed-specific mutations to the RAS-GRP2 gene. DNA testing is available for some breed-specific variants.

Breeds: 🐕 **Basset hound, Border terrier, Finnish spitz, Greater Swiss mountain dog, Landseer, Newfoundland**

Thymic Atrophy

Description: Thymic atrophy is a tardive condition in which the dogs are born with a normal thymus, which undergoes significant atrophy by several weeks of age. The result is chronic, recurring infections.

Breeds: 🐕 **Xoloitzcuintli (Mexican hairless)**

Tooth Resorption

Description: Also referred to as feline odontoclastic resorptive lesion (FORL), this disorder results in the destruction of dentin in one or more teeth. It is a common issue in cats, although the cause is not yet known with certainty. Some breed predisposition is reported, but a mode of inheritance has not been determined.

Breeds: 🐈 **Abyssinian, Siamese**

Tracheal Collapse

Description: Tracheal collapse results from reduction in the luminal diameter of the cervical or intrathoracic trachea or both, and the pathogenesis is still a matter of debate. It has been considered to be a congenital or inherited problem, and breed predisposition is recognized.

Breeds: 🐕 **Affenpinscher, bolonka zwetna, bull terrier, Chihuahua, Norwich terrier, Pekingese, Pomeranian, (miniature) poodle, pug, schipperke, shih tzu, (Australian) silky terrier, Yorkshire terrier**

Tracheal Hypoplasia

Description: Tracheal hypoplasia is a congenital malformation that results in narrowing of the trachea, and a congenital or inherited pathogenesis is suspected. In some cases, it is associated with brachycephalic syndrome.

Breeds: 🐕 **Boston terrier, boxer, English bulldog, Labrador retriever**

Trance-Like Syndrome

Description: A condition in which affected animals display a hypokinetic gait with pacing. Currently it has not been determined if this is a form of seizure or a compulsive behavior.

Breeds: 🐕 **Bull terrier**

Trapped Neutrophil Syndrome

Description: An inherited condition in which neutrophils are produced by the bone marrow, but these leukocytes are unable to be effectively released into the bloodstream. This is an autosomal recessive trait resulting from a mutation on the VPS13B gene and breed-specific DNA testing is available. The result is an impaired immune system that leads to secondary infections.

Breeds: 🐕 **Border collie, koolie**

Tremor Syndromes

Description: A family of disorders associated with breed-specific tremors. Both autosomal recessive and x-linked recessive inheritance is recognized. The condition in the Weimaraner seems to be associated with a mutation in the FNIP2 gene. See also hypomyelination and shaker syndrome.

Breeds: 🐕 **Chow chow, Dalmatian, Doberman pinscher, English bulldog, Labrador retriever, Samoyed, (English) springer spaniel, Weimaraner**

Tricuspid Valve Dysplasia

Description: A congenital abnormality of the right atrioventricular valve, characterized by anomalies of the chordae tendineae, papillary muscles, and valvular tissue. There may be some similarity to Ebstein anomaly in humans. A breed predisposition is noted.

Breeds: 🐕 **Airedale terrier, borzoi, boxer, dogue de Bordeaux, German shepherd dog, golden retriever, Great Dane, Great Pyrenees, Irish setter, Labrador retriever, Newfoundland, old English sheepdog, saluki, shih tzu, Weimaraner**

Tubulointerstitial Nephropathy

Description: A noninflammatory progressive renal disease. Although the mode of inheritance is not known, there is a strong familial tendency. The kidneys of affected dogs are normal at birth but undergo advancing irreversible interstitial fibrosis. The course is highly variable.

Breeds: 🐕 **Norwegian elkhound**

Tyrosinase Deficiency

Description: A rare pigmentary disorder in which the tyrosinase enzyme is deficient, which is needed to produce melanin. The result is loss of pigment in the tongue, buccal mucosa, and fur. The cause is not known for certain, but a breed predisposition is recognized.

Breeds: 🐕 **Chow chow**

Tyrosinemia II

Description: A rare metabolic condition associated with a deficiency of hepatic tyrosine aminotransferase. Clinically, the condition presents as erosions and ulcerations of the footpads and nose, as well as exudative ophthalmic lesions.

Breeds: 🐕 **German shepherd dog**

Ulcerative Dermatosis

Description: Ulcerative dermatosis is a poorly understood condition seen in the collie and Shetland sheepdog. It is thought to possibly represent a variant of dermatomyositis or perhaps a vesicular subset of cutaneous lupus erythematosus (see vesicular cutaneous lupus erythematosus).

Breeds: 🐕 **Collie, Shetland sheepdog**

Ulcerative Keratitis

Description: Refractory corneal ulcers may result in visual impairment and seem to have a discernible breed predisposition although a mode of inheritance has not been determined. It may represent inadequate function of basement membrane complexes necessary for epithelial adhesion

Breeds: 🐕 **Alaskan malamute, Boston terrier, boxer, Brussels griffon, Dandie Dinmont terrier, French bulldog, golden retriever, Japanese chin, Lhasa apso, Pekingese, pug, Rottweiler, Samoyed, shih tzu and many more;** 🐈 **Himalayan, Persian**

Upper Airway Syndrome

Description: A condition that seems clinically similar to brachycephalic obstructive airway syndrome (BOAS) and associated with respiratory distress in the Norwich terrier. There is obstruction of air flow in the upper airways. The mode of inheritance has not been determined but is presumed to be complex (like BOAS). An ADAMTS3 missense variant is associated with the condition and DNA testing can help predict risk for developing this condition.

Breeds: 🐕 **Norwich terrier**

Urea Cycle Enzyme Deficiencies

Description: Congenital disorders resulting from complete or partial functional deficiency in one of the enzymes of the urea cycle. When ammonia is not sufficiently metabolized into urea, urea cycle intermediates and ammonia can accumulate in the bloodstream.

Breeds: 🐕 **Irish wolfhound**

Urinary Incontinence

Description: The situation that arises when well-housetrained animals have bladder leaks or loss of control. There are many causes, including increased prevalence in older spayed females, but a breed predisposition has also been recognized.

Breeds: 🐕 **Dalmatian, Doberman pinscher, Greater Swiss mountain dog, Irish setter, (giant) schnauzer, vizsla, Weimaraner**

Urolithiasis

Description: Urolithiasis is the condition caused when crystals combine to form stones in the urinary tract. Uroliths can form in any part of the urinary tract and can be found in the kidneys, ureters, bladder, or urethra. They may contain magnesium ammonium phosphate hexahydrate, ammonium acid urate (also called urate stones), cystine, calcium oxalate (CaOx), and others.

Breeds: 🐕 **Basset hound, (American) cocker spaniel, English bulldog, dachshund, Dalmatian, Pekingese, poodle, pug, schnauzer, shih tzu, (Pembroke) Welsh corgi, Yorkshire terrier, and many others**

Urolithiasis (Apatite)

Description: A relatively rare form of urolithiasis in which the stones are composed of calcium phosphate, hydroxyapatite, or carbonite-apatite. These can be seen with a variety of underlying disorders, such as hypercalcemia, and breed predisposition has been recognized.

Breeds: 🐕 **Pekingese, (miniature) schnauzer, shih tzu**

Urolithiasis (Calcium Oxalate)

Description: CaOx uroliths are usually associated with metabolic factors promoting hypercalciuria. For example, dogs with hyperadrenocorticism are much more likely to have calcium-containing uroliths. Hypercalciuria, however, does not imply hypercalcemia, and normocalcemic hypercalciuria is to be expected in most cases

Breeds: 🐕 **Bichon frisé, cairn terrier, Chihuahua, Dalmatian, Doberman pinscher, Jack Russell terrier, keeshond, Lhasa apso, Norfolk terrier, papillon, phalene, Pomeranian, poodle (miniature, toy), Samoyed, miniature schnauzer, standard schnauzer, Parson Russell terrier, shih tzu, Tibetan terrier, West Highland white terrier, Yorkshire terrier;** 🐈 **British shorthair, Burmese, Devon Rex, Exotic, Havana brown, Highland fold, Himalayan, Persian, Ragdoll, Scottish fold, Siamese, Tonkinese**

Urolithiasis (Cystine)

Description: Not all cases of cystine urolithiasis have a hereditary cause, but there are several genetic varieties that have been characterized, including those with mutations of the SLC3A1 (rBAT) and SLC7A9 genes, which are autosomal recessive traits. The disorder is one of an inherited defect in the renal proximal tubular transport system, which allows excessive urinary excretion of cystine (and, to a lesser extent, ornithine, lysine, and arginine) in the urine. Although cystinuria occurs in both male and female dogs, cystine calculi develop almost exclusively in males. DNA testing for types IA, IIA, and IIB cystinuria is available.

Breeds: 🐕 **American pit bull terrier, Australian cattle dog, Australian shepherd dog, basenji, basset hound, bichon frisé, bullmastiff, Chihuahua, dachshund, English bulldog, Irish terrier, Jack Russell terrier, Labrador retriever, Landseer, (English) mastiff, (large) Münsterländer, miniature pinscher, Newfoundland, Rottweiler, Scottish deerhound, Scottish terrier,** (Australian) silky terrier, Staffordshire bull terrier, (Pembroke) Welsh corgi

Urolithiasis (Magnesium Ammonium Phosphate)

Description: Frequently referred to as struvite or triple phosphate stones, these uroliths are the most common type of stones seen in dogs. Although struvite urolithiasis is common, not much is known about the genetics of the condition although breed predisposition is recognized.

Breeds: 🐕 **Beagle, bichon frisé, dachshund, (English) cocker spaniel, Lhasa apso, (miniature) poodle, (miniature) schnauzer, Scottish terrier, shih tzu, (Pembroke) Welsh corgi, Yorkshire terrier;** 🐈 **Chartreux, Himalayan, Manx, Oriental shorthair**

Urolithiasis (Silica)

Description: Silica uroliths are most often associated with diets containing substantial quantities of corn gluten feed or soybean hulls. A mode of inheritance has not been determined, and it is quite likely that the condition is not heritable.

Breeds: 🐕 **(American) cocker spaniel, German shepherd dog, golden retriever, Labrador retriever, Lhasa apso, old English sheepdog, Pekingese, Samoyed, (miniature) schnauzer, shih tzu, Yorkshire terrier**

Urolithiasis (Urate)

Description: Predisposing factors for urate urolith formation include hyperuricemia, hyperuricosuria, hyperammonemia, hyperammonuria, aciduria, and genetic predisposition. The vast majority of urate uroliths are diagnosed in male Dalmatians. DNA testing is now available for hyperuricosuria, a predisposing factor.

Breeds: 🐕 **Black Russian terrier, Bolognese, Dalmatian, English bulldog, Pekingese, (miniature) schnauzer, shih tzu, Yorkshire terrier;** 🐈 **Bengal, Birman, Egyptian Mau, European shorthair, Ocicat, Ragdoll, Siamese, Snowshoe, Sphynx**

Urolithiasis (Xanthine)

Description: Primary xanthinuria can be seen in many breeds, associated with a variety of mutations in either xanthine dehydrogenase (XDH, type 1 xanthinuria) or molybdenum co-factor sulfurase (MOCOS, type 2 xanthinuria). Nongenetic causes also occur. In most cases of primary xanthinuria, there is an autosomal recessive pattern of inheritance.

Breeds: 🐕 **Cavalier King Charles spaniel, Chihuahua, (English) cocker spaniel, dachshund, Manchester terrier, and mixed breed dogs**

Urticaria Pigmentosa

Description: A rare skin condition characterized by mast cell and eosinophil accumulation in the skin, in which degranulation of the mast cells can be triggered by a number of mechanisms. It has been reported in both dogs and cats, but no genetic characterization of the disorder has been reported.

Breeds: 🐈 **Devon Rex, Himalayan, Sphynx**

Uveal Cysts

Description: Cysts that appear on the iris and ciliary body. They may be congenital or acquired, and single or multiple. Most occur spontaneously and are benign. A genetic basis has not been determined, but breed predisposition has been recognized.

Breeds: 🐕 **Boston terrier, golden retriever, Labrador retriever;** 🐈 **Burmese**

Uveal Hypopigmentation

Description: Blue irides, heterochromia iridis, and iris hypoplasia are related to coat color genetics and they may be associated with deafness. White or merle coats are inherited as autosomal dominant traits, and heterochromia iridis and deafness are autosomal dominant with incomplete penetrance.

Breeds: 🐕 **Alaskan malamute, Australian shepherd, beagle, (blue merle) collie, Dalmatian, (harlequin) Great Dane, Shetland sheepdog, Siberian husky**

Uveodermatologic Syndrome

Description: Also known as Vogt–Koyanagi–Harada-like syndrome, this may represent an autoimmune attack against melanocytes. Thus, heavily pigmented tissues such as the uveal tract, skin, and mucous membranes are primarily involved. There are known breed predispositions, but a mode of inheritance is not known.

Breeds: 🐕 **Akita, Alaskan malamute, chow chow, dachshund, German shepherd dog, Hokkaido, Irish terrier, old English sheepdog, Samoyed, Shetland sheepdog, shiba inu, Siberian husky**

Van Den Ende–Gupta Syndrome

Description: An autosomal recessive musculoskeletal disorder in which there are multiple sites of involvement, including the maxilla and often patellar luxation, elbow luxation, and spinal arthritis. It results from a mutation in the SCARF2 gene and DNA testing is available.

Breeds: 🐕 **Wire fox terrier**

Vasculitis

Description: Cutaneous vasculitis is a collection of disorders in which the underlying problem includes destructive and inflammatory changes in the blood vessels. Most syndromes are associated with immune complex deposition in the walls of blood vessels. Breed predispositions are noted for many varieties, but actual genetic mutations and modes of inheritance have not been determined in most instances. Urticarial vasculitis may be associated with adverse food reactions.

Breeds: 🐕 **Beagle, Bernese mountain dog, boxer, dachshund, greyhound, Jack Russell terrier, (miniature) poodle, Rottweiler**

Ventricular Ectopy

Description: Also known as inherited lethal ventricular arrhythmia, this includes premature ventricular complexes, ventricular bigeminal or trigeminal rhythms, ventricular couplets, and ventricular tachycardia. An inherited ectopy that results in sudden cardiac death has been reported, but the mode of inheritance has not been identified.

Breeds: 🐕 **German shepherd dog**

Ventricular Septal Defect

Description: This refers to a collection of congenital disorders characterized by an abnormal opening or hole in the wall between the left and right ventricles of the heart. It is quite likely that these presentations reflect breed-specific mutations, and potentially different modes of inheritance.

Breeds: 🐕 **Airedale terrier, Alaskan malamute, bichon frisé, bloodhound, Border terrier, Brittany spaniel, chow chow, English bulldog, (smooth) fox terrier, French bulldog, German shepherd dog, keeshond, Maltese, Newfoundland, Samoyed, shiba inu, Siberian husky, (English) springer spaniel**

Vertebral Stenosis

Description: Vertebral stenosis is a rare narrowing of the spine present at birth. It can occur alone or in association with other congenital anomalies of the spinal cord.

Breeds: 🐕 **Beagle, Doberman pinscher, German shepherd dog, Labrador retriever, Lhasa apso, (toy) poodle**

Vestibular Disease (Congenital)

Description: Congenital peripheral vestibular disease is presumed to be inherited. Clinical presentation includes head tilt, ataxia, circling, and deafness without nystagmus, seen in pups younger than 4 months of age.

Breeds: 🐈 **Akita, beagle, (English) cocker spaniel, Doberman pinscher, German shepherd dog, Shetland sheepdog, Tibetan terrier**

Vitamin A-Responsive Dermatosis

Description: A skin disease of scaling and crusting, centered on the hair follicle rather than the skin surface. It responds to supplementation with large doses of vitamin A. The mode of inheritance is unknown, but breed predisposition has been recognized.

Breeds: 🐈 **Cairn terrier, (American) cocker spaniel, Labrador retriever**

Vitamin K-Dependent Multifactor Coagulopathy

Description: A rare feline condition associated with abnormal vitamin K-dependent enzyme deficiency that results in clotting defects similar to vitamin K deficiency. The genetic

defect has not yet been characterized, but the condition is presumed to be autosomal recessive in nature.

Breeds: 🐈 **Devon Rex**

Vitiligo

Description: A patchy loss of pigment that may be inherited or acquired. In general, it refers to white patches that appear on the surface of the skin rather than whitening of the hairs (leukotrichia). A mode of inheritance is not known.

Breeds: 🐕 **Belgian sheepdog, Belgian Tervuren, Doberman pinscher, German shepherd dog, Labrador retriever, Rottweiler**

Vitreous Degeneration

Description: Vitreous degeneration refers to liquefaction of the vitreous gel, which can predispose to retinal detachment and blindness. The three major forms of vitreous degeneration are synchysis scintillans, syneresis, and asteroid hyalosis. A mode of inheritance has not been characterized but breed predisposition is recognized.

Breeds: 🐕 **Bichon frisé, Border terrier, Boston terrier, bouvier des Flandres, Brittany spaniel, Brussels griffon, (miniature) bull terrier, Cavalier King Charles spaniel, Chihuahua, Chinese crested, Chinook husky, coton de Tulear, German pinscher, greyhound, Havanese, Italian greyhound, Jack Russell terrier, Japanese chin, Kerry blue terrier, kuvasz, Labrador retriever, löwchen, mi-ki, miniature pinscher, Norfolk terrier, Norwich terrier, papillon, Parson Russell terrier, petit basset griffon Vendeen, Pomeranian, pug, Russian tsvetnaya bolonka (bolonka), schipperke, Scottish terrier, shiba inu, shih tzu, (Australian) silky terrier, (Welsh) springer spaniel, Swedish vallhund, whippet**

Von Willebrand Disease

Description: Von Willebrand disease (vWD) is the most common inherited bleeding disorder of dogs and the genetic mutations (types 1, 2, and 3) result in a platelet function defect and prolonged bleeding times. For breeds in which a DNA test for vWD is not available, the disease is suspected by measuring levels of von Willebrand factor (vWF) in the blood.

Breeds: 🐈 **Many**

Von Willebrand Disease Type I (VWD1)

Description: The most common inherited bleeding disorder and has been reported in many breeds. It is associated with a mutation on the VWF gene and is inherited as an autosomal recessive trait. Many cases are subclinical or are associated with a bleeding tendency after following surgery or trauma. The condition is very rare in cats.

Breeds: Bernese mountain dog, cockapoo, coton de Tulear, Doberman pinscher, Drentsche patrijschond, German pinscher, goldendoodle, Irish red and white setter, Kerry blue terrier, Kromfohrlander, Labradoodle, Manchester terrier, papillon, poodle (all varieties), stabyhoun, (Pembroke) Welsh corgi, and many others; Himalayan

Von Willebrand Disease Type II (VWD2)

Description: An inherited form of von Willebrand disease associated with a particular genetic variant of the VWD gene. It is also inherited as an autosomal recessive trait. Type 2 vWD is clinically severe and quite rare. It is characterized by structurally abnormal vWF, resulting in severe bleeding episodes. DNA testing is available for breed-specific variants.

Breeds: Boykin spaniel, collie, Chinese crested, German shorthaired pointer, German wirehaired pointer, (English) pointer, poodle (miniature, moyen, standard, toy)

Von Willebrand Disease Type III (VWD3)

Description: An inherited form of von Willebrand disease associated with a particular genetic variant of the VWD gene. It is also inherited as an autosomal recessive trait. Typically, the most severe form of the disease. DNA testing is available for some breed-specific variants. The condition is very rare in cats.

Breeds: Chesapeake Bay retriever, Dutch Kooiker dog, Scottish terrier, Shetland sheepdog; Domestic longhair

Weimaraner Immunodeficiency

Description: A poorly understood entity characterized by impaired phagocytic and humoral immune functions. Affected dogs are prone to suppurative and granulomatous

disease processes. A mode of inheritance has not been determined.

Breeds: Weimaraner

Wool Sucking

Description: An abnormal behavior in cats that is thought to be compulsive in nature. A genetic basis has not been determined, but breed predisposition has been recognized.

Breeds: Birman, Burmese, Siamese

Zinc-Responsive Dermatosis

Description: Zinc-responsive dermatosis is a scaling and crusting disorder that is probably caused by an inherited impairment in zinc absorption or metabolism. There are clear breed predispositions, but the mode of inheritance is not known. An unusual manifestation of a localized parakeratotic hyperkeratosis has been reported in the Boston terrier although only some of the affected animals responded to zinc supplementation. There is also a zinc-related disorder that is seen in rapidly growing large-breed puppies that likely results from a dietary deficiency of zinc or diets that include ingredients that impact zinc absorption.

Breeds: Alaskan malamute, American Eskimo, American pit bull terrier, Boston terrier, Doberman pinscher, Great Dane, Samoyed, Siberian husky

Recommended Reading

Ackerman, L: *The Genetic Connection*, 2, AAHAPress, Lakewood, CO, 2011.

Bell, JS; Cavanagh, KE; Tilley, LP; Smith, FWK: *Veterinary Medical Guide to Dog and Cat Breeds*, Teton NewMedia, Jackson, WY, 2012.

Ackerman, L. *Proactive Pet Parenting: Anticipating pet health problems before they happen.* Problem Free Publishing, 2020.

Gough, A, Thomas, A; O'Neill, D: *Breed Predispositions to Disease in Dogs and Cats*, 3, Wiley, Ames, IA, 2018.

University of Prince Edward Island. Canine Inherited Disorders Database. http://cidd.discoveryspace.ca

University of Sydney. Online Mendelian Inheritance in Animals. http://omia.org

World Small Animal Veterinary Association. Canine and Feline Hereditary Disease (DNA)Testing Laboratories. www.vet.upenn.edu/research/academic-departments/clinical-sciences-advanced-medicine/research-labs-centers/penngen/tests-worldwide

11.4

Heritable Health Conditions by Breed

Lowell Ackerman, DVM, DACVD, MBA, MPA, CVA, MRCVS

Global Consultant, Author, and Lecturer, MA, USA

The following are just some of the conditions recognized in purebred dogs and cats and considered predisposed in certain breeds. Not all conditions are defined here, and some definitions are purposefully excluded to save space, especially different forms of neoplasia (e.g., mast cell tumor), conditions that are relatively common and well known (e.g., dental "bites"), or those that are poorly characterized or ill defined (e.g., myelin deficiency in cats).

To a certain extent, the number of disorders attributed to breeds reflects their popularity, so a long list of genetic disorders does not indicate that the breed is necessarily more prone to genetic disorders. In many cases, the relative risk is not known for individual conditions, so it is anticipated that conditions might be reported preferentially in breeds that are most commonly seen in practice.

Use the material here as a source of conditions reported in breeds within the veterinary literature, and not an indication that any individual is predisposed or likely susceptible to any or all of the conditions listed. Also, there is likely to be some duplication of conditions, since they may be reported differently in the literature. For example, a breed may be listed as predisposed to elbow dysplasia in one reference, but listed as predisposed to fragmented coronoid process in another. Typically, both would be listed here. It is also possible that a condition is linked to a breed in one geographic location, but not necessarily everywhere. This is to be expected since most genetic problems run in families rather than the entire breed. On the other hand, some references cite a breed disposition broadly (e.g., poodle), without specifying the variety (toy, miniature, moyen, standard, etc.), making it difficult to attribute the condition appropriately.

Similarly, the occasion also arises when breeds becomes highly segmented, with very specific susceptibility based on genetic testing and susceptibilities (e.g., dachshund, miniature longhaired dachshund, miniature wirehaired dachshund, standard wirehaired dachshund, miniature smooth dachshund, standard longhaired dachshund, standard smooth dachshund, etc.), whereas most of the veterinary literature ascribes breed predisposition to "dachshund." Such listings will likely evolve as genetic testing becomes more commonplace.

Sometimes, there is even confusion about what breed names signify. For example, domestic shorthair may be confused with American shorthair. A domestic shorthair is any nonpedigreed cat with short fur, while the American shorthair is a recognized pure breed (the two were not distinguished until 1966, helping to explain the confusion). Pit bull is an ambiguous term used for a variety of dog breeds descended from bulldogs and terriers, while the American pit bull terrier is a recognized breed, at least by some registries.

Finally, even some conditions with strong breed predispositions may be rare and infrequently seen in primary care practice. They might still be listed here as a breed predisposition (even if rare) so it is important for veterinary healthcare teams to consider what is most likely to affect pets in their care, the impact those conditions have on quality of life, and the things that can be influenced by early-detection programs. Thus, the information here is just an imperfect attempt to help veterinary teams be aware of potential conditions that could be associated with specific breeds. More specific attribution is not implied, nor should it be inferred.

Abyssinian

Amyloidosis, Arterial thromboembolism, Atopic dermatitis, Cardiomyopathy (dilated), Cardiomyopathy (hypertrophic), Diabetes mellitus, Excessive grooming, Feline hyperesthesia syndrome, Feline infectious peritonitis (FIP) susceptibility, Feline lower urinary tract disease (FLUTD), Myasthenic syndrome, Mycobacterial susceptibility, Patellar luxation, Progressive Retinal Atrophy (rdAc), Progressive retinal atrophy (Rdy), Pyruvate kinase deficiency, Tooth resorption

Abyssinian Sand Terrier 🐕
Hairlessness

Affenpinscher 🐕
Anasarca, Atopic dermatitis, Cataracts, Cleft lip/palate, Corneal dystrophy, Cryptorchidism, Dermoid, Distichiasis, Elbow dysplasia, Elongated soft palate, Hip dysplasia, Hypothyroidism, Keratoconjunctivitis sicca, Legg–Calvé–Perthes disease, Oligodontia, Patellar luxation, Patent ductus arteriosus, Persistent pupillary membranes, Polydontia (retained primary teeth), Progressive retinal atrophy, Recurrent flank alopecia, Retinal dysplasia, Tracheal collapse

Afghan Hound 🐕
Amyloidosis, Atrioventricular heart block, Brachygnathism, Cataracts, Cervical vertebral instability, Chylothorax, Corneal dystrophy, Deafness, Demodicosis, Distichiasis, Elbow dysplasia, Exocrine pancreatic insufficiency, Fanconi syndrome, Gastric dilation/volvulus, Glaucoma, Hereditary myelopathy, Hernia (perineal), Hernia (umbilical), Hip dysplasia, Hypothyroidism, Intervertebral disk disease, Laryngeal paralysis, Leukoencephalomyelopathy, Lung lobe torsion, Malocclusion, Megaesophagus, Mitral valve disease, Narcolepsy, Necrotizing myelopathy, Oligodontia, Optic nerve hypoplasia and micropapilla, Osteochondritis dissecans (shoulder), Panosteitis, Patellar luxation, Persistent pupillary membranes, Prognathism, Progressive retinal atrophy, Pulmonic stenosis, Retinal dysplasia, Seborrhea, von Willebrand disease

Airedale Terrier 🐕
Atopic dermatitis, Atrial septal defect, Cardiomyopathy (dilated), Cataracts, Cerebellar abiotrophy, Cerebellar hypoplasia, Chromosomal intersex, Corneal dystrophy, Cryptorchidism, Degenerative lumbosacral stenosis, Degenerative myelopathy, Demodicosis, Distichiasis, Elbow dysplasia, Entropion, Epilepsy, Exocrine pancreatic insufficiency, Factor VII deficiency, Factor IX deficiency (hemophilia B), Follicular dysplasia, Gastric dilation/volvulus, Hernia (umbilical), Hip dysplasia, Hyperlipoproteinemia, Hypoadrenocorticism, Hypothyroidism, Immune-mediated hemolytic anemia, Immune-mediated thrombocytopenia, Interstitial lung disease, Intervertebral disk disease, Laryngeal paralysis, Lymphoproliferative disease (T-cell), Melanoma, Myasthenia gravis, Narcolepsy, Oligodontia, Pancreatitis, Pannus, Panosteitis, Patellar luxation, Persistent pupillary membranes, Polycystic kidney disease, Portosystemic shunts, Progressive retinal atrophy, Protein-losing nephropathy, Pulmonic stenosis, Recurrent flank alopecia, Retinal dysplasia, Sebaceous adenitis, Seborrhea, Subaortic stenosis, Transitional cell carcinoma, Tricuspid valve dysplasia, Ventricular septal defect, von Willebrand disease type I

Akbash Dog (Turkish Shepherd Dog) 🐕
Cardiomyopathy, Entropion, Epilepsy, Gastric dilation/volvulus, Hernia (umbilical), Hip dysplasia, Hypertrophic osteodystrophy, Hypothyroidism, Panosteitis, Prognathism, Retinal dysplasia

Akita 🐕
Acanthomatous ameloblastoma, Amelogenesis imperfecta, Atopic dermatitis, Brachygnathism, Cataracts, Cruciate ligament disease, Deafness, Elbow dysplasia (fragmented coronoid process), Enamel hypoplasia, Entropion, Epidermolysis bullosa, Epidermolysis bullosa (dystrophic), Exocrine pancreatic insufficiency, Factor VIII deficiency (hemophilia A), Gastric dilation/volvulus, Glaucoma, Glycogen storage disease III, Hip dysplasia, Hypothyroidism, Immune-mediated polyarthritis, Immunoglobulin A (IgA) deficiency, Microcytosis, Microphthalmia, Myasthenia gravis, Osteochondritis dissecans (shoulder), Osteochondritis dissecans (stifle), Osteochondrodysplasia, Panosteitis, Patellar luxation, Pemphigus foliaceus, Persistent pupillary membranes, Portosystemic shunts, Prognathism, Progressive retinal atrophy, Pseudohyperkalemia, Renal dysplasia, Retinal dysplasia, Sebaceous adenitis, Sebaceous adenitis, Uveodermatologic syndrome, Vestibular disease (congenital), von Willebrand disease

Alaskan Husky 🐕
Achromatopsia, Alaskan husky encephalopathy, GM-2 gangliosidosis, Hyperuricosuria, Hypothyroidism, Laryngeal paralysis, Laryngeal paralysis-polyneuropathy, Necrotizing encephalopathy, Peripheral neuropathy (Warburg), Polyneuropathy, Progressive retinal atrophy

Alaskan Klee Kai 🐕
Factor VII deficiency, Hypothyroidism, Patellar luxation

Alaskan Malamute 🐕
Achromatopsia, Alopecia X, Cataracts, Chondrodysplasia/Stomatocytosis, Ciliary dyskinesia, Corneal dystrophy, Cruciate ligament disease, Cryptorchidism, Degenerative myelopathy, Diabetes mellitus, Distichiasis, Elbow dysplasia, Elbow dysplasia (fragmented coronoid process), Epilepsy, Factor VII deficiency, Factor VIII deficiency (hemophilia A), Factor IX deficiency (hemophilia B), Follicular dysplasia, Follicular dysplasia (wooly syndrome), Gastric dilation/volvulus, Glaucoma, Hemivertebra, Hemolytic anemia, Hip dysplasia, Hypothyroidism, Keratoconjunctivitis sicca, Lupus erythematosus (discoid), Megaesophagus, Muscular dystrophy, Myelodysplasia, Narcolepsy, Necrotizing encephalopathy, Optic nerve

hypoplasia and micropapilla, Osteochondritis dissecans (shoulder), Osteochondrodysplasia, Pancreatitis, Panosteitis, Patellar luxation, Peripheral neuropathy (Alaskan malamute), Persistent pupillary membranes, Polydontia (retained primary teeth), Polyneuropathy, Portosystemic shunts, Progressive retinal atrophy, Pulmonic stenosis, Renal dysplasia, Retinal dysplasia, Spinal dysraphism, Stomatocytosis, Ulcerative keratitis, Uveal hypopigmentation, Uveodermatologic syndrome, Ventricular septal defect, von Willebrand disease, Zinc-responsive dermatosis

Alpine Dachsbracke 🐕
Intervertebral disk disease, Neuronal ceroid lipofuscinosis 8, Spinocerebellar ataxia

American Bobtail 🐈
Deafness, Hip dysplasia, Taillessness

American Bulldog 🐕
Cardiomyopathy (dilated), Cystinuria, Degenerative myelopathy, Hip dysplasia, Hyperuricosuria, Hypothyroidism, Ichthyosis, Iris cysts, Multifocal retinopathy (CMR1), Nemaline myopathy, Neuronal ceroid lipofuscinosis 10, Progressive retinal atrophy (crd2)

American Bully 🐕
Demodicosis, Hip dysplasia, Hyperuricosuria, Hypothyroidism, Merling, Multifocal retinopathy (CMR1), Patellar luxation, Progressive retinal atrophy (crd1), Progressive retinal atrophy (crd2)

American Curl 🐈
Deafness, Progressive retinal atrophy (rdAc)

American Eskimo Dog 🐕
Anasarca, Cataracts, Cryptorchidism, Deafness, Degenerative myelopathy, Elbow dysplasia, Epilepsy, Hemivertebra, Hip dysplasia, Hypoadrenocorticism, Hypothyroidism, Immune-mediated polyarthritis, Laryngeal paralysis, Legg–Calvé–Perthes disease, Lens luxation, Megaesophagus, Methemoglobin reductase deficiency, Narcolepsy, Patellar luxation, Patent ductus arteriosus, Prognathism, Progressive retinal atrophy (prcd), Pyruvate kinase deficiency, Sebaceous adenitis, Signal transduction disorder, Thrombopathia, Zinc-responsive dermatosis

American Hairless Terrier 🐕
Degenerative myelopathy, Hairlessness, Hypothyroidism (congenital, with goiter), Lens luxation, Muscular dystrophy, Patellar luxation, Progressive retinal atrophy (prcd)

American Pit Bull Terrier 🐕
Atopic dermatitis, Babesiosis, Cerebellar ataxia, Cleft lip/palate, Degenerative myelopathy, Demodicosis,

Endocardial fibroelastosis, Hip dysplasia, Hyperuricosuria, Hypothyroidism, Ichthyosis, Merling, Neuronal ceroid lipofuscinosis 4A, Patellar luxation, Progressive retinal atrophy (crd1), Progressive retinal atrophy (crd2), Progressive retinal atrophy (rcd1b), Retinal dysplasia, Urolithiasis (cystine), Zinc-responsive dermatosis

American Shorthair 🐈
Cardiomyopathy (hypertrophic), Craniofacial deformity, Hip dysplasia, Polycystic kidney disease

American Staffordshire Terrier 🐕
Arrhythmia, Atopic dermatitis, Cataracts, Cerebellar abiotrophy, Cerebellar ataxia, Cervical vertebral instability, Cleft lip/palate, Color dilution alopecia, Compulsive tail chasing, Craniomandibular osteopathy, Cruciate ligament disease, Cryptorchidism, Cystinuria, Deafness, Degenerative myelopathy, Demodicosis, Distichiasis, Elbow dysplasia, Elbow dysplasia (fragmented coronoid process), Gastric carcinoma, Hip dysplasia, Hyperuricosuria, Hypothyroidism, Ichthyosis, Lymphoma, Mast cell tumor, Merling, Necrotizing encephalopathy, Neuronal ceroid lipofuscinosis 4A, Osteochondromatosis, Panosteitis, Patellar luxation, Patent ductus arteriosus, Persistent pupillary membranes, Progressive retinal atrophy (crd1), Progressive retinal atrophy (crd2), Progressive retinal atrophy (rcd1b), Prostate disorders, Pulmonary fibrosis, Pulmonic stenosis, Retinal degeneration, Retinal dysplasia, Subaortic stenosis, Tail chasing

American Water Spaniel 🐕
Cataracts, Cleft lip/palate, Cryptorchidism, Degenerative myelopathy, Diabetes mellitus, Distichiasis, Elbow dysplasia, Epilepsy, Follicular dysplasia, Growth hormone-responsive dermatosis, Hernia (inguinal), Hip dysplasia, Hypothyroidism, Mitral valve disease, Osteochondrodysplasia, Patellar luxation, Patent ductus arteriosus, Persistent pupillary membranes, Progressive retinal atrophy, Pulmonic stenosis, Retinal dysplasia

American Wirehair 🐈
Cardiomyopathy (hypertrophic), Deafness, Hip dysplasia, Progressive retinal atrophy (rdAc)

Asian Shorthair Cat (Malayan) 🐈
GM-1 gangliosidosis, GM-2 gangliosidosis

Australian Cattle Dog (Queensland Blue Heeler) 🐕
Achromatopsia, Cataracts, Cystinuria, Deafness, Degenerative myelopathy, Dermatomyositis, Dysautonomia, Elbow dysplasia, Elbow dysplasia (fragmented coronoid process), Glaucoma, Hip dysplasia, Hyperuricosuria, Hypothyroidism, Lens luxation, Leukodystrophy (spongiform leukoencephalopathy), Mast cell tumor, Multidrug resistance-1, Myotonia congenita, Necrotizing

encephalopathy, Neuronal ceroid lipofuscinosis 5, Neuronal ceroid lipofuscinosis 12, Osteochondritis dissecans (hock), Patellar luxation, Pelger–Huet Anomaly, Persistent pupillary membranes, Portosystemic shunts, Progressive retinal atrophy (prcd), Progressive retinal atrophy (rcd4), Short Tail, Urolithiasis (cystine), von Willebrand disease

Australian Cobber Dog (Labradoodle) 🐕

Centronuclear myopathy, Cystinuria, Elliptocytosis, Exercise-induced collapse, Hyperuricosuria, Macrothrombocytopenia, Myasthenia gravis, Nasal parakeratosis, Progressive retinal atrophy (crd4), Progressive retinal atrophy (prcd)

Australian Kelpie 🐕

Cerebellar abiotrophy, Choroidal hypoplasia (collie eye anomaly), Cutaneous asthenia, Degenerative myelopathy, Globoid cell leukodystrophy, Hernia (perineal), Hip dysplasia, Hypothyroidism, Neuronal ceroid lipofuscinosis 12, Pannus, Progressive retinal atrophy

Australian Mist 🐈

Feline infectious peritonitis (FIP) susceptibility, Hypokalemic periodic polymyopathy

Australian Shepherd 🐕

Achromatopsia, Anterior cross-bite, Brachygnathism, Cardiomyopathy (dilated), Cataracts, Cerebellar vermian hypoplasia, Choroidal hypoplasia (collie eye anomaly), Cobalamin malabsorption (amnionless), Color dilution alopecia, Craniomandibular osteopathy, Cryptorchidism, Cystinuria, Deafness, Degenerative myelopathy, Diabetes mellitus, Distichiasis, Elbow dysplasia, Elbow dysplasia (fragmented coronoid process), Epidermolysis bullosa (junctional epidermolysis bullosa), Epilepsy, Factor VIII deficiency (hemophilia A), Hip dysplasia, Hyperadrenocorticism, Hyperuricosuria, Hypothyroidism, Legg–Calvé–Perthes disease, Lupus erythematosus (discoid), Lymphoproliferative disease (T-cell), Malocclusion, Merling, Microphthalmia, Multidrug resistance-1, Multifocal retinopathy (CMR1), Multiple skeletal defect syndrome, Myotonia congenita, Neuronal ceroid lipofuscinosis 6, Neuronal ceroid lipofuscinosis 8, Optic nerve colobomas, Optic nerve hypoplasia and micropapilla, Osteochondrodysplasia, Panniculitis, Pannus, Panosteitis, Patellar luxation, Patent ductus arteriosus, Pelger–Huet anomaly, Persistent hyaloid artery, Persistent pupillary membranes, Persistent right aortic arch, Polydactyly, Portosystemic shunts, Prognathism, Progressive retinal atrophy (prcd), Pulmonic stenosis, Retinal dysplasia, Short tail, Urolithiasis (cystine), Uveal hypopigmentation, von Willebrand disease type I

Australian Shepherd, Miniature (Miniature Australian Shepherd) 🐕

Achromatopsia, Cardiomyopathy (dilated), Cataracts, Choroidal hypoplasia (collie eye anomaly), Cobalamin deficiency (amnionless), Color dilution alopecia, Degenerative myelopathy, Hyperuricosuria, Multidrug resistance-1, Multifocal retinopathy, Myotonia congenita, Neuronal ceroid lipofuscinosis 6, Progressive retinal atrophy (prcd), Short tail

Australian Stumpy-Tail Cattle Dog 🐕

Deafness, Degenerative myelopathy, Hip dysplasia, Lens luxation, Multidrug resistance-1, Myotonia congenita, Neuronal ceroid lipofuscinosis 5, Neuronal ceroid lipofuscinosis 12, Progressive retinal atrophy (prcd), Progressive retinal atrophy (rcd4), Short tail, von Willebrand disease type II

Australian Terrier 🐕

Atopic dermatitis, Cataracts, Cleft lip/palate, Cruciate ligament disease, Cryptorchidism, Deafness, Degenerative myelopathy, Diabetes mellitus, Distichiasis, Elbow dysplasia, Epilepsy, Glucocerebrosidosis, Hip dysplasia, Hyperadrenocorticism, Hypothyroidism, Juvenile cellulitis, Keratoconjunctivitis sicca, Legg–Calvé–Perthes disease, Mast cell tumor, Megaesophagus, Pancreatitis, Patellar luxation, Patent ductus arteriosus, Persistent pupillary membranes, Portosystemic shunts, Progressive retinal atrophy, Retinal dysplasia, von Willebrand disease type I

Austrian Pinscher (Österreichischer Pinscher) 🐕

Demodicosis, Elbow dysplasia, Hip dysplasia, Short tail

Azawakh 🐕

Cervical vertebral instability, Demodicosis, Epilepsy, Gastric dilation/volvulus, Hypothyroidism, von Willebrand disease

Balinese 🐈

Amyloidosis (hepatic), Cardiomyopathy (dilated), Cardiomyopathy (hypertrophic), Chronic obstructive pulmonary disease, Feline hyperesthesia syndrome, GM-1 gangliosidosis, Hydrocephalus, Mucopolysaccharidosis VI, Myelin deficiency, Niemann–Pick C, Progressive retinal atrophy (rdAc), Retinal degeneration, Strabismus

Barbet 🐕

Cataracts, Color dilution alopecia, Cryptorchidism, Elbow dysplasia, Entropion, Epilepsy, Hip dysplasia, Progressive retinal atrophy (prcd), von Willebrand disease type I

Basenji 🐕

Cataracts, Corneal dystrophy, Cystinuria, Demodicosis, Elbow dysplasia, Epilepsy, Fanconi syndrome, Hip dysplasia, Hypothyroidism, Immunoproliferative enteropathy, Lymphangiectasia, Optic nerve colobomas, Patellar luxation, Pelger–Huet anomaly, Persistent pupillary membranes, Progressive retinal atrophy (PRA-BAS), Protein-losing enteropathy, Pyruvate kinase deficiency, Renal glucosuria, Retinal dysplasia, Spinocerebellar ataxia (myokymia and neuromyotonia), Urolithiasis (cystine)

Basset Fauve de Bretagne 🐕
Cataracts, Glaucoma (POAG), Ulcerative keratitis

Basset Hound 🐕
Black hair follicular dysplasia, Brachygnathism, Cardiomyopathy (dilated), Cataracts, Cervical vertebral instability, Chondrodysplasia, Chondrodystrophy, Corneal dystrophy, Craniomandibular osteopathy, Cruciate ligament disease (caudal), Cystinuria, Dermatomyositis, Distichiasis, Ectodermal dysplasia (x-linked), Ectropion, Elbow dysplasia, Elbow dysplasia (ununited anconeal process), Elbow dysplasia (fragmented coronoid process), Elongated soft palate, Epilepsy (Lafora body disease), Factor VII deficiency, Gastric dilation/volvulus, Glaucoma (PACG), Glaucoma (POAG), Globoid cell leukodystrophy, Hemivertebra, Hernia (inguinal), Hip dysplasia, Hypoadrenocorticism, Hypothyroidism, Hypotrichosis, Intersex (gonadal), Intervertebral disk disease, Lymphoma, Malassezia dermatitis, Malocclusion, Mycobacterial susceptibility, Nasal arteritis, Panosteitis, Patellar luxation, Persistent hyaloid artery, Persistent Mullerian duct syndrome, Persistent pupillary membranes, Progressive retinal atrophy, Prolapsed gland of nictitans, Pulmonic stenosis, Retinal dysplasia, Sebaceous adenitis, Seborrhea, Severe Combined immunodeficiency, Signal transduction disorder, Subaortic stenosis, Temporomandibular joint dysplasia, Thrombopathia, Urolithiasis (cystine), von Willebrand disease type I

Bavarian Mountain Hound (Bayerischer Gebirgsschweißhund) 🐕
Cerebellar abiotrophy, Demodicosis, Ectropion, Elbow dysplasia, Entropion, Hip dysplasia, Progressive retinal atrophy, Retinal dysplasia

Beagle 🐕
Amyloidosis, Amyloidosis (renal), Black hair follicular dysplasia, Brachygnathism, Cardiomyopathy (dilated), Catalase deficiency, Cataracts, Cerebellar abiotrophy, Cerebellar ataxia (hound), Cerebellar cortical degeneration, Cervical vertebral instability, Chondrodystrophy, Cleft lip/palate, Cobalamin malabsorption (cubilin), Color dilution alopecia, Congenital stationary night blindness, Copper hepatopathy, Corneal dystrophy, Cryptorchidism, Cutaneous asthenia, Deafness, Degenerative myelopathy, Demodicosis, Diabetes mellitus, Distichiasis, Dysfibrinogenemia,

Ectodermal defect, Elbow dysplasia, Elongated soft palate, Epilepsy (Lafora body disease), Exocrine pancreatic insufficiency, Factor VII deficiency, Factor VIII deficiency (hemophilia A), Familial nephropathy, Familial vasculopathy, Glaucoma (POAG), Globoid cell leukodystrophy, GM-2 gangliosidosis, Hip dysplasia, Hyperadrenocorticism, Hyperlipidemia (Hypertriglyceridemia), Hyperuricosuria, Hypoadrenocorticism, Hypothyroidism, Hypotrichosis, Immune-mediated polyarthritis, Immunoglobulin A (IgA) deficiency, Intersex (gonadal), Intervertebral disk disease, Leishmania susceptibility, Lens luxation, Lissencephaly, Microphthalmia, Mitral valve disease, Musladin–Leuke syndrome, Narcolepsy, Nonspherocytic hemolytic anemia, Optic nerve hypoplasia and micropapilla, Osteogenesis imperfecta, Osteosarcoma, Pain syndrome, Panosteitis, Patellar luxation, Persistent pupillary membranes, Polycystic kidney disease, Polycystic liver disease, Prognathism, Progressive retinal atrophy, Progressive retinal atrophy (cord1), Progressive retinal atrophy (crd4), Prolapsed gland of nictitans, Pulmonic stenosis, Pyruvate kinase deficiency, Renal agenesis, Retinal dysplasia, Shaker syndrome, Small intestinal bacterial overgrowth, Spina bifida, Spinocerebellar ataxia, Stationary night blindness, Tapetal degeneration, Urolithiasis (magnesium ammonium phosphate; struvite), Uveal hypopigmentation, Vasculitis, Vertebral stenosis, Vestibular disease (congenital)

Bearded Collie 🐕
Black hair follicular dysplasia, Brachygnathism, Cataracts, Choroidal hypoplasia (collie eye anomaly), Cleft lip/palate, Corneal dystrophy, Cryptorchidism, Elbow dysplasia, Elbow dysplasia (fragmented coronoid process), Epilepsy, Hip dysplasia, Hypoadrenocorticism, Hypothyroidism, Lens luxation, Lupoid onychopathy, Lupus erythematosus (SLE), Oligodontia, Osteochondritis dissecans (elbow), Patellar luxation, Patent ductus arteriosus, Pemphigus foliaceus, Persistent pupillary membranes, Prognathism, Progressive retinal atrophy, Progressive retinal atrophy (prcd), Recurrent flank alopecia, Retinal dysplasia, Subaortic stenosis, von Willebrand disease

Beauceron (Berger de Beauce) 🐕
Atopic dermatitis, Dermatomyositis, Elbow dysplasia, Epidermolysis bullosa, Epidermolysis bullosa (dystrophic), Gastric dilation/volvulus, Hip dysplasia, Hypothyroidism, Mast cell tumor, Merling, Patellar luxation, Squamous cell carcinoma (toes)

Bedlington Terrier 🐕
Atopic dermatitis, Cataracts, Chronic inflammatory hepatic disease, Copper hepatopathy, Corneal dystrophy, Cryptorchidism, Deafness, Distichiasis, Elbow dysplasia, Entropion, Epilepsy, Exocrine pancreatic insufficiency,

Glaucoma, Hip dysplasia, Hyperadrenocorticism, Hypothyroidism, Imperforate nasolacrimal puncta, Keratoconjunctivitis sicca, Microphthalmia, Oligodontia, Osteogenesis imperfecta, Patellar luxation, Persistent pupillary membranes, Progressive retinal atrophy, Renal dysplasia, Retinal dysplasia

Belgian Shepherd (Belgian Sheepdog, Chien de Berger Belge), Groenendael

Cardiomyopathy (dilated), Cataracts, Cerebellar ataxia (spongy degeneration), Congenital nystagmus, Degenerative myelopathy, Ectodermal defect, Elbow dysplasia, Elbow dysplasia (fragmented coronoid process), Epilepsy, Gastric carcinoma, Gracilis or semitendinosus myopathy, Hip dysplasia, Hypothyroidism, Hypotrichosis, Macroblepharon, Mucopolysaccharidosis VII, Muscular dystrophy, Optic nerve hypoplasia and micropapilla, Pannus, Patellar luxation, Persistent pupillary membranes, Prognathism, Progressive retinal atrophy, Retinal dysplasia, Subaortic stenosis, Vitiligo

Belgian Shepherd (Belgian Sheepdog, Chien de Berger Belge), Laekenois

Cardiomyopathy (dilated), Cataracts, Cerebellar ataxia (spongy degeneration), Degenerative myelopathy, Elbow dysplasia, Elbow dysplasia (fragmented coronoid process), Epilepsy, Hip dysplasia, Hypothyroidism, Mucopolysaccharidosis VII, Progressive retinal atrophy

Belgian Shepherd (Belgian Sheepdog, Chien de Berger Belge), Malinois

Cardiomyopathy (dilated), Cataracts, Cerebellar ataxia (spongy degeneration), Degenerative myelopathy, Ectodermal dysplasia (x-linked), Elbow dysplasia, Elbow dysplasia (fragmented coronoid process), Epilepsy, Exertional myositis, Gastric dilation/volvulus, Hip dysplasia, Hypothyroidism, Leukodystrophy (spongiform encephalopathy), Lumbosacral stenosis, Mucopolysaccharidosis VII, Pannus, Patellar luxation, Persistent pupillary membranes, Prognathism, Progressive retinal atrophy, Retinal dysplasia, Spinocerebellar ataxia (myokymia and neuromyotonia)

Belgian Shepherd (Belgian Sheepdog, Chien de Berger Belge), Tervuren

Anasarca, Anterior cross-bite, Atopic dermatitis, Atrial septal defect, Cardiomyopathy (dilated), Cataracts, Cerebellar ataxia (spongy degeneration), Cryptorchidism, Degenerative myelopathy, Demodicosis, Dermatomyositis, Elbow dysplasia, Elbow dysplasia (fragmented coronoid process), Epilepsy, Gastric carcinoma, Hip dysplasia, Hypothyroidism, Level bite, Lymphedema, Macroblepharon, Malocclusion, Mucopolysaccharidosis VII, Muscular dystrophy, Oligodontia, Optic nerve hypoplasia and

micropapilla, Pannus, Patellar luxation, Persistent pupillary membranes, Prognathism, Progressive retinal atrophy, Retinal dysplasia, Vitiligo, Wry mouth

Bengal

Cardiomyopathy (hypertrophic), Cataracts, Feline infectious peritonitis (FIP) susceptibility, Polyneuropathy, Progressive retinal atrophy (PRA-b), Progressive retinal atrophy (rdAc), Pyruvate kinase deficiency, Urolithiasis (urate)

Bergamasco Sheepdog

Elbow dysplasia, Hip dysplasia, Merling

Berger Blanc Suisse (White Swiss Shepherd Dog)

Cleft lip/palate, Degenerative lumbosacral stenosis, Degenerative myelopathy, Ectodermal dysplasia (x-linked), Factor VIII deficiency (hemophilia A), Hip dysplasia, Hyperuricosuria, Leukocyte adhesion deficiency type III, Lumbosacral transitional vertebrae, Mucopolysaccharidosis VII, Multidrug resistance-1, Nodular dermatofibrosis, Scott syndrome, von Willebrand disease type I

Berger Picard

Cataracts, Degenerative myelopathy, Ectropion, Elbow dysplasia, Entropion, Hip dysplasia, Multidrug resistance-1, Progressive retinal atrophy, Retinal dysplasia

Bern Running Dog (Chien Courant Bernois)

Cataracts, Cerebellar abiotrophy, Ectropion, Elbow dysplasia, Entropion, Hip dysplasia, Patellar luxation, Progressive retinal atrophy

Bernese Mountain Dog

Alexander disease, Aseptic meningitis, Atopic dermatitis, Borrelia susceptibility, Cataracts, Cerebellar abiotrophy, Cervical vertebral instability, Cleft palate, Color dilution alopecia, Cruciate ligament disease, Degenerative myelopathy, Dysmyelinogenesis, Elbow dysplasia, Elbow dysplasia (ununited anconeal process), Elbow dysplasia (fragmented coronoid process), Entropion, Epilepsy, Factor I (fibrinogen) deficiency, Factor VII deficiency, Gastric dilation/volvulus, Glomerulonephritis (membranoproliferative), Hepatocerebellar degeneration, Hernia (umbilical), Hip dysplasia, Histiocytosis, Hypertrophic osteodystrophy, Hypoadrenocorticism, Hypomyelination, Hypothyroidism, Immune-mediated polyarthritis, Leptospirosis susceptibility, Leukodystrophy (fibrinoid), Lymphoma, Mast cell tumor, Meningitis (aseptic), Osteochondritis dissecans (shoulder), Panosteitis, Patellar luxation, Persistent pupillary membranes, Portosystemic shunts, Progressive retinal atrophy, Protein-losing nephropathy, Renal dysplasia, Sebaceous adenitis, Vasculitis, von Willebrand disease type I

Bichon Frisé

Atlantoaxial instability, Atopic dermatitis, Brachygnathism, Cataracts, Caudal occipital malformation, Chondrodystrophy, Ciliary dyskinesia, Corneal dystrophy, Cruciate ligament disease, Cryptorchidism, Cystinuria, Deafness, Degenerative myelopathy, Diabetes mellitus, Distichiasis, Ectodermal dysplasia (x-linked), Elbow dysplasia, Elbow dysplasia (fragmented coronoid process), Entropion, Epilepsy, Factor IX deficiency (hemophilia B), Glaucoma, Hernia (umbilical), Hip dysplasia, Hyperadrenocorticism, Hypothyroidism, Hypotrichosis, Immune-mediated hemolytic anemia, Legg–Calvé–Perthes disease, Macrothrombocytopenia, Paroxysmal dyskinesia, Patellar luxation, Patent ductus arteriosus, Persistent pupillary membranes, Portosystemic shunts, Prognathism, Progressive retinal atrophy, Pulmonary fibrosis, Renal dysplasia, Retinal dysplasia, Shaker syndrome, Thrombopathia, Urolithiasis (calcium oxalate), Urolithiasis (cystine), Urolithiasis (magnesium ammonium phosphate, struvite), Ventricular septal defect, Vitreous degeneration, von Willebrand disease

Biewer Terrier

Degenerative myelopathy, L2-hydroxyglutaric aciduria, Legg–Calvé–Perthes syndrome, Lens luxation, Patellar luxation, Portosystemic shunting, Progressive retinal atrophy (prcd), Tracheal collapse

Birman (Sacred Birman)

Arterial thromboembolism, Audiogenic reflex seizures, Chediak–Higashi-like syndrome, Corneal sequestrum, Feline infectious peritonitis (FIP) susceptibility, Hypotrichosis, Mucopolysaccharidosis VI, Neonatal isoerythrolysis, Neutrophil granulation anomaly, Polycystic kidney disease, Polyneuropathy, Progressive retinal atrophy (PRA-pd), Urolithiasis (urate), Wool-sucking behavior

Black and Tan Coonhound

Amyloidosis, Blastomycosis susceptibility, Cataracts, Cryptorchidism, Distichiasis, Ectropion, Elbow dysplasia, Entropion, Factor IX deficiency (hemophilia B), Gastric dilation/volvulus, Hip dysplasia, Hypothyroidism, Patellar luxation, Pelger–Huet anomaly, Persistent pupillary membranes, Polyradiculoneuritis, Progressive retinal atrophy, Progressive retinal atrophy (central), Retinal dysplasia

Black Russian Terrier

Cataracts, Elbow dysplasia, Hip dysplasia, Hyperuricosuria, Hypothyroidism, Laryngeal Paralysis, Laryngeal paralysis-polyneuropathy, Microphthalmia, Patellar luxation, Peripheral neuropathy (Warburg), Polyendocrinopathy (immune-mediated), Polyneuropathy, Progressive retinal atrophy (prcd), Subaortic stenosis, Urolithiasis (silica)

Bloodhound

Brachygnathism, Cataracts, Cryptorchidism, Degenerative myelopathy, Ectropion, Elbow dysplasia, Elbow dysplasia (ununited anconeal process), Entropion, Gastric dilation/volvulus, Hip dysplasia, Hypothyroidism, Keratoconjunctivitis sicca, Macropalpebral fissure, Pannus, Patellar luxation, Persistent pupillary membranes, Prolapsed gland of nictitans, Retinal dysplasia, Spinal muscular atrophy, Ventricular septal defect

Bluetick Coonhound

Cataracts, Degenerative myelopathy, Elbow dysplasia, Gastric dilation/volvulus, Globoid cell leukodystrophy, Hip dysplasia, Hock luxation, Hypothyroidism, Patellar luxation, Pelger–Huet anomaly, Polyradiculoneuritis

Boerboel

Cardiomyopathy, Cervical vertebral instability, Elbow dysplasia, Epilepsy (psychomotor), Gastric dilation/volvulus, Hip dysplasia, Hyperuricosuria, Hypothyroidism, Multifocal retinopathy (CMR1)

Bolognese

Cataracts, Patellar luxation, Progressive retinal atrophy, Progressive retinal atrophy (prcd), Retinal dysplasia, Urolithiasis (urate)

Bolonka Zwetna (Tsvetnaya Bolonka)

Legg–Calvé–Perthes disease, Lens luxation (secondary), Patellar luxation, Portosystemic shunts, Progressive retinal atrophy (prcd), Tracheal collapse, Vitreous degeneration

Bombay

Craniofacial deformity, Hypokalemic periodic polymyopathy, Polycystic kidney disease

Border Collie

Black hair follicular dysplasia, Border collie collapse, Cataracts, Cerebellar abiotrophy, Choroidal hypoplasia (collie eye anomaly), Ciliary dyskinesia, Cobalamin malabsorption (cubilin), Color dilution alopecia, Corneal dystrophy, Cyclic hematopoiesis, Cyclic hematopoiesis, Deafness, Degenerative myelopathy, Diabetes mellitus, Dysautonomia, Elbow dysplasia, Elbow dysplasia (fragmented coronoid process), Epilepsy, Epilepsy – phenobarbital resistant, Goniodysgenesis and Glaucoma, Hemangiosarcoma (tongue), Hip dysplasia, Hyperuricosuria, Hypothyroidism, Inflammatory bowel disease, Klippel–Trenaunay syndrome, Lens luxation, Lupus erythematosus (vesicular cutaneous), Malignant hyperthermia, Meningitis/arteritis, Merling, Microphthalmia, Multidrug resistance-1, Musculotendinopathy, Myotonia congenita, Neuroaxonal dystrophy, Neuronal ceroid lipofuscinosis 5, Organic aciduria (methylmalonic aciduria), Osteochondritis dissecans (shoulder), Osteochondritis dissecans (stifle), Pannus, Patellar luxation, Patent ductus arteriosus, Pelger–Huet anomaly, Peripheral neuropathy (sensory), Persistent pupillary membranes, Portosystemic shunts, Progressive retinal atrophy, Progressive retinal atrophy (central), Progressive retinal atrophy (XLPRA3), Proliferative episcleritis, Raine syndrome, Retinal dysplasia, Sensory neuropathy, Superficial necrolytic dermatitis, Trapped neutrophil syndrome, von Willebrand disease type II

Border Terrier 🐾

Brachury, Cataracts, Conotruncal defect, Craniomandibular osteopathy, Cryptorchidism, Degenerative myelopathy, Diabetes mellitus, Ectopic ureters, Elbow dysplasia, Epilepsy, Epileptoid cramping syndrome, Fanconi syndrome, Gallbladder mucocele, Hip dysplasia, Hypothyroidism, Hypothyroidism (congenital) with goiter, Legg–Calvé–Perthes disease, Leukodystrophy (spongiform leukoencephalomyelopathy), Oligodontia, Paroxysmal dyskinesia, Patellar luxation, Peripheral neuropathy (progressive axonopathy), Persistent atrial standstill, Persistent pupillary membranes, Polydontia (retained primary teeth), Prognathism, Progressive retinal atrophy, Pulmonic stenosis, Retinal dysplasia, Sebaceous gland hyperplasia, Tetralogy of Fallot, Thrombopathia, Ulcerative keratitis, Ventricular septal defect, Vitreous degeneration

Borzoi (Russian Wolfhound) 🐕

Anesthetic metabolism (CYP2B11), Cardiomyopathy (dilated), Cataracts, Cervical vertebral instability, Chorioretinitis, Deafness, Degenerative myelopathy, Dysfibrinogenemia, Elbow dysplasia, Factor I (fibrinogen) deficiency, Focal retinal degeneration, Gastric dilation/volvulus, Hip dysplasia, Hypertrophic osteodystrophy, Hypothyroidism, Lens luxation (secondary), Lymphedema, Malocclusion, Methemoglobin reductase deficiency, Microphthalmia, Multifocal retinopathy, Oligodontia, Optic nerve hypoplasia and micropapilla, Osteochondritis dissecans (stifle), Osteosarcoma, Patellar luxation, Persistent pupillary membranes, Posterior cross-bite, Progressive retinal atrophy, Retinal degeneration, Retinal dysplasia, Tricuspid valve dysplasia

Boston Terrier 🐕

Anasarca, Atopic dermatitis, Atresia ani, Brachycephalic obstructive airway syndrome, Calcinosis circumscripta, Cataracts, Cerebellar vermian hypoplasia, Chemodectoma, Cleft lip/palate, Color dilution alopecia, Corneal dystrophy, Craniomandibular osteopathy, Cryptorchidism, Deafness, Degenerative myelopathy, Demodicosis, Distichiasis, Dystocia, Elbow dysplasia, Elongated soft palate, Entropion, Fold dermatitis, Glaucoma, Hemivertebra, Hernia (perineal), Hip dysplasia, Hydrocephalus,

Hyperadrenocorticism, Hyperuricosuria, Hypospadias, Hypothyroidism, Iris cysts, Keratoconjunctivitis sicca, Legg–Calvé–Perthes disease, Lens luxation (secondary), Malocclusion, Mast cell tumor, Mitral valve disease, Muscular dystrophy, Nasodigital hyperkeratosis, Patellar luxation, Pelger–Huet anomaly, Persistent pupillary membranes, Persistent right aortic arch, Progressive retinal atrophy, Prolapsed gland of nictitans, Pyloric stenosis, Sacrocaudal dysgenesis, Spina bifida, Strabismus, Tracheal hypoplasia, Ulcerative keratitis, Uveal cysts, Vitreous degeneration, Wry mouth, Zinc-responsive dermatosis

Bouvier des Flandres 🐕

Atopic dermatitis, Brachygnathism, Cataracts, Cleft lip/palate, Degenerative myelopathy, Elbow dysplasia, Elbow dysplasia (fragmented coronoid process), Entropion, Exercise-induced collapse, Gastric carcinoma, Gastric dilation/volvulus, Glaucoma/goniodysplasia, Hernia (perineal), Hip dysplasia, Hypothyroidism, Intestinal villus atrophy, Laryngeal paralysis-polyneuropathy, Megaesophagus, Muscular dystrophy, Osteochondritis dissecans (shoulder), Patellar luxation, Peripheral neuropathy (distal sensorimotor), Persistent primary vitreous, Persistent pupillary membranes, Polyneuropathy, Portosystemic shunts, Prognathism, Prostate carcinoma, Recurrent flank alopecia, Squamous cell carcinoma (toe), Subaortic stenosis, Vitreous degeneration

Boxer 🐾

Acne, Arrhythmogenic right ventricular cardiomyopathy, Atopic dermatitis, Atrial septal defect, Brachycephalic obstructive airway syndrome, Calcinosis circumscripta, Cardiomyopathy (dilated), Cataracts, Cervical vertebral instability, Chemodectoma, Chondrosarcoma, Cleft palate, Corneal dystrophy, Cruciate ligament disease, Cryptorchidism, Cutaneous asthenia, Cystinuria, Deafness, Degenerative myelopathy, Demodicosis, Dermoid sinus, Diffuse idiopathic skeletal hyperostosis, Distichiasis, Dysrhythmia, Dystocia, Eccentrocytosis, Ectropion, Elbow dysplasia, Elongated soft palate, Endocardial fibroelastosis, Epilepsy, Factor I (fibrinogen) deficiency, Factor II (prothrombin) deficiency, Factor VII deficiency, Factor VIII deficiency (hemophilia A), Familial nephropathy, Folate (decreased levels), Fold dermatitis, Follicular dysplasia, Gastric dilation/volvulus, Gingival hyperplasia, Hemangiosarcoma, Hernia (perineal), Hip dysplasia, Histiocytic ulcerative colitis, Hyperadrenocorticism, Hypertrophic osteodystrophy, Hyperuricosuria, Hypoplastic trachea, Hypothyroidism, Immune-mediated polyarthritis, Inflammatory bowel disease, Inflammatory myopathy, Leishmania susceptibility, Leproid granuloma, Lupoid onychopathy, Lymphoma, Macrothrombocytopenia, Malocclusion, Mast cell tumor, Meningitis (aseptic), Mitral valve dysplasia,

Nasodigital hyperkeratosis, Neuroaxonal dystrophy, Niemann–Pick disease, Nodular dermatofibrosis, Ocular melanosis, Osteochondritis dissecans (lumbosacral), Osteochondritis dissecans (shoulder), Osteochondritis dissecans (stifle), Osteosarcoma, Pancreatitis, Panosteitis, Patellar luxation, Peripheral neuropathy (progressive axonopathy), Peripheral neuropathy (Warburg), Piebaldism, Polydontia (supernumerary teeth), Polymyositis, Progressive retinal atrophy, Progressive retinal atrophy (central), Prolapsed gland of nictitans, Pulmonic stenosis, Pyloric stenosis, Radial carpal bone fracture, Recurrent flank alopecia, Renal dysplasia, Short tail, Spina bifida, Spondylosis deformans, Spontaneous chronic corneal epithelial defects, Subaortic stenosis, Tracheal hypoplasia, Transmissible venereal tumor susceptibility, Tricuspid valve dysplasia, Ulcerative keratitis, Vaginal prolapse, Vasculitis, von Willebrand disease

Boykin Spaniel

Atopic dermatitis, Cataracts, Choroidal hypoplasia (collie eye anomaly), Corneal dystrophy, Degenerative myelopathy, Distichiasis, Elbow dysplasia, Elbow dysplasia (fragmented coronoid process), Exercise-induced collapse, Factor VIII deficiency (hemophilia A), Hip dysplasia, Hypothyroidism, Patellar luxation, Persistent hyaloid artery, Persistent pupillary membranes, Phosphofructokinase deficiency, Progressive retinal atrophy, Progressive retinal atrophy (crd4), Progressive retinal atrophy (prcd), Pulmonic stenosis, Retinal dysplasia, von Willebrand disease type II

Braque du Bourbonnais (Bourbonnais Pointer)

Ectropion, Entropion, Hip dysplasia, Lupus erythematosus (exfoliative cutaneous), Patellar luxation, Pulmonic stenosis, Short tail

Brazilian Terrier

Atopic dermatitis, Deafness, Epilepsy, Mucopolysaccharidosis VII, Multifocal retinopathy (CMR1), Patellar luxation, Short tail, von Willebrand disease type I

Briard

Atopic dermatitis, Cataracts, Corneal dystrophy, Ectopic ureters, Elbow dysplasia, Elbow dysplasia (fragmented coronoid process), Gastric dilation/volvulus, Hip dysplasia, Hyperlipidemia (Hypertriglyceridemia), Hyperuricosuria, Hypothyroidism, Lymphoma, Open bite, Patellar luxation, Persistent pupillary membranes, Progressive retinal atrophy, Progressive retinal atrophy (central), Recurrent flank alopecia, Squamous cell carcinoma (toe), Stationary night blindness

British Longhair

Autoimmune lymphoproliferative syndrome, Deafness, Polycystic kidney disease, Progressive retinal atrophy (PRA-pd)

British Shorthair

Autoimmune lymphoproliferative syndrome, Cardiomyopathy (hypertrophic), Deafness, Factor IX deficiency (hemophilia B), Feline infectious peritonitis (FIP) susceptibility, Heterochromia iridis, Intervertebral disk disease, Neonatal isoerythrolysis, Polycystic kidney disease, Progressive retinal atrophy (PRA-pd), Urolithiasis (calcium oxalate)

Brittany Spaniel (Brittany)

Amyloidosis, Brachygnathism, Cataracts, Cerebellar abiotrophy, Cerebellar ataxia (spinocerebellar degeneration), Cleft palate, Complement (C3) deficiency, Cryptorchidism, Distichiasis, Elbow dysplasia, Elbow dysplasia (incomplete ossification of humeral condyle), Elbow dysplasia (fragmented coronoid process), Epilepsy, Factor VIII deficiency (hemophilia A), Glaucoma, Hip dysplasia, Histoplasmosis susceptibility, Hyperlipidemia (hypertriglyceridemia), Hypothyroidism, Lens luxation, Lupus erythematosus (discoid), Muscular dystrophy, Oligodontia, Osteochondritis dissecans (shoulder), Otitis externa, Panniculitis, Patellar luxation, Persistent pupillary membranes, Prognathism, Progressive retinal atrophy, Retinal dysplasia, Sensory neuropathy, Short tail, Spinal muscular atrophy, Sudden acquired retinal degeneration, Ventricular septal defect, Vitreous degeneration, Wry mouth

Brussels Griffon (Griffon Bruxellois)

Atopic dermatitis, Cataracts, Chiari-like malformation, Cleft palate, Corneal dystrophy, Cryptorchidism, Distichiasis, Ectopic ureters, Elbow dysplasia, Epilepsy, Hip dysplasia, Hypothyroidism, Legg–Calvé–Perthes disease, Optic nerve colobomas, Patellar luxation, Persistent hyaloid artery, Persistent pupillary membranes, Polydontia (retained primary teeth), Progressive retinal atrophy, Progressive retinal atrophy (PAP1), Syringomyelia, Ulcerative keratitis, Vitreous degeneration

Bulldog (English Bulldog)

Acne, Anasarca, Arrhythmogenic right ventricular cardiomyopathy, Atopic dermatitis, Brachycephalic obstructive airway syndrome, Cardiomyopathy (ventricular tachycardia), Cataracts, Cerebellar abiotrophy, Chemodectoma, Cleft palate, Cruciate ligament disease, Cryptorchidism, Cystinuria, Deafness, Degenerative myelopathy, Degenerative myelopathy, Demodicosis, Diskospondylitis, Distichiasis, Dystocia, Ectopic ureters, Elbow dysplasia, Endocardial fibroelastosis, Entropion, Factor VII deficiency, Factor VIII deficiency (hemophilia A), Fold dermatitis, Head tremor syndrome, Hemivertebra, Hernia (Hiatal), Hip dysplasia, Hydrocephalus, Hydrocephalus (ventriculomegaly), Hyperuricosuria, Hypomagnesemia, Hypoplastic trachea, Hypothyroidism, Keratoconjunctivitis sicca, Laryngeal paralysis, Lymphedema, Malocclusion, Multifocal retinopathy (CMR1), Myelodysplasia, Nasodigital hyperkeratosis, Osteochondritis dissecans (stifle), Pannus, Panosteitis, Paroxysmal dyskinesia, Patellar luxation, Perianal gland tumors, Persistent pupillary membranes, Polydontia, Polydontia (supernumerary teeth), Prolapsed gland of nictitans, Pulmonic stenosis, Recurrent flank alopecia, Recurrent flank alopecia, Retinal dysplasia, Sacrocaudal dysgenesis, Spina bifida, Splenic torsion, Sterile pyogranuloma, Subaortic stenosis, Tetralogy of Fallot, Tracheal hypoplasia, Tremor syndrome, Ulcerative keratitis, Urethral prolapse, Urolithiasis (cystine), Urolithiasis (urate), Ventricular septal defect, von Willebrand disease, Wry mouth

Bull Terrier

Actinic keratosis, Albinism (Waardenburg), Atopic dermatitis, Cataracts, Cerebellar abiotrophy, Cerebellar vermian hypoplasia, Compulsive tail chasing, Deafness, Deep pyoderma, Demodicosis, Ectropion, Elbow dysplasia, Entropion, Factor IX deficiency (hemophilia B), Hereditary nephritis, Hip dysplasia, Hypothyroidism, Keratoconjunctivitis sicca, Laryngeal paralysis, Lens luxation, Lethal acrodermatitis, Lymphoma, Malocclusion, Mast cell tumor, Mitral valve disease, Mitral valve dysplasia, Neuronal ceroid lipofuscinosis 4A, Osteochondritis dissecans (hock), Osteochondritis dissecans (stifle), Panosteitis, Patellar luxation, Persistent pupillary membranes, Piebaldism, Polycystic kidney disease, Polycystic liver disease, Polydontia (retained primary teeth), Prognathism, Progressive retinal atrophy, Prolapsed gland of nictitans, Pulmonary fibrosis, Retinal dysplasia, Squamous cell carcinoma, Subaortic stenosis, Tail chasing, Tracheal collapse, Trance-like syndrome, Vitreous degeneration, Wry mouth

Bull Terrier, Miniature (Miniature Bull Terrier)

Cataracts, Compulsive tail chasing, Corneal dystrophy, Deafness, Hereditary nephritis, Hypothyroidism, Laryngeal paralysis, Lens luxation, Lethal Acrodermatitis, Neuronal ceroid lipofuscinosis 4A, Persistent pupillary membranes, Polycystic kidney disease, Tail chasing, Vitreous degeneration

Bullmastiff

Calvarial hyperostotic syndrome, Cardiomyopathy (dilated), Cataracts, Cerebellar abiotrophy, Cerebellar ataxia (familial), Cervical vertebral instability, Cruciate ligament disease, Cystinuria, Degenerative myelopathy, Distichiasis, Ectropion, Elbow dysplasia, Elbow dysplasia (ununited anconeal process), Elbow dysplasia (fragmented coronoid process), Entropion, Familial nephropathy, Gastric dilation/volvulus, Hip dysplasia, Hydrocephalus, Hypothyroidism, Leukodystrophy, Leukodystrophy (oligodendroglial dysplasia), Lymphosarcoma, Malocclusion, Multifocal retinopathy (CMR1), Neuroaxonal dystrophy, Optic nerve hypoplasia and micropapilla, Osteochondritis dissecans (hock), Osteochondritis dissecans (shoulder), Osteochondritis dissecans (stifle), Osteosarcoma, Panosteitis, Patellar luxation, Persistent pupillary membranes, Polydontia (supernumerary teeth), Progressive retinal atrophy (dominant), Recurrent flank alopecia, Retinal dysplasia, Urolithiasis (cystine), Vaginal prolapse

Burmese

Cardiomyopathy (dilated), Corneal sequestrum, Craniofacial deformity, Cutaneous asthenia, Dermoids (epibulbar), Diabetes mellitus, Endocardial fibroelastosis, Feline hyperesthesia syndrome, Feline infectious peritonitis (FIP) susceptibility, Feline leukemia virus susceptibility, Feline orofacial pain syndrome, Glaucoma, GM-1 gangliosidosis, GM-2 gangliosidosis, Hypertriglyceridemia, Hypokalemic periodic polymyopathy, Iris cysts, Mast cell tumor, Meningoencephalocele, Prolapse of gland of nictitans, Urolithiasis (calcium oxalate), Wool-sucking behavior

Burmilla

GM-2 gangliosidosis, Hypokalemic periodic polymyopathy, Polycystic kidney disease

Cairn Terrier

Atopic dermatitis, Base-narrow canines, Cataracts, Chondrodysplasia, Chromatolytic neuronal degeneration, Chronic inflammatory hepatic disease, Cleft lip/palate, Craniomandibular osteopathy, Cryptorchidism, Diabetes mellitus, Ectopic ureters, Elbow dysplasia, Factor IX deficiency (hemophilia B), Gallbladder mucocele, Glaucoma, Globoid cell leukodystrophy, Hemivertebra (tail), Hip dysplasia, Hydrocephalus, Hyperadrenocorticism, Hypoadrenocorticism, Hypothyroidism, Immune-mediated hemolytic anemia, Legg–Calvé–Perthes disease, Macrothrombocytopenia, Malocclusion, Mitral valve disease, Ocular melanosis, Pancreatitis, Patellar luxation, Persistent hyaloid artery, Persistent pupillary membranes, Polycystic liver disease, Portal vein hypoplasia, Portosystemic shunts, Progressive retinal atrophy, Pulmonary fibrosis, Pyruvate kinase deficiency, Renal dysplasia, Retinal dysplasia, Seborrhea, Sertoli cell tumor, Spinal muscular atrophy, Urolithiasis (calcium oxalate), Vitamin A-responsive dermatosis, von Willebrand disease type I, Wry mouth

California Spangled Cat

Insufficient information available

Canaan Dog 🐕

Cataracts, Cryptorchidism, Degenerative myelopathy, Distichiasis, Elbow dysplasia, Epilepsy, Hip dysplasia, Hypothyroidism, Osteochondritis dissecans, Patellar luxation, Persistent pupillary membranes, Progressive retinal atrophy, von Willebrand disease type II

Cane Corso (Italian Mastiff) 🐕

Demodicosis, Ectropion, Elbow dysplasia, Entropion, Epilepsy, Gastric dilation/volvulus, Hip dysplasia, Hypothyroidism, Multifocal retinopathy (CMR1), Neuroaxonal dystrophy, Neuronal ceroid lipofuscinosis I, Patellar luxation, Prolapsed gland of nictitans

Carlin Pinscher 🐕

Cystinuria, Degenerative myelopathy, Glaucoma (POAG), Hypothyroidism (congenital, with goiter), Lens luxation, May–Hegglin anomaly, Patellar luxation, Progressive retinal atrophy (crd4), Pyruvate kinase deficiency, Spinocerebellar ataxia

Catahoula Leopard Dog 🐕

Cataracts, Deafness, Degenerative myelopathy, Demodicosis, Elbow dysplasia, Exercise-induced collapse, Factor VII deficiency, Heart block, Hip dysplasia, Hyperuricosuria, Merling, Short tail

Cavalier King Charles Spaniel 🐕

Anal sac adenocarcinoma, Atopic dermatitis, Black hair follicular dysplasia, Brachycephalic OBSTRUCTIVE AIRWAY SYNDROME, Brachygnathism, Cataracts, Chiari-like malformation, Chondrodystrophy, Chronic inflammatory hepatic disease, Collagenolytic (eosinophilic) granuloma, Corneal dystrophy, Curly coat/dry eye, Deafness, Degenerative myelopathy, Diabetes mellitus, Distichiasis, Dystocia, Elbow dysplasia, Epilepsy, Episodic falling, Exocrine pancreatic insufficiency, Femoral artery occlusion, Fly catching behavior, Hernia (inguinal), Hernia (umbilical), Hip dysplasia, Hypothyroidism, Ichthyosis, Intervertebral disk disease, Keratoconjunctivitis sicca, Legg–Calvé–Perthes disease, Lymphoproliferative disease (T-cell), Macrothrombocytopenia, Masticatory myositis, Microphthalmia, Mitral valve disease, Muscular dystrophy, Organic aciduria, Pancreatitis, Paroxysmal dyskinesia, Patellar luxation, Persistent pupillary membranes, Pneumocystosis, Primary secretory otitis media, Prognathism, Progressive retinal atrophy, Retinal dysplasia, Skeletal dysplasia 2, Syringomyelia, Temporomandibular joint dysplasia, Ulcerative keratitis, Urolithiasis (xanthine), Vitreous degeneration, Wry mouth

Central Asian Shepherd Dog 🐕

Deafness, Elbow dysplasia, Epidermolysis bullosa (dystrophic), Gastric dilation/volvulus, Glaucoma, Hip dysplasia, Progressive retinal atrophy

Cesky Terrier 🐕

Hip dysplasia, Lens luxation, Patellar luxation, Scottie cramp

Chartreux 🐈

Cardiomyopathy (hypertrophic), Polycystic kidney disease, Progressive retinal atrophy (PRA-pd), Urolithiasis (magnesium ammonium phosphate)

Chausie 🐈

Insufficient information available

Cheetoh 🐈

Patellar luxation

Chesapeake Bay Retriever 🐕

Anterior cross-bite, Atopic dermatitis, Brachygnathism, Cataracts, Chondrodystrophy, Cruciate ligament disease, Degenerative myelopathy, Distichiasis, Ectodermal dysplasia (skin fragility syndrome), Ectropion, Elbow dysplasia, Entropion, Epilepsy, Exercise-induced collapse, Follicular dysplasia, Gastric dilation/volvulus, Hernia (umbilical), Hip dysplasia, Hypothyroidism, Malocclusion, Osteochondritis dissecans (shoulder), Panosteitis, Patellar luxation, Peripheral neuropathy (distal sensorimotor), Persistent pupillary membranes, Prognathism, Progressive retinal atrophy (central), Progressive retinal atrophy (prcd), Retinal dysplasia, Skeletal dysplasia, von Willebrand disease, Wry mouth

Chihuahua 🐕

Alexander disease, Atlantoaxial instability, Brachygnathism, Cataracts, Chiari-like malformation, Chondrodystrophy, Color dilution alopecia, Corneal dystrophy, Cryptorchidism, Cystinuria, Deafness, Demodicosis, Dystocia, Eclampsia, Elbow dysplasia, Epilepsy (Lafora body disease), Factor VIII deficiency (hemophilia A), Follicular dysplasia, Gallbladder mucocele, Glaucoma, Hernia (inguinal), Hip dysplasia, Hydrocephalus, Hypothyroidism, Keratoconjunctivitis sicca, Legg–Calvé–Perthes disease, Macrothrombocytopenia, Meningoencephalitis (necrotizing), Merling, Methemoglobin reductase deficiency, Mitral valve disease, Muscular dystrophy, Myasthenia gravis, Myelodysplasia, Narcolepsy, Neuroaxonal dystrophy, Neuronal ceroid lipofuscinosis, Neuronal ceroid lipofuscinosis 7, Osteochondritis dissecans (shoulder), Panniculitis, Patellar luxation, Patent ductus arteriosus, Persistent pupillary membranes, Polydontia, Polydontia (retained primary teeth), Portosystemic shunts, Prognathism, Progressive retinal atrophy (crd4/cord1), Progressive retinal atrophy (prcd), Pulmonic stenosis, Spina bifida, Spinocerebellar ataxia (myokymia and neuromyotonia),

Syringomyelia, Tracheal collapse, Ulcerative keratitis, Urolithiasis (calcium oxalate), Urolithiasis (cystine), Urolithiasis (xanthine), Vitreous degeneration, von Willebrand disease type II, Wry mouth

Chinese Crested Dog 🐕

Cataracts, Cerebellar abiotrophy, Chondrodystrophy, Comedo syndrome, Deafness, Degenerative myelopathy, Hairlessness, Keratoconjunctivitis sicca, Legg–Calvé–Perthes disease, Lens luxation, Neuronal ceroid lipofuscinosis 7, Neuronal degeneration, Oligodontia, Patellar luxation, Persistent pupillary membranes, Progressive retinal atrophy (prcd), Progressive retinal atrophy (rcd3), Vitreous degeneration, von Willebrand disease type II

Chinook 🐕

Atopic dermatitis, Cataracts, Chondrodysplasia (ITGA), Choroidal hypoplasia (collie eye anomaly), Cryptorchidism, Elbow dysplasia, Epilepsy, Hip dysplasia, Hypothyroidism, Multidrug resistance-1, Paroxysmal dyskinesia, Patellar luxation, Persistent pupillary membranes, Retinal dysplasia, Vitreous degeneration

Chow Chow 🐕

Adrenal sex hormone imbalance, Alopecia X, Atopic dermatitis, Atrioventricular heart block, Cataracts, Cerebellar hypoplasia, Cervical vertebral instability, Ciliary dyskinesia, Color dilution alopecia, Cor triatriatum, Corneal dystrophy, Cruciate ligament disease, Deafness, Degenerative myelopathy, Dermatomyositis, Dermoid sinus, Diabetes mellitus, Dysmyelinogenesis, Ectropion, Elbow dysplasia, Elbow dysplasia (ununited anconeal process), Elbow dysplasia (fragmented coronoid process), Elliptocytosis, Entropion, Exocrine pancreatic insufficiency, Familial nephropathy, Gastric carcinoma, Gastric dilation/volvulus, Glaucoma, Growth hormone-responsive dermatosis, Heart block, Hip dysplasia, Hypothyroidism, Immunoglobulin A (IgA) deficiency, Keratoconjunctivitis sicca, Melanoma (oral), Myotonia congenita, Osteochondritis dissecans (elbow), Osteochondritis dissecans (stifle), Osteogenesis imperfecta, Pannus, Panosteitis, Patellar luxation, Pemphigus foliaceus, Persistent pupillary membranes, Pituitary dwarfism, Progressive retinal atrophy, Pulmonic stenosis, Renal dysplasia, Sebaceous adenitis, Tremor syndrome, Tyrosinase deficiency, Uveodermatologic syndrome, Ventricular septal defect

Cirneco dell'Etna 🐕

Atopic dermatitis, Demodicosis

Clumber Spaniel 🐕

Anasarca, Atopic dermatitis, Cataracts, Cryptorchidism, Degenerative myelopathy, Distichiasis, Dystocia, Ectropion, Elbow dysplasia, Entropion, Exercise-induced collapse, Hemangiosarcoma, Hip dysplasia, Hypothyroidism, Inflammatory bowel disease, Intervertebral disk disease, Keratoconjunctivitis sicca, Mitochondrial myopathy, Oligodontia, Patellar luxation, Persistent pupillary membranes, Portosystemic shunts, Prognathism, Pyruvate dehydrogenase phosphatase 1 deficiency, Retinal dysplasia, Wry mouth

Cocker Spaniel, American (American Cocker Spaniel) 🐕

Anal sac adenocarcinoma, Atopic dermatitis, Babesiosis susceptibility, Bernard Soulier syndrome, Black hair follicular dysplasia, Brachygnathism, Bradyarrhythmia, Bronchiectasis, Cardiomyopathy (dilated), Cataracts, Chondrodystrophy, Chronic inflammatory hepatic disease, Cleft lip/palate, Corneal dystrophy, Cruciate ligament disease, Cyclic hematopoiesis, Deafness, Degenerative myelopathy, Distichiasis, Ectodermal defect, Ectodermal dysplasia (x-linked), Ectropion, Elbow dysplasia, Elbow dysplasia (incomplete ossification of humeral condyle), Entropion, Epilepsy, Episcleritis, Exercise-induced collapse, Factor II (prothrombin) deficiency, Factor VIII deficiency (hemophilia A), Factor IX deficiency (hemophilia B), Factor X deficiency, Familial nephropathy, Fold dermatitis, Gallbladder mucocele, Glaucoma, Hernia (umbilical), Hip dysplasia, Hyperadrenocorticism, Hypoadrenocorticism, Hypothyroidism, Hypotrichosis, Immune-mediated hemolytic anemia, Immune-mediated thrombocytopenia, Immunoglobulin A (IgA) deficiency, Intersex (gonadal), Intervertebral disk disease, Iron deficiency anemia, Keratoconjunctivitis sicca, Lymphoma, Macrothrombocytopenia, Malassezia dermatitis, Malignant hyperthermia, Melanoma (oral), Merling, Microphthalmia, Muscular dystrophy, Myotonia congenita, Nasodigital hyperkeratosis, Neuronal ceroid lipofuscinosis, Neuronal degeneration, Obesity (POMC), Optic nerve colobomas, Optic nerve hypoplasia and micropapilla, Otitis externa, Pancreatitis, Pannus, Panosteitis, Patellar luxation, Patent ductus arteriosus, Pelger–Huet anomaly, Perianal gland tumors, Persistent right aortic arch, Phosphofructokinase deficiency, Plasmacytoma, Platelet D-storage pool disease, Portal vein hypoplasia, Portosystemic shunts, Prognathism, Progressive retinal atrophy (central), Progressive retinal atrophy (prcd), Prolapsed gland of nictitans, Proliferative episcleritis, Pulmonic stenosis, Renal dysplasia, Retinal detachment, Retinal dysplasia, Sebaceous adenitis, Seborrhea, Skeletal dysplasia 2, Superficial necrolytic dermatitis, Temporomandibular joint dysplasia, Ulcerative keratitis, Urolithiasis (silica), Vestibular disease (congenital), Vitamin A-responsive dermatosis, von Willebrand disease

Cocker Spaniel, English (English Cocker Spaniel) 🐕

Acral mutilation syndrome, Bernard Soulier syndrome, Brachygnathism, Cardiomyopathy (dilated), Cataracts, Degenerative myelopathy, Entropion, Exercise-induced collapse, Factor II (prothrombin) deficiency, Familial nephropathy, Gallbladder mucocele, Glaucoma, Hip dysplasia, Intersex (gonadal), Keratoconjunctivitis sicca, Neuronal ceroid lipofuscinosis, Optic nerve hypoplasia and micropapilla, Persistent pupillary membranes, Phosphofructokinase deficiency, Polydontia, Polydontia (retained primary teeth), Prognathism, Progressive retinal atrophy (central), Progressive retinal atrophy (prcd), Renal dysplasia, Retinal dysplasia, Urolithiasis (magnesium ammonium phosphate, struvite), Urolithiasis (xanthine), Vestibular disease (congenital), von Willebrand disease

Collie, Rough, Smooth (Rough Collie, Smooth Collie) 🐕

Albinism (Waardenburg), Amyloidosis, Atopic dermatitis, Brachygnathism, Cataracts, Cerebellar abiotrophy, Choroidal hypoplasia (collie eye anomaly), Colorectal polyps, Corneal dystrophy, Cutaneous lupus erythematosus, Cyclic hematopoiesis, Deafness, Degenerative myelopathy, Demodicosis, Dermatomyositis, Diabetes mellitus, Distichiasis, Dysfibrinogenemia, Elbow dysplasia, Entropion, Epilepsy, Exocrine pancreatic insufficiency, Factor I (fibrinogen) deficiency, Factor VIII deficiency (hemophilia A), Gastric carcinoma, Gastric dilation/volvulus, Hernia (perineal), Hip dysplasia, Hyperlipidemia (hypercholesterolemia), Hyperuricosuria, Hypomagnesemia, Hypothyroidism, Immune-mediated hemolytic anemia, Inflammatory pulmonary disease, Lupus erythematosus, Lupus erythematosus (discoid), Lupus erythematosus (vesicular cutaneous), Malignant hyperthermia, Malocclusion, Merling, Microphthalmia, Multidrug resistance-1, Myopia, Nasal cavity tumors, Neuroaxonal dystrophy, Optic nerve colobomas, Optic nerve hypoplasia and micropapilla, Osteochondritis dissecans (stifle), Pancreatitis, Panniculitis, Patellar luxation, Patent ductus arteriosus, Pemphigoid (bullous), Pemphigus (erythematosus), Pemphigus foliaceus, Persistent hyaloid artery, Persistent pupillary membranes, Piebaldism, Polydontia, Polydontia (supernumerary teeth), Posterior cross-bite, Prognathism, Progressive retinal atrophy (central), Progressive retinal atrophy (rcd2), Proliferative episcleritis, Renal dysplasia, Retinal dysplasia, Sebaceous adenitis, Sterile pyogranuloma, Testicular cancer, Ulcerative dermatosis, Uveal hypopigmentation, von Willebrand disease type II

Colorpoint Shorthair 🐈

Corneal sequestrum, Polycystic kidney disease, Progressive retinal atrophy (PRA-pd), Progressive retinal atrophy (rdAc)

Corgi, Cardigan Welsh (Cardigan Welsh Corgi) 🐕

Cataracts, Chondrodystrophy, Color dilution alopecia, Cystinuria, Degenerative myelopathy, Distichiasis, Elbow dysplasia, Epilepsy (Lafora body disease), Exercise-induced collapse, Glaucoma, Hernia (perineal), Hip dysplasia, Hypothyroidism, Intervertebral disk disease, Merling, Patellar luxation, Persistent pupillary membranes, Progressive retinal atrophy (central), Progressive retinal atrophy (prcd), Progressive retinal atrophy (rcd3), Retinal dysplasia, Severe combined Immunodeficiency

Corgi, Pembroke Welsh (Pembroke Welsh Corgi) 🐕

Brachygnathism, Cataracts, Chondrodysplasia, Chondrodystrophy, Corneal dystrophy, Cutaneous asthenia, Cystinuria, Degenerative myelopathy, Dermatomyositis, Distichiasis, Elbow dysplasia, Epilepsy, Epilepsy (Lafora body disease), Exercise-induced collapse, Familial nephropathy, Hernia (perineal), Hip dysplasia, Histiocytic sarcoma, Immune-mediated inflammatory myopathy, Intervertebral disk disease, Lymphoma, Meningitis/arteritis, Methemoglobin reductase deficiency, Mucopolysaccharidosis VI, Muscular dystrophy, Narcolepsy, Patent ductus arteriosus, Persistent pupillary membranes, Polymyositis, Prognathism, Progressive retinal atrophy, Progressive retinal atrophy (rcd3), Renal telangiectasia, Retinal dysplasia, Sensory neuropathy, Severe combined Immunodeficiency, Short tail, Telangiectasia, Urolithiasis (cystine), Urolithiasis (magnesium ammonium phosphate, struvite), von Willebrand disease type I

Cornish Rex 🐈

Cardiomyopathy (hypertrophic), Deafness, Feline infectious peritonitis (FIP) susceptibility, Heterochromia iridis, Hypokalemic periodic polymyopathy, Neonatal isoerythrolysis, Patellar luxation, Polycystic kidney disease, Progressive retinal atrophy (rdAc)

Coton de Tulear 🐕

Cerebellar ataxia (neonatal), Chondrodystrophy, Degenerative myelopathy, Exercise-induced collapse, Hyperoxaluria, Multifocal retinopathy (CMR2), Progressive retinal atrophy (prcd), Vitreous degeneration, von Willebrand disease type I

Croatian Sheepdog 🐕

Patellar luxation, Short tail

Curly-Coated Retriever 🐕

Cataracts, Color dilution alopecia, Distichiasis, Elbow dysplasia, Entropion, Exercise-induced collapse, Follicular dysplasia, Gastric dilation/volvulus, Glycogen storage disease IIIa, Hip dysplasia, Hypothyroidism, Optic nerve colobomas, Patellar luxation, Persistent pupillary membranes,

Progressive retinal atrophy, Progressive retinal atrophy (crd4/cord1), Subaortic stenosis, Vitreous degeneration

Cymric 🐈

Fecal incontinence, Taillessness

Czechoslovak Wolfdog 🐕

Degenerative myelopathy, Elbow dysplasia, Epilepsy, Exocrine pancreatic insufficiency, Hip dysplasia, Lens luxation, Pituitary dwarfism

Dachshund (Teckel, Dackel) 🐕

Acanthosis nigricans, Achromatopsia, Atopic dermatitis, Black hair follicular dysplasia, Brachygnathism, Calcinosis circumscripta, Cataracts, Cholecystitis, Chondrodysplasia, Chondrodystrophy, Ciliary dyskinesia, Cleft lip/palate, Color dilution alopecia, Colorectal polyps, Corneal dystrophy, Cryptorchidism, Cutaneous asthenia, Cystinuria, Deafness, Demodicosis, Dermoid, Diabetes mellitus, Dystocia, Ectodermal dysplasia (x-linked), Elbow dysplasia (ununited anconeal process), Entropion, Epilepsy, Epilepsy (Lafora body disease), Factor VIII deficiency (hemophilia A), Follicular dysplasia (lipidosis), Glaucoma, Glycogen storage disease IIIa, Hemangiosarcoma (cardiac), Hernia (inguinal), Heterochromia iridis, Hip dysplasia, Hyperadrenocorticism, Hyperparathyroidism, Hypothyroidism, Immunoglobulin A (IgA) deficiency, Intersex (gonadal), Intervertebral disk disease, Juvenile cellulitis, Keratoconjunctivitis sicca, Legg–Calvé–Perthes disease, Macroblepharon, Malocclusion, Merling, Microphthalmia, Mitral valve disease, Mucopolysaccharidosis IIIa, Myasthenia gravis, Narcolepsy, Nasopharyngeal dysgenesis, Neuronal ceroid lipofuscinosis 1, Neuronal ceroid lipofuscinosis 2, Optic nerve colobomas, Optic nerve hypoplasia and micropapilla, Osteogenesis imperfecta, Pancreatitis, Panniculitis, Pannus, Patellar luxation, Pemphigoid (bullous), Peripheral neuropathy (sensory), Persistent hyaloid artery, Persistent pupillary membranes, Pes varus, Pneumocystosis, Portal vein hypoplasia, Portosystemic shunts, Progressive retinal atrophy (crd1), Progressive retinal atrophy (crd2), Progressive retinal atrophy (crd SWD), Progressive retinal atrophy (crd4), Recurrent flank alopecia, Retinal dysplasia, Sebaceous adenitis, Seborrhea, Sensory neuropathy, Shaker syndrome, Sialocele, Squamous cell carcinoma (toes), Sudden acquired retinal degeneration, Urolithiasis (cystine), Urolithiasis (magnesium ammonium phosphate, struvite), Urolithiasis (xanthine), Uveodermatologic syndrome, Vasculitis, von Willebrand disease type I

Dachshund, Miniature Longhaired (Miniature Longhaired Dachshund) 🐕

Chondrodystrophy, Glycogen storage disease IIIa, Mucopolysaccharidosis IIIa, Narcolepsy, Neuronal ceroid lipofuscinosis 1 & 2, Osteogenesis imperfecta (SERPINH1), Progressive retinal atrophy (crd4/cord1), Progressive retinal atrophy (crd SWD)

Dachshund, Miniature Smooth-haired (Miniature Smooth-haired Dachshund) 🐕

Chondrodystrophy, Factor VII deficiency, Glycogen storage disease IIIa, Narcolepsy, Neuronal ceroid lipofuscinosis 1 & 2, Osteogenesis imperfecta (SERPINH1), Progressive retinal atrophy (crd4/cord1), Progressive retinal atrophy (crd SWD)

Dachshund, Miniature Wirehaired (Miniature Wirehaired Dachshund) 🐕

Chondrodystrophy, Epilepsy (Lafora body disease), Glycogen storage disease IIIa, Mucopolysaccharidosis IIIa, Neuronal ceroid lipofuscinosis 1 & 2, Osteogenesis imperfecta (SERPINH1), Progressive retinal atopy (crd SWD), Progressive retinal atrophy (crd4/cord1)

Dachshund, Standard Longhaired (Standard Longhaired Dachshund) 🐕

Chondrodystrophy, Mucopolysaccharidosis IIIa, Neuronal ceroid lipofuscinosis 1 & 2, Osteogenesis imperfecta (SERPINH1), Progressive retinal atopy (crd SWD), Progressive retinal atrophy (crd4/cord1)

Dachshund, Standard Smooth-Haired (Standard Smooth-Haired Dachshund) 🐕

Chondrodystrophy, Mucopolysaccharidosis IIIa, Narcolepsy, Neuronal ceroid lipofuscinosis 1 & 2, Osteogenesis imperfecta (SERPINH1), Progressive retinal atopy (crd SWD), Progressive retinal atrophy (crd4/cord1)

Dachshund, Standard Wirehaired (Standard Wirehaired Dachshund) 🐕

Chondrodystrophy, Mucopolysaccharidosis IIIa, Narcolepsy, Neuronal ceroid lipofuscinosis 1 & 2, Osteogenesis imperfecta (SERPINH1), Progressive retinal atopy (crd SWD), Progressive retinal atrophy (crd4/cord1)

Dalmatian 🐕

Actinic keratosis, Acute respiratory distress syndrome, Albinism (Waardenburg), Atopic dermatitis, Brachygnathism, Bronzing syndrome, Cardiomyopathy, Chronic inflammatory hepatic disease, Ciliary dyskinesia, Deafness, Deep pyoderma, Degenerative myelopathy, Demodicosis, Dermoid, Dysmyelinogenesis, Entropion, Epilepsy, Familial nephropathy, Familial nephropathy, Glaucoma, Globoid cell leukodystrophy, Hereditary nephritis, Hyperuricosuria, Hypothyroidism, Immunoglobulin A (IgA) deficiency, Iris sphincter dysplasia, Laryngeal paralysis-polyneuropathy, Leukodystrophy, Leukoencephalomyelopathy, Microphthalmia, Myelodysplasia, Neuronal ceroid lipofuscinosis, Osteochondritis dissecans (shoulder), Panniculitis, Pannus, Panosteitis, Peripheral neuropathy, Prognathism, Progressive retinal atrophy, Sebaceous adenitis, Spina bifida, Spinal dysraphism, Squamous cell carcinoma, Tremor syndrome, Urinary incontinence, Urolithiasis (calcium oxalate), Urolithiasis (urate), Uveal hypopigmentation, Wry mouth

Dandie Dinmont Terrier 🐕

Brachygnathism, Chondrodysplasia, Chondrodystrophy, Glaucoma (PACG), Hyperadrenocorticism, Oligodontia, Portosystemic shunts, Prognathism, Ulcerative keratitis

Danish Farmdog (Swedish Farmdog) 🐕

Atopic dermatitis, Dystocia, Hyperuricosuria, Lens luxation, Short tail, Spondyloepiphyseal dysplasia tarda

Devon Rex 🐈

Bowenoid *in situ* carcinoma, Cardiomyopathy (hypertrophic), Deafness, Hereditary myopathy, Heterochromia iridis, Hip dysplasia, Hypokalemic periodic polymyopathy, Hypotrichosis, Malassezia dermatitis, Muscular dystrophy (x-linked), Myasthenic syndrome, Neonatal isoerythrolysis, Patellar luxation, Polycystic kidney disease, Urolithiasis (calcium oxalate), Urticaria pigmentosa, Vitamin K-dependent coagulopathy

Doberman Pinscher (Dobermann) 🐕

Acne, Acral lick dermatitis, Albinism (oculocutaneous), Atherosclerosis, Atrial fibrillation, Atrial septal defect, Avulsion of tibial tuberosity, Brachygnathism, Cardiomyopathy (dilated), Carpal laxity syndrome, Cataracts, Cervical vertebral instability, Chromosomal intersex, Chronic inflammatory hepatic disease, Ciliary dyskinesia, Color dilution alopecia, Cutaneous asthenia, Dancing Doberman disease, Darier disease, Deafness, Degenerative myelopathy, Demodicosis, Dermoid, Diabetes mellitus, Diskospondylitis, Ectodermal defect (x-linked), Factor IX deficiency (hemophilia B), Familial nephropathy, Fanconi syndrome, Flank sucking, Follicular dysplasia, Gastric dilation/volvulus, Head tremor syndrome, Hemivertebra, Histiocytosis, Hyperlipidemia (hypercholesterolemia), Hypertrophic osteodystrophy, Hypothyroidism, Ichthyosis, Intersex (chromosomal), Intervertebral disk disease, Leproid granuloma, Lupoid onychopathy, Lymphoma, Macroblepharon, Malignant hyperthermia, Masticatory myositis, Melanoma, Microphthalmia, Mucinosis, Myositis ossificans, Myxoma (synovial), Narcolepsy, Neutrophil bactericidal defect, Oculocutaneous albinism, Oligodontia, Osteochondritis dissecans (shoulder), Osteochondritis dissecans (stifle), Osteosarcoma, Panosteitis, Paroxysmal dyskinesia, Parvovirus susceptibility, Patent ductus arteriosus, Pemphigoid (bullous), Pemphigus foliaceus,

Peripheral neuropathy (dancing Doberman), Persistent primary vitreous, Persistent pupillary membranes, Polydontia, Polydontia (supernumerary teeth), Prognathism, Progressive retinal atrophy, Prostate disorders, Recurrent flank alopecia, Renal agenesis, Renal dysplasia, Retinal dysplasia, Sebaceous adenitis, Seborrhea, Sulfa sensitivity, Tremor syndrome, Urinary incontinence, Urolithiasis (calcium oxalate), Vertebral stenosis, Vestibular disease (congenital), Vitiligo, von Willebrand disease type I, Wry mouth, Zinc-responsive dermatosis

Dogo Argentino 🐕

Deafness, Degenerative myelopathy, Elbow dysplasia, Gastric dilation/volvulus, Glaucoma, Hip dysplasia, Hypothyroidism, Laryngeal paralysis, Mast cell tumor

Dogue de Bordeaux (Bordeaux Mastiff) 🐕

Cardiomyopathy (dilated), Familial nephropathy, Familial nephropathy, Footpad hyperkeratosis, Hypothyroidism, Multifocal retinopathy (CMR1), Subaortic stenosis, Thoracic spinal stenosis, Tricuspid valve dysplasia

Domestic Longhair 🐈

Deafness, Factor XII deficiency, Hyperoxaluria, Leukocyte adhesion deficiency I, Lipoprotein lipase deficiency, Mannosidosis (alpha), Mucopolysaccharidosis VI, Pemphigus foliaceus, Porphyria, Pyruvate kinase deficiency, von Willebrand disease type III

Domestic Shorthair 🐈

Acne, Cerebellar abiotrophy, Cerebellar degeneration, Chronic obstructive pulmonary disease, Craniofacial deformity, Cutaneous asthenia, Deafness, Dihydropyrimidase deficiency, Epidermolysis bullosa simplex, Factor IX deficiency (hemophilia B), Factor XII deficiency, Fibrodysplasia ossificans, GM-1 gangliosidosis, GM-2 gangliosidosis, Hyperoxaluria, Hypothyroidism (congenital), Inflammatory linear verrucous epidermal nevus, Junctional epidermolysis bullosa, Lipoprotein lipase deficiency, Mannosidosis (alpha), Methemoglobin reductase deficiency, Mucolipidosis II, Mucopolysaccharidosis I, Mucopolysaccharidosis VI, Mucopolysaccharidosis VII, Muscular dystrophy (x-linked), Neuronal ceroid lipofuscinosis 6, Neuronal ceroid lipofuscinosis 7, Niemann–Pick C, Pemphigus foliaceus, Porphyria, Pyruvate kinase deficiency, Rickets

Drentse Patrijshond (Dutch Partridge Dog) 🐕

Hypertrophic gastritis, Hyperuricosuria, Progressive retinal atrophy, Stomatocytosis, von Willebrand disease type I

Dunker (Norwegian Hound) 🐕

Deafness, Hip dysplasia, Merling

Dutch Kooiker dog (Kooikerhondje) 🐕
Cataracts, Degenerative myelopathy, Epilepsy, Leukoencephalomyelopathy, Necrotizing myelopathy, Patellar luxation, Renal dysplasia, von Willebrand disease type III

Dutch Shepherd 🐕
Atopic dermatitis, Cerebellar ataxia (spongy degeneration), Cryptorchidism, Degenerative myelopathy, Inflammatory bowel disease, Inflammatory myopathy, Masticatory myositis, Pannus

Egyptian Mau 🐈
Cardiomyopathy (hypertrophic), Dysmyelinogenesis, Feline leukemia virus susceptibility, Pyruvate kinase deficiency, Urolithiasis (urate)

Elf 🐈
Hairlessness, Myasthenic syndrome, Progressive retinal atrophy (rdAc)

English Coonhound (American English Coonhound, Redtick Coonhound) 🐕
Degenerative myelopathy

English Setter 🐕
Atopic dermatitis, Brachygnathism, Cutaneous asthenia, Darier disease, Deafness, Eccentrocytosis, Ectropion, Elbow dysplasia, Elbow dysplasia (ununited anconeal process), Exocrine pancreatic insufficiency, Factor VIII deficiency (hemophilia A), Familial benign pemphigus, Hip dysplasia, Hypothyroidism, Keratoconjunctivitis sicca, Lupoid onychopathy, Malassezia dermatitis, Mast cell tumor, Methemoglobin reductase deficiency, Neuronal ceroid lipofuscinosis 8, Osteochondritis dissecans (shoulder), Panosteitis, Prognathism, Progressive retinal atrophy (central), Progressive retinal atrophy (rcd4), von Willebrand disease, Wry mouth

English Shepherd 🐕
Cataracts, Choroidal hypoplasia (collie eye anomaly), Degenerative myelopathy, Elbow dysplasia, Hip dysplasia, Hyperuricosuria, Multidrug resistance-1, Patellar luxation, Progressive retinal atrophy (prcd)

English Toy Spaniel (King Charles Spaniel) 🐕
Cataracts, Chiari-like malformation, Cleft palate, Corneal dystrophy, Degenerative myelopathy, Macrothrombocytopenia, Malocclusion, Microphthalmia, Mitral valve disease, Oligodendroglioma, Persistent hyaloid artery, Persistent primary vitreous, Retinal dysplasia, Syringomyelia, Ulcerative keratitis, von Willebrand disease type I

Entlebucher Mountain Dog (Entlebucher Sennenhund) 🐕
Cataracts, Cruciate ligament disease, Ectopic ureters, Glaucoma, Hip dysplasia, Progressive retinal atrophy (prcd)

Eurasier 🐕
Dandy–Walker malformation, Degenerative myelopathy, Distichiasis, Ectropion, Elbow Dysplasia, Entropion, Epidermolysis bullosa simplex, Hip dysplasia, Hypothyroidism, Patellar luxation, Progressive retinal atrophy

European Shorthair 🐈
Urolithiasis (urate)

Exotic 🐈
Brachycephalic airway obstructive syndrome, Deafness, Dental anomalies, Neonatal isoerythrolysis, Polycystic kidney disease, Progressive retinal atrophy (PRA-pd), Urolithiasis (calcium oxalate)

Field Spaniel 🐕
Cataracts, Hip dysplasia, Hypothyroidism, Progressive retinal atrophy, Progressive retinal atrophy (cord1), Progressive retinal atrophy (crd4), Retinal dysplasia, Subaortic stenosis

Fila Brasileiro 🐕
Elbow dysplasia, Gastric dilation/volvulus, Glaucoma, Hip dysplasia, Patellar luxation, Progressive retinal atrophy

Finnish Hound 🐕
Cerebellar ataxia (hound), Demodicosis, Diabetes mellitus, Factor VII deficiency, Hip dysplasia

Finnish Lapphund 🐕
Cataracts, Degenerative myelopathy, Glycogen storage disease II, Hip dysplasia, Hyperuricosuria, Multifocal retinopathy (CMR3), Persistent pupillary membranes, Progressive retinal atrophy (prcd)

Finnish Spitz 🐕
Atresia ani, Cataracts, Degenerative myelopathy, Diabetes mellitus, Epilepsy, Hip dysplasia, Immune-mediated hemolytic anemia, Lupus erythematosus, Pemphigus foliaceus, Pituitary dwarfism, Shaker syndrome, Signal transduction disorder, Thrombopathia

Flat-Coated Retriever 🐕
Cataracts, Degenerative myelopathy, Distichiasis, Ectropion, Elbow dysplasia, Entropion, Exercise-induced collapse, Glaucoma, Hip dysplasia, Histiocytosis, Hypothyroidism, Obesity (POMC), Optic nerve hypoplasia and micropapilla, Osteosarcoma, Patellar luxation, Spondylosis deformans

Fox Terrier, Smooth (Smooth Fox Terrier) 🐾

Atopic dermatitis, Brachygnathism, Cataracts, Cervical vertebral instability, Cystinuria, Deafness, Degenerative myelopathy, Diabetes mellitus, Ectopic ureters, Glaucoma, Hip dysplasia, Hypothyroidism (congenital) with goiter, Lens luxation, Leproid granuloma, Leukoencephalomyelopathy, Megaesophagus, Mitral valve disease, Myasthenia gravis, Oligodontia, Pancreatitis, Persistent pupillary membranes, Prognathism, Progressive retinal atrophy, Pulmonic stenosis, Spinocerebellar ataxia, Spinocerebellar ataxia (myokymia and neuromyotonia), Ventricular septal defect, Vitreous degeneration, von Willebrand disease

Fox Terrier, Toy (Toy Fox Terrier) 🐾

Cataracts, Chondrodystrophy, Cryptorchidism, Deafness, Demodicosis, Degenerative myelopathy, Glaucoma, Hypothyroidism, Hypothyroidism (congenital) with goiter, Lens luxation, Mitral valve disease, Patellar luxation, Spinocerebellar ataxia, von Willebrand disease

Fox Terrier, Wire (Wire Fox Terrier) 🐾

Atopic dermatitis, Brachygnathism, Cataracts, Cerebellar abiotrophy, Cerebellar hypoplasia, Cervical vertebral instability, Cholesterol ester storage disease, Cystinuria, Deafness, Degenerative myelopathy, Demodicosis, Ectopic ureters, Epilepsy, Glaucoma, Hip dysplasia, Hypothyroidism (congenital) with goiter, Lens luxation, Leproid granuloma, Lissencephaly, Megaesophagus, Mitral valve disease, Oligodontia, Patellar luxation, Persistent pupillary membranes, Prognathism, Progressive retinal atrophy (central), Pulmonic stenosis, Sensory neuropathy, Spinocerebellar ataxia (myokymia and neuromyotonia), Tetralogy of Fallot, Van den Ende-Gupta syndrome, von Willebrand disease

Foxhound, American (American Foxhound) 🐾

Amyloidosis, Catalase deficiency, Cerebellar ataxia (hound), Cricopharyngeal dysphagia, Cryptorchidism, Deafness, Degenerative myelopathy, Elbow dysplasia, Factor VII deficiency, Hip dysplasia, Hypothyroidism (congenital) with goiter, Leishmania susceptibility, Patellar luxation, Pelger–Huet anomaly

Foxhound, English (English Foxhound) 🐾

Amyloidosis (renal), Brachygnathism, Cerebellar ataxia (hound), Epilepsy, Hip dysplasia, Prognathism

French Bulldog 🐾

Arachnoid cyst, Atopic dermatitis, Brachycephalic obstructive airway syndrome, Cataracts, Chondrodystrophy, Cleft lip/palate, Cystinuria, Degenerative myelopathy, Demodicosis, Distichiasis, Elbow dysplasia (ununited anconeal process), Entropion, Epilepsy (Lafora body disease), Factor VIII deficiency (hemophilia A), Factor IX deficiency (hemophilia B), Fold dermatitis, Fracture of humeral condyle, Hemivertebra, Hip dysplasia, Histiocytic ulcerative colitis, Hyperuricosuria, Hypothyroidism (congenital) with goiter, Hypotrichosis, Intervertebral disk disease, Malocclusion, Meningoencephalitis (necrotizing), Multifocal retinopathy (CMR1), Oligodendroglioma, Patellar luxation, Progressive retinal atrophy (cord1), Progressive retinal atrophy (crd4), Pulmonic stenosis, Recurrent flank alopecia, Spina bifida, Ulcerative keratitis, Ulcerative keratitis, Ventricular septal defect, von Willebrand disease

French Spaniel (Epagneul Français) 🐾

Acral mutilation syndrome, Elbow dysplasia, Hip dysplasia

Frisian Water Dog (Wetterhoun) 🐾

Hip dysplasia, Patellar luxation, Severe combined immunodeficiency

Gammel Dansk Honsehund (Old Danish Pointer) 🐾

Ectropion, Elbow dysplasia, Entropion, Hip dysplasia, Myasthenia gravis, Progressive retinal atrophy (rcd4)

Garafian Shepherd (Pastor Garafiano) 🐾

Cutaneous asthenia, Dermatomyositis, Hip dysplasia, Progressive retinal atrophy

German Hunting Terrier (Jagdterrier) 🐾

Centronuclear myopathy, Exercise-induced metabolic myopathy, Footpad hyperkeratosis, Hyperuricosuria, Lens luxation

German Longhaired Pointer 🐾

Epidermolysis bullosa (junctional), Hip dysplasia

German Pinscher (Deutscher Pinscher) 🐾

Cataracts, Color dilution alopecia, Degenerative myelopathy, Persistent hyperplastic tunica vasculosa lentis, Persistent right aortic arch, Vitreous degeneration, von Willebrand disease type I

German Rex 🐱

Insufficient information available

German Shepherd Dog (German Shepherd, Deutscher Schäferhund, Alsatian) 🐾

Achromatopsia, Acral lick dermatitis, Acromegaly, Atopic dermatitis, Base-narrow canines, Brachygnathism, Calcinosis circumscripta, Cataracts, Cauda equina syndrome, Cerebellar abiotrophy, Cervical vertebral instability, Cleft lip/palate, Cobalamin malabsorption, Corneal dystrophy, Cryptorchidism, Cutaneous asthenia, Deafness, Degenerative myelopathy, Demodicosis, Dermatomyositis, Dermoid, Diskospondylitis, Ectodermal dysplasia (skin fragility syndrome), Ectodermal dysplasia (x-linked), Elbow dysplasia,

Elbow dysplasia (ununited anconeal process), Elbow dysplasia (fragmented coronoid process), Epilepsy, Exocrine pancreatic insufficiency, Factor VIII deficiency (hemophilia A), Factor IX deficiency (hemophilia B), Familial vasculopathy, Gastric dilation/volvulus, German shepherd dog pyoderma, Giant axonal neuropathy, Glycogen storage disease III, Gracilis or semitendinosus myopathy, Hemangiosarcoma, Hemivertebra, Hip dysplasia, Hyperadrenocorticism, Hyperparathyroidism, Hypertrophic osteodystrophy, Hyperuricosuria, Hypospadias, Ichthyosis, Immune-mediated polyarthritis, Immunoglobulin A (IgA) deficiency, Intervertebral disk disease, Leishmania susceptibility, Leptospirosis susceptibility, Leukocyte adhesion deficiency type III, Lumbosacral transitional vertebrae, Lupoid onychopathy, Lupus erythematosus, Lupus erythematosus (discoid), Lupus erythematosus (mucocutaneous), Lymphedema, Lymphoma, Macroblepharon, Malocclusion, Mannosidosis (beta), Masticatory myositis, Megaesophagus, Melanoma (limbal), Metatarsal fistula, Mitochondrial myopathy, Mitral valve disease, Mitral valve dysplasia, Mucocutaneous pyoderma, Mucopolysaccharidosis VII, Multidrug resistance-1, Myasthenia gravis, Myopia, Neuroaxonal dystrophy, Nodular dermatofibrosis, Oligodontia, Optic nerve hypoplasia and micropapilla, Osteochondritis dissecans (elbow), Osteochondritis dissecans (shoulder), Osteochondritis dissecans (stifle), Osteochondrodysplasia, Osteogenesis imperfecta, Otitis externa, Panniculitis, Panniculitis (pedal), Pannus, Panosteitis, Parvovirus susceptibility, Patent ductus arteriosus, Pelger–Huet anomaly, Pemphigoid (mucous membrane), Pemphigus (erythematosus), Pemphigus foliaceus, Perianal adenocarcinoma, Perianal fistulae, Peripheral neuropathy (giant axonal), Persistent right aortic arch, Pituitary dwarfism, Progressive retinal atrophy, Progressive retinal atrophy (central), Pulmonic stenosis, Renal cystadenocarcinoma (dermatofibrosis), Renal dysplasia, Retinal dysplasia, Scott syndrome, Sebaceous adenitis, Seborrhea, Sialocele, Small intestinal bacterial overgrowth, Spinal dysraphism, Spinal muscular atrophy, Splenic torsion, Spondylosis deformans, Subaortic stenosis, Tricuspid valve dysplasia, Tyrosinemia II, Urolithiasis (silica), Uveodermatologic syndrome, Ventricular ectopy, Ventricular septal defect, Vertebral stenosis, Vestibular disease (congenital), Vitiligo, von Willebrand disease type I, Wry mouth

German Shorthaired Pointer

Achromatopsia, Acral mutilation syndrome, Amaurotic idiocy, Brachygnathism, Cataracts, Chronic inflammatory hepatic disease, Cruciate ligament disease, Cutaneous lupus erythematosus, Deafness, Degenerative myelopathy, Entropion, Epidermolysis bullosa (junctional), Everted cartilage of third eyelid, Factor I (fibrinogen) deficiency,

Factor VII deficiency, Factor VIII deficiency (hemophilia A), Factor XII deficiency, Gastric dilation/volvulus, GM-2 gangliosidosis, Hemivertebra, Hip dysplasia, Hyperuricosuria, Immune-mediated polyarthritis, Intersex (gonadal), Lupus erythematosus (discoid), Lupus erythematosus (exfoliative cutaneous), Lymphedema, Meningoencephalitis, Muscular dystrophy, Myasthenia gravis, Osteochondritis dissecans (shoulder), Overshot jaw, Panosteitis, Persistent hyaloid artery, Prognathism, Recurrent flank alopecia, Sensory neuropathy, Subaortic stenosis, von Willebrand disease type II

German Spitz (Deutscher Spitz)

Albinism (oculocutaneous), Progressive retinal atrophy (prcd), Thrombopathia, von Willebrand disease type I and II

German Wirehaired Pointer (Deutsch Drahthaar)

Atopic dermatitis, Atrioventricular heart block, Brachygnathism, Cataracts, Degenerative myelopathy, Elbow dysplasia, Entropion, Epidermolysis bullosa (junctional), Exercise-induced collapse, Factor VII deficiency, Factor IX deficiency (hemophilia B), Hip dysplasia, Hyperuricosuria, Hypothyroidism, Osteochondritis dissecans (shoulder), Osteochondritis dissecans (stifle), Patellar luxation, Prognathism, Retinal dysplasia, von Willebrand disease type II

Glen of Imaal Terrier

Atopic dermatitis, Cataracts, Distichiasis, Elbow dysplasia, Hip dysplasia, Hypothyroidism, Optic nerve colobomas, Patellar luxation, Progressive retinal atrophy (crd3), Subaortic stenosis

Golden Retriever

Acanthomatous ameloblastoma, Acral lick dermatitis, Anesthetic metabolism (CYP2B11), Atopic dermatitis, Cardiomyopathy, Cataracts, Cervical vertebral instability, Ciliary dyskinesia, Corneal dystrophy, Cricopharyngeal dysfunction, Cruciate ligament disease, Degenerative myelopathy, Dermoid, Diabetes mellitus, Distichiasis, Ectopic ureters, Elbow dysplasia, Elbow dysplasia (ununited anconeal process), Elbow dysplasia (fragmented coronoid process), Elliptocytosis, Entropion, Epidermolysis bullosa (dystrophic), Epilepsy, Factor VIII deficiency (hemophilia A), Factor IX deficiency (hemophilia B), Fibrosarcoma (oral, tongue), Folate (decreased levels), Gastric dilation/volvulus, Glaucoma, GM-2 gangliosidosis, Hemangiosarcoma, Hip dysplasia, Histiocytosis, Horner's syndrome, Hyperparathyroidism, Hypertrophic osteodystrophy, Hypothyroidism, Ichthyosis, Immunoglobulin A (IgA) deficiency, Iris cysts, Juvenile cellulitis, Lymphoma, Mast cell tumor, Masticatory myositis, Megaesophagus, Melanoma (oral, limbal, cutaneous), Meningitis-arteritis, Mitral valve dysplasia, Multidrug resistance-1, Muscular dystrophy, Myasthenia gravis, Neuronal ceroid lipofuscinosis 5,

Nodular dermatofibrosis, Ophthalmic malformations, Optic nerve hypoplasia and micropapilla, Osteochondritis dissecans (elbow), Osteochondritis dissecans (hock), Osteochondritis dissecans (shoulder), Osteogenesis imperfecta, Osteosarcoma, Pannus, Panosteitis, Patellar luxation, Peripheral neuropathy (golden retriever), Peripheral neuropathy (hypomyelinating), Peripheral neuropathy (progressive axonopathy), Peripheral neuropathy (sensory ataxic neuropathy), Peripheral neuropathy (sensory ataxic), Persistent pupillary membranes, Pigmentary uveitis, Polydontia, Polydontia (supernumerary teeth), Portosystemic shunts, Progressive retinal atrophy (central), Progressive retinal atrophy (GR1), Progressive retinal atrophy (GR2), Progressive retinal atrophy (prcd), Proliferative episcleritis, Protein-losing nephropathy, Recurrent flank alopecia, Renal dysplasia, Retinal dysplasia, Sebaceous adenitis, Seborrhea, Skeletal dysplasia, Spherocytosis, Spinal dysraphism, Spontaneous chronic corneal epithelial defects, Subaortic stenosis, Tetralogy of Fallot, Tricuspid valve dysplasia, Trigeminal neuropathy, Urolithiasis (silica), Uveal cysts, von Willebrand disease

Gordon Setter 🐕

Black hair follicular dysplasia, Cataracts, Cerebellar abiotrophy, Cerebellar ataxia (autophagy), Degenerative myelopathy, DUNGd, Ectropion, Elbow dysplasia, Elbow dysplasia (fragmented coronoid process), Entropion, Gastric dilation/volvulus, Hereditary ataxia, Hip dysplasia, Hypothyroidism, Juvenile cellulitis, Keratoconjunctivitis sicca, Lethal astrocytosis, Lupoid onychopathy, Lymphoma, Melanoma (oral), Neuronal ceroid lipofuscinosis 8, Optic nerve hypoplasia and micropapilla, Patellar luxation, Patent ductus arteriosus, Persistent hyaloid artery, Persistent pupillary membranes, Progressive retinal atrophy (rcd4), Renal dysplasia, Retinal dysplasia, Temporomandibular joint dysplasia

Great Dane 🐕

Achromatopsia, Acne, Acral lick dermatitis, Albinism (oculocutaneous), Albinism (Waardenburg), Atrial fibrillation, Brachygnathism, Calcium phosphate deposition, Cardiomyopathy (dilated), Cataracts, Centronuclear myopathy, Cervical vertebral instability, Chronic inflammatory hepatic disease, Ciliary body cysts, Color dilution alopecia, Deafness, Demodicosis, Diffuse idiopathic skeletal hyperostosis, Diskospondylitis, Dystocia, Elbow dysplasia, Elbow dysplasia (ununited anconeal process), Endocardial fibroelastosis, Entropion, Epidermolysis bullosa acquisita, Everted cartilage of third eyelid, Gastric dilation/volvulus, Glaucoma (goniodysgenesis), Hip dysplasia, Hypertrophic osteodystrophy, Hypoadrenocorticism, Hypothyroidism, Ichthyosis, Inherited myopathy, Leukoencephalomyelopathy, Lymphedema, Megaesophagus, Microphthalmia,

Mitral valve disease, Mitral valve dysplasia, Mucopolysaccharidosis VI, Myotonia congenita, Necrotizing myelopathy, Oligodontia, Osteochondritis dissecans (elbow), Osteochondritis dissecans (shoulder), Osteochondritis dissecans (stifle), Osteosarcoma, Panosteitis, Patellar luxation, Peripheral neuropathy (distal sensorimotor), Persistent pupillary membranes, Persistent right aortic arch, Piebaldism, Prognathism, Progressive retinal atrophy, Prolapse of gland of nictitans, Retinal dysplasia, Splenic torsion, Sterile pyogranuloma, Subaortic stenosis, Tricuspid valve dysplasia, Uveal hypopigmentation, von Willebrand disease type I, Wry mouth, Zinc-responsive dermatosis

Great Pyrenees 🐕

Atopic dermatitis, Brachygnathism, Cataracts, Cervical vertebral instability, Chondrodysplasia, Choroidal hypoplasia (collie eye anomaly), Corneal dystrophy, Craniomandibular osteopathy, Deafness, Degenerative myelopathy, Distichiasis, Elbow dysplasia, Elbow dysplasia (ununited anconeal process), Entropion, Factor XI deficiency, Gastric dilation/volvulus, Glanzmann's thrombasthenia I, Hip dysplasia, Hyperlipidemia (hypercholesterolemia), Hyperuricosuria, Hypoadrenocorticism, Hypothyroidism, Laryngeal paralysis-polyneuropathy, Multifocal retinopathy (CMR1), Neuronal degeneration, Optic nerve hypoplasia and micropapilla, Osteochondritis dissecans (shoulder), Osteochondrodysplasia, Osteosarcoma, Panosteitis, Patellar luxation, Peripheral neuropathy (progressive axonopathy), Persistent pupillary membranes, Polydactyly, Prognathism, Progressive retinal atrophy, Short tail, Thrombasthenic thrombopathia, Tricuspid valve dysplasia, von Willebrand disease

Greater Swiss Mountain Dog (Grosser Schweizer Sennenhund) 🐕

Cataracts, Distichiasis, Elbow dysplasia, Epilepsy, Fibroma/fibrosarcoma, Gastric dilation/volvulus, Hernia (umbilical), Hip dysplasia, Hypothyroidism, Leukocyte adhesion deficiency type III, Lumbosacral transitional vertebrae, Lymphoma, Mast cell tumor, Osteochondritis dissecans (shoulder), Panosteitis, Patellar luxation, Persistent pupillary membranes, Postoperative hemorrhage, Procoagulant expression disorder, Thrombopathia (P2Y12), Urinary incontinence, von Willebrand disease

Greyhound 🐕

Anesthetic metabolism (CYP2B11), Arteriosclerosis (renal), Atopic dermatitis, Avulsion of tibial tuberosity, Babesiosis susceptibility, Bald thigh syndrome, Brachygnathism, Cataracts, Cruciate ligament disease, Cryptorchidism, Cutaneous and renal glomerular vasculopathy, Cutaneous asthenia, Deafness, Degenerative myelopathy, Dystocia, Epilepsy, Exocrine pancreatic insufficiency,

Factor VIII deficiency (hemophilia A), Follicular dysplasia, Gastric dilation/volvulus, Glomerulonephritis, Greyhound alopecia, Hemangiosarcoma, Hip dysplasia, Hyperhomocysteinemia, Hyperkalemia during anesthesia, Hypertension, Hypothyroidism, Inflammatory bowel disease, Intervertebral disk disease, Keratoma (digital corns), Lens luxation, Lumbosacral stenosis, Lupoid onychopathy, Lymphoma, Malignant hyperthermia, Megaesophagus, Meningoencephalitis, Metatarsal fistula, Mitral valve disease, Nasal parakeratosis, Optic nerve hypoplasia and micropapilla, Osteochondritis dissecans (shoulder), Osteochondritis dissecans (stifle), Osteosarcoma, Pannus, Patellar luxation, Peripheral neuropathy (greyhound), Persistent right aortic arch, Polydontia, Polydontia (supernumerary teeth), Polyneuropathy, Postoperative hemorrhage, Retinal degeneration, Sesamoid disease, Startle disease, Vasculitis, Vitreous degeneration, von Willebrand disease

Harrier 🐕

Cataracts, Cerebellar abiotrophy, Cerebellar ataxia (hound), Degenerative myelopathy, Epilepsy, Hernia (inguinal), Hip dysplasia, Persistent pupillary membranes, Progressive retinal atrophy, Renal dysplasia

Havana Brown 🐈

Factor VIII deficiency, Urolithiasis (calcium oxalate)

Havanese 🐕

Cataracts, Chondrodystrophy, Deafness, Distichiasis, Elbow dysplasia, Factor VIII deficiency (hemophilia A), Hip dysplasia, Hypothyroidism, Macrothrombocytopenia, Multifocal retinopathy (CMR1), Oligodontia, Osteochondrodysplasia, Patellar luxation, Persistent pupillary membranes, Portosystemic shunts, Progressive retinal atrophy, Renal dysplasia, Retinal dysplasia, Sebaceous adenitis, Vitreous degeneration

Highland Fold 🐈

Deafness, Neonatal isoerythrolysis, Osteochondrodysplasia, Urolithiasis (calcium oxalate)

Highlander (Highland Lynx) 🐈

GM-1 gangliosidosis, Pyruvate kinase deficiency

Himalayan 🐈

Asthma, Basal cell tumor, Cataracts, Corneal sequestrum, Facial dermatitis, Feline hyperesthesia syndrome, Feline infectious peritonitis (FIP) susceptibility, Hernia (peritoneopericardial), Hip dysplasia, Pemphigus foliaceus, Polycystic kidney disease, Portosystemic shunts, Progressive retinal atrophy (PRA-pd), Strabismus, Ulcerative keratitis, Urolithiasis (calcium oxalate), Urolithiasis (magnesium ammonium phosphate), Urticaria pigmentosa, von Willebrand disease type I

Hokkaido (Ainu) 🐕

Choroidal hypoplasia (collie eye anomaly), Epilepsy, Hip dysplasia, Patellar luxation, Uveodermatologic syndrome

Hovawart 🐕

Degenerative myelopathy, Factor IX deficiency (hemophilia B), Hypothyroidism, Immunoglobulin A (IgA) deficiency, Intestinal adenocarcinoma, Sebaceous adenitis

Ibizan Hound 🐕

Atopic dermatitis, Axonal dystrophy, Brachygnathism, Cataracts, Deafness, Elbow dysplasia, Epilepsy, Hip dysplasia, Hypothyroidism, Patellar luxation, Persistent pupillary membranes, Prognathism, Retinal dysplasia

Icelandic Sheepdog 🐕

Cataracts, Cryptorchidism, Deafness, Distichiasis, Elbow dysplasia, Entropion, Hip dysplasia, Patellar luxation, Persistent pupillary membranes, Retinal dysplasia

Irish Red and White Setter 🐕

Cataracts, Color dilution alopecia, Degenerative myelopathy, Distichiasis, Gastric dilation/volvulus, Globoid cell leukodystrophy, Hip dysplasia, Hypothyroidism, Iris cysts, Leukocyte adhesion deficiency type I, Neuronal ceroid lipofuscinosis 8, Pannus, Patellar luxation, Persistent pupillary membranes, Progressive retinal atrophy (rcd1), Progressive retinal atrophy (rcd4), Retinal dysplasia, von Willebrand disease type I

Irish Setter 🐕

Acral lick dermatitis, Amblyopia and quadriplegia, Atopic dermatitis, Brachygnathism, Cataracts, Cerebellar abiotrophy, Cerebellar hypoplasia, Cervical vertebral instability, Color dilution alopecia, Cutaneous asthenia, Degenerative myelopathy, Distichiasis, Ectropion, Elbow dysplasia, Entropion, Epilepsy, Factor VIII deficiency (hemophilia A), Gastric dilation/volvulus, Globoid cell leukodystrophy, Gluten-sensitive enteropathy, Hernia (umbilical), Hip dysplasia, Hypertrophic osteodystrophy, Hypochondroplastic dwarfism, Hypothyroidism, Ichthyosis, Immunoglobulin A (IgA) deficiency, Insulinoma, Laryngeal paralysis-polyneuropathy, Leukocyte adhesion deficiency type I, Lissencephaly, Lupoid onychopathy, Megaesophagus, Melanoma, Narcolepsy, Neuronal ceroid lipofuscinosis 8, Optic nerve hypoplasia and micropapilla, Osteochondritis dissecans (hock), Osteochondritis dissecans (shoulder), Osteochondrodysplasia, Osteosarcoma, Perianal fistulae, Persistent hyaloid artery, Persistent pupillary membranes, Persistent right aortic arch, Polydontia, Polydontia (retained primary teeth), Prognathism, Progressive retinal atrophy, Progressive retinal atrophy (central), Progressive retinal atrophy (rcd1), Progressive retinal atrophy (rcd4), Sebaceous adenitis, Seborrhea, Temporomandibular joint dysplasia, Tricuspid valve dysplasia, Urinary incontinence, von Willebrand disease type I

Irish Terrier 🐕

Cystinuria, Degenerative myelopathy, Familial nephropathy, Footpad hyperkeratosis, Hypothyroidism, Ichthyosis, Microphthalmia, Muscular dystrophy, Progressive retinal atrophy, Subaortic stenosis, Urolithiasis (cystine), Uveodermatologic syndrome

Irish Water Spaniel 🐕

Cataracts, Color dilution alopecia, Distichiasis, Elbow dysplasia, Entropion, Epilepsy, Factor VII deficiency, Follicular dysplasia, Hip dysplasia, Hypotrichosis, Persistent pupillary membranes, Progressive retinal atrophy

Irish Wolfhound 🐕

Atrial fibrillation, Cardiomyopathy (dilated), Cataracts, Cervical vertebral instability, Corneal dystrophy, Degenerative myelopathy, Distichiasis, Dystocia, Elbow dysplasia, Elbow dysplasia (ununited anconeal process), Elbow dysplasia (fragmented coronoid process), Entropion, Epilepsy, Everted cartilage of third eyelid, Fanconi syndrome, Gastric dilation/volvulus, Hip dysplasia, Hypothyroidism, Iris cysts, Irish wolfhound respiratory disorder, Lymphoproliferative disease (T-cell), Malignant hyperthermia, Optic nerve hypoplasia and micropapilla, Osteochondritis dissecans (shoulder), Osteochondritis dissecans (stifle), Osteosarcoma, Panosteitis, Patellar luxation, Portosystemic shunts, Progressive retinal atrophy, Retinal dysplasia, Rhinitis/bronchopneumonia, Startle disease, Urea cycle enzyme deficiencies, von Willebrand disease type I

Italian Greyhound 🐕

Amelogenesis imperfecta, Brachygnathism, Cataracts, Color dilution alopecia, Corneal dystrophy, Cryptorchidism, Deafness, Demodicosis, Epilepsy, Hemangioma/hemangiosarcoma, Hyperuricosuria, Hypothyroidism, Lens luxation, Patellar luxation, Persistent hyaloid artery, Persistent pupillary membranes, Piebaldism, Polydontia, Polydontia (retained primary teeth), Polyendocrinopathy (immune-mediated), Prognathism, Progressive retinal atrophy (IG-PRA1), Vitreous degeneration, von Willebrand disease

Jack Russell Terrier 🐕

Black hair follicular dysplasia, Brachygnathism, Cataracts, Cerebellar ataxia (Jack Russell), Chondrodystrophy, Choroidal hypoplasia (collie eye anomaly), Chronic inflammatory hepatic disease, Compulsive tail chasing, Deafness, Degenerative myelopathy, Demodicosis, Epilepsy, Factor IX deficiency (hemophilia B), Factor X deficiency, Glaucoma,

Hyperadrenocorticism, Hyperuricosuria, Ichthyosis, Intersex (gonadal), Juvenile encephalopathy, Late-onset ataxia, Legg–Calvé–Perthes disease, Lens luxation, Leukoencephalomyelopathy, Macrothrombocytopenia, Meningitis/arteritis, Mitochondrial myopathy, Myasthenia gravis, Neuroaxonal dystrophy, Oligodontia, Paroxysmal dyskinesia, Polyps, Portosystemic shunts, Prognathism, Progressive retinal atrophy (prcd), Pulmonary fibrosis, Sensory neuropathy, Severe combined immunodeficiency, Short tail, Spinocerebellar ataxia, Spinocerebellar ataxia (myokymia and neuromyotonia), Tail chasing, Urolithiasis (calcium oxalate), Urolithiasis (cystine), Vasculitis, Vitreous degeneration

Japanese Bobtail 🐈

Deafness, Heterochromia iridis, Neonatal isoerythrolysis, Taillessness, Transitional vertebrae

Japanese Chin (Japanese Spaniel) 🐕

Atlantoaxial instability, Cataracts, Distichiasis, Entropion, GM-2 gangliosidosis, GM-2 gangliosidosis type I, Hypothyroidism, Legg–Calvé–Perthes disease, Lens luxation, Mitral valve disease, Patellar luxation, Persistent hyaloid artery, Persistent hyperplastic tunica vasculosa lentis, Persistent pupillary membranes, Progressive retinal atrophy (prcd), Ulcerative keratitis, Vitreous degeneration

Japanese Domestic 🐈

GM-2 gangliosidosis

Japanese Spitz (Nihon Supittsu) 🐕

Factor VII deficiency, Muscular dystrophy, Patellar luxation, Progressive retinal atrophy (rcd4), Thrombopathia

Javanese 🐈

GM-1 gangliosidosis, Mucopolysaccharidosis VI, Progressive retinal atrophy (rdAc)

Kangal Shepherd Dog (Anatolian Shepherd Dog) 🐕

Angulation deformities, Ankyloglossia, Atopic dermatitis, Carpal laxity syndrome, Cryptorchidism, Degenerative myelopathy, Distichiasis, Elbow luxation, Entropion, Gastric dilation/volvulus, Hip dysplasia, Hypothyroidism, Malocclusion, Renal dysplasia, Retinal dysplasia, Short tail, Tail chasing

Karelian Bear Dog 🐕

Cataracts, Chondrodysplasia (ITGA), Hip dysplasia, Hypophosphatasia, Persistent primary vitreous, Pituitary dwarfism, Progressive retinal atrophy (prcd), Retinal dysplasia, Short tail

Keeshond (Wolfspitz) 🐕

Adrenal sex hormone imbalance, Alopecia X, Atopic dermatitis, Cataracts, Cutaneous asthenia, Degenerative myelopathy, Diabetes mellitus, Distichiasis, Elbow dysplasia, Epilepsy, Glaucoma, Growth hormone-responsive dermatosis, Hip dysplasia, Histiocytosis, Hyperparathyroidism, Hypothyroidism, Oligodontia, Optic nerve hypoplasia and micropapilla, Patellar luxation, Patent ductus arteriosus, Progressive retinal atrophy, Progressive retinal atrophy (central), Progressive retinal atrophy (prcd), Pulmonic stenosis, Renal dysplasia, Spontaneous chronic corneal epithelial defects, Tetralogy of Fallot, Ulcerative keratitis, Urolithiasis (calcium oxalate), Ventricular septal defect, von Willebrand disease type I

Kerry Blue Terrier 🐕

Cataracts, Cerebellar abiotrophy, Cerebellar ataxia, Degenerative myelopathy, Dermoid sinus, Distichiasis, Elbow dysplasia, Entropion, Factor XI deficiency, Footpad hyperkeratosis, Hip dysplasia, Hypothyroidism, Intersex (gonadal), Keratoconjunctivitis sicca, Neuronal degeneration, Oligodontia, Patellar luxation, Patent ductus arteriosus, Persistent pupillary membranes, Pilomatrixoma, Progressive retinal atrophy, Sebaceous gland hyperplasia/cysts, Spiculosis, Vitreous degeneration, von Willebrand disease type I

Komondor 🐕

Cataracts, Cobalamin malabsorption (cubilin), Degenerative myelopathy, Elbow dysplasia, Entropion, Gastric dilation/volvulus, Hip dysplasia, Hypothyroidism, Oligodontia, Patellar luxation, Persistent pupillary membranes, Polydontia, Polydontia (retained primary teeth), Prognathism

Koolie 🐕

Choroidal hypoplasia (collie eye anomaly), Cobalamin malabsorption (cubilin), Degenerative myelopathy, Epilepsy – phenobarbital resistant, Hyperuricosuria, Lens luxation, Merling, Multidrug resistance-1, Multifocal retinopathy (CMR1), Neuronal ceroid lipofuscinosis 5, Neuronal ceroid lipofuscinosis 12, Progressive retinal atrophy (prcd), Sensory neuropathy, Trapped neutrophil syndrome

Korat 🐈

GM-1 gangliosidosis, GM-2 gangliosidosis

Kromfohrländer 🐕

Cystinuria, Epilepsy, Footpad hyperkeratosis, Hyperuricosuria, Patellar luxation, von Willebrand disease type I

Kuvasz 🐕

Anesthetic sensitivity, Atopic dermatitis, Cataracts, Corneal dystrophy, Cruciate ligament disease, Deafness, Degenerative myelopathy, Dermatomyositis, Distichiasis, Elbow dysplasia, Gastric dilation/volvulus, Hip dysplasia, Hypertrophic osteodystrophy, Hypothyroidism, Lumbosacral disease, Osteochondritis dissecans (shoulder), Patellar luxation, Persistent pupillary membranes, Prognathism, Progressive retinal atrophy (prcd), Vitreous degeneration, von Willebrand disease

Labrador Retriever 🐕

Accessory pathway arrhythmia, Achromatopsia, Acral lick dermatitis, Alexander disease, Atopic dermatitis, Atrioventricular heart block, Blaschko's lines disorders, Calcinosis circumscripta, Cataracts, Central axonopathy, Centronuclear myopathy, Cerebellar abiotrophy, Cervical vertebral instability, Chronic inflammatory hepatic disease, Cleft lip/palate, Color dilution alopecia, Copper hepatopathy, Corneal dystrophy, Corneal dystrophy (macular), Cruciate ligament disease, Cutaneous asthenia, Cystinuria, Deafness, Degenerative myelopathy, Diabetes mellitus, Diskospondylitis, Distichiasis, Ectodermal dysplasia (x-linked), Ectopic ureters, Ectropion, Elbow dysplasia, Elbow dysplasia (ununited anconeal process), Elbow dysplasia (fragmented coronoid process), Elliptocytosis, Endocardial fibroelastosis, Entropion, Epilepsy, Exercise-induced collapse, Facial dysmorphia, Factor VIII deficiency (hemophilia A), Factor IX deficiency (hemophilia B), Fanconi syndrome, Follicular dysplasia, Gastric dilation/volvulus, Hemangioma/hemangiosarcoma, Hereditary centronuclear myopathy, Hip dysplasia, Histiocytosis, Hypertension, Hypertrophic osteodystrophy, Hyperuricosuria, Hypothyroidism, Hypotrichosis, Ichthyosis, Immune-mediated hemolytic anemia, Immune-mediated polyarthritis, Iris cysts, Juvenile cellulitis, Laryngeal paralysis-polyneuropathy, Leukodystrophy (fibrinoid), Leukodystrophy (spongiform encephalopathy), Lumbosacral transitional vertebrae, Lymphedema, Lymphoma, Macrothrombocytopenia, Malignant hyperthermia, Mast cell tumor, Masticatory myositis, Megaesophagus, Melanoma (limbal), Menkes' syndrome, Microphthalmia, Mucinosis, Mucopolysaccharidosis II, Multidrug resistance-1, Muscular dystrophy (autosomal), Muscular dystrophy (x-linked), Musculotendinopathy, Myasthenia gravis, Myelodysplasia, Myoclonus, Myotonia congenita, Myotubular myopathy (x-linked), Narcolepsy, Nasal parakeratosis, Neuroaxonal dystrophy, Obesity (POMC), Ocular melanosis, Oculoskeletal dysplasia, Oligodontia, Optic nerve colobomas, Optic nerve hypoplasia and micropapilla, Organic aciduria (methylmalonic aciduria), Ossification of infraspinatus tendon-bursa, Osteochondritis dissecans (elbow), Osteochondritis dissecans (hock), Osteochondritis dissecans (shoulder), Osteochondritis dissecans (stifle), Osteochondrodysplasia, Osteosarcoma, Otitis externa, Panosteitis, Paroxysmal dyskinesia, Patellar luxation, Pemphigus foliaceus, Persistent pupillary membranes, Polydontia, Polydontia (supernumerary teeth), Progressive retinal atrophy (central), Progressive

Malassezia dermatitis, Patellar luxation, Persistent pupillary membranes, Prognathism, Progressive retinal atrophy (prcd), Vitreous degeneration, von Willebrand disease retinal atrophy (cord1), Progressive retinal atrophy (crd4), Progressive retinal atrophy (GR2), Progressive retinal atrophy (prcd), Protein-losing nephropathy, Pyruvate kinase deficiency, Recurrent flank alopecia, Retinal dysplasia, Sebaceous adenitis, Seborrhea, Skeletal dysplasia, Squamous cell carcinoma (digital/lingual), Stargardt disease, Tetralogy of Fallot, Thymoma, Tracheal hypoplasia, Tremor syndrome, Tricuspid valve dysplasia, Urolithiasis (cystine), Urolithiasis (silica), Uveal cysts, Vertebral stenosis, Vitamin A-responsive dermatosis, Vitiligo, Vitreous degeneration, von Willebrand disease

Lagotto Romagnolo

Cerebellar abiotrophy, Cerebellar ataxia (autophagy), Epilepsy, Hyperuricosuria, Lysosomal storage disease, Noise sensitivity, Progressive retinal atrophy (prcd)

Lakeland Terrier

Cataracts, Cryptorchidism, Degenerative myelopathy, Dermatomyositis, Glaucoma, Hypothyroidism, Legg–Calvé–Perthes disease, Lens luxation, Microphthalmia, Persistent pupillary membranes, Prognathism, von Willebrand disease

Lancashire Heeler

Chondrodysplasia, Choroidal hypoplasia (collie eye anomaly), Craniomandibular osteopathy, Degenerative myelopathy, Lens luxation, Progressive retinal atrophy (prcd)

Landseer

Cystinuria, Degenerative myelopathy, Muscular dystrophy, Signal transduction disorder, Thrombopathia, Urolithiasis (cystine)

LaPerm

Cardiomyopathy (hypertrophic), Deafness, Pyruvate kinase deficiency

Lapponian Herder

Choroidal hypoplasia (collie eye anomaly), Degenerative myelopathy, Glycogen storage disease II, Multifocal retinopathy (CMR3), Progressive retinal atrophy (prcd)

Leonberger

Albinism (Oculocutaneous), Anesthetic sensitivity, Cardiomyopathy (dilated), Cataracts, Cruciate ligament disease, Diffuse idiopathic skeletal hyperostosis, Distichiasis, Ectropion, Elbow dysplasia, Entropion, Everted cartilage of third cyclid, Familial aortic aneurysm, Gastric carcinoma, Gastric dilation/volvulus, Hernia (umbilical), Hip dysplasia, Hypoadrenocorticism, Hypothyroidism, Laryngeal paralysis-polyneuropathy, Leukoencephalomyelopathy, Osteochondritis dissecans, Osteosarcoma, Panosteitis, Pectinate ligament dysplasia, Perianal fistulae, Peripheral neuropathy (LPN1), Peripheral neuropathy (LPN2), Persistent pupillary membranes, Polyneuropathy (LPN1), Polyneuropathy (LPN2)

Lhasa Apso

Albinism (Oculocutaneous), Atopic dermatitis, Brachycephalic obstructive airway syndrome, Cataracts, Chondrodystrophy, Corneal dystrophy, Demodicosis, Distichiasis, Ectodermal defect, Entropion, Factor VIII deficiency (hemophilia A), Factor IX deficiency (hemophilia B), Glaucoma, Hip dysplasia, Hydrocephalus, Hypotrichosis, Intervertebral disk disease, Juvenile cellulitis, Keratoconjunctivitis sicca, Legg–Calvé–Perthes disease, Lissencephaly, Oligodontia, Pancreatitis, Patellar luxation, Persistent pupillary membranes, Portal vein hypoplasia, Portosystemic shunts, Progressive retinal atrophy (GR1), Progressive retinal atrophy (PRA4), Prolapsed gland of nictitans, Proptosis, Recurrent flank alopecia, Renal dysplasia, Retinal dysplasia, Sebaceous adenitis, Superficial necrolytic dermatitis, Ulcerative keratitis, Urolithiasis (calcium oxalate), Urolithiasis (magnesium ammonium phosphate, struvite), Urolithiasis (silica), Vertebral stenosis, von Willebrand disease

Lowchen

Cataracts, Distichiasis, Hip dysplasia, Pannus, Patellar luxation, Persistent pupillary membranes, Progressive retinal atrophy, Vitreous degeneration

Lucas Terrier

Degenerative myelopathy, Ichthyosis, Lens luxation, Patellar luxation

Lurcher

Dysmyelinogenesis, Gastric dilation/volvulus, Hypothyroidism, Osteosarcoma

Maine Coon

Cardiomyopathy (hypertrophic), Hernia (peritoneopericardial), Hip dysplasia, Intussusception, Middle ear polyps, Patellar luxation, Pemphigus foliaceus, Polycystic kidney disease, Polydactyly, Pyruvate kinase deficiency, Spinal muscular atrophy

Maltese

Atresia ani, Brachygnathism, Cataracts, Chondrodystrophy, Cryptorchidism, Deafness, Distichiasis, Dystocia, Glaucoma, Glycogen storage disease 1a, Hemorrhagic gastroenteritis, Hydrocephalus, Hypothyroidism, Immune-mediated hemolytic anemia, Ligneous membranitis, Macrothrombocytopenia, Mast cell tumor (gastrointestinal), Meningoencephalitis (necrotizing), Mitral valve disease, Oligodontia, Organic aciduria (methylmalonic aciduria), Patellar luxation, Patent ductus arteriosus, Persistent pupillary membranes, Polydontia, Polydontia (retained primary teeth), Portal vein hypoplasia, Portosystemic shunts, Prognathism, Progressive retinal atrophy, Protein-losing enteropathy, Pyloric stenosis, Retinal dysplasia, Sebaceous adenitis, Shaker syndrome, Syringomyelia, Urolithiasis (calcium oxalate), Ventricular septal defect, Wry mouth

Manchester Terrier

Cardiomyopathy (juvenile), Cataracts, Cryptorchidism, Cutaneous asthenia, Deafness, Demodicosis, Diabetes mellitus, Factor VIII deficiency (hemophilia A), Glaucoma, Hernia (umbilical), Hydrocephalus, Hypothyroidism, Legg–Calvé–Perthes disease, Oligodontia, Patellar luxation, Polydontia, Polydontia (retained primary teeth), Progressive retinal atrophy, Recurrent flank alopecia, Urolithiasis (xanthine), von Willebrand disease type I

Manx

Deafness, Fecal incontinence, Sacrocaudal dysgenesis, Spina bifida, Taillessness, Urolithiasis (magnesium ammonium phosphate)

Maremma Sheepdog

Degenerative myelopathy, Gastric dilation/volvulus, Hip dysplasia, Panosteitis, Retinal dysplasia

Markiesje (Dutch Tulip Hound)

Paroxysmal dyskinesia, Progressive retinal atrophy (prcd)

Mastiff (English Mastiff)

Atopic dermatitis, Atrial fibrillation, Cataracts, Caudal cervical spondylomyelopathy, Cerebellar abiotrophy, Corneal dystrophy, Cruciate ligament disease, Cystinuria, Degenerative myelopathy, Ectropion, Elbow dysplasia, Elbow dysplasia (ununited anconeal process), Elbow dysplasia (fragmented coronoid process), Entropion, Epilepsy, Gastric dilation/volvulus, Hip dysplasia, Hyperuricosuria, Hypothyroidism, Macroblepharon, Microphthalmia, Multifocal retinopathy (CMR1), Oligodendroglioma, Osteochondritis dissecans (shoulder), Osteochondritis dissecans (stifle), Osteosarcoma, Panosteitis, Patellar luxation, Persistent pupillary membranes, Prognathism, Progressive retinal atrophy (dominant), Progressive retinal atrophy (prcd), Pulmonic stenosis, Retinal dysplasia, Urolithiasis (cystine)

McNab Shepherd (McNab Dog)

Multidrug resistance-1, Lens luxation

Mi-Ki

Progressive retinal atrophy (prcd), Vitreous degeneration

Miniature American Shepherd

Achromatopsia, Cataracts, Choroidal hypoplasia (collie eye anomaly), Cobalamin malabsorption (amnionless), Color dilution alopecia, Cone degeneration, Degenerative myelopathy, Hyperuricosuria, Multidrug resistance-1, Multifocal retinopathy, Myotonia congenita, Neuronal ceroid lipofuscinosis 6, Progressive retinal atrophy (prcd), Short tail

Miniature Pinscher (Zwergpinscher)

Cataracts, Color dilution alopecia, Corneal dystrophy, Cystinuria, Deafness, Demodicosis, Diabetes mellitus, Eclampsia, Epilepsy, Glaucoma, Hemorrhagic gastroenteritis, Immune-mediated hemolytic anemia, Legg–Calvé–Perthes disease, Mitral valve disease, Mucopolysaccharidosis VI, Optic nerve hypoplasia and micropapilla, Pannus, Patellar luxation, Persistent pupillary membranes, Pituitary dwarfism, Portosystemic shunts, Progressive retinal atrophy, Sebaceous adenitis, Shaker syndrome, Urolithiasis (calcium oxalate), Urolithiasis (cystine), Vitreous degeneration

Mudi

Cataracts, Elbow dysplasia, Epilepsy, Hip dysplasia, Merling, Patellar luxation, Short tail

Munchkin

Chondrodysplasia, Heterochromia iridis, Lordosis, Pectus excavatum, Polycystic kidney disease, Progressive retinal atrophy (rdAc)

Münsterländer, Large (Large Münsterländer)

Black hair follicular dysplasia, Color dilution alopecia, Hip dysplasia, Hyperuricosuria, Osteochondritis dissecans (shoulder), Progressive retinal atrophy (rcd4), Urolithiasis (cystine)

Münsterländer, Small (Small Münsterländer)

Hyperuricosuria, Progressive retinal atrophy (rcd4)

Native American Indian Dog

Hip dysplasia, Hyperuricosuria

Neapolitan Mastiff

Cardiomyopathy (dilated), Cataracts, Cruciate ligament disease, Distichiasis, Ectropion, Elbow dysplasia, Entropion, Fold dermatitis, Gastric dilation/volvulus, Hip dysplasia, Hypothyroidism, Macroblepharon, Panosteitis, Patellar luxation, Prolapsed gland of nictitans

Nebelung

Insufficient information available

New Zealand Huntaway

Cardiomyopathy (dilated), Mucopolysaccharidosis IIIa, Neuronal ceroid lipofuscinosis 6

Newfoundland

Atopic dermatitis, Atrial fibrillation, Cardiomyopathy (dilated), Cataracts, Ciliary dyskinesia, Color dilution alopecia, Cruciate ligament disease, Cystinuria, Degenerative myelopathy, Ectopic ureters, Ectropion, Elbow dysplasia, Elbow dysplasia (ununited anconeal process), Elbow dysplasia (fragmented coronoid process), Entropion, Everted cartilage of third eyelid, Exocrine pancreatic insufficiency, Gastric dilation/volvulus, Glaucoma, Glomerulosclerosis/glomerulofibrosis, Hip dysplasia, Hypothyroidism, Inflammatory myopathy, Iris cysts, Laryngeal paralysis, Megaesophagus, Myasthenia gravis, Nasal arteritis, Osteochondritis dissecans (elbow), Osteochondritis dissecans (shoulder), Osteochondritis dissecans (stifle), Osteosarcoma, Panosteitis, Patellar luxation, Patent ductus arteriosus, Pemphigus foliaceus, Persistent pupillary membranes, Polymyositis, Prognathism, Prolapsed gland of nictitans, Retinal dysplasia, Skeletal dysplasia, Subaortic stenosis, Thrombopathia, Tricuspid valve dysplasia, Urolithiasis (cystine), Ventricular septal defect

Norfolk Terrier

Brachygnathism, Cataracts, Degenerative myelopathy, Glaucoma, Hip dysplasia, Ichthyosis, Lens luxation, Macrothrombocytopenia, Mitral valve disease, Muscular dystrophy, Optic nerve colobomas, Optic nerve hypoplasia and micropapilla, Patellar luxation, Persistent pupillary membranes, Portosystemic shunts, Prognathism, Progressive retinal atrophy, Retinal dysplasia, Urolithiasis (calcium oxalate), Vitreous degeneration

Norrbottenspets

Cerebellar ataxia (hound), Progressive retinal atrophy (prcd)

Norwegian Buhund

Cataracts, Cerebellar ataxia, Hip dysplasia, Noise sensitivity

Norwegian Elkhound

Atopic dermatitis, Brachygnathism, Cataracts, Chondrodysplasia (ITGA), Ciliary dyskinesia, Diabetes mellitus, Distichiasis, Entropion, Epilepsy, Familial nephropathy, Fanconi syndrome, Gastric carcinoma, Glaucoma (POAG), Hip dysplasia, Immunoglobulin A (IgA) deficiency, Inflammatory bowel disease, Intersex (gonadal), Intracutaneous cornifying epithelioma, Lens luxation (secondary), Mast cell tumor, Oligodontia, Osteochondrodysplasia, Osteogenesis imperfecta, Persistent pupillary membranes, Prognathism, Progressive retinal atrophy (erd), Progressive retinal atrophy (prcd), Progressive retinal atrophy (rod dysplasia), Renal dysplasia, Renal glucosuria, Retinal dysplasia, Tubulointerstitial nephropathy

Norwegian Forest Cat

Cardiomyopathy (hypertrophic), Deafness, Diabetes mellitus, Glycogen storage disease type IV, Neonatal isoerythrolysis, Pyruvate kinase deficiency

Norwegian Lundehund

Atrophic gastritis, Follicular dysplasia, Gastric carcinoma, Lundehund syndrome, Lymphangiectasia, Patellar luxation, Polydactyly, Protein-losing enteropathy, Small intestinal bacterial overgrowth

Norwich Terrier

Atopic dermatitis, Brachycephalic obstructive airway syndrome, Brachygnathism, Cataracts, Chondrodysplasia, Corneal dystrophy, Cystic renal dysplasia/hepatic fibrosis, Deafness, Degenerative myelopathy, Elongated soft palate, Epilepsy, Epileptoid cramping syndrome, Glaucoma, Hip dysplasia, Lens luxation, Macrothrombocytopenia, Oligodontia, Paroxysmal dyskinesia, Patellar luxation, Persistent pupillary membranes, Portosystemic shunts, Prognathism, Renal dysplasia/hepatic fibrosis, Tracheal collapse, Upper airway syndrome, Vitreous degeneration

Nova Scotia Duck Tolling Retriever

Cataracts, Chondrodystrophy, Choroidal hypoplasia (collie eye anomaly), Cleft palate, Cleft palate and syndactyly, Color dilution alopecia, Corneal dystrophy, Cryptorchidism, Deafness, Degenerative encephalopathy, Degenerative myelopathy, Distichiasis, Elbow dysplasia, Epilepsy, Familial nephropathy (x-linked), Gastric carcinoma, Hernia (umbilical), Hip dysplasia, Hypoadrenocorticism, Hypothyroidism, Immune-mediated rheumatic disease, Immunoglobulin A (IgA) deficiency, Lupus erythematosus (SLE), Lymphoma, Meningitis (aseptic), Meningitis/arteritis, Optic nerve hypoplasia and micropapilla, Patellar luxation, Persistent pupillary membranes, Progressive retinal atrophy (prcd), Pulmonic stenosis, Skeletal dysplasia

Ocicat

Progressive retinal atrophy (rdAc), Progressive retinal atrophy (Rdy), Pyruvate kinase deficiency, Urolithiasis (urate)

Ojos Azules

Cranial deformities

Old English Sheepdog

Atopic dermatitis, Atrial fibrillation, Atrial septal defect, Brachygnathism, Cardiomyopathy, Cataracts, Cerebellar abiotrophy, Cerebellar ataxia (autophagy), Cervical vertebral instability, Ciliary dyskinesia, Cryptorchidism, Deafness, Degenerative myelopathy, Demodicosis, Diabetes mellitus, Distichiasis, Elbow dysplasia, Entropion, Exercise-induced collapse, Factor VIII deficiency (hemophilia A), Factor IX deficiency (hemophilia B), Gastric dilation/volvulus, Hernia (perineal), Hip dysplasia, Hypothyroidism, Immune-mediated hemolytic anemia, Immune-mediated thrombocytopenia, Lymphedema, Lymphoma, Macroblepharon, Merling, Microphthalmia, Mitochondrial myopathy, Multidrug resistance-1, Muscular dystrophy, Optic nerve hypoplasia and micropapilla, Osteochondritis dissecans (shoulder), Osteosarcoma, Patellar luxation, Persistent pupillary membranes, Portosystemic shunts, Prognathism, Progressive retinal atrophy, Retinal dysplasia, Sebaceous adenitis, Tricuspid valve dysplasia, Urolithiasis (silica), Uveodermatologic syndrome, von Willebrand disease

Oriental Longhair
Insufficient information available

Oriental Shorthair
Amyloidosis, Deafness, GM-1 gangliosidosis, Lymphosarcoma, Mucopolysaccharidosis VI, Progressive retinal atrophy (rdAc), Urolithiasis (magnesium ammonium phosphate)

Otterhound
Atopic dermatitis, Brachygnathism, Cataracts, Epilepsy, Factor II (prothrombin) deficiency, Gastric dilation/volvulus, Glanzmann thrombasthenia, Hip dysplasia, Prognathism, Sebaceous cysts, Thrombasthenic thrombopathia

Papillon (Phalene)
Black hair follicular dysplasia, Cataracts, Cleft palate, Cryptorchidism, Deafness, Distichiasis, Epilepsy, Factor VII deficiency, Hydrocephalus, Intervertebral disk disease, Meningoencephalitis (necrotizing), Mitral valve disease, Neuroaxonal dystrophy, Patellar luxation, Persistent pupillary membranes, Polydontia, Polydontia (retained primary teeth), Portosystemic shunts, Progressive retinal atrophy (crd4), Progressive retinal atrophy (PAP1), Syringomyelia, Urolithiasis (calcium oxalate), Vitreous degeneration, von Willebrand disease type I

Parson Russell Terrier
Amelogenesis imperfecta, Cataracts, Cerebellar ataxia (Jack Russell), Choroidal hypoplasia (collie eye anomaly), Craniomandibular osteopathy, Deafness, Degenerative myelopathy, Distichiasis, Elbow dysplasia, Epilepsy, Exercise-induced collapse, Glaucoma, Hip dysplasia, Hyperuricosuria, Ichthyosis, Immune-mediated hemolytic anemia, Intersex (gonadal), Juvenile encephalopathy, Late-onset ataxia, Legg–Calvé–Perthes disease, Lens luxation, Macrothrombocytopenia, Mast cell tumor, Mitochondrial myopathy, Myasthenia gravis, Neuroaxonal dystrophy, Patellar luxation, Persistent pupillary membranes, Portosystemic shunts, Progressive retinal atrophy (prcd), Pulmonic stenosis, Severe combined immunodeficiency, Short tail, Spinocerebellar ataxia, Spinocerebellar ataxia (myokymia and neuromyotonia)

Patterdale Terrier
Cruciate ligament disease, Degenerative myelopathy, Hip dysplasia, Hypothyroidism, Intervertebral disk disease, Lens luxation

Pekingese
Albinism (oculocutaneous), Atlantoaxial instability, Brachycephalic obstructive airway syndrome, Cataracts, Chondrodysplasia, Chondrodystrophy, Cleft lip/palate, Cryptorchidism, Distichiasis, Dystocia, Entropion, Fold dermatitis, Glaucoma, Hemivertebra, Hernia (perineal), Hip dysplasia, Hydrocephalus, Intersex (gonadal), Intervertebral disk disease, Intervertebral disk extrusion, Keratoconjunctivitis sicca, Malocclusion, Meningoencephalitis (necrotizing), Mitral valve disease, Pannus, Patellar luxation, Portosystemic shunts, Prognathism, Progressive retinal atrophy, Proptosis, Sertoli cell tumor, Tracheal collapse, Ulcerative keratitis, Urolithiasis, Urolithiasis (apatite), Urolithiasis (silica), Urolithiasis (urate), Wry mouth

Perro de Presa Canario
Cryptorchidism, Demodectic mange, Epilepsy, Multifocal retinopathy (CMR1), Osteochondrodysplasia, Patellar luxation

Persian
Acne, Brachycephalic airway obstructive syndrome, Cardiomyopathy (hypertrophic), Cerebellar degeneration, Chediak–Higashi syndrome, Corneal sequestrum, Cryptorchidism, Deafness, Dental anomalies, Dermatophytosis susceptibility, Entropion, Facial dermatitis, Feline hyperesthesia syndrome, Feline infectious peritonitis (FIP) susceptibility, Feline leukemia virus susceptibility, Feline lower urinary tract disease (FLUTD), Hernia (peritoneopericardial), Heterochromia iridis, Hip dysplasia, Intervertebral disk disease, Mannosidosis (alpha), Neonatal isoerythrolysis, Patent ductus arteriosus, Pemphigus foliaceus, Polycystic kidney disease, Polycystic liver disease, Portosystemic shunts, Progressive retinal atrophy (PRA-pd), Pulmonary carcinoma, Pyruvate kinase deficiency, Strabismus, Ulcerative keratitis, Urolithiasis (calcium oxalate)

Peruvian Inca Orchid (Peruvian Hairless Dog)
Degenerative myelopathy, Epilepsy, Hairlessness, Inflammatory bowel disease

Peterbald
GM-1 gangliosidosis, Mucopolysaccharidosis VI, Progressive retinal atrophy (rdAc)

Petit Basset Griffon Vendeen
Atopic dermatitis, Cataracts, Chondrodysplasia, Elbow dysplasia, Epilepsy, Glaucoma (POAG), Hip dysplasia, Hypothyroidism, Lens luxation, Mast cell tumor, Meningitis/arteritis, Patellar luxation, Persistent pupillary membranes, Retinal dysplasia, Vitreous degeneration

Pharaoh Hound
Atopic dermatitis, Degenerative myelopathy, Demodicosis, Elbow dysplasia, Epilepsy, Gastric dilation/volvulus, Hip dysplasia, Patellar luxation

Pixie-Bob 🐾
Pancreatitis, Taillessness

Plott Hound 🐕
Degenerative myelopathy, Gastric dilation/volvulus, Hip dysplasia, Hyperuricosuria, Mucopolysaccharidosis I, Progressive retinal atrophy (prcd)

Pointer (English Pointer) 🐕
Acral mutilation syndrome, Black hair follicular dysplasia, Cataracts, Cerebellar ataxia (x-linked), Chondrodysplasia (dwarfism), Ciliary dyskinesia, Cleft lip/palate, Corneal dystrophy, Deafness, Degenerative myelopathy, Demodicosis, Elbow dysplasia, Elbow dysplasia (ununited anconeal process), Entropion, Hemangiosarcoma, Hip dysplasia, Hypothyroidism, Juvenile cellulitis, Malignant hyperthermia, Mast cell tumor, Osteochondritis dissecans (shoulder), Pannus, Prognathism, Progressive retinal atrophy, Progressive retinal atrophy (central), Retinal dysplasia, Sensory neuropathy, Spinal muscular atrophy, von Willebrand disease, von Willebrand disease type II

Polish Lowland Sheepdog (Owczarek Nizinny) 🐕
Atrioventricular heart block, Cataracts, Corneal dystrophy, Hip dysplasia, Hypothyroidism, Neuronal ceroid lipofuscinosis, Patent ductus arteriosus, Persistent pupillary membranes, Progressive retinal atrophy (central), Progressive retinal atrophy (rcd4), Short tail

Pomeranian 🐕
Adrenal sex hormone imbalance, Albinism (oculocutaneous), Alopecia X, Atlantoaxial instability, Cataracts, Cryptorchidism, Cyclic hematopoiesis, Deafness, Degenerative myelopathy, Demodicosis, Distichiasis, Eclampsia, Elbow dysplasia, Elbow dysplasia (ununited anconeal process), Entropion, Gallbladder mucocele, Globoid cell leukodystrophy, Growth hormone-responsive dermatosis, Hydrocephalus, Hyperuricosuria, Hypoadrenocorticism, Hypothyroidism, Intervertebral disk disease, Meningoencephalitis (necrotizing), Merling, Methemoglobin reductase deficiency, Mitral valve disease, Oligodontia, Panniculitis, Patellar luxation, Patent ductus arteriosus, Persistent pupillary membranes, Portosystemic shunts, Prognathism, Progressive retinal atrophy (prcd), Progressive retinal atrophy (rcd3), Rickets, Sebaceous adenitis, Stomatocytosis, Tracheal collapse, Urolithiasis (calcium oxalate), Vitreous degeneration, von Willebrand disease type I

Poodle, Miniature (Miniature Poodle) 🐕
Achromatopsia, Adrenal sex hormone imbalance, Anterior cross-bite, Atlantoaxial instability, Atopic dermatitis, Atresia ani, Atrial septal defect, Base-narrow canines, Bronchiectasis, Cataracts, Cerebellar abiotrophy, Chondrodystrophy, Cleft lip/palate, Corneal dystrophy, Cruciate ligament disease, Cryptorchidism, Deafness, Degenerative myelopathy, Diabetes mellitus, Distichiasis, Eclampsia, Ectodermal defect, Ectopic ureters, Elbow dysplasia, Entropion, Epilepsy, Epilepsy (Lafora body disease), Factor VIII deficiency (hemophilia A), Factor XII deficiency, Gallbladder mucocele, Glaucoma, Globoid cell leukodystrophy, GM-2 gangliosidosis, Growth hormone-responsive dermatosis, Hernia (perineal), Hip dysplasia, Hydrocephalus, Hyperadrenocorticism, Hypoadrenocorticism, Hypothyroidism, Hypotrichosis, Intersex (gonadal), Intervertebral disk disease, Keratoconjunctivitis sicca, Legg–Calvé–Perthes disease, Lens luxation, Leukodystrophy, Leukodystrophy (fibrinoid), Leukoencephalomyelopathy, Lupus erythematosus (SLE), Lymphedema, Macrocytosis/dyshematopoiesis, Macrothrombocytopenia, Malassezia dermatitis, Malocclusion, Methemoglobin reductase deficiency, Microphthalmia, Mitral valve disease, Mucopolysaccharidosis VI, Narcolepsy, Neonatal encephalopathy with seizures, Neuronal ceroid lipofuscinosis, Niemann–Pick disease, Nonspherocytic hemolytic anemia, Oligodontia, Optic nerve hypoplasia and micropapilla, Osteochondritis dissecans (shoulder), Osteochondrodysplasia, Osteogenesis imperfecta, Otitis externa, Pancreatitis, Panniculitis, Patellar luxation, Patent ductus arteriosus, Persistent pupillary membranes, Portal vein hypoplasia, Portosystemic shunts, Prekallikrein deficiency, Progressive retinal atrophy (prcd), Progressive retinal atrophy (rcd4), Prolapsed gland of nictitans, Proliferative episcleritis, Renal dysplasia, Retinal dysplasia, Sebaceous adenitis, Shaker syndrome, Sialocele, Squamous cell carcinoma (digital), Tracheal collapse, Urolithiasis (calcium oxalate), Urolithiasis (magnesium ammonium phosphate, struvite), Vasculitis, Vitreous degeneration, von Willebrand disease type I, von Willebrand disease type II, Wry mouth

Poodle, Moyen/Medium (Moyen Poodle, Medium Poodle) 🐕
Degenerative myelopathy, GM-2 gangliosidosis, Macrothrombocytopenia, Mucopolysaccharidosis VI, Neonatal encephalopathy with seizures, Progressive retinal atrophy (prcd), Progressive retinal atrophy (rcd4), von Willebrand disease type II

Poodle, Standard (Standard Poodle) 🐕
Achromatopsia, Brachygnathism, Cardiomyopathy (dilated), Cataracts, Color dilution alopecia, Cryptorchidism, Day blindness/retinal degeneration, Degenerative myelopathy, Ectodermal dysplasia (x-linked), Epilepsy, Epilepsy (Lafora body disease), Factor XII deficiency, Gastric carcinoma, Gastric dilation/volvulus, Glaucoma, GM-2 gangliosidosis, Hypoadrenocorticism, Ichthyosis, Macrothrombocytopenia, Microphthalmia, Mucopolysaccharidosis VI, Neonatal encephalopathy with seizures, Oligodontia, Optic nerve hypoplasia and micropapilla, Organic aciduria,

Osteochondritis dissecans (shoulder), Osteochondritis dissecans (stifle), Patellar luxation, Persistent pupillary membranes, Polymicrogyria, Portosystemic shunts, Prognathism, Progressive retinal atrophy (prcd), Progressive retinal atrophy (rcd4), Renal dysplasia, Retinal dysplasia, Sebaceous adenitis, Seborrhea, Squamous cell carcinoma (toes), Stationary night blindness, von Willebrand disease type I, von Willebrand disease type II, Wry mouth

Poodle, Toy (Toy Poodle) 🐕

Atlantoaxial instability, Cataracts, Chondrodystrophy, Cleft lip/palate, Corneal dystrophy, Cryptorchidism, Deafness, Degenerative myelopathy, Diabetes mellitus, Distichiasis, Ectopic ureters, Epilepsy, Glaucoma, GM-2 gangliosidosis, Growth hormone-responsive dermatosis, Hydrocephalus, Hypoparathyroidism, Intervertebral disk disease, Legg–Calvé–Perthes disease, Lens luxation, Macrothrombocytopenia, Microphthalmia, Mitral valve disease, Mucopolysaccharidosis VI, Myopia, Neonatal encephalopathy with seizures, Optic nerve hypoplasia and micropapilla, Patellar luxation, Patent ductus arteriosus, Portal vein hypoplasia, Portosystemic shunts, Progressive retinal atrophy (prcd), Progressive retinal atrophy (rcd4), Retinal dysplasia, Sebaceous adenitis, Tetralogy of Fallot, Urolithiasis (calcium oxalate), Vertebral stenosis, von Willebrand disease type I, von Willebrand disease type II

Portuguese Podengo 🐕

Cerebellar degeneration, Degenerative myelopathy, Demodicosis, Elbow dysplasia, Hip dysplasia, Patellar luxation, Progressive retinal atrophy (prcd)

Portuguese Podengo Pequeno 🐕

Degenerative myelopathy, Progressive retinal atrophy (crd4), Progressive retinal atrophy (prcd)

Portuguese Water Dog 🐕

Atopic dermatitis, Cardiomyopathy (juvenile), Cataracts, Chondrodystrophy, Cleft palate, Color dilution alopecia, Cryptorchidism, Dermatomyositis, Distichiasis, Elbow dysplasia, Epilepsy, Follicular dysplasia, GM-1 gangliosidosis, Hemangiosarcoma, Hernia (umbilical), Hip dysplasia, Hypoadrenocorticism, Improper coat, Inflammatory bowel disease, Keratoconjunctivitis sicca, Microphthalmia, Patellar luxation, Persistent pupillary membranes, Progressive retinal atrophy (prcd), Renal dysplasia

Pudelpointer 🐕

Epilepsy, Hip dysplasia

Pug 🐕

Acne, Arachnoid cyst, Atopic dermatitis, Brachycephalic obstructive airway syndrome, Brachygnathism, Cataracts, Cleft palate, Corneal pigmentation, Degenerative myelopathy, Demodicosis, Dentigerous cysts, Diabetes mellitus,

Distichiasis, Ectopic cilia, Elbow dysplasia, Entropion, Fold dermatitis, Hemivertebra, Hip dysplasia, Hydrocephalus, Hydrops fetalis, Hypothyroidism, Intersex (gonadal), Intervertebral disk disease, Iris hypoplasia, Keratoconjunctivitis sicca, Legg–Calvé–Perthes disease, Lens luxation, Lentigo, Lung lobe torsion, Macroblepharon, Mast cell tumor, May–Hegglin anomaly, Meningoencephalitis (necrotizing), Optic nerve hypoplasia and micropapilla, Pannus, Patellar luxation, Persistent pupillary membranes, Portosystemic shunts, Progressive retinal atrophy, Proptosis, Pyruvate kinase deficiency, Sacrocaudal dysgenesis, Spina bifida, Squamous–cell carcinoma (corneal), Sudden acquired retinal degeneration, Syringomyelia, Thoracic vertebral malformations, Tracheal collapse, Ulcerative keratitis, Urolithiasis, Vitreous degeneration, von Willebrand disease type I

Puli 🐕

Bardet–Biedl syndrome, Cataracts, Corneal dystrophy, Deafness, Degenerative myelopathy, Diabetes mellitus, Elbow dysplasia, Hip dysplasia, Lens luxation, Optic nerve hypoplasia and micropapilla, Patellar luxation, Persistent hyaloid artery, Persistent pupillary membranes, Progressive retinal atrophy (Bardet–Biedl), Progressive retinal atrophy (prcd), Retinal dysplasia, von Willebrand disease type I

Pumi 🐕

Degenerative myelopathy, Hip dysplasia, Lens luxation

Pyrenean Shepherd (Berger des Pyrénées) 🐕

Cataracts, Choroidal hypoplasia (collie eye anomaly), Cleft lip/palate, Elbow dysplasia, Epilepsy, Hip dysplasia, Lens luxation, Merling, Patellar luxation, Patent ductus arteriosus, Persistent pupillary membranes, Progressive retinal atrophy, Short tail

Ragdoll 🐈

Arterial thromboembolism, Cardiomyopathy (hypertrophic), Deafness, Feline gastrointestinal eosinophilic sclerosing fibroplasia, Feline infectious peritonitis (FIP) susceptibility, Mast cell tumor, Mucopolysaccharidosis VI, Polycystic kidney disease, Progressive retinal atrophy (PRA-pd), Urolithiasis (calcium oxalate), Urolithiasis (magnesium ammonium phosphate), Urolithiasis (urate)

Rat Terrier 🐕

Deafness, Degenerative myelopathy, Demodicosis, Hypothyroidism (congenital) with goiter, Lens luxation, Patellar luxation, Progressive retinal atrophy (prcd)

Redbone Coonhound 🐕

Glaucoma, Hip dysplasia, Hypothyroidism, Pelger–Huet anomaly, Polyradiculoneuritis, Progressive retinal atrophy (central)

Rhodesian Ridgeback

Arrythmia (familial), Atopic dermatitis, Cataracts, Cerebellar abiotrophy, Cervical vertebral instability, Color dilution alopecia, Deafness, Degenerative myelopathy, Dermoid sinus, Distichiasis, Dystocia, Elbow dysplasia, Entropion, Epilepsy – myoclonic, Exercise-induced collapse, Factor IX deficiency (hemophilia B), Glaucoma (secondary), Hip dysplasia, Hypothyroidism, Laryngeal paralysis-polyneuropathy, Lumbosacral transitional vertebrae, Mast cell tumor, Myotonia congenita, Osteochondritis dissecans (shoulder), Osteosarcoma, Panosteitis, Patellar luxation, Persistent pupillary membranes, Ridgelessness

Rottweiler

Acne, Albinism (oculocutaneous), Atopic dermatitis, Atrial fibrillation, Atrophic membranous glomerulopathy, Avulsion of tibial tuberosity, Blaschko's lines disorders, Brachygnathism, Calcinosis circumscripta, Cataracts, Cervical vertebral instability, Ciliary dyskinesia, Corneal dystrophy, Cruciate ligament disease, Cryptorchidism, Deafness, Degenerative myelopathy, Demodicosis, Dermatomyositis, Diabetes mellitus, Diskospondylitis, Elbow dysplasia, Elbow dysplasia (incomplete ossification of humeral condyle), Elbow dysplasia (ununited anconeal process), Elbow dysplasia (fragmented coronoid process), Entropion, Epilepsy, Familial nephropathy, Fibroma/fibrosarcoma, Follicular dysplasia (lipidosis), Footpad hyperkeratosis, Gastric dilation/volvulus, Gastroduodenal perforation, Hemivertebra, Hernia (umbilical), Hip dysplasia, Histiocytosis, Hyperlipidemia (hypercholesterolemia), Hypertrophic osteodystrophy, Hyperuricosuria, Hypoadrenocorticism, Hypothyroidism, Ichthyosis, Immunodeficiency syndrome, Immunoglobulin A (IgA) deficiency, Inflammatory bowel disease, Intervertebral disk disease, Laryngeal paralysis, Laryngeal paralysis-polyneuropathy, Leishmania susceptibility, Leukodystrophy, Leukoencephalomyelopathy, Lupus erythematosus (discoid), Lymphangiectasia, Lymphedema, Lymphoma, Macroblepharon, Mast cell tumor, Melanoma, Microphthalmia, Multidrug resistance 1, Muscular dystrophy, Myelodysplasia, Myopia, Myositis ossificans, Myotubular myopathy (x-linked), Narcolepsy, Neuroaxonal dystrophy, Oligodontia, Osteochondritis dissecans (elbow), Osteochondritis dissecans (hock), Osteochondritis dissecans (shoulder), Osteochondritis dissecans (stifle), Osteosarcoma, Panosteitis, Parvovirus susceptibility, Patellar luxation, Patent ductus arteriosus, Peripheral neuropathy (Rottweiler), Peripheral neuropathy (Warburg), Persistent pupillary membranes, Polydontia, Polyneuropathy, Prognathism, Progressive retinal atrophy, Recurrent flank alopecia, Retinal dysplasia, Seborrhea, Spinal dysraphism, Spinal muscular atrophy, Spinal subarachnoid cysts, Squamous cell carcinoma (toes), Subaortic stenosis, Tibial valgus deformity, Ulcerative keratitis, Urolithiasis (cystine), Vasculitis, Vitiligo, von Willebrand disease type I, Wry mouth

Russian Blue

Diabetes mellitus, Mast cell tumor, Polycystic kidney disease, Progressive retinal atrophy (PRA-pd), Pyruvate kinase deficiency

Ryukyu Inu

Choroidal hypoplasia (collie eye anomaly), Elbow dysplasia, Glaucoma, Hip dysplasia, Hypothyroidism, Multidrug resistance-1, Patellar luxation

Saarloos Wolf Dog

Degenerative myelopathy, Hip dysplasia, Pituitary dwarfism

Saint Bernard

Cardiomyopathy (dilated), Cataracts, Cerebellar cortex dysplasia, Corneal dystrophy, Cruciate ligament disease, Cutaneous asthenia, Deafness, Degenerative myelopathy, Dermoid, Dermoid sinus, Distichiasis, Ectropion, Elbow dysplasia, Elbow dysplasia (ununited anconeal process), Elbow dysplasia (fragmented coronoid process), Entropion, Epilepsy, Factor I (fibrinogen) deficiency, Factor IX deficiency (hemophilia B), Fibrocartilaginous embolic myelopathy, Gastric dilation/volvulus, Hemangiosarcoma, Hip dysplasia, Hypoadrenocorticism, Hypoparathyroidism, Hypothyroidism, Laryngeal paralysis, Lymphoma, Malignant hyperthermia, Microphthalmia, Narcolepsy, Nasal arteritis, Optic nerve hypoplasia and micropapilla, Osteochondritis dissecans (shoulder), Osteochondritis dissecans (stifle), Osteosarcoma, Panosteitis, Patellar luxation, Peripheral neuropathy (LPN1), Persistent pupillary membranes, Polydactyly, Polyneuropathy (LPN1), Polyneuropathy (LPN2), Prolapsed gland of nictitans, Retinal dysplasia, Sebaceous adenitis

Saluki

Black hair follicular dysplasia, Brachygnathism, Cardiomyopathy (dilated), Cataracts, Cerebellar abiotrophy, Color dilution alopecia, Degenerative myelopathy, Glaucoma, Hemangiosarcoma (cardiac), Hip dysplasia, Hypothyroidism, Immune-mediated hemolytic anemia, Mitral valve disease, Neuronal ceroid lipofuscinosis, Persistent pupillary membranes, Prognathism, Progressive retinal atrophy, Spinal muscular atrophy, Tricuspid valve dysplasia, Vitreous degeneration

Samoyed

Adrenal sex hormone imbalance, Alopecia X, Alport syndrome (hereditary nephritis), Amelogenesis imperfecta,

Atrial septal defect, Cataracts, Cerebellar abiotrophy, Chronic inflammatory hepatic disease, Corneal dystrophy, Degenerative myelopathy, Diabetes mellitus, Distichiasis, Dysmyelinogenesis, Elbow dysplasia, Factor VIII deficiency (hemophilia A), Familial nephropathy, Familial nephropathy (x-linked), Gastric dilation/volvulus, Glaucoma, Growth hormone-responsive dermatosis, Hereditary nephritis (x-linked), Hip dysplasia, Hypothyroidism, Leukodystrophy (spongiform encephalopathy), Microphthalmia, Muscular dystrophy, Myasthenia gravis, Myelodysplasia, Myotonia congenita, Oculoskeletal dysplasia, Osteochondritis dissecans (shoulder), Osteochondritis dissecans (stifle), Osteochondrodysplasia, Patellar luxation, Pelger–Huet anomaly, Persistent pupillary membranes, Portosystemic shunts, Progressive retinal atrophy (XLPRA1), Pulmonic stenosis, Renal dysplasia, Retinal dysplasia, Sebaceous adenitis, Shaker syndrome, Spina bifida, Squamous cell carcinoma (lingual), Subaortic stenosis, Tremor syndrome, Ulcerative keratitis, Urolithiasis (calcium oxalate), Urolithiasis (silica), Uveodermatologic syndrome, Ventricular septal defect, von Willebrand disease, Zinc-responsive dermatosis

Savannah

Deafness, Cardiomyopathy (hypertrophic), Progressive retinal atrophy (PRA-b), Pyruvate kinase deficiency

Schapendoes

Elbow dysplasia, Hip dysplasia, Hyperuricosuria, Progressive retinal atrophy, Progressive retinal atrophy (PRA-DS)

Schipperke

Black hair follicular dysplasia, Cataracts, Color dilution alopecia, Demodicosis, Diabetes mellitus, Distichiasis, Dystocia, Elbow dysplasia, Epilepsy, Galactosialidosis, Hip dysplasia, Hypothyroidism, Legg–Calvé–Perthes disease, Mucopolysaccharidosis IIIb, Pancreatitis, Patellar luxation, Pemphigus foliaceus, Persistent pupillary membranes, Prognathism, Progressive retinal atrophy (prcd), Retinal dysplasia, Short tail, Tracheal collapse, Vitreous degeneration, von Willebrand disease type I

Schnauzer, Giant (Giant Schnauzer)

Brachygnathism, Cardiomyopathy (dilated), Cataracts, Cobalamin malabsorption (amnionless), Cruciate ligament disease, Deafness, Degenerative myelopathy, Elbow dysplasia, Epilepsy, Factor VII deficiency, Gastric dilation/volvulus, Glaucoma, Hemangioma, Hip dysplasia, Hyperuricosuria, Hypothyroid dwarfism, Hypothyroidism, Lupoid onychopathy, Narcolepsy, Nasal arteritis, Neuroaxonal dystrophy, Osteochondritis dissecans (stifle), Osteosarcoma, Panosteitis, Patellar luxation, Persistent pupillary membranes, Prognathism, Progressive retinal atrophy (NECAP1), Progressive

retinal atrophy (prcd), Retinal dysplasia, Squamous cell carcinoma (digital), Urinary incontinence

Schnauzer, Miniature (Miniature Schnauzer)

Acquired aurotrichia, Anterior cross-bite, Atherosclerosis, Atopic dermatitis, Avian tuberculosis susceptibility, Base-narrow canines, Brachygnathism, Cataracts, Charcot–Marie–Tooth disease, Cleft lip/palate, Color dilution alopecia, Cryptorchidism, Cutaneous asthenia, Deafness, Degenerative myelopathy, Diabetes mellitus, Distichiasis, Dystocia, Epilepsy, Factor VII deficiency, Factor VIII deficiency (hemophilia A), Familial nephropathy, Fanconi syndrome, Fibrocartilaginous embolic myelopathy, Gallbladder mucocele, Glaucoma, Histiocytic sarcoma, Histiocytosis, Hyperadrenocorticism, Hyperlipidemia (hypertriglyceridemia), Hypoparathyroidism, Hypothyroidism, Immune-mediated hemolytic anemia, Immunoglobulin A (IgA) deficiency, Intersex (gonadal), Intervertebral disk disease, Keratoconjunctivitis sicca, Lentigo, Leukoencephalomyelopathy, Malocclusion, Megaesophagus, Melanoma (cutaneous), Meningioma, Microphthalmia, Mitral valve disease, Mucopolysaccharidosis VI, Muscular dystrophy, Mycobacterial susceptibility, Myopia, Myotonia congenita, Neuronal ceroid lipofuscinosis, Odontogenic parakeratinized cyst, Optic nerve hypoplasia and micropapilla, Osteochondritis dissecans (stifle), Pancreatitis, Patent ductus arteriosus, Persistent hyperplastic primary vitreous, Persistent Mullerian duct syndrome, Persistent pupillary membranes, Photoreceptor dysplasia, Portosystemic shunts, Prognathism, Progressive retinal atrophy (A), Progressive retinal atrophy (B), Progressive retinal atrophy (photoreceptor dysplasia), Progressive retinal atrophy (XLPRA2), Pulmonic stenosis, Recurrent flank alopecia, Renal dysplasia, Retinal dysplasia, Schnauzer comedo syndrome, Sick sinus syndrome, Spondylocostal dysostosis, Stomatocytosis, Sudden acquired retinal degeneration, Superficial necrolytic dermatitis, Urolithiasis (apatite), Urolithiasis (calcium oxalate), Urolithiasis (magnesium ammonium phosphate, struvite), Urolithiasis (silica), Urolithiasis (urate), von Willebrand disease type I, Wry mouth

Schnauzer, Standard (Standard Schnauzer)

Anterior cross-bite, Base-narrow canines, Cardiomyopathy (dilated), Cataracts, Corneal dystrophy, Degenerative myelopathy, Diabetes mellitus, Distichiasis, Elbow dysplasia, Hemangiosarcoma, Hip dysplasia, Hyperadrenocorticism, Hypothyroidism, Leukodystrophy, Leukoencephalomyelopathy, Malocclusion, Myotonia congenita, Osteosarcoma, Pancreatitis, Persistent Mullerian duct syndrome, Persistent primary vitreous, Portosystemic shunts, Prognathism, Progressive retinal atrophy, Retinal dysplasia, Stomatocytosis, Urolithiasis (calcium oxalate), Wry mouth

Schweizer Laufhund (Swiss Hound) 🐾
Hip dysplasia, Progressive retinal atrophy

Scottish Deerhound 🐾
Anesthetic metabolism (CYP2B11), Atopic dermatitis, Cardiomyopathy (dilated), Cervical vertebral arthrosis, Cystinuria, Factor VII deficiency, Gastric dilation/volvulus, Osteochondrodysplasia, Osteosarcoma, Portosystemic shunts, Urolithiasis (cystine)

Scottish Fold 🐱
Deafness, Heterochromia iridis, Neonatal isoerythrolysis, Osteochondrodysplasia, Polycystic kidney disease, Urolithiasis (calcium oxalate)

Scottish Terrier 🐾
Alexander disease, Atopic dermatitis, Brachygnathism, Cataracts, Central axonopathy, Cerebellar abiotrophy, Chondrodysplasia, Chondrodystrophy, Chronic inflammatory hepatic disease, Corneal dystrophy, Craniomandibular osteopathy, Cystinuria, Deafness, Demodicosis, Distichiasis, Dystocia, Epilepsy, Factor IX deficiency (hemophilia B), Hemivertebra (caudal), Hyperadrenocorticism, Hyperphosphatemia, Hypoparathyroidism, Leukodystrophy (fibrinoid), Ligneous membranitis, Lymphoma, Malocclusion, Melanoma (cutaneous), Myasthenia gravis, Nasal vasculopathy, Paroxysmal dyskinesia, Patellar luxation, Persistent pupillary membranes, Portosystemic shunts, Progressive retinal atrophy, Pulmonary fibrosis, Recurrent flank alopecia, Renal glucosuria, Retinal dysplasia, Scottie cramp, Sebaceous adenitis, Superficial necrolytic dermatitis, Transitional cell carcinoma, Urolithiasis (cystine), Urolithiasis (magnesium ammonium phosphate, struvite), Vitreous degeneration, von Willebrand disease type I, von Willebrand disease type III

Sealyham Terrier 🐾
Albinism (Waardenburg), Atopic dermatitis, Brachygnathism, Cataracts, Deafness, Degenerative myelopathy, Distichiasis, Factor VII deficiency, Glaucoma, Keratoconjunctivitis sicca, Lens luxation, Persistent pupillary membranes, Prognathism, Progressive retinal atrophy, Retinal dysplasia, Vitreous degeneration

Selkirk Rex 🐱
Deafness, Polycystic kidney disease

Shar-Pei (Chinese Shar-Pei) 🐾
Amyloidosis, Atopic dermatitis, Brachycephalic obstructive airway syndrome, Brachygnathism, Cataracts, Ciliary dyskinesia, Cobalamin malabsorption, Corneal dystrophy, Demodicosis, Ectropion, Elbow dysplasia, Elbow dysplasia (ununited anconeal process), Entropion, Factor XII deficiency, Familial benign pemphigus, Familial shar-pei fever, Fold dermatitis, Gastric dilation/volvulus, Glaucoma (POAG), Hernia (hiatal), Hernia (perineal), Hip dysplasia, Histiocytic sarcoma, Hypothyroidism, Immunodeficiency syndrome, Immunoglobulin A (IgA) deficiency, Keratoconjunctivitis sicca, Lens luxation, Lymphangiectasia, Lymphoma (gastrointestinal), Lymphoproliferative disease (T-cell), Malassezia dermatitis, Mast cell tumor, Megaesophagus, Melanoma (tongue), Mucinosis, Otitis externa, Pannus, Panosteitis, Patellar luxation, Pemphigus foliaceus, Persistent pupillary membranes, Prognathism, Prolapsed gland of nictitans, Pseudohyperkalemia, Retinal dysplasia, Seborrhea, Shar-pei immunodeficiency

Shetland Sheepdog (Sheltie) 🐾
Atherosclerosis, Atrial rupture, Brachygnathism, Cataracts, Choroidal hypoplasia (collie eye anomaly), Color dilution alopecia, Corneal dystrophy, Craniomandibular osteopathy, Cryptorchidism, Deafness, Degenerative myelopathy, Dermatomyositis, Distal tibial valgus deformity, Distichiasis, Ectodermal dysplasia (x-linked), Elbow dysplasia, Epilepsy, Epulis, Factor VIII deficiency (hemophilia A), Factor IX deficiency (hemophilia B), Fanconi syndrome, Gallbladder mucocele, Hip dysplasia, Hyperlipidemia (hypercholesterolemia), Hypothyroidism, Immune-mediated hemolytic anemia, Intervertebral disk disease, Leukodystrophy, Leukodystrophy (spongiform leukoencephalomyelopathy), Lupus erythematosus, Lupus erythematosus (discoid), Lupus erythematosus (vesicular cutaneous), Malocclusion, Merling, Mucinosis, Multidrug resistance-1, Oligodontia, Optic nerve colobomas, Optic nerve hypoplasia and micropapilla, Organic aciduria, Osteochondrodysplasia, Otitis externa, Pannus, Patellar luxation, Patent ductus arteriosus, Pemphigoid (vullous), Pemphigus (erythematosus), Persistent pupillary membranes, Piebaldism, Portosystemic shunts, Posterior cross-bite, Progressive retinal atrophy (central), Progressive retinal atrophy (CNGA1), Proliferative episcleritis, Renal agenesis, Renal dysplasia, Retinal dysplasia, Rostrally displaced maxillary canine, Stationary night blindness, Superficial digital flexor tendon luxation, Superficial necrolytic dermatitis, Tibial valgus deformity, Ulcerative dermatosis, Uveal hypopigmentation, Uveodermatologic syndrome, Vestibular disease (congenital), von Willebrand disease type III

Shiba Inu 🐾
Atopic dermatitis, Base-narrow canines, Cataracts, Distichiasis, Elbow dysplasia, Epulis, Glaucoma, GM-1 gangliosidosis, GM-2 gangliosidosis, Hip dysplasia, Hyperkalemia, Intervertebral disk disease, Malocclusion, Microcytosis, Patellar luxation, Persistent pupillary membranes, Pseudohyperkalemia, Rostrally displaced maxillary canine, Tail chasing, Uveodermatologic syndrome, Ventricular septal defect, Vitreous degeneration, von Willebrand disease, Wry mouth

Shih Tzu 🐕

Arachnoid cyst, Atlantoaxial instability, Atopic dermatitis, Brachycephalic obstructive airway syndrome, Cataracts, Chondrodysplasia, Chondrodystrophy, Chronic hypertrophic pyloric gastropathy, Cleft lip/palate, Corneal dystrophy, Cryptorchidism, Degenerative myelopathy, Demodicosis, Dentigerous cysts, Dermoid sinus, Distichiasis, Dystocia, Eclampsia, Entropion, Familial nephropathy, Glaucoma, Hernia (umbilical), Hip dysplasia, Hydrocephalus, Hypothyroidism (congenital) with goiter, Intervertebral disk disease, Keratoconjunctivitis sicca, Legg–Calvé–Perthes disease, Leukodystrophy (spongiform leukoencephalomyelopathy), Lymphoproliferative disease (T-cell), Macroblepharon, Macrothrombocytopenia, Malassezia dermatitis, Malocclusion, Mast cell tumor, Meningoencephalitis (necrotizing), Mitral valve disease, Oligodontia, Optic nerve hypoplasia, and micropapilla, Pannus, Panosteitis, Patellar luxation, Portal vein hypoplasia, Portosystemic shunts, Prekallikrein deficiency, Prognathism, Progressive retinal atrophy, Prolapsed gland of nictitans, Proptosis, Pulmonary fibrosis, Renal dysplasia, Retinal dysplasia, Sebaceous adenitis, Shaker syndrome, Tracheal collapse, Tricuspid valve dysplasia, Ulcerative keratitis, Urolithiasis (apatite), Urolithiasis (calcium oxalate), Urolithiasis (silica), Urolithiasis (urate), Vitreous degeneration, von Willebrand disease

Shiloh Shepherd 🐕

Degenerative myelopathy, Ectodermal dysplasia (x-linked), Factor VIII deficiency (hemophilia A), Gastric dilation/volvulus, Hip dysplasia, Hyperuricosuria, Leukocyte adhesion deficiency type III, Megaesophagus, Mucopolysaccharidosis VII, Multidrug resistance-1, Nodular dermatofibrosis, Panosteitis, Perianal fistulae

Shropshire Terrier 🐕

Deafness

Siamese 🐈

Albinism (oculocutaneous), Amyloidosis, Asthma, Cardiomyopathy (dilated), Cerebellar abiotrophy, Cerebellar degeneration, Chronic obstructive pulmonary disease, Corneal sequestrum, Endocardial fibroelastosis, Excessive grooming, Factor IX deficiency, Factor XII deficiency, Feline hyperesthesia syndrome, Feline lower urinary tract disease (FLUTD), Glaucoma, GM-1 gangliosidosis, Heterochromia iridis, Hyperparathyroidism, Lens luxation, Lymphosarcoma, Mast cell tumor, Megaesophagus, Mitral stenosis, Mucopolysaccharidosis VI, Myasthenic syndrome, Mycobacterial susceptibility, Niemann–Pick C,

Pancreatitis, Patellar luxation, Pemphigus foliaceus, Polycystic kidney disease, Porphyria, Progressive retinal atrophy (rdAc), Pyloric stenosis, Rickets, Strabismus, Tooth resorption, Urolithiasis (calcium oxalate), Urolithiasis (urate), Wool-sucking behavior

Siberian Forest Cat 🐈

Cardiomyopathy (hypertrophic), Deafness, Pyruvate kinase deficiency

Siberian Husky 🐕

Achromatopsia, Alopecia X, Bronchiectasis, Cataracts, Collagenolytic (eosinophilic) granuloma, Corneal dystrophy, Cryptorchidism, Cutaneous lupus erythematosus, Deafness, Degenerative myelopathy, Ectopic ureters, Entropion, Epilepsy, Factor VIII deficiency (hemophilia A), Familial hyperphosphatemia, Follicular dysplasia, Follicular dysplasia (wooly syndrome), Glaucoma, GM-1 gangliosidosis, Hip dysplasia, Hyperphosphatemia, Hypertension, Hypothyroidism, Laryngeal paralysis, Lupus erythematosus (discoid), Lymphoproliferative disease (T-cell), Microphthalmia, Myelodysplasia, Osteochondritis dissecans (shoulder), Otitis externa, Pannus, Persistent hyaloid artery, Persistent primary vitreous, Persistent pupillary membranes, Portosystemic shunts, Progressive retinal atrophy (XLPRA1), Retinal dysplasia, Schwannoma (uveal), Sensory neuropathy, Spontaneous pneumothorax, Tetralogy of Fallot, Thyroid carcinoma/adenocarcinoma, Uveal hypopigmentation, Uveodermatologic syndrome, Ventricular septal defect, von Willebrand disease, Zinc-responsive dermatosis

Silken Windhound 🐕

Choroidal hypoplasia (collie eye anomaly), Degenerative myelopathy, Hip dysplasia, Multidrug resistance-1

Silky Terrier, Australian (Australian Silky Terrier) 🐕

Atopic dermatitis, Brachygnathism, Cataracts, Color dilution alopecia, Cryptorchidism, Cystinuria, Degenerative myelopathy, Diabetes mellitus, Elliptocytosis, Epilepsy, Glucocerebrosidosis, Hyperadrenocorticism, Legg–Calvé–Perthes disease, Leukodystrophy (spongiform encephalopathy), Malassezia dermatitis, Patellar luxation, Persistent pupillary membranes, Portosystemic shunts, Prognathism, Progressive retinal atrophy (prcd), Retinal dysplasia, Sialocele, Tracheal collapse, Urolithiasis (cystine), Vitreous degeneration, von Willebrand disease type I

Singapura 🐈

Cardiomyopathy (hypertrophic), Hypokalemic periodic polymyopathy, Progressive retinal atrophy (PRA-pd), Progressive retinal atrophy (rdAc), Pyruvate kinase deficiency

Skye Terrier

Atopic dermatitis, Chondrodysplasia, Chronic inflammatory hepatic disease, Copper hepatopathy, Ectopic ureters, Elbow dysplasia, Hypothyroidism, Lens luxation, Oligodontia, von Willebrand disease

Sloughi

Color dilution alopecia, Factor VIII deficiency (hemophilia A), Hypoadrenocorticism, Inflammatory bowel disease, Low thyroxine levels, Progressive retinal atrophy (rcd1a)

Snowshoe

Axonal neuropathy, Polycystic kidney disease, Polyneuropathy, Urolithiasis (urate)

Soft-Coated Wheaten Terrier

Anterior cross-bite, Atopic dermatitis, Brachygnathism, Cataracts, Cutaneous asthenia, Deafness, Degenerative myelopathy, Distichiasis, Ectopic ureters, Elbow dysplasia, Familial nephropathy, Glomerulonephritis, Hip dysplasia, Hypoadrenocorticism, Ichthyosis, Intersex (gonadal), Lymphangiectasia, Malocclusion, Microphthalmia, Noise sensitivity, Optic nerve hypoplasia and micropapilla, Paroxysmal dyskinesia, Patellar luxation, Persistent hyaloid artery, Persistent pupillary membranes, Prognathism, Progressive retinal atrophy, Protein-losing enteropathy, Protein-losing nephropathy, Renal dysplasia, Retinal dysplasia, von Willebrand disease

Somali

Amyloidosis, Cardiomyopathy (hypertrophic), Myasthenic syndrome, Neonatal isoerythrolysis, Progressive retinal atrophy (PRA-pd), Progressive retinal atrophy (rdAc), Progressive retinal atrophy (Rdy), Pyruvate kinase deficiency

Spanish Water Dog

Hip dysplasia, Hyperuricosuria, Hypothyroidism (congenital) with goiter, Myasthenia gravis, Neuroaxonal dystrophy, Portal vein hypoplasia, Progressive retinal atrophy (prcd), Progressive retinal atrophy (SWD), Short tail

Sphynx

Cardiomyopathy (hypertrophic), Deafness, Hairlessness, Hereditary myopathy, Heterochromia iridis, Hypokalemic periodic polymyopathy, Mitral valve dysplasia, Myasthenic syndrome, Polycystic kidney disease, Urolithiasis (urate), Urticaria pigmentosa

Spinone Italiano (Italian Spinone)

Atopic dermatitis, Cataracts, Cerebellar abiotrophy, Cerebellar ataxia (Italian spinone), Ectropion, Elbow dysplasia, Entropion, Epilepsy, Gastric dilation/volvulus, Hip dysplasia, Hypothyroidism, Peripheral neuropathy, Persistent pupillary membranes, Polyneuropathy

Springer Spaniel, English (English Springer Spaniel)

Acral mutilation syndrome, Aggression (rage syndrome), Atopic dermatitis, Bronchiectasis, Cataracts, Cerebellar abiotrophy, Chondrodystrophy, Chronic inflammatory hepatic disease, Ciliary dyskinesia, Cutaneous asthenia, Deafness, Degenerative myelopathy, Diabetes mellitus, Dysmyelinogenesis, Ectropion, Elbow dysplasia, Elbow dysplasia (incomplete ossification of humeral condyle), Endocardial fibroelastosis, Entropion, Epilepsy, Factor XI deficiency, Familial nephropathy, Follicular dysplasia (wooly syndrome), Fucosidosis, Generalized tremor (shaking puppy), Glaucoma, GM-2 gangliosidosis, Hip dysplasia, Hypoadrenocorticism, Hypomyelination, Immune-mediated hemolytic anemia, Lichenoid-psoriasiform dermatitis, Long QT syndrome, Malignant hyperthermia, Meningitis-arteritis, Microphthalmia, Myasthenia gravis, Myopia, Narcolepsy, Odontogenic parakeratinized cyst, Otitis externa, Panosteitis, Patent ductus arteriosus, Pectinate ligament dysplasia, Pemphigus foliaceus, Persistent atrial standstill, Persistent hyaloid artery, Phosphofructokinase deficiency, Progressive retinal atrophy (central), Progressive retinal atrophy (cord1), Progressive retinal atrophy (crd4), Protein-losing nephropathy, Retinal dysplasia, Sebaceous adenitis, Seborrhea, Sudden acquired retinal degeneration, Tremor syndrome, Ventricular septal defect, von Willebrand disease

Springer Spaniel, Welsh (Welsh Springer Spaniel)

Atopic dermatitis, Cardiomyopathy (dilated), Cataracts, Corneal dystrophy, Distichiasis, Dysmyelinogenesis, Elbow dysplasia, Entropion, Epilepsy, Factor VII deficiency, Familial nephropathy, Glaucoma, Hip dysplasia, Hypothyroidism, Pectinate ligament dysplasia, Persistent pupillary membranes, Prognathism, Progressive retinal atrophy, Retinal dysplasia, Sebaceous adenitis, Ulcerative keratitis, Vitreous degeneration

Stabyhoun (Stabijhoun, Stabyhound)

Cerebral dysfunction, Degenerative myelopathy, Elbow dysplasia, Epilepsy, Hip dysplasia, Patent ductus arteriosus, von Willebrand disease type I

Staffordshire Bull Terrier

Atopic dermatitis, Brachycephalic obstructive airway syndrome, Cataracts, Caudally displaced canine teeth, Ciliary dyskinesia, Cobalamin malabsorption, Compulsive tail chasing, Cryptorchidism, Cystinuria, Degenerative myelopathy, Demodicosis, Distichiasis, Dystocia, Elbow dysplasia, Epilepsy, Gastric carcinoma, Hip dysplasia,

Laryngeal paralysis, Leproid granuloma, Mast cell tumor, Myotonia congenita, Organic aciduria (L-2 hydroxyglutaric aciduria), Osteochondritis dissecans (stifle), Patellar luxation, Persistent hyaloid artery, Persistent primary vitreous, Persistent pupillary membranes, Prognathism, Progressive retinal atrophy (crd1), Progressive retinal atrophy (crd2), Pulmonary fibrosis, Tibial tuberosity avulsion fracture, Urolithiasis (cystine)

Sussex Spaniel 🐕
Atopic dermatitis, Cataracts, Deafness, Distichiasis, Ectropion, Elbow dysplasia, Hip dysplasia, Iris hypoplasia, Mitochondrial myopathy, Persistent hyaloid artery, Persistent pupillary membranes, Prognathism, Pulmonic stenosis, Pyruvate dehydrogenase Phosphatase 1 deficiency, Retinal dysplasia, Skeletal dysplasia 2

Swedish Elkhound 🐕
Diabetes mellitus, Epilepsy, Progressive retinal atrophy

Swedish Lapphund 🐕
Cerebellar cortical degeneration, Degenerative myelopathy, Diabetes mellitus, Glycogen storage disease II, Multifocal retinopathy (CMR3), Progressive retinal atrophy (prcd), Spinal muscular atrophy

Swedish Vallhund 🐕
Cataracts, Chondrodystrophy, Cryptorchidism, Distichiasis, Elbow dysplasia, Hip dysplasia, Hyperuricosuria, Oligodontia, Persistent pupillary membranes, Progressive retinal atrophy, Progressive retinal atrophy (vallhund), Retinal dysplasia, Short tail, Vitreous degeneration

Teddy Roosevelt Terrier 🐕
Atopic dermatitis, Degenerative myelopathy, Elbow dysplasia, Hypothyroidism (congenital) with goiter, Lens luxation, Patellar luxation, von Willebrand disease

Tenterfield Terrier 🐕
Degenerative myelopathy, Hypothyroidism (congenital) with goiter, Lens luxation, Patellar luxation, Spinocerebellar ataxia, Spinocerebellar ataxia (myokymia and neuromyotonia)

Thai 🐈
GM-1 gangliosidosis, Mucopolysaccharidosis VI, Progressive retinal atrophy (rdAc)

Thai Ridgeback 🐕
Color dilution alopecia, Dermoid sinus, Ridgelessness

Tibetan Mastiff 🐕
Cataracts, Demodicosis, Elbow dysplasia, Epilepsy, Hip dysplasia, Hypertrophic neuropathy, Hypothyroidism, Osteochondritis dissecans (shoulder), Panosteitis, Peripheral neuropathy (hypertrophic), Progressive retinal atrophy

Tibetan Spaniel 🐈
Atopic dermatitis, Brachycephalic obstructive airway syndrome, Brachygnathism, Cataracts, Chondrodystrophy, Cryptorchidism, Cystinuria, Deafness, Degenerative myelopathy, Demodicosis, Distichiasis, Elbow dysplasia, Entropion, Hernia (inguinal), Hernia (umbilical), Hip dysplasia, Hyperoxaluria, Intervertebral disk disease, Lens luxation, Mast cell tumor, Microphthalmia, Neuronal ceroid lipofuscinosis, Optic nerve hypoplasia and micropapilla, Pannus, Patellar luxation, Persistent pupillary membranes, Polydontia (retained primary teeth), Portosystemic shunts, Prognathism, Progressive retinal atrophy (PRA3), Prolapsed gland of nictitans

Tibetan Terrier 🐕
Atopic dermatitis, Brachygnathism, Cataracts, Corneal dystrophy, Deafness, Degenerative myelopathy, Diabetes mellitus, Distichiasis, Elbow dysplasia, Epilepsy, Hemophagocytic syndrome, Hernia (umbilical), Hip dysplasia, Hypothyroidism, Lens luxation, Neuronal ceroid lipofuscinosis A, Oligodontia, Patellar luxation, Persistent pupillary membranes, Prognathism, Progressive retinal atrophy (PRA3), Progressive retinal atrophy (prcd), Progressive retinal atrophy (rcd4), Renal dysplasia, Retinal dysplasia, Urolithiasis (calcium oxalate), Vestibular disease (congenital), von Willebrand disease

Tiffanie 🐈
Hypokalemic periodic polymyopathy

Tonkinese 🐈
Diabetes mellitus, Hypokalemic periodic polymyopathy, Mucopolysaccharidosis VI, Patellar luxation, Progressive retinal atrophy (rdAc), Urolithiasis (calcium oxalate)

Tosa Inu 🐕
Pseudohyperkalemia

Treeing Walker Coonhound 🐕
Amyloidosis, Degenerative myelopathy, Hip dysplasia

Turkish Angora 🐈
Deafness, Heterochromia iridis, Neonatal isoerythrolysis, Polycystic kidney disease, Progressive retinal atrophy (PRA-pd)

Turkish Naked Dog 🐕
Hairlessness

Turkish Van 🐈
Deafness, Heterochromia iridis, Neonatal isoerythrolysis, Polycystic kidney disease

Vizsla (Hungarian Vizsla) 🐕
Atopic dermatitis, Cataracts, Cerebellar cortical degeneration, Corneal dystrophy, Cryptorchidism, Demodicosis,

Distichiasis, Elbow dysplasia, Entropion, Epilepsy, Exercise-induced collapse, Factor I (fibrinogen) deficiency, Factor VIII deficiency (hemophilia A), Glaucoma, Hemangiosarcoma, Hernia (umbilical), Hip dysplasia, Hyperuricosuria, Hypothyroidism, Immune-mediated hemolytic anemia, Immune-mediated inflammatory myopathy, Lupus erythematosus (exfoliative cutaneous), Lymphoma, Mast cell tumor, Melanoma, Osteochondritis dissecans (shoulder), Persistent pupillary membranes, Polymyositis, Progressive retinal atrophy, Sebaceous adenitis, Urinary incontinence, von Willebrand disease

Volpino Italiano

Lens luxation, Patellar luxation, von Willebrand disease type I

Wachtelhund (German Spaniel)

Atopic dermatitis, Degenerative myelopathy, Hypoadrenocorticism, Phosphofructokinase deficiency

Weimaraner (Vorstehhund)

Cataracts, Cervical vertebral instability, Color dilution alopecia, Corneal dystrophy, Diskospondylitis, Distichiasis, Dysmyelinogenesis, Elbow dysplasia, Elbow dysplasia (ununited anconeal process), Epidermolysis bullosa (junctional), Everted cartilage of third eyelid, Exocrine pancreatic insufficiency, Factor VIII deficiency (hemophilia A), Factor XI deficiency, Follicular dysplasia, Gastric dilation/volvulus, Hernia (peritoneopericardial), Hip dysplasia, Hypertrophic osteodystrophy, Hyperuricosuria, Hypomyelination, Immune-mediated polyarthritis, Immunodeficiency syndrome, Inflammatory bowel disease, Intersex (gonadal), Lupoid onychopathy, Mast cell tumor, Metatarsal fistulae, Muscular dystrophy, Myelodysplasia, Panosteitis, Patellar luxation, Persistent pupillary membranes, Pituitary dwarfism, Prognathism, Progressive retinal atrophy (XLPRA), Pulmonary artery dissection, Recurrent flank alopecia, Renal dysplasia, Sebaceous adenitis, Spinal dysraphism, Tremor syndrome, Tricuspid valve dysplasia, Urinary incontinence, von Willebrand disease type II, Weimaraner immunodeficiency

Welsh Terrier

Atopic dermatitis, Cataracts, Corneal dystrophy, Degenerative myelopathy, Distichiasis, Epilepsy, Glaucoma, Hip dysplasia, Keratoconjunctivitis sicca, Lens luxation, Pectus excavatum, Persistent pupillary membranes

West Highland White Terrier

Atopic dermatitis, Atrioventricular heart block, Bronchiectasis, Cataracts, Chondrodysplasia, Chondrodystrophy, Chronic inflammatory hepatic disease, Chronic interstitial lung disease, Copper hepatopathy, Craniomandibular osteopathy, Cruciate ligament disease, Deafness, Demodicosis,

Diabetes mellitus, Ectopic ureters, Epidermal dysplasia, Exocrine pancreatic insufficiency, Glaucoma, Globoid cell leukodystrophy, Hyperadrenocorticism, Hypoadrenocorticism, Ichthyosis, Immunoglobulin A (IgA) deficiency, Inflammatory bowel disease, Keratoconjunctivitis sicca, Legg–Calvé–Perthes disease, Leukoencephalomyelopathy, Lymphoma, Malassezia dermatitis, Microphthalmia, Mitral valve disease, Myotonia congenita, Oligodontia, Organic aciduria (L-2 hydroxyglutaric aciduria), Panosteitis, Patellar luxation, Persistent pupillary membranes, Polycystic kidney disease, Polycystic liver disease, Polydontia, Polydontia (retained primary teeth), Polyradiculoneuritis, Portal vein hypoplasia, Portosystemic shunts, Prognathism, Progressive retinal atrophy, Pulmonary fibrosis, Pulmonic stenosis, Pyruvate kinase deficiency, Renal dysplasia, Retinal dysplasia, Shaker syndrome, Sick sinus syndrome, Spinal dysraphism, Stiff skin syndrome, Superficial necrolytic dermatitis, Ulcerative keratitis, Urolithiasis (calcium oxalate), von Willebrand disease type I

Whippet

Anesthetic metabolism (CYP2B11), Atopic dermatitis, Brachygnathism, Cataracts, Choroidal hypoplasia (collie eye anomaly), Color dilution alopecia, Corneal dystrophy, Cryptorchidism, Deafness, Degenerative myelopathy, Demodicosis, Eccentrocytosis, Ectodermal defect, Ectodermal dysplasia (x-linked), Epilepsy, Factor VII deficiency, Follicular dysplasia, Hemangioma/hemangiosarcoma, Hip dysplasia, Hypotrichosis, Lens luxation, Meningitis-arteritis, Mitral valve disease, Multidrug resistance-1, Myostatin deficiency (double muscling), Optic nerve hypoplasia and micropapilla, Osteochondritis dissecans (shoulder), Persistent pupillary membranes, Phosphofructokinase deficiency, Prognathism, Progressive retinal atrophy, Vitreous degeneration, von Willebrand disease

Wirehaired Pointing Griffon

Atopic dermatitis, Cataracts, Corneal dystrophy, Cryptorchidism, Degenerative myelopathy, Elbow dysplasia, Entropion, Epilepsy, Hernia (umbilical), Hip dysplasia, Meningitis-arteritis, Osteochondritis dissecans (shoulder), Recurrent flank alopecia

Xoloitzcuintli (Mexican Hairless)

Comedo syndrome, Contact dermatitis, Cryptorchidism, Hairlessness, Oligodontia, Progressive retinal atrophy (prcd), Sunburn, Thymic atrophy, von Willebrand disease type II

Yakutian Laika

Degenerative myelopathy, Elbow dysplasia, Gastric dilation/volvulus, Hip dysplasia, Progressive retinal atrophy (prcd)

Yorkshire Terrier 🐕

Atlantoaxial instability, Atopic dermatitis, Cataracts, Chronic inflammatory hepatic disease, Cleft lip/palate, Color dilution alopecia, Congenital alacrima, Corneal dystrophy, Cruciate ligament disease, Cryptorchidism, Deafness, Degenerative myelopathy, Dermoid sinus, Diabetes mellitus, Distichiasis, Dystocia, Epilepsy, Fanconi syndrome, Glaucoma, Hernia (perineal), Hip dysplasia, Hydrocephalus, Hyperadrenocorticism, Hypoglycemia, Hypotrichosis, Inflammatory bowel disease, Intersex (gonadal), Intervertebral disk disease, Keratoconjunctivitis sicca, Legg–Calvé–Perthes disease, Lens luxation, Lymphangiectasia, Lymphoproliferative disease (T-cell), Meningoencephalitis (necrotizing), Mitral valve disease, Necrotizing encephalopathy, Organic aciduria (L-2 hydroxyglutaric aciduria), Pancreatitis, Patellar luxation, Patent ductus arteriosus, Persistent pupillary membranes, Plasmacytoma (cutaneous), Polydontia, Polydontia (retained primary teeth), Portal vein hypoplasia, Portosystemic shunts, Progressive retinal atrophy (prcd), Protein-losing enteropathy, Pulmonary fibrosis, Retinal dysplasia, Shaker syndrome, Sinus tachycardia, Syringomyelia, Tracheal collapse, Ulcerative keratitis, Urolithiasis (calcium oxalate), Urolithiasis (magnesium ammonium phosphate, struvite), Urolithiasis (silica), Urolithiasis (urate), von Willebrand disease

Yugoslavian Shepherd Dog (Sarplaninac) 🐕

Neuronal ceroid lipofuscinosis

Recommended Reading

Ackerman, L: *The Genetic Connection*, 2, AAHA Press, Lakewood, CO, 2011

Ackerman, L: Proactive Pet Parenting: Anticipating pet health problems before they happen. Problem Free Publishing, 2020. problemfreepets.com

Bell, JS; Cavanagh, KE; Tilley, LP; Smith, FWK: *Veterinary Medical Guide to Dog and Cat Breeds*, Teton NewMedia, Jackson, WY, 2012

Gough, A, Thomas, A; O'Neill, D: *Breed Predispositions to Disease in Dogs and Cats*, 3, Wiley, 2018.

University of Prince Edward Island. Canine Inherited Disorders Database, http://cidd.discoveryspace.ca

University of Sydney. Online Mendelian Inheritance in Animals. http://omia.org.

World Small Animal Veterinary Association. Canine and Feline Hereditary Disease (DNA) Testing Laboratories. www.vet.upenn.edu/research/academic-departments/clinical-sciences-advanced-medicine/research-labs-centers/penngen/tests-worldwide

11.5

Life Planning by Breed

Lowell Ackerman, DVM, DACVD, MBA, MPA, CVA, MRCVS

Global Consultant, Author, and Lecturer, MA, USA

The table presented here provides useful information on the great variability inherent in different dog breeds, relative to weight, height (at the withers), typical lifespan, the age at which individual breeds could be considered senior, and even a target healthspan.

The intent was not to include all breeds of dogs, but to give preference to those breeds included in other tables in this book, especially those for which a breed predisposition to disease has been recognized. It is important to realize that the information presented here reflects generalizations, but the goal of pet-specific care is to appreciate that pets need to be considered on an individual basis.

While this appendix is limited to dog breeds, this is only because there is much less variability in cat breeds related to weight, height, lifespan, and healthspan. Certainly some cats, such as the Savannah and the Maine Coon, are larger than most other cat breeds, and others, such as the Singapura and Munchkin, are smaller than typical for the species, but the average lifespan is relatively consistent across most breeds (14–16 years) and as far as healthspan goes, with proper pet-specific care, it is not unusual for most cats to make it to 20 years and beyond. Most cats approach senior status between 7 and 10 years of age, and the AAFP/AAHA guidelines consider cats to be mature by 7 years of age, and senior by 11 years of age.

Name	Also Known As	Country of Origin	Male Height range (cm)	Female Height Range (cm)	Male Weight Range (kg)	Female Weight Range (kg)	Typical Lifespan (years)	Senior status (years)	Healthspan Target (years)
Abyssinian Sand Terrier	African Hairless Dog	Africa	39–52	39–52	9–18	9–18	12–14	7	18
Affenpinscher	Monkey Dog	Germany	18–30	18–30	3–4	3–4	12–14	7	18
Afghan Hound	Afghan, Tazi Spay	Afghanistan	68–74	60–69	26–34	26–34	12–14	7	18
Airedale Terrier	Airedale, Bingley Terrier, Waterside Terrier	United Kingdom	58–61	56–59	23–29	18–20	10–12	6	16
Akbash Dog	Akbaş Çoban Köpeği	Turkey	71–81	71–81	40–59	38–57	10–12	6	16
Akita	Akita Inu	Japan	66–71	61–66	45–59	32–45	10–12	6	16
Alaskan Husky		United States of America	58–66	58–66	18–27	16–22	10–12	6	16
Alaskan Klee-Kai	Klee Kai	United States of America	33–43	33–43	3–10	3–10	12–14	7	18
Alaskan Malamute	Malamute	United States of America	61–66	56–61	36–43	32–38	10–12	6	16

(Continued)

Pet-Specific Care for the Veterinary Team, First Edition. Edited by Lowell Ackerman.
© 2021 John Wiley & Sons, Inc. Published 2021 by John Wiley & Sons, Inc.

Name	Also Known As	Country of Origin	Male Height range (cm)	Female Height Range (cm)	Male Weight Range (kg)	Female Weight Range (kg)	Typical Lifespan (years)	Senior status (years)	Healthspan Target (years)
Alpine Dachsbracke	Alpenländische Dachsbracke	Austria	34–41	33–40	15–17	15–18	11–13	7	17
American Bulldog	Old Southern White Bulldog	United States of America	55–80	52–65	32–54	27–45	12–14	6	16
American Bully	Bully	United States of America	33–53	33–53	31–54	31–54	10–12	6	16
American Eskimo, Miniature	American Eskimo Dog, Cloud Spitz, American Spitz	United States of America	30–40	30–40	5–8	5–8	13–15	8	19
American Eskimo, Standard	American Eskimo Dog, Cloud Spitz, American Spitz	United States of America	40–50	40–50	8–16	8–16	12–14	7	18
American Eskimo, Toy	American Eskimo Dog, Cloud Spitz, American Spitz	United States of America	22–30	22–30	3–5	3–5	13–15	8	19
American Hairless Terrier		United States of America	18–41	18–41	3–7	3–7	14–16	8	20
American Pit Bull Terrier	American Pitbull Terrier	United States of America	35–60	35–60	10–35	10–35	11–13	7	17
American Shepherd, Miniature	Berger Miniature Américain, Miniatur Amerikanischer Schäferhund	United States of America	36–46	33–43	11–14	9–13	13–15	8	18
American Staffordshire Terrier	AmStaff	United States of America	46–48	43–46	28–40	28–40	10–12	6	16
American Water Spaniel	American Brown Spaniel, American Brown Water Spaniel	United States of America	38–46	38–46	14–20	11–18	10–12	6	16
Anatolian Shepherd Dog	Kangal, Karabash, Turkish Shepherd Dog, Kangal Shepherd Dog	Turkey	74–81	71–79	50–65	40–55	10–12	6	16
Australian Cattle Dog (Queensland Blue Heeler)	Blue Heeler, Red Heeler, Queensland Heller, Queensland Blue Heeler	Australia	46–51	43–48	15–16	14–16	9–11	6	15
Australian Cobberdog	Australian Cobber Dog, Australian Labradoodle	Australia	35–58	33–56	8–35	6–33	12–14	7	16
Australian Kelpie	Kelpie, Barb, Farmer Dog	Australia	40–51	39–50	15–20	14–19	12–14	7	16
Australian Shepherd	Aussie	Australia	51–58	46–54	25–32	16–25	12–14	7	17
Australian Stumpy-Tail Cattle Dog	Stumpy Tail Cattle Dog, Stumpy	Australia	47–51	46–50	16–23	16–23	13–15	8	17
Australian Terrier		Australia	23–28	23–28	6.4–7.3	5.4–6.4	12–14	7	18

Name	Also Known As	Country of Origin	Male Height range (cm)	Female Height Range (cm)	Male Weight Range (kg)	Female Weight Range (kg)	Typical Lifespan (years)	Senior status (years)	Healthspan Target (years)
Austrian Pinscher	Österreichischer Kurzhaarpinscher, Austrian Shorthaired Pinscher	Austria	44–50	42–48	12–18	12–18	12–14	7	17
Azawakh	Idi, Hanshee, Oska, Rawondu, Bareeru, Wulo	Mali	64–74	60–70	20–25	15–20	10–12	6	15
Barbet	French Water Dog	France	58–65	53–61	17–28	14–23	13–15	8	20
Basenji	African Bush Dog, African Barkless Dog, Ango Angari, Congo Dog, Zande Dog	Democratic Republic of Congo	41–43	38–41	12–Oct	43719	11–13	7	17
Basset Fauvre de Bretagne	Fawn Brittany Basset	France	32–38	32–38	15–19	15–17	12–14	7	17
Basset Hound		France	30–39	28–36	25–34	20–29	9–11	6	15
Bavarian Mountain Hound	Bayerischer Gebirgsschweißhund	Germany	47–52	44–48	20–25	20–25	10–12	6	16
Beagle	English Beagle	United Kingdom	33–41	33–41	10–11	9–10	12–14	7	18
Bearded Collie	Beardie, Highland Collie, Mountain Collie, Hairy Mou'ed Collie	United Kingdom	53–56	51–56	18–27	18–27	12–14	7	17
Beauceron	Beauceron Shepherd, Berger de Beauce, Beauce sheepdog, Beace Shepherd, Bas Rouge	France	66–71	64–66	32–50	32–50	10–12	6	16
Bedlington Terrier	Rothbury Terrier, Rodbery Terrier, Rothbury's Lamb	United Kingdom	41–44	38–42	7.7–10.4	7.7–10.4	12–14	7	18
Belgian Laekenois	Laekonois, Belgian Shepherd Dog, Laeken, Chien de Berger Belge	Belgium	61–66	56–61	25–30	20–25	10–12	6	15
Belgian Malinois	Malinois, Mechelaar, Mechelse Herder, Mechelse Scheper, Pastor Belga Malinois, Mechelse schaper	Belgium	61–66	56–61	25–30	20–25	10–12	6	16
Belgian Shepherd (Groenendael)	Belgian Sheepdog, Chien de Berger Belge, Groenendael	Belgium	60–66	56–61	25–30	20–25	10–12	6	16
Belgian Tervuren	Belgian Tervueren	Belgium	60–66	56–62	25–30	20–25	10–12	6	16
Bergamasco Shepherd	Bergamasco Sheepdog, Pastore Bergamasco, Bergamasco	Italy	59–61	55–57	32–38	26–32	12–14	7	18

(Continued)

Name	Also Known As	Country of Origin	Male Height range (cm)	Female Height Range (cm)	Male Weight Range (kg)	Female Weight Range (kg)	Typical Lifespan (years)	Senior status (years)	Healthspan Target (years)
Berger Blanc Suisse (White Swiss Sheepdog)	White Swiss Sheepdog, White Swiss Shepherd Dog, Weisser Schweizer Schäferhund, Pastore Svizzero Bianco, Swiss Sheepdog	Switzerland	60–66	55–61	30–40	25–35	11–13	7	16
Berger Picard	Picard, Berger de Picardie, Picardy Shepherd, Picardy Sheepdog	France	60–65	56–60	23–32	23–32	12–14	7	17
Bern Running Dog (Chien Courant Bernois)	Chien Courant Bernois, Chien Courant Suisse	Switzerland	48–60	46–58	13–20	13–20	12–14	7	17
Bernese Mountain Dog	Berner, Berner Sennenhund, Bernese Cattle Dog	Switzerland	64–70	58–66	35–55	35–45	6–8	5	12
Bichon Frisé	Bichon, Bichón Tenerife, Bichon à poil frisé	Spain	23–30	23–28	5-Mar	3–5	12–14	7	18
Black Russian Terrier	Tchornyi Terrier	Russia	72–76	68–74	50–60	45–50	10–12	6	16
Bloodhound	Chien de Saint-Hubert, St Hubert Hound, Sleuth Hound	Belgium	64–72	23–26 in.	46–54	40–48	7–9	5	13
Boerboel	South African Mastiff	South Africa	64–70	59–65	70–90	70–90	10–12	6	16
Bolognese	Bichon Bolognese, Bologneser, Bolo, Botoli	Italy	27–30	25–28	3–5	3–4	13–15	8	19
Bolonka Zwetna	Bolonka, Tsvetnaya Bolonka	Russia	22–27	18–24	3.5–5	2–4	13–15	8	19
Border Collie	Scottish Sheepdog	United Kingdom	48–56	46–53	14–20	12–19	12–14	7	18
Border Terrier		United Kingdom	33–40	28–36	6–7	5–6.5	12–14	7	18
Borzoi (Russian Wolfhound)	Russian Wolfhound, Russkaya psovaya borzaya, Russian Hunting Sighthound	Russia	75–100	68–78	34–48	27–41	8–10	5	14
Boston Terrier	Boston Bull, Boston Bull Terrier	United States of America	38.1–43	38.1–43	4.5–11.3	4.5–11.3	13–15	8	19
Bouvier des Flandres	Flanders Cattle Dog, Vlaamse Koehond	Belgium	58–71	56–69	36–54	27–36	10–12	6	16
Boxer	Deutscher Boxer, German Boxer	Germany	57–63	53–60	30–32	25–27	9–11	6	15
Boykin Spaniel	Boykin Swamp Poodle	United States of America	38–46	38–46	15–18	11–18	12–14	7	18
Braque du Bourbonnais	Bourbonnais Pointer, Bourbonnais Pointing Dog	France	51–57	48–55	18–25	16–22	11–13	7	16

Name	Also Known As	Country of Origin	Male Height range (cm)	Female Height Range (cm)	Male Weight Range (kg)	Female Weight Range (kg)	Typical Lifespan (years)	Senior status (years)	Healthspan Target (years)
Brazilian Terrier	Fox Paulistinha, Terrier Brasileiro	Brazil	35–40	33–38	8–12	8–12	12–14	7	18
Briard	Berger de Brie, Berger Briard	France	61–69	58–65	30–40	25–35	10–12	6	16
Brittany	Brittany Spaniel, Brittany Wiegref, Epagneul Breton, French Brittany	France	47–52	46–51	14–18	14–18	10–12	6	16
Brussels Griffon	Griffon Bruxellois, Belgium Griffon, Petit Brabançon, Griffon Belge, Brabançon Griffon	Belgium	18–20	18–20	2.5–5.5	2.5–5.5	12–14	7	18
Bull Terrier	English Bull Terrier, Varkhond	United Kingdom	51–61	51–61	20–36	20–36	11–13	7	16
Bull Terrier, Miniature	Mini Bull	United Kingdom	25–33	25–33	11–15	11–15	12–14	7	17
Bullmastiff		United Kingdom	63–69	61–66	50–60	45–54	8–10	5	14
Cairn Terrier		United Kingdom	25–33	23–30	6–8	6–8	12–14	7	18
Canaan Dog	Canaanite Dog	Israel	50–60	45–50	18–25	18–25	12–14	7	18
Cane Corso	Italian Mastiff, Cane Corso Italiano, Italian Corso Dog	Italy	64–68	60–64	45–50	40–45	10–12	6	16
Catahoula Leopard Dog	Louisiana Catahoula Leopard Dog, Catahoula Cur, Catahoula Hog Dog	United States of America	56–58	51–68	16–37	16–37	12–14	7	18
Cavalier King Charles Spaniel	Blenheim	United Kingdom	30–33	30–33	5–8	5–8	10–12	6	16
Central Asian Shepherd Dog	Central Asian Ovtcharka, Alabai, Aziat	Afghanistan	70–95	65–78	60–100	45–65	12–14	7	16
Cesky Terrier	Český Teriér, Bohemian Terrier	Czech Republic	25–32	25–32	6–10	6–10	12–14	7	18
Chesapeake Bay Retriever	Chesapeake, Chessie	United States of America	58–66	53–61	29–36	25–32	10–12	6	16
Chihuahua		Mexico	15–25	15–25	1.8–2.7	1.8–2.7	14–16	8	20
Chinese Crested Dog	Crested, Puff	China	27–33	27–33	4.5–5.5	4.5–5.5	14–16	8	20
Chinese Shar-Pei	Shar-pei, Cantonese Shar-pei	China	46–56	46–56	25–29	18–25	9–11	6	14
Chinook		United States of America	58–69	53–64	25–32	25–32	11–13	7	17
Chow Chow	Chow, Chowdron	Tibet	43–51	43–51	25–32	20–27	9–11	6	15
Cirneco dell'Etna	Cirneco	Italy	46–52	42–50	10–12	8–10	12–14	7	18
Clumber Spaniel		United Kingdom	41–51	41–51	25–39	25–39	10–12	6	16

(Continued)

Name	Also Known As	Country of Origin	Male Height range (cm)	Female Height Range (cm)	Male Weight Range (kg)	Female Weight Range (kg)	Typical Lifespan (years)	Senior status (years)	Healthspan Target (years)
Cocker Spaniel, American	Cocker, Cocker Spaniel, Merry Cocker	United States of America	37–39	34–37	11–14	11–14	11–13	7	17
Cocker Spaniel, English	Cocker, Cocker Spaniel	United Kingdom	38–43	35–41	13–16	12–15	11–13	7	17
Collie (Rough, Smooth)	Rough Collie, Smooth Collie	United Kingdom	61–66	56–61	27–34	23–29	12–14	7	18
Coonhound, Black and Tan	American Black and Tan Coonhound	United States of America	58–69	53–66	23–34	18–29	10–12	6	16
Coonhound, Bluetick	Bluetick Coonhound	United States of America	56–69	53–64	25–36	20–29	12–14	7	16
Coonhound, English (American)	American English Coonhound, Redtick Coonhound	United States of America	56–69	53–64	18–30	18–30	10–12	6	16
Coonhound, Redbone	Redbone Coonhound	United States of America	56–69	53–66	20–32	20–32	10–12	6	16
Coonhound, Treeing Walker	Walker, Walker Treeing Coonhound	United States of America	51–69	51–69	23–32	23–32	11–13	7	17
Coton de Tulear	Coton, Cotie	Madagascar	23–28	23–28	4–6	4–6	14–16	8	20
Croatian Sheepdog	Hrvatski ovčar, Kroatischer Schäferhund	Croatia	38–48	40–53	14–20	13–18	12–14	7	17
Curly-Coated Retriever	Curly	United Kingdom	64–69	58–64	29–36	29–36	10–12	6	16
Czechoslovakian Wolf Dog	Československý vlčák, Československý vlčiak, Czechoslovak Vlcak, Czechoslovakian Wolfdog	Czech Republic	65–70	60–68	26–30	25–28	12–14	7	17
Dachshund	Teckel, Dackel, Doxie, Bassotto, Perro Salchicha, Worshond, Taksa	Germany	20–27	20–27	7.3–15	7.3–15	12–14	7	18
Dalmatian	Carriage Dog, Spotted Coach Dog, Firehouse Dog, Leopard Carriage Dog	Croatia	50–60	50–55	21–25	21–25	10–12	6	16
Dandie Dinmont Terrier	Dandie, Hindlee Terrier	United Kingdom	20–28	20–28	8.2–10.9	8.2–10.9	13–15	8	19
Danish/Swedish Farmdog	Dansk/Svensk Gårdshund, Scanian Terrier	Denmark, Sweden	32–39	30–37	9–12	7–11	12–14	7	17
Doberman Pinscher	Doberman, Dobermann, Dobie	Germany	68–72	63–68	34–45	30–40	11–13	7	17
Dogo Argentino	Argentine Dogo, Dogo	Argentina	65–68	60–65	40–44	40–42	10–12	6	15
Dogue de Bordeaux	Bordeaux Mastiff, French Mastiff, Bordeauxdog	France	61–69	58–66	54–68	54–68	6–8	5	13
Drentse Patrijshond	Dutch Partridge Dog, Drentsche Patrijshond, Drent	Netherlands	58–63	55–60	22–33	21–31	11–13	7	16

Name	Also Known As	Country of Origin	Male Height range (cm)	Female Height Range (cm)	Male Weight Range (kg)	Female Weight Range (kg)	Typical Lifespan (years)	Senior status (years)	Healthspan Target (years)
Dunker	Norwegian Dunker Hound, Norwegian Hound	Norway	50–55	47–52	16–18	16–18	12–14	7	17
Dutch Kooiker Dog (Kooikerhondje)	Kooikerhondje, Kooiker	Netherlands	38–41	36–39	10–14	8–13	12–14	7	17
Dutch Shepherd	Dutch Herder, Hollandse Herder	Netherlands	57–62	55–60	32–40	30–38	11–13	7	16
English Bulldog	Bulldog, British Bulldog	United Kingdom	31–40	31–40	24–25	22–23	8–10	5	14
English Setter	Lawerack, Laverack, Llewellin Setter, Llewellyn Setter	United Kingdom	61–69	58–66	25–36	20–32	10–12	6	16
English Shepherd	Farm Collie	United Kingdom	46–58	46–58	22–30	20–28	11–13	7	16
English Toy Spaniel	King Charles Spaniel, Toy Spaniel, Ruby Spaniel, Blenheim Spaniel	United Kingdom	23–28	23–28	3.6–6.4	3.6–6.4	12–14	7	18
Entlebucher Mountain Dog	Entlebucher Sennenhund, Entlebucher Cattle Dog, Entlebuch Mountain Dog	Switzerland	48–51	48–51	25–30	25–30	11–13	7	17
Eurasier	Eurasian Dog	Germany	52–60	48–56	23–32	18–26	12–14	7	17
Field Spaniel		United Kingdom	43–46	43–46	18–25	18–25	10–12	6	16
Fila Brasiliero (Brazilian Mastiff)	Brazilian Mastiff, Onceiro, Cabeçudo	Brazil	62–75	60–70	50–60	40–52	9–11	5	15
Finnish Lapphund	Finnish Lapponian Dog, Lapinkoira, Suomenlapinkoira	Finland	46–52	41–47	15–24	17–19	12–14	7	18
Finnish Spitz	Finnish Hunting Dog, Finnish Spets, Finsk Spets, Suomenpystykorva, Loulou Finois, Suomalainen Pystykorva	Finland	44–50	39–45	12–13	7–10	12–14	7	18
Flat-Coated Retriever	Flatte, Flattie, Flatcoat	United Kingdom	59–61.5	56.5–59	27–36	25–32	10–12	6	16
Fox Terrier, Smooth	Smooth Fox Terrier	United Kingdom	36–41	33–38	7–9	6–8	12–14	7	18
Fox Terrier, Toy	Toy Fox Terrier, American Toy Terrier, AmerToy	United States of America	21.5–29.2	21.5–29.2	1.5–3	1.5–3	12–14	7	18
Fox Terrier, Wire	Wire Fox Terrier	United Kingdom	36–41	33–38	7–9	6–8	12–14	7	18
Foxhound, American	Foxhound, American Foxhound	United States of America	56–64	53–61	29–34	20–29	11–13	7	17

(Continued)

Name	Also Known As	Country of Origin	Male Height range (cm)	Female Height Range (cm)	Male Weight Range (kg)	Female Weight Range (kg)	Typical Lifespan (years)	Senior status (years)	Healthspan Target (years)
Foxhound, English	Foxhound, English Foxhound	United Kingdom	56–63 in.	53–61	29–32	29–32	11–13	7	17
French Bulldog	Bouledogue Français, Frenchie	France	27–30	27–30	9–13	7–11	10–12	6	16
French Spaniel	French Setter, Epagneul Français, Canadian Setter	France	55–63	54–61	21–27	20–25	12–14	7	17
Frisian Water Dog (Wetterhoun)	Wetterhoun, Otterhoun, Dutch Spaniel	Netherlands	56–59	55–58	25–35	25–33	11–13	7	16
Gammel Dansk Honsehond (Old Danish Pointer)	Gammel Dansk Hønsehund, Old Danish Pointer, Old Danish Bird Dog	Denmark	54–60	50–56	30–35	26–31	12–14	7	17
Garafian Shepherd (Pastor Garafiano)	Pastor Garafiano, Garafian Shepherd Dog, Pastor de Garafía	Spain	57–70	55–62	28–40	25–35	11–13	7	16
German Hunting Terrier (Jagdterrier)	Jagdterrier, Deutscher Jagdterrier, German Jagdterrier	Germany	34–40	33–38	89	7.5–8.5	13–15	8	19
German Longhaired Pointer	Deutscher Langhaariger Vorstehhund	Germany	60–70	58–66	28–32	27–31	12–14	7	17
German Pinscher	Deutscher Pinscher	Germany	43–51	43–51	11–20	11–20	12–14	7	18
German Shepherd Dog	German Shepherd, Alsatian, Alsatian Wolf Dog, Deutscher Schäferhund, Berger Allemand	Germany	60–65	55–60	30–40	22–32	10–12	6	16
German Shorthaired Pointer	Deutscher Kurzhaariger Vorstehhund, Deutsch Kurzhaar	Germany	59–64	53–58	25–32	20–27	12–14	7	18
German Spitz (Klein)	German Spitz Klein, Deutscher Spitz	Germany	25–29	23–28	4–5	4–5	12–14	7	18
German Wirehaired Pointer	Deutsch Drahthaar, Deutscher Drahthaariger Vorstehhund, Drahthaar	Germany	60–67	56–62	27–32	27–32	12–14	7	18
Glen of Imaal Terrier	Irish Glenn of Imaal Terrier, Wicklow Terrier	Ireland	30–36	30–36	15–17	15–17	11–13	7	17
Golden Retriever	Golden	United Kingdom	56–61	51–56	27–36	25–32	10–12	6	16
Gordon Setter	Gordon	United Kingdom	61–69	58–66	25–36	20–32	10–12	6	16
Great Dane	Deutsche Dogge, German Mastiff	Germany	76–86	71–81	54–90	45–59	8–10	5	14

Name	Also Known As	Country of Origin	Male Height range (cm)	Female Height Range (cm)	Male Weight Range (kg)	Female Weight Range (kg)	Typical Lifespan (years)	Senior status (years)	Healthspan Target (years)
Great Pyrenees	Pyrenean Mountain Dog, Patou, Perro de Montaña de los Pirineos, Chien de Montagne des Pyrénées	France	69–81	63–74	50–54	39–45	10–12	6	16
Greater Swiss Mountain Dog	Grosser Schweizer Sennenhund, Grand Bouvier Suisse	Switzerland	65–72	60–69	60–70	50–60	9–11	6	15
Greyhound	English Greyhound	United Kingdom	71–76	Jun-71	27–40	27–34	10–12	6	16
Harrier		United Kingdom	48–50	48–50	18–27	18–27	10–12	6	16
Havanese	Havanese Cuban Bichon, Bichón Havanés, Havaneser, Havanezer, Bichon Habanero	Cuba	20–28	20–027	3–6	3–6	12–14	7	18
Hokkaido (Ainu)	Ainu, Ainu-Ken, Dō-Ken, Seta, Hokkaido-Ken	Japan	48–52	46–48	20–30	20–30	11–13	7	17
Hovawart	Hovie	Germany	58–70	58–70	25–51	25–51	11–13	7	17
Ibizan Hound	Ibizan Warren Hound, Ca Eivissenc, Podenco Ibicenco	Spain	56–74	56–74	20–29	19–25	10–12	6	16
Icelandic Sheepdog	Iceland Dog, Icelandic Spitz, Íslenskur Fjárhundur, Islandsk Fårehund, Friaar Dog	Iceland	31–46	31–42	9.1–13.6	9.1–13.6	11–13	7	17
Irish Red and White Setter	An Sotar Rua agus Bán	Ireland	62–66	56–61	25–34	25–34	11–13	7	17
Irish Setter	Red Setter, Sotar Rua	Ireland	61–71	55–62	29–24	25–29	11–13	7	17
Irish Terrier	Irish Red Terrier, Brocaire Rua	Ireland	45–50	45–50	11–12	11–12	13–15	8	19
Irish Water Spaniel	Whiptail, An Spáinnéar Uisce, Shannon Spaniel, Rat Tail Spaniel, Bog Dog	Ireland	56–61	56–61	25–30	25–30	10–12	6	16
Irish Wolfhound		Ireland	71–90	71–90	40–69	40–69	7–9	5	13
Italian Greyhound	Italian Sighthound, Piccolo Levriero Italiano, Galgo Italiano, Levrette d'Italie, Italienisches Windspiel, Italiaans Windhondje	Italy	33–38	33–38	3.6–8.2	3.6–8.2	13–15	8	19
Jack Russell Terrier	Jack Russell	United Kingdom	25–38	25–38	6.4–78.2	6.4–78.2	13–15	8	19
Japanese Chin	Japanese Spaniel	China	20–27	20–27	1.4–6.8	1.4–6.8	12–14	7	18
Japanese Spitz	Nihon Supittsu	Japan	30–38	29–37	6–10	5–9	12–14	7	17

(Continued)

Name	Also Known As	Country of Origin	Male Height range (cm)	Female Height Range (cm)	Male Weight Range (kg)	Female Weight Range (kg)	Typical Lifespan (years)	Senior status (years)	Healthspan Target (years)
Kangal Shepherd Dog	Anatolian Shepherd Dog, Sivas Kangal, Anadolu Çoban Köpeği, Kangal, Karabash, Turkish Shepherd Dog	Turkey	74–81	71–79	50–63	41–59	10–12	6	16
Karelian Bear Dog	Karjalankarhukoira, Karelsk Björnhund	Finland	54–60	49–55	20–23	20–23	11–13	7	16
Keeshond	Dutch Barge Dog, Wolfspitz	Germany	44–48	40–46	15–20	15–20	12–14	7	18
Kerry Blue Terrier	Irish Blue Terrier	Ireland	46–48	44–46	12–15	10–13	12–14	7	18
Komondor	Hungarian Sheepdog	Hungary	70–80	65–70	50–60	40–50	10–12	6	16
Koolie	Australian Koolie, Coulie	Australia	40–60	40–58	15–24	15–24	11–13	7	16
Kromfohrländer	Länder Kromi	Germany	40–46	38–44	11–14	10–13	11–13	7	16
Kuvasz	Hungarian Kuvasz	Hungary	70–76	65–70	45–52	32–41	9–11	6	15
Labrador Retriever	Labrador, Lab	Canada	57–62	55–60	29–36	25–32	10–12	6	16
Lagotto Romagnolo	Romagna Water Dog, Water Dog of Romagna	Italy	43–48	41–46	13–16	11–14	12–14	7	17
Lakeland Terrier		United Kingdom	33–38	33–38	7–8	7–8	12–14	7	18
Lancashire Heeler	Ormskirk Heeler, Ormskirk Terrier	United Kingdom	25–30	25–30	6–8	6–8	12–14	7	17
Landseer	Landseer-ECT	Canada	72–80	67–72	65–80	60–75	10–12	6	15
Lapponian Herder	Lapinporokoira, Lappland Reindeer Dog, Lapsk Vallhund	Finland	51–53	46–50	25–30	25–28	12–14	7	17
Leonberger		Germany	71–80	65–75	54–77	45–61	8–10	5	14
Lhasa Apso	Lhasa	Tibet	25–28	25–28	5–7	5–7	13–15	8	19
Löwchen	Little Lion Dog, Petit Chien Lion	France	30–36	28–33	4–7	4–7	12–14	7	18
Lurcher		United Kingdom	60–71	55–68	29–32	27–30	12–14	7	17
Maltese		Malta	20–25	20–23	2–3.6	1–3	12–14	7	18
Manchester Terrier		United Kingdom	38–40	38–40	5–10	5–10	13–15	8	19
Maremma Sheepdog	Maremmano-Abruzzese Sheepdog, Cane da Pastore Maremmano-Abruzzese, Maremmano, Abruzzese Sheepdog, Pastore Abruzzese, Pastore Maremmano	Italy	65–73	60–68	35–45	30–40	10–12	6	15
Markiesje	Dutch Tulip Hound	Netherlands	36–41	34–39	5–7	5–6	13–15	8	19

Name	Also Known As	Country of Origin	Male Height range (cm)	Female Height Range (cm)	Male Weight Range (kg)	Female Weight Range (kg)	Typical Lifespan (years)	Senior status (years)	Healthspan Target (years)
Mastiff		United Kingdom	70–91	70–91	68–113	54–84	10–12	6	16
Mastiff (English)	Old English Mastiff	United Kingdom	76–86	70–80	68–100	54–82	9–11	6	15
McNab Shepherd	McNab, McNab Dog, McNab Collie, McNab Herding Dog, McNab Sheepdog	United States of America	45–64	40–54	16–30	14–23	13–15	8	16
Mi-Ki	MiKi	United States of America	25–28	25–28	4–5	4–5	13–15	8	18
Miniature Pinscher	Zwergpinscher, Min Pin	Germany	25–30	25–28	4–5	3.5–4	12–14	7	18
Mixed Breed	Mutt, Mongrel				< 5	< 5	13–15	8	20
Mixed Breed	Mutt, Mongrel				5–10	5–10	12–14	7	19
Mixed Breed	Mutt, Mongrel				10–20	10–20	11–13	7	18
Mixed Breed	Mutt, Mongrel				20–30	20–30	10–12	6	17
Mixed Breed	Mutt, Mongrel				30–40	30–40	10–12	6	16
Mixed Breed	Mutt, Mongrel				40–50	40–50	9–11	6	15
Mixed Breed	Mutt, Mongrel				>50	>50	8–10	5	14
Mudi	Hungarian Mudi	Hungary	40–48	38–46	10–13	9–12	11–13	7	16
Münsterländer, Large	Großer Münsterländer	Germany	60–65	58–63	27–33	26–32	11–13	7	15
Münsterländer, Small	Kleiner Münsterländer, Heidewachtel	Germany	52–56	50–54	17–26	17–24	12–14	7	17
Neapolitan Mastiff	Mastino, Mastino Napoletano, Italian Molosso, Can'e presa	Italy	66–79	61–74	60–70	50–60	8–10	5	14
New Zealand Huntaway	Huntaway, New Zealand Sheepdog, New Zealand Huntadog	New Zealand	58–66	56–64	27–45	25–43	12–14	7	17
Newfoundland		Canada	69–74	63–69	59–68	54–54	8–10	5	14
Norbottenspets	Nordic Spitz, Norrbottenspitz, Pohjanpystykorva	Sweden	42–46	42–46	11–15	8–12	12–14	7	17
Norfolk Terrier		United Kingdom	23–25	23–25	5–5.4	5–5.4	12–14	7	18
Norwegian Buhund	Norsk Buhund, Norwegian Sheepdog	Norway	43–47	41–45	14–18	12–16	12–14	7	18
Norwegian Elkhound	Norsk Elghund, Norwegian Moose Dog, Harmaa norjanhirvikoira	Norway	48–53	46–51	23–27	18–25	12–14	7	18
Norwegian Lundehund	Norsk Lundehund, Norwegian Puffin Dog	Norway	30–40	30–40	6–7	6–7	12–14	7	18
Norwich Terrier		United Kingdom	24–25.5	24–25.5	5–5.5	5–5.5	12–14	7	18

(Continued)

Name	Also Known As	Country of Origin	Male Height range (cm)	Female Height Range (cm)	Male Weight Range (kg)	Female Weight Range (kg)	Typical Lifespan (years)	Senior status (years)	Healthspan Target (years)
Nova Scotia Duck Tolling Retriever	Yarmouth Toller, Toller	Canada	48–51	45–48	20–23	17–20	12–14	7	18
Old English Sheepdog	Bob-Tail, Bobtail	United Kingdom	56–61	51–56	29–45	29–45	10–12	6	16
Otterhound		United Kingdom	60–65	60–65	30–52	30–52	10–12	6	16
Papillon	Continental Toy Spaniel, Epagneul Nain Continental, Phalène	Belgium	20–28	20–28	4–5	3–4	12–14	7	18
Parson Russell Terrier	Parson Jack Russell Terrier, Parson	United Kingdom	31–36	31–36	6–8	6–8	13–15	8	19
Patterdale Terrier		United Kingdom	27–38	25–36	5–6	5–6	13–15	8	19
Pekingese	Peke, Beijingese, Lion Dog, Chinese Spaniel, Pelchie, Peking Palasthund	China	15–23	15–23	3.2–6.4	3.2–6.4	12–14	7	18
Perro de Presa Canario	Canary Mastiff, Canarian Molosser, Dogo Canario, Presa Canario	Spain	61–66	57–62	45–57	40–50	10–12	6	15
Peruvian Inca Orchid	Inca Hairless Dog, Perro Sin Pelo de Perú, Viringo, Peruvian Hairless Dog, Calato, Dielmatian	Peru	30–65	25–62	6–25	4–23	12–14	7	18
Petit Basset Griffon Vendéen		France	34–38	34–38	14–18	14–18	12–14	7	18
Pharaoh Hound	Kelb tal-Fenek	Malta	59–63	53–61	20–25	20–25	11–13	7	17
Plott Hound	Plott, Plotthund	United States of America	55–71	53–63	23–27	18–25	11–13	7	17
Pointer (English)	Pointer, English Pointer	United Kingdom	55–62	54–60	20–30	20–30	11–13	7	17
Polish Lowland Sheepdog	Polski Owczarek Nizinny, Valee Sheepdog	Poland	45–50	42–47	14–23	14–23	11–13	7	17
Pomeranian	Pom, Zwergspitz, Dwarf-Spitz, Deutscher Spitz	Germany	13–28	13–28	1.9–3.5	1.9–3.5	13–15	8	19
Poodle, Miniature	Caniche, Pudelhund	France	30–38	28–36	7–9	6–8	13–15	8	20
Poodle, Moyen	Caniche, Pudelhund	France	37–45	35–43	10–15	9–13	11–13	7	17
Poodle, Standard	Caniche, Pudelhund	France	45–60	45–60	20–32	20–27	12–14	7	18
Poodle, Toy	Caniche, Pudelhund	France	24–28	24–28	2–4	2–4	13–15	8	19
Portuguese Podengo Grande	Podengo Portugues, Portuguese Warren Hound	Portugal	55–71	54–70	20–30	20–30	12–14	7	18

Name	Also Known As	Country of Origin	Male Height range (cm)	Female Height Range (cm)	Male Weight Range (kg)	Female Weight Range (kg)	Typical Lifespan (years)	Senior status (years)	Healthspan Target (years)
Portuguese Podengo Pequeno	Podengo Portugues, Portuguese Warren Hound	Portugal	20–31	20–31	4–6	4–6	12–14	7	18
Portuguese Water Dog	Cão de água Português, Cão de Água Algarvio, Algarvian Water Dog, Portuguese Fishing Dog	Portugal	50–57	43–52	19–25	16–22	11–13	7	17
Pudelpointer		Germany	60–68	55–63	20–30	20–30	11–13	7	16
Pug	Chinese pug	China	30–36	25–30	6–9	6–8	12–14	7	18
Puli	Hungarian Puli	Hungary	41–46	36–41	13–15	10–13	12–14	7	18
Pumi	Hungarian Pumi, Hungarian Herding Terrier	Hungary	43–45	40–42	12–13	10–11	12–14	7	17
Pyrenean Shepherd	Berger des Pyrénées, Pastor de Los Pirineos, Pyrenees Sheepdog	France	39–53	38–52	7–15	7–15	11–13	7	17
Rat Terrier	American Rat Terrier, Ratting Terrier	United States of America	33–45	33–45	4.5–11.3	4.5–11.3	14–16	8	20
Rhodesian Ridgeback	African Lion Dog, African Lion Hound	South Africa	63–69	61–66	36–41	29–35	10–12	6	16
Rottweiler	Rottie	Germany	61–69	56–63	50–60	35–48	8–10	5	14
Ryukyu Inu	Ryukyu Dog, Okinawa Native Dog, Tora Inu	Japan	46–50	43–47	17–25	15–23	12–14	7	17
Saarloos Wolf Dog	Saarloos Wolfdog, Saarloos Wolfhound, Saarloos-Wolfhond	Netherlands	65–75	60–70	40–45	37–43	11–13	7	15
Saint Bernard	St Bernhardshund	Switzerland	70–90	70–90	65–120	65–120	8–10	5	14
Saluki	Persian Hound	Iran	58–71	58–71	18–27	18–27	12–14	7	18
Samoyed	Bjelkier, Samoiedskaya Sobaka	Russia	53–60	48–53	20.5–30	16–20.5	12–14	7	18
Schapendoes	Dutch Shapendoes, Nederlandse Schapendoes, Dutch Sheepdog	Netherlands	40–50	37–47	20–25	18–23	11–13	7	16
Schipperke		Belgium	21–33	21–33	5.5–8	5.5–8	13–15	8	19
Schnauzer, Giant	Riesenschnauzer	Germany	66–71	58–66	27–48	25–34	12–14	7	18
Schnauzer, Miniature	Zwergschnauzer	Germany	30–36	30–36	5–8.2	4.5–6.8	12–14	7	18
Schnauzer, Standard	Mittelschnauzer	Germany	46–51	43–48	16–26	14–20	12–14	7	18
Schweizer Laufhund (Swiss Hound)	Swiss Hound, Jura Hound	Switzerland	49–59	47–57	18–22	17–20	11–13	7	16
Scottish Deerhound	Deerhound	United Kingdom	75–80	70–80	40–50	35–43	8–10	5	14

(Continued)

Name	Also Known As	Country of Origin	Male Height range (cm)	Female Height Range (cm)	Male Weight Range (kg)	Female Weight Range (kg)	Typical Lifespan (years)	Senior status (years)	Healthspan Target (years)
Scottish Terrier	Scottie, Aberdeen Terrier, Abhag Albannach	United Kingdom	25–28	25–28	8.5–10.5	8.5–10.5	12–14	7	18
Sealyham Terrier	Welsh Border Terrier, Cowley Terrier, Daeargi Sealyham	United Kingdom	26–30	26–30	10–11	10–11	12–14	7	18
Shetland Sheepdog	Sheltie	United Kingdom	33–41	33–41	5–10.9	5–10.9	11–13	7	17
Shiba Inu	Shiba Ken, Japanese Shiba Inu, Japanese Brushwood Dog, Japanese Turf Dog	Japan	36–41	33–38	8–11	7–9	12–14	7	18
Shih Tzu	Chinese Lion Dog, Chrysanthemum Dog	China	20–28	20–28	4–7.25	4–7.25	12–14	7	18
Shiloh Shepherd Dog	Shiloh, Shiloh Shepherd	United States of America	71–76	66–71	54–65	45–54	10–12	6	15
Siberian Husky	Sibirskiy Khaski, Chukcha	Russia	53–61	51–56	20–27	16–23	10–12	6	16
Silken Windhound	Silken, Windhound	United States of America	45–60	45–58	15–25	10–20	12–14	7	18
Silky Terrier	Australian Silky Terrier	Australia	23–25	23–25	4–5	4–5	12–14	7	18
Skye Terrier		United Kingdom	23–25	23–25	16–18	11.5–14	12–14	7	18
Sloughi	Arabian Greyhound, Sloughi Moghrebi	Morocco	66–72	61–68	22–28	18–23	12–14	7	17
Soft-Coated Wheaten Terrier	Wheaten, Irish Soft-Coated Wheaten Terrier, An Brocaire Buí	Ireland	46–51	43–48	16–20	14–18	12–14	7	18
Spanish Water Dog	Perro de Agua Español	Spain	44–50	40–45	18–22	14–18	10–12	6	16
Spinone Italiano	Spinone, Italian Spinone, Italian Griffon, Italian Wirehaired Pointer, Italian Coarsehaired Pointer	Italy	60–70	60–70	34–39	34–39	12–14	7	18
Springer Spaniel, English	English Springer Spaniel, Springer Spaniel	United Kingdom	48–56	46–51	20–25	18–23	11–13	7	17
Springer Spaniel, Welsh	Welsh Spaniel, Llamgi Cymru	United Kingdom	43–48	41–46	18–20	16–20	12–14	7	18
Stabyhoun	Stabij, Beike, Stabijhoun, Fryske Stabij	Netherlands	50–55	48–53	23–25	18–23	10–12	6	15
Staffordshire Bull Terrier	Stafford, Staffy	United Kingdom	36–41	36–41	13–17	11–15.4	12–14	7	18
Sussex Spaniel	Sussex	United Kingdom	38–40	38–40	18–20	18–20	11–13	7	17
Swedish Elkhound	Jämthund	Sweden	57–65	52–60	30–35	25–30	10–12	6	15

Name	Also Known As	Country of Origin	Male Height range (cm)	Female Height Range (cm)	Male Weight Range (kg)	Female Weight Range (kg)	Typical Lifespan (years)	Senior status (years)	Healthspan Target (years)
Swedish Lapphund	Svensk Lapphund	Sweden	45–51	40–46	19–21	19–21	11–13	7	16
Swedish Vallhund	Västgötaspets, Swedish Cow Dog	Sweden	30–40	30–40	11–15	11–15	12–14	7	18
Teddy Roosevelt Terrier		United States of America	20–38	20–38	4.5–11	4.5–11	14–16	8	20
Tenterfield Terrier		Australia	23–31	22–30	3.5–5	3.5–4.5	12–14	7	18
Tibetan Mastiff	Wylie, Zàng Áo	Tibet	61–71	61–71	64–78	64–78	10–12	6	16
Tibetan Spaniel	Simkhyi	Tibet	23–25	23–25	4.1–6.8	4.1–6.8	12–14	7	18
Tibetan Terrier	Tsang Apso, Dokhi Apso	Tibet	36–43	36–43	8.2–13.6	8.2–13.6	13–15	8	19
Tosa Inu	Tosa, Tosa-Ken, Tosa Tōken, Japanese Mastiff	Japan	65–82	62–78	40–90	36–86	8–10	5	14
Vizsla	Hungarian Vizsla, Hungarian Pointer, Magyar Vizsla	Hungary	56–64	53–61	20–30	18–25	11–13	7	17
Volpino Italiano	Volpino, Cane del Quirinale, Florentine Spitz, Italian Spitz	Italy	27–30	25–28	4.5–5.5	4.1–4.5	12–14	7	17
Wachtelhund (German Spaniel)	German Spaniel, Deutscher Wachtelhund, German Quail Dog	Germany	48–54	45–52	20–25	18–23	11–13	7	16
Weimaraner	Weimaraner Vorstehhund	Germany	63–68	58–63	32–37	25–32	10–12	6	16
Welsh Corgi, Cardigan	Cardigan Welsh Corgi	United Kingdom	25–33	25–33	11–14	11–14	12–14	7	18
Welsh Corgi, Pembroke	Pembroke Welsh Corgi	United Kingdom	25–30	25–30	10–14	11–13	12–14	7	18
Welsh Terrier	Daeargi Cymreig	United Kingdom	38–40	38–40	9–9.5	9–9.5	12–14	7	18
West Highland White Terrier	Westie, Poltalloch Terrier, Roseneath Terrier, White Roseneath Terrier	United Kingdom	25–30	23–28	7–10	6–7	13–15	8	19
Whippet	English Whippet, Snap Dog	United Kingdom	47–57	44–55	9.1–19.1	9.1–19.1	12–14	7	18
Wirehaired Pointing Griffon	Korthals Griffon, Griffon d'Arrêt à Poil dur Korthals	Netherlands	56–61	51–56	23–27	23–27	10–12	6	16
Xoloitzcuintli	Xoloitzcuintle, Xolo, Mexican Hairless Dog, Mexican Hairless	Mexico	25–60	24–58	4–25	4–22	13–15	8	19
Yorkshire Terrier	Yorkie	United Kingdom	15–17.5	15–17.5	1.8–2.8	1.8–2.8	13–15	8	19
Yugoslavian Shepherd Dog (Sarplaninac)	Šarplaninac, Šarplaninec, Yugoslavia Sheepdog	Serbia	60–64	56–60	35–45	30–40	9–11	6	15

Recommended Reading

AAFP/AAHA. 2010. Feline Life Stage Guidelines. https://catvets.com/guidelines/practice-guidelines/life-stage-guidelines.

AAHA. 2019. Canine Life Stage Guidelines. www.aaha.org/aaha-guidelines/life-stage-canine-2019/life-stage-canine-2019/.

www.dogbreedinfo.com/a-z.htm

https://dogtime.com/dog-breeds

www.worldlifeexpectancy.com/dog-life-expectancy

11.6

Glossary

Lowell Ackerman, DVM, DACVD, MBA, MPA, CVA, MRCVS

Global Consultant, Author, and Lecturer, MA, USA

Below is a glossary of terms useful to a discussion of pet-specific care. These definitions may differ slightly from the terms defined within individual topics, which might have more topic-specific explanations as well as potentially providing more detail.

10-Minute Flex	Scheduling system that allows the user to determine the appropriate amount of time for the appointment based on the number of 10-minute blocks that are combined. Therefore, an appointment could be 10 minutes, 20 minutes, 30 minutes, or 40 minutes, as needed.
360 Evaluation	Performance appraisal information collected from peers, supervisors, subordinates, and even customers to get a broader perspective on an employee's performance.
Abandonment	The relinquishing of a right or interest with the intention of never again claiming it.
ABC Analysis	An assessment of inventory items based on their economic value with usage, sales, and cost. An ABC analysis is an extension of the Pareto Principle and a method of grading products based on their usage and turnover.
Abnormal Behaviors	Behaviors rooted in abnormal anxiety, stress, or fear, such as compulsive disorders, picas, thunder phobias, separation anxiety, etc.
Absenteeism	The practice of regularly missing work without good reason.
Abuse, Animal	Traditionally reserved for acts causing unnecessary injury or death to an animal, such as overworking, torturing, traumatizing, or mutilating.
Accessibility	The ease of reaching and approaching.
Accountability	The obligation to be responsible and to act in the best interest of the organization and its mission.
Accounts Payable	Monies owed by a practice to its creditors (laboratories, distributors, etc.).
Accounts Receivable	Monies owed to a company for goods sold or services rendered for which payment has not yet been received.
Acquisition Cost	The wholesale unit cost at which a product or service can be purchased, including any delivery fees and/or taxes.
Acquisition Marketing	Marketing to pet owners that are not your clients to get them to choose your practice for their veterinary care.
Activities of Daily Living (ADL)	Daily activities that a client or pet normally performs (related to hygiene, exercise, play, eating and drinking, etc.) and which may require support in order to maintain quality of life.
Acupuncture	A form of medical treatment in which thin needles are inserted into the body at very specific locations in order to exert a neuromodulatory effect.

Pet-Specific Care for the Veterinary Team, First Edition. Edited by Lowell Ackerman.
© 2021 John Wiley & Sons, Inc. Published 2021 by John Wiley & Sons, Inc.

Acute Kidney Injury (AKI)	A sudden insult to renal function that results in inadequate to absent urine production and the subsequent accumulation of nitrogenous waste products within the bloodstream.
Adaptive Coping	Positive coping strategies that provide long-term stress management.
Adaptive Leadership	Incorporating change by challenging the status quo, and adapting leadership styles to yield success.
Adherence	The extent to which clients administer medications prescribed, including administering the correct dose, timing and use, and completing the prescribed course.
Adolescence	The period between puberty and social maturity.
Adoption	An action that permanently alters the relationship between a pet and its prior guardian. As contrasted with guardianship, which od a legal relationship between guardian and ward.
Adverse Drug Event (ADE)	Any adverse event associated with the use of an animal drug, whether or not considered to be drug related, and whether or not the drug was used in accordance with the approved purpose.
Adverse Event	When patients come to harm as a result of their veterinary treatment journey.
Adverse Event, Serious	Any adverse event which results in death, is life-threatening or results in persistent or significant disability/incapacity, or a congenital anomaly or birth defect.
Adverse Incident	A medical error that harms the patient.
Adverse Outcome	Unanticipated harm that was induced by appropriate veterinary medical care.
Advertising	A marketing effort to promote or sell a product, service or idea
Advocate	Someone who speaks or takes action on behalf of another.
After-Hours Emergency Practice	This type of facility provides emergency services when regular primary care (first opinion) practices are presumed to be closed.
Aggression	Behavior intended to harm, or at least threaten to harm, another.
Aging	A complex set of biological changes occurring in older individuals that result in a progressive reduction of the ability to maintain homeostasis when exposed to internal physiological and external environmental stresses.
Allele	A variant or alternative form of a gene, found at the same location on a chromosome, and which can result in different observable traits.
Allergen	A substance capable of inducing an allergic reaction.
Allodynia	A pain response to nonnoxious stimuli such as touch and light pressure.
Ambulatory Practice	Generally used to refer to work out of a vehicle, with or without additional equipment such as a portable ultrasound, x-ray unit, or dental equipment.
Ambulatory Services	Services provided by a veterinarian at an owner's premises, away from the clinic.
Analytics	Techniques and processes used to enhance productivity through data analysis.
Anesthesia	The rendering of a patient insensitive to pain, typically by means of gas inhalation or the administration of injectable drugs.
Animal Dietary Supplement	A substance for oral consumption intended for specific benefit to an animal by means other than provision of nutrients recognized as essential.
Animal Drug	Any article intended for use in the diagnosis, cure, mitigation, treatment, or prevention of disease in animals other than humans.
Animal Hospice	A philosophy and/or a program of care that addresses the physical, emotional, and social needs of animals in the advanced stages of a progressive, life-limiting illness or disability as well as the mental health of the human caregivers in preparation for the death of the pet and subsequent grief.
Antecedent	Anything that happens before the target behavior, such as a cue or a trigger. Antecedents can be environmental, gesture, sound, smell, person, etc.
Anthropomorphism	Attributing human characteristics to nonhuman entities, such as animals.

Antibody	A large, Y-shaped protein that is produced by the body to inactivate pathogens, including viruses and bacteria. An antibody is antigen specific, meaning that it only binds to the substance that it was primed to attack.
Antigen	A specific substance that has the potential to trigger an immune response by activating the body's lines of defense.
Antimicrobial Resistance	The property of a bacterial population to survive exposure to an antimicrobial that previously would have been an effective treatment. Resistance can be conferred by mutation or gene transfer.
Antiseptic	Antimicrobial agents that are applied to living tissues (e.g., skin) to decrease the number of microorganisms present.
Antivirus Software	Used to prevent, detect, and remove malware (of all descriptions), such as computer viruses, adware, backdoors, malicious BHOs, dialers, fraudtools, hijackers, keyloggers, malicious LSPs, rootkits, spyware, Trojan horses, and worms.
Anxiety	A diffuse generalized feeling of apprehension, unease, and/or nervousness regarding a potential threat, uncertain outcome, or danger.
Anxiety Disorder	A persistent state of negative emotional state without identifiable trigger or stimulus. Interferes with the individual's daily life and causes significant distress.
Anybody	Generic term used by many practices to identify a client who scheduled an appointment but did not request a specific doctor. Therefore, "anybody" can see this client.
Apathy	Lack of interest, lack of feeling; not caring.
Application, Insurance	A form that insurance companies collect and use to decide if they want to provide insurance.
Approximation	A step toward the desired behavior.
Archetype	A recurrent symbol or motif in literature, art, or mythology.
Asepsis	A state where no living organisms are present.
Assessment	The gathering of data about a patient.
Assets	Things of value, such as cash, equipment, inventory, or buildings.
Associate Veterinarians	Those veterinarians who work for the practice, but do not have any ownership in the business. Also known as employed veterinarians.
Association of American Feed Control Officials (AAFCO)	Nongovernmental organization in the United States that creates model animal feed laws, regulations, and ingredient definitions, which then may be adopted by individual state agencies charged with regulation of animal feed.
Atopic Dermatitis	The preferred term for a genetically predisposed inflammatory and pruritic skin disease with characteristic clinical presentation. Previously known by several terms, including atopy, inhalant allergies, eczema, and hay fever.
Atopic March	The natural progression and evolution of allergic manifestations that occurs over time.
Attachment	The enduring emotional bond between individuals. It is characterized by behaviors such as seeking proximity to the individual and being attentive to their needs.
Attachment Loss, Dental	Loss of any periodontal tissues around the tooth (gingiva, bone, periodontal ligament, cementum).
Audiences/Stakeholders	The individuals that have the potential to be impacted by business situations and that represent the front line of accountability for a business.
Audit	Methodical examination and review of practice records to assess accuracy and completeness.
Autocratic Leadership	A style of leadership whereby one person has sole influence over a group of people within an organization
Automated Clearing House (ACH)	The national automated bank payment clearing system in the United States.

Autonomic Shifts	Physiological manifestations that reflect individual response, emotion, and reaction (for example, flushing, blanching, tearing, sweating, piloerection, changes in breathing and pupil size, swallowing, and dry mouth).
Average Transaction Charge (ATC)	Total revenue over a period of time divided by the total number of transactions during that same period; this represents the average amount spent by clients at the practice.
Azotemia	Elevated levels of nitrogenous compounds in the bloodstream, in particular, blood urea nitrogen (urea) and creatinine.
Baby Boom Generation	Commonly called "Boomers," this generation of people was born after the end of World War II, between the years 1946 and 1964.
Back-Up	In information technology, a back-up, or the process of backing up, refers to the copying and archiving of computer data so it may be used to restore the original after a data loss event.
Backyard Breeder	An amateur animal breeder whose breeding is considered substandard, with little or misguided effort toward ethical, selective breeding
Beacons	The technology enables smartphones, tablets and other devices to perform actions (such as receive push notifications, open web pages and social media activities) when in close proximity to a beacon.
Bedside Manner	Perception of how well a physician relates to a client or patient
Behavioral Counseling	The systematic approach to discovering, diagnosing, and treating behavioral issues, encouraging better client compliance and success.
Behavioral Interviewing	A job interviewing technique in which the applicant is asked to describe past behavior and experiences to help determine appropriateness for an available position.
Benchmarking	Process by which a practice compares itself to others (especially those known for outstanding performance) in an attempt to improve performance.
Benchmarks	Numbers, percentages, dollars, or some type of measurable quantity for a given period of time that are industry standards.
Benchmarks, Historical	Data from a practice that represent various time periods. The most common historical data are collected at the end of each operating year, although other periods of time may be used depending on the specific focus of the research.
Beneficiary	The individual who benefits from a trust agreement.
Benefit Schedule	Summary of covered services, benefit limitations, and applicable co-payments provided in an insurance policy.
Benefit Stream	Any level of revenue (income), cash flow or earnings (profit) generated by a business entity.
Beta-Blockers	A group of medications that can be utilized in cases of glaucoma to reduce intraocular pressure by decreasing aqueous humor formation.
Bias	Any systematic deviation of research results from the true state of the subject being studied. Most often, bias is an unintentional result of how research studies are designed and conducted. Also, prejudice in favor of or against one thing, person, or group compared with another, usually in a way considered to be unfair.
Big Picture	The larger context of a situation, not just what is immediately apparent.
Bioavailability	The degree to which a substance is actually available to be absorbed into the body and is utilized.
Biofilm	A collection of microorganisms and extracellular matrix that adheres to the surface of inanimate or living beings.
Biological Response Modifier	A type of treatment that mobilizes the body's immune system to fight disease.
Biopharmaceutical	Also known as biologicals, these are pharmaceutical drugs derived from biological sources.
Biophilic Design	Design inspired by humans' inherent need to connect with the natural world.

Biosecurity	Procedures used to reduce the risk of the introduction or internal spread of infectious organisms in a facility or operation. Cleaning, disinfection, quarantine, limiting access by unauthorized personnel, and limiting the introduction of potentially contaminated materials are essential practices.
Biosimilars	Approved versions of innovator biopharmaceutical products.
Bioterrorism	A premeditated attack on people, animals, or plants using infectious biological agents as a weapon.
Blockchain	A database that is shared across a network of computers.
Blog	A discussion or informational site published on the World Wide Web and consisting of discrete entries (posts) typically displayed in reverse chronological order (the most recent posts appearing first).
Blood Pressure (BP)	The force of blood moving through the arteries as produced by myocardial contractility, represented most typically in medicine as two numbers. The first number represents systolic pressure and it occurs immediately after the heart contracts; the second number represents diastolic pressure and it is the lowest number that is seen throughout the cardiac cycle.
Blood Pressure (BP) Measurement, Direct	The placement of an arterial line where a catheter is fed into the lumen of an artery, so that, once connected to a transducer, the actual BP of the patient can be recorded.
Blood Pressure (BP) Measurement, Indirect	The use of Doppler ultrasonic devices or oscillometric tools to determine BP indirectly.
Blood-Borne Pathogens	Generally refers to disease-causing organisms present in blood, but could refer to any organism capable of infecting a human from blood or body fluid contact.
Bluetooth®	A low-power wireless technology that allows devices to communicate.
Board Certification	The recognition of a veterinarian's expertise in a particular specialty or subspecialty of veterinary medicine, as determined by a certifying body within the profession. Board certification typically follows an approved residency program in the specialty as well as passing certifying examinations in the specialty.
Body Condition Score (BCS)	System of assigning a number to indicate a pet's degree of adiposity (fat) based on visual and tactile cues.
Body Language	Communicating nonverbally through movements or position.
Bonding Philosophy	There are two primary bonding philosophies in multidoctor practices. The first is to bind clients to the practice. The second binds the client to a specific doctor.
Bonding Rate	A measure of the client bond with a specific doctor, calculated as the percentage of appointments with a doctor in which that doctor was specifically requested.
Bottom Line	Typically, a synonym for profit, referring to the bottom line in financial statements that indicates net profit or loss In calculations, Bottom line = Revenues − Cost of Goods Sold − Operating Expenses − Professional Salaries − Taxes.
Brachycephalic	A term used to refer to breeds with flat faces, such as pugs and Himalayans.
Brachycephalic Syndrome	A pathological condition of respiratory distress affecting dogs and cats with short noses. Also referred to as brachycephalic airway syndrome and brachycephalic obstructive airway syndrome.
Brand	A brand is made up of the name, symbol, design, messages, and ethos that together form the identity of a practice, differentiating it from its competitors. A brand allows those familiar with it to distinguish it among its competitors.
Brand Champion	Someone who advocates for and embodies a brand; enthusiastically promotes a practice with passion.
Brand Equity	The value of a brand.
Brand Identity	Unique set of associations that the brand strategiest aspires to create or maintain.
Brand Promise	The spoken or unspoken expression of the continuing, important, and specific benefits clients connect with a firm, service or product.

Branding	The practice of creating a consistent image for a brand.
Breakeven Point	The level of sales that will just cover all costs, both fixed and variable. It can be expressed in dollars or units sold (or, in a veterinary practice, the number of patients treated with a specific service).
Breed Clubs	Organization of like-minded individuals concerned about the issues and interest of specific breeds.
Breed-Specific Marketing	Educating clients about the pertinent risks relevant to their specific pet in order to encourage proactive engagement. Breed-specific marketing also refers to programs created to educate and inform clients about their pet's risks based upon that breed's associated risk factors.
Broadband	An internet connection with a much larger capacity than dial-up (e.g., cable, DSL, or fiberoptics).
Brochure	A pamphlet or handout bound or folded in booklet form.
Budget	Quantitative expression of a financial plan of action for the practice.
Buphthalmia or Buphthalmos	Increased size of the globe (eye).
Burden of Proof	Level of proof that must be provided by the plaintiff in order to prevail in a legal action. In negligence actions, the plaintiff must usually prove that the probability of negligence and harm is "more likely than not." The legal term often applied to this burden of proof is "by a preponderance of the evidence," a much lower burden than the "beyond reasonable doubt" required in criminal cases.
Burnout	The endpoint of chronic exposure to a stressful work environment.
Business Contingency (Continuity) Planning	Process of developing, communicating, practicing, and evaluating a comprehensive emergency plan to keep a business operating in the face of adverse conditions and to recover quickly from a disaster.
Business Intelligence (BI)	Business intelligence is the accumulation, analysis, reporting, budgeting, and presentation of business financial and operational data. The goal of utilizing business intelligence for a veterinary hospital is to increase the visibility of hospital operations and financial status to better lead and manage the hospital.
Buyer Journey	A framework that acknowledges a buyer's progression through a research and decision process ultimately culminating in a purchase.
Buy-In	In management and decision making, buy-in signifies the commitment of interested or affected parties to a decision to "buy in" to the action specified; that is, to agree to give it support, often by having been involved in the process.
Calculus Index (CI)	A measurement of the accumulation of calculus on the tooth surface.
Call to Action (CTA)	A request within a communication for the recipient to initiate a desired behavior, e.g., phone, email, visit the practice to make a purchase or book an appointment.
Call-to-Action Button	A call-to-action (CTA) button directs visitors to do something specific, like visit your website, call your practice or book an appointment.
Campaign	An organized effort that involves a connected series of initiatives designed to bring about a particular result.
Cannabidiol (CBD)	Cannabidiol (CBD) is a compound found in the flower of the *Cannabis* plant. CBD is nonintoxicating and thought to have certain medical benefits.
Carbon Footprint	A measure of the global warming potential of a given project, system, or activity using carbon dioxide equivalents (CO_2E).
Carbonic Anhydrase Inhibitors	A group of medications used for glaucoma which inhibit the enzyme carbonic anhydrase which leads to decreased aqueous humor formation and thereby decreases intraocular pressure.
Carcinogen	Substance or agent that is known to cause cancer.
Care Bundle	A group of evidence-based interventions related to a disease, set of clinical signs or clinical procedure that when implemented together result in better outcomes than when implemented separately.

Care Guidelines (Care Recommendations)	The set of processes and practices that meet the needs of both the pet and the pet owner.
Care Pathway	Also known as clinical pathways and care maps, care pathways are evidence-based practices for specific groups of patients with a predictable clinical course in which professional intervention can be defined, optimized and sequenced, and in which the outcomes can be measured, contributing further to evidence-based evaluation.
Care Plan	An alternative term for "estimate" with a focus more on care than cost.
Care Planning	The process of recognizing an animal's problems and making decisions about clinical interventions to assist in addressing them.
Care Plans, Personalized	Long-term outline of the examinations, diagnostics, procedures, monitoring, and other care that a pet will need and most benefit from throughout its life.
Care Team	The veterinarian(s), technicians, assistants, and customer service representatives (CSRs) that regularly and consistently care for and interact with a particular patient and client.
Career Pathing	Scheduled progression of responsibilities that helps an employee achieve a higher position. For example, a technician could become a shift manager, then a technician manager, and then a practice manager.
Carrier	In genetics, the situation where an individual has one typical and one atypical copy of a gene; that is, it is heterozygous for that phene.
Cascade of Care	The increasing array of tests that may be attempted when trying to understand an abnormal laboratory result that may be spurious. The term is also used to describe the different sequential aspects of care in the management of a complex disorder.
Castration	Surgical excision of the testicles.
Cataract	Any opacity of the crystalline lens.
Catchment Area	Area from which a business draws its clientele. Also known as a *trade area*.
Cat-Friendly Practices	Veterinary clinics where attention to the processes of transporting, attending to the examination, testing, and treatment of clients' cats has been planned and orchestrated to minimize distress to feline patients.
Central Sensitization	A condition within the nervous system in which there is the development and maintenance of a chronic pain state. This is sometimes referred to as *wind-up* and reflects a state of abnormal nervous system reactivity.
Change	To make or become different.
Change Agent	An individual that serves as a catalyst for change within the organization.
Change Management	Managing the people side of change to achieve a desired business outcome of change.
Charitable Corporation	A corporation that has been organized under state law as a nonprofit corporation and that meets the criteria under US Internal Revenue Code Section 501(c)(3) to have its income exempted from Federal income taxes and its donations tax deductible for the donors.
Chart of Accounts	An organized listing of all the income, expense, asset, liability, and equity categories used to record a practice entity's transactions that are monetarily measured.
Checklist	A tool that is intended to reduce human failure by drawing the user's attention to key tasks that must be performed in a particular order and allowing the user to mark off each task as it is performed to prevent missed steps.
Chemotherapeutic	Medication used to treat cancer.
Chemotherapy	The introduction of drugs into the body primarily used to treat cancers. Chemotherapy drugs are carcinogenic in long-term exposures outside therapeutic treatments. Chemotherapy drugs are often referred to as cytotoxic drugs because they are toxic at the cellular level.
Chiropractic	A form of medical treatment that relies on the restoration of normal movement throughout the musculoskeletal system, especially in the spine, by way of small-amplitude, high-velocity adjustments.

Choroidal Hypoplasia	Underdevelopment of the choroid, which is a tissue layer located beneath the retina.
Chromosome	The physical structure of DNA in pairs, one from the sire and one from the dam. The number of chromosomes varies between species.
Churn	The percentage of customers who cease their patronage of a given service.
Classical Conditioning	Also known as Pavlovian or respondent conditioning, this describes the pairing of a neutral stimulus with an unconditioned stimulus; through repeated pairing, the neutral stimulus becomes a conditioned stimulus and elicits a conditioned response.
Classical Counterconditioning	Changing a patient's conditioned emotional response (CER) to a perceived stimulus from an unpleasant emotion to a pleasant emotion.
Cleaning	Physical removal of microbial contaminants.
Click-Through Rate (CTR)	Number of clicks a website has received, particularly in reference to advertising.
Client	An individual or group who engages in a professional working relationship with a veterinarian or veterinary practice for the delivery of veterinary services.
Client Communications	Information shared between the client, the client's agents and the veterinarian and veterinarian's agents in pursuit of a diagnosis, treatment or prognosis.
Client Engagement	Refers to the communication connection and relationship between a client and the veterinary business.
Client Lifetime Value	Often referred to as CLV or LTV, client lifetime value is a prediction of the net profit attributed to the entire future relationship with a customer.
Client or Market Niche	A subset of a client or market segment that possesses like characteristics. An example of a client or market niche might be pet owners who go camping with their dogs.
Client Persona	A semi-fictional representation of an ideal client based on market research and real data about existing clients.
Client Profiling	Understanding a practice's existing client (and patient) base by grouping together pet owners based on a variety of like traits and attributes. These resulting client "segments" are then assumed to have similar needs and wants based on these attributes.
Client Segmentation	Using client profile data to categorize existing clients (and patients) into groups with similar characteristics.
Client Service	Refers to meeting the needs of individuals with whom you hope to maintain a long-standing relationship.
Client Service Representative	Employee who works at the front reception desk with primary responsibilities interacting with clients during the check-in and check-out process and ensuring their needs have been met.
Client-Centered Communication	An interaction with a focus on the client's needs, concerns, ideas, expectations, and preferences for the purpose of achieving a shared understanding between veterinarian and client.
Clinical Governance	The process of checking that care being given is to the highest possible standard, usually compared to contemporary evidence-based practice and/or previously agreed practice benchmarks.
Clinical Practice Guidelines	Systematically developed statements to assist practitioner and patient decisions about appropriate medical care for specific clinical circumstances.
Clone	Derivative of an animal with which it is genetically identical.
Closed-Ended Question	Question that can be answered with a "no" or "yes" response or a single word.
Cloud	A communications network that often refers to the internet, and more precisely to a datacenter full of services that is connected to the internet.
Cloud Computing	The use of computing resources (hardware and software) that are delivered as a service over a network (typically the internet).

Coaching	An ongoing approach to managing people by creating a motivating environment. It improves employee performance and increases their success by providing timely feedback, recognition, clarity, and support.
Code of Conduct	A set of rules defining acceptable behavior within the hospital, some of which might apply to clients as well as staff.
Codon	A sequence of three nucleotides that represents amino acids or start and stop commands as DNA constituents
Cognitive Decline	Normal age-related reduction in memory, learning, and reasoning skills.
Cognitive Dissonance	Mental discomfort experienced when an individual's beliefs or expectations clash with new information perceived by the individual.
Cognitive Impairment	Problems with concentration, making decisions, learning, and memory that affect the individual's everyday life.
Cognitive Limitations	Veterinary medical mistakes that result from distraction or absent-mindedness. For example, failing to count sterile gauze squares prior to closure of a laparotomy is a cognitive limitation.
Cognitive Skills/Abilities	Brain-related skills such as memory, learning, and reasoning that are needed for most tasks.
Co-Insurance	Payments for medical services shared by insurance companies and individuals, usually expressed in percentages, such as 80% paid by the insurance company and 20% paid by the individual.
Coloboma	A hole in one of the structures of the eye, such as the retina, choroid, or optic disk.
Commensal	A relationship in which one organism benefits from another organism without helping or hurting it.
Commodity	An item that is considered interchangeable, and whose price is a reflection of supply and demand. For example, one 500 mg capsule of cephalexin is much like any other to a client, regardless of brand name and whether they get it at a veterinary hospital, at their local drug store, or through an online pharmacy.
Common Law	A product of judicial evolution, a sort of gap-filling established over generations by judges; compare to "statutory or code law," which is set forth by legislative ordinance.
Communication Channels	The vehicles by which audiences/stakeholders can be reached.
Communicative Medicine	Involvement of the family in the discussions surrounding patient care and the development of a treatment plan to assure that the family's needs and preferences are appropriately being met.
Community Pricing	Establishing a price for a good or service based on the prices charged by others.
Community Relations	Continuing, planned, and active participation with and within a community to maintain and enhance its environment to the benefit of both an organization and the community.
Co-Morbidities	More than one disease or condition occurring at the same time, often complicating treatments and responses.
Companion Diagnostics	A method to test safety and efficacy of a drug specific to a target patient group, breed, or otherwise identified individual (biomarkers, genetic markers, etc.).
Companioning	The act of helping someone through the process of grief, without having the education or designation of counselor or therapist.
Compassion Fatigue	Also known as secondary traumatic stress disorder, this is the gradual loss of compassion by people who work with individuals that are ill, suffering, or victims of trauma. This includes veterinary staff working with worried clients with sick or injured animals.
Compassion Fatigue-Induced Burnout	Burnout as a result of unidentified and unmanaged compassion fatigue.
Compassion Satisfaction	Deriving pleasure from being a caregiver, and feeling good about the ability to help and make a positive contribution.

Compelling	Motivating to the point that the target is likely to act – or is compelled to do something.
Competition	The process of two or more businesses vying for the same group or a fixed pool of customers.
Complementary Therapies	Those therapies used to augment conventional medical and surgical remedies vs alternative therapies, those therapies used instead of conventional medical and surgical remedies.
Complete Dental Therapy	Includes dental cleaning, thorough dental examination and charting, dental radiographs, polishing and treatment (periodontal treatment, extractions), performed under general anesthesia.
Compliance	The extent to which pets receive a treatment, screening, or procedure in accordance with veterinary healthcare recommendations.
Compliance Reminders	A reminder for a pet owner to apply a treatment (usually for prevention of parasites) when due rather than to simply repurchase it.
Compounding	Customized manipulation of an approved drug(s) by a veterinarian or pharmacist to meet the needs of a particular patient.
Compromise Fatigue	An extreme sense of stress associated with repeated requests to make compromises on the basis of the medical or financial management of patient care.
Concentration-Dependent Antimicrobials	Antimicrobials whose efficacy is associated with achieving high concentrations at the site of infection.
Concierge Medicine	A doctor–client–patient relationship in which medical care is provided for an agreed-upon fee and array of services.
Conditioned Response	After classical conditioning has taken place, it is the response to a conditioned stimulus. It is also the response of an organism after learning has occurred.
Conditioned Stimulus	After classical conditioning has taken place, it is the stimulus that creates the conditioned response.
Conditioning	A reaction to an event modified by learning or experience.
Confidential Information	Information intended to be kept secret and not disclosed to others.
Confidentiality	The duty of keeping secret or private information pertaining to a patient's health that was obtained during the formation of a diagnosis, treatment or prognosis of the animal.
Conformation	The shape or dimensions of an animal.
Connected Care	Another term for telehealth or virtual care.
Consent	Giving permission for something to happen. In animal training, it is a behavior that has been taught to allow the trainer to touch or perform a procedure on the animal.
Consequences	Anything that happens immediately after the target behavior. The process by which these consequences influence behavior is called *operant conditioning*.
Considerate Approach	A specific form of interaction between the veterinary team and the patient designed to minimize the negative emotional responses that may arise during patient care.
Consumer	A person who purchases goods and services
Contagious or Communicable Disease	A disease caused by an infectious agent that is transmissible between hosts.
Content	Broad category of substance conveyed through customer interactions. Content can be information or the customer's experience. In all cases, to be effective, content should be compelling and deliver customer value.
Continuity of Care	The cooperative efforts of the healthcare team and clients to ensure quality of care and beneficial outcomes over time, even when multiple healthcare professionals are involved.
Continuous Quality Improvement (CQI)	An ongoing process of seeking small improvements in processes that have an overall effect of improving efficiency and productivity while reducing waste within an organization.

Continuum of Care	The delivery of healthcare over a period of time, such that intervention at any point on the timeline affects quality of life in the periods afterwards
Contraception	The intentional use of physical barriers, pharmaceutical agents, or other techniques to prevent pregnancy.
Convergence Schedule	In veterinary medicine, the coming together of different processes into the same continuum of care
Cookies	A cookie is a small amount of data generated by a website and saved by a web browser. Its purpose is to recall information or preferences about the user.
Cooperative Care	System of management teaching, using positive reinforcement, and animals' behaviors that make examination and treatment easier.
Co-Pay or Co-Payment	Specified amount of covered services that is the insurance policyholder's responsibility.
Core Values	Belief system of the practice – the cultural values that give team members the broad vision to make decisions for the practice.
Corporate Practice	A veterinary hospital owned and managed by a group of investors, rather than by private veterinarians.
Cost Driver	Quantifiable measure used to assign costs to activities; reflects the consumption of costs by activities. Examples include labor, supplies, equipment, and associated depreciation.
Cost Object	Any activity for which a separate measurement of costs is desired. Examples include services, service lines, products, product lines, processes, and responsibility centers (surgery, pharmacy).
Cost of Goods Sold	Variable expenses associated with revenue generation.
Cost of Professional Services (COPS)	Direct costs of patient care and product retailing, including drug and pharmacy costs, professional and hospital supplies costs, laboratory supplies and reference laboratory fees, radiology and imaging supply costs, surgery and anesthesia supply costs, dietary product costs, mortuary costs.
Cost–Benefit Analysis (CBA)	An organized approach to clinical practice in which the clinician helps the client to consider the pros and cons of each diagnostic and/or treatment plan to decide the best course of action for proceeding with patient care.
Credibility	The extent to which a clinician is perceived as believable, expert, genuine, and trustworthy.
Credit Policy	Written guidelines to assist in deciding to extend credit to a customer. A good credit policy should help retain good relationships without jeopardizing cash flow.
Credit Report	Listing of all outstanding debt and the history of paying on that debt.
Credit Terms	Time limits set for customers' promises to pay for the merchandise or services purchased from the practice. Credit terms affect the timing of cash collections.
Criminal Negligence	A person acts negligently when inadvertently creating a substantial and unjustifiable risk of which one ought to be aware. The fault is *inattentiveness*.
Crisis	A situation, often unexpected, that has the potential to cause physical or reputational damage or harm to a facility, its personnel and constituents.
Crisis Management	A proactive approach to anticipating crisis situations and taking responsibility for how the situation is handled.
Crisis Plan	A written document that anticipates possible crisis situations and details how such situations will be managed from operational and communication perspectives.
Critical Path	The succession of connected tasks that will take the longest to complete. The critical path is the longest path to complete the project. Therefore, to complete the project on schedule, it is the critical path and the tasks that are part of it that must be managed most closely.
Critical Care Facility	A facility that is open 24 hours a day, seven days a week, and is able to handle emergencies and the critical care needs of patients, similar to the Urgent Care facilities available for people.

Critically Appraised Topic	A brief summary and appraisal of the evidence concerning a narrow clinical topic which resembles a systematic review but is shorter and less comprehensive.
Criticism	Negative feedback that is generally destructive in nature. Often focuses on the person rather than the behavior or the task. Delivered in this way, many recipients feel attacked, reject the feedback, and hence no behavioral change tends to ensue.
Cross-Selling	Encouraging a buyer to purchase related or complementary products or services.
Culture	The set of shared attitudes, morals, values, and goals that characterizes an organization.
Curettage, Dental	Removal of calculus, debris, and diseased soft tissue from a tooth surface using a hand instrument (curette)
Customer	Someone who pays for goods or services.
Customer Acquisition Cost	This is the total cost of acquiring a client.
Customer Insights	A window into how consumers think and the motivation behind their needs and wants for a given product or service category. Used to predict future customer behaviors.
Customer Relationship Management (CRM)	A strategy for managing all a practice's relationships and interactions with customers and potential customers. It helps to improve customer satisfaction and a practice's profitability.
Customer Relationship Management Platforms	Customer relationship management (CRM) is used by veterinary practices to manage and analyze client interactions and data throughout the pet lifecycle to improve relationships with clients, deliver personalized healthcare, assist in client retention, and drive sales growth.
Customer Service	Refers to assistance to individuals who are purchasing a product. Typically, the interaction involves a transaction.
Customer Success	The business methodology of ensuring customers achieve their desired outcomes while using your product or service.
Customer Value	How well a service provider or product manufacturer does at satisfying customers' needs at any point in a transaction. A customer can assign value beginning with prepurchase information to postpurchase service and follow-up.
Cybersecurity	The protection against the unauthorized or unlawful use of electronic data.
Cycle Counting	An inventory management tool in which select products are counted on a periodic basis to detect inventory errors and for continuous quality improvement, so process problems can be detected before official inventory counts or audits.
Cylindruria	The state of having casts in the urine.
Cytotoxic Waste	Waste that is associated with cytotoxic drugs (often chemotherapeutics) that is toxic to cells.
Daily Energy Requirement (DER)	The energy requirement needed for activities beyond just remaining completely at rest (e.g., activity, life-stage or physiological condition, dealing with environmental conditions). These total daily energy requirements can be approximated by multiplying the resting energy requirement (RER) by an appropriate factor given likely activity levels.
Data	Information collected for reference or analysis. Practice management software allows practices to establish data collection variables and to analyze data using these variables.
Decedent	A person who has died.
Decibel (dB)	A measure of the intensity of sound, based on the human ear.
Decisional Conflict	An experience whereby a client has ambivalent thoughts and feelings, which tend to both accept and reject a given course of action.
Decisional Support	Skills and behaviors of the veterinary team to assist clients who are in decisional conflict.

Deductible	Amount an individual must pay for health services before the individual's insurance company starts to pay.
Defalcation	Misappropriation of money or funds by someone entrusted with their care or management.
Defections	Clients who choose to leave the practice during a specific unit of time (e.g., one year).
Deferred Payment Plan	A written document stating amount owed, dates, and amounts for expected future payment installments.
Definitive Diagnosis	Determination of the nature or cause of a disease.
Degenerative Joint Disease (DJD)	The umbrella term for damage to and degradation of hyaline cartilage and its negative consequences on joint function and comfort.
Delegating	Entrusting a task or a skill to another person.
Democratic Leadership	A style of leadership that encourages opinion and input from everyone involved within an organization.
Democratization	The process of making something accessible to everyone.
Demographics	Description of objective and quantifiable characteristics of an audience or population such as age, marital status, household income, and pet-spending index.
Dental Calculus (Tartar)	Hardened dental plaque, often caused by the accumulation of minerals from saliva.
Dental Plaque	A biofilm consisting of bacteria, mucus, and food particles that adheres to the surface of teeth.
Dental Prophy	Less than optimal term commonly used for the complete dental therapy experience.
Deoxyribonucleic Acid (DNA)	The chemical structure of the genetic instruction set containing coding and regulatory genes.
Desensitization	The decrease of an emotional response to a stimulus after gradual exposure.
Diabetes Mellitus	A medical condition that is characterized by persistent high blood glucose (sugar) levels, due to either inadequate production of insulin or inadequate sensitivity of cells to the action of insulin.
Diabetic Ketoacidosis (DKA)	A metabolic complication of uncontrolled or poorly regulated diabetes mellitus, in which rapid breakdown of fat leads to an accumulation of ketones in the bloodstream and urine. Body fluids become dangerously acidic, and the condition is fatal if acid–base and electrolyte imbalances cannot be corrected in a timely fashion.
Diagnostic Local Blockade	The use of local and regional perineural block and peri/intraarticular techniques to confirm pain's presence by the reduction of pain response once administered.
Diastole	The phase of the cardiac cycle in which the heart relaxes.
Dietary Supplement	A product intended to supplement the diet that bears or contains one or more of the following dietary ingredients – a vitamin, a mineral, an herb or other botanical, an amino acid, a dietary substance used to supplement the diet by increasing the total daily intake.
Differential Diagnosis	Conditions with common features that are being considered as potential diagnoses. Also known as "rule-outs."
Differentiation	The process of distinguishing your hospital, products, and services from others, to make them more attractive to your target market.
Digital Imaging	Any imaging that captures image data in a digital format, for storage, manipulation, viewing, and distribution. All imaging modalities are capable of producing digital images, either inherently or through analogue to digital converters built into their hardware.
Digital Imaging and Communications in Medicine (DICOM)	Image standard that allows communication between image capture devices, viewing software, storage, and print devices.
Disaster and Emergency	These terms are often used interchangeably when departments, agencies, or private entities are unexpectedly torn from their standard operating procedures or are required to obtain resources outside their normal authority.

Disaster Declaration	An official designation of an event as a disaster by local, tribal, state, or federal authorities. An official declaration may often trigger economic or resource assistance.
DISC	DISC is a behavior assessment tool based on the DISC theory of psychologist William Moulton Marston, the original process focusing on four different behavioral traits– dominance, inducement, submission, and compliance. In more contemporary applications, the letters can also signify basic tendencies such as directing, influencing, steadiness and compliant, or they can also stand for the following personality types: Dominant, Inspiring, Supportive, and Cautious (or conscientious). DiSC® is a branded form of the DISC assessment.
Discipline	Training people to obey rules and codes of behavior, using punishment as a deterrent for misconduct. Also used to define a branch of knowledge.
Discount	A deduction from the usual cost of something typically given for prompt or advanced payment or for a special category of buyers.
Discount Plans	Not insurance. Instead, this is a service by which pet owners pay a fee to receive discounted services from participating veterinarians.
Disease Liability Genes	The genetic factors that contribute to the manifestation of complex heritable conditions.
Dishonorable Conduct	This term is referred to by some state practice acts to be the same as unprofessional conduct.
Disinfectant	An antimicrobial agent that is used to decrease the numbers of microorganisms present on the surface on inanimate objects.
Disinfection	Using physical or chemical approaches to ensure the destruction of pathogens from nonliving objects.
Disintermediation	Giving the user or the consumer direct access to information that otherwise would require a mediator. This is often done through technological innovation.
Disposable Income	Income remaining after all taxes and mandatory expenses have been deducted, that can be spent or saved at one's prerogative.
Distraction Techniques	Utilizing things the individual pet finds desirable, such as treats, brushing, toys, petting, etc. to focus their attention away from a perceived negative experience and alleviate fear, anxiety, and stress (FAS).
Diversification	A manner of attempting to gain increased sales through offering new products or services or by selling products or services into new markets.
Doggy Daycare	A service for dogs to play together in supervised group settings. This may be a drop-off day service, or it may be offered as an enhancement to overnight boarding.
Dolichocephalic	A term used to refer to breeds with a long, narrow muzzle, such as collies and greyhounds.
Dominant	Heritable characteristics, traits, phenes, or diseases that are expressed when inherited even from one parent
Driver	An aspect of a business that leads to change in other aspects of a business, usually in a positive fashion.
Drug	A medication intended for use in the diagnosis, cure, mitigation, treatment, or prevention of disease or that affects the structure or function of the body.
Due Diligence	The process by which persons conduct inquiries for the purposes of timely, sufficient, and accurate disclosure of all material statements/information or documents that may influence the outcome of the transaction.
Dynamic Laboratory Testing	A testing format in which multiple samples are collected over a period of time to assess function (e.g., ACTH stimulation testing).
Dysbiosis	An imbalance of microbial communities with potential negative consequences on host health.
Dysthesia	Unpleasant or abnormal sensation, such as tingling, burning, itching, numbness.

Early Detection	Evaluating patients for early evidence of issues, ideally before they become problematic.
Earned Media	Publicity gained through invitation to participate in media events, rather than paying for them.
Economic Euthanasia	A situation in which euthanasia is selected principally on the basis of a pet owner's unwillingness or inability to pay for needed veterinary care.
Economic Life	The number of years over which cash is expected to be returned from an investment in property.
Economic Value-Added	Monetary value of an entity at the end of a time period minus the monetary value of that same entity at the beginning of that time period; that is, after-tax earnings minus the opportunity cost of capital.
Economy of Scale	The reduction in cost per unit that results when operational efficiencies allow increased production. Thus, there is an increase in savings because as production increases, the cost of producing each additional unit decreases.
Economy of Scope	The reduction in cost that results when delivering two or more distinct goods or services, when the cost of doing so is less than that of delivering each separately. It is the efficiency attributed to variety and diversification rather than volume.
Ecosystem	A system that includes all the organisms and their interactions with each other and the environment around them.
Ectoparasite	A parasite that lives on the outside of its host. e.g., flea, tick, mosquito.
Electronic Funds Transfer (EFT)	The process of moving transaction funds from one bank to another via the Automated Clearing House of the Federal Reserve Network. An EFT processes preauthorized debits or credits from one bank account to another without using a physical check/cheque.
Electronic Health Record (EHR)	A comprehensive report of a patient's overall health. It may or may not include electronic medical records from one or more practices and is intended to be shared among authorized providers, staff, and other users.
Electronic Medical Record (EMR)	The systematized collection of patient health information in a digital format.
Electronic Prescribing (E-Prescribing)	The use of digital electronic prescriptions rather than providing a printed prescription or faxing a prescription.
Email	Electronic mail, commonly referred to as email or e-mail, is a method of exchanging digital messages from an author to one or more recipients. Modern email operates across the internet or other computer networks.
Email Automation System	Software which allows you to automate email sending. It is the most effective way to engage in email marketing, enabling you to send out emails at specific times, or when a customer takes a specific action.
Emergency	An unplanned event that is likely to cause significant harm to people or animals or property damage. Some emergencies require immediate action (such as a fire) whereas others provide warnings and possible reaction time (such as a wildfire or hurricane).
Emergency Action Plan (EAP)	A specific written plan on how the practice will respond to a given emergency situation.
Emerging Disease	A new disease or new strain of known disease that may impact human, animal, or plant health.
Emotional Branding	The practice of building a brand that appeals directly to a consumer's emotional state, needs, and aspirations.
Emotional Intelligence	The capacity to perceive, assess, and positively influence one's own and other people's emotions.
Emotion-Focused Coping	Coping strategies that address the emotional response to a problem.

Empathy	The ability to appreciate the feelings of others.
Employee Handbook (Policy Manual)	The document that describes the employment policies of a specific employer, describing what the employer expects of the employee, and what the employee can expect from the employer.
Employee Manuals	Written manuals running from a few pages to many pages explaining the terms and conditions employees must operate under while working for a given business.
Employee Policy Book	The policy book should be separate from the employee manual in that it can include many operating policies giving more detail on the day-to-day operations than an employee manual can. The employee manual primarily directs behavior, attendance, and/or absences.
Employee Relations	Responding to concerns and informing and motivating employees.
Empowerment	Authority of power given to someone to do something (carry out a task that has been delegated).
End of Life Care	Care provided to attend to the physical, emotional, and social needs of patients in the final hours or days of their lives, and, more broadly, of all patients with a terminal condition that has become advanced, progressive, and incurable.
Endolaser Cyclophotocoagulation	A vision-sparing surgical procedure utilized to reduce intraocular pressure.
Endoparasite	A parasite that lives inside its host, e.g., roundworm, whipworm, tapeworm.
Engage	Obtain someone's interest or attention as a result of some form of interaction.
Engaged	Involved in and committed to a specific activity.
Engaged Employee	An employee who is actively involved in his/her work, and highly committed to duties and the company mission.
Engagement	The ongoing active interaction between a practice and a customer.
Enteropathogen	A microorganism that causes disease of the gastrointestinal tract.
Entropion	An eyelid that turns inwards and rubs on the eyeball.
Enucleation	Removal of the eye, third eyelid, and conjunctival tissue.
Environmental Enrichment	Modifications that improve the quality of one's surroundings.
Environmental Needs	Requirements related to the pet's surroundings that are essential for the maintenance of the its physical and emotional well-being.
Enzyme-Linked Immunosorbent Assay (ELISA)	A type of diagnostic test that detects the presence or absence of antibodies related to a specific infectious agent.
Epidemiology	The study of how diseases occur in given patient populations and why.
Epigenetics	The study of heritable changes in genetic expression caused by mechanisms other than those attributable to underlying DNA sequences.
Epiphora	Increased tearing.
Epistasis	The situation in which the action of one gene depends on the action of another gene.
E-Slots or Same Days	These are two of the many terms practices use to describe appointments that are held open until that day to accommodate emergencies, walk-ins, or other situations that require a doctor's immediate attention.
Estimate	An opinion of probable cost prepared prior to the completion of an interaction. Also known as a *care plan*.
Ethics Exhaustion	Fatigue, emotional distress, and lack of will to continue to act in a way that is consistent with what you believe is the ethical thing to do.
Ethos	The distinguishing character, sentiment, moral nature, or guiding beliefs of a person, group, or institution. An ethical appeal using credibility and character.
Euthanasia	The intentional humane termination of life.

Evidence-Based Medicine	An approach to medical practice intended to optimize decision making by emphasizing the use of evidence from well-designed and -conducted research.
Evidence-Based Practice	Use of the best currently available resources (research and clinical expertise) in making decisions about patient care.
Evolution	The gradual development of something, especially from a simple to a more complex form.
Exclusion	In insurance, a condition that is not covered under an insurance policy.
Executive Dashboard	A reporting tool that provides visual displays of an organization's financial and operational metrics, and data. The objective of developing an executive dashboard is to give healthcare executives an instant summarized visibility into business performance across all business lines.
Executor	A person or entity appointed by a testator to carry out the terms of their will.
Exome	The protein-coding part of the genome
Exon	A segment of nucleic acid (DNA or RNA) that codes for specific proteins or peptides.
Exophthalmos	Abnormal bulging or protrusion of the eyeball.
Expectancy Theory	The theory that motivation is increased when employees believe that increased effort leads to desired results.
Expectation	A strong belief that something will happen or will be the case in the future.
Expressivity	The extent to which a genetic variant (genotype) expresses the so-called clinical abnormality (phenotype) on an individual level.
External Crisis	A crisis that originates due to outside factors, in most cases outside the practice's control.
External Marketing	Written or verbal communication aimed at attracting new clients.
Extraction, Tooth	The removal of a tooth from the surrounding periodontal tissue, often through surgical means.
Extra-Label Drug Use (ELDU)	The use of an approved drug in a manner that is not in accordance with the approved labeling (for example, the use of the product for another species, different indication, or dose).
Facebook Boost	Advertising created from posts on a Facebook page. Boosting a post may get more people to react, share, and comment on it.
Facebook Pixel	An analytics tool that allows one to measure the effectiveness of advertising by understanding the actions people take on a website.
Facilitated Compliance	Efforts by the veterinary team to help ensure that pets receive the care they need according to recommended schedules.
Facilitator	The facilitator has the task of leading a group to a reasonable consensus.
False-Negative	A test result that erroneously reports that a particular patient does not have a particular disease state, when in fact s/he does.
False-Positive	A test result that erroneously reports that a particular patient has a particular disease state, when in fact s/he does not.
Fear	An aversive emotional state involving physical and psychological responses to a stimulus that is perceived as a threat or danger.
Fear Free Homes and Clinics	A broad group of recommendations that encompass the environment and husbandry of pets in the home and in the veterinary clinic. The concepts are based on the view of the pets rather than the human participants and are designed to improve the welfare of pets in all places.
Feasibility Study	A study to objectively and rationally uncover the strengths and weaknesses of an existing business or proposed venture, and ultimately the prospects for success.
Features	The characteristics of products, services, or programs you offer. Features answer the question "What does it do?"

Fecal–Oral Transmission	Disease transmission that occurs due to ingestion of organisms from another animal's feces.
Feline Friendly Care (FFC)	Quiet, calm, controlled cat care, respecting the individual cat's preferences and health parameters. FFC also involves the use of in-home and outpatient management of the most important feline diseases and disabilities.
Fill Rate	Percentage of available appointment slots that were scheduled during a specific period of time.
Finance Charges	The amount of money charged for payments that extend beyond an agreed-upon time limit. The amount charged is governed by the usury laws in the state within which you practice. The amount of finance fee charged must be clearly reflected on the invoices rendered.
Finance Risk	One approach to risk management involves purchasing enough insurance to transfer responsibility for losses to an insurer. Insurance is an essential aspect of risk management.
Five Freedoms	Internationally recognized and accepted standards of care detailing the need for freedom from hunger/thirst, discomfort, fear/distress, pain/injury/disease, and the freedom to express normal behavior.
Five Stages of Grief	Created by Elisabeth Kübler-Ross, the five stages are known as denial, anger, bargaining, depression, and acceptance. They do not necessarily happen in sequence, and a person doesn't necessarily experience all of these stages.
Fixed Cost	A consistent and predetermined cost (e.g., rent).
Fixed Schedule	The scheduling of staff members, their duties, their workday, and workweek are the same (fixed) week after week and do not change.
Floor Workers	The floor workers are those people on the veterinary team who are doing the hands-on work of a veterinary practice; these people are not involved in the management of the business, but instead are the first line for taking care of the patients and clients.
Flora	Also known as microbiota, this refers to the community of microorganisms present on/in people or animals.
Flowchart	Graphic representation of the stages in a process or of the steps required to solve a problem.
Focus Group	A group of clients who are asked to participate in a discussion about a particular topic or issue. The information from the group is used to develop programs, improve service, or solve problems in the practice.
Folliculitis	Inflammation of the hair follicles. The term is often used to imply not only inflammation, but the involvement of bacteria.
Follower	An adherent or devotee of a particular person, cause, business, or activity.
Fomite	Any nonliving surface or object that can harbor microorganisms and transfer them from one individual to another.
Food and Drug Administration (FDA)	The FDA is an agency within the US Department of Health and Human Services that is responsible for protecting the public health by regulating the manufacturing, marketing, and distribution of human biological products, human and veterinary drugs and medical devices, cosmetics, and products that emit radiation.
Food and Drug (FDA) Center for Veterinary Medicine (FDA/CVM)	The FDA Center for Veterinary Medicine (FDA/CVM) is a branch of the FDA dedicated to ensuring the safety and efficacy of animal drugs, devices, medicated feed for companion and food-producing animals, and safety of food products made from treated animals. In addition, the FDA/CVM monitors the safety and effectiveness of animal drugs on the market, and ensures the safety of pet foods and food additives.
Foreign Animal Disease	A disease of great concern that is currently not endemic to the country. This may also be referred to as a *transboundary disease*.
Forming	A team stage in which members may be uncertain about rules, roles, and expectations.

Forward Booking	This is the process of scheduling a client's next visit to the practice before they leave so a client always knows when they need to return, instead of waiting for a reminder notification.
Four Cs of Onboarding	A memory tool used to recall four important content areas to include in the onboarding process: Compliance, Clarification, Culture, and Connection.
Fraud	An intentional misrepresentation of the truth to mislead another to bargain or act in reliance upon the misrepresentation.
Fraud Triangle	Three key factors that identify individuals who may be susceptible to committing fraud: situational pressures, opportunities to commit fraud, and (lack of) personal integrity.
Frequently Asked Questions (FAQ)	A collection of common queries and their correct responses.
Full-Time Equivalent	A method of comparing practices based on a full-time schedule of 40 hours a week. If a practice has two veterinarians, one working 50 hours a week and one working 20 hours a week, that practice has 1.75 full-time equivalent veterinary positions ((50 + 20)/40).
Functional Food	Food alleged to have a health-promoting or disease-preventing property beyond the basic function of supplying nutrients.
Functionally Illiterate	Lacking basic reading and writing skills.
Fungibility	The property of a good or commodity to have individual units that are essentially interchangeable. For example, in currency, bills and coins of equal value are considered interchangeable, and are thus fungible.
Furcation Exposure (FE)	Exposure of the space in between roots of a multirooted tooth that is normally covered by periodontal tissues (gingiva and bone).
Furunculosis	Literally, the development of furuncles (boils) in the skin, but often signifying a deep folliculitis, typically with hair follicle rupture into the dermis or panniculus.
Gain Sharing Program	Cost-savings commission programs in which a compensation plan is self-funding. Employees strive to improve the hospital's patient satisfaction scores, which in turn would increase employees' payouts and their own connection to how they impact total practice success.
Gamification	The integration of game dynamics and design to nongame applications, such as learning tools, to make them more engaging.
Gastric Dilation-Volvulus (GDV or Bloat)	Life-threatening medical condition in dogs in which the stomach becomes distended (dilation/bloat) and twists on itself (volvulus).
Gender Predisposition	A predilection for a condition to occur predominantly but not exclusively in one gender over another.
Gene	A length of DNA that codes for a specific protein, enzyme or cellular event.
General Anesthesia	Drug-induced loss of consciousness induced to conduct invasive medical or surgical procedures.
Generally Recognized As Safe (GRAS)	Substance generally recognized, among experts qualified by scientific training and experience to evaluate its safety, as having been adequately shown through scientific procedures to be safe under the conditions of its intended use.
Generation X	People in this generation were born between 1965 and 1981, but more generally this includes anyone born in the 1960s and 1970s.
Generation Y or Millennials	This generation includes anyone born between 1982 and 1999.
Generation Z	Also known as the iGeneration or Net Generation, these are individuals born after 1999. They have always had familiarity with communications and media technology.
Generic Drugs	Generic drugs require a demonstration of bioequivalence of safety and efficacy with the pioneer drug product.
Genetics	The study of genes and how traits or conditions are passed from one generation to the next.

Genome	All the hereditary information encoded in the DNA, including the genes and the noncoding sequences of DNA.
Genomics	The study of the entire genome, and its combined influence on complex diseases and the impact of environmental factors such as diet, exercise, medications, and toxins on genes.
Genotoxic Waste	Waste that may have the potential to damage genetic information, typically derived from drugs used in chemotherapy or radiation oncology.
Genotype	The underlying genetic constitution of an individual. Usually pertaining to the two versions of a single phene (i.e., AA, aa, or Aa).
Genotypic Testing	Testing that determines actual genetic mutations (variants) or markers of traits, phenes, or conditions.
Gentle Control	Handling method that allows the veterinary team to comfortably and safely position patients for veterinary care without causing fear, anxiety, and stress (FAS).
Geriatric	A pet's life stage defined when the pet has reached its expected life span and beyond.
Gingival Index (GI)	A measurement of the extent of gingival inflammation.
Gingival Recession (GR)	Loss of gingival tissue that, together with accompanying bone loss, can expose the root of the tooth and even the furcation of a multirooted tooth.
Gingivitis	Inflammation of the soft tissue immediately surrounding the tooth – the attached gingiva.
Glaucoma	A group of ocular diseases that exhibit increased levels of intraocular pressure that are detrimental to the maintenance of vision and health of the eye.
Glaucoma, Primary	Glaucoma in dogs thought to have a genetic predisposition.
Glaucoma, Secondary	Glaucoma occurring due to any other condition except having a genetic predisposition.
Global Positioning System (GPS)	A space-based satellite navigation system that provides location and time information in all weather, anywhere on Earth.
Glucosuria	The state of having glucose present in the urine.
Goals of Care	Desired results for a particular clinical situation.
Gold Standard	That which is considered the best available diagnostic test, treatment plan, or other benchmark that is available to manage patient care.
Gold Standard Care	Focusing on the most successful, most complete course of action for a given health condition, irrespective of cost.
Gonadectomy	Technically, surgical removal of ovaries or testes; colloquially, this term often refers to excision of the reproductive tract and is therefore synonymous with ovariohysterectomy or castration.
Gonioimplant	A surgically placed device utilized to provide an alternate aqueous humor outflow pathway to reduce intraocular pressure.
Goodhart's Law	The observation that when a metric becomes a target for control, it often ceases to remain a good measure.
Goodwill	An intangible asset resulting from a business's reputation, name, location, products, services, customer base, and so on.
Google AdWords	Google's search advertising platform.
Grantor	An individual who transfers or conveys ownership.
Grief	The constellation of internal thoughts and feelings we have when someone we love dies.
Gross Ignorance	An act or omission that reaches a level of incompetence or error much greater than that of a more common negligent or mistaken action or omission.
Guardian	One who has legal authority and duty to care for another's person (ward) or property because of the other's infancy, incapacity or disability.

Guardian *Ad Litem*	A guardian, appointed to the court to appear in a lawsuit on behalf of an incompetent or minor party.
Guardianship	The fiduciary relationship between a guardian and a ward, whereby the guardian assumes the role of owner to make decisions about the ward's person or property. Guardianship implies a fiduciary duty in the relationship.
Guidelines	Routine or sound practices, often formed by consensus within veterinary organizations. A general rule intended to make the actions of its followers more predictable.
Hacker	Someone who accesses a computer system by circumventing its security system.
Hand Curette	Hand instrument with a rounded tip and curved back that can be safely introduced into a periodontal pocket to help dislodge or curette away calculus, debris, and even soft tissue from the surfaces in a periodontal pocket.
Hand Scaler	Hand instrument with a sharp tip that can be used to help dislodge or scale calculus and debris from an exposed tooth/root surface; never to be used under the gum line.
Handling	The manner by which pets are visualized, approached, and touched. The term and mindset which should replace the concept and the word "restraint" in all veterinary practices.
Hard Costs	Cost of tangible items. This typically includes material costs, laboratory costs, and medications, etc.
Hard Skills	These are teachable and quantifiable skills. This means they produce quantifiable results and you can be graded and/or evaluated for your ability.
Hardware	The collection of physical elements that comprise a computer system. Computer hardware refers to the physical parts or components of the computer such as monitor, keyboard, hard disk, mouse, and so on.
Harmless Hit	A medical error that occurs, but does not harm the patient.
Hash Code	A form of cryptographic security that, unlike encryption, cannot be reversed or decrypted.
Hazard	Any threat that could impact a nation, region, community, facility, or individual household. Hazards may be natural, man-made, accidental, intentional, low-impact, high-impact, low-probability, high-probability, local, or regional.
Hazard Assessment	A review and analysis of the facility and the procedures of a practice with the goal of identifying potential hazards to the staff. Often referred to as a "physical exam" of the practice.
Hazardous Chemical	Any chemical product that can cause physical harm to a person or the environment, including seemingly mild products that can be irritating to the eyes or cause skin reactions.
Hazardous Waste	Waste products harmful or toxic to humans, animals, or the environment. Chemotherapy drugs fall under this category.
Health Education Methods and Strategies	Various ways for delivering health education to clients, such as providing written information sheets, showing educational videos in the waiting room, providing verbal information during the visit, and so forth.
Health Information Portability and Protection Act 1996 (HIPPA)	A Federal law that governs medical privacy and contains provisions for safeguarding medical information. HIPPA specifically defines protected health information as being geared towards individuals, and therefore does not specifically regulate veterinary medical information.
Health Literacy	Level of understanding that is required by the client to access, utilize, and follow through on recommendations to maintain the health of an animal in their care.
Health Registry	Database containing health screening information and identifying characteristics such as breed, sex, age, and pedigree of individuals.
Health Risk Assessment (HRA)	A comprehensive system for helping to determine a specific patient's risks for developing particular diseases and conditions, or suffering from toxicities and other emergencies.

Health Screening	The use of tests to identify individuals that do not exhibit overt clinical signs but that have risk factors or early stages of disease.
Healthspan	The portion of a pet's life in which it is considered generally healthy, in contradistinction to *lifespan* which is the quantity of time a pet is alive.
Hedonic Adaptation	Sometimes referred to as the hedonic treadmill, this refers to the observed tendency of individuals to return to a relatively stable level of happiness despite major positive or negative events or life changes.
Heightened Arousal	Arousal is a state of heightened activity in mind and body that makes individuals more alert. It manifests along a spectrum from low to high.
Held Checks	Checks dated the day they are written, with a verbal agreement that you will hold them for deposit until an agreed-upon date.
Hemizygous	The situation when only one copy of a gene is present, such as in males when a condition is x linked (since males only have one X chromosome).
Herd Immunity	Concept that if a sufficient proportion of a population is immune to a pathogen, there will be resistance to the spread of infection despite not reaching a 100% immunization rate.
Herzberg's Motivator–Hygiene Theory	The theory that meeting basic needs results in motivation and increased performance.
Heterozygous	A gene pair where the two copies have different alleles (i.e., Aa).
Hierarchy	Classification of people in accordance to their professional standing or position of authority.
High-Density Scheduling	Refers to any scheduling system where the doctor has access to more than one examination room. It requires a well-trained and well-choreographed staff that can leverage the available doctor's time and expertise, resulting in increased productivity.
High Tech	Refers to practicing on the cutting edge, using highly technical or advanced equipment and procedures.
High Touch	Refers to high-quality service and ambiance.
Holacracy	A flat organizational structure in which authority and decision making are controlled by self-organizing teams rather than by a management hierarchy
Holding (Carrying) Costs	All costs associated with maintaining inventory on the premises.
Home Care, Dental	Any effort a pet parent can provide to help decrease the amount of plaque and calculus from forming on tooth surfaces; daily effective tooth brushing is optimal, with other methods including dental wipes and appropriate dental food, treats, and chews.
Homeostasis	A "steady-state" condition in which the body attempts to maintain itself in spite of external influences, so that core body functions and vital signs remain relatively constant.
Homozygous	A gene pair where both copies have the same allele (i.e., AA or aa).
Horizontal Bone Loss	Loss of alveolar bone in a horizontal manner, lowering the ridge of alveolar bone across several roots or several teeth
Horizontal Transmission	Passage of an infectious agent between two organisms that do not share a parent–offspring relationship, through either direct contact or indirectly, as through exposure to respiratory droplets from coughing or sneezing.
Hospice	A philosophy or program of care that addresses the physical, emotional, and social needs of animals in the advanced stages of a progressive, life-limiting illness or disability. Also addresses the emotional, social, and spiritual needs of the human caregivers in preparation for the death of the animal and the grief experience.
Hospice-Supported Natural Death	Use of palliative care measures during a patient's terminal life stage, including the treatment of pain and other signs of discomfort under veterinary supervision until the natural death of the individual.

Hospital-Acquired Infection (HAI)	Also known as nosocomial infections, these are infections that are contracted within a healthcare facility or hospital setting.
Hospital Administrator	Similar to practice manager, with more responsibility for veterinary doctors and technicians. This is an unregulated position in that credentials are not needed to use this term.
Hospital Safety Manual (HSM)	A collection of all the safety rules and policies of the facility. It should contain the set training schedule for the staff, a written safety plan, Safety Data Sheet (SDS) Library, and evacuation plans for emergencies.
House Call Fee (or Trip Fee)	An additional fee added to an invoice to reflect the veterinarian traveling to the client.
House Call Practice	A veterinary practice operated from a vehicle, where services are provided at a client's residence or place of business.
Human Capital	The value of the skills, knowledge, and experience of persons within an organization.
Human Factors	The organizational, individual, and environmental characteristics that influence behaviors that can impact patient safety.
Human Resources	Hiring, training, firing, and supervising the activities of the entire healthcare team while maintaining the legal requirements of the management of people.
Human–Animal Bond (HAB)	A mutually beneficial and dynamic relationship between people and animals that is influenced by behaviors that are essential to the health and well-being of both.
Humane Euthanasia	The intentional termination of life by human intervention utilizing approved methods that cause minimal pain, discomfort, and anxiety for the purpose of relieving an animal's suffering.
Humanization of Pets	The societal trend of treating pets more like human family members than as property or with lesser status than people.
Hybrid	Also known as a designer breed, this is a cross between two or more purebreds. In most cases, the cross is intentional.
Hybrid Schedule	This schedule has characteristics of both a fixed and rotating schedule. A typical hybrid schedule may include a fixed weekday schedule with a weekend rotation.
Hybrid Vigor	Biological enhancements that may result from outbreeding. Also known as *heterosis*.
Hyperalgesia	An exaggerated pain response to a noxious stimulus.
Hypercarnivore	This term refers to specialized digestion and metabolism requiring elements only available from animal (meat) sources. Cats share this designation with dolphins, spiders, ferrets, owls, and alligators.
Hyperglycemia	An elevation in blood sugar that may be transitory, as occurs during times of stress, or chronic, as in cases of diabetes mellitus.
Hypersensitization	The molecular and cellular "wind-up" in peripheral tissue and dorsal horn of the spinal cord, characterized by decreased neuron-firing threshold, decreased descending inhibition, recruitment of bystanding neurons and more; results in maladaptive pain.
Hyperthermia	Sustained elevation of core body temperature beyond that which is considered the normal reference range for the patient.
Hyphema	Blood in the anterior chamber of the eye.
Hypopyon	An accumulation of inflammatory cells found in the anterior chamber of the eye.
Hypothermia	Sustained depression of core body temperature below that which is considered the normal reference interval for the patient.
Iatrogenic	Caused by the medical team during either the process of examination or treatment.
Ideal Customer Profile	A description of the customers that are a perfect fit for your services.
Identity Elements	The various ways in which a practice conveys who it is. This includes everything from the facility in which a practice is housed, to the behaviors of its people, to its manner of service delivery, to its visual identity (logo, icons, and symbols), to its messaging.

Identity Theft	A third party's fraudulent taking and use of another person's or business's uniquely identifiable information (Social Security/Employer Identification number, copied signatures, credit card numbers and holder's name) for the third party's financial gain.
Immunity	Resistance to infection by a pathogen due to the action of the immune system including pathogen-specific antibodies and sensitized immune system cells.
Inbreeding	The breeding of closely related individuals.
Incidence	The rate of newly diagnosed cases of a given disease process in a specified period of time.
Incident Command System (ICS)	Defined command and control system to manage an emergency. Activities of all responding agencies and people are coordinated through the ICS.
Incremental Care	The philosophy of providing all options for treating or diagnosing a specific condition, along with the costs of those options. This is contrasted with providing only the best option and then negotiating "down" to what the client can afford.
Indemnity Insurance	System of health insurance in which the insurance carrier reimburses the insured individual for medical expenses after care has been provided.
Independent Contractors	Nonemployee workers who are contracted by veterinary practice owners to perform certain jobs for the practice.
Individual Development Plan	A staff member's individual plan for self-development that is then approved by a manager to ensure it is aligned with the organization's goals.
Industry Norms	Values derived from the analysis of a large number of practices. Most of the national groups that represent organized veterinary medicine publish some variety of industry norms.
Informatics	The process of using data to improve health and the delivery of healthcare services.
Information Technology (IT)	Concerned with the development, management, and use of computer-based information systems.
Informed Consent	Person's agreement to allow something to happen, such as a medical diagnostic or surgical procedure, that is based on full disclosure of the facts necessary to make an intelligent decision.
In-House Laboratory Services	All laboratory testing that can be readily completed at the hospital by the hospital team. This includes chemistry profiles, complete blood cell counts, urinalysis, intestinal parasite testing, cytology, in-house testing kits, and so on.
Inner Leadership Qualities	Qualities an individual must have as inner strengths to be an effective leader – vision, self-belief, integrity, courage, and being results focused.
Instagram Stories	Instagram feature that lets users post photos and videos that vanish after 24 hours.
Insurance	A form of risk management in which reimbursement for specified veterinary expenses is guaranteed in exchange for premium payments.
Insurance Coverage	Insurance coverage, or cover, is the amount of risk or liability that is protected in an insurance contract.
Insurance Policy	A legal contract between an individual and an insurance company. The insurance company agrees to pay for claims in exchange for payment of premium.
Integrated Diagnostic Systems	Diagnostic tests that are linked to practice software. Often entering the diagnostic code will both order the test (in-house or outside) and input the charge for the test. Results typically are downloaded into the medical record and manual entry is not required.
Integration	Specialized tools to simplify the sharing of medical and related data between medical equipment and electronic health records.
Integrative Medicine	The use of complementary and conventional diagnostics and therapies in health and disease.
Integrity	A sense of commitment to open and honest communication, inclusiveness, and high standards in discharge of professional responsibilities and actions.

Intensive Care Unit (ICU) Flow Sheets	These are records of treatments, observations, and nursing notes that are often kept with the patient while in the hospital. Also known at *treatment sheets*.
Intentionally	A conscious decision to perform an action.
Interdisciplinary Team (IDT)	A transdisciplinary approach crosses disciplinary boundaries to create a holistic, collaborative, and unified team.
Interest	The cost of borrowing money assessed by the lender over time and usually expressed as a percentage of the principal amount of borrowings. The percentage is expressed as a rate over a time period, and can change (variable rate) or stay the same over the term of the loan (fixed rate).
Internal Crisis	A crisis that originates as a result of the actions of a practice employee or facility malfunction.
Internal Marketing	In veterinary medicine, this refers to efforts to increase the utilization of services by existing clients. Internal marketing also refers to efforts by the practice to train and motivate staff to work together as a team to better meet client needs.
Internet	Worldwide network of computer networks.
Internet Marketing	Also known as web marketing, online marketing, web advertising, or e-marketing, the marketing (generally promotion) of products or services over the internet.
Internet of Things (IOT)	Physical devices containing hardware, software, and sensors which are connected to a network, enabling these objects to connect and exchange data.
Interoperability	The ability for data or information to be consumed by disparate systems or processes.
Interventional Pain Management Techniques	The use of invasive interventions such as joint injections, epidural or spinal injections, perineural or local/regional blocks, and infusion therapies usually preceded by or using advanced imaging techniques (CT, fluoroscopy, MRI, ultrasound).
Intraocular Silicone Prosthesis	Removal of the uvea, lens, and retina and placement of an intraocular silicone sphere in cases of advanced glaucoma.
Intron	A segment of nucleic acid (DNA or RNA) that interrupts the sequence within genes but doesn't code for proteins.
Inurement	Inappropriate benefit of a private person or company from a charitable organization.
Inventory	Goods ready to be sold.
Inventory Turnover	Also known as inventory turns, merchandise turnover, stockturn, stock turns, turns, and stock turnover, this refers to the cost of goods sold divided by the average inventory. It is a measure of the number of times inventory is sold or used within a time period.
Invitee	Anyone who enters the premises by invitation and whose entry is connected with or may in some way enhance the business of the owner.
Iridodonesis	Abnormal movement or vibration of the iris typically seen in patients with lens subluxation or luxation.
Job	A task or series of tasks that are performed to accomplish one's occupation.
Job Description	A written summary listing elements of a particular job that should include responsibilities, purpose, duties, qualifications, training, physical and mental demands, and working conditions associated with a specific job.
Job Enlargement	Assignment of additional tasks similar to those the employee is already trained to accomplish. For example, asking an employee who is trained to do callbacks for one doctor to begin doing callbacks for all the doctors.
Job Enrichment	A method of making work more satisfying by expanding the tasks to increase not only their variety but also the employee's responsibility and accountability.
Just-in-Time (JIT) Inventory	Receiving product as it is needed, rather than storing product as inventory.
Juvenile	Young, immature, looking like the adult except in size and reproductive ability.

Juvenile Period	The time after the socialization period and before puberty.
Key Performance Indicators (KPIs)	Key metrics (financial and operational) used to measure performance of an organization.
Kinesics	Individual communication through facial expressions, body tension, gestures, use of touch, body position, posture, and angulation.
Kitten	Young cat aged 8–16 weeks.
Lead Position (Shift Lead)	This refers to the first level of management, the person who is responsible for providing the closest observation of floor workers.
Leadership	The ability to influence a group of people to behave in a particular way to achieve a shared goal.
Leadership Fatigue	An extreme sense of stress associated with managing expectations regarding policies and procedures in the hospital.
Learning	The process by which a behavior is acquired, omitted, or changed as a result of experience.
Learning Curve	The relationship between efficiency of the activity and length of experience with the activity. More experience is expected to result in better outcomes.
Legal Duty	Any duty that is defined or regulated by laws in the jurisdiction where the veterinarian is licensed to practice.
Legend Drug	A drug that can be dispensed to a client only with an order from a properly authorized individual (such as a veterinarian). Legend drugs are often more commonly referred to as prescription drugs.
Legend Pharmaceuticals	Another term for prescription drugs.
Leukocytes	Also known as white blood cells, these are immune cells derived from progenitor cells in the bone marrow. These cells play an important role in host defense systems and help to fight off infection.
Level of Care	The intensity, appropriateness or competence of care provided.
Liability	The state of being legally responsible for something.
Libel	Defamation of another's character, appearing in written form.
Life Plan	A proactive personalized schedule of care and intervention for pets, based on risk factors identified and prioritized.
Life Stage	One of several predetermined phases of life that the patient experiences as s/he grows and matures.
Lifestage Nutrition	Feeding animals foods designed to meet their optimum nutritional needs at a specific age or physiological state (e.g., maintenance, reproduction, growth or senior) is known as lifestage nutrition.
Lifetime Value (LTV)	Lifetime value (LTV) is a metric that represents the total net profit a veterinary practice makes from any given pet over its lifespan.
Lineage	Series of generations (ancestors or descendants). Relationship that is established through kinship, of common ancestors, the members of a family, genealogy, race.
Link Nurse	A member of the nursing team who takes on extra responsibility to develop their knowledge and skills in a particular area of nursing care with the aim of sharing their learning with their colleagues.
Linked Test	A test that targets the region of DNA that is generally associated with a disease.
Literacy Sensitive	Providing health information in a manner that considers the health literacy level of the client.
Local or Regional Anesthesia	Drug-induced analgesia that targets one or more body parts without rendering the patient unconscious.
Local Search	Search queries involving localized keywords such as "near me" or "nearby."
Locus	A fixed position on a chromosome for a gene or marker.

Log, Hybrid	These logs are a combination of patient and procedure logs.
Log, Patient	Any record or list of patients that have received a particular service or product.
Log, Procedure	Procedure logs help ensure that tasks have been completed and/or completed in a specific manner.
Logo	A symbol or other small design that identifies your products, uniform, vehicles, and so forth. Logos often include the company name and meaningful icons or images.
Loss Leader	Products or services sold at a loss to attract customers to potentially purchase other products or services.
Low-Income	Typically living at between 100% and 200% of the Federal poverty threshold.
Loyalty Programs	Structured and long-term marketing efforts that reward and encourage loyal buying behavior from the client.
Macrothrombocytopenia	The condition of having fewer platelets than is considered normal. Platelets that are present are abnormally enlarged.
Maladaptive Coping	Negative coping strategies that provide only short-term stress relief.
Malice	The intentional and wrongful doing of an act without lawful justification and with evil motivation.
Malpractice	A professional's failure to practice the quality of medicine set by similarly situated veterinarians.
Malware	Short for malicious software. A general term used to refer to a variety of forms of hostile or intrusive software.
Managed Care	Healthcare system under which healthcare professionals are organized into a group or "network" to manage the cost, quality, and access to healthcare.
Management	The responsibility for the administration of an organization
Manager	Administrative staff member who oversees the daily operations of the veterinary practice.
Manual, Disaster Recovery	A disaster recovery manual covers simple tasks such as how to function when the internet goes down or when the electricity goes out.
Manual, Doctor	A guide to help ensure that all doctors in a multidoctor practice are following the same basic protocols so as to avoid client confusion that will undermine client trust in the practice.
Manual, Exam Room Assistant	A resource for those veterinary assistants responsible for assisting veterinarians in appointments and other exam room procedures ranging from pedicures to emergency triage.
Manual, Laboratory	A complete reference guide for technicians and doctors who may be working in the laboratory or processing samples through the laboratory.
Manual, Policy (Employee Handbook)	The document that describes the employment policies of a specific employer, describing what the employer expects of the employee, and what the employee can expect from the employer.
Manual, Receptionist or Customer Service	Outlines all front desk procedures in a step-by-step manner.
Manual, Safety	A guide that identifies hazards within the practice and delineates procedures for dealing with them.
Manual, Technician	Document designed to support the technicians/nurses in accomplishing their daily tasks in the back of the practice. It includes step-by-step instructions on how to operate and maintain all technical aspects in the practice.
Margin Pricing	Also known as cost-plus pricing, this involves taking all the direct and indirect costs in providing a good or service and adding a set amount or percentage that corresponds to a gross profit margin to arrive at a retail price.
Marginally Literate	Possesses only the most basic of reading and writing skills.

Market	Your customers, prospective customers, and other consumers or providers of your products and service. Competition is central to the concept of market – clients can choose you, or other options, or not buy at all.
Market Development	Promoting existing products to new markets.
Market Identity	The results of positioning; the way in which a practice is perceived or understood by pet owners and in the marketplace.
Market Maturation	As a growth market for services or products begins to transition into a more stable market, this often marks a time when customer needs or demand are not evolving or growing rapidly. As a market shifts from growth to maturation, businesses need to adopt different strategies due to the nature of competition and the demands of the customer.
Market Penetration	The extent of sales of existing products and services to existing clients.
Market Research	Determining attitudes and behaviors of various public segments and their causes in order to plan, implement, and measure activities to influence or change those attitudes and behaviors.
Market Segment	A piece or part of the overall market that shares similarities in its demographic traits, attitudes or views, that lead it to experience similar needs or desires.
Market Segmentation	The process of splitting or segmenting the pet owner market into identifiable parts or segments that share similar traits. Market segmentation makes it easier for any business to identify and reach out to its most likely and/or desirable targets.
Market Viability	Determination of the probable success of a business venture based on an evaluation of demand, price, and quality of goods or services.
Marketing	The process of developing and delivering services and/or products matched to the needs of consumers with the ability, desire, and means to acquire them. Marketing includes service/product development, pricing, distribution, and promotion.
Marketing Communications	Combination of activities designed to sell a product, service, or idea, including advertising, collateral (printed) materials, publicity, promotion, packaging, point-of-sale display, trade shows, and special events.
Marketing Goals	The ultimate measurable outcome – or series of outcomes – that a business desires to achieve based on marketing opportunities and the realities of the marketplace.
Marketing Mix	The unique blend of product, pricing, promotion, and place (distribution channel) designed to reach a specific group of consumers.
Marketing Plan	Involves establishing marketing objectives, defining target markets, and deciding on the marketing mix.
Marketing Process	The steps involved in developing, producing, and delivering products and/or services to a targeted group.
Marketplace	A collective term for the representation of numerous market segments that span a wide range of consumer demographic and lifestyle traits.
Marketplace Opportunity	An identified reason to pursue and reach out to a particular market segment as a result of unmet needs, dissatisfaction, inadequate delivery systems or other weaknesses affecting the segment.
Mark-Up Pricing	Pricing based on taking the acquisition cost and increasing it by percentage or factor to arrive at a retail price.
Maslow's Hierarchy of Needs	People seek to satisfy basic needs, and satisfying a lower-level need results in the next level being a motivating factor.
Materials	Costs associated with providing products used for a service, including both direct and indirect costs.
Mean Arterial Pressure (MAP)	A measurement of the average pressure in the arteries at one moment in time.
Means Test	A determination as to whether an individual, family or group has the ability to pay for services without assistance (i.e., literally do they have the financial *means* to afford care without being subsidized?).

Media Relations	Outreach to news media in seeking publicity or responding to their interest in an organization.
Medical Error	An adverse effect of patient care that may or may not be harmful to the patient but could have been prevented.
Medical Massage	The application of specific massage techniques to a specific issue the patient is exhibiting.
Medical Model of Nursing	An approach to nursing whereby only the signs and symptoms that are presenting are treated, usually linked to a specific diagnosis.
Medical Record	A chronological written account of a patient's examination and treatment that includes the patient's medical history and complaints, the veterinarian's physical findings, the results of diagnostic tests and procedures, definitive or differential diagnoses, medications and therapeutic procedures, prognoses, and follow-up plans.
Medicalese	Terminology used within the profession that may not be familiar to the client.
Medicalization	In veterinary medicine, this term has come to represent the percentage of total owned animals that have been seen by a veterinarian at least once in a 12-month period. This is different from the sociological use of the term to describe nonmedical issues that are described in medical terms of prevention, diagnosis, and treatment.
Medically Important Antibiotics	Antibiotics that are used in both veterinary and human medicine and are characterized by the World Health Organization (WHO) and the FDA as important for therapeutic use in humans. For example, macrolides and tetracyclines are "medically important" but ionophores are not, because they are not used therapeutically in humans.
Mental Health	An individual's condition with regard to their emotional, cognitive, and psychological well-being.
Mental Illness	Condition which causes serious disorder in an individual's behavior, emotions or thinking.
Mentor	An experienced individual assigned to help new employees navigate the culture and flow of the workplace, as well as manage office personalities and professional relationships.
Mentoring	An informal relationship where, on an ongoing basis, a more experienced individual offers guidance and/or career advice to a less experienced colleague.
Merchant	A business which accepts payments from consumers. Also, a type of bank account that allows businesses to accept payments by payment cards, typically debit or credit cards.
Meta Description	A snippet of text that summarizes a page's content, used primarily for search engine results purposes.
Metabolism	The physical and biochemical processes that make or use energy in the body.
Methicillin-Resistant Staphylococci	Related species of *Staphylococcus* bacteria that have acquired antimicrobial resistance to beta-lactam antibiotics.
Microbiome	The collective populations of microorganisms inhabiting a particular environment, including body surfaces and tissues.
Microbiota	The population of microbes in a specific location.
Microcytosis	The presence of smaller than normal erythrocytes, as evidenced by a decreased mean corpuscular volume (MCV).
Microsatellite	A tract of DNA in which certain base pairs are repeated. They are sometimes referred to as short tandem repeats.
Microwave Thinking	The mistaken perception that if changes are made, then results will be quickly evident. Most changes made will yield gradual improvement, which can be difficult to appreciate in times when instant gratification is expected.
Minimum Database	A set of diagnostic tests that is recommended to be performed on every patient to provide the attending clinician with sufficient data to either confirm a diagnosis or narrow down the possibilities of what may be ailing the patient.

Minimum Inhibitory Concentration	The lowest drug concentration that inhibits bacterial growth.
Minimum Order Point	The level below which you don't want your inventory stock to fall.
Mission Statement	A formal summary of the aims and values of a company, organization, or individual.
Mixed Breed	An animal of unknown or mixed parentage. Mixed-breed dogs are sometimes referred to as mutts or mongrels; mixed-breed cats are sometimes referred to as moggies or mutt-cats.
Mobile Health (mHealth)	Subclassification of telehealth in which mobile applications (apps) and wearables are used to provide healthcare information for pets
Mobility, Tooth (M)	An assessment of the degree of mobility of a tooth.
Modified Triadan System	A tooth-numbering system used in veterinary dentistry.
Mom-and-Pop	A colloquial term for a small, closely held company in which the principals owning the business are also the principals working in the business.
Monoamine Neurotransmitters	Noradrenaline/norepinephrine, dopamine, and serotonin.
Moral Distress	When (i) you know the ethically appropriate action to take, but you are unable to act upon it, and (ii) you act in a manner contrary to your personal and professional values, which undermines your integrity and authenticity.
Moral Turpitude	The act of baseness, vileness, or depravity in private and social duties which people owe to their fellows or society in general, contrary to accepted and customary rules of right and duty to others. It also includes acts or behaviors that gravely violate moral sentiment or accepted moral standards of a community.
Morbidity	Having a disease, or the clinical signs associated with a disease.
Motivation	The desire to accomplish things for the sake of achievement.
Motivators	Factors that create change in an employee's behavior, making his or her actions more consistent with or complementary to the practice's needs.
Mourning	When you take the grief you have on the inside and express it outside yourself; the outward expression of grief.
Multidisciplinary Team	A team that consists of clinicians from multiple specialties that are involved with a given patient's care.
Multidrug Resistant (MDR)	A classification of antimicrobial resistance in a microorganism characterized by resistance to three or more classes of antimicrobial drugs.
Multimedia	Media and content that use a combination of different content forms. Multimedia includes a combination of text, audio, still images, animation, video, or interactivity content forms.
Multimodal Pain Management	An approach to pain that considers the source of the pain as well as the mechanism of action of available drug choices, often combining several drugs at lower doses.
Muscle Condition Score (MCS)	Assessment of a patient's muscle mass graded as normal, mild, moderate, or severe muscle loss.
Mutation	Permanent alterations in the DNA sequence. These can occur due to mistakes that can happen during the DNA replication process, environmental factors (e.g., UV light), or infections (e.g., viruses).
Mutation Test	A test that targets the actual DNA change that causes the disease; sometimes referred to as a direct genetic test.
Mycobiota	The population of fungal microbes in a specific location.
Myers-Briggs Type Indicator (MBTI)	A well-established test instrument that measures the personality traits and preferences of normal, healthy people. The test is a personality inventory, not a test of skills or abilities.
Myers-Briggs Type Indicator (MBTI) Personality Types	The MBTI Personality Types (16 in all) are the result of individual preferences on the four MBTI scales. An individual's personality type does not change over time; however, people may express their type in somewhat different ways at different times, and at different ages and stages of life.

Myofascial Trigger Point Diagnosis and Therapy	The diagnosis and treatment of hyperirritable soft tissue (fascial, tendon, ligament, muscle) areas which are a source of pain, decreased healing, and altered function.
Mystery Shoppers	Individuals known to management but unknown to the team, who call or visit the practice and report back to management about their experience. Mystery shoppers can be used to assess the practice's client service efforts from the client's perspective.
Narrative Nutritional History Taking	Using narrative veterinary medicine techniques to obtain a more accurate nutritional and lifestyle history.
Narrative Veterinary Medicine	Clinical communication technique utilizing open-ended questions to facilitate more open, thorough, truthful, and sensitive medical conversations.
Natural Disaster	A tornado, hurricane, blizzard, earthquake, wildfire, or even severe weather such as lightning storms.
Near Miss	Any circumstance in which the patient would have been harmed had the medical error reached the patient.
Near-Field Communication (NFC)	A wireless technology that allows devices to communicate by touching or "tapping" them, or by holding them in close proximity to each other.
Need	Require something because it is essential or very important.
Negative Feedback	Feedback pointing out what someone has done incorrectly so that they can change it. This form of feedback should still be framed positively; however, in many cases it isn't and becomes criticism.
Negative Punishment	Subtraction of a pleasurable stimulus to decrease the likelihood that an animal will perform a behavior again.
Negative Reinforcement	Subtraction of an aversive stimulus to increase the likelihood the animal will perform a behavior again.
Negative Stress	Also known as distress, this refers to the body's response to stress that lacks positive attributes and outcomes. Not all stress is bad, and negative stress refers to those stressors that cause anxiety or concern, are perceived as outside our coping abilities, can decrease performance, and can lead to mental and physical problems.
Neglect	Often used of negative acts causing unnecessary injury or death to an animal, such as deprivation of medical attention, ventilation, shelter, space, and sustenance.
Negligence	Doing an act that a person of ordinary prudence would not have done under similar circumstances, or the failure to do what a person of ordinary prudence would have done under the same or similar circumstances.
Negotiation	Any communication process between individuals that is intended to reach a compromise or agreement to the satisfaction of both parties; a discussion aimed at reaching an agreement.
Nephrotoxin	A substance that damages the kidneys.
Net Promoter or Net Promoter Score (NPS)	A management tool that can be used to gauge the loyalty of a practice's client relationships.
Network	A collection of computers and other hardware components interconnected by communication channels that allow sharing of resources and information.
Neuropharmacology	Utilizing substances to influence the nervous system and behavior.
Neutral Stimulus	Anything that has an effect on behavior before conditioning occurs.
New Client Target	The number of new clients each practice needs to maintain its transaction volume. If a practice wishes to grow, it must exceed this number.
News Media	Any number of news and information outlets that might have an interest in covering a practice's news situation.
Nocebo	A negative type of placebo effect in which being informed that there could be adverse effects associated with a therapy increases the likelihood that adverse effects will be experienced and reported.
Nociception	Pain processing with peripheral neuronal activation, transmission in the primary afferent neuron, modulation in the spinal cord, and perception in various centers throughout the brain.

No-kill	Having or being a policy that prohibits or severely limits the euthanizing of animals in a shelter.
Noncompliance	This describes the veterinarian's lack of maintaining adequate medical records to meet the minimum requirements stated in a veterinary practice act.
Noncore vaccines	Vaccines that offer protection against less serious infections or those that provide a regional risk.
Nonlinearity	A relationship between *x* and *y*, wherein a unit change in *x* will not always bring about an equal unit change in *y*. The graphic representation of this relationship is a curve rather than a straight line.
Nonprofit	An entity that is not conceived for the purposes of earning a profit, but rather to serve a public good.
Nonverbal Communication	Aspects of communication, such as gestures and facial expressions or body postures, that do not involve verbal communication; this may include aspects of speech (accent, tone of voice, speed of speaking, etc.).
Normalizing	Providing a verbal message to the client that indicates the acceptance and normalcy of their preferences, thoughts, feelings, ideas, concerns, behaviors, and/or responses.
Norming	A team stage in which working styles are agreed to and systems are set up.
Not for Profit	Any activity that is conducted without purposes of earning a profit. Often used interchangeably with *nonprofit*.
Nursing Care Plans	The written record of the care planning process.
Nursing Process	A systematic approach to nursing comprising a four-stage cycle of assessment, planning, implementation, and evaluation.
Nutraceuticals	Dietary supplements intended for health benefits beyond prevention of essential nutrient deficiencies.
Nutrigenomics	Also known as nutritional genomics, this is the interaction of genetics and nutrition and the role the two play in the prevention and treatment of disease.
Nutritional Evaluation	An in-depth evaluation of objective and subjective data related to the patient's food and nutrient intake, lifestyle, and medical history.
Obesity	An increase in fat tissue mass sufficient to contribute to disease. Defined as 30% above ideal body weight, equivalent to 8 to 9/9 using the 9-point Body Condition Score system.
Objective Data	Data obtained by performing procedures that result in measurements that can usually be compared to an expected value, e.g., body temperature, blood pressure.
Occupational Stress	The particular stress that arises from working in a specific occupation.
Odds Ratio	The ratio of the odds of an event in a select group (e.g., breed) to the odds of an event in a control group.
Office Manager	Administrative staff primarily responsible for reception, clerical, and nonmedical staff in a practice. There is no standard definition for this term, and it is unregulated, so anyone can refer to himself or herself as an office manager.
Office Politics	When an individual or group tries to circumvent the system to gain privileges or power by manipulating events or other people to their advantage, usually in an underhand manner. This works against teamwork and fairness in the workplace.
Off-Label	Pharmaceuticals prescribed, dispensed, or administered for an unapproved indication. Also referred to as extra-label drug use.
Omnichannel Consumer	Consumer exposure to information and marketing messages, preferably seamlessly, through a variety of different channels, including bricks-and-mortar stores, the internet, apps, etc.
Onboarding	The process of helping new employees become productive more quickly by providing them with documentation and training related to practice culture, vision, policies, protocols, and expectations.

One Health	One Health is a concept that recognizes the interconnection between people, animals, and the environment and has a goal of optimal health for each.
On-the-Job Training	Method of training that focuses on employees acquiring skills within the work environment under normal working conditions. Through on-the-job training, team members acquire both general skills that they can transfer from one job to another and specific skills that are unique to a particular job.
Open Reading Frame	A continuous stretch of amino acid-forming codons that has the ability to be translated into a protein or peptide.
Open-Book Management	The premise that employers should share with employees the measures of the practice's business success so that employees better understand the efforts that impact the success of the business.
Open-Ended Question	A question that cannot be answered with a "yes" or "no" but requires a developed answer. These questions help identify opinions, attitudes, and beliefs.
Operant Conditioning	Also called Skinnerian conditioning or instrumental conditioning, this is a method of learning through trial and error that creates associations between behavior and consequence.
Operant Counterconditioning	Also called response substitution, this is a form of behavior modification performed by changing the animal's behavioral response from an unwanted behavior to a desired behavior in response to the same stimulus.
Opportunity Cost	A benefit that could have been realized, but wasn't, because an alternative was selected instead.
Optimization	In online terms, the strategy and tactics used to make a website favored in online searches.
Orchiectomy	Surgical excision of both testicles; synonymous with the term *castration*.
Ordering Costs	Costs associated with employee time used for shopping, ordering, receiving, and documenting purchased products.
Organizational Behavior	The values and behaviors that contribute to the unique social environment within an organization.
Organizational Chart	Overview of who reports to whom within an organization.
Organizational Compassion Fatigue	As a result of employing those with compassion fatigue, the effect on the organization where the personal symptoms of compassion fatigue are incorporated into the culture of the corporation.
Organizational Pyramid	A charted structure that usually puts the frontline workers at the bottom or base of the pyramid, with increasing tiers of management levels ascending to the owners or executives of the company at the apex.
Orientation Training	Introductory training that all new employees should receive. It is informational and typically covers hours of operation, confidentiality, pay and compensation, dress code, practice mission and philosophy, overview of how the hospital works and expected interaction between the departments, hospital policy and goals, grounds for dismissal, and the "trial period" for new employees.
Osteoarthritis	A subset of degenerative joint disease that occurs when the protecting cartilage on the ends of bones wears down over time.
Otitis Externa	Inflammation of the external ear canal.
Outbound Telephone Calls	Telephone calls to clients that are initiated by the practice. Their purpose is to increase the purchases of veterinary services, improve client service, and salvage lost accounts.
Outer Leadership Qualities	Qualities an individual must possess as outer signs that he or she can be an effective leader – communication skills, visibility, teamwork, attentiveness, and commitment.
Outreach	A means of connecting with and communicating with a target; part of the promotion phase of marketing.

Outsourcing (Laboratory Testing)	Laboratory testing that is sent out to be completed by an outside company, typically a reference laboratory.
Ovariectomy	Surgical removal of one or both ovaries, leaving the uterus intact.
Ovariohysterectomy	Surgical excision of the ovaries and uterus.
Overcapacity	Situation in which there is capacity available to perform services, but inadequate demand to perform those services at capacity.
Overhead	Costs of operating a business, even if no clients avail themselves of any services.
p27 Protein	Feline leukemia virus (FeLV) soluble antigen.
P4 Medicine	The clinical face of systems medicine, P4 medicine is Predictive, Preventive, Personalized, and Participatory. Its two major objectives are to quantify wellness and demystify disease.
Pain	Multidimensional unpleasant sensory and emotional experience associated with actual or potential tissue damage.
Pain Score	The application of an objective rating to a subjective acute physiological and/or psychological hurtful experience.
Pain, Acute	Pain experienced during the expected time of posttrauma inflammation and healing.
Pain, Adaptive	Normal and protective pain.
Pain, Chronic	Pain experienced past the expected time of posttrauma inflammation and healing (in humans, defined as pain still present 2–3 months or longer after initial tissue damage).
Pain, Maladaptive	Maladaptive pain is a chronic pain state in which the pain is out of proportion to tissue damage and that persists long after tissues have healed. This is "pain as disease."
Pain, Neuropathic	Hypersensitization and maladaptive pain that have progressed to gene expression and permanent morphological and functional changes in the peripheral and central nervous system; pain as a disease at this point.
Palliative Care	Treatment that supports or improves the quality of life (QOL) for patients and caregivers by relieving suffering; this applies to treating curable or chronic conditions as well as end of life (EOL) care.
Paper-Light Practice	A practice that uses practice information management software but continues to use some paper forms in the workflow of the practice.
Paperless Practice	Complete digital utilization of the practice management software such that paper medical records are no longer needed or used.
Paralanguage	Range of voice tone, rhythm, volume of speech, degree of emphasis, and rate of speech.
Parasite	An organism that lives in (endoparasite) or on (ectoparasite) another organism (its host) and benefits by deriving nutrients at the host's expense.
Parasympathomimetics	A group of medications used in glaucoma treatment that cause miosis, leading to a decrease in intraocular pressure by opening the iridocorneal angle.
Paraverbal Communication	The pitch, tone, inflection, and pace of a communication. Often referred to as "it's not what you said, it's *how* you said it." The "how" is the paraverbal.
Pareto Principle	The concept that 80% of outcomes come from 20% of causes. For example, 80% of pharmacy revenues come from 20% of products.
Pathogen or Infectious Agent	Organism causing disease, typically referring to microorganisms or microbes such as prion, virus, bacterium, protozoan, or fungus.
Patient Safety Incident	An umbrella term for an episode of failed or substandard healthcare that causes or has the potential to cause an adverse event.
Patient-Centered Care	Human-centered healthcare concept that strives to ensure all decisions are made with the involvement of the patient and their chosen support network.
Patient-First Language	Communication technique that emphasizes the pet patient first, not the disease or medical condition, in order to decrease bias and judgment by veterinary professionals.

Payment Plan	A bundled medical plan in which specified veterinary services are provided and paid for in installments or prepaid, rather than at time of service. Sometimes referred to as wellness plans or concierge plans.
Payment Plan Management Services	Companies that set up in-house payment plans for veterinary practices. These companies typically assess credit, set up automatic bank withdrawals from the pet owner's account, and follow up if payments aren't made.
Pediatric Gonadectomy	Surgical excision of the canine/feline male/female reproductive tract between 6 to 16 weeks of age.
Pedigree	Recorded ancestry.
Pedigreed	An animal whose ancestry is recorded by a registry organization.
Penetrance	The likelihood of individuals in a population with a given genetic variant (genotype) fully displaying the clinical manifestations (phenotype) of that variant.
Perceived Value	What someone feels they have gotten in return (not always financial) in return for money they have paid.
Perception Gap	The difference between what a practice believes is the perception of clients and what clients actually perceive. The result is a *perception gap* – the desired reality and the actual reality may not be in alignment.
Performance Appraisal	A system of determining how well an individual employee has performed during a period of time.
Performance Review	A formal individual performance appraisal and/or review process. Generally performed by a more senior staff member on or about a more junior employee.
Performing	A team stage where members are functioning at a high level.
Periodontal disease (PD)	Infection, inflammation, and loss of the tissues surrounding and supporting the teeth, including attached gingiva, bone, the periodontal ligament and cementum covering the root.
Periodontal Disease Index (PD or PDI)	The degree of severity of periodontal disease of a particular tooth (stage).
Periodontal Ligament (PDL)	Connective tissue that runs between the tooth and bone (alveolar socket), supporting and keeping the tooth in the alveolus (socket).
Periodontal Pocket (PP)	The deepening of a sulcus depth due to the attachment loss of periodontal tissues, measured in millimeters.
Periodontal Probe	A hand instrument used to measure the depth of a pocket or amount of root exposure; marked in various millimeter increments, depending on type of probe.
Periodontitis	Inflammation of the periodontal structures.
Perpetual Inventory	System of inventory control in which the number and value of inventory items can be determined directly by stock records and are updated directly as transactions occur.
Personal Property	Movable assets.
Personal Protective Equipment (PPE)	Any type of clothing or items used to protect an animal handler (and potentially the animal itself) from physical and health hazards. PPE includes specialized/disposable clothing, gloves, masks, protective eyewear, catchpoles, restraints, nets, prods, and other items.
Personally Identifiable Information (PII)	Any information that can be used to identify an individual. Regulatory definitions vary by location.
Personalty	Personal property; compare "realty," which is real property.
Pesticide	Any substance or mixture of substances intended for preventing, destroying, repelling, or mitigating pests.
Pet Information Management System (PIMS)	The software used by the practice to record appointments, notes, prescriptions, vaccines, reminders, invoices, and more. Also known as *practice management software* (PMS).
Pet Parent	A term used to designate that the relationship between individuals and their pets is more than just ownership. Such individuals endeavor to do what is best for their pets and seek to maximize the benefits of the human–animal bond for both parties.

Pet-Specific	Pertaining to, and relevant to, the needs and concerns of different pet types based on variables such as breed, size, color, lifestyle, geographic region, health risks, and so on.
Pet-Specific Care	An approach that tailors veterinary care to individual pets based on their predicted risk of disease, likely response to intervention, and client needs.
Pharmacodynamics	The effects of drugs and their mechanisms of action.
Pharmacogenetics	The study of inherited genetic differences in drug pharmacokinetics and pharmacodynamics, which can affect individual responses to drugs, both in terms of therapeutic effect as well as adverse effects.
Pharmacogenomics	The study of how genes affect the response to drugs.
Pharmacokinetics	What the body does to a drug, including absorption, distribution, metabolism, and excretion.
Pharmacovigilance	The science and activities relating to the detection, assessment, understanding, and prevention of adverse effects or any other drug-related problem.
Phene	A trait or characteristic that is genetically determined.
Phenotype	The outward observable characteristics of an individual, resulting from the interaction of its underlying genetic constitution with environmental factors.
Phenotypic Testing	Testing that determines observable features of traits, phenes or conditions and compares them to normal or typical values.
Phishing	Attempting to acquire such information as passwords, user names, and credit card details through electronic communication by posing as a trustworthy entity.
Phobia	Persistent and excessive fear of certain things or situations that are usually out of proportion to the actual threat that they present. Examples include fear of fireworks, thunderstorms, and fire alarms.
Physiotherapy	Physiotherapy (also referred to as physical therapy) involves the use of physical medicine techniques and modalities (such as therapeutic laser, neuromuscular electrical stimulation, etc.) to restore mobility and function.
Pica	The persistent ingestion of nonfood items.
Pioneer Drug	The brand name or patented version of a drug, later copied to make generic drugs after the patent expires.
Placebo	The beneficial effect perceived for a product without actual physiological impact.
Plan B	An alternate strategy, often considered as a second choice to a preferred strategy.
Plaque Index (PI)	A measurement of the accumulation of plaque on the tooth surface.
Polymorphism	Genetic variation within a population and with which selection pressures can operate.
Polypharmacy	The simultaneous use of multiple drugs in an individual patient.
Portal, Patient	Healthcare-related online applications that allow clients to interact and communicate with their pet's healthcare providers, such as veterinarians.
Positioning Strategy	Defining a practice and creating a market identity in alignment with the needs and desires of the practice's targets.
Positive Feedback	Feedback that is supportive of what someone has done, and framed positively.
Positive Reinforcement	Rewarding a pet for a desired behavior in order to increase the frequency of that behavior
Postantibiotic Effect (PAE)	The period of time for which bacterial growth remains suppressed after antimicrobial concentration has decreased below the minimum inhibitory concentration (MIC).
Postdated Checks	Checks written on the current day, but dated for a future date.
Posttraumatic Stress Disorder (PTSD)	The impact of experiencing a traumatic event first-hand.
Poverty	Living with an income below an amount determined to provide a basic standard of living.

Practice App	Application used on smartphones that allows easy access to a business and improves the client experience.
Practice Culture	Refers to the attitudes, motivation, values, role expectations, and beliefs that employees have about their daily work environment.
Practice Information Management Software (PIMS)	The software that tracks client and patient data and interactions in a veterinary hospital. Also known as practice management software (PMS) and pet information management system.
Practice Management Software (PMS)	Software that deals with the day-to-day operations of a medical practice. Also known as practice information management software (PIMS) and pet information management system.
Practice Manager	Similar to an office manager, but typically with more responsibility for staff supervision and human resource issues.
Practice Models	The array of various aspects of ownership and management of veterinary practices including the practice size, and the scope and breadth of services or markets served.
Practice Positioning	Defining how a practice wants to be understood in the marketplace; the *space* the practice seeks to occupy in the minds of pet owners.
Precision Cancer Medicine	An emerging field in oncology and molecular biology through which a patient's cancer is analyzed to a molecular level with the goal of identifying unique characteristics (most often specific mutations) that may respond more favorably to specific (targeted) treatments.
Preiridal Fibrovascular Membrane	A network of fibrovascular membrane that forms on the anterior surface of the iris and extends into and over the iridocorneal angle.
Premium, Insurance	Amount paid to an insurance company in exchange for insurance coverage.
Presenteeism	The concept that describes being present at work but ineffective due to poor physical or mental health.
Prevalence	The number of cases of a disease process that occur in a specified period of time.
Primary Literature	Published reports of original research studies.
Primary Care Veterinarian	A veterinarian who is the primary contact for a pet owner and manages the medical needs of the pet. Also known as a first-opinion veterinarian or general practitioner.
Principles of Veterinary Medical Ethics	A code of ethical conduct to which veterinarians are expected to adhere.
Privacy Policy	A written or legal statement that discloses how a practice uses or intends to use a client or customer's data. Generally pertains to nonmedical information such as name and demographic data, but may also include purchasing data, credit card information, data gathered online, and other potentially sensitive information.
Private Foundation	A nonprofit organization which is usually created via a single primary donation from an individual or a business and whose funds and programs are managed by its own trustees or directors.
Probate	The court process by which a will is proved valid or invalid.
Probiotic	A substance or preparation that stimulates proliferation of beneficial microorganisms.
Problem Behavior	Any behavior by a pet that the owner considers to be undesirable. The behavior may or may not be normal for the species.
Problem-Focused Coping	Coping strategies that address the underlying cause of a problem.
Product Development	Developing new products or services for sale to existing clients.
Production	A form of commission paid to veterinarians on the basis of their revenue generation.
Production Report	Report produced by practice management software which shows fees by service code, i.e., surgery, examinations, vaccinations, retail sales, etc.
Productivity	The rate at which goods or services are produced per unit of labor.
Professional Development Plan	A plan assembled by an organization's management for the purpose of enriching its employees' skills and enhancing their careers, while at the same time aligning the employees' motives with the organization's business needs and goals.

Professional Liability Insurance	Insurance that protects against claims arising from acts, errors, or omissions in rendering services of a professional nature.
Profit Center	A section of a practice that can be assessed in terms of its revenues and expenses (e.g., surgery, imaging, laboratory, etc.).
Profit Center Report	Report that tracks income from related service codes (all dentistry codes, for example) and expenses related to producing that income (doctor and tech time, dental supplies, dental equipment, etc.), arriving at the profit (or loss) for those practice areas.
Profit Margin	The (gross) profit margin is the difference between the total cost to the practice of delivering a product or service and the final price to the client. It is typically expressed as a percentage.
Profitability	The revenue for a practice once all expenses are paid, a fair market facility rent is paid, and the owner is compensated at a rate similar to what employees in the same position are paid.
Pro-Forma Budget	Budget that charts a course of future action for the practice by outlining and defining the plans of the practice in financial terms.
Prognosis	A forecasting of the probable course and outcome of a disease, especially of the chances of recovery.
Project	A project is a temporary endeavor with a defined beginning and end (usually time-constrained, and often constrained by funding or deliverables), undertaken to meet unique goals and objectives, typically to bring about beneficial change or added value.
Project Management	The discipline of planning, organizing, securing, managing, leading, and controlling resources to achieve specific goals.
Promotion	The act of encouraging a trial or persuading an action to contribute to the growth and advancement of a business.
Prophy	Colloquial term for a dental prophylaxis procedure.
Pros/Cons Analysis	A decision-making tool that weighs advantages (pros) and disadvantages (cons) of a contemplated change. Weighting may be assigned to various pros and cons.
Prospect	An identified potential client who can be targeted for business.
Prostaglandin Analogues	A group of glaucoma medications which decrease intraocular pressures and are typically used in cases of primary glaucoma. These medications reduce intraocular pressure by increasing uveoscleral outflow.
Proteinuria	The condition by which protein appears in the urine.
Protocol	The form and etiquette observed for a specific event or procedure.
Pro-Veterinary	Content that supports the message and recommendations of veterinarians and the veterinary profession.
Proxemics	Spatial relationships or distance between individuals when communicating, including barriers that may inhibit the communication process.
Psychographics	Research that attempts to explain behavior by analyzing people's personality traits and values.
Puberty	Period in development characterized by the onset of reproductive system activity.
Public Relations	The art of developing reciprocal understanding and good will between a business and the public.
Publicity	The act of delivering information of news value as a means of gaining public attention or support.
Publics	Any group with some common characteristic with which an organization needs to communicate, including the media, government bodies, financial institutions, pressure groups, and so on, as well as customers and suppliers.
Pull Marketing	The opposite of "push" marketing in which marketers seek to engage and connect with consumers through relevant and compelling content with the goal of consumer engagement leading to sales.

Pulse Pressure	The change in the force of blood moving through the arteries between systole and diastole; the greater the pulse pressure, the greater the difference between the systolic and diastolic blood pressures.
Punishment	The removal or addition of something in order to attempt to decrease a behavior (positive punishment = yelling, leash corrections, physical reprimands; negative punishment = removing something desired, e.g., attention or food).
Puppy	Young dog aged between 8 and 16 weeks.
Puppy Mill	Derogatory term for an indiscriminate breeding facility, where pets are commodities for sale, sometimes with little concern for animal welfare or genetic health.
Purebred	An animal bred from parents of the same breed or variety; one whose ancestry contains members of the same breed.
Purposefully Bred	A description indicating the intentional breeding of two animals, compared to the random matings that tend to occur in nature.
Push Marketing	Promotional efforts that rely on advertising campaigns to promote products and services with the goal of increasing consumer sales.
Push Notifications	This allows a smartphone to receive and display alerts even when the device's screen is locked and the application that is pushing the notification is closed.
Pyoderma	A skin condition associated with the production of pus. Often used synonymously with any bacterial issue involving the skin.
Qualitative Research	Qualitative research generates nonnumerical data.
Quality of Life (QOL)	Quality of life refers to the total well-being of an individual animal, taking into account the physical, social, and emotional components of the animal's life.
Quality of Life Assessment	The assessment a caregiver makes about how well or poorly an animal is doing, considering the totality of an animal's feelings, experiences, and preferences, as demonstrated by the animal.
Quality of Life Score	An objective rating of criteria that determine how well an animal lives and daily functions long term, usually with a chronic disease, impairment, or pain.
Quantitative Research	Quantitative research generates numerical data or information that can be converted into numbers.
Query	Precise request for information. A question.
Ransomware	Malware that encrypts the files on the computer, making them unreadable unless a ransom is paid.
Rate of Return	The amount an investment appreciates or depreciates over time, often expressed as a decimal (e.g., 0.06) or a percentage (6%).
Reach	The total number of different people or households exposed to a medium during a given period.
Real-Time Laboratory Testing	Laboratory testing performed at the hospital (in-house), by the hospital team, for immediate results.
Reasonableness	The subjective standard by which the actions of a veterinarian with similar qualifications, skills, and knowledge are assessed.
Recessive	Heritable characteristics, traits or diseases that are expressed only when inherited from both parents.
Recklessly	Consciously creating a risk that injury might result with some probability, but disregarding that risk due to indifference.
Recommendation	A suggestion or proposal as to the best course of action, especially one put forward by an authoritative body.
Recurring Revenues	The portion of a company's revenue that is highly likely to continue in the future. This is revenue that is predictable, stable, and can be counted on in the future with a high degree of certainty, and usually doesn't require the major costs of new customer acquisition.

Red Flag Rules	A set of Federal regulations that require certain businesses and organizations to develop and implement plans to keep client information secure in efforts to discourage identity theft.
Reference Interval (RI)	A range that has been ascribed to a population of healthy adult animals for a given diagnostic test. Synonymous with reference range or normal range.
Reference Laboratory	Offsite laboratory where tests are done on clinical specimens in order to obtain information about the health of a patient as pertaining to the diagnosis, treatment, and prevention of disease.
Referral	The transfer of patient care from one clinician or hospital to another, upon request.
Referral Marketing	Marketing to clients and other local businesses to get them to refer their friends, family, and co-workers to your practice for veterinary and other care that your practice provides.
Referring Veterinarian	The referring veterinarian is generally the primary care veterinarian for the pet, typically the veterinarian who requested the referral.
Referring Veterinarian Liaison	A staff member such as a technician who works with the hospital manager and specialists to facilitate improved relationships with area practitioners.
Reflective Listening	Communication technique that demonstrates to the client that his or her interests and concerns have been heard. It focuses completely on what the client is saying and confirms understanding of the message content and the underlying emotions to ensure an accurate understanding.
Regenerative Medicine	The process of creating and implanting living, functional tissues to repair or replace tissue or organ function lost due to age, disease, damage, or congenital defects.
Regulated Medical Waste	A subcategory of solid waste covering biohazardous or infectious waste produced by the diagnosis, treatment, or vaccination of animals.
Rehabilitation Modalities and Therapies	Techniques and tools used to enhance and restore functional ability and quality of life to those with physical impairments or disabilities via focus on connective and nervous tissues.
Relative Age	The age in "people years" that corresponds to a dog's or cat's age.
Relative Risk	The ratio of the probability of a phene, condition or trait occurring in a specific group (e.g., breed), compared to the probability of it happening in a nonaffiliated group.
Relinquishment	Giving up a pet for adoption or euthanasia.
Reorder Point	Inventory level at which additional product is ordered.
Responsibility	The duty to perform or complete an assigned task.
Resting Energy Requirement (RER)	The daily energy needed to sustain essential bodily functions (e.g., respiration, circulation, digestion, metabolism) while the dog/cat is at rest in a thermoneutral environment.
Retail-Anchored Practice	A veterinary practice affiliated with a retail entity.
Retention Marketing	Marketing specifically to existing clientele to get them to continue to utilize services.
Retrovirus	An infectious agent that converts its RNA into DNA after infecting a host cell. This DNA is integrated into the genetic material of the host cell, allowing the virus to replicate. When the host cell divides, each daughter cell carries copies of proviral DNA, thus spreading the infection.
Return on Investment (ROI)	Income that an investment generates compared to the cost of the investment. ROI is a measure of how effectively a firm uses its assets to generate profit.
Revenues	All sales of the practice for goods and services. Also referred to as income, and in some countries as turnover.
Reversible Contraception	A method of preventing pregnancy that does not result in permanent sterilization, such that if pregnancy is desired at a later point, removal of this method makes this physiological state possible.
Risk	An exposure to danger, harm or loss.
Risk Management	The identification and assessment of risks and minimization of their impact, such as with insurance or reducing risk factors.

Risk-Averse	Less likely to take risks.
Root Cause Analysis	A systemic approach to establishing the fundamental cause or causes of a problem.
Root Exposure (RE)	Exposure of the root of a tooth that is normally covered by periodontal tissues (gingiva and bone).
Root Planing, Closed (RP/C)	Scaling, curettage or debridement of a root without making a gingival flap to expose the area; calculus, debris, and diseased soft tissue are removed from the periodontal pocket area.
Root Planing, Open (RP/O)	Making a gingival flap with incisions and elevation (lifting the gingival tissue off the surface of the tooth and bone) for scaling or debridement of the exposed/visible portion of a root; calculus, debris, and diseased soft tissue are removed from the periodontal pocket area.
Rule of Thumb	A rough approximation that is not intended to be strictly accurate or reliable for every situation.
Safety Data Sheet (SDS)	A document prepared by the manufacturer of a product that contains detailed technical and safety information about the product.
Safety Stock	Inventory remaining past the reorder point.
Sales Funnel	The system or process that companies lead customers through when purchasing a product or service.
Sanitization	Reducing microbial populations to safe levels.
Scaling (Dental)	Removal of calculus and debris from a tooth surface using hand instruments (hand scaler or curette) or mechanical instruments (ultrasonic scaler).
Scienter	A legal term implying that the offender had knowledge of wrongdoing before the act was committed.
Screening	Testing for disease or disease precursors in seemingly well individuals for the purposes of early detection of subclinical disease.
Search Engine Optimization (SEO)	The process of affecting the visibility of a website or web page in a search engine's "natural" or unpaid ("organic") search results.
Secondary Traumatic Stress	An indirect exposure to trauma through a firsthand account or narrative of a traumatic event; compassion fatigue is a form of secondary traumatic stress.
Secretome	Proteins expressed by an organism and secreted into the extracellular space.
Sedation	The administration of one or more drugs to reduce anxiety and improve patient tolerance of a medical or diagnostic procedure.
Segmentation	A marketing term referring to the aggregating of prospective buyers into groups (segments) that have common needs and will respond similarly to a marketing action.
Self-Awareness	The ability to know one's emotions, strengths, and weaknesses and their impact on others.
Self-Directed Teams	Self-managed group of employees who work together to produce a product or service. They are empowered to effectively make "operational" decisions without deferring to a supervisor or other manager for their area.
Self-Regulation	The ability to control or redirect one's disruptive emotions and adapt to changing circumstances.
Senior	A pet's life stage defined as the fourth quartile of a pet's expected lifespan (from 75% to 100% of its lifespan).
Sensitive Period	Time in the development of young where the brain is more sensitive to environmental stimuli.
Sensitivity	A statistical measure that examines how many actual positive test results are correctly identified as such.
Sensory Marketing	Marketing that engages the consumers' senses and as a result affects their perception, judgment, and behavior.
Seroprevalence	The number of individuals within a population who have a positive result for a specific disease when using a blood-based diagnostic test.

Service	The action of helping or doing work for someone.
Service Mix	The selection of services a practice offers that should be in alignment with, and reflective of, the needs of its targets.
Service Standards	Standards that help define the level of service that clients should expect to receive, whether it be in person, on the phone, or in writing, and provide a foundation for management and employee expectations and obligations.
Settlor	A person who has created a trust. Also known as a trustor or grantor.
Sex-Limited Trait	A trait that can be only seen in one gender, even though it is not transmitted on the sex chromosomes.
Sex-Linked Trait	A trait that is transmitted on the X chromosome.
Shaping	Teaching a new behavior through selectively reinforcing small criteria toward the desired behavior.
Shared Decision Making	Shared decision making addresses the ethical need to fully inform clients about the risks and benefits of treatments, as well as the need to ensure that clients' values and preferences play a prominent role.
Shared Leadership	Sharing wisdom, knowledge, and influence through empowerment.
Short Interspersed Element	Noncoding sequences of DNA that are useful markers of divergent evolution between species.
Short Message Service (SMS)	Commonly referred to as text messages. Limited to 160 characters per message, including spaces.
Shortage Costs	The costs of not maintaining sufficient inventory so that the sale is lost when consumers go elsewhere.
Shrinkage	The loss of product from inventory not resulting from sale, including product lost to employee theft, shoplifting, administrative and paperwork errors, and vendor errors/issues.
Signalment	That part of the veterinary medical history dealing with the animal's age, sex, and breed.
Single Nucleotide Polymorphism (SNP)	Genetic variation in a single DNA building block (nucleotide) that occurs at a specific position in the genome and is present within the population. Most have little or no impact on health and disease, but some can predict an individual's risk of developing particular diseases, an individual's likely response to certain drugs, or susceptibility to environmental factors.
Situational Analysis	Review of the current environment, including competitors as well as social, political, economic, and legal conditions. For established veterinary practices, the situational analysis includes looking carefully at the current state of affairs for the practice in terms of its ability to meet client needs.
Skill Hog	Employee who has mastered a skill, but refuses to train others.
Skill-Based Scheduling	A method of scheduling based on the known skill sets of individual employees and the needs of the practice. The more skill sets an employee has developed, the more flexible their scheduling options.
SMART	Goal-based acronym for Specific, Measurable, Attainable, Related to Mission, and Time limited.
Smart Device	An electronic device that is cordless (unless while being charged), mobile (easily transportable), always connected (via Wi-Fi, 3G, 4G, 5G, etc.) and is capable of voice and video communication, internet browsing, "geo-location" (for search purposes), and that can operate to some extent autonomously.
Smartphone	Mobile telephone built on a mobile operating system, with more advanced computing capability and connectivity than a feature phone.
SOAP	An acronym that identifies the most common data entry format used by veterinary practices. The data are generally located in the progress notes portion of a problem-oriented medical record. The letters stand for Subjective, Objective, Assessment, and Plan.

Social Media	Interactive platforms that allow individuals and communities to create and share user-generated content.
Social Skills	The ability to manage relationships and direct others in a desired direction.
Soft Costs	Cost of intangible items that may include fees to regulatory agencies, any legal fees, financing costs, design fees, insurance costs, and relocation expenses.
Soft Skills	Personal attributes that enhance an individual's interactions, job performance, and career prospects. Soft skills relate to a person's ability to interact effectively with co-workers and customers; these skills are broadly applicable both inside and outside the workplace.
Software	A collection of computer programs and related data that provide the instructions for telling a computer what to do and how to do it. Software refers to one or more computer programs and data held in the storage of the computer.
Solid Waste	A term that covers a broad range of solid and liquid waste products. Most of the waste that is produced by a veterinary hospital is solid waste. Solid waste is then broken down into many different categories and subcategories.
Spam	The use of electronic messaging systems to send unsolicited bulk messages, especially advertising, indiscriminately.
Specialist	A clinician highly skilled in a specific medical discipline.
Specialty/Emergency Practice	A facility that operates an emergency facility to ensure 24-hour care for all hospitalized patients, as well as specialty practice.
Specificity	A statistical measure that examines how many actual negative test results are correctly identified as such.
Spectrum of Care	The availability and accessibility of veterinary medical care regardless of the socioeconomic status of the pet owner.
Spoliation	The intentional destruction of documents meant to be saved.
Spyware	A type of malware (malicious software) installed on computers that collects information about users without their knowledge. The presence of spyware is typically hidden from the user and can be difficult to detect.
Staff Turnover	The rate at which workers leave a workplace and need to be replaced by new employees.
Stakeholder	An individual or a group with an interest in a particular business; the individual or group has something at risk (at stake).
Stand-Alone Specialty Practice	A facility that does not have an emergency facility present on site and would send critical cases to an emergency practice for observation during the evenings and/or weekends.
Standard of Care	Customized directives within a practice, organization or locality that promote and guide clinical practice. In veterinary medicine, the term *standard of care* is often used synonymously with *protocol*. Also, the legal level of medical care that is expected for a competent veterinary professional to deliver to a patient.
Standard Operating Procedures (SOP)	Preferred methods of doing a procedure or protocol in the practice.
Standards of Performance	Written protocols regarding patient care, customer service, and team professionalism.
Standing	The legal requirement for a party to prove that they can participate in a lawsuit. Simply put, standing is the legal right and ability to sue and be sued.
Stationary Practice	A traditional "bricks and mortar" veterinary practice, as compared to a mobile practice.
Sterilization	A process by which *all* microorganisms are removed, deactivated or eliminated from an object.
Sticker Shock	Surprise as a result of a bill due to lack of communication and not being prepared for the amount.

Stockout	A stockout, or out-of-stock event, is a situation in which the demand for an item cannot be met from the supply in inventory; the amount on hand is insufficient for the amount needed or wanted.
Storming	A team stage in which members come into conflict over goals and personalities.
Straight 15s	Historically the most common scheduling system. The staff would schedule a steady stream of appointments at 15-minute intervals (e.g., 8.00, 8.15, 8.30, etc.). Currently, it is estimated that 10–15% of companion animal practices still use this system.
Straight 20s	A popular expansion of the straight 15s approach. Appointments are scheduled at 20-minute intervals (e.g., 8.00, 8.20, 8.40, etc.). Currently, it is estimated that approximately 40% of companion animal practices use this system.
Straight 30s	A popular time-scheduling option in very competitive markets and perhaps the schedule of choice for new practices trying to bond clientele. It is estimated that less than 5% of companion animal practices use this system.
Strategy	A plan or action to achieve a specific end, typically within a long time frame (usually greater than a year). Often, strategies are achieved by utilizing various tactics to achieve specific aspects of the overall strategy.
Stratified Medicine	An approach to medical care designed to segment or stratify patients into grouping with similar disease profiles, attributes, or presumed response to specific therapies.
Stress	Physiological changes experienced when the animal's emotional state is disrupted by an aversive trigger or event. The response exists along a spectrum from mild to extreme stress, which is called distress.
Subclinical	Referring to a condition which has not yet advanced to the stage where there are readily evident clinical signs.
Subjective Data	Data obtained through qualitative descriptive reports from an owner or healthcare professional after assessing an animal, e.g., coat condition or level of pain.
Subsidized Care	Programs in which all or part of the cost of veterinary care is paid by an entity other than the pet's owner.
Suffering	An unpleasant or painful experience, feeling, emotion, or sensation, which may be acute or chronic in nature. Suffering is an umbrella term that covers the range of negative subjective experiences which may be experienced by humans and by animals.
Sulcus	The space that naturally exists between the tooth/root surface and the unattached edge of gingiva (free gingival margin).
SWOT Analysis	A strategic planning method used to evaluate the Strengths, Weaknesses/Limitations, Opportunities, and Threats involved in a project or business venture.
Sympathy	Feelings of sorrow for someone else's misfortune.
Synthetic Literature	Published summaries and critical analyses of primary research studies.
System Failure	Any circumstance in which one or more components of the workplace alter an employee's ability to act under pressure, resulting in medical error.
Systematic Review	A comprehensive summary and critical appraisal of primary research studies conducted according to established procedures for minimizing bias.
Systemic Hypertension	A condition that is characterized by a persistent increase in blood pressure within systemic vessels; that is, those that carry blood from the heart to the rest of the body, with the exception of the lungs.
Systole	The phase of the cardiac cycle in which the heart beats, forcing blood through a network of vasculature.
Tactic	A plan or action to achieve a specific end, typically within a short time frame (usually less than a year, but occasionally spanning a few years).
Talent Acquisition	The process of finding and acquiring skilled human labor for organizational needs and to meet any labor requirement.

Target	The particular market segment that is the focus or intended recipient of campaign efforts and messages.
Target Audience	A target audience is a specific group of people within a target market at which a product or the marketing message of a product/service is aimed.
Target Market	A particular type of client that the practice wants to attract.
Target Marketing	Identifying select target markets and directing marketing efforts to these targets. The opposite of mass marketing in which all customers and prospects are treated the same.
Target Organs	Organs and organ systems that are prone to injury from a specific threat. For example, if systemic hypertension is unchecked, target organs for damage include the central nervous system (CNS), cardiovascular system, kidneys, and eyes.
Team	Trained and focused group of people working synergistically toward a goal.
Team/Group Stages	A team grows and changes markedly during its lifetime. The process of development has been described as having four stages – forming, storming, norming, and performing.
Teamship	The collective standard of behavior that is understood and appreciated by everyone participating on a team.
Teamwork	The collaborative efforts of individuals to complete tasks effectively and efficiently.
Teleadvice	Subclassification of telehealth in which only general advice is provided that is not specific to a particular patient's situation.
Teleconsulting	Subclassification of telehealth in which the consulting takes place between a primary care veterinarian and a specialist.
Telehealth	Broad term to describe healthcare consulting delivered remotely. Also referred to as virtual care and connected care.
Telemedicine	Telehealth delivered between a veterinarian and an animal-owning client, under the auspices of a veterinary–client–patient relationship.
Telemonitoring	A form of telehealth in which patients are monitored remotely.
Teletriage	Subclassification of telehealth in which assessment is made remotely regarding the need for urgent veterinary visitation. Teletriage does not include rendering any diagnosis, just advising regarding the potential urgency of the situation based on the information provided.
Telomere	Structure at the end of a chromosome that protects DNA data. Telomere shortening is associated with aging.
Testator	A person who has made a will.
Text (SMS) Messaging	The act of typing and sending a brief, electronic message between two or more mobile phones or fixed or portable devices over a phone network.
Theranostics	A combination of diagnostics and therapy in which specific targeted therapy is based on specific targeted diagnostic tests.
Therapeutic Exercise	Therapeutic exercise refers to physical activities that are used to restore function and build physical strength, balance, and endurance.
Therapeutic Relationship	A series of interactions between team member and pet owner that supports the clinical treatment of an animal.
Thin Slicing	The ability to find patterns in events based only on "thin slices," or narrow windows, of experience.
Third-Party Payment	Financial reimbursement for the delivery of medical care by an institution or individual other than the client.
Thrombocytopenia	The condition of having a reduced platelet count.
Time Management	The process of organizing and planning how to divide time between specific activities and tasks.

Time-Dependent Antimicrobials	Antimicrobials whose efficacy is associated with keeping concentrations above the bacterial minimal inhibitory concentration (MIC) for some proportion of the dosage interval.
Tip Sheet	A document containing the latest information or "tips" for a particular topic.
Tonic Immobility	A state of motionlessness caused by fear or a sense of being overwhelmed with stimulus to the point of freezing.
Tonometer	Instrument used to measure intraocular pressure.
Tooth Resorption (TR)	Resorption of hard dental tissues – enamel, cementum, dentin.
Tort	A wrongful act or an infringement of a right leading to civil legal liability.
Total Quality Management	Consistent performance, expectations, and consequences of nonperformance from all staff and doctors.
Touch Gradient	Initiating and maintaining continual physical contact and gradually increasing intensity when administering treatments that involve contact with the body such as injections, nail trimming, and others.
Toxgnostics	The identification of genetic variants that predict adverse reactions to specific drugs.
Toxicosis	Illness that stems from absorption, ingestion, or inhalation of a toxin.
Toxin	Plant- or animal-based poison or venom that causes disease if present at low levels within the body.
Trade Area	The geographic area from which the organization draws most of its customers and within which the organization's market penetration is the highest. A trade area is also known as a "region of influence" or "catchment area."
Traditionalists, Silent, Greatest Generation	Born before 1945, the "Depression Babies." Influenced by the Depression and WWII.
Trainer	Someone in the practice who has mastered a specific skill well enough to be entrusted with the responsibility of teaching it to others.
Transactional Leadership	A style of leadership that involves offering a reward for the adherence to instructions.
Transcleral Cyclophotocoagulation	A vision-sparing surgical procedure utilized to reduce intraocular pressure.
Transferrable Soft Skills	These are skills that involve the way a person interacts with other people that can be transferred between positions and even between industries.
Transformational Leadership	A style of leadership that influences people to decide to adhere to instructions.
Travel Sheet	Also known as a tracking sheet, this is a document that accompanies the patient and on which is detailed the services to be provided and (typically) the fees for those goods and services to ensure that nothing is missed when being recorded in the medical record and the invoice.
Travel Surcharge	An additional fee added to an invoice to reflect travel-related expenses of the visit.
Trigger	Anything that exacerbates or causes clinical signs to occur.
Trust	A relationship whereby property is held by one individual for the benefit of another.
Trustee	The individual or organization who receives the settlor's property for the benefit of the beneficiaries.
Unconditioned Stimulus	Anything that elicits a reaction from an animal without prior conditioning.
Underwriting	The review of a risk with the purpose of approving, declining, and pricing a new insurance policy.
United States Department of Agriculture (USDA)	Government agency that regulates animal vaccines and biologics under the Federal Virus, Serum, and Toxin Act.
United States Pharmacopeia (USP)	A nongovernmental organization that sets quality standards for medicines, food ingredients, and dietary supplements for the US and other countries.
Universal Waste	A subcategory of hazardous waste that includes, but is not limited to, pesticides, mercury-containing equipment, fluorescent bulbs, and batteries. Most veterinary hospitals fall under the Federal designation for small-quantity handlers of this material.

Unprofessional Conduct	The finding of a veterinary license board where the behavior of a veterinarian is below the standards of behavior set for a licensee.
Unsafe Condition	Any circumstance that puts a patient's safety in jeopardy.
Upselling	Encouraging a buyer to purchase a higher level of items or services.
Uveitis	Inflammation of the anterior chamber.
Vaccination	Inoculation with a killed or attenuated microbe with the purpose of preventing disease caused by that microbe.
Vaccine	Substance used to stimulate a prolonged immune response against an infectious agent prepared from killed microorganism, live attenuated microorganisms or a portion of the microorganisms.
Vaccine, Core	A vaccine that is considered standard and recommended for all pets of a certain species.
Vaccine, DNA or Recombinant DNA	Contains protein antigens from the virus that stimulate an immune response.
Vaccine, Killed/Inactivated	Does not contain a weakened form of the live virus, but contains the antigen with an adjuvant to help stimulate the immune response.
Vaccine, Modified Live Virus (MLV)	Also known as live attenuated vaccine, it contains a weakened or attenuated form of the infectious agent to stimulate an immune response.
Vaccine, Noncore	Vaccines that are optional and should be administered if there is exposure risk for the individual.
Valuation	The determination of the economic value of an asset or liability.
Value	Determined by what is important, desirable, and useful to clients.
Value-Added	The increase in real or perceived value of a product or service is the value to the client after intervention less the value before the intervention.
Value Proposition	Description of the value that a product, service or process will provide to the pet owner, hospital, and staff.
Variable	An element, feature or factor, such as patient traits and characteristics, health conditions, treatment options, outcomes, and other factors that can be measured and analyzed.
Variable Cost	A fluctuating cost, typically reflecting changes in usage (e.g., utility charges).
Vector	An organism or agent that does not cause disease itself but which spreads infection by conveying pathogens from one host to another.
Vertical Bone Loss	Loss of alveolar bone in a vertical manner, causing a wide separation between the root and adjacent bone.
Vertical Transmission	Passage of an infectious agent from parent to progeny, as through the placenta, direct contact after birth, or via consumption of mother's milk.
Veterinarian–Client–Patient Relationship	A legal relationship between veterinarian and animal owner in which the veterinarian has assumed responsibility for making clinical judgments and the client has agreed to follow the veterinarian's instructions, the veterinarian has sufficient knowledge of the patient to make such judgments, continuing care is provided or available, the veterinarian provides oversight of treatment, compliance and outcome, and patient records are maintained.
Veterinary Assistant	A title sometimes used for individuals who have received training less than that required for identification as a credentialed veterinary technician, technologist, or nurse.
Veterinary Medical Error	Unintentional harm that was induced by inappropriate veterinary medical care. For example, the accidental administration of one medication instead of another due to the similarity of their trade names or their packaging constitutes a veterinary medical error.
Veterinary Psychiatry	The arm of veterinary medicine that diagnoses and treats mental health disorders in animals.

Veterinary Reference Laboratory	A laboratory which performs comprehensive diagnostic testing for veterinary medicine.
Veterinary Technician/ Technologist/Nurse	A veterinary paraprofessional, often equated to a nurse, and referred to as a veterinary nurse in some countries.
Veterinary Time Equivalent (VTE)	Method of assigning labor expenses on the basis of veterinary staffing expense. This allows a practice to calculate approximate labor expenses for procedures using veterinary expense as a standard.
Victory Visits	A veterinary hospital visit designed to reinforce the idea that the veterinary clinic is somewhere where good things happen rather than one where painful treatments or procedures are performed.
Viremia	A condition in which a viral infectious agent is present and detectable within the bloodstream.
Virtual Care	See Telehealth.
Vision	Description of what an organization aspires to be.
Vision Statement	Statement that identifies where the organization intends to be in the future or where it should be to best meet the needs of its stakeholders.
Waiver	A client may sign a form explaining that they have declined to accept (or have waived) the doctor's recommendations or advice.
Waste Anesthetic Gas (WAG)	Inhalation anesthetic gas that is not metabolized by the patient and subsequently exhausted from the machine or from the animal, preferably into a scavenging system.
Wayfinding	People's ability to find their way through a facility and to their selected destination.
Wearables	Electronic devices that are worn by a person or animal that gather, store, and share data. For pets, these often include collars or tags that have sensors.
Wellness	The pursuit of good health.
Whale Eye	A body language signal where the dog shows the whites of its eyes. This is a warning signal of anxiety and, potentially, aggression.
Wholistic approach	Looks at healthcare for the whole pet, including factors related to exercise, diet, well-being and the environment rather than just focusing on diagnoses and treatments.
Will	Also known as a testament, the legal declaration by which a person names one or more persons to manage aspects of the estate after the testator's death.
Willingness to Pay	Amount of money a consumer thinks a product or service is worth and that they would be prepared to pay.
Word of Mouth Marketing	Recommendation of an organization by a satisfied customer to prospective customers.
Workflow	The consistent series of steps by which processes are completed within the organization.
Workflow Dynamics	How the flow of work is organized to occur at the business place/hospital.
Workstream	The step-by-step process by which tasks are completed by teams working within the hospital.
Zoonosis	Disease that is transmissible between animals and humans.
Zoonotic	Pertaining to a zoonosis; a disease that can be transmitted from animals to people or, more specifically, a disease that normally exists in animals but that can infect humans.

Index

Pet-Specific Care for the Veterinary Team, First Edition. Edited by Lowell Ackerman.
© 2021 John Wiley & Sons, Inc. Published 2021 by John Wiley & Sons, Inc.